Parkinson's Disease and Movement Disorders

FIFTH EDITION

Parkinson's Disease and Movement Disorders

FIFTH EDITION

■ **JOSEPH JANKOVIC, M.D.**

Professor of Neurology
Director, Parkinson's Disease Center and Movement Disorders Clinic
Department of Neurology
Baylor College of Medicine
Houston, Texas

■ **EDUARDO TOLOSA, M.D.**

Professor of Neurology
Director, Parkinson's Disease and Movement Disorder Unit
Department of Neurology
Hospital Clinic Universitari
University of Barcelona
Barcelona, Spain

Lippincott Williams & Wilkins
a Wolters Kluwer business
Philadelphia · Baltimore · New York · London
Buenos Aires · Hong Kong · Sydney · Tokyo

Acquisitions Editor: Frances DeStefano
Managing Editor: Julia Seto
Project Manager: Fran Gunning
Senior Manufacturing Manager: Benjamin Rivera
Marketing Manager: Kimberly Schonberger
Design Coordinator: Rita Clow
Cover Designer: Lou Fuiano
Production Service: GGS Book Services
Printer: Maple-Vail

© 2007 by LIPPINCOTT WILLIAMS & WILKINS, a WOLTERS KLUWER business
530 Walnut Street
Philadelphia, PA 19106 USA
LWW.com

Printed in the USA

Library of Congress Cataloging-in-Publication Data
Parkinson's disease and movement disorders / editors, Joseph Jankovic, Eduardo
Tolosa.—5th ed.
     p. ; cm.
   Includes bibliographical references and index.
   ISBN 13: 978-0-7817-7881-7
   ISBN 10: 0-7817-7881-6
     1. Parkinson's disease. 2. Movement disorders. I. Jankovic, Joseph.
   II. Tolosa, Eduardo.
     [DNLM: 1. Parkinson Disease. 2. Movement Disorders. WL 359 P2473 2007]
RC382.P257 2007
616.8'33—dc22

                                                                        2006018969

To purchase additional copies of this book, call our customer service department at
(800) 638-3030 or fax orders to (301) 223-2320. International customers should call
(301) 223-2300.

Visit Lippincott Williams & Wilkins on the Internet: at LWW.com. Lippincott Williams &
Wilkins customer service representatives are available from 8:30 am to 6 pm, EST.

                                        10 9 8 7 6 5 4 3 2

This book is dedicated to our loving families
in acknowledgment of their understanding and support.

Contents

Contributing Authors

ALBERTO ALBANESE, M.D. Professor, Department of Neurology, Catholic University of Milan, Milan, Italy; Chief, First Department of Neurology, National Neurological Institute "Carlo Besta," Milan, Italy

SERGEY V. ANISIMOV, M.D., PH.D. Postdoctoral Fellow, Department of Experimental Medical Sciences, Wallenberg Neuroscience Center, Neuronal Survival Unit, Lund University, Lund, Sweden

YACOV BALASH Clinic of Neurology, 1st Medical Faculty, Charles University, Prague, Czech Republic

ANNA RITA BENTIVOGLIO University Researcher, Università Cattolica del Sacro Cuore, Rome, Italy

CATHERINE BERGERON, M.D., F.R.C.P.C. Professor, Department of Laboratory Medicine and Pathobiology, Centre for Research in Neurodegenerative Diseases, University of Toronto, Toronto, Ontario

KAILASH P. BHATIA, M.D., D.M., F.R.C.P. Professor, Department of Neurology, Sobell Department of Motor Neuroscience and Movement Disorders, Institute of Neurology, University College London, London, United Kingdom; Consultant Neurologist, Clinical Neurology, National Hospital for Neurology and Neurosurgery, London, United Kingdom

BRADLEY F. BOEVE, M.D. Department of Neurology, Mayo Clinic College of Medicine, Rochester, Minnesota

DAVID J. BROOKS, M.D., D.SC., F.R.C.P., F.MED.SCI. Hartnett Professor of Neurology, Department of Neuroscience, Imperial College London, London, United Kingdom; Professor, Department of Neurology, Hammersmith Hospital, London, United Kingdom

PATRIK BRUNDIN, M.D., PH.D. Group Leader, Department of Experimental Medical Sciences, Wallenberg Neuroscience Center, Neuronal Survival Unit, Lund University, Lund, Sweden

FRANCISCO CARDOSO, M.D., PH.D. Associate Professor, Department of Clinical Medicine–Neurology, The Federal University of Minas Gerais, Belo Horizonte, MG, Brazil; Chief, Sector of Abnormal Movements–Neurology, Hospital of the Clinics of The Federal University of Minas Gerais, Belo Horizonte, MG, Brazil

CYNTHIA L. COMELLA, M.D., F.A.A.N. Associate Professor, Department of Neurological Sciences, Rush University Medical Center, Chicago, Illinois

ANA SOFIA CORREIA, M.S. Doctoral Student, Department of Experimental Medical Sciences, Wallenberg Neuroscience Center, Neuronal Survival Unit, Lund University, Lund, Sweden

GÜNTHER DEUSCHL, M.D. Director, Clinic for Neurology, Christian-Albrechts-Universität zu Kiel, Kiel, Germany

DENNIS W. DICKSON, M.D. Department of Pathology, Mayo Clinic College of Medicine, Jacksonville, Florida

BRUNO DUBOIS, M.D. Professor, Department of Neurology, INSERM V 610; Neurologist, Fédération de Neurologie, Hôpital de la Salpêtrière, Paris, France

ALEXANDRA DURR, M.D., PH.D. Medical Director, Department of Genetics, Cytogenetics, and Embryology, Clinical Researcher, INSERM Unit 679, Pitié-Salpêtrière Hospital, Paris, France

MURAT EMRE, M.D. Professor, Department of Neurology, Chief, Behavioral Neurology and Movement Disorders Unit, Istanbul Faculty of Medicine, Istanbul University, Istanbul, Turkey

STANLEY FAHN, M.D. H. Houston Merritt Professor of Neurology, Department of Neurology, Columbia University, New York, New York

JOSEPH H. FRIEDMAN, M.D. Department of Neurology, Brown University, Providence, Rhode Island

VICTOR S.C. FUNG, PH.D., F.R.A.C.P. Director, Movement Disorders Unit, Department of Neurology, Westmead Hospital, Sydney, Australia

THOMAS GASSER, M.D. Professor of Neurology, Department of Neurodegenerative Disorders, Hertie Institute for Clinical Brain Research, Tübingen, Germany; Director, Department of Neurodegenerative Disorders, University Hospital Tübingen, Tübingen, Germany

FELIX GESER, M.D., PH.D. Department of Pathology and Laboratory Medicine, University of Pennsylvania School of Medicine, Hospital of the University of Pennsylvania, Philadelphia, Pennsylvania

NIR GILADI, M.D. Director, Movement Disorders Unit, NPF Parkinson Center, Department of Neurology, Tel-Aviv Sourasky Medical Center, Sackler School of Medicine, Tel-Aviv University, Tel-Aviv, Israel

MICHEL GOEDERT Medical Research Council Laboratory of Molecular Biology, Cambridge, United Kingdom

CHRISTOPHER G. GOETZ, M.D. Professor, Department of Neurological Sciences, Rush University Medical Center, Chicago, Illinois

LAWRENCE I. GOLBE, M.D. Professor, Department of Neurology, Robert Wood Johnson Medical School, New Brunswick, New Jersey; Neurology Service, Robert Wood Johnson University Hospital, New Brunswick, New Jersey

LEV G. GOLDFARB, M.D. Medical Officer, National Institute of Neurological Disorders and Stroke, National Institutes of Health, Bethesda, Maryland

ROBERT G. GROSSMAN, M.D. Professor and Chairman, Department of Neurosurgery, Baylor College of Medicine, Houston, Texas

YADOLLAH HARATI, M.D. Professor, Department of Neurology, Director, Neuromuscular Disease Center, Baylor College of Medicine, Houston, Texas

STACY HORN, D.O. Clinical Assistant Professor, Department of Neurology, University of Pennsylvania, Philadelphia, Pennsylvania

JOSEPH JANKOVIC, M.D. Professor, Department of Neurology, Director, Parkinson's Disease Center and Movement Disorders Clinic, Baylor College of Medicine, Houston, Texas

PETER JENNER, D.SC., PH.D. Professor, Neurodegenerative Diseases Research Centre, Head, Pharmacology and Therapeutics Division, King's College, University of London, London, United Kingdom

REGINA KATZENSCHLAGER, M.D. Consultant Neurologist, Department of Neurology, Donauspital/SMZ-Ost, Vienna, Austria

THOMAS KLOCKGETHER, M.D. Full Professor, Department of Neurology, University of Bonn, Bonn, Germany

KATIE KOMPOLITI, M.D. Associate Professor and Attending Physician, Neurological Sciences, Rush University Medical Center, Chicago, Illinois

PAUL KRACK, M.D., PH.D. Department of Neurology, University Hospital of Grenoble, Joseph Fourier University, Grenoble, France

JOACHIM K. KRAUSS, M.D. Professor and Director, Department of Neurosurgery, Medical University of Hannover, Hannover, Germany

JUSTIN KWAN, M.D. Assistant Professor, Department of Neurology, Baylor College of Medicine, Houston, Texas

ANTHONY E. LANG, M.D., FRCPC Professor, Division of Neurology, Department of Medicine, University of Toronto, Toronto, Ontario; Director, Movement Disorders Unit, Toronto Western Hospital, Toronto, Ontario

ANDREW JOHN LEES, M.D., F.R.C.P. Director of Research, RLW Institute of Neurological Studies, Reta Lila Weston Institute, London, United Kingdom; Professor, Department of Neurology, The National Hospital for Neurology and Neurosurgery, University College London, London, United Kingdom

RICHARD LEVY, M.D., PH.D. INSERM V 610, Fédération de Neurologie, Hôpital de la Salpêtrière, Paris, France

PETER A. LEWITT, M.D. Professor, Departments of Neurology and of Psychiatry and Behavioral Neuroscience, Clinical Neuroscience Center, Wayne State University School of Medicine, Southfield, Michigan

JIA-YI LI, M.D., PH.D. Assistant Group Leader, Department of Experimental Medical Sciences, Wallenberg Neuroscience Center, Neuronal Survival Unit, Lund University, Lund, Sweden

KEVIN ST. P. MCNAUGHT, PH.D. Department of Neurology, Mt. Sinai Medical Center, New York, New York

JONATHAN W. MINK, M.D., PH.D. Associate Professor, Departments of Neurology, of Neurobiology and Anatomy, and of Pediatrics, University of Rochester, Rochester, New York; Chief of Child Neurology, Departments of Neurology and of Pediatrics, Golisano Children's Hospital at Strong, Rochester, New York

JOHN C. MORGAN, M.D., PH.D. Assistant Professor, Movement Disorders Program, Department of Neurology, Medical College of Georgia, Augusta, Georgia; Staff Neurologist, Department of Veterans Affairs Medical Center, Augusta, Georgia

C. WARREN OLANOW, M.D. Professor and Chair, Department of Neurology, Professor, Department of Neuroscience, Mount Sinai School of Medicine, New York, New York

WILLIAM G. ONDO, M.D. Associate Professor, Department of Neurology, Baylor College of Medicine, Houston, Texas

RONALD PFEIFFER, M.D., PH.D. Professor, Department of Neurology, University of Tennessee, Memphis, Tennessee

BERNARD PILLON, PH.D. Director of Research, INSERM V 610; Psychologist, Fédération de Neurologie, Hôpital de la Salpêtrière, Paris, France

WERNER POEWE, M.D. Professor and Chairman, Department of Neurology, Innsbruck Medical University, Innsbruck, Austria

PIERRE POLLAK, M.D., PH.D. Professor, Department of Neurology, Joseph Fourier University, Grenoble, France; Responsible for the Movement Disorders Unit, Department of Neurology, University Hospital of Grenoble, Grenoble, France

MICHAEL R. PRANZATELLI, M.D. Professor, Departments of Neurology and of Pediatrics, Head, Division of Child and Adolescent Neurology, Southern Illinois University School of Medicine, Springfield, Illinois

SERGE PRZEDBORSKI, M.D., PH.D. Professor, Departments of Neurology, of Pathology, and of Cell Biology, Columbia University, New York, New York; Attending Neurologist, Department of Neurology, New York Presbyterian Hospital, New York, New York

JAN RAETHJEN Clinic for Neurology, Kiel, Germany

OLIVIER RASCOL, M.D., PH.D. Professor, Department of Clinical Pharmacology, Faculty of Medicine, Toulouse, France; Chief, Clinical Investigation Center, University Hospital, Toulouse, France

EVŽEN RŮŽIČKA, M.D., D.SC. Clinic of Neurology, 1st Medical Faculty, Charles University, Prague, Czech Republic

SHINJI SAIKI, M.D. Research Associate, Department of Medical Genetics, Cambridge Institute for Medical Research, University of Cambridge, Cambridge, United Kingdom

KOICHIRO SAKAI, M.D., PH.D. Chief, Department of Internal Medicine, Tokyo Rinkai Hospital, Tokyo, Japan

CRISTINA SAMPAIO, M.D., PH.D. Professor, Department of Clinical Pharmacology and Therapeutics, Institute of Molecular Medicine, University of Lisbon, Lisbon, Portugal

ANTHONY H.V. SCHAPIRA, M.D., D.SC., F.R.C.P., F.MED.SCI. Professor and Chairman, University Department of Clinical Neurosciences, Royal Free and University College Medical School, London, United Kingdom; Professor, Department of Clinical Neurology, National Hospitals for Neurology and Neurosurgery, London, United Kingdom

SUSANNE ANNIKA SCHNEIDER, M.D. Research Fellow and Ph.D. Candidate, Sobell Department of Motor Neuroscience and Movement Disorders, Institute of Neurology, University College London, London, United Kingdom; Clinical Assistant, Department of Movement Disorders, National Hospital for Neurology and Neurosurgery, London, United Kingdom

ANETTE SCHRAG, M.D., PH.D. Senior Lecturer, Department of Clinical Neurosciences, Royal Free and University College Medical School, London, United Kingdom; Consultant Neurologist, Department of Neurology, Royal Free Hospital and Luton & Dunstable Hospital, London, United Kingdom

KAPIL D. SETHI, M.D., F.R.C.P. Professor and Director, Movement Disorders Program, Department of Neurology, Medical College of Georgia, Augusta, Georgia

HIROSHI SHIBASAKI, M.D., PH.D. Emeritus Professor, Department of Neurology, Human Brain Research Center, Kyoto University, Kyoto, Japan

HARVEY S. SINGER, M.D. Haller Professor of Pediatric Neurology and Director of Child Neurology, Departments of Neurology and of Pediatrics, Johns Hopkins University School of Medicine, Baltimore, Maryland

MARIA GRAZIA SPILLANTINI, PH.D. Centre for Brain Repair, Department of Clinical Neurosciences, University of Cambridge, Cambridge, United Kingdom

MADHAVI THOMAS, M.D. Medical Director, Movement Disorders and Parkinson's Disease Clinic and Research Institute, Neurologist and Associate Attending, Department of Internal Medicine, Baylor University Medical Center, Dallas, Texas

PHILIP D. THOMPSON, M.D., PH.D. Professor, Department of Neurology, University Department of Medicine, University of Adelaide, Adelaide, South Australia; Head, Department of Neurology, Royal Adelaide Hospital, Adelaide, South Australia

EDUARDO TOLOSA, M.D. Professor, Department of Neurology, Director, Parkinson's Disease and Movement Disorder Unit, Hospital Clinic Universitari, University of Barcelona, Barcelona, Spain

JOSEP VALLS-SOLÉ, M.D., PH.D. Associate Professor, Department of Medicine, School of Medicine, University of Barcelona, Barcelona, Spain; Senior Consultant, EMG Unit, Neurology Service, Institute of Neurosciences, Hospital Clinic, Barcelona, Spain

JENS VOLKMANN, M.D., PH.D. Privatdozent, Department of Neurology, Christian-Albrechts-Universität zu Kiel, Kiel, Germany; Leitender Oberarzt, Department of Neurology, Universitätsklinikum Schleswig-Holstein, Campus Kiel, Kiel, Germany

GREGOR K. WENNING, M.D., PH.D. Professor, Clinical Department of Neurology, Innsbruck Medical University, Innsbruck, Austria

Preface

Since the first edition of *Parkinson's Disease and Movement Disorders*, published in 1988, extraordinary advances have been made in Parkinson's disease and other movement disorders. The primary goal of this fifth edition is to highlight and critically review this progress.

Functional, biochemical, or structural abnormalities of the basal ganglia, the cerebellum, and their connections are responsible for the vast majority of the disorders discussed in this volume. The traditional models of the basal ganglia and their role in motor control, somatosensory function, and behavior, however, are continuously being refined. Our understanding of mechanisms underlying cell death and their relevance to neurodegeneration has also improved markedly as a result of new knowledge about cell biology and molecular genetics in certain forms of parkinsonism, dystonia, cerebellar ataxias, and other movement disorders. It is now generally accepted that there is no single cause of Parkinson's disease, and the concept of "Parkinson's diseases" is now emerging to indicate multiple etiologies for a group of diseases with overlapping clinical and pathological features. New classes of diseases, such as synucleinopathies (e.g., Parkinson's disease, multiple system atrophy, dementia with Lewy bodies) and tauopathies (e.g., progressive supranuclear palsy, corticobasal degeneration, frontotemporal dementia with parkinsonism) have evolved. As a result of these studies and new insights into the mechanisms of neuronal death, many neurodegenerative diseases, including Parkinson's disease, are now considered proteinopathies caused by abnormal protein processing in the affected cells.

In addition to the motor abnormalities associated with the various basal ganglia disorders, cognitive, emotional, and other behavioral aspects are increasingly recognized as important clinical features. More and more studies draw attention to the non–levodopa-responsive and nonmotor aspects of Parkinson's disease. Obsessive–compulsive disorders and abnormalities of attention are not only features of Tourette's syndrome but also of a variety of other basal ganglia disorders. The overlap between psychiatric disorders and movement disorders is a subject of several topics reviewed in this new edition.

Advances in understanding mechanisms of neurodegeneration are now being translated into therapies that are not merely symptomatic but also potentially disease modifying. Although levodopa continues to be the most effective symptomatic treatment for Parkinson's disease, the emergence of motor fluctuations and dyskinesias limits the usefulness of the drug. Strategies designed to prevent and treat these levodopa-related complications are addressed in one of many new chapters. Other advances in the symptomatic therapy of dystonia, tremor, tics, myoclonus, painful rigidity, and other movement disorders are also highlighted in this volume. Considerable attention is devoted to surgical treatments, including deep-brain stimulation. We were encouraged to highlight advances in experimental therapeutics and to review relevant drugs and other treatments in the pipeline, and we have.

One of the major additions in this fifth edition is the inclusion of *Video Atlas of Movement Disorders*. Since the diagnosis of movement disorders is based on phenomenology and pattern recognition, these instructive videos clearly enhance the educational value of the book. The atlas consists of a compilation of videos of movement disorders from more than 100 patients evaluated at the Baylor College of Medicine Movement Disorders Clinic. The atlas illustrates the broad spectrum of common, as well as unusual, movement disorders. All patients in these videos gave their permission to use the videos to expand knowledge about this range of disorders and to educate professionals and trainees.

It is the hope and wish of the editors that this new edition will serve as a testimony to the extraordinary progress that has been made in the area of Parkinson's disease, related neurodegenerative disorders, and movement disorders. Although not meant to be encyclopedic, this comprehensive volume highlights recent advances in basic and clinical sciences related to movement disorders and as such should be of interest not only to clinicians concerned with the care of those afflicted with Parkinson's disease and other movement disorders but also to clinical and basic investigators pursuing answers to some of the unanswered questions about the pathogenesis of this challenging group of disorders. In addition to neurologists and neuroscientists, this book should be of value to neurosurgeons, psychiatrists, physiatrists, neurophysiologists, primary care physicians, nurses, and all other health care professionals caring for patients with movement disorders.

We are extremely grateful to all the distinguished contributors for their scholarly reviews. We also wish to express our deep appreciation to the professional staff of Lippincott Williams and Wilkins, particularly Scott M. Scheidt and Frances R. DeStefano. Without their tireless efforts, this volume could not have been delivered in such a timely and professional way.

Joseph Jankovic, MD (Houston)
Eduardo Tolosa, MD (Barcelona)

Parkinson's Disease and Movement Disorders

FIFTH EDITION

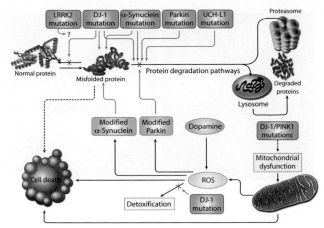

Figure 7.3

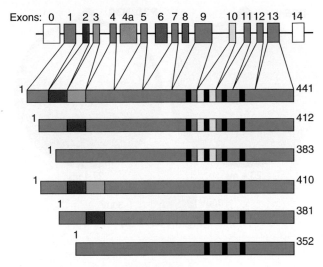

Figure 16.1

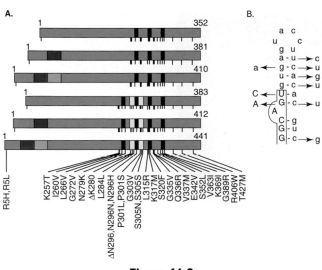

Figure 16.3

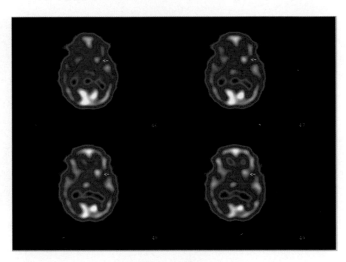

Figure 19.1

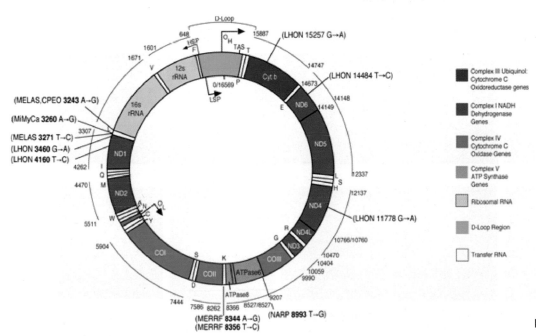

Figure 23.1

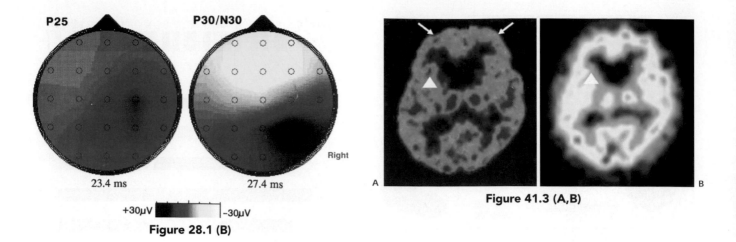

P25

P30/N30

Right

23.4 ms

27.4 ms

+30µV ▬▬▬ −30µV

Figure 28.1 (B)

Figure 41.3 (A,B)

^{18}F-Dopa PET

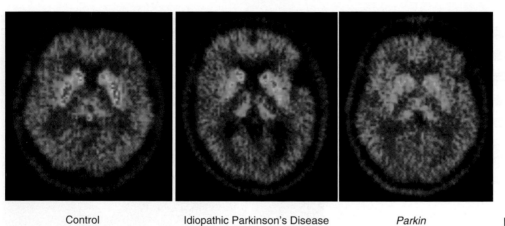

Control

Idiopathic Parkinson's Disease

Parkin

Figure 43.1

Imaging Dopamine Terminal Function

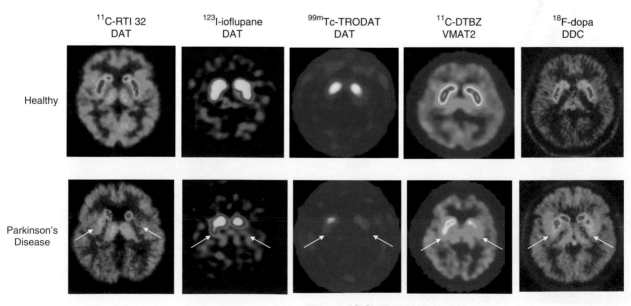

| ^{11}C-RTI 32 DAT | ^{123}I-ioflupane DAT | ^{99m}Tc-TRODAT DAT | ^{11}C-DTBZ VMAT2 | ^{18}F-dopa DDC |

Healthy

Parkinson's Disease

Figure 43.2

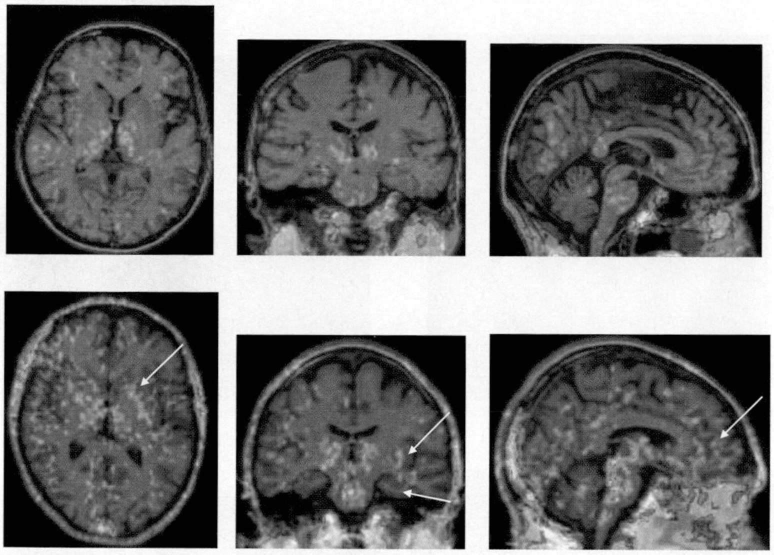

Microglial Activation in Parkinson's Disease
Healthy volunteer
PD patient

Figure 43.3

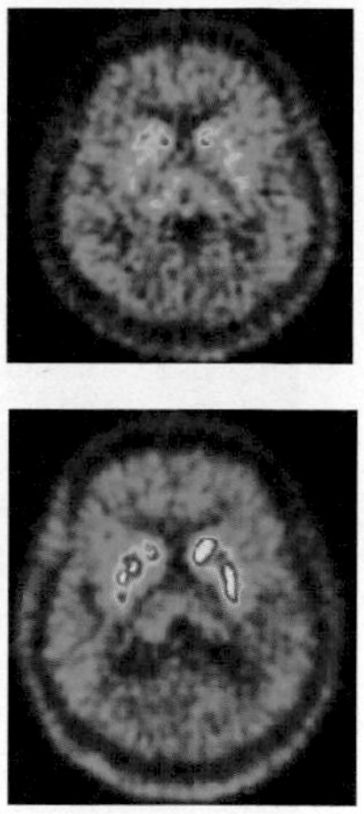

Pre-graft
Post-graft

Figure 43.4

11C-raclopride Binding at Baseline and Following 250 Mg Oral L-Dopa
Baseline
L-dopa
T-42
T-39
T-33
T-42
T-39
T-33

Figure 43.5

Diffusion-Weighted MRI
Normal
Parkinson's Disease
Multiple System Atrophy

Figure 43.6

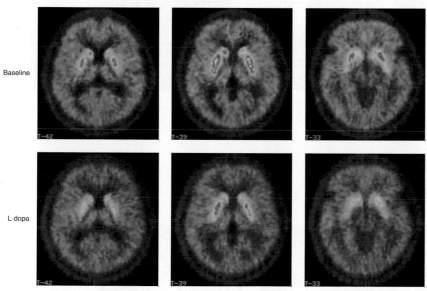

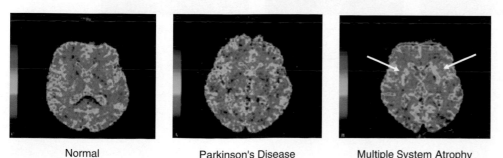

^{18}FDG PET

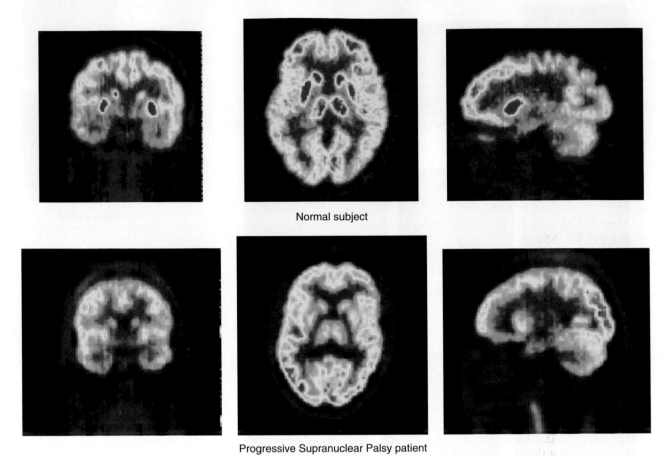

Normal subject

Progressive Supranuclear Palsy patient

Figure 43.7

^{11}C-raclopride PET: D2 Binding

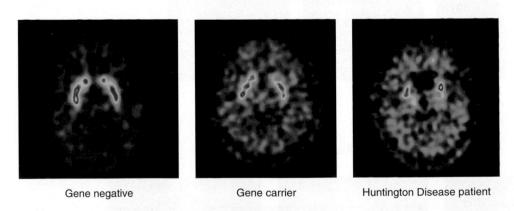

Gene negative   Gene carrier   Huntington Disease patient

Figure 43.8

Functional Organization of the Basal Ganglia

Jonathan W. Mink

The basal ganglia have all the aspects of a "clearing house" that accumulates samples of ongoing projected activity and, on a competitive basis, can facilitate any one and suppress all others."—D. Denny-Brown and N. Yanagisawa (1)

We propose that this circuit is organized anatomically and neurochemically so that the striatum can select and maintain motor behaviors. . . . Furthermore, the basal ganglia function to suppress other conflicting activities while reinforcing ongoing behaviors."—J. B. Penney and A. B. Young (2)

The basal ganglia are large subcortical structures comprising several interconnected nuclei in the forebrain, diencephalon, and midbrain. Historically, the basal ganglia have been viewed as a component of the motor system. However, there is now substantial evidence that the basal ganglia interact with all of the frontal cortex and with the limbic system. Thus, the basal ganglia likely have a role in cognitive and emotional function in addition to their role in motor control. Indeed, diseases of the basal ganglia often cause a combination of movement, affective, and cognitive disorders. The motor circuits of the basal ganglia are better understood than the other circuits, but because of similar organization of the circuitry, conceptual understanding of basal ganglia motor function also can provide a useful framework for understanding cognitive and affective function.

The basal ganglia include the striatum (caudate, putamen, nucleus accumbens), the subthalamic nucleus, the globus pallidus (internal segment, external segment, ventral pallidum), and the substantia nigra (pars compacta and pars reticulata) (Fig. 1.1). The striatum and subthalamic nucleus receive the majority of inputs from outside the basal ganglia. Most of those inputs come from the cerebral cortex, but the thalamic nuclei also provide strong inputs to striatum. The bulk of the outputs from the basal ganglia arise from the globus pallidus internal segment, ventral pallidum, and substantia nigra pars reticulata. These outputs are inhibitory to the pedunculopontine area in the brainstem and to the thalamic nuclei that in turn project to the frontal lobe.

The striatum receives the bulk of extrinsic input to the basal ganglia, including excitatory input from virtually all of the cerebral cortex (3). In addition, the ventral striatum (nucleus accumbens and rostroventral extensions of the caudate and putamen) receive inputs from the hippocampus and amygdala (4). The cortical input uses glutamate as its neurotransmitter and terminates largely on the heads of the dendritic spines of medium spiny neurons (5). The projection from the cerebral cortex to the corpus striatum has a roughly topographic organization. It has been suggested that this topography provides the basis for a segregation of functionally different circuits in the basal ganglia (6). Although the topography implies a certain degree of parallel organization, there is also evidence for convergence and divergence in the corticostriatal projection. The large dendritic fields of medium spiny neurons (7) allow them to receive input from adjacent projections, which arise from different areas of the cortex. Inputs to the striatum from several functionally related cortical areas overlap, and a single cortical area projects divergently to multiple striatal zones (8,9). Thus, there is a multiply convergent and divergent

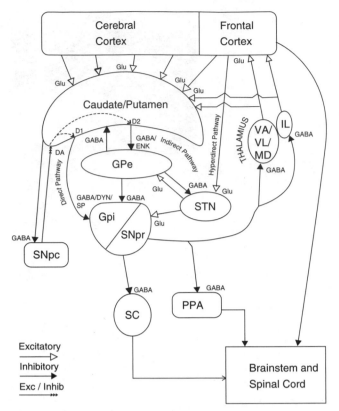

Figure 1.1 Simplified schematic diagram of basal ganglia–thalamocortical circuitry. Excitatory connections are indicated by open arrows, inhibitory connections by filled arrows. The modulatory dopamine projection is indicated by a three-headed arrow. dyn, dynorphin; enk, enkephalin; GABA, gamma-aminobutyric acid; glu, glutamate; GPe, globus pallidus pars externa; GPi, globus pallidus pars interna; IL, intralaminar thalamic nuclei; MD, mediodorsal nucleus; PPA, pedunculopontine area; SC, superior colliculus; SNpc, substantia nigra pars compacta; SNpr, substantia nigra pars reticulata; SP substance P; STN, subthalamic nucleus; VA, ventral anterior nucleus; VL, ventral lateral nucleus.

organization within a broader framework of functionally different parallel circuits. This organization provides an anatomical framework for the integration and transformation of cortical information in the striatum.

Medium spiny striatal neurons make up about 95% of the striatal neuron population. They project outside of the striatum and receive a number of inputs, in addition to the important cortical input, including (a) excitatory glutamatergic inputs from the thalamus; (b) cholinergic input from striatal interneurons; (c) gamma-aminobutyric acid (GABA), substance P, and enkephalin input from adjacent medium spiny striatal neurons; (d) GABA input from small interneurons; (e) a large input from dopamine-containing neurons in the substantia nigra pars compacta (SNpc); and (f) a more sparse input from the serotonin-containing neurons in the dorsal and median raphe nuclei.

In recent years, there has been increasing recognition of the importance of the fast-spiking GABAergic striatal interneurons. These cells make up less than 2% of the striatal neuron population, but they exert powerful inhibition

on medium spiny neurons. Like medium spiny neurons, they receive excitatory input from the cerebral cortex. They appear to play an important role in focusing the spatial pattern of medium spiny neuron activation (10).

The dopamine input to the striatum terminates largely on the shafts of the dendritic spines of medium spiny neurons, where it is in a position to modulate transmission from the cerebral cortex to the striatum (11). The action of dopamine on striatal neurons depends on the type of dopamine receptor involved. Five types of G protein–coupled dopamine receptors have been described (D1–D5) (12) and grouped into two families based on their linkage to adenylcyclase activity and response to agonists. The D1 family includes D1 and D5 receptors, and the D2 family includes D2, D3, and D4 receptors. The conventional view has been that dopamine acts at D1 receptors to facilitate the activity of postsynaptic neurons and at D2 receptors to inhibit postsynaptic neurons (13). Indeed, this is a fundamental concept for currently popular models of basal ganglia pathophysiology (14,15). However, the physiologic effect of dopamine on striatal neurons is more complex. While activation of dopamine D1 receptors potentiates the effect of cortical input to striatal neurons in some states, it reduces the efficacy of cortical input in others (16). Activation of D2 receptors more consistently decreases the effect of cortical input to striatal neurons (17). Dopamine contributes to focusing the spatial and temporal patterns of striatal activity.

In addition to short-term facilitation or inhibition of striatal activity, there is evidence that dopamine can modulate corticostriatal transmission by mechanisms of long-term depression (LTD) and long-term potentiation (LTP). Through these mechanisms, dopamine strengthens or weakens the efficacy of corticostriatal synapses and can thus mediate reinforcement of specific discharge patterns. LTP and LTD are thought to be fundamental to many neural mechanisms of learning and may underlie the hypothesized role of the basal ganglia in habit learning (18). SNpc dopamine neurons fire in relation to behaviorally significant events and reward (19). These signals are likely to modify the responses of striatal neurons to inputs that occur in conjunction with the dopamine signal resulting in the reinforcement of motor and other behavior patterns. Striatal lesions or focal striatal dopamine depletion impairs the learning of new movement sequences (20), supporting a role for the basal ganglia in certain types of procedural learning.

Medium spiny striatal neurons contain the inhibitory neurotransmitter GABA and co-localized peptide neurotransmitters (21). Based on the type of neurotransmitters and the predominant type of dopamine receptor they contain, the medium spiny neurons can be divided into two populations. One population contains GABA, dynorphin, and substance P and primarily expresses D1 dopamine receptors. These neurons project to the basal ganglia output nuclei, globus pallidus pars interna (GPi), and substantia nigra pars reticulata (SNpr). The second population contains GABA and enkephalin and primarily expresses D2 dopamine receptors. These neurons project to the external segment of the globus pallidus para externa (GPe) (14).

Although no apparent regional differences in the striatum are based on cell type, an intricate internal organization has been revealed with special stains. When the striatum is stained for acetylcholinesterase (AChE), there is a patchy distribution of lightly staining regions within more heavily stained regions (22). The AChE-poor patches have been called *striosomes*, and the AChE-rich areas have been called the *extrastriosomal matrix*. The matrix forms the bulk of the striatal volume and receives input from most areas of the cerebral cortex. Within the matrix are clusters of neurons with similar inputs that have been termed *matrisomes*. The bulk of the output from cells in the matrix is to both segments of the GP, to ventral pallidum (VP), and to SNpr. The striosomes receive input from the prefrontal cortex and send output to the SNpc (23). Immunohistochemical techniques have demonstrated that many substances, such as substance P, dynorphin, and enkephalin, have a patchy distribution that may be partly or wholly in register with the striosomes. The striosome-matrix organization suggests a level of functional segregation within the striatum that may be important in understanding the variety of symptoms in TS.

The subthalamic nucleus receives an excitatory, glutamatergic input from many areas of the frontal lobes with especially large inputs from motor areas of the cortex [reviewed by (24)]. The subthalamic nucleus (STN) also receives an inhibitory GABA input from the GPe. The output from the STN is glutamatergic and excitatory to the basal ganglia output nuclei, GPi, VP, and SNpr. STN also sends an excitatory projection back to the GPe. There is a somatopic organization in STN (25) and a relative topographic separation of "motor" and "cognitive" inputs to STN.

The primary basal ganglia output arises from the GPi, a GPi-like component of the VP, and the SNpr. As previously described, GPi and SNpr receive excitatory input from the STN and inhibitory input from the striatum. They also receive an inhibitory input from the GPe. The dendritic fields of GPi, VP, and SNpr neurons span up to 1 mm diameter and thus have the potential to integrate a large number of converging inputs (26). The output from GPi, VP, and SNpr is inhibitory and uses GABA as its neurotransmitter. The primary output is directed to the thalamic nuclei that project to the frontal lobes: the ventrolateral, ventroanterior, and mediodorsal nuclei. The thalamic targets of the GPi, VP, and SNpr project, in turn, to the frontal lobe, with the strongest output going to motor areas. Collaterals of the axons projecting to the thalamus project to an area at the junction of the midbrain and pons near the pedunculopontine nucleus (27). Other output neurons (20%) project to intralaminar nuclei of the thalamus, to the lateral habenula, or to the superior colliculus (28).

The basal ganglia motor output has a somatotopic organization such that the body below the neck is largely represented in the GPi and the head and eyes are largely represented in the SNpr. The separate representation of different body parts is maintained throughout the basal ganglia. Within the representation of an individual body part, it also appears that there is segregation of outputs to different motor areas of the cortex and that an individual GPi neuron sends output via the thalamus to just one area of the cortex (29). Thus, GPi neurons that project via the thalamus to the motor cortex are adjacent to, but separate from, those that project to the premotor cortex or supplementary motor area. GPi neurons that project via the thalamus to the prefrontal cortex are also separate from those projecting to motor areas and from VP neurons projecting via the thalamus to the orbitofrontal cortex. The anatomic segregation of basal ganglia–thalamocortical outputs suggests functional segregation at the output level, but other anatomic evidence suggests interactions between circuits within the basal ganglia (see previous text) (30).

The GPe, and the GPe-like part of the VP may be viewed as intrinsic nuclei of the basal ganglia. Like the GPi and SNpr, the GPe receives an inhibitory projection from the striatum and an excitatory projection from the STN. Unlike the GPi, the striatal projection to the GPe contains GABA and enkephalin but not substance P (14). The output of the GPe is different from the output of the GPi. The output is GABAergic and inhibitory, and the majority of the output projects to STN. The connections from the striatum to the GPe, from the GPe to the STN, and from the STN to the GPi form the "indirect" striatopallidal pathway to the GPi (31) (Fig. 1.1). In addition, there is a monosynaptic GABAergic inhibitory output from the GPe directly to the GPi and to the SNpr and a GABAergic projection back to the striatum (32). Thus, GPe neurons are in a position to provide feedback inhibition to neurons in the striatum and STN and feedforward inhibition to neurons in the GPi and SNpr. This circuitry suggests that GPe may act to oppose, limit, or focus the effect of the striatal and STN projections to the GPi and SNpr as well as to focus activity in these output nuclei.

Dopamine input to the striatum arises from the SNpc and the ventral tegmental area (VTA). The SNpc projects to most of the striatum; the VTA projects to the ventral striatum. The SNpc and VTA are made up of large dopamine-containing cells. The SNpc receives input from the striatum, specifically from the striosomes. This input is GABAergic and inhibitory. The SNpc and VTA dopamine neurons project to caudate and putamen in a topographic manner (30), but with overlap. The nigral dopamine neurons receive inputs from one striatal circuit and project back to the same and to adjacent circuits. Thus, they appear to be in a position to modulate activity across functionally different circuits.

Although the basal ganglia intrinsic circuitry is complex, the overall picture is of two primary pathways through the basal ganglia from the cerebral cortex with the output directed via the thalamus at the frontal lobes. These pathways consist of two disynaptic pathways from the cortex to the basal ganglia output (Fig. 1.1). In addition, there are several multisynaptic pathways involving GPe. The two disynaptic pathways are from the cortex through (a) the striatum (the *direct pathway*) and (b) the STN (the *hyperdirect pathway*) to the basal ganglia outputs. These pathways show important anatomical and functional differences. First, the cortical input to the STN comes only from frontal lobe, whereas the input to the striatum arises from virtually all areas of the cerebral cortex. Second, the output from the STN is excitatory, whereas the output from the striatum is inhibitory. Third, the excitatory route through the STN is faster than the inhibitory route through the striatum (33). Finally, the STN projection to the GPi is divergent, and the striatal projection is more focused (34). Thus, the two disynaptic pathways from the cerebral cortex to the basal ganglia output nuclei, GPi and SNpr, provide fast, widespread, divergent excitation through the STN and slower, focused, inhibition through the striatum. This organization provides an anatomical basis for focused inhibition and surround excitation of neurons in the GPi and SNpr (Fig. 1.2). Because the output of the GPi and SNpr is inhibitory, this would result in focused facilitation and surround inhibition of basal ganglia thalamocortical targets.

We have developed a scheme of normal basal ganglia motor function based on the results of anatomical, physiological, and lesion studies (24,35). In this scheme, the tonically active inhibitory output of the basal ganglia acts

as a "brake" on motor pattern generators (MPGs) in the cerebral cortex (via the thalamus) and brainstem. When a movement is initiated by a particular MPG, basal ganglia output neurons projecting to competing MPGs increase their firing rate, thereby increasing inhibition and applying a "brake" on those generators. Other basal ganglia output neurons projecting to the generators involved in the desired movement decrease their discharge, thereby removing tonic inhibition and releasing the "brake" from the desired motor patterns. Thus, the intended movement is enabled, and competing movements are prevented from interfering with the desired one.

The anatomical arrangement of the STN and striatal inputs to the GPi and SNpr form the basis for a functional center-surround organization (Fig. 1.3). When a voluntary movement is initiated by cortical mechanisms, a separate signal is sent to the STN, exciting it. The STN projects in a widespread pattern and excites the GPi. The increased GPi activity causes inhibition of thalamocortical motor mechanisms. In parallel to the pathway through the STN, signals are sent from all areas of the cerebral cortex to the striatum. The cortical inputs are transformed by the striatal integrative circuitry to a focused, context-dependent output that inhibits specific neurons in the GPi. The inhibitory striatal input to the GPi is slower, but more powerful, than the excitatory STN input. The resulting focally decreased activity in the GPi selectively disinhibits the desired thalamocortical MPGs. Indirect pathways from the striatum to the GPi (striatum → GPe → GPi and

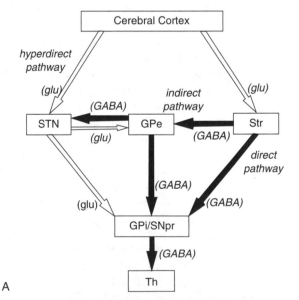

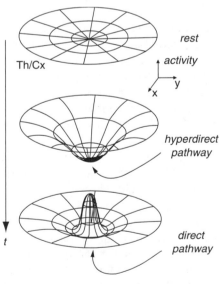

Figure 1.2 A: A schematic diagram of the hyperdirect cortico–subthalamo–pallidal, direct cortico–striato–pallidal, and indirect cortico–striato–GPe–subthalamo–GPi pathways. White and black arrows represent excitatory glutamatergic (glu) and inhibitory GABAergic projections, respectively. GPe, external segment of the globus pallidus; GPi, internal segment of the globus pallidus; SNr, substantia nigra pars reticulata; STN, subthalamic nucleus; Str, striatum; Th, thalamus. **B:** A schematic diagram explaining the activity change over time (*t*) in the thalamocortical projection (Th/Cx) following the sequential inputs through the hyperdirect cortico–subthalamo–pallidal (*middle*) and direct cortico–striato–pallidal (*bottom*) pathways. Modified from (33).

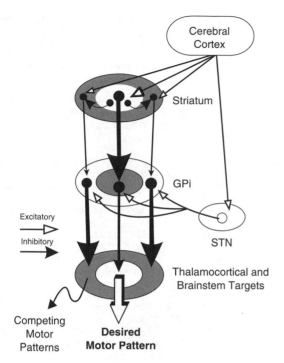

Figure 1.3 Schematic of normal functional organization of the basal ganglia output. Excitatory projections are indicated with open arrows; inhibitory projections are indicated with filled arrows. Relative magnitude of activity is represented by line thickness. Modified from (44).

striatum → GPe → STN → GPi) (Fig. 1.1) result in further focusing of the output. The net result of basal ganglia activity during a voluntary movement is the inhibition ("braking") of competing motor patterns and focused facilitation (releasing the "brake") from the selected voluntary movement pattern generators.

This scheme provides a framework for understanding both the pathophysiology of parkinsonism (24,36) and involuntary movements (24,35). Different involuntary movements such as parkinsonism, chorea, dystonia, or tics result from different abnormalities in the basal ganglia circuits. Loss of dopamine input to the striatum results in a loss of normal pauses of GPi discharge during voluntary movement. Hence, there is excessive inhibition of motor pattern generators and ultimately bradykinesia (36). Furthermore, loss of dopamine results in abnormal synchrony of GPi neuronal discharge and loss of the normal spatial and temporal focus of GPi activity (36–38). Broad lesions of the GPi or SNpr disinhibit both desired and undesired motor patterns leading to inappropriate activation of competing motor patterns but normal generation of the desired movement. Thus, lesions of the GPi cause co-contraction of multiple muscle groups and difficulty in turning off unwanted motor patterns, similar to what is seen in dystonia, but they do not affect movement initiation (39). Lesions of the SNpr cause unwanted saccadic eye movements that interfere with the ability to maintain visual fixation but do not impair the initiation of voluntary

saccades (40). Lesions of the putamen may cause dystonia due to the loss of focused inhibition in the GPi (35). Lesions of the STN produce continuous involuntary movements of the contralateral limbs (hemiballism or hemichorea) (35). Despite the involuntary movements, voluntary movements can still be performed. Although structural lesions of the putamen, GPi, SNpr, or STN produce certain types of unwanted movements or behaviors, they do not produce tics. Tics are more likely to arise from abnormal activity patterns, most likely in the striatum (35).

Our scheme of the basal ganglia function was developed specifically for the motor circuits of the basal ganglia–thalamocortical system (24). However, it is likely that the fundamental principles of function in the somatomotor, oculomotor, limbic, and cognitive basal ganglia circuits are similar. If the basic scheme of facilitation and inhibition of competing movements is extended to encompass more complex behaviors and thoughts, many features of basal ganglia disorders can be explained as failures to facilitate desired behaviors and simultaneously inhibit unwanted behaviors due to abnormal basal ganglia output patterns.

The scheme presented here differs in emphasis from the now classic model of basal ganglia circuitry that emphasizes opposing *direct and indirect pathways* from the striatum to the GPi/SNpr (14,15). These models have contributed substantially to advances in basal ganglia research over the past 15 years. If the success of a model is measured by the amount of research it stimulates, these schemes have been extraordinarily successful. In simple terms, these models proposed that hypokinetic movement disorders (e.g., parkinsonism) are distinguished from hyperkinetic movement disorders (e.g., chorea, dystonia, tics) based on the magnitude of basal ganglia output. Both clinical and basic research findings have required revision of the classic model (24,35,41–43). New emphasis on (a) the importance of timing cortical input to the STN and the timing of STN input to the GPi/SNpr (24,33); (b) the temporal–spatial organization of activity patterns in the different basal ganglia nuclei (24,35); and (c) the importance of spike train patterns (37,43) reflects our improved understanding of basal ganglia function and dysfunction. It is our expectation that knowledge will continue to expand at an impressive rate with future revisions of the models to follow.

ACKNOWLEDGMENTS

Supported by NIH R01NS39821 and R21NS40086

REFERENCES

1. Denny-Brown D, Yanagisawa N. The role of the basal ganglia in the initiation of movement. In: Yahr, MD, ed. *The Basal Ganglia.* New York: Raven Press, 1976;115–149.
2. Penney JB, Young AB. Speculations on the functional anatomy of basal ganglia disorders. *Ann Rev Neurosci* 1983;6:73–94.

3. Kemp JM, Powell TPS. The corticostriate projection in the monkey. *Brain* 1970;93:525–546.
4. Fudge J, Kunishio K, Walsh C, et al. Amygdaloid projections to ventromedial striatal subterritories in the primate. *Neuroscience* 2002;110:257–275.
5. Cherubini E, Herrling PL, Lanfumey L, et al. Excitatory amino acids in synaptic excitation of rat striatal neurones in vitro. *J Physiol* 1988;400:677–690.
6. Alexander GE, DeLong MR, Strick PL. Parallel organization of functionally segregated circuits linking basal ganglia and cortex. *Ann Rev Neurosci* 1986;9:357–381.
7. Wilson CJ, Groves PM. Fine structure and synaptic connections of the common spiny neuron of the rat neostriatum: a study employing intracellular injection of horseradish peroxidase. *J Comp Neurol* 1980;194:599–614.
8. Selemon LD, Goldman-Rakic PS. Longitudinal topography and interdigitation of corticostriatal projections in the rhesus monkey. *J Neurosci* 1985;5:776–794.
9. Flaherty AW, Graybiel AM. Corticostriatal transformations in the primate somatosensory system. Projections from physiologically mapped body-part representations. *J Neurophysiol* 1991;66:1249–1263.
10. Mallet N, Le Moine C, Charpier S, et al. Feedforward inhibition of projection neurons by fast-spiking GABA interneurons in the rat striatum in vivo. *J Neurosci* 2005;25:3857–3869.
11. Bouyer JJ, Park DH, Joh TH, et al. Chemical and structural analysis of the relation between cortical inputs and tyrosine hydroxylase-containing terminals in rat neostriatum. *Brain Res* 1984;302:267–275.
12. Sibley DR, Monsma FJ. Molecular biology of dopamine receptors. *Trends Pharm Sci* 1992;13:61–69.
13. Gerfen CR, Engber TM, Mahan LC, et al. D_1 and D_2 dopamine receptor-regulated gene expression of striatonigral and striatopallidal neurons. *Science* 1990;250:1429–1432.
14. Albin RL, Young AB, Penney JB. The functional anatomy of basal ganglia disorders. *Trends Neurosci* 1989;12:366–375.
15. DeLong MR. Primate models of movement disorders of basal ganglia origin. *Trends Neurosci* 1990;13:281–285.
16. Hernandez-Lopez S, Bargas J, Surmeier DJ, et al. D1 receptor activation enhances evoked discharge in neostriatal medium spiny neurons by modulating an L-type Ca2+ conductance. *J Neurosci* 1997;17:3334–3342.
17. Nicola S, Surmeier J, and Malenka R. Dopaminergic modulation of neuronal excitability in the striatum and nucleus accumbens. *Ann Rev Neurosci* 2000;23:185–215.
18. Jog M, Kubota Y, Connolly C, et al. Building neural representations of habits. *Science* 1999;286:1745–1749.
19. Schultz W, Romo R, Ljungberg T, et al. Reward-related signals carried by dopamine neurons. In: Houk JC, Davis JL, Beiser DG, eds. *Models of Information Processing in the Basal Ganglia.* Cambridge, MA: MIT Press, 1995:233–249.
20. Matsumoto N, Hanakawa T, Maki S, et al. Role of nigrostriatal dopamine system in learning to perform sequential motor tasks in a predictive manner. *J Neurophysiol* 1999;82:978–998.
21. Penny GR, Afsharpour S, Kitai ST. The glutamate decarboxylase-, leucine enkephalin-, methionine enkephalin- and substance P-immunoreactive neurons in the neostriatum of the rat and cat: evidence for partial population overlap. *Neuroscience* 1986;17:1011–1045.
22. Graybiel AM, Aosaki T, Flaherty AW, et al. The basal ganglia and adaptive motor control. *Science* 1994;265:1826–1831.
23. Gerfen CR. The neostriatal mosaic: multiple levels of compartmental organization in the basal ganglia. *Ann Rev Neurosci* 1992;15:285–320.
24. Mink JW. The basal ganglia: focused selection and inhibition of competing motor programs. *Prog Neurobiol* 1996;50:381–425.
25. Nambu A, Takada M, Inase M, et al. Dual somatotopical representations in the primate subthalamic nucleus: evidence for ordered but reversed body-map transformations from the primary motor cortex and the supplementary motor area. *J Neurosci* 1996;16:2671–2683.
26. Percheron G, Yelnik J, Francois C. A Golgi analysis of the primate globus pallidus. III. Spatial organization of the striato-pallidal complex. *J Comp Neurol* 1984;227:214–227.
27. Parent A. Extrinsic connections of the basal ganglia. *Trends Neurosci* 1990;13:254–258.
28. Francois C, Percheron G, Yelnik J, et al. A topographic study of the course of nigral axons and of the distribution of pallidal axonal endings in the centre median-parafascicular complex of macaques. *Brain Res* 1988;473:181–186.
29. Hoover JE, Strick PL. Multiple output channels in the basal ganglia. *Science* 1993;259:819–821.
30. Haber SN, Fudge JL, McFarland NR. Striatonigrostriatal pathways in primates form an ascending spiral from the shell to the dorsolateral striatum. *J Neurosci* 2000;20:2369–2382.
31. Alexander GE, Crutcher MD. Functional architecture of basal ganglia circuits: neural substrates of parallel processing. *Trends Neurosci* 1990;13:266–271.
32. Bolam JP, Hanley JJ, Booth PA, et al. Synaptic organisation of the basal ganglia. *J Anat* 2000;196:527–542.
33. Nambu A, Tokuno H, Hamada I, et al. Excitatory cortical inputs to pallidal neurons via the subthalamic nucleus in the monkey. *J Neurophysiol* 2000;84:289–300.
34. Parent A, Hazrati L-N. Anatomical aspects of information processing in primate basal ganglia. *Trends Neurosci* 1993;16:111–116.
35. Mink J. The basal ganglia and involuntary movements: impaired inhibition of competing motor patterns. *Arch Neurol* 2003;60:1365–1368.
36. Boraud T, Bezard E, Bioulac B, et al. From single extracellular unit recording in experimental and human Parkinsonism to the development of a functional concept of the role played by the basal ganglia in motor control. *Prog Neurobiol* 2002;66:265–283.
37. Raz A, Vaadia E, Bergman H. Firing the patterns and correlations of spontaneous discharge of pallidal neurons in the normal and the tremulous 1-methyl-4-phenyl-1,2,3,6-tetrahydropyridine Vervet model of parkinsonism. *J Neurosci* 2000;20:8559–8571.
38. Tremblay L, Filion M, Bedard PJ. Responses of pallidal neurons to striatal stimulation in monkeys with MPTP-induce parkinsonism. *Brain Res* 1989;498:17–33.
39. Mink JW, Thach WT. Basal ganglia motor control. III. Pallidal ablation: normal reaction time, muscle cocontraction, and slow movement. *J Neurophysiol* 1991;65:330–351.
40. Hikosaka O, Wurtz RH. Modification of saccadic eye movements by GABA-related substances. II. Effects of muscimol in monkey substantia nigra pars reticulata. *J Neurophysiol* 1985;53:292–308.
41. Hutchison WD, Lang AE, Dostrovsky JO, et al. Pallidal neuronal activity: implications for models of dystonia. *Ann Neurol* 2003;53:480–488.
42. Hutchison WD, Dostrovsky JO, Walters JR, et al. Neuronal oscillations in the basal ganglia and movement disorders: evidence from whole animal and human recordings. *J Neurosci* 2004;24:9240–9243.
43. Vitek JL. Pathophysiology of dystonia: a neuronal model. *Mov Disord* 2002;17:S49–S62.
44. Mink JW. Basal ganglia dysfunction in Tourette's syndrome: a new hypothesis. *Pediatr Neurol* 2001;25:190–198.

Neurophysiology of Motor Control and Movement Disorders

Josep Valls-Solé

ABSTRACT

The study of the motor system and its disorders has always been an important subject for neurophysiology. One of the goals of clinical neurophysiology is to try to understand the physiological mechanisms underlying functions and dysfunctions of the motor system. Neurophysiology contributes not only to the study of the physiology of motor control and the pathophysiology of movement disorders but also to their diagnosis, quantitation, and documentation. In this chapter, clinical neurophysiology is used as the main conductor for a review of some physiological aspects of human motor activities and for the assessment of the main characteristics of diseases presenting with movement disorders.

INTRODUCTION

The physiology of human motor control and movement disorders is still not completely understood. Little is known about the basic mechanisms put to work in a normal human brain to permit the desired movement performance in a given situation. It is completely clear, however, that some natural stimuli, such as muscle stretch, sensory inputs, or even gravity forces, cause muscle contraction and movements. Therefore, in the execution of a motor program, the central nervous system has to consider not only the activation of the muscles that will act as prime movers and those involved in associated postural activity but also the control of sensory inputs generated in muscle and skin receptors being activated by the change induced in the human body during movement performance. The characteristic ability of human beings to perform very fine movements has likely brought additional complexity to the mechanisms of motor programming and execution. Controlled movements require a larger amount of inhibitory actions over unwanted interferences from sensory inputs or from concomitantly preactivated muscles. It is not surprising, therefore, that some dysfunctions may arise in the overactivated systems used to control human movement performance. Disorders of motor control ensue from dysfunctions in one or many of the excitatory and inhibitory circuits working in parallel to reach the ultimate goal of a precise movement. Disorders may be caused by a degenerative disease specifically or predominantly involving movement-related structures or by systemic disorders, traumatic injuries, or vascular lesions.

Cortical motor areas are relatively accessible to study with noninvasive neurophysiological techniques such as cortical electrical or magnetic stimulation. This is not the case with subcortical motor structures, either those involved in movement preparation, such as the basal ganglia, the cerebellum, or the thalamus, or those involved mainly in movement execution, such as the brainstem nuclei and tracts, and some spinal cord centers. The role of the basal ganglia and the cerebellum in motor control and movement programming has been defined mainly theoretically, after studies in experimentation animals and learning from disease states in humans. Recently, the advent of treatment with implanted electrodes for chronic deep brain stimulation in patients with Parkinson's disease, tremor, or dystonia has led to new possibilities for assessing some of the characteristics of basal ganglia nuclei, their connections, and the surrounding structures (1,2). Classically, the role of the descending motor tracts generating in the brainstem has been considered accessory for the performance of programmed voluntary movements, and mainly related to postural control or lateral actions. However, the vestibulospinal, reticulospinal, rubrospinal, and tectospinal tracts are important vehicles for execution of specific actions, as subsystems used by the motor cortex, not only in animals but also in humans (3,4).

Neurophysiological techniques can be used to document and quantify the physiological mechanisms involved in movement execution, both in health and disease. One of the most valuable pieces of information brought by electrodiagnostic techniques is the conduction time. We are able to know the conduction velocity in motor and sensory fibers of peripheral nerves and, also, the motor conduction time from the brain to the muscle and the sensory conduction time from the skin to the brain. The event-related potentials even may tell us something about the electrical change that takes place in some neurons when a sensory input is being processed, and the premotor potentials indicate that general processes of movement preparation are taking place. However, the exact link between a sensory input and a motor action is still a subject of speculation. Neuroimaging techniques and, specifically, functional magnetic resonance imaging (fMRI) and positron emission tomography (PET) furnish good localization information in the brain, but these techniques are not yet adequate to examine the timing of sensorimotor integration processes. Sensorimotor integration is surely an important part in the study of movement control. Many of the movements performed are responses to sensory stimuli. Sensorimotor integration may actually occur at various levels of the central nervous system, including the spinal cord, the brainstem, and the sensorimotor cortex. Certain features of sensorimotor integration are suitable for neurophysiological recording. These are, for example, the change in excitability occurring before movement in motor pathways, the presynaptic modulation of reflexes, or the cerebral events that follow sensory stimulation. Some of these events can be quantified in a reliable manner. Other features of motor control and movement performance are still not well understood and are currently being studied. Future advances in understanding sensorimotor integration and movement preparation and performance should come from a combination of clinical neurophysiology and neuroimaging techniques. This chapter provides an overview of the physiological mechanisms underlying motor control and its disturbances in diseases presenting with movement disorders, from the basis of the neurophysiological information available today.

STRUCTURES INVOLVED IN MOVEMENT PROGRAMMING AND SENSORIMOTOR INTEGRATION

Theoretical and animal-based experimental evidence indicates that the basal ganglia are related to movement initiation and programming, while the cerebellum deals mainly with the practicalities of movement preparation by feedforward control of peripheral constraints. In any case, although there are no direct connections between the basal ganglia and the cerebellum, these structures should work in parallel, being confronted with common input and output circuits from the motor cortex, and thalamic and brainstem nuclei. It is the combined and well-orchestrated activation of multiple functional circuits that underlies accurate movement execution.

Basal Ganglia and Their Connections

In humans, clinical neurophysiology procedures can indirectly inform only on the function and dysfunction of the basal ganglia. There is no universal agreement on the connectivity between nuclei of the basal ganglia (5,6). However, the most accepted views indicate that the putamen and caudate (the striatum) are the nuclei receiving most inputs entering the basal ganglia. These inputs come from other nuclei of the basal ganglia, the cerebral cortex, thalamic nuclei, and in part from brainstem nuclei. An important contingent of inputs to the striatum is the dopaminergic projection originating in the substantia nigra pars compacta, which innervates striatal neurons expressing D1 and D2 receptors, with opposite effects. Striatal D1 receptor neurons initiate the direct pathway by sending inhibitory inputs to the globus pallidus pars interna (GPi). Striatal D2 receptor neurons initiate the indirect pathway by sending inhibitory inputs to the globus pallidus pars externa (GPe). The GPe sends inhibitory projections to the subthalamic nucleus (STN), and the STN sends excitatory inputs to the GPi. The GPi, together with the substantia nigra pars reticulata, (GPi/SNpr) comprise the main output nucleus of the basal ganglia. This output is inhibitory for the thalamocortical excitatory projections that would mediate corticospinal activation for voluntary movements.

Simultaneous activation of direct and indirect pathways seems to be adequate for an effective control of thalamocortical inputs. The net result of activity in the direct pathway is decreased inhibition, which would help in the initiation of a movement. By contrast, the net result of activity in the indirect pathway is increased inhibition, which will be helpful in avoiding unnecessary and unwanted movements. Nevertheless, this scheme is too simple. Far more complicated connections and circuits have been proposed that are probably closer to reality than the simplified diagrams usually depicting the main flow of inputs in the basal ganglia circuits. Competing influences exist in the excitatory projections from STN to GPi and GPe. STN neurons excite neurons in GPi, but they also indirectly inhibit the same neurons through excitation of GPe neurons that are inhibitory for the GPi. There are also interconnections among GPe, GPi/SNpr, and STN, which are organized in associative, sensorimotor, and limbic territories (7). The associative, sensorimotor, and limbic areas of GPi/SNpr project, respectively, to ventralis anterior (VA) and medialis dorsalis (MD) (associative), ventralis lateralis (VL) and VA (sensorimotor), and posteromedial MD (limbic). These pathways are channels through which emotion and environment can influence motor function and may drive some of the abnormalities in those aspects of human behavior that are present in patients with basal ganglia disorders (7,8).

Basal ganglia output is directed not only to thalamocortical projections but also to brainstem nuclei following at least two pathways (Fig. 2.1). Through one of them, the basal ganglia are thought to control the excitability of brainstem interneurons and is destined to regulate eye and eyelid movements (9,10). The superior colliculus (SC) receives inhibitory inputs from the SNpr and sends excitatory inputs to the nucleus raphe magnus (nRM), which, in turn, inhibits the neurons of the trigeminal spinal nuclei. Abnormalities in facial expression, blinking, and some eye and eyelid movements seen in certain movement disorders may be due to a dysfunction in this basal ganglia–brainstem circuit. Through another circuit, the basal ganglia send

inputs to the pedunculopontine tegmental nucleus (PPn) that stem from various nuclei. The PPn is a poorly understood multifunctional structure, with relevant influences on locomotion, regulation of sleep cycle, attention, arousal, startle, prepulse inhibition, and many other behavioral reactions (11–13). The basal ganglia–PPn circuit may participate in locomotor control and in the integration of motor, associative, and limbic functions (12). Abnormalities in gait and in the control of the startle reaction and prepulse inhibition seen in certain basal ganglia disorders may be due to a dysfunction in the basal ganglia–PPn circuit.

The Cerebellum and Its Connections

The physiology of the cerebellum and its connections is simpler than that of the basal ganglia. However, the exact effect of the cerebellar output on motor control and movement disorders is less clear. The cerebellar and cerebral motor cortex are not directly interconnected, but projections from both structures actually reach their targets through intermediate structures, such as the pontine nuclei, reticular formation, red nucleus, inferior olive, and brainstem nuclei and thalamus (14). The cerebellum receives inputs from many sensory afferents and brainstem nuclei (Fig. 2.2). They are conveyed through climbing fibers, which project contralaterally to the Purkinje cells via the inferior olive and the cerebellar peduncle, and mossy fibers, generated in brainstem nuclei, which also make synaptic connections with the Purkinje cells via the granule cells and the parallel fibers. The Purkinje cells are inhibitory for the deep cerebellar output nuclei, where they modulate the direct excitatory inputs from climbing and mossy fibers. Therefore, the mechanism by which the cerebellum participates in movement control is again a competing circuit of excitation and inhibition.

When reaching for an object, feed-forward control of movement utilizes current sensory information and prior experience to launch the hand in the correct direction and to decelerate the hand smoothly, as it approaches the target. The nervous system must initiate movement with appropriate force and direction, and this must be accomplished with due consideration of the complex mechanical properties of the limb. The segments and joints of an extremity have inertial, elastic, and viscous properties, and the motion of one limb segment influences other segments. Interaction torques and forces can facilitate or impede a desired movement, so the nervous system must generate muscle forces that are in harmony with the biomechanical properties of the body. Somatosensory and visual input are required to accomplish this feat, but a purely feedback mode of control would not have sufficient speed and sensitivity for rapid movements. Fortunately, the central nervous system learns the biomechanical characteristics of the body, and this knowledge is used to predict how body segments will interact during a particular movement.

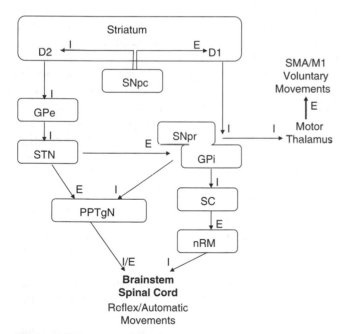

Figure 2.1 Schematic representation of the basal ganglia circuit and its output pathways. D1/D2, Dopaminergic receptors; E, excitation; GPe, globus pallidum externum; GPi, globus pallidum internum; I, inhibition; nRM, nucleus Raphe Magnus; PPTgN, pedunculopontine nucleus; SC, superior colliculus; SNpc, substantia nigra pars compacta; SNpr, substantia nigra pars reticulata; STN, subthalamic nucleus.

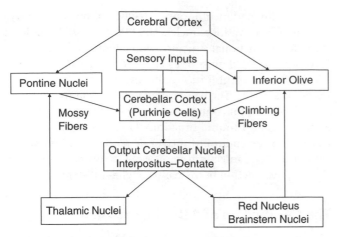

Figure 2.2 Schematic representation of the cerebellar circuits involved in motor control.

The cerebellum plays an important role in formulating and employing this model (15). Olivary neurons are capable of rhythmic discharge at 0.5–12 Hz, but they fire irregularly at roughly 1 Hz during arrhythmic movements and rest (16). By contrast, cerebellar mossy fibers fire at rates as high as 100 per second. The effect of climbing fiber discharge on Purkinje cells is to reduce the strength of the parallel-Purkinje cell synapse, thereby reducing Purkinje cell inhibition of the cerebellar nuclei. This synaptic interaction is believed to facilitate motor learning (15).

An oscillatory circuit generated between the cerebellum, the red nucleus, and the inferior olive—the Guillain-Mollaret triangle—is involved in many disorders featuring tremor. The cerebellar output nuclei send excitatory projections to the red nucleus which, in turn, sends excitatory projections to the inferior olive, and this to the cerebellar cortex to begin the circuit again (15,17). The parvicellular division of the red nucleus sends most of its output to the inferior olive. The rubro-olivary and olivocerebellar projections are also excitatory. Thus, the Guillain-Mollaret triangle works as a positive feedback system. This triangle and other positive feedback loops between the cerebellar nuclei and brainstem nuclei are prone to reverberation, and it is hypothesized that this reverberation plays a role in sustaining loop activity related to motor commands (17). The magnocellular division of the red nucleus, which is the origin of the rubrospinal tract, is very sparse in humans.

The Motor Cortex and the Subcortical Motor Structures and Pathways Involved in Execution of Voluntary Movements

The primary motor cortex and the corticospinal tract are typically considered as the executing part of the motor system. Inputs from many subcortical and cortical sources impinge on neurons of the primary motor cortex. When the large pyramidal cells of the motor cortex reach a threshold level of excitability, they generate a propagated action potential running downward to the cranial nerve and spinal motoneurons. The descending bundle of cortical axons run in the posterior limb of the internal capsule and through the cerebral peduncle to the pons. At this level, the axons are interspersed between the pontine nuclei. However, they converge again afterward to form the bulbar pyramids, where the majority cross to the contralateral side. Although most of the axons innervating cranial nerve nuclei have already left the tract before reaching the pyramids, the concept of pyramidal tract is commonly used to describe together the descending fibers that, being generated in the motor cortex, reach the cranial nerve and spinal cord motoneurons, the very last integrating step before the actual execution of the intended movement. It is to note that only a few axons have direct synapsis with spinal motoneurons. The majority of them reach the motoneurons through spinal interneurons that modulate the corticomotoneuronal input and integrate them with other inputs.

Control of Subcortical Reflex Motor Circuits

As previously noted, cortical motoneurons project to the brainstem nuclei where subcortical motor tracts originate. Also, they act over sensory afferents and over reflex pathways of the brainstem and spinal cord. The simplest reflex, the spinal monosynaptic stretch reflex, can actually be modulated voluntarily or automatically in preparation for a movement. More complex reflex circuits, such as those activating the vestibulospinal, the reticulospinal, and other subcortical motor tracts are also centrally modulated. The difference is that the motor consequences of a stretch reflex are circumscribed to a single muscle or limb segment, whereas activation of subcortical descending motor tracts gives rise to a widespread, sometimes purposeful, movement or behavior.

One of the most interesting complex reflex responses generated in the brainstem is the startle reaction (SR). Unexpected high-intensity auditory stimuli are commonly used for triggering the SR in humans. The acoustic SR is actually the fastest of all organized movements performed by human subjects. Davis and coworkers (18) reported that the SR in the rat could be generated by electrical stimulation of the nucleus reticularis pontis caudalis (nRPC), and they proposed a circuit for the acoustic SR consisting of the cochlear nucleus, the nucleus of the lateral lemniscus, the nRPC, and the brainstem and spinal motoneurons. Later, Lingenhohl and Friauf (19) further simplified the circuit and showed that the nRPC received direct inputs from the cochlear nucleus. The nRPC projects to the brainstem and spinal cord alpha motoneurons via the medial reticulospinal tract. Currently, the simplest circuit of the auditory SR is believed to involve the cochlear nucleus, the nRPC, and the alpha motoneurons (20–22). The giant neurons of the nRPC are not modality specific (23), likely responding to inputs other than those generated by acoustic stimuli. It is conceivable that somatosensory, visual, and vestibular inputs induce SRs through activation of the same efferent circuit.

Control of Subcortical Pattern Generators for Posture and Locomotion

Posture and locomotion are semiautomatic tasks that also depend in part on the activity of subcortical structures. Gait-related structures are located in the upper brainstem (24,25). The mesencephalic locomotor region (MLR), identified as a center where stimulation induces locomotion in experimentation animals, may exist also in humans, probably corresponding to the PPn. Cats with high cervical cord transections can walk on a treadmill with rudimentary locomotor activity that emerges from spinal cord networks, or central pattern generators (CPGs). Similar functional capacity is assumed to exist in patients with spinal cord lesions (26,27). However, activity of the CPG alone is not sufficient for recovery of postural or locomotor functions. The spinal CPG receives important connections from the reticulospinal, rubrospinal, vestibulospinal, and other descending motor tracts (24,28). The integrity of these subcortical pathways determines the possibilities for recovery in patients with spinal cord injuries (28). The ventrolateral spinal quadrant, containing the reticulospinal and vestibulospinal pathways, is important for the activation of spinal locomotor networks and for the recovery of locomotion after spinal cord injury (28). The vestibulospinal tract is involved in the control of antigravity muscle tone, and this control of tone is shared by the reticulospinal tract. These bulbospinal pathways are modulated in harmony with the support and swing (stepping) phases of the gait cycle, and this modulation is accomplished through connections with the cerebellar vermis and fastigial nuclei (29). Lesions of the vermis produce truncal ataxia, as is seen in alcoholics with anterior vermis degeneration. Similarly, inactivation of the fastigium with muscimol causes severe truncal disequilibrium with frequent falls to the side of the lesion (29). Damage to the flocculonodular lobe (vestibulocerebellum) and its connections with the vestibular nucleus produces truncal disequilibrium and impaired head–eye coordination (vestibulo-ocular reflex).

Gait initiation requires the subject to integrate postural and movement control. In normal adults, the key events occurring in gait initiation are ankle dorsiflexion, flexion and abduction of the hip, and flexion of the knee. These events propel the body forward and laterally, so that the swing foot can leave the ground and ultimately reach a forward step. Similar transient disequilibrium stages also happen in maneuvers such as rising on tiptoes, rising from a chair, and quickly bending forward (30). Each of these tasks entails postural shifts that move the body from one steady-state posture or movement to another, and they are often the first to be impaired in patients with vestibular or cerebellar disorders.

NEUROPHYSIOLOGICAL METHODS USED IN STUDIES OF MOTOR CONTROL AND MOVEMENT DISORDERS

Neurophysiological techniques used in the study of motor control and movement disorders are somewhat different from those used in conventional electrodiagnosis. Some of them are listed in Table 2.1. They require no sophisticated equipment and are readily available in all electromyography (EMG) laboratories. Simple EMG recording of muscle activation is the most basic method. It is used for measuring the characteristics of normal or abnormal muscle activation, the relationship between agonist and antagonist muscles, or the pattern of activation in ballistic movements. Single-axis accelerometers, which are rather simple bar electrodes containing a strain gauge, are very useful for recording the movement-related signal and analyzing the results together with those of the EMG surface recording. Needle recording is used very rarely, even though needle EMG of the anal sphincter is still considered in the diagnosis of parkinsonism. Eye-movement recording can be done easily with a pair of electrodes attached at the main axis of eye movements (vertical and horizontal) and recording with a low-filter bandpass. Nerve conduction studies are of little use, but brainstem reflexes can bring indirect information on the excitability of structures receiving some control from the basal ganglia. Assessment of autonomic dysfunction by all available means is certainly an important tool. Least sophisticated and available to most laboratories are the study of the sympathetic skin response and the evaluation of the changes in the heartbeat interval with various stress maneuvers. Specific methods more directly related to the study of motor control include the study of premotor potentials, the analysis of paradigms of reaction time, and the assessment of responses induced by transcranial stimulation of the motor cortex.

Premotor Potentials

The cerebral activity preceding voluntary or involuntary movement can be recorded using electroencephalographic methods and special features of modern oscilloscopes that make it possible to delay the trigger of the sweep in order to examine the epochs before the event employed as trigger (back-averaging techniques). In this way, the EMG or the movement signal generated when performing a phasic discrete voluntary movement can be used to trigger the system while recording the brain activity that precedes the movement. Different types of premotor potentials precede different types of movement.

In normal subjects, self-initiated movements are preceded by a slow negative shift of the baseline that may start about one and a half seconds before the actual movement, known as the Bereitschaftpotential (BSP) or readiness potential (31). A steeper negativity, known as the negative slope (NS), occurs in the last part of the premovement phase.

TABLE 2.1

NEUROPHYSIOLOGICAL TECHNIQUES USED IN THE STUDY OF MOTOR CONTROL AND MOVEMENT DISORDERS

Behavioral physiology	Surface recording of EMG and Movement Reaction time Startle Conditioning
Eye and eyelid movements	Blink rate Saccades

Brainstem reflexes	Trigemino-facial reflexes
	(Blink reflex; Perioral reflex)
	Trigemino-trigeminal reflexes
	(Jaw-jerk; Masseter inhibitory reflex)
	Other brainstem reflexes (Sternocleidomastoid
	  inhibition; Facial responses to peripheral nerve
	  stimuli)

Long latency and spinal reflexes	Cutaneo-muscular and stretch reflexes Propriospinal inhibitory circuits
Evoked potentials	Somatosensory, visual, auditory Event-related potentials
Transcranial magnetic stimulation	Central conduction time Threshold Cortical excitability
Needle electromyography	Anal and vesical sphincter EMG
Autonomic nervous system	Sympathetic skin response Heartbeat frequency modulation Urodynamic/rectal pressure studies

The premotor potential is not present when movements are made in the context of a reaction-time task paradigm. In a warned reaction-time task, a forewarning and an imperative stimulus, separated by a certain interval, are present. The subject is asked to react to the presentation of the second (imperative) stimulus. In this paradigm, there is a slow-rising negative shift, a contingent negative variation (CNV), that appears between the first and the second stimulus. The CNV is likely related to planning and programming of the movement to be executed and is, therefore, an indication of sensorimotor integration. The early part of the CNV is probably more related to arousal, whereas the second part is likely related to motor preparation (32).

Transcranial Cortical Stimulation

Noninvasive stimulation of the human brain is possible using electrical or magnetic stimuli (33). The interest in knowing the consequences of brain stimulation come from the beginning of the last century, when in 1909 Harvey Cushing began localizing sensory functions to the post-central gyrus in two patients undergoing brain surgery under local anesthesia. Later on, Wilder Penfield mapped the motor strip in patients undergoing neurosurgery (34). Merton and Morton (35) were the first to develop a technique appropriate for electrical stimulation of the human

brain through the scalp in intact humans. However, electrical stimulation is painful and uncomfortable, which makes it unsuitable for clinical purposes. Barker et al. (36) showed for the first time the possibility for activation of the human brain using nonpainful magnetic stimulation. Since then, transcranial magnetic stimulation (TMS) has been used in many studies on the physiology of motor control and is currently admitted as a helpful neurophysiological technique for the diagnosis of disorders affecting the motor pathway.

Cortical stimulation, either electrical or magnetic, activates the corticobulbar and the corticospinal tracts, sending volleys of inputs downstream that can be recorded at the spinal cord level. In experimentation animals, Patton and Amassian (37) showed for the first time that a single electrical cortical stimulus induced multiple descending volleys in corticospinal axons. This has been confirmed to be the case also with electrical stimulation in humans. The first part of the descending volley is defined as the D wave, assuming that it is the consequence of direct activation of corticospinal axons. This is followed by a few indirect (I) waves, separated between each other by intervals of 1.5 to 2.5 milliseconds. TMS induces descending volleys with a latency slightly longer than those induced by electrical stimulation (38,39), which is believed to be due to the lack of direct activation of the corticospinal axons and absence of a D wave. Therefore, it is believed that TMS does not activate corticospinal axons directly but rather cortical motoneurons through depolarization of premotoneuronal cortico-cortical axons.

TMS induces an excitatory postsynaptic potential (EPSP) in the spinal motoneurons either directly or through activation of interneurons. The actual strength of the EPSP varies according to the muscles and may be measured indirectly in humans using techniques such as the peri-stimulus time histogram (39). The motoneurons may be made to fire in response to a single cortical stimulus that is able to generate a suprathreshold EPSP. The response of muscles activated by TMS is the motor-evoked potential (MEP). The latency of the MEP to TMS in hand muscles is about 20 milliseconds, and the central conduction time from the motor cortex to the cervical spinal cord varies depending on the authors and the exact methodology applied between 5.5–9.5 milliseconds (33). While early reports were mainly devoted to the study of the corticospinal conduction time, new methodologies have brought other possibilities (Table 2.2), ranging from the study of the inhibition induced during voluntary contraction to paired stimulation and sensory modulation of the response to TMS. However, even though the functional assessment provided by application of TMS techniques is increasing, the clinical correlate of the results is not always clear.

Reaction Time

Reaction-time task paradigms have been used for a long time in the assessment of sensorimotor integration and behavior. Usually, subjects are requested to perform a movement at the perception of a sensory stimulus or imperative signal (IS). The characteristics of the required movement could be completely specified beforehand, which defines a paradigm of simple reaction time (SRT). Alternatively, the exact characteristics of the movement may be made available only to the subject at the presentation of the IS, which defines the paradigm of choice reaction time (CRT). In the first condition, subjects can prepare

their motor circuitry and have it ready for motor performance upon perception of the IS. In the second condition, subjects still can make some kind of preparation, albeit only partial because the ultimate instruction is unknown until presentation of the IS. As a consequence, SRT is shorter than CRT. Stimulus perception is an obvious prerequisite for the initiation of the voluntary action in a reaction-time task experiment. This does not mean necessarily that there should be a conscious perception of the sensory stimulus used as an imperative signal, but rather just that there is an awareness of it (40,41). The time required for such a process in a SRT experiment has been defined as the "time for recognition" (42). According to Pascual-Leone et al. (42), once the sensory signal has been recognized, subjects may start the "time of initiation" in which the motor program is transferred to the execution channel for development of the action "time for execution"). There is no universal agreement on how to measure reaction time, but the most common outcome measures are the execution of a task (43,44), the ending of an action (45,46), the onset of limb displacement (47,48), and the onset of EMG activity (49,50).

The execution of ballistic movements in a reaction-time task paradigm involves activation of many descending motor tracts, but the relative role of each one of them in the accurate performance of fast movements is mostly unknown (51). That the corticospinal tract is involved in the execution of fast ballistic movements in humans is assumed in part from the observations of a progressive increase in the excitability of the motor pathway (52). Using TMS (42) showed that an otherwise subthreshold TMS was able to induce an MEP in the agonist muscle for the incoming reaction when applied a short time after the IS. The amplitude of the MEP increased progressively, starting at about 80 milliseconds before onset of the EMG activity.

When testing such an effect, Pascual-Leone et al. (42) also observed that subthreshold TMS induced acceleration of the voluntary reaction. Reaction-time shortening by subthreshold TMS was interpreted as the consequence of an externally induced acceleration in the process of motor cortex energization to reach the level of excitability appropriate for activation of the execution channel. However, alternative explanations were given, such as the possibility that TMS activated subcortical motor structures through cortico-subcortical connections. Valls-Solé et al. (53,54) found out later that a startling auditory stimulus, which is supposed to directly activate the reticulospinal tract, induced even more acceleration of the reaction time than TMS. Furthermore, the shortening effect involved the whole three-burst pattern constituting the motor program for ballistic movements (55). In such a study, the authors asked healthy volunteers to perform a ballistic wrist movement. They were trained to produce the triphasic agonist–antagonist–agonist EMG pattern in a vigorous movement of the wrist. In some trials, a startling stimulus was delivered together with the IS. In test trials, the latency of the first agonist EMG burst was significantly shorter than in control trials, but the configuration of

TABLE 2.2

TRANSCRANIAL MAGNETIC STIMULATION IN THE STUDY OF MOVEMENT DISORDERS

Techniques	Assessment
Threshold at rest	Level of cortical excitability
MEP facilitation with contraction	"Energization" of motor cortex
MEP increase with stimulus intensity	Recruitment of motor neurons
Mapping of motor cortex	Cortical synaptic plasticity
Contralateral silent period	Cortical inhibitory function
Ipsilateral silent period	Transcallosal inhibition
Paired stimulation ISIs 3–4 ms	Cortico-cortical inhibition
Paired stimulation ISIs 12–15 ms	Cortico-cortical facilitation
Modulation of reflexes	Effects at a spinal level
Somatosensory modulation of MEP	Sensorimotor integration

the triphasic pattern did not change between control and test trials. These findings indicate that the whole programmed three-bursts pattern of the ballistic movement was moved to a shorter latency, as if it were triggered by the startle itself. The interpretation of these findings is that the excitability of the pathways involved in the SR was modulated according to the patterned response during preparation for the execution of the ballistic movement. If this were not the case, one should have expected a significant change in the configuration of the three-burst pattern. The consequence is that the reticulospinal tract is actively involved and plays a most important role in the execution of ballistic movements (54).

The excitability of the startle pathways is enhanced during motor preparation (56). Therefore, according to the observations described, the subcortical motor tracts are already in a state of hyperexcitability with respect to resting conditions at the time of the IS, while the motor cortex increases its excitability only after the IS, just about 80 milliseconds before onset of EMG activity (41,42). When a startling auditory stimulus is used to test the excitability of the subcortical motor pathways after the IS, the responses of the orbicularis oculi and sternocleidomastoid muscles remain unchanged, larger than at rest in a similar percentage in intervals ranging from 20–100 milliseconds after the IS (Fig. 2.3). The hypothesis underlying these observations is that execution of a ballistic movement requires a certain enhancement of the excitability of subcortical motor pathways. Such enhancement would probably have been established after the forewarning and before the IS and would remain stable until the motor cortex sends a release command after the perception of the IS. This hypothesis requires that the central nervous system exerts an inhibitory action over the hyperexcitable subcortical motor tracts to prevent unwanted precipitated execution of the task.

MOVEMENT DISORDERS

Typically, movement disorders are classified in two large groups: hypokinetic and hyperkinetic. The pathophysiological mechanisms of both types can at least in part be attributed to a dysfunction in the basal ganglia circuits. In hypokinetic states the activity in the indirect pathway predominates over that of the direct pathway, giving rise to an increase in GPi inhibitory output, which results in decreased motor activity. The most classic example of hypokinetic movement disorders is Parkinson's disease (PD). In hyperkinetic states the activity in the indirect pathway is decreased, giving rise to a decreased inhibitory output, which results in excess motor activity. The typical example of a hyperkinetic movement disorder is Huntington's disease. However, apart from these paradigmatic abnormalities, other dysfunctions in the basal ganglia and in the other subcortical motor circuits contribute to the pathophysiology of movement disorders.

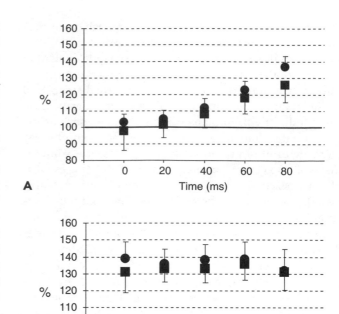

Figure 2.3   Size of the responses of the agonist wrist flexor muscles (*circles*) and the postural sternocleidomastoid muscle (*squares*) to threshold transcranial magnetic stimulation **(A)**, and startling auditory stimuli **(B)**, applied in the context of a reaction-time task experiment, at the time interval with respect to the IS shown in the X axis. The response sizes are represented as percentages of baseline, determined as the mean of the responses obtained out of three consecutive stimuli given at rest. Note the differences in excitability of the two circuits, indicating that the subcortical motor tract is in a state of relatively high excitability before the increase observed in the corticospinal tract.

Parkinsonism

Parkinson's disease (PD) is a degenerative disorder characterized by a constellation of symptoms and signs known as *parkinsonism*. According to current diagnostic criteria (57,58,59), patients can be considered to have PD when they have bradykinesia and at least one of the following: rigidity, tremor, or postural instability with no other known causes. They should also not have any of the signs considered atypical for PD, such as dementia, cerebellar or pyramidal signs, or oculomotor abnormalities. Apart from parkinsonism, patients with PD may also present with cognitive disorders, depression, sleep disorders, autonomic dysfunction, and so on. Other degenerative diseases featuring parkinsonism that should be differentiated from idiopathic PD are progressive supranuclear palsy (PSP), multisystem atrophy (MSA), cortico-basal ganglionic degeneration (CBGD), and secondary causes of parkinsonism. The similarities among these disorders regarding their clinical presentation are probably the basis of diagnostic errors (59). Neurophysiological examinations can be of some help to the clinician in reaching a more accurate differentiation among parkinsonisms, on the basis of the characterization of their specific symptoms and signs (for a review, see 60).

Functional abnormalities of basal ganglia activation could explain the abnormalities reported in PD patients on premotor potentials. The BSP that precedes self-initiated movements is abnormally reduced (61), as it occurs with the CNV observed with a "Go/NoGo" finger-movement task (62). Cunnington et al. (62) found that the premovement cortical activity was shifted toward the side of the impairment in patients with predominantly unilateral disease, suggesting that a compensatory mechanism was operating predominantly on the side of greatest basal ganglia impairment. Several other functional studies demonstrated abnormalities that are directly or indirectly related to the basal ganglia disorders. Indirect evidence for the implication of nigrostriatal dopaminergic dysfunction in the generation of some of the neurophysiological abnormalities reported so far comes from the improvement seen with L-dopa treatment. This is the case, for example, with the BSP (63), motor cortex excitability (64,65), and SEPs (66).

Treatments based on stereotactic neurosurgery procedures have been reintroduced for advanced PD with quite successful results (67,68). Surgery is aimed at the destruction or inactivation of hyperfunctioning nuclei, such as the STN and the GPi. At present, the most common target structure is the STN. The clinical improvement reported by the great majority of patients after surgery in most laboratories is outstanding evidence in favor of the implication of the target nuclei in the pathophysiology and pathogenesis of parkinsonian motor symptoms (68,69). Direct recording of the firing characteristics of neurons in basal ganglia nuclei, such as the elevated neuronal activity of the STN reported by Hutchison et al. (70), speaks also in favor of the excitability abnormalities that can be suspected from the model.

As previously stated, the basal ganglia dysfunction in PD leads not only to consequences at the level of the motor cortex but also at the level of the brainstem. The increased SNpr inhibition of the SC ultimately causes fewer inhibitory inputs to reach the spinal trigeminal nucleus and leads to an enhancement of the excitability recovery curve of the reflexes mediated by the trigeminal spinal nucleus, such as the blink reflex, the masseteric inhibitory reflex, and others. Another dysfunctional pathway in PD is the circuit linking the basal ganglia and the brainstem through the PPn (71). The PPn cholinergic neurons regulate the excitability of startle-related structures of the reticular formation. We can only speculate on what would be the net effect of the abnormal inputs to, and abnormal function of, PPn in PD patients. In experimentation animals, PPn lesions cause enhancement of the amplitude of the startle reaction and reduction of prepulse inhibition (72,73).

Although the motor cortex is typically not damaged in idiopathic PD and the motor conduction time was reported as normal in an early work with cortical stimulation (74),

subsequent studies have shown several functional abnormalities of the motor cortex. The MEP amplitude is enhanced at rest (75,76) but does not grow as much as in normal subjects with progressive increase of voluntary contraction of the target muscle (77). The silent period induced by TMS during voluntary contraction is shorter in PD patients than in normal subjects (76,77) but lengthens with L-dopa treatment (64,78). The facilitation of the MEP occurring just before onset of voluntary contraction in a reaction time paradigm is reduced in IPD patients with respect to control subjects (50), meaning that there is probably reduced excitability of the motor cortex. The same mechanisms may also be responsible for the observation made by Berardelli et al. (79) of reduced MEP amplitude recovery with paired stimuli at long intervals. Another abnormality observed with TMS is reduced cortico-cortical inhibition (80), when conditioning TMS is applied between 1–5 milliseconds before a subsequent suprathreshold stimulus. The reduced percentage inhibition found in IPD patients compared to control subjects is interpreted as the consequence of an imbalance of inhibitory and facilitatory motor cortical circuits.

Tremor

Tremor is an intrinsic aspect of movements made by normal individuals, although it is of so small an amplitude that it is usually not visible to the naked eye. Physiologic tremor, at frequencies of 8–12 Hz, can have many causes. Mechanical properties of joints determine the presence of some oscillations, which frequency would depend on the inertia and stiffness of the joint. It is lower in proximal joints (3–5 Hz at the elbow) than in distal joints (20–30 Hz at the metacarpophalangeal joint (81). Cardioballistic impulse is another source of mechanical tremor, although its exact contribution to physiological tremor is unlikely because of the relatively low frequency of heartbeat in relation to tremor frequencies. Neurogenic causes of physiologic tremor have to take into account the fact that the motoneuronal firing rate is about 10 Hz (82). This rhythmic behavior would not necessarily have to cause oscillations during contraction because of the nonsynchronized firing of motoneurons. However, there may be central oscillatory circuits driving the motoneurons to some synchronization, such as the inferior olive and other brain structures.

The neurophysiological study of tremor is usually carried out using surface EMG recordings from antagonistic forearm muscles. The actual movement can also be recorded using an accelerometer attached over the moving segment. Accelerometer recording with a rather low-frequency band-pass filter can be submitted to Fast Fourier transformation analysis, to determine the dominant frequency peak. The degree of rhythmicity of the oscillation can be indirectly appreciated by analyzing the relative power of the dominant peak with respect to the total power of the spectrum. This is a nice piece of information to add to the studies of tremor, since it permits an objective distinction between rhythmic and nonrhythmic movements (83). The analysis of tremor oscillations during performance of a contralateral ballistic movement may also be of help for the identification of patients with psychogenic tremor (84). Tremor is the most frequent type among all abnormal movements in psychogenic disorders. When a tremor requires voluntary drive, such as in healthy subjects requested to mimic tremor or patients with psychogenic tremor, this drive stops transiently during execution of a ballistic movement with the contralateral hand (Fig. 2.4). This may be due to the movement-related generation of inhibitory commands for the contralateral motor pathway. Interestingly, the effect is absent in patients with Parkinsonian tremor or essential tremor.

Physiologic tremor may be enhanced in conditions such as fatigue, anxiety, strenuous muscle contractions, the use of beta-adrenergic drugs, or other conditions. In these situations, the amplitude of tremor increases and, consequently, the frequency decreases. This aspect is useful in distinguishing tremors depending at least partly on peripheral mechanisms, such as physiological tremor and enhanced physiological tremor, from those that depend more on central oscillatory circuits, such as Parkinsonian

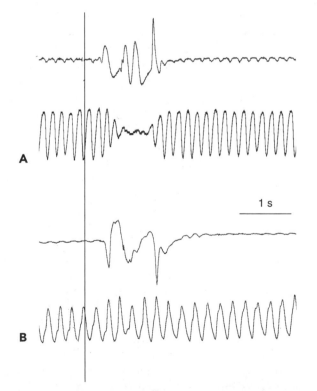

Figure 2.4 Recording of tremor during performance of a ballistic movement in the context of a reaction-time task paradigm in a patient with psychogenic tremor **(A)** and in a patient with parkinsonian tremor **(B)**. Reaction is performed with the right hand (*upper traces in* **A** and **B**), while tremor oscillations are recorded from the left hand (*lower traces in* **A** and **B**). Note the transient stop of tremor oscillations in **A** beginning a few hundred milliseconds after movement onset.

tremor and essential tremor. Tremor is a feature of many central nervous system disorders. An abnormal functioning of the inferior olive is the recognized cause of a particular tremor: palatal tremor (85). Lesions in the vicinity of the red nucleus may be responsible for rubral tremor, which is a low-frequency rest, postural, and kinetic tremor (86) that characteristically appears weeks or months after a lesion. Essential tremor is an action tremor that affects predominantly the hands and also may involve the head and other body parts, at a frequency that is usually 5–8 Hz (87). Even though the cerebellum is likely to be involved, postmortem examinations have revealed no structural damage (88,89). Stereotactic surgery targeting the thalamic ventralis intermedius nucleus (VIM) reduces considerably the tremor and has become a treatment option in patients in whom tremor markedly impairs quality of life (90). VIM is a cerebellar receiving nucleus and a relay for short-latency proprioceptive feedback to the motor cortex (91). Therefore, VIM thalamotomy or repetitive stimulation could interrupt a hypothetically unstable transthalamocortical sensorimotor loop.

Tremor is probably the most apparent motor dysfunction in PD. It is usually a low-frequency, rhythmic ("pill-rolling") oscillation at rest that disappears transiently when the patient is performing a movement (92). Tremor-related phasic activity has been seen in the STN, the GPi, the striatum, and the ventral lateral nucleus of the thalamus (93). The motor cortex is also involved, at least as part of the execution pathway of the rhythmic activity. This can be demonstrated by the fact that TMS but not electrical cortical stimulation reset tremor oscillations (94). Studies of coherence also have helped in identifying a motor-cortex–muscle-oscillations relationship (95). The tremor frequency is capable of attracting other voluntary, repetitive movements (96). In most instances, parkinsonian patients initiate contractions during the descending phase of the oscillation and produce the agonist burst after the midpoint of the EMG tremor cycle (97). Action tremor may be present also in parkinsonian patients and could be contributing to bradykinesia in PD, since a direct correlation has been found between slowness of reaction time and the presence of tremor bursts during the acceleration phase of the movement (98).

Chorea

Chorea is the term used to describe abnormal movements with unpredictable timing, which are asymmetric, asynchronous, and randomly changing from one body part to another. Chorea (and hemiballism) are hypothesized to occur when subthalamic activation of the inhibitory pallidothalamic pathway is reduced, which is precisely opposite to the situation in parkinsonism. A critical balance between the direct and indirect pathways is needed to produce normal movement and avoid hypo- or hyperkinesias. Many diseases are present with chorea, but the most paradigmatic is Huntington's disease, in which there is degeneration of the GABAergic striatal neurons. However, the neurons of the indirect pathway projecting to the GPe seem to degenerate before those of the direct pathway projecting to the GPi (99). This differential degeneration provides a plausible pathophysiological explanation for many symptoms and signs seen in Huntington's disease (99,100).

While the excitability of the blink reflex is enhanced in PD, it is reduced in Huntington's disease (101,102). Interestingly, however, prepulse inhibition of the startle reflex or of the blink reflex is equally reduced in patients of both diseases (103). Patients with Huntington's disease also have other noticeable abnormalities, such as a decrease in the size of the somatosensory-evoked potentials (SEPs) and of the long latency stretch reflexes, a reduction in the size of the premotor potentials in self-generated or externally cued movements, and an increase in the duration of the silent period of hand muscles to TMS (104).

Dystonia

Dystonia is an abnormal co-contraction of antagonistic muscles. The multiple forms of dystonia have different etiology and pathophysiology. Primary or idiopathic dystonia may be of genetic cause (a deletion in the *DYT1* gene). Secondary dystonia may be due to focal lesions, usually localized in the striatum, pallidum, or thalamus (105,106), peripheral nerve injuries such as trauma, overuse, or repetitive strain injuries (107), or the use of neuroleptics or other related drugs. Dystonia is considered a basal ganglia disorder (108). Internal pallidal recordings in dystonic patients have revealed reduced mean firing rates and altered firing patterns (109). This association between reduced GPi activity and dystonia fits with the notion that dystonia is a hyperkinetic movement disorder. However, internal pallidotomy or the implantation of electrodes for chronic electrical stimulation of the GPi has been used with some success as a treatment for dystonia, which is at odds with the notion that dystonia is simply the result of reduced GPi activity (110). The precise pathophysiological mechanisms underlying dystonia remain elusive. There is evidence for a sensory base of the disorder (111–114). However, how the sensory inputs are abnormally gated at basal ganglia level is not known (115,116).

Several neurophysiological abnormalities have been reported in patients with dystonia that slightly vary with the form of dystonia (117). The paradigmatic feature is that of a co-contraction between antagonistic muscles in attempts to perform a discrete movement (Fig. 2.5). Such co-contraction also can be demonstrated by a decrease in reciprocal inhibition between antagonistic muscles of the forearm. In brainstem reflexes, patients with dystonia show a decrease of the normal inhibition of the blink reflex after trigeminal nerve stimulation (an increase in the excitability recovery). With transcranial magnetic

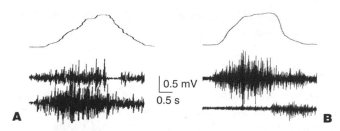

Figure 2.5 Co-contraction between antagonistic muscles of the forearm when performing an oscillatory wrist movement in a patient with dystonia **(A)** compared to the well-defined alternation of EMG activity in a control subject **(B)**.

stimulation, a decrease of short-latency cortico-cortical inhibition has been shown (80), together with a decrease in the duration of the silent period (104).

Tics

Tics are jerklike, simple or coordinated, stereotyped movements that look like normal movements. Most of them are brief and quick, but some tics may be prolonged (*dystonic tics*). Although tics are classified as abnormal involuntary movements, they cannot always be considered involuntary. Most tics are easily suppressed for short periods, but continued suppression causes anxiety and an urge to let the tic happen (119). Tics may be preceded by sensory symptoms, called premonitory sensations (also called *sensory tics* in the past). In these cases, patients may explain the motor act as if it were directed to deal with the sensory symptom.

The most paradigmatic disease presenting with tics is Gilles de la Tourette's syndrome, in which the motor tics are accompanied by a variety of simple or complex vocalizations, a requisite for the diagnosis. Patients with Tourette's syndrome often have obsessive–compulsive behavior, hyperactivity, inattentiveness, impulsivity, and emotional lability. These abnormalities are consistent with dysfunction of lateral prefrontal, orbitofrontal, and limbic cortices and their subcortical connections. Patients with Tourette's syndrome have many motor dysfunctions to show in a neurophysiological exam. However, no single test is specific for the disorder. In a reaction-time task experiment in which subjects had to make a sequence of movements along a path with variable amounts of advance information, patients with Tourette's syndrome were significantly slower in performing a movement if advance information was not available, but they were similar to those of healthy subjects when advance information was available (120). The conclusion of this and similar studies is that patients with Tourette's syndrome have some difficulty generating movements from internal storage and are more dependent than normals on external stimuli. Premovement potentials are abnormally short or absent before tics (121), which is in line with the idea that the movement of the tic is not made with the same preparatory cortical activity as self-generated voluntary movements. This may be in line with the manifestation of some patients that their tics are made to respond to sensory signals.

Myoclonus

Myoclonus are sudden, brief, shocklike, involuntary movements caused by muscular contractions or inhibitions. Clinical neurophysiology is often required in the assessment of myoclonus, since it may help in etiological and pathophysiological classifications (122). According to their etiology, myoclonus are classified as physiologic, essential, epileptic, and symptomatic (123). Pathophysiological classifications are of more interest to clinical neurophysiology. According to the results of clinical and neurophysiological studies, myoclonus can be classified as cortical, subcortical, segmental, and peripheral. In spontaneous myoclonus, the abnormal bursts of EMG activity appear at rest. However, the most frequent types of myoclonus are the action and postural myoclonus. In these types the EMG bursts interrupt the ongoing EMG activity, typically with a synchronized burst followed by a short silence. It is not always easy to distinguish myoclonic bursts from variations in the ongoing activity. Sensory stimulation such as touch or passive change of joint position may help with triggering some bursts or silences. The most common cause of cortical myoclonus is hypoxia (Lance-Adams syndrome). In cortical reflex myoclonus (124), the EMG bursts are preceded by a time-locked cortical potential at less than 40 milliseconds and are accompanied by reflex cortical phenomena such as enlarged cortical (SEPs) or reflex-induced myoclonus. Back-averaging of the EEG activity time-locked to the myoclonic burst is the preferred method for recording the cortical spike. If this is present, it is usually more clearly picked up at the centroparietal contralateral region. In some cases of posthypoxic myoclonus, the damage may be subcortical rather than cortical. This is the case in reticular reflex myoclonus

(125). In these patients, EEG activity may be present, but it is not time-locked to the myoclonic jerk.

Many diseases may present with myoclonus originated at the cortical level. This is the case with Creutzfeldt-Jakob disease, subacute sclerosing panencephalitis, cortico-basal ganglionic degeneration, Alzheimer's disease, multisystem atrophy, and a few disorders. In some instances, the myoclonic jerks are very small and may mimic tremor. The term "cortical tremor" was introduced by Ikeda et al. (126) to describe patients with irregular individual finger movements who had EEG spikes revealed with back-averaging. Many authors have used the term *minipolymyoclonus* to describe these small isolated finger movements that may actually be present in diseases not involving cortical dysfunction (Table 2.3).

Stiffness and Neuromyotonia

Continuous firing of motor units or muscle fibers can cause abnormal postures and movements. The most commonly known situations are the stiff-person syndrome and the continuous muscle fiber activity syndrome. The stiff-person syndrome (127) is characterized by axial rigidity, involving the paraspinal and abdominal muscles. Muscular spasms may appear with emotions, stress, peripheral nerve stimulation, startle, and other types of stimuli (128). Patients may develop fear to certain stress-inducing situations and may be seen by psychiatrists with the suspicion of social phobias or other kinds of abnormal behavior. In the classical stiff-person syndrome, 70% of patients are diabetic, and 90% have high titers of antibodies against glutamic acid decarboxylase (GAD), an enzyme necessary for the synthesis of GABA. The absence of GABA-mediated inhibition of motoneuronal firing may be a likely pathophysiological mechanism to account for the repetitive firing of motor unit action potentials and the spasms that characterize the syndrome. In a neurophysiological study of different inhibitory circuits for alpha motoneurons, Floeter et al. (129) found that most patients

TABLE 2.3
DISORDERS FEATURING MINIPOLYMYOCLONUS

Disorder	Dominant clinical sign	EMG bursts	EEG	"C" wave
Motoneuron disease	Fasciculation atrophy	Asynchronous (1–20 Hz)	Not described	Not described
Polyneuropathy	Absent tendon jerks Severe sensory deficit	Slow and asynchronous	Not described	Not described
Alzheimer's disease	Dementia	Multifocal	Slow waves Epileptiform activity Negative frontal wave	Present
Myoclonic epilepsy	Seizures	Synchronized or irregular	Slow negative frontal wave	Present
Syringomyelia	Weakness Spasticity Sensory deficit	Asynchronous and irregular	Not described	Not described

had abnormally reduced presynaptic inhibition, which is a GABA-mediated inhibitory mechanism. However, glycine-mediated inhibitory circuits, such as homonymous, reciprocal, or recurrent inhibition, were also impaired in a few cases. In these cases, inhibitory circuit dysfunctions likely would have to be attributed to abnormalities in the supraspinal control of the spinal mechanisms of inhibition.

Another mechanism by which there may be involuntary muscle contractions is the presence of *myokymia* or *neuromyotonia*. These terms refer to the clinical observation of involuntary muscle contraction or movement or involuntary delay of muscle relaxation after a voluntary contraction. There is an electromyographic counterpart of the disorders, defined respectively as myokymic or neuromyotonic discharges. This peculiar activity consists in the abnormal firing of action potentials usually generated in the axon terminals (Fig. 2.6). Isaac's syndrome is a rare, genetically mediated disorder presenting with myokymia and neuromyotonia. The Schwartz-Jampel syndrome, or chondrodystrophic myotonica, is an autosomal recessive disease, characterized by clinical myotonia and osteoarticular deformities. The most commonly seen form of neuromyotonia is the acquired one, in which immune-mediated ion channel disturbances occur, principally in the voltage-gated potassium channels (130). Some of these cases are paraneoplastic and associated with thymoma or small-cell lung cancer. Needle electromyography and nerve stimulation may help in identifying the nature of the disorder and may sometimes be the first unexpected sign of a paraneoplastic syndrome in a patient complaining of weakness and cramps. The EMG activity is typically that of fasciculations, myokymic discharges, and neuromyotonic activity,

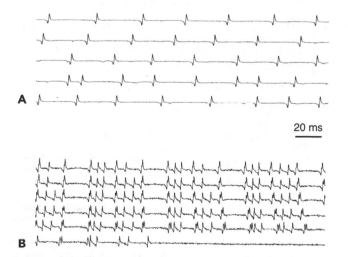

20 ms

Figure 2.6 Needle EMG recordings of abnormal firing of motor unit action potentials in dorsal paraspinal muscles in a woman with a stiff-person syndrome **(A)** and of a neuromyotonic discharge in the quadriceps in a patient with neuromyotonia in the context of a paraneoplastic syndrome **(B)**. Note the difference in the firing pattern and in the shape of the action potential, identical to a motor unit action potential in the stiff-person syndrome and compatible with a group of muscle fibers in the neuromyotonic discharge.

clearly different from the motor unit action potentials seen in the stiff-person syndrome.

Control of Posture and Gait

Somatosensory, vestibular, and visual inputs to the central nervous system are utilized in the control of posture and balance. Somatosensory proprioception is the most important modality for generating protective postural reactions (131). Patients with somatosensory loss (e.g., due to peripheral neuropathy) exhibit increased reliance on vestibular, visual, and predictive mechanisms of postural control. Modest mechanical perturbations of quiet stance (e.g., a nudge to the sternum) produce a synergistic distal-to-proximal activation of muscles in the lower extremities and torso. This coordinated sequence of reflex responses in muscles of the limbs and trunk has been called the *"ankle strategy"* of postural control and is preprogrammed by the nervous system, based on current sensory information, previous experience, and motor intent (131). The ankle strategy is not adequate for strong perturbations or a precarious base of support (e.g., a balance beam or slippery surface). Under these circumstances, hip rotation with appropriate arm motion (*hip strategy*) may be necessary to keep the body's center of mass over the base of support, or it may be necessary to establish an entirely new base of support through the execution of a so-called *rescue response*. The nervous system may generate postural activity in advance of a predictable perturbation, based on sensory feedback and previous experience. For example, muscles in the extremities are activated *before* impact during a fall (132).

Rescue responses require strength and agility that can easily exceed the neurological and musculoskeletal capabilities of patients with neurological disorders (133). A common manifestation of general failure of this complex neurological and musculoskeletal link is the disorders of gait. Nutt et al. (133) grouped the gait disorders in highest-, middle-, and lowest-level gait disorders. Highest-level gait disorders would be those generated in dysfunctions of the frontal lobes and their connections with other cortical and subcortical structures. Middle-level gait disorders would be those caused by ascending or descending sensorimotor tract lesions, cerebellar ataxia, bradykinesia, hyperkinesia, and dystonia. Lowest-level gait disorders would be those related to diseases of muscle, bone peripheral nerves, visual pathway, or the vestibular system.

REFERENCES

1. Ashby P, Kim YJ, Kumar R, Lang AE, Lozano AM. Neurophysiological effects of stimulation through electrodes in the human subthalamic nucleus. *Brain* 1999;122:1919–1931.
2. Kuhn AA, Brandt SA, Kupsch A, et al. Comparison of motor effects following subcortical electrical stimulation through electrodes in the globus pallidus internus and cortical transcranial magnetic stimulation. *Exp Brain Res* 2004;155:48–55.
3. Nathan PW, Smith MC. The rubrospinal and central tegmental tracts in man. *Brain* 1982;105:233–269.
4. Rothwell JC. Control of human voluntary movement. 2nd edition. London: Chapman and Hall, 1994.

5. Alexander GE, Crutcher MD. Functional architecture of basal ganglia circuits: neural substrates of parallel processing. *Trends Neurosci* 1990;13:266–271.
6. Parent A, Cicchetti F. The current model of basal ganglia organization under scrutiny. *Mov Disord* 1998;13:199–202.
7. Nakano K, Kayahara T, Tsutsumi T, et al. Neural circuits and functional organization of the striatum. *J Neurol* 2000;247[Suppl 5]:V1–15.
8. Bolam JP, Hanley JJ, Booth PA, et al. Synaptic organisation of the basal ganglia. *J Anat* 2000;196:527–542.
9. Basso MA, Powers AS, Evinger C. An explanation for reflex blink hyperexcitability in Parkinson's disease. I. Superior colliculus. *J Neurosci* 1996;16,7308–7317.
10. Basso MA, Evinger C. An explanation for reflex blink hyperexcitability in Parkinson's disease. II. Nucleus raphe magnus. *J Neurosci* 1996;16,7318–7330.
11. Garcia-Rill E. The pedunculopontine nucleus. *Progress in Neurobiology* 1991;36:363–389.
12. Inglis WL, Winn P. The pedunculopontine tegmental nucleus: where the striatum meets the reticular formation. *Prog Neurobiol* 1995;47:1–29.
13. Reese NB, Garcia-Rill E, Skinner RD. The pedunculopontine nucleus: auditory input, arousal and pathophysiology. *Prog Neurobiol* 1995;42:105–133.
14. Haines DE, Mihailoff GA, Bloedel JR. The cerebellum. In: Haines DE, ed. *Fundamental Neuroscience.* New York: Churchill Livingstone, 1997:379–398.
15. Thach WT. On the specific role of the cerebellum in motor learning and cognition: clues from PET activation and lesion studies in man. *Behav Brain Sc* 1996;19:411–431.
16. Smith SS. Step cycle-related oscillatory properties of inferior olivary neurons recorded in ensembles. *Neuroscience* 1998;82:69–81.
17. De Zeeuw CI, Simpson JI, Hoogenraad CC, et al. Microcircuitry and function of the inferior olive. *Trends Neurosci* 1998;21:391–400.
18. Davis M, Gendelman DS, Tischler MD, Gendelman PM. A primary acoustic startle circuit: lesion and stimulation studies. *J Neurosci* 1982;2,791–805.
19. Lingenhohl K, Friauf E. Giant neurons in the rat reticular formation: a sensorimotor interface in the elementary acoustic startle circuit? *J Neurosci* 1994;14:1176–1194.
20. Yeomans JS, Frankland PW. The acoustic startle reflex: neurons and connections. *Brain Res Rev* 1996;21:301–314.
21. Davis M. Differential roles of the amygdala and bed nucleus of the stria terminalis in conditioned fear and startle enhanced by corticotropin-releasing hormone. In: Ono T, McNaughton BL, Molotchnikoff S, Rolls ET, Nishijo H, eds. *Perception, Memory and Emotion.* Oxford: Elsevier Ltd., 1996: 525–548.
22. Koch M. The neurobiology of startle. *Progr Neurobiol* 1999;59:107–128.
23. Wu MF, Suzuki SS, Siegel JM. Anatomical distribution and response patterns of reticular neurons active in relation to acoustic startle. *Brain Res* 1988;457:399–406.
24. Mori S, Matsuyama K, Mori F, et al. Supraspinal sites that induce locomotion in the vertebrate central nervous system. *Adv Neurol* 2001;87:25–40.
25. Kinjo N, Atsuta Y, Webber M, et al. Medioventral medulla-induced locomotion. *Brain Res Bull.* 1990;24:509–516.
26. Armstrong DM. The supraspinal control of mammalian locomotion. *J Physiol* 1988;405:1–37.
27. Dietz V, Colombo G, Jensen L, et al. Locomotor capacity of spinal cord in paraplegic patients. *Ann Neurol* 1995;37:574–582.
28. Eidelberg E, Walden JG, Nguyen LH. Locomotor control in macaque monkeys. *Brain* 1981;104:647–663.
29. Thach WT, Goodkin HP, Keating JG. The cerebellum and the adaptive coordination of movement. *Annu Rev Neurosci* 1992;15:403–442.
30. Schultz AB, Alexander NB, Ashton-Miller JA. Biomechanical analyses of rising from a chair. *J Biomech* 1992;25:1383–1391.
31. Shibasaki H, Barrett G, Halliday E, Halliday A. Components of the movement-related cortical potential and their scalp topography. *Electroenceph Clin Neurophysiol* 1980;49:213–226.
32. Ikeda A. Electrocorticography in motor control and movement disorders. In: Hallett M, ed. *Handbook of Clinical Neurophysiology,* vol 1. Amsterdam: Elsevier, 2003:31–44.
33. Rothwell JC, Thompson PD, Day BL, Boyd S, Marsden CD. Stimulation of the human motor cortex through the scalp. *Experimental Phsyiology* 1991;76:159–200.
34. Penfield W. The excitable cortex in conscious man. Liverpool: Liverpool University Press, 1967;1–5.
35. Merton PA, Morton HB. Stimulation of the cerebral cortex in the intact human subject. *Nature* 1980;285:277.
36. Barker AJ, Jalinous R, Freeston IL. Non-invasive stimulation of human motor cortex. *Lancet* 1985;ii:1106–1107.
37. Patton HD, Amassian VE. Single and multiple unit analysis of cortical stage of pyramidal tract activation. *J Neurophysiol* 1954;17:345–363.
38. Boyd SG, Rothwell JC, Cowan JMA, et al. A method of monitoring function in cortical pathways during scoliosis surgery with a note on motor conduction velocities. *J Neurol Neurosurg Psych* 1986;49:251–257.
39. Day BL, Dressler D, Maertens de Noordhout A, et al. Electric and magnetic stimulation of human motor cortex: surface EMG and single motor unit responses. *J Physiol* 1989;412:449–473.
40. Taylor JL, McCloskey DI. Triggering of preprogrammed movements as reactions to masked stimuli. *J Neurophysiol* 1990;63:439–446.
41. Super H, Spekreijse H, Lamme VA. Two distinct modes of sensory processing observed in monkey primary visual cortex (V1). *Nat Neurosci* 2001;4:304–310.
42. Pascual-Leone A, Valls-Solé J, Wassermann EM, Brasil-Neto J, Cohen LG, Hallett M. Effects of focal transcranial magnetic stimulation on simple reaction time to acoustic, visual and somatosensory stimuli. *Brain* 1992;115:1045–1059.
43. Bloxham CA, Mindel TA, Frith CD. Initiation and execution of predictable and unpredictable movements in Parkinson's disease. *Brain* 1984;107:371–384.
44. Rafal RD, Posner MI, Walker JA, Friedrich FJ. Cognition and the basal ganglia. *Brain* 1984;107:1083–1094.
45. Godaux E, Koulischer D, Jacquy J. Parkinsonian bradykinesia is due to depression in the rate of rise of muscle activity. *Ann Neurol* 1992;31:93–100.
46. Brown P, Corcos DM, Rothwell JC. Does parkinsonian action tremor contribute to muscle weakness in Parkinsonís disease? *Brain* 1997;120:401–408.
47. Evarts EV, Teravainen H, Calne DB. Reaction time in Parkinson's disease. *Brain* 1981;104:167–186.
48. Pullman SL, Watts RL. Dopaminergic effects on simple and choice reaction time performance in Parkinson's Disease. *Neurology* 1988;38:249–254.
49. Berardelli A, Dick JPR, Rothwell JC, Day BL, Marsden CD. Scaling of the size of the first agonist EMG burst during rapid wrist movements in patients with Parkinson's disease. *J Neurol Neurosurg Psychiatry* 1986;49:1273–1279.
50. Pascual-Leone A, Valls-Solé J, Brasil-Neto JP, Cohen LG, Hallett M. Akinesia in Parkinson's disease. I. Shortening of simple reaction time with focal, single pulse transcranial magnetic stimulation. *Neurology* 1994;44,884–891.
51. Porter R, Lemon R. *Corticospinal function and voluntary movement.* Oxford, England: Oxford Science Publications, Clarendon Press. 1993;428.
52. Starr A, Caramia M, Zarola F, Rossini PM. Enhancement of motor cortex excitability in humans by non-invasive electrical stimulation appears prior to voluntary movement. *Electroenceph Clin Neurophysiol* 1988;70:26–32.
53. Valls-Solé J, Solé A, Valldeoriola F, Muñoz E, González LE, Tolosa ES. Reaction time and acoustic startle. *Neuroscience Letters* 1995;195:97–100.
54. Valls-Solé J, Rothwell JC, Goulart F, Cossu G, Muñoz JE. Patterned ballistic movements triggered by a startle in healthy humans. *J Physiol* 1999;516:931–938.
55. Hallett M, Shahani BW, Young RR. EMG analysis of stereotyped voluntary movements in man. *J Neurol Neurosurg Psych* 1975;38:1154–1162.
56. Valls-Solé J, Valldeoriola F, Tolosa E, Nobbe F. Habituation of the startle reaction is reduced during preparation for execution of a motor task in normal human subjects. *Brain Research* 1997;751:155–159.

57. Koller WC. How accurately can Parkinson's disease be diagnosed? *Neurology* 1992;42(Suppl 1):6–16.
58. Calne DB, Snow BJ, Lee C. Criteria for diagnosing Parkinson's disease. *Ann Neurol* 1992;42:1142–1146.
59. Hughes AJ, Daniel SE, Kilford L, Lees AJ. Accuracy of the clinical diagnosis of idiopathic Parkinson's disease: a clinicopathological study of 100 cases. *J Neurol Neurosurg Psychiatry* 1992;55:181–184.
60. Valls-Solé J. Neurophysiological characterization of parkinsonian syndromes. *Neurophysiol Clin* 2000;30:352–367.
61. Deecke L, Englitz HG, Kornhuber HH, Schmitt G. Cerebral potential preceding voluntary movement in patients with bilateral or unilateral Parkinson akinesia. In: Desmedt JE, ed. *Progress in Clinical Neurophysiology.* Basel: Karger, 1977;(1):151–163.
62. Cunnington R, Lalouschek W, Dirnberger G, Walla P, Lindinger G, Asenbaum S, Brucke T, Lang W. A medial to lateral shift in premovement cortical activity in hemi-Parkinson's disease. *Clin Neurophysiol* 2001;112:608–618.
63. Feve AP, Bathien N, Rondot P. Chronic administration of L-dopa affects the movement-related cortical potentials of patients with Parkinson's disease. *Clin Neuropharmacol* 1992;15:100–108.
64. Ziemann U, Tergau F, Bruns D, Baudewig J, Paulus W. Changes in human motor cortex excitability induced by dopaminergic and anti-dopaminergic drugs. *Electroenceph Clin Neurophysiol* 1997;105:430–437.
65. Strafella AP, Valtzania F, Nassetti SA, Tropeani A, Bisulli A, Santangelo M, Tassinari CA. Effects of chronic levodopa and pergolide treatment on cortical excitability in patients with Parkinson's disease: a transcranial magentic stimulation study. *Clin Neurophysiol* 2000;111:1198–1202.
66. Rossini PM, Babiloni F, Bernardi G, Cecchi L, Johnson PB, Malentacca A, Stanzione P, Urbano A. Abnormalities of short-latency somatosensory evoked potentials in parkinsonian patients. *Electroenceph Clin Neurophysiol* 1989;74:277–289.
67. Limousin P, Krack P, Pollack P, Banazzouz A, Ardouin C, Hoffman D, Benabid AL. Electrical stimulation of the subthalamic nucleus in advanced Parkinson's disease. *N Engl J Med* 1998;339:1105–1111.
68. Kumar R, Lozano AM, Kim YJ, Hutchison WD, Sime E, Halket E, Lang AE. Double-blind evaluation of subthalamic nucleus deep brain stimulation in advanced Parkinson's disease. *Neurology* 1998;51:850–855.
69. Benazzouz A, Piallat B, Ni ZG, Koudsie A, Pollak P, Benabid AL. Implication of the subthalamic nucleus in the pathophysiology and pathogenesis of Parkinson's disease. *Cell Transplant* 2000;9:215–221.
70. Hutchison WD, Allan RJ, Opitz H, Levy R, Dostrovsky JO, Lang AE, Lozano AM. Neurophysiological identification of the subthalamic nucleus in surgery for Parkinson's disease. *Ann Neurol* 1998;44:622–628
71. Pahapill PA, Lozano AM. The pedunculopontine tegmental nucleus and Parkinson's disease. *Brain* 2000;123:1767–1783.
72. Koch M, Kungel M, Herbert H. Cholinergic neurons in the pedunculopontine tegmental nucleus are involved in the mediation of prepulse inhibition of the acoustic startle response in the rat. *Exp Brain Res* 1993;97:71–82.
73. Swerdlow NR, Geyer MA. Prepulse inhibition of acoustic startle in rats after lesions of the pedunculopontine tegmental nucleus. *Behav Neurosci* 1993;107:104–117.
74. Dyck JPR, Cowan JMA, Day BL, Berardelli A, Kachi T, Rothwell JC, Marsden CD. The corticomotoneurone connection is normal in Parkinson's disease. *Nature* 1984;310:407–409.
75. Eisen A, Siejka S, Schulzer M, Calne D. Age-dependent decline in motor evoked potential (MEP) amplitude: with a comment on changes in Parkinson's disease. *Electroenceph Clin Neurophysiol* 1991;81:209–215.
76. Cantello R, Gianelli M, Bettucci D, Civardi C, De Angelis MS, Mutani R. Parkinson's disease rigidity: magnetic MEPs in a small hand muscle. *Neurology* 1991;41:1449–1456.
77. Valls-Solé J, Pascual-Leone A, Brasil-Neto JP, McShane L, Hallett M. Abnormal facilitation of the response to transcranial magnetic stimulation in patients with Parkinson's disease. *Neurology* 1994;44:735–741.
78. Priori A, Berardelli A, Inghilleri M, Accornero N, Manfredi M. Motor cortical inhibition and the dopaminergic system.

79. Berardelli A, Rona S, Inghilleri M, Manfredi M. Cortical inhibition in Parkinson's disease. a study with paired magnetic stimulation. *Brain* 1996;119:71–77.
80. Ridding MC, Inzelberg R, Rothwell JC. Changes in excitability of motor cortical circuitry in patients with Parkinson's disease. *Ann Neurol* 1995;37:181–188.
81. Elble RJ. Physiologic and enhanced physiologic tremor. In: Hallett M, ed. *Handbook of Clinical Neurophysiology,* vol 1. Amsterdam: Elsevier, 2003;357–364.
82. Wessberg J, Kakuda N. Single motor unit activity in relation to pulsatile motor output in human finger movements. *J Physiol* 1999;517:273–285.
83. Salazar G, Valls-Solé J, Martí MJ, Chang H, Tolosa ES. Postural and action myoclonus in patients with parkinsonian type multiple system atrophy. *Mov Disord* 2000;15:77–83.
84. Kumru H, Valls-Solé J, Valldeoriola F, Marti MJ, Sanegre MT, Tolosa E. Transient arrest of psychogenic tremor induced by contralateral ballistic movements. *Neurosci Lett* 2004;370:135–139.
85. Deuschl G, Mischke G, Schenck E, et al. Symptomatic and essential rhythmic palatal myoclonus. *Brain* 1990;113:1645–1672.
86. Remy P, de Recondo A, Defer G, et al. Peduncular "rubral" tremor and dopaminergic denervation: a PET study. *Neurology* 1995;45:472–477.
87. Deuschl G, Raethjen J, Lindemann M, Krack P. The pathophysiology of tremor. *Muscle Nerve* 2001;24:716–735.
88. Elble RJ. Origins of tremor [comment]. *Lancet* 2000;355:1113–1114.
89. Elble RJ. Animal models of action tremor. *Mov Disord* 1998;13[Suppl 3]:35–39.
90. Limousin P, Speelman JD, Gielen F, Janssens M. Multicenter European study of thalamic stimulation in parkinsonian and essential tremor. *J Neurol Neurosurg Psych* 1999;66:289–296.
91. Hirai T, Jones EG. A new parcellation of the human thalamus on the basis of histochemical staining. *Brain Res Brain Res Rev* 1989;14:1–34.
92. Shahani BT, Young RR. Physiological and pharmacological aids in the differential diagnosis of tremor. *J Neurol Neurosurg Psychiatry* 1976;39:772–783.
93. Elble RJ. The pathophysiology of tremor. In: Watts RL, Koller WC, ed. *Movement Disorders:. Neurologic Principles and Practice.* New York: McGraw Hill, 1996;405–417.
94. Pascual-Leone A, Valls-Solé J, Toro C, Wassermann EM, Hallett M. Resetting of essential tremor and postural tremor in Parkinson's disease with transcranial magnetic stimulation. *Muscle Nerve* 1994;17:800–807.
95. Ben-Pazi H, Bergman H, Goldber JA, Giladi N, Hansel D, Reches A, Simon ES. Synchrony of rest tremor in multiple limbs in Parkinson's disease: evidence for multiple oscillators. *J Neural Transm* 2001;108:287–296.
96. Logigian E, Hefter H, Reiners K, Freund HJ. Does tremor pace repetitive voluntary motor behavior in Parkinson's disease? *Ann Neurol* 1991;30:172–179.
97. Wierzbicka MM, Staude G, Wolf W, Dengler R. Relationship between tremor and the onset of rapid voluntary contraction in Parkinson's disease. *J Neurol Neurosurg Psychiatry* 1993;56:782–787.
98. Carboncini MC, Manzoni D, Strambi S, Bonuccelli U, Pavese N, Andre P, Rossi B. The relation between EMG activity and kinematic parameters strongly supports a role of the action tremor in parkinsonian bradykinesia. *Mov Disord* 2001;16:47–57.
99. Hedreen JC, Folstein SE. Early loss of neostriatal striosome neurons in Huntington's disease. *J Neuropathol Exp Neurol* 1995;54:105–120.
100. Crossman AR. Functional anatomy of movement disorders. *J Anat* 2000;196:519–525.
101. Esteban A, Giménez-Roldan S. Blink reflex in Huntington's chorea and Parkinson's disease. *Acta Neurol Scand* 1975;2:145–157.
102. Agostino R, Berardelli A, Cruccu G, Pauletti G, Stocchi F, Manfredi M. Correlation between facial involuntary movements

and abnormalities of blink and corneal reflexes in Huntington's chorea. *Mov Disord* 1988;3:281–289.

103. Valls-Solé J, Muñoz JE, Valldeoriola F. Abnormalities of prepulse inhibition do not depend on blink reflex excitability: a study in Parkinson's disease and Huntington's disease. *Clinical Neurophysiology* 2004;115:1527–1536.

104. Berardelli A, Noth J, Thompson PD, Bollen EL, Currà A, Deuschl G, Van Dijk JG, Topper R, Schwarz M, Roos RA. Pathophysiology of chorea and bradykinesia in Huntington's disease. *Movement Disorders* 1999;14:398–403.

105. Bhatia KP, Marsden CD. The behavioural and motor consequences of focal lesions of the basal ganglia in man. *Brain* 1994;117:859–876.

106. Lee MS, Marsden CD. Movement disorders following lesions of the thalamus or subthalamic region. *Mov Disord* 1994;9: 493–507.

107. Jankovic J. Post-traumatic movement disorders: central and peripheral mechanisms. *Neurology* 1994;44:2006–2014.

108. Fahn S. Concepts and classification of dystonia. *Adv Neurol* 1988;50:1–8.

109. Hashimoto T, Tada T, Nakazato F, et al. Abnormal activity in the globus pallidus in off-period dystonia. *Ann Neurol* 2001;49: 242–245.

110. Yoshor D, Hamilton WJ, Ondo W, et al. Comparison of thalamotomy and pallidotomy for the treatment of dystonia. *Neurosurgery* 2001;48:818–824.

111. Hallett M. Is dystonia a sensory disorder? *Ann Neurol* 1995;38: 139–140.

112. Kaji R, Rothwell JC, Kanayama M, Ikeda T, Kubori T, Kohara N, Mezaki T, Shibasaki H, Kimura J. Tonic vibration reflex and muscle afferent block in writer's cramp. *Ann Neurol* 1995;38:155–162.

113. Bara-Jimenez W, Shelton P, Sanger TD, Hallett M. Sensory discrimination capabilities in patients with focal hand dystonia. *Ann Neurol* 2000;47:377–380.

114. Gomez-Wong E, Marti MJ, Tolosa E, Valls-Solé. J Sensory modulation of the blink reflex in patients with blepharospasm. *Arch Neurol* 1998;55:1233–1237

115. Tinazzi M, Priori A, Bertolasi L, Frasson E, Mauguière F, Fiaschi A. Abnormal central integration of a dual somatosensory input in dystonia: evidence for sensory overflow. *Brain* 2000;123:42–50.

116. Murase N, Kaji R, Shimazu H, Katayama-Hirota M, Ikeda A, Kohara N, et al. Abnormal premovement gating of somatosensory input in writer's cramp. *Brain* 2000;123:1813–1829.

117. Rothwell JC, Obeso J, Day B, Marsden CD. Pathophysiology of dystonia. *Adv Neurol* 1983;39:851–863.

118. Chen R, Wassermann EM, Canos M, Hallett M. Impaired inhibition in writer's cramp during voluntary muscle activation. *Neurology* 1997;49:1054–1059.

119. Hallett M. Tics. In: Hallett M, ed. *Handbook of Clinical Neurophysiology*, vol 1. Amsterdam: Elsevier, 2003;549–558.

120. Georgiu N, Bradshaw JL, Phillips JG, Bradshaw JA, Chiu E. Advance information and movement sequencing in Gilles de la Tourette's syndrome. *J Neurol Neurosurg Psych* 1995;58: 184–191.

121. Obeso JA, Rothwell JC, Marsden CD. Simple tics in Gilles de la Tourette's syndrome are not prefaced by a normal premovement potential. *J Neurol Neurosurg Psych* 1981;44:735–738.

122. Shibasaki H. Electrophysiologic studies of myoclonus. AAEE Minimonograph 30. *Muscle Nerve* 2000;23:321–335.

123. Marsden CD, Hallett M, Fahn S. The nosology and pathophysiology of myoclonus. In: CD Marsden and S Fahn, eds. *Movement Disorders*. London: Butterworth, 1982;196–248.

124. Hallett M, Chadwick D, Marsden CD. Cortical reflex myoclonus. *Neurology* 1977;29:1107–1125.

125. Hallett M, Chadwick D, Adam J, Marsden CD. Reticular reflex myoclonus: a physiological type of human post-hypoxic myoclonus. *J Neurol Neurosurg Psych* 1977;40:253–264.

126. Ikeda A, Kakigi R, Funai N, Kuorda Y, Shibasaki H. Cortical tremor: a variant of cortical reflex myoclonus. *Neurology* 1990;40:1561–1565.

127. Moersch FP, Woltman HW. Progressive fluctuating muscular rigidity and spasm ("stiff-man syndrome"): report of a case and some observations in 13 other cases. *Mayo Clinic Proc* 1956;31:421–427.

128. Meinck HM, Ricker K, Hulser PJ, Schmid E, Peiffer J, Solimena M. Stiff man syndrome: clinical and laboratory findings in eight patients. *J Neurol* 1994;24:157–166.

129. Floeter MK, Valls-Solé J, Toro C, Jacobowitz D, Hallett M. Physiologic studies of spinal inhibitory circuits in patients with stiff-person syndrome. *Neurology* 1998;51:85–93.

130. Newsom-Davis J. Autoimmune neuromyotonia (Isaacs' syndrome): an antibody-mediated potassium channelopathy. *Ann N Y Acad Sci* 1997;835:111–119.

131. Horak FB. Postural ataxia related to somatosensory loss. *Adv Neurol* 2001;87:173–182.

132. Dietz V, Noth J. Pre-innervation and stretch responses of triceps brachii in man falling with and without visual control. *Brain Res* 1978;142:576–579.

133. Nutt JG, Marsden CD, Thompson PD. Human walking and higher-level gait disorders, particularly in the elderly. *Neurology* 1993;43:268–279.

Neurobehavioral Disorders Associated with Basal Ganglia Lesions

3

Richard Levy

Focal lesions affecting the basal ganglia are often followed by behavioral disorders that are, in many cases, more predominant than the motor syndrome. This review describes the neurobehavioral disorders encountered after lesions of the basal ganglia, explains why such disorders occur, and considers what lessons can be learned about the role and function of the basal ganglia.

THE GENERAL FRAMEWORK: BEHAVIOR AND ANATOMY

Neurobehavioral changes are every observable behavior accounting for cognitive or affective dysfunctions. For example, apathy may be related to cognitive changes (cognitive inertia) or to affective disorders (lack of motivation) or to both (auto-activation deficit). When behavioral disturbances occur after basal ganglia lesions, they are frequently associated with an impairment of executive functions (planning, working memory, allocation of attention resources, temporal ordering, self-generation of cognitive strategies, set-shifting, etc.), supporting the concept of a functionally essential neural network linking the prefrontal cortex to the basal ganglia (1,2). The scope of *behavioral*

changes can be extended to include the consequences of motor dysfunctions, if these abnormalities are translated into observable behaviors. Indeed, the clinical signs usually included in akinesia, such as delayed initiation or freezing, should be included within the general framework of behavioral disorders. However, for the sake of clarity, the motor aspects will not be discussed within the scope of this review.

Nonmotor neurobehavioral changes occur only when specific subcortical nuclei or portions of these nuclei are affected. This could be interpreted with regard to the anatomical and functional heterogeneity of the basal ganglia. This obvious heterogeneity exists at different levels. The basal ganglia are organized in closed loops with the cerebral cortex (1,3,4): the striatum (putamen, caudate nucleus, and ventral striatum) represents the input structure, that is, it receives cortical projections. The internal portion of the globus pallidus pars interna (GPi) and the substantia nigra pars reticulata (SNpr) are the two output structures. Other basal ganglia nuclei include the external portion of the globus pallidus pars externa (GPe) and the subthalamic nucleus (STN), located in intermediate anatomical positions between the input and output structures of the basal ganglia (5). The substantia nigra pars compacta (SNpc) is the dopaminergic modulating system. Lastly, in view of their subcortical locations and connections, the thalamic nuclei can be considered to belong to the basal ganglia. As there is no direct projection from the output structures of the basal ganglia to the cerebral cortex, the thalamic nuclei, which receive inputs from the GPi/SNpr, may be considered as the *true* output structures of the basal ganglia as the thalamocortical pathways close the cerebral cortex–basal ganglia–cerebral cortex loops. From this organization and the fact that the intrinsic anatomical and cellular organization is clearly different among all of these structures, it is reasonable to expect the clinical consequences of basal ganglia lesions to differ depending on which of the structures, striatum, GPi/SNpr, GPe, STN, thalami, or SNpc, is affected.

In addition, within each of the preceding structures, there is a topographical distribution of extrinsic connections. Thus, within the striatum, the sensorimotor and premotor cortical areas project to the dorsal putamen, whereas projections arising from the cognitive associative cortical areas project to the dorsal caudate nucleus and to the posterior and ventral putamen (6–9). Projections from the limbic brain regions terminate in the more ventral portion of the striatum (6,8,10). The topographical distribution of connecting fibers is relatively well maintained throughout the basal ganglia, from the striatum to the thalamic nuclei (although concentration and convergence exist throughout the basal ganglia funneling) (1,11). It should also be noted that there may be significant differences in the intrinsic architecture of each territory. For example, one may separate subregions within the ventral striatum into shells and cores, according to biochemical and connectivity parameters (12), whereas a different type of differentiation exists within the dorsal striatum (striosomes, matrix, matrisomes), based on other biochemical and connectivity parameters (9,13). These data clearly suggest that, within each ordered level, there could be different functional territories according to the nature of the extrinsic connecting fibers and also according to the differences in the intrinsic architecture and biochemistry.

These preliminary considerations are important because they indicate that, according to the location of the lesions, the clinical disorders are likely to be different. Thus, within the basal ganglia, not all the sites are likely to produce behavioral problems and the pattern of disturbances may vary from one location to another. It follows, therefore, that far more information can be obtained from restricted lesions to the areas defined according to the above distinction (e.g., caudate nucleus, ventral striatum, putamen, GPi, paramedian thalamus) than from large lesions that unfortunately (both for the patients and for the advancement of knowledge) are the most frequent (e.g., lenticular lesions affecting the putamen and the globus pallidus, large striatal lesions encompassing the caudate nucleus, the putamen, and the internal capsule). Therefore, we focus in this review on data obtained from well-defined focal lesions of the basal ganglia, in both humans and monkeys. It is important to note that small lesions are difficult to locate and to relate to a specific territory, especially downstream to the striatum where the concentration of fibers makes it difficult to discriminate the different functional territories. In addition, one should keep in mind that the neuroanatomy of the cortico-basal ganglia circuits largely relies on knowledge acquired from connection studies in animals. Therefore, a linear transfer of this knowledge from animals to human remains largely speculative, though a 2004 study using the in vivo MRI diffusion tensor fiber tracking method provides evidence in support of similarities between cortico-striatal connectivity in humans and in monkeys (14).

Striatal Lesions

As suggested, focal striatal lesions produce a variety of clinical signs depending on the location of the lesions.

Caudate and Ventral Striatum Lesions

Small and isolated lesions of the caudate nucleus rarely induce motor disturbances, although lesion to the most anterodorsal portion of the caudate nucleus may contribute to movement disorders, in particular to contralateral choreic movements or focal dystonia (15). By contrast, unilateral or bilateral caudate lesions often produce isolated neurobehavioral disturbances similar to those observed after prefrontal lesions.

When the lesion is sudden (e.g., a stroke), patients often exhibit acute confusion and fluctuating arousal followed by more permanent behavioral deficits (15,16). Bhatia and Marsden (15), in a meta-analysis of 240 patients with focal basal ganglia lesions (including 43 patients with small, isolated caudate nucleus lesions), separated behavioral changes into two broad categories: apathy and disinhibition (Fig. 3.1).

Apathy (often called *aboulia* or *psychic akinesia* when it is intense), the more frequent (28%) of the two syndromes, can be seen after unilateral or bilateral caudate lesions (15,17,18). Apathy refers to an intense quantitative reduction of goal-directed behaviors: Patients exhibit a lack of initiative for usual daily activities, leading to a drastic decrease in their spontaneous behaviors, which may be partially reversed by external and strong solicitation (15,18,19). It is associated with a slowness and a latency of responses after stimulation. This behavior cannot be related to depressive disorders, but it could be associated with flattened affect and emotional blunting. *Cognitive inertia* refers to the expression of this apathy in the sphere of executive functions, especially difficulty in generating new rules or strategies or difficulty in shifting from one mental and behavioral set to another. Indeed, in patients with caudate lesions, impairment of executive functions, including planning, working memory, set-shifting, failure to activate, or generate cognitive strategies (for example,

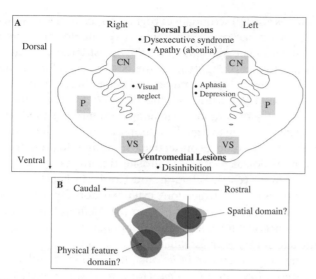

Figure 3.1   Relationship between specific clinical features and the location of the lesions within the striatum. **A:** Frontal section at the level of the anterior striatum. CN, caudate nucleus; P, putamen; VS, ventral section. **B:** Sagittal view of striatum along the rostral-caudal axis.

those used to retrieve semantic or episodic information from memory), and temporal ordering, is consistently found when behavioral disturbances are present (16,19). Almost every pattern of language impairment can be observed after direct striatal lesions, including fluent aphasia with semantic paraphasia (20). However, in most cases, language dysfunctions occurring after left caudate lesions could be included within the framework of a dysexecutive syndrome. Indeed, aphasia is often described as being frontal in type and consisting of nonfluent speech associated with word-finding difficulties, dysarthria, and stuttering contrasting with normal word comprehension and repetition and the absence of verbal paraphrasias (17,19,21). In all described cases, aphasic disorders are mild and patients often recover rapidly (17). Among other cognitive dysfunctions, one should note impairments in procedural learning tasks, such as mirror reading or the Tower of Hanoi puzzle (22). Contralateral spatial neglect is observed after right-sided caudate lesions (17,19). It is described as supramodal, affecting visual and auditory stimuli (17). Finally, cognitive decline may be delayed after caudate stroke. Indeed, Bokura and Robinson (23) have shown that a significant number of patients with a caudate stroke may exhibit a cognitive deterioration 1 to 2 years after the stroke. The authors suggest that this cognitive decline is related to a progressive degeneration of corticostriatal fibers.

Disinhibition [11% of the patients with caudate lesions in Bhatia and Marsden's (15) meta-analysis] is characterized by a massive deficit in the regulation of personal behavior and social cognition. In some cases, it resembles the behavioral syndrome observed after direct ventromedial prefrontal lesions and the pattern of behavioral changes observed in the frontal type of frontotemporal dementia (24,25). For example, Richfield and colleagues described a 25-year-old woman, suffering from a bilateral ischemic stroke affecting the head of the caudate nuclei, who had undergone alterations in affect and motivation associated with disinhibited behaviors (vulgarity, impulsiveness, easy frustration, violent outbursts, increased appetite, hypersexuality, poor hygiene, enuresis, etc.) (24).

Hyperactivity is also encountered after caudate stroke (17). Patients overreact to environmental stimuli and have difficulty focusing and maintaining their attention when faced with an environmental flood of information. Hyperactivity should be dissociated from disinhibition in terms of the underlying mechanisms. Indeed, it seems to be secondary to a cognitive and attentional deficit rather than to a dysregulation of social cognition and personal conduct. Indeed, hyperactivity can be regarded as a failure to maintain information or goals in working memory, as well as difficulty in focusing or allocating attention to relevant information (26,27). However, in some cases, disinhibited behavior, hyperactivity and abulia may coexist (15,17).

In vascular stroke, depression has often been associated with subcortical lesions of the left hemisphere that in most cases encompass the caudate nucleus (28). There are also reports of bipolar disease revealed or induced by lesions of the caudate nuclei [see cases 10 and 12 of Mendez et al. (16)]. These observations suggest that the occurrence of a depressive state may be at least partly related to a dysfunction of the prefrontal–basal ganglia–prefrontal loops affecting the limbic and cognitive territories of the basal ganglia. Obsessive–compulsive behaviors have been described after a lesion restricted to the caudate nucleus (18,29). Penisson-Besnier and colleagues reported the case of a woman who developed severe arithmomania (pathological mental counting) associated with behavioral disinhibition (30). Neuropathological examination showed caudate nuclei gliosis in the absence of pathological abnormalities in other brain regions, including the frontal cortex. Other neuropsychiatric states, such as anxiety, agoraphobia, auditory hallucinations, and paranoia, have also been reported after right or left caudate lesions (16).

Relationship Between the Clinical Signs and the Functional Neuroanatomy of the Caudate Nucleus and the Ventral Striatum

From the first studies of Kemp and Powell using fiber degeneration techniques (31) to the most recent and sophisticated techniques of pathway labeling using viral polysynaptic retrograde tracers (3), all the evidence suggests that almost every associative cortex projects to the caudate nucleus and the ventral striatum (Fig. 3.2). However, there is in particular a strong linkage between the prefrontal cortex (PFC) and the caudate nucleus/ventral striatum, supporting the existence of a coherent PFC–caudate nucleus/ventral striatum functional network. Indeed, lesions of the basal ganglia affecting the limbic or the associative territories often

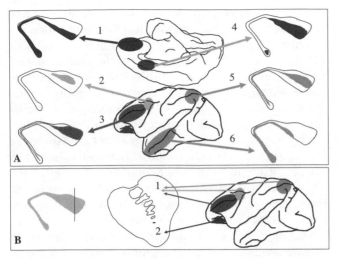

Figure 3.2 Anatomical connections between association cortical areas and the caudate nucleus in the rhesus monkey. **A:** Cortical-caudate connections at the level of the head of the caudate nucleus. Connections from 1, ventromedial PFC; 2, Frontal Eye Field (FEF) 3, dorsolateral PFC (principal sulcus region); 4, dorsal ACC; 5, posterior parietal cortex (superior parietal lobule); 6, inferior temporal cortex. **B:** Projections from selected cortical areas: 1, projections from regions involved in spatial cognition (posterior parietal cortex, FEF, and the principal sulcus within the PFC) converge toward the centro-dorsal portion of the head of the caudate nucleus; 2, inputs from the limbic portion of the PFC (ventromedial PFC) terminate in the limbic striatum (ventral striatum).

produce a prefrontal-like syndrome. This concept is supported by lesion and electrophysiological studies in monkeys showing the similarity in neuronal activation and behavioral changes whether the target is the PFC or a specific location in the caudate nuclei (32–38). However, there are multiple PFC–caudate nucleus/ventral striatum anatomical and functional networks, according to the anatomical and functional organization of the PFC (26,27,39) and also to the relative segregation of PFC–basal ganglia–PFC circuits (1,4). The different anatomical– functional areas of the PFC project into the striatum in a relatively segregated but interdigitated manner, and this relative segregation is maintained throughout the basal ganglia funneling to the PFC from which these circuits originated (1,3,4,6,7,40). How can the anatomical and functional organization of the prefrontal–striatal connections explain the clinical abnormalities observed after focal lesions of the caudate nuclei and the ventral striatum?

A more precise clinical–radiological analysis of the signs and symptoms observed with regard to the location of the lesions suggests a differential clinical impact of the lesions, depending on their location. At first glance, the most obvious differences are related to the lateralization of the lesion, right caudate nucleus lesions being associated with spatial neglect, whereas left lesions are associated with aphasic and mood disorders. However, it appears that the most interesting functional and anatomical difference concerns the dorsal–ventral axis (Fig. 3.1):

1. Lesions in the dorsal area of the head of the caudate nucleus seem to be associated with behavioral abnormalities

(such as apathy) secondary to cognitive alterations, in particular to a dysexecutive syndrome (16). The dorsal portion of the caudate nucleus (i.e., the neostriatum) receives its most massive inputs from the dorsolateral (Brodmann areas 9/lateral 10/46) and ventrolateral (Brodmann areas 12/44/45/47) portions of the PFC. Within the caudate nucleus, the projections originating from the lateral PFC terminate according to a gradient from the dorsal to the ventral portion of the caudate nuclei that corresponds to projections from the dorsolateral and ventrolateral portions of the PFC, respectively (6–9). Selemon and Goldman-Rakic (1985) found that these projections extended dorsally along the rostral–caudal axis of the striatum (6). Neuropsychological and functional imaging studies in humans have pinpointed the lateral PFC as an essential node in the neural network of many of the cognitive functions often gathered under the concept of *executive functions* (for a review, see references 26,27). Executive functions refer to "the capacity to plan and carry out complex goal-directed behaviors" (41) and include distinct functions and processes, such as planning, working memory, rule finding, set-shifting, and reasoning. In functional imaging in humans, activation in the dorsal portion of the head of the caudate nuclei was found during working memory tasks and, more importantly, during planning tasks (42). In monkeys, lesions of the dorsal portion of the caudate nucleus induce impairments in tasks that are also altered after dorsolateral lesions, such as spatial delayed and delayed alternation tasks (32,34–36,43). Moreover, electrophysiological studies focusing on the head of the caudate nuclei have demonstrated patterns of neural activation similar to those observed in the dorsolateral PFC during working memory or sequencing tasks (38,44,45). In addition, the pattern of cortical–striatal connectivity also suggests distinct functional domains within the caudate nuclei (Fig. 3.1 and 3.2). For example, in monkeys, inputs from the dorsolateral PFC (Walker area 46, the principal sulcus), the visual–spatial posterior parietal regions (Walker area 7), the frontal eye field (Walker area 8B), and the supplementary eye field (SEF) terminate in the central portion of the dorsal and rostral caudate nucleus (6–8,40,46,47), suggesting that this particular subarea within the caudate nuclei may have a preeminent role in visual–spatial cognition (37). It is thus expected (but not yet demonstrated) that lesions in the anterior and dorsal caudate nucleus may be associated with some of the deficits occurring in the field of spatial cognition (spatial working memory, spatial neglect), whereas more posterior and ventral lesions may be associated with disturbances in the sphere of visual discrimination of physical features. Indeed, in monkeys, lesions of the tail of the caudate nucleus produce a visual pattern discrimination deficit (34,36). Likewise, in early stages of Parkinson's disease (PD) and in presymptomatic (motor-free) 1-methyl-4-phenyl-1,2,3,6-tetrahydropyridine (MPTP)-intoxicated monkeys, visual spatial impairments are often observed (48–50) and may be interpreted as the result of a dopaminergic depletion in the dorsal and anterior striatum (including the dorsal caudate nuclei) (51). By contrast, tasks that usually assess cognition based on visual feature discrimination are in general well performed at the early stages of the disease (50), and this could be interpreted as the result of a relative sparing of dopaminergic innervation of the more ventral and posterior striatal areas (including the ventral caudate nucleus and the putamen, which receive projections from visual temporal association cortices) (51). Taken together, these data indicate that the dorsal portion of the caudate nuclei (in particular the head) should be considered as a key structure in an anatomical–functional network, in combination with the dorsolateral PFC, which mostly contributes to executive functions. Therefore, most of the behavioral changes included in abulia may be interpreted as the consequence of a cognitive inertia secondary to the disruption of the PFC–caudate nucleus network, subserving the cognitive aspect of the executive processing (e.g., activation of strategies to retrieve information or generate thoughts and rules, shifting from one mental set to another, maintaining subgoals and goals in working memory, and allocating attention resources to several tasks simultaneously). Hyperactivity can also be viewed as a consequence of the disruption of the same network that, in the normal state, is necessary to maintain focused attention toward relevant stimuli or thoughts and to maintain information in working memory.

2. Lesions of the ventral portion of the caudate nucleus and in the ventral striatum are associated with disinhibited behaviors (16) and affective and emotional dysfunctions. A 2004 study reports that patients with lesions restricted to the ventral striatum are impaired in recognition of emotions useful for survival, such as anger (52). The medial and ventral portion of the head, body, and tail of the caudate nuclei, as well as the core structure of the ventral striatum, receive massive inputs from the orbital and medial PFC (Brodmann areas 10 ventral, 11, 13, 14) and from the anterior cingulate cortex (ACC) (Brodmann areas 24–32) (6,8,10). Lesions of the orbital and medial PFC induce failure to decode the motivational value of a given context and use this information to generate and control goal-directed behaviors, leading to a reduction of the willingness to perform them (loss of will, loss of goals, emotional blunting) and to maintain actions to their completion, or to a reduction of the ability to evaluate the consequences of future actions (53). These striatal regions also receive projections from the medial temporal lobe and, in particular, from the amygdala (54). Lesions to the amygdala are associated with emotional and affective impairments such as the inability to decode emotions such as fear or to learn to associate affective and emotional signals with a given behavior (such as the inability to learn fear conditioning) (55,56). In addition, dopaminergic innervation of the ventral regions of the striatum is mostly provided by the ventral tegmental area (A10), which gives rise to the mesocorticolimbic dopaminergic ascending pathway, also involved in reward processing in the normal state and leading to addictive behavior when lesioned (57).

According to this particular connectivity, the ventral portion of the striatum (ventral caudate nuclei and the ventral striatum) could be considered as a node of a limbic functional system, involved in affective, emotional, and motivational processing. Several behavioral and electrophysiological studies in monkeys have indeed confirmed the involvement of the ventral portion of the striatum in integrating the affective or emotional value of a given stimulus into the ongoing behavior (58,59). The main patterns of neural discharge are an anticipatory response to a forthcoming reward and double coding (reward and motor preparation). In addition, it seems that dopamine depletion within the ventral striatum (but not in the dorsal striatum) is associated with failure impairments in reward processing (60). In rats, ventral striatal lesions or dysfunctions result in a failure to learn adaptive behavior in response to conditioned reinforcers (61). In monkeys, direct ventral striatal lesions are associated with pathological responses to changes in task contingencies (object alternation task and inhibition paradigms) and in reward processing, such as aggressive behaviors when the reward in response to the expected response is no longer delivered (32,34,35,62). Based on these data, it has been hypothesized that the ventral striatum contributes to behavior by decoding the incentive value of a reward or punishment and integrating these learned incentives into the behavioral program (60).

Putaminal Lesions

Putaminal lesions are rarely associated with behavioral disturbances. In most cases, such problems occur because the lesions extended to other contiguous structures (such as the white matter or the caudate nucleus). For example, Pramstaller and Marsden (63) described a series of patients with lenticular lesions who presented various degrees and types of apraxia. However, when the lesions spared the subcortical white matter (internal capsule and peristriatal white matter), no apraxia was observed, leading the authors to conclude that putaminal lesions alone are not sufficient to produce apraxia. In a similar way, although language impairment (aphemia) has been described after lesions encompassing the left putamen, it is not in general related to isolated putaminal lesion but to more diffuse lesions affecting the caudate nucleus, other basal ganglia structures, or periventricular or peristriatal white matter (21). However, there are reports of visual neglect following pure right putaminal lesions (64). Furthermore, in monkeys, lesions of the ventral putamen are associated with impairments in learning tasks based on visual discrimination (65). A possible explanation is that the posterior and ventral portion of the putamen receives direct input from association temporal cortices, in particular from the superior temporal gyrus (Brodmann area 22) (66). A 2004 clinical–radiological correlation study suggests that visual neglect is mostly due to lesions centered on the superior temporal gyrus (67). It is, therefore, likely that the right putamen forms part of a cortical–basal ganglia network essential for visual–spatial integration.

It should also be mentioned that a study performed in 25 children who had suffered a stroke found that 15 of them presented attention deficit/hyperactivity disorder (ADHD) (68). Superimposition of the lesions demonstrated that the lesions responsible for ADHD overlapped in the posterior and ventral putamen.

Intermediate Structures of the Basal Ganglia

Lesions of the External Portion of the Globus Pallidus

The behavioral impact of pure GPe lesions in humans is not well-known. Information can, however, be obtained from monkey and rodent studies focusing on the effect of GPe lesions or inhibition of GPe neural activity (69,70). In particular, a set of experiments performed in monkeys showed that behavioral changes may occur after GPe dysfunction and that these changes depend on the location of GPe disactivation (70,71): Bicuculline (a GABAergic antagonist) was injected locally in different portions of the GPe. The injections produced different patterns of abnormal behaviors: Microinjections in cognitive territories (anterior and dorsal GPe) induced attention deficit and hyperactivity. Injections of retrograde tracers in these sites labeled neurons in dorsal areas of the head of the caudate nuclei. Bicuculline injections in the limbic territories (ventral and anterior GPe) were associated with stereotyped and complex movements resembling compulsive behaviors. Injections of retrograde tracers in these sites labeled neurons in the ventral striatum. By contrast, bicuculline microinjections in the sensorimotor territories (in a site subsequently demonstrated, using retrograde tracers, to be connected with the putamen) induced elementary dyskinesia. Taken together, these data suggest that, like other basal ganglia nuclei, there is an anatomical and functional organization in territories according to their connectivity (sensorimotor, cognitive, and limbic). However, to achieve a better understanding of the functional role of the GPe within the global framework of basal ganglia functions, more data are needed, particularly in humans.

Subthalamic Lesions

STN lesions are classically associated with contralateral hemiballism. However, limbic and cognitive territories also exist within this structure (72). It is thus very likely that STN lesions affect cognition and emotion–affect. Although such impairments have not yet been described in isolated STN lesions in humans, data from animal studies indicate their involvement in motivation (73) and cognitive or protocognitive functions (74). However, data from PD indicate that STN stimulation does not affect cognition performance (75). This absence of changes could, according to the authors, be interpreted as being related to the positioning of the electrodes, confined to the sensorimotor circuits.

Output Structures

Lesions of the Internal Portion of the Globus Pallidus Pars Interna

Athymhormia—also called psychic akinesia or self-activation deficit (SAD)—is one of the most intense forms of apathy and has been reported after bilateral or unilateral lesions that in most cases affected the GPi. These lesions are generally due to anoxia secondary to cardiovascular collapse, or intoxication by carbon monoxide and other substances (disulfuram, carbon disulfide, potassium cyanide, etc.). They are followed by a necrosis of the GPi neurons (76–79). This syndrome consists in a loss of spontaneous activation in three different domains: behavior, cognition, and emotion. Patients tend to remain quietly in the same place or position all day, without speaking or taking any spontaneous initiative. When questioned, patients express the feeling that their mind is empty when they are not stimulated. Affect is usually flattened with anhedonia, and emotional responses are blunted; Any reactivity to emotional situations is poor and short-lived (80). Although quite similar in some aspects, depression can be ruled out in SAD patients. One of the most important features of this syndrome is that it can be partially and temporarily reversed by external stimulation and, when solicited, SAD patients can produce relevant answers and behaviors. In other words, there is a sharp contrast between the drastic quantitative reduction of self-generated actions and the relatively normally executed externally driven behaviors. Although global intellectual efficiency is preserved (81), SAD patients exhibit a dysexecutive syndrome in which cognitive inertia (decreased ability to generate and activate cognitive strategies, slowness, delayed initiation of responses, and decreased mental flexibility) is predominant (79,80,82). Stereotypic and pseudocompulsive behaviors or thoughts (such as arithmomania) are frequently associated with SAD (83). Unlike the usual obsessive–compulsive disorders, it is not associated with anxiety and rituals and personality is considered normal (78). In some cases, patients are unable to stop repetitive movements (for example, when asked to clap three times as quickly as possible, some patients have difficulty interrupting this motor sequence and execute an automatic program of applause that they cannot stop spontaneously). It is also worthy of note that pallidal lesions may be followed by obsessive–compulsive behaviors that are in accordance with the Diagnostic and Statistical Manual of Mental Disorders (DSM) or by more elementary stereotyped movements or thoughts without the presence of SAD (84). Finally, in the vast majority of patients with GPi lesions, no elementary motor dysfunction is observed (in particular, no motor akinesia or rigidity).

How can one explain the occurrence of SAD after GPi lesions? First, an identical or very similar syndrome can be observed after unilateral or bilateral lesions of the head of the caudate nucleus (it is very difficult clinically to dissociate SAD from the apathetic syndrome, often referred to as *abulia*, that follows caudate lesions) and paramedian thalamic lesions (affecting medial-dorsal [MD] and anterior nuclei) (18,76,85,86) (Fig. 3.3A). Second, a significant prefrontal hypometabolism has been found in SAD using PET scan, suggesting a frontal diaschisis induced by the pallidal lesions (83). Third, the impact of GPi lesions is very similar to the cognitive and behavioral state observed in progressive supranuclear palsy (PSP), in which the prefrontal-like syndrome consists of an intense apathy mostly affecting the self-generation of behaviors, a strong cognitive inertia, and pseudocompulsive and stereotyped behavior (87). In PSP, lesions are particularly dense in the output structure of the basal ganglia (GPi/SNpr) (88). In addition, in PSP one may observe a massive hypometabolism of the anterior portion of the frontal lobes (89). Fourth, direct lesions of the prefrontal white matter and the medial wall of the PFC (including the ACC) result in SAD (82,90,91) or clinical states that are clinically and conceptually very close to SAD (in that there is a dissociation between decreased self-generated behavior and relatively spared externally driven ones) such as akinetic mutism (92,93), motor transcortical aphasia (94), and motor neglect (patients exhibit an underutilization of the contralateral arm in spontaneous conditions even though they do not suffer from any sensory-motor deficit) (95). In monkeys, a clinical syndrome of this type was induced by experimental

lesions of the medial wall (including the dorsal portion of the ACC): The monkeys exhibited a sharp decrease in self-initiation of voluntary movements, contrasting with the total sparing of externally triggered actions (96). Taken together, these data suggest that lesions of the dorsal–medial PFC are associated with an apathetic syndrome largely explained by the subject's inability to self-activate (or generate) actions, whereas these actions can clearly be elaborated and performed under strong and sustained external stimulation.

Taken together, this set of clinical and behavioral data strongly suggests that (a) SAD results in lesions affecting the limbic and cognitive territories of the basal ganglia (including the GPi but also the caudate nuclei and the MD and anterior thalamic nuclei); (b) SAD is likely a consequence of the disruption of the basal ganglia–PFC system, supporting the existence of a functional basal ganglia–PFC axis; and (c) the pattern of behavioral changes following lesions in the limbic and cognitive territories of the GPi shares similarities with the pattern following lesions of the medial PFC, suggesting that both structures are associated in a functional network dedicated to the internal generation of voluntary behaviors.

In accord with the preceding point, SAD may be due to an impairment of elementary processing devoted to auto-activation. According to this hypothesis, auto-activation may represent a central function of the basal ganglia, and the fact that the lesions responsible for this syndrome are located in cognitive and limbic territories could be interpreted as the nonmotor expression of

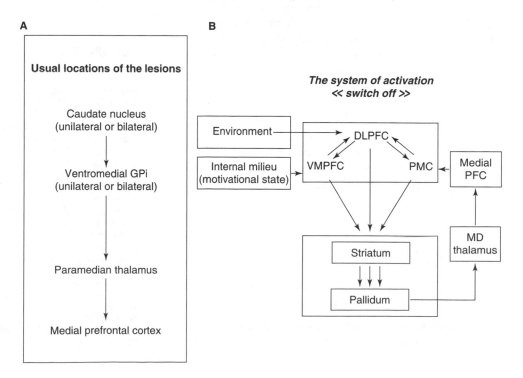

Self-Activation Deficit (SAD)
(Severe apathy, partially reversed by external stimulation)

Figure 3.3 **A:** Locations of the lesions responsible for SAD. GPi, internal segment of the globus pallidus. **B:** A model for self-activation deficit after direct lesions of the basal ganglia. DLPFC, dorsolateral PFC; MD, medial-dorsal; PMC, premotor cortex; VMPFC, ventromedial PFC. Hatched boxes indicate damage to the corresponding structure.

an auto-activation deficit (the same auto-activation deficit may arise in the field of motor functions and may be represented by some of the signs usually classified as motor signs, such as a diminished number of movements, delayed initiation, and freezing). SAD suggests that basal ganglia lesions induce a failure to activate the output structures, in particular the frontal lobes, when behavior depends upon internalized guidance (Fig. 3.3B). It is thus possible to propose that the disruption of the PFC–basal ganglia–PFC loops at the level of the basal ganglia may lead to apathy because basal ganglia processing is no longer able to generate the relevant neural signal at the level of its output targets in the prefrontal cognitive and limbic territories (particularly in the dorsal-medial PFC). SAD strongly suggests that one of the main functions of the basal ganglia is to set the threshold for the signals returning to the PFC and, therefore, that it helps, through a validation processing, to favor, at the level of the medial-frontal regions, the most relevant neural signals. One may thus hypothesize that if there is a focal destruction within the basal ganglia subregions involved in affective–cognitive processing, the signal emerging from the basal ganglia will be diminished and the ongoing behavior will not be validated (i.e., will not be amplified) at the level of the PFC and could be difficult to maintain, and the forthcoming behavior (if it is not reflexive) will not be activated (Fig. 3.3B). Above all, if the destruction is massive in these areas, no signal will ultimately be transferred to the PFC. Because the medial PFC may be considered an essential node to self-generate action (i.e., in the absence of external drive), a GPi lesion or diminished activation may switch off the medial PFC (based on the hypothesis that the main functional route of output fibers terminates in the medial PFC) and lead to an auto-activation deficit, contrasting with a relative sparing of externally driven behavior. It may be hypothesized that, because the system that generates voluntary behaviors based on internal guidance is strongly affected, it may favor the occurrence of automatic and stereotyped behavior. In other words, it can be hypothesized that, in the normal state, there is a form of hierarchical processing that favors purposeful and self-generated actions (presumably via an inhibition of nonadaptive automatic and repetitive responses).

CONCLUSION

The main conclusions that can be drawn from the study of focal lesions of the basal ganglia are the following:

1. Neurobehavioral changes are common features of basal ganglia lesions.

2. They occur when specific regions (i.e., the cognitive and limbic territories) are affected.

3. The pattern of these changes shares similarities with the behavioral disturbances observed after direct lesions of the PFC.

4. The clinical profile of the behavioral deficits varies according to the location of the lesions within the cognitive–limbic territories of the basal ganglia.

5. The latter observation can be explained by the relative topographical segregation of cortical–basal ganglia–cortical loops, which is maintained in each structure of the basal ganglia even though concentration and convergence increase throughout the basal ganglia funneling.

6. One of the dominant syndromes is apathy, which in some very severe cases is called *auto-activation deficit*.

7. This syndrome is in general associated with unilateral or bilateral lesions of the GPi, the head of the caudate nucleus, and the MD thalamic nucleus.

8. Taken as a mirror of the normal functioning of the basal ganglia, this syndrome sheds light on one of the essential roles of the basal ganglia–PFC circuit: It can be hypothesized that it serves as a selective amplifier of the relevant signals, useful in disambiguating decision making when behavior is voluntary and based on internal guidance.

9. It is clearly apparent that more studies are required to elucidate the specific role of the basal ganglia as compared to the PFC, to clarify the functional differences within the basal ganglia between each of the nodes involved in cognition and behavior in support of the above hypothesis, and to determine the involvement in cognition and behavior of structures such the GPe, STN, or SNpr.

REFERENCES

1. Alexander GE, Delong MR, Strick PL. Parallel organization of functionally segregated circuits linking basal ganglia and cortex. *Annual Review of Neurosciences* 1986;9:357–381.
2. Pillon B, Boller F, Levy R, et al. Cognitive deficits in Parkinson's disease. In: Boller F, Grafman J, eds. *Handbook of Neuropsychology.* Amsterdam: Elsevier Science Publishers, 2002.
3. Middleton FA, Strick PL. Basal-ganglia "projections" to the prefrontal cortex of the primate. *Cereb Cortex* 2002;12:926–935.
4. Haber SN. The primate basal ganglia: parallel and integrative networks. *J Chem Neuroanat* 2003;26:317–330.
5. Wichmann T, DeLong MR. Pathophysiology of parkinsonian motor abnormalities. In: Narabayashi H, Nagatsu T, Yanagisawa N, Muzino Y, eds. *Advances in Neurology.* New York: Raven Press, 1993.
6. Selemon LD, Goldman-Rakic PS. Longitudinal topography and interdigitation of corticostriatal projections in the rhesus monkeys. *J Neurosci* 1985;5:776–794.
7. Saint-Cyr JA, Ungerleider LG, Desimone R. Organization of visual cortical inputs to the striatum and subsequent outputs to the pallido-nigral complex in the monkey. *J Comp Neurol* 1990;298:129–156.
8. Yeterian EH, Pandya DN. Prefrontostriatal connections in relation to cortical architectonic organization in rhesus monkeys. *J Comp Neurol* 1991;312:43–67.

9. Eblen F, Graybiel AM. Highly restricted origin of prefrontal cortical inputs to striosomes in the macaque monkey. *J Neurosci* 1995;15:5999–6013.
10. Haber SN, Kunishio K, Mizobuchi M, et al. The orbital and medial prefrontal circuit through the primate basal ganglia. *J Neurosci* 1995;15:4851–4867.
11. Yelnik J. Functional anatomy of the basal ganglia. *Mov Disord* 2002;17 Suppl 3:S15–21.
12. Haber SN, McFarland NR. The concept of the ventral striatum in nonhuman primates. *Ann N Y Acad Sci* 1999;877:33–48.
13. Graybiel AM, Ragsdale CW Jr. Histochemically distinct compartments in the striatum of human, monkeys, and cat demonstrated by acetylthiocholinesterase staining. *Proc Natl Acad Sci USA* 1978;75:5723–5726.
14. Lehericy S, Ducros M, Krainik A, et al. 3-D diffusion tensor axonal tracking shows distinct SMA and Pre-SMA projections to the human striatum. *Cereb Cortex* 2004;14:1302–1309.
15. Bhatia KP, Marsden CD. The behavioural and motor consequences of focal lesions of the basal ganglia in man. *Brain* 1994;117:859–876.
16. Mendez MF, Adams NL, Lewandowski KS. Neurobehavioral changes associated with caudate lesions. *Neurology* 1989;39:349–354.
17. Caplan LR, Schmahmann JD, Kase CS, et al. Caudate Infarcts. *Arch Neurol* 1990;47:133–143.
18. Trillet M, Croisile B, Tourniaire D, et al. Disorders of voluntary motor activity and lesions of caudate nuclei. *Rev Neurol* (Paris) 1990;146:338–344.
19. Kumral E, Evyapan D, Balkir K. Acute caudate vascular lesions. *Stroke* 1999;30:100–108.
20. Nadeau SE, Crosson B. Subcortical aphasia. *Brain Lang* 1997;58:355–402.
21. Mega MS, Alexander MP. Subcortical aphasia: the core profile of capsulostriatal infarction. *Neurology* 1994;44:1824–1829.
22. Vakil E, Blachstein H, Soroker N. Differential effect of right and left basal ganglionic infarctions on procedural learning. *Cogn Behav Neurol* 2004;17:62–73.
23. Bokura H, Robinson RG. Long-term cognitive impairment associated with caudate stroke. *Stroke* 1997;28:970–975.
24. Richfield EK, Twyman R, Berent S. Neurological syndrome following bilateral damage to the head of the caudate nuclei. *Ann Neurol* 1987;22:768–771.
25. Nishio Y, Nakano Y, Matsumoto K, et al. Striatal infarcts mimicking frontotemporal dementia: a case report. *Eur J Neurol* 2003;10:457–460.
26. Goldman-Rakic PS. Circuitry of primate prefrontal cortex and regulation of behaviour by representational memory. In: Plum F, Mouncastle U, eds. *Handbook of Physiology.* Washington: The American Physiological Society; 1987:373–417.
27. Fuster JM. *The Prefrontal Cortex.* 2nd ed. New York: Raven Press, 1997.
28. Starkstein SE, Robinson RG, Berthier ML, et al. Differential mood changes following basal ganglia vs thalamic lesions. *Arch Neurol* 1988;45:725–730.
29. Kwak CH, Jankovic J. Tourettism and dystonia after subcortical stroke. *Mov Disord* 2002;17:821–825.
30. Penisson-Besnier I, Le Gall D, Dubas F. Obsessive-compulsive behavior (arithmomania): atrophy of the caudate nuclei. *Rev Neurol* (Paris) 1992;148:262–267.
31. Kemp JM, Powell TPS. The cortico-striate projections in the monkey. *Brain* 1970;93:525–546.
32. Battig K, Rosvold HE, Mishkin M. Comparison of the effect of frontal and caudate lesions on delayed response and alternation in monkeys. *J Comp Physiol Psychol* 1960;53:400–404.
33. Rosvold HE, Szwarbach MK. Neural structures involved in delayed response performance. In: Warren JM, Akert K, eds. *The Frontal Granular Cortex and Behavior.* New York: McGraw-Hill; 1964:1–15.
34. Divac I, Rosvold HE, Scwarcbart MK. Behavioural effects of selective ablation of the caudate nucleus. *J Comp Physiol Psych* 1967;63:184–190.
35. Butters N, Rosvold HE. Effect of caudate and septal nuclei lesions on resistance to extinction and delayed alternation. *J Comp Physiol Psychol* 1968;65:397–403.
36. Iversen SD. Behaviour after neostriatal lesions in animals. In: Divac I, Oberg RGE, eds. *The Neostriatum.* Oxford: Pergamon; 1979:195–210.
37. Levy R, Friedman HR, Davachi L, et al. Differential activation of the caudate nucleus in primates performing spatial and nonspatial working memory tasks. *J Neurosci* 1997;17:3870–3882.
38. Kimura M, Matsumoto N, Okahashi K, et al. Goal-directed, serial and synchronous activation of neurons in the primate striatum. *Neuroreport* 2003;14:799–802.
39. Petrides M, Pandya DN. Dorsolateral prefrontal cortex: comparative cytoarchitectonic analysis in the human and the macaque brain and corticocortical connection patterns. *Eur J Neurosci* 1999;11:1011–1036.
40. Yeterian EH, Pandya DN. Corticostriatal connections of extrastriate visual areas in rhesus monkeys. *J Comp Neurol* 1995;352:436–457.
41. Stuss DT, Van Reekum R, Murphy KJ. Differentiation of states and causes of apathy. Chapter 14. In: Borod JC, ed. *The Neuropsychology of Emotion.* Oxford: University Press, 2000:340–363.
42. Owen AM, Doyon J, Petrides M, et al. Planning and spatial working memory: a positron emission tomography study in humans. *Eur J Neurosci* 1996;8:353–364.
43. Rosvold HE, Mishkin M, Szwarbach MK. Effects of subcortical lesions in monkeys on visual-discrimination and single-alternation performance. *J Comp Physiol Psychol* 1958;51:437–444.
44. Rolls ET, Thorpe SJ, Maddison SP. Responses of striatal neurons in the behaving monkey. I. Head of the caudate nucleus. *Behav Brain Res* 1983;7:179–210.
45. Hikosaka O, Sakamoto M, Usui S. Functional properties of monkey caudate neurons. III. Activities related to expectation of target and reward. *J Neurophysiol* 1989;61:814–832.
46. Stanton GB, Goldberg ME, Bruce CJ. Frontal eye field efferents in the macaque monkey: I. Subcortical pathways and topography of striatal and thalamic terminal fields. *J Comp Neurol* 1988;271:473–492.
47. Parthasarathy HB, Schall JD, Graybiel AM. Distributed but convergent ordering of striatal projections: the frontal eye field and the supplementary eye field in monkey. *J Neurosci* 1992;12:4468–4488.
48. Schneider JS, Kovelowski CJ. Chronic exposure to low doses of MPTP. I. Cognitive deficits in motor asymptomatic monkeys. *Brain Res* 1990;519:122–128.
49. Taylor JR, Elsworth JD, Roth RH, et al. Cognitive and motor deficit in acquisition of an object retrieval/detour task in MPTP-treated monkeys. *Brain* 1990;113:617–637.
50. Owen AM, James M, Leigh PN, et al. Fronto-striatal cognitive deficits at different stages of Parkinson's disease. *Brain* 1992;115:1727–1751.
51. Javoy-Agid F, Agid Y. Is the mesocortical dopaminergic system involved in Parkinson's disease? *Neurology* 1980;30:1326–1330.
52. Calder AJ, Keane J, Lawrence AD, et al. Impaired recognition of anger following damage to the ventral striatum. *Brain* 2004;127:1958–1969.
53. Bechara A, Damasio H, Damasio AR. Emotion, decision making and the orbitofrontal cortex. *Cereb Cortex* 2000;10:295–307.
54. Fudge JL, Kunishio K, Walsh P, et al. Amygdaloid projections to ventromedial striatal subterritories in the primate. *Neuroscience* 2002;110:257–275.
55. Adolphs R, Tranel D, Damasio AR, et al. Impaired recognition of emotion in facial expression following bilateral damage to human amygdala. *Nature* 1994;372:669–672.
56. LeDoux JE. Emotion: clues from the brain. *Annu Rev Psychol* 1995;46:209–235.
57. Koob GF, Le Moal M. Drug abuse: hedonic homeostatic dysregulation. *Science* 1997;278:52–58.
58. Schultz W, Apicella P, Scarnati E, et al. Neuronal activity in monkey ventral striatum related to the expectation of reward. *J Neurosci* 1992;12:4595–4610.
59. Hollerman JR, Tremblay L, Schultz W. Influence of reward expectation on behavior-related neuronal activity in primate striatum. *J Neurophysiol* 1998;80:947–963.
60. Rolls ET. The brain and emotion. Oxford: Oxford University Press, 1999.

61. Everitt BJ, Robbins TW. Amygdala-ventral striatal interactions and reward-related processes. In: Aggleton JP, ed. *The Amygdala.* Chichester, England: Wiley; 1992:401–429.

62. Stern CE, Passingham RE. The nucleus accumbens in monkeys (Macaca fascicularis): II. Emotion and motivation. *Behav Brain Res* 1996;75:179–193.

63. Pramstaller PP, Marsden CD. The basal ganglia and apraxia. *Brain* 1996;119:319–340.

64. Karnath HO, Himmelbach M, Rorden C. The subcortical anatomy of human spatial neglect: putamen, caudate nucleus and pulvinar. *Brain* 2002;125:350–360.

65. Buerger AA, Gross CG, Rocha-Miranda CE. Effects of ventral putamen lesions on discrimination learning by monkeys. *J Comp Physiol Psychol* 1974;86:440–446.

66. Webster MJ, Bachevalier J, Ungerleider LG. Subcortical connections of inferior temporal areas TE and TEO in macaque monkeys. *J Comp Neurol* 1993;335:73–91.

67. Karnath HO, Fruhmann Berger M, Kuker W, et al. The anatomy of spatial neglect based on voxelwise statistical analysis: a study of 140 patients. *Cereb Cortex* 2004;14:1164–1172.

68. Max JE, Fox PT, Lancaster JL, et al. Putamen lesions and the development of attention-deficit/hyperactivity symptomatology. *J Am Acad Child Adolesc Psychiatry* 2002;41:563–571.

69. Jeljeli M, Strazielle C, Caston J, et al. Effects of electrolytic lesions of the lateral pallidum on motor coordination, spatial learning, and regional brain variations of cytochrome oxidase activity in rats. *Behav Brain Res* 1999;102:61–71.

70. Grabli D, McCairn K, Hirsch EC, et al. Behavioural disorders induced by external globus pallidus dysfunction in primates: I. Behavioural study. *Brain* 2004;127:2039–2054.

71. Francois C, Grabli D, McCairn K, et al. Behavioural disorders induced by external globus pallidus dysfunction in primates II. Anatomical study. *Brain* 2004;127:2055–2070.

72. Parent A, Hazrati LN. Functional anatomy of the basal ganglia. II. The place of subthalamic nucleus and external pallidum in basal ganglia circuitry. *Brain Res Rev* 1995;20:128–154.

73. Baunez C, Amalric M, Robbins TW. Enhanced food-related motivation after bilateral lesions of the subthalamic nucleus. *J Neurosci* 2002;22:562–568.

74. Desbonnet L, Temel Y, Visser-Vandewalle V, et al. Premature responding following bilateral stimulation of the rat subthalamic nucleus is amplitude and frequency dependent. *Brain Res* 2004;1008:198–204.

75. Ardouin C, Pillon B, Peiffer E, et al. Bilateral subthalamic or pallidal stimulation for Parkinson's disease affects neither memory nor executive functions: a consecutive series of 62 patients. *Ann Neurol* 1999;46:217–223.

76. Pulst SM, Walshe TM, Romero JA. Carbon monoxide poisoning with features of Gilles de la Tourette's syndrome. *Arch Neurol* 1983;40:443–444.

77. Ali-Cherif A, Royere ML, Gosset A, et al. Behavior and mental activity disorders after carbon monoxide poisoning: bilateral pallidal lesions. *Rev Neurol* (Paris) 1984;140:401–405.

78. Laplane D, Baulac M, Widlocher D, et al. Pure psychic akinesia with bilateral lesions of basal ganglia. *J Neurol Neurosurg Psychiatry* 1984;47:377–385.

79. Strub RL. Frontal lobe syndrome in a patient with bilateral globus pallidus lesions. *Arch Neurol* 1989;46:1024–1027.

80. Habib M, Poncet M. Loss of vitality, of interest and of the affect (athymhormia syndrome) in lacunar lesions of the corpus striatum. *Rev Neurol* (Paris) 1988;144:571–577.

81. Dubois B, Defontaines B, Deweer B, et al. Cognitive and behavioral changes in patients with focal lesions of the basal ganglia. In: Lang AE, Weiner WJ, eds. *Behavioral Neurology of Movement Disorders.* New York: Raven Press; 1995:29–41.

82. Laplane D, Dubois B, Pillon B, et al. Loss of psychic self-activation and stereotyped mental activity caused by a frontal lesion: relation of the obsessive-compulsive disorder. *Rev Neurol* (Paris) 1988;144:564–570.

83. Laplane D, Levasseur M, Pillon B, et al. Obsessive-compulsive and other behavioural changes with bilateral basal ganglia lesions: A neuropsychological, magnetic resonance imaging and positron tomography study. *Brain* 1989;112:699–725.

84. Laplane D. Obsessive-compulsive disorders caused by basal ganglia diseases. *Rev Neurol* (Paris) 1994;150:594–598.

85. Laplane D, Widlocher D, Pillon B, et al. Obsessional-type compulsive behavior caused by bilateral circumscribed pallidostriatal necrosis: encephalopathy caused by a wasp sting. *Rev Neurol* (Paris) 1981;137:269–276.

86. Godefroy O, Rousseaux M, Leys D, et al. Frontal lobe dysfunction in unilateral lenticulo-striate infarcts. *Arch Neurol* 1992;49:1285–1289.

87. Litvan I, Mega MS, Cummings JL, et al. Neuropsychiatric aspects of progressive supranuclear palsy. *Neurology* 1996;47:1184–1189.

88. Litvan I, Paulsen JS, Mega MS, et al. Neuropsychiatric assessment of patients with hyperkinetic and hypokinetic movement disorders. *Arch Neurol* 1998;55:1313–1319.

89. Leenders KL, Frackowiak R, Lees AJ. Steele-Richardson-Olszewsky syndrome: brain energy metabolism, blood flow and fluorodopa uptake measured by positron emission tomography. *Brain* 1988;111:615–630.

90. Bogousslavsky J, Regli F, Delaloye B, et al. Loss of psychic self-activation with bithalamic infarction: neurobehavioural, CT, MRI and SPECT correlates. *Acta Neurol Scand* 1991;83:309–316.

91. Van Domburg PH, ten Donkelaar HJ, Notermans SL. Akinetic mutism with bithalamic infarction: neurophysiological correlates. *J Neurol Sci* 1996;139:58–65.

92. Kumral E, Bayulkem G, Evyapan D, et al. Spectrum of anterior cerebral artery territory infarction: clinical and MRI findings. *Eur J Neurol* 2002;9:615–624.

93. Nagaratnam N, Nagaratnam K, Ng K, et al. Akinetic mutism following stroke. *J Clin Neurosci* 2004;11:25–30.

94. Ardila A, Lopez MV. Transcortical motor aphasia: one or two aphasias? *Brain Lang* 1984;22:350–353.

95. von Giesen HJ, Schlaug G, Steinmetz H, et al. Cerebral network underlying unilateral motor neglect: evidence from positron emission tomography. *J Neurol Sci* 1994;125:29–38.

96. Thaler DE, Rolls ET, Passingham RE. Neuronal activity of the supplementary motor area (SMA) during internally and externally triggered wrist movements. *Neurosci Lett* 1988;93:264–269.

Protein Mishandling: Role of the Ubiquitin Proteasome System in the Pathogenesis of Parkinson's Disease

4

Kevin St. P. McNaught   *Peter Jenner*   *C. Warren Olanow*

INTRODUCTION

The etiology of Parkinson's disease (PD) remains obscure but continues to attract much investigation. Approximately 10%–15% of PD cases are inherited, and a specific linkage and gene product has been identified in a small proportion of these cases (1–3). The vast majority of PD cases occur sporadically with no obvious cause. Several concepts have been proposed to account for the etiology of sporadic PD, and most hypotheses have implicated environmental toxins, possibly in individuals who have been rendered susceptible by their genetic profile, poor ability to metabolize toxins, and/or advancing age (4). Identifying a specific environmental agent, however, has proven challenging, and despite the many toxins, occupations, and infectious agents that have been reported to have an association with PD, none has been established to play a causative role.

The sequence or network of cellular, biochemical, and molecular changes that underlie the pathogenesis of neuronal death in PD also has not been determined, although here there are many clues based on changes that have been identified in the brains of PD patients. Factors that have been implicated include oxidative stress (5), mitochondrial dysfunction (6), inflammation (7), excitotoxicity (8), and signal alterations indicative of apoptosis (9). However, it remains unclear which if any of these abnormalities is primary, how these defects relate to each other, precisely what role each plays in the neurodegenerative process, and what percentage of cells in PD die by means of signal-mediated apoptosis.

In recent years, several lines of genetic, postmortem and experimental evidence have converged to suggest that defects in the ubiquitin-proteasome system (UPS) and in its capacity to clear unwanted proteins play a major role in the etiopathogenesis of both the familial and sporadic forms of PD (Table 4.1) (1,3,10). In this chapter, we critically examine the evidence supporting a relationship between defects in the UPS and PD. We begin with a brief overview of the mechanisms responsible for protein clearance within normal cells. We then consider how the different familial and sporadic forms of PD that have been identified to date might result from interference with normal UPS function and a consequent impairment in protein handling. Finally, we consider how defects in the UPS might relate to the various pathologic and biochemical alterations that have been found in the brains of patients with PD.

INTRACELLULAR PROTEIN HANDLING

The life cycle of cells is associated with the generation of a variety of abnormal proteins, including those that are mutant, misfolded, denatured, incomplete, misdirected, oxidized, and otherwise damaged (11,12). This is of particular importance in the brain because of the relatively high utilization of oxygen and elevated rate of metabolism of neurons; the enzymatic- and auto-oxidation of neurotransmitters such as dopamine, which promote the production of reactive oxygen species and other free radicals that can damage proteins; and the fact that nerve cells do not turn over and persist for

the life span of the indivdiuals (13,14). Abnormal proteins that accumulate can misfold, aggregate, disrupt key intracellular processes, and induce cytotoxicity (15,18). Thus, it is important that an accumulation of abnormal proteins be limited by rapid clearance to maintain the integrity and viability of cells (11,12). Indeed, in the brain, a balance between the generation of abnormal proteins and their clearance is crucial since these neurons have a limited ability for repair and regeneration (13).

The degradation of unwanted proteins within eukaryocytic cells is primarily mediated by the UPS (Fig. 4.1) (11,19,21). This pathway not only plays a role in the clearance of abnormal proteins but is also involved in the turnover of short-lived regulatory/functional proteins that mediate a variety of additional cellular activities (11,19,21).

The UPS clearance of proteins comprises two steps that occur in sequence; ubiquitination (Fig. 4.1) and

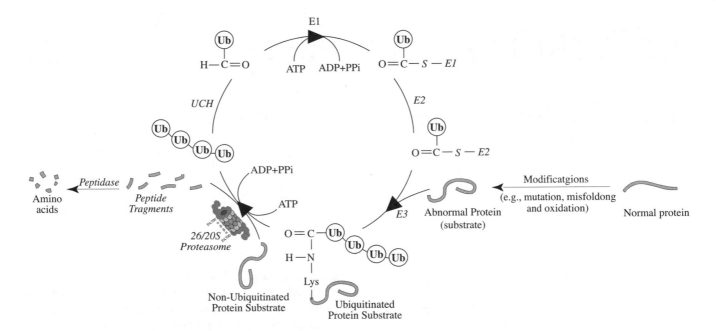

Figure 4.1 The ubiquitin-proteasome system. The ubiquitin-proteasome system (UPS) is the primary system in eukaryocytic cells responsible for the degradation and clearance of unwanted proteins that otherwise have a high tendency to aggregate, interfere with cellular processes, and induce cytotoxicity (UPS) (11,19,21). This process generally occurs in two sequential steps: ubiquitination/deubiquitination and proteolysis. In the first step, unwanted proteins are labeled for degradation by a series of one or more polyubiquitin chains in a series of ATP-dependent reactions. In this process, a ubiquitin-activating enzyme (E1) activates ubiquitin monomers (a 76 amino acid, 8.5 kDa, polypeptide) by forming a thioester; a conjugating enzyme (E2) carries the activated ubiquitin–thioester; and a ubiquitin ligase (E3) transfers activated ubiquitin to the substrate protein. The ubiquitin molecule is attached to the unwanted protein via a covalent isopeptide bond between the carboxy group of the C-terminal residue (Gly) of ubiquitin and an internal Lys residue of the substrate protein. Additional ubiquitin molecules are attached to the previously conjugated ubiquitin (at a Lys residue) in a sequential manner to form a polyubiquitin chain. Polyubiquitinated proteins are then transported to the proteasome for degradation by a molecular chaperone. In the second step, polyubiquitinated proteins are deubiquitinated by deubiquitination enzymes (ubiquitin C-terminal hydrolases), unfolded, and translocated into the core of the 26S proteasome complex where they are degraded in an ATP-dependent manner. The degradation products are small peptide fragments (2–25 residues) that undergo hydrolysis by peptidases to produce their constituent amino acids, which can then be reused in protein synthesis (23). Monomeric ubiquitin, which is detached from protein conjugates, is reused in the ubiquitination cycle to facilitate the clearance of other unwanted proteins. Some proteins (e.g., oxidatively damaged proteins and possibly α-synuclein) can be degraded directly by the 20S proteasome, the catalytic core of the 26S proteasome, without the need for ubiquitination (17,92,94).

TABLE 4.1

GENE MUTATIONS THAT IMPLICATE ALTERED PROTEIN HANDLING IN FAMILIAL PARKINSON'S DISEASE

Locus	Chromosome Location	Gene Product and Properties	Mutations	Inheritance Pattern	Age of Onset (yr)	Clinical Spectrum	Pathological Features
PARK 1 & 4	4q21–4q23	α-Synuclein 140 amino acids/14 kDa protein Localized to synaptic terminals Function: Unknown. Possibly a role in synaptic activity	Point mutations (A53T, A30P, and E46K) Duplication Triplication	Autosomal dominant	Range: 30–60 Mean: 45	Levodopa-responsive; rapid progression; prominent dementia E46K and multiplication cases demonstrate overlap with dementia with Lewy bodies	Neuronal loss in the SNpc, LC, and DMN Lewy bodies are rare, and tau accumulation occurs in some A53T cases. Extensive Lewy bodies in E46K and multiplication cases. Triplication cases demonstrate degeneration in the hippocampus, vacuolation in the cortex, and glial cytoplasmic inclusions.
PARK 2	6q25.2–6q27	Parkin 465 amino acids/ 52 kDa protein Expressed in cytoplasm, golgi complex, nuclei, and processes Function: E3 ubiquitin ligase	Deletions Point mutations Multiplications	Autosomal recessive Rarely autosomal dominant	Range: 7–58 Mean: 26.1	Levodopa-responsive and severe dyskinesias; foot dystonia; diurnal fluctuations; hyperreflexia; slow progression	Selective and severe destruction of the SNpc and LC Generally, Lewy body-negative
PARK 5	4p14	Ubiquitin C-terminal hydrolase L1 230 amino acids/26 kDa protein Neuron-specific protein Function: Deubiquitinating enzyme (possible E3 activity also)	Missense mutation (I93M)	Autosomal dominant	49 and 50	Typical PD	Lewy bodies reported in a single case
PARK 6	1p35–1p36	PINK 1 581 amino acids/62.8 kDa protein Localized to mitochondria Function: Unknown. May be a protein kinase.	Missense Truncating	AR	Range: 32–48	Levodopa- responsive; slow progression	Neuropathology not yet determined

(Continued)

TABLE 4.1
CONTINUED

Locus	Chromosome Location	Gene Product and Properties	Mutations	Inheritance Pattern	Age of Onset (yr)	Clinical Spectrum	Pathological Features
PARK 7	1p36	DJ-1 189 amino acids/20 kDa protein More prominent in the cytoplasm and nucleus of astrocytes compared to neurons Function: Unknown. Possible antioxidant, molecular chaperone, and protease.	Deletion Truncating Missense	AR	Range: 20–40s Mean: mid 30s	Levodopa responsive; dystonia; psychiatric disturbance; slow progression	Neuropathology not yet determined
PARK 8	12p11.2–12q31.1	Dardarin/LRRK2 2482/2527 amino acids Function: Unknown. May be a protein kinase	Missense	AD	Range: 35–79 Mean: 57.4	Typical PD features; slow progression; dementia present; features of motor neuron disease reported	SNpc degeneration Some cases show extensive Lewy bodies; some do not have Lewy bodies. Also, intranuclear inclusions, tau-immunoreactive inclusions, and neurofibrillary tangles are present.

proteasomal degradation (Fig. 4.2) (11,19,21). In the first step, a 76 amino acid ubiquitin molecule is conjugated to unwanted proteins via a covalent isopeptide bond between the C-terminal Gly residue of ubiquitin and an internal Lys residue of the substrate protein. Thereafter, additional ubiquitin molecules are attached to the previously conjugated ubiquitin (at Lys residues) in a sequential manner to form a polyubiquitin chain. Ubiquitination is an ATP-dependent process. It is mediated by three different enzymes acting in sequence, namely ubiquitin-activating enzyme (E1), which activates ubiquitin by forming a thioester; a ubiquitin-conjugating enzyme (E2), which carries activated ubiquitin as a thioester; and a ubiquitin ligase (E3), which transfers activated ubiquitin to the substrate protein (Fig. 4.1). The selectivity of protein ubiquitination is ensured by the fact that each E3 enzyme is specific for one or a limited number of different proteins. Thus, while there is just a single E1 enzyme, there are hundreds if not thousands of E3 enzymes. Further, some proteins require post-translational modification (e.g., phosphorylation of IκB) before they can undergo ubiquitination, and this provides a further degree of selectivity in the ubiquitination process (22). In the second step, ubiquitin-protein conjugates are transferred to the proteasome by molecular chaperones and translocated into the chamber of the 26S proteasome complex, where they are degraded in an ATP-dependent manner (Fig. 4.2). The degradation products of 26/20S proteasomes are 2–25 residue peptide fragments that are further hydrolyzed by peptidases to produce their constituent amino acids, which can then be reused in new protein synthesis (23). Following recognition of the ubiquitinated proteins, but before entry into the proteasome, the polyubiquitin chains are separated from protein conjugates to permit entry of the protein into the proteasome. Ubiquitin chains are disassembled by deubiquitinating enzymes (ubiquitin C-terminal hydrolases), which yield monomeric ubiquitin molecules that can then be reused in the ubiquitination cycle to facilitate the clearance of additional unwanted proteins. It is noteworthy that short peptides and some proteins (e.g., oxidatively damaged proteins) can be degraded by the 20S proteasome (the catalytic core of the 26S proteasome) without prior ubiquitination and in an ATP-independent manner (17). UPS-mediated protein degradation occurs diffusely throughout the cell, including in the cytoplasm, nucleus, and endoplasmic reticulum (ER) (Fig. 4.3) (11,19,21).

Several compensatory mechanisms protect against the development of proteolytic stress. Heat shock proteins (HSPs), such as HSP70 and HSP90, upregulate in the presence of excess levels of misfolded proteins and promote refolding of proteins to their native state. They also facilitate protein degradation by acting as chaperones to transport abnormal proteins to the proteasome (11,24,25). HSPs also activate phosphatases that prevent the formation of pro-apoptotic proteins such as Jun-Kinase (11). High levels of

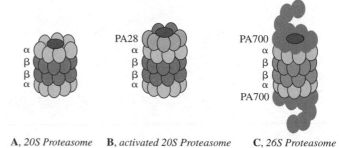

A, *20S Proteasome*   **B,** *activated 20S Proteasome*   **C,** *26S Proteasome*

Figure 4.2 Proteasomal organization. **A:** The 20S proteasome (670 kDa) that is assembled from two outer (α) and two inner (β) heptameric rings stacked axially to form a barrel structure in which proteolysis occurs. Enzymatic activities are localized to the two inner β-rings, which are composed of seven different β-subunits, three of which host different catalytic sites on the inner surface of the complex. These proteolytically active sites mediate the hydrolysis of proteins at the C-terminus of hydrophobic, basic, and acidic residues and are referred to as the chymotrypsin-, trypsin-, and peptidyl glutamyl peptide hydrolytic (PGPH) activities, respectively. The two outer α-rings are each comprised of seven different α-subunits, none of which contains catalytic activity but which serve as an anchor for the 20S proteasome and the multi-subunit PA28 and PA700 proteasome activators. **B:** The PA28/11S regulatory complex (200 kDa) is a hetero- or homoheptameric ring of PA28α-, PA28β-, or PA28γ-subunits. It binds to the 20S proteasome and promotes the opening of the channel through the complex. This process is ATP-independent and mediates the degradation of nonubiquitinated proteins or peptides and is particularly important for clearing oxidized proteins and for antigen presentation in the immune system (173). **C:** The PA700/19S regulator (700 kDa) binds to either or both ends of the 20S proteasome to form the 26S proteasome complex. PA700 is assembled from two sub-complexes: a base that contains six ATPase plus two non-ATPase subunits and an attached lid that comprises several non-ATPase subunits. PA700 performs several ATP-dependent functions: It recognizes polyubiquitinated proteins (via the Rpn10/S5a and Rpt5/S6' subunits), unfolds proteins to allow them entry into the catalytic core, and opens the channel through the 20S proteasome, which is normally gated by the N-termini of the α-subunits (20,174).

protein aggregates bind HSPs and thereby prevent them from exerting these protective effects. In the presence of protein accumulation and aggregation, cells can also activate a protective response involving the formation of inclusions known as *aggresomes*. Here, poorly degraded/undegraded proteins and aggregates that cannot be cleared regionally are transported by way of the microtube system to the centrosome, which expands to form an inclusion body/aggresome where proteins are sequestered and compartmentalized (16,26,31). Simultaneously, components of the UPS are recruited to the centrosome/aggresome to facilitate the clearance of these abnormal proteins. In neurodegenerative disorders, where proteolytic stress is a key factor, protein aggregates and inclusion bodies can be seen within different compartments of the cell (32). We have speculated that Lewy bodies and Lewy neurites, found at different sites of neurodegeneration in PD, are types of aggresomes that serve a protective role (see the following) (26,33).

Normally, cells maintain a dynamic balance between the production of abnormal proteins and their clearance

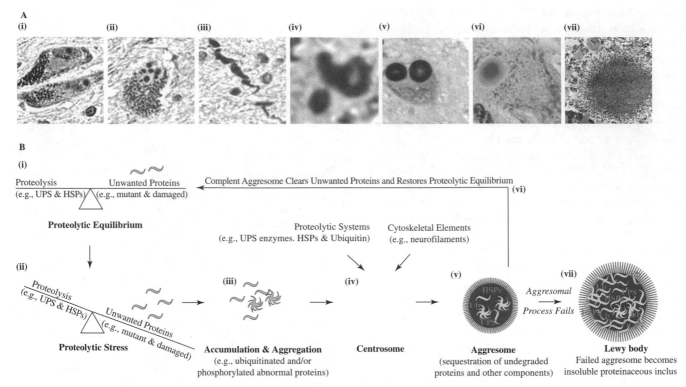

Figure 4.3 **A:** Lewy bodies and protein aggregates in PD. Brain sections immunostained using a standard Vector ABC protocol with 3,3'-diaminobenzidine/H_2O_2 as a brown chromogen and novel antibodies that are highly sensitive for detecting ubiquitin–protein conjugates (UPC) but have little or no immunoreactivity to free ubiquitin. Panel **(i)** demonstrates a melanized dopamine neuron with poor UPC staining in the normal control SNpc. Panels **(ii–iv)** demonstrate numerous discrete aggregates of ubiquitinated proteins (arrows) in the soma **(ii)** and processes **(iii)** of neuromelanin-pigmented neurons in the SNpc in PD. Panel **(iv)** shows what could represent the transport and coalescing of ubiquitinated protein aggregates to form a Lewy body in an aggresome-like manner. Panel **(v)** demonstrates two Lewy bodies staining for α-synuclein. Note that α-synuclein staining is primarily in the periphery of the Lewy body. Panel **(vi)** shows a Lewy body with prominent staining for the protein-binding dye eosin, particularly in the central core. Panel **(vii)** illustrates the dense proteinaceous core and the fibrillary nature of the periphery of Lewy bodies when examined using an electron microscope. **B:** Hypothesis: An aggresome-related concept for Lewy body formation. Normally, there is a dynamic balance between the production of unwanted proteins and their degradation by the ubiquitin-proteasome system (UPS) within cells **(i)**. Proteolytic stress results from impaired degradation and/or excess production of unwanted proteins (mutant, misfolded, denatured, and damaged proteins) **(ii)**. Under these circumstances, unwanted and undegraded proteins begin to accumulate and aggregate **(iii)**. Proteins that are not degraded locally, are actively transported along microtubules to the perinuclear centrosome, which expands to become an aggresome **(iv)**. Simultaneously, UPS components such as UPS enzymes, proteasome components, proteasome activators, HSPs, and ubiquitin (Ub) are recruited to the centrosome/aggresome to facilitate the degradation of sequestered proteins (d). The centrosome/aggresome is identified by specific staining for γ-tubulin and pericentrin. Sequestered proteins within the aggresome are encased by cytoskeletal elements such as neurofilaments to form a distinct proteinaceous core with a peripheral halo **(v)**. If sequestered proteins are successfully degraded, proteolytic equilibrium is restored **(vi)**. However, if proteolysis fails as a result of defects in the protein degradation machinery or the overwhelming production of abnormal proteins, the aggresome continues to expand and forms an insoluble mass of proteins that is identified as a Lewy body **(vii)**.

by the UPS or other proteolytic pathways. Disturbance of this equilibrium, either by the excess production of abnormal proteins or reduced proteasomal degradation, leads to an adverse state called *proteolytic stress* (3,26). During proteolytic stress, poorly degraded or undegraded proteins tend to accumulate and aggregate with each other and with normal proteins (11,17,27). Such protein aggregates can promote oxidative stress, disrupt fundamental intracellular processes, and induce apoptosis (15,18).

PARKINSON'S DISEASE AND THE UBIQUITIN-PROTEASOME SYSTEM

In this section, we consider the different forms of hereditary and sporadic PD that have been linked to a specific defect in the UPS or a propensity to generate abnormal proteins that are prone to misfold and aggregate. We also consider how other familial forms of PD might theoretically be related to a defect in the capacity of the UPS to clear proteins.

Parkinson's Disease Associated with a Defect in Protein Ubiquitination: Parkin Mutations

An autosomal recessive juvenile parkinsonism (AR-JP) has been described in association with mutations in the gene that encodes for the protein parkin. It is characterized clinically by a very early age of onset (average 26.1 years), although older cases have been described. (34,35). Patients typically have a slow rate of disease progression and demonstrate foot dystonia at disease onset, diurnal fluctuations, hyperreflexia, transient improvement in motor disability after rest, infrequent rest tremor, a dramatic response to levodopa, and a propensity to develop dyskinesias (35). Pathologically, neurodegeneration is characterized by severe cell loss that is confined to the substantia nigra pars compacta (SNpc) and the locus coeruleus (LC) (36). Lewy bodies are rarely seen in the brain of patients with AR-JP36, 37, although they have been reported in older individuals who carry this mutation.

The mutations responsible for AR-JP are various deletions, multiplications, and point mutations in the gene (6q25.2-q27; PARK2) that encodes for a 465 amino acid/52 kDa protein called *parkin* (34,38,40). It has been estimated that parkin mutations could be responsible for as many as 50% of early-onset cases of PD (35), although these cases are still quite rare. Parkin is diffusely expressed in the cytoplasm, nucleus, golgi apparatus, and processes of neurons (41). It is now appreciated that parkin is a ubiquitin ligase that attaches ubiquitin molecules to substrate proteins (42)-46. Parkin acts in conjunction with the E2 enzymes Ubc6, UbcH7, and UbcH8 to ubiquitinate a variety of target proteins. Specific substrates, are thought to include synphilin-1, CDCrel-1, parkin-associated endothelin-like receptor (Pael-R), O-glycosylated isoform of α-synuclein (αSp22), cyclin E α/β-tubulin, p38 subunit of aminoacyl-tRNA synthetase complex, and synaptotagmin X1(1,42,44,45). Parkin also interacts with Rpn10/S5a, a subunit of the PA700 regulator of the 26S proteasome subunit, which along with the Rpt5/S6′ subunit plays a role in the recognition of ubiquitinated substrates (20,47) and can bind to the heat shock protein complex CHIP/HSP70 and may thereby promote its activity (48,49).

It is not clear precisely how mutations in parkin lead to neurodegeneration. However, it likely relates to a loss of ubiquitin ligase activity and a reduced capacity to label misfolded substrate proteins for proteasomal degradation. Consistent with this hypothesis, patients with AR-JP have markedly reduced parkin protein and enzyme activity in areas that degenerate (SNpc and LC) (36,42,43,50) and accumulate nonubiquitinated parkin substrates (e.g., Pael-R, αSp22) in these regions (43,45). This concept is further supported by the demonstration that parkin protein prevents cell death induced by overexpression of Pael-R in both cultured cells and *Drosophila* (44,45,51). Thus, parkin mutations could cause cell death in PD by impairing ubiquitination and degradation of target proteins that

then accumulate, aggregate, and cause neurodegeneration. Interestingly, parkin also protects against cell death induced by overexpression of α-synuclein, even though this is not thought to be a parkin substrate. This suggests that parkin might act through additional mechanisms such as enhanced chaperone function (52), failure of which contributes to cell death.

Notably, neither transgenic mice that express parkin mutations nor parkin knockout mice develop nigrostriatal degeneration (53,56). Further, the frequency of parkin point mutations is similar in PD patients (3.8%) and control subjects (3.1%) (57). These observations raise the possibility that patients with parkin mutations require other factors, such as additional genetic alterations or exposure to environmental toxins, to trigger neurodegeneration and the development of a PD syndrome.

Parkinson Disease's Associated with Altered Protein Deubiquitination: UCHL1 Mutation

A familial form of PD has been described in two German siblings associated with a I93M missense mutation in the gene (4p14; PARK5), which encodes for the protein ubiquitin C-terminal hydrolase-L1 (UCH-L1) (58). The affected patients had a relatively early age of onset (49 and 51 years) and a clinical picture that closely resembled sporadic PD, including a good response to levodopa. Postmortem study in one of these individuals noted the presence of Lewy bodies (59). Subsequent genetic screenings have failed to detect UCH-L1 mutations in other PD patients (60), which leads to questioning of the importance of this mutation as a cause of PD. There is, however, evidence that the UCH-L1 gene is a susceptibility locus, and that polymorphisms, particularly an S18Y substitution, confer some degree of protection against developing PD (61).

UCH-L1 is a 230 amino acid/26 kDa protein. It is confined to neurons in many areas of the central nervous system (CNS) (62) and is thought to constitute 1%–2% of soluble proteins in the brain (62,64). UCH-L1 is a deubiquitinating enzyme that removes and dismantles polyubiquitin chains from protein adducts. Alterations in UCH-L1 cause a reduction in deubiquitinating activity and reduced ubiquitin levels in vitro (58,65,66). Inhibition of ubiquitin C-terminal hydrolases in rat ventral midbrain cell cultures leads to degeneration of dopaminergic neurons with the formation of Lewy-bodylike inclusions that stain positively for ubiquitin and α-synuclein (67). Transgenic mice with gracile axonal dystrophy (GAD), resulting from a mutation in UCH-L1, have reduced deubiquitinating activity, neuronal degeneration, and inclusion body formation, although cell loss occurs in the cerebellum and not the substantia nigra (66,68). It is not known how alterations in UCH-L1 cause neurodegeneration in PD patients. However, one can hypothesize that failure to deubiquitinate might prevent ubiquitinated proteins from entering the proteasome for degradation and reduce the supply of ubiquitin monomers necessary for UPS-mediated clearance of additional proteins.

Parkinson's Disease Associated with Excess Production and Aggregation of Proteins: α-Synuclein Mutations

The first gene mutation to be associated with hereditary PD was described in familial patients with an autosomal dominant form of the disorder and linked to chromosome 4q21–q23 (PARK1) (69,73). Subsequent analyses have found A53T, A30P, and E46K mutations in the gene that encodes for the 140 amino acid/14 kDa protein called α-synuclein (71). More recently, PD has been described in patients with duplication or triplication of the wild type α-synuclein protein (74,79).

PD linked to α-synuclein mutations share similar clinical features with standard idiopathic PD, but there is a relatively early age of onset (approximately 40 years) and a high occurrence of dementia. Indeed, some patients with multiplication of the normal α-synuclein gene demonstrate clinical features consistent with a diagnosis of dementia with Lewy bodies (74,79). Pathologically, patients with the A53T mutation show a marked increase in α-synuclein positive protein aggregates in various brain regions, but Lewy bodies are rare and prominent accumulations of α-synuclein and tau deposits are found in the cerebral cortex and striatum (77,80,81). Unlike typical sporadic PD, patients with triplication of the α-synuclein gene also show vacuolization in the cortex, neurodegeneration in the hippocampus, and glial cytoplasmic inclusions (77).

The protein α-synuclein, so called because of its localization to synapses and the nuclear envelope (82,83), belongs to a family of related proteins that include the β- and γ-synucleins (84). It is expressed throughout the CNS and is particularly enriched in presynaptic terminals, lipid membranes, and vesicles (62,84). Its normal function is unknown, but there are indications that it plays a role in synaptic functions such as plasticity and neurotransmission (84,85).

The discovery of α-synuclein-linked familial PD has led to much effort aimed at determining how mutations in this protein lead to its accumulation and neuronal death. The observations that α-synuclein-linked PD is transmitted in a dominant manner and that PD develops in patients who have multiple copies of wild-type α-synuclein point to a gain of function mutation. Wild-type α-synuclein is monomeric and intrinsically unstructured/natively unfolded at low concentrations, but in high concentration it has a propensity to oligomerize and aggregate into β-pleated sheets (86,87). Mutations in α-synuclein increase its potential for misfolding, oligomerization, and aggregation (86,88,91). Oligomerization of α-synuclein produces

intermediary species (protofibrils) that form annular structures with porelike properties that can permeabilize and directly damage cell membranes (88,90). It has been suggested that these protofibrils are the toxic α-synuclein species responsible for Lewy body formation and cell death (91), but this concept is largely based on studies of the in vitro biophysical and conformational properties of α-synuclein.

An alternate hypothesis suggests that cell death associated with α-synuclein mutations/overproduction involves defective clearance of the protein by the proteasome. Wild-type α-synuclein is a substrate for both the 26S and 20S proteasome and is preferentially degraded in a ubiquitin-independent manner (92,94). It has been shown that mutant α-synuclein resists proteasomal degradation and also can inhibit proteasomal function, possibly by blocking the canal and preventing its capacity to degrade other misfolded proteins (95,97). This may account for why mutations in α-synuclein are associated with the accumulation of a wide range of intracellular proteins in addition to α-synuclein. Additionally, high levels of undegraded or poorly degraded normal α-synuclein have a tendency to self-aggregate, induce aggregation of other proteins, and interfere with intracellular functions leading to cell death (15). Studies have shown that α-synuclein can be broken down by the proteasome through endoproteolytic degradation that does not involve entry into the proteasome by way of the –N or –C terminus (92,94). This type of degradation produces truncated α-synuclein fragments that are particularly prone to aggregate and promote aggregation of both the full-length protein and other normal proteins (98). It is therefore possible that excess production or mutant forms of α-synuclein could lead to a cycle of events that include α-synuclein misfolding and aggregation, proteasomal dysfunction, generalized protein aggregation, and neuronal death.

Many studies have examined the effects of α-synuclein mutations or overexpression in cell culture and transgenic animal models (99). Overexpression of mutant α-synuclein can induce degeneration of dopaminergic neurons and accelerate cell death induced by other toxins (100). Overexpression of mutant (A53T, A30P) or wild-type α-synuclein in *Drosophila* results in motor impairment, relatively selective loss of SNpc dopamine neurons and inclusion body formation (101). Similarly, SNpc dopamine cell loss occurs following adenovirus delivery of A53T mutant or wild-type α-synuclein into the SNpc of common marmosets (102). However, overexpression of wild-type or mutant α-synuclein does not lead to neurodegeneration or parkinsonism in transgenic mice (99), raising the possibility that α-synuclein may be degraded differently in this species or that additional factors, such as gene changes or toxins in the environment, might be required to trigger neurodegeneration. This hypothesis is in line with observations that PD does not develop in all individuals who carry a mutation in α-synuclein gene.

Other Mutations in Familial Parkinson's Disease: Theoretical Relationship to the Ubiquitin-Proteasome System

Several additional gene mutations (DJ-1, PINK1, and LRRK2) have recently been described in patients with familial forms of PD where a relationship to the UPS is less clearly evident. The normal function of these proteins is still unclear, and it is not yet known if or how these mutations lead to cell death and PD. Nevertheless, available evidence does permit one to speculate on how the pathogenic process in these familial forms of the illness might involve altered protein handling.

DJ-1 Mutations

An autosomal recessive, early-onset form of parkinsonism has been linked to chromosome 1p36 (PARK7) (103). Genetic analyses patients with this chromosome has identified deletion, truncating, and missense mutations in the gene that encodes for DJ-1, a 189 amino acid/20 kDa protein (104,106). It has been suggested that these mutations might underlie as many as 1%–2% of early-onset PD cases (107). The disorder is characterized by an early onset (mid-30s), slow rate of progression, dystonia, good levodopa response, and psychiatric disturbances (104,105). The pathology in DJ-1-linked PD is not yet known.

In the CNS, DJ-1 is widely expressed in the cytosol and nucleus of cells and is more prominent in astrocytes than neurons (108,109). The normal function of DJ-1 is not known, but evidence suggests that it acts as an antioxidant or a sensor of oxidative stress (110, 111). Further, its molecular structure and in vitro properties suggest that it could have molecular chaperone and protease activity (112,114). Interestingly, DJ-1 has been shown to interact with parkin and CHIP/HSP70, indicating a possible link to these UPS-related systems (115). The mechanism whereby mutant DJ-1 induces cell death in PD is unknown, but the recessive pattern of inheritance raises the possibility of a loss of function of the mutant protein. PD-related mutations in DJ-1 destabilize the protein, inactivate and impair its proteolytic activity, and promote its rapid degradation by the proteasome (112,116). In cell culture studies, expression of DJ-1 protects cells from oxidative stress, while knockdown of DJ-1 increases susceptibility to a variety of insults including proteasomal inhibition, oxidative stress, and endoplasmic reticulum stress (110,111). Interestingly, wild-type DJ-1 inhibits the aggregation of α-synuclein, and this effect is lost when DJ-1 is mutated, as in PD (117). Thus, there are several theoretical means whereby DJ-1 mutations could be linked to altered UPS functions. Recent studies have shown that deletion of DJ-1 in transgenic mice does not induce neurodegeneration (118), suggesting that here too other factors might be involved in the pathogenic process.

PINK1 Mutations

An autosomal recessive early-onset form of PD was found to be associated with missense and truncating mutations in a gene located at chromosome 1p35 (PARK6) that encodes for a 581 amino acid/62.8 kDa protein designated PINK1 (PTEN [phosphatase and tensin homolog deleted on chromosome 10]-induced kinase1) that is primarily located within mitochondria (119,122). Clinically, these patients experience an early onset form of PD (32–48 years), with slow progression and a good response to levodopa (119,122).

The normal function of PINK1 is not known, but its structure suggests that it might be a serine/threonine protein kinase that phosphorylates proteins involved in signal transduction pathways (121). Wild-type PINK1 prevents the development of mitochondrial dysfunction and cell death induced by proteasome inhibitors in cultured nerve cells, but this protection is lost with PD-related mutations (121). These findings raise the possibility that mutations in PINK1 could render neurons susceptible to toxic agents that act on proteasomes to induce cytotoxicity. In addition, mutations in PINK1 might interfere with mitochondrial activity and diminish the ATP production necessary for the normal functioning of the UPS. Interestingly, familial PD-related mutations in PINK1 have been found in normal control subjects without clinical features of parkinsonism or other neurodegenerative disorders (123). Again, this finding raises the possibility that multiple factors may be necessary for the development of PD linked to mutations in PINK1.

LRRK2/Dardarin

An autosomal dominant form of PD with incomplete penetrance has been linked to a mutation on chromosome 12p11.2-q13.1 (PARK8) (51–58,124,125). These patients have missense mutations in the gene encoding for LRRK2, a leucine-rich repeat kinase 2 protein (126,127). The protein has also been referred to as dardarin, the Basque word for "tremor." Interestingly, not all carriers of this mutation develop PD (128), suggesting once again that other etiological factors might be involved in the development of PD in these patients.

The clinical phenotype of patients with LRRK2 mutations is similar to sporadic PD with an age of onset ranging from 35 to 78 years. Pathologically, a variety of phenotypes have been observed even in patients in the same family with the same mutation. All patients have evidence of SNpc dopaminergic cell loss (124,127,129), but Lewy bodies are only found in some. In addition, some patients have extensive cortical Lewy bodies consistent with a diagnosis of dementia with Lewy bodies, while others have tau-immunoreactive glial and neuronal inclusions (124,127,129). It is noteworthy that in contrast to other genetic forms of PD, some patients with LRRK2 mutations have a late-onset clinical syndrome with a clinical and pathologic picture identical to patients with sporadic PD. Indeed, it has been estimated that LRRK2 mutation might account for 7% of familial cases and as many as 1.5%–3% of cases of patients diagnosed with sporadic PD.

The LRKK2 protein is widely expressed throughout the brain (126), but its normal function is not known. LRKK2 resembles the family of tyrosine-like kinases and, based on sequence homology with other proteins, might be a cytoplasmic kinase (126,127). Early predictions suggest that PD-related mutations might lead to increased kinase activity that could promote altered phosphorylation and misfolding of substrates. In addition, some proteins, such as IκB, require phosphorylation as a prerequisite to their ubiquitination and proteasomal degradation (22). Thus, it will be interesting to determine if mutations in LRRK2 lead to altered formation or clearance of UPS substrates.

PD Associated with Proteasomal Dysfunction: Sporadic PD

Sporadic PD is characterized pathologically by neuronal loss in the SNpc, LC, nucleus basalis of Meynert, and various other brain regions. Neuronal death at these sites is associated with protein accumulation, aggregation, and the formation of Lewy-body proteinaceous inclusions. Thus, it is reasonable to consider that impairment in the capacity to clear proteins and/or their propensity to accumulate and aggregate might play a role in the pathogenic process of cell death in sporadic PD. Several studies have now shown that proteasome structure and function are altered in the SNpc in PD. Levels of the proteasomal α-subunits, but not β-subunits, are significantly reduced by approximately 40% in the SNpc of PD patients (130). In contrast, there is an increase in the level of expression of α-subunits in the cerebral cortex (~9%) and striatum (~29%) in patients with sporadic PD. Immunostaining studies confirm these findings, demonstrating reduced expression of the α-subunits, but not β-subunits, of the 20S proteasome in SNpc dopaminergic neurons in PD subjects compared to age-matched controls (130). Although all enzyme activity of the proteasome is located within the β-subunits, α-subunits are required for normal proteasomal assembly and function. Consistent with this observation, there is a 45%–55% reduction in each of the chymotrypsin-like, trypsin-like and peptidyl glutamyl peptide hydrolytic (PGPH) activities of the proteasome in the SNpc in PD patients (130,133). In contrast, there is a compensatory *increase* in proteasomal enzyme activity in regions that do not degenerate in PD, such as the frontal cortex, striatum, hippocampus, pons, and cerebellum (130,132). Interestingly, proteasomal enzyme levels are equally affected in patients with mild and advanced PD, suggesting that altered proteasomal function occurs early in the pathogenic process (132).

Expression of the PA700 and PA28 proteasome activators is also altered in PD. The PA700 is comprised of more than 20 different subunits of various molecular weights (20). In the SNpc in PD, there was either *no change* (42 kDa, 46 kDa, and 95 kDa bands) or *a loss* of up to 33% (52.5 kDa, 75 kDa, and 81 kDa bands) in these specific subunits (130). In contrast, there was a marked compensatory *increase* in the levels of the 81 kDa, 75 kDa, 52.5 kDa, and 42 kDa subunits in the frontal cortex and/or the striatum of PD subjects compared to controls. Levels of the PA28 regulator are also very low in the SNpc in PD patients and significantly less than found in normal controls (130). Interestingly, levels of the PA28 proteasome activator in control subjects are much lower in the SNpc than in other brain regions examined, perhaps accounting for the specific vulnerability of this region in PD (130). Taken together, these studies indicate that proteasomal function is impaired in patients with sporadic PD, and that there is a compensatory upregulation of proteasomal expression in brain regions that are not affected in PD and might account for why these regions are spared.

Several lines of laboratory investigation support the concept that proteasomal dysfunction may play a primary role in the pathogenesis of cell death in PD. In vitro and in vivo studies show that administration of proteasome inhibitors induces a relatively selective degeneration of dopamine neurons coupled with the formation of inclusion bodies that stain positively for both α-synuclein and ubiquitin (52,67,134,135). Recently, we have shown that systemic administration of a proteasome inhibitor recapitulates key features of PD in the rat (136). Following a latency of several weeks, animals developed a gradually progressive, levodopa/apomorphine-responsive, PD-like syndrome. Positron emission tomography (PET) imaging demonstrated a progressive loss of dopaminergic nerve terminals in the striatum, and postmortem analyses showed progressive neurodegeneration with inclusion bodies in the SNpc and the LC, dorsal motor nucleus of the vagus nerve (DMN), and nucleus basalis of Meynert (NMB). At sites of neurodegeneration, there was a 43%–82% inhibition of proteasomal enzyme function while enzyme activity was upregulated in areas that did not degenerate, similar to what is found in PD patients. Many groups have had difficulty reproducing this model, and an intensive search for an explanation of why this is so is currently underway. If it is confirmed that proteasome inhibition generates a model that mirrors the behavioral, imaging, pathologic, and biochemical features of PD, it would strongly support the concept that proteasomal dysfunction is a key factor in the pathogenesis of the disorder.

The basis of the proteasomal dysfunction found in sporadic PD is not known. It could occur secondary to the other biochemical defects that occur in PD, such as oxidative stress or mitochondrial dysfunction (137,139). It could also result from as yet undiscovered gene mutations. Most exciting is the possibility that proteasomal dysfunction in PD could result from exposure to toxins in the environment that inhibit proteasomal function (140). Toxins that inhibit the proteasome can be manufactured by bacteria (e.g., actinomycetes that infect the below-ground parts of crops) (141,142), fungi (e.g., *Apiospora montagne*, which infests wheat/flour) (143), plants (144,146), and the chemical/pharmaceutical industry (140,147). Lactacystin and epoxomicin are among the most potent proteasome inhibitors and are naturally produced by actinomycetes *(Streptomyces)* bacteria, which are found globally in the soil and aquatic habitats of gardens and farmland and have the potential to infect root vegetables (e.g., carrots and potatoes causing "scab" formation) (148,149). Thus, exposure to proteasome inhibitors could occur through living in a rural environment and by consumption of contaminated drinking water or food.

Ubiquitin-Proteasome System Dysfunction May Account for Other Key Features of Parkinson's Disease

If UPS dysfunction is a key factor in the etiopathogenesis of PD, it should explain the other key features of the disease. In particular, UPS failure should then account for Lewy body formation, the age-related vulnerability of the SNpc, and the occurrence of the other biochemical defects found in PD, such as oxidative stress and mitochondrial dysfunction. In the following section, we consider how a defect in UPS function might relate to each of these.

The Ubiquitin-Proteasome System and Lewy Body Formation

Lewy bodies are characteristic pathologic hallmarks of PD and consist of intacytoplasmic proteinaceous inclusions 8–30 μm in diameter found at sites of neurodegeneration. In the SNpc, the Lewy body has a dense central core surrounded by a light halo when stained with haemotoxylin and eosin (Fig. 4.3A). Morphological studies show that the core is comprised of punctate aggregates of ubiquitinated proteins, while the outer region consists of radiating filaments (7–20 nm in diameter) of fibrillar α-synuclein and neurofilaments (26,150). The mechanism underlying the formation of Lewy bodies and their role in the neurodegenerative process have been the focus of considerable debate. It has been suggested that α-synuclein is fundamental to Lewy body formation (86,91). However, not all Lewy bodies stain positively for α-synuclein (151), and not all PD cases have Lewy bodies (36,127).

An alternative hypothesis for Lewy body formation suggests that these inclusions form and function in an aggresome-related manner (Fig. 4.3B). Aggresomes are cytoprotective inclusions that form at the centrosome (a perinuclear structure linked to the microtubular system) in response to excess levels of misfolded proteins (33). In this process, misfolded and aggregated proteins that cannot be cleared by the UPS regionally are delivered via the microtubular system to the centrosome, which enlarges to become an aggresome (16,28,31). At the same time, proteasomal components and HSPs are recruited to the aggresome to facilitate the clearance of these sequestered proteins. Under normal circumstances, if the protein load has been satisfactorily addressed, the aggresome regresses and protein equilibrium is restored. Consistent with the hypothesis that Lewy bodies are a form of aggresome, they share structural similarities. Lewy bodies contain the centrosome/aggresome-specific markers γ-tubulin and pericentrin, and they stain positively for the various components of the UPS, as does the aggresome (26). It is possible that Lewy bodies persist in PD because they cannot adequately clear proteins because of an intrinsic proteasomal dysfunction and/or because there is an overwhelming production of abnormal proteins (26,33). If the aggresomal concept of Lewy body formation is correct, it implies that Lewy body formation is a cytoprotective event aimed at combating proteolytic stress. Indeed, inhibition of inclusion body formation in laboratory models of proteolytic stress is associated with more rapid and more severe cell death (152,153). Failure to ubiquitinate proteins might preclude their transport to the centrosome/aggresome and explain the absence of Lewy bodies in patients with parkin mutations. Lack of this protective response might also account for why parkin patients experience such an early onset of severe neuronal degeneration.

The Ubiquitin-Proteasome System and the Age-Related Susceptibility of the Substantia Nigra Pars Compacta

PD has long been appreciated to be an age-related neurodegenerative disorder. Aging is associated with a progressive increase in the production of abnormal/damaged proteins and a decline in proteasomal function (13,154,155). Specifically, with aging there are increased levels of protein carbonyls (oxidatively damaged proteins) and a reduction in mRNA expression for the various components of the 26/20S proteasome and proteasomal enzymatic activity (13,154,157). Thus, with aging there is an increased risk that hereditary or environmental stresses that cause protein misfolding/proteasomal damage will lead to proteolytic stress and cell death.

In the CNS, neurons are particularly prone to accumulate abnormal proteins with aging as they have a long lifespan and do not regenerate. SNpc dopaminergic neurons in particular might be vulnerable to age-related proteolytic stress because of the oxidative metabolism of dopamine, which generates free radicals that can damage proteins (156), cause a decline in proteasomal activity (155), and create the potential for dopamine to interact with α-synuclein and promote the formation of toxic protofibrils with protein aggregation (158,159). Further, levels of the

TABLE 4.2

ALTERATIONS IN UPS-LINKED CELLULAR PROCESSES IN SPORADIC PARKINSON'S DISEASE

Cellular Processes Linked to the UPS	Alterations in Sporadic Parkinson's Disease
Degradation and clearance of abnormal proteins (11)	YES: Protein accumulation and aggregation (161,175)
Antioxidant defense mechanisms (162,163,168,170)	YES: Oxidative stress (5,139)
Mitochondrial function (138,164,176,177)	YES: Complex I activity impaired (6,179)
Inflammatory response (166,169)	YES: Microglial activation and gliosis (7,220)
Immune processes (173)	YES: Complement activation (6)
Apoptotic signaling (12,167)	YES: Apoptotic cell death (9,180)
Synaptic function and neurotransmission (181)	YES: Altered basal ganglia compensation (182,183)
Signal transduction (184)	YES: Altered neuronal activity (185,186)
Protein transport/trafficking (187)	YES: Lewy neurites and inclusions (126,133,161,175)
Gene transcription (188)	YES: Altered gene expression (189)

PA28 proteasome activator, which is critical to the clearance of oxidatively damaged proteins, are markedly reduced in the SNpc in comparison to other brain regions in normal controls (130). Similar studies in other regions that degenerate in PD remain to be performed.

Thus, the normal aging process, particularly in the SNpc, is associated with an increase in the formation of damaged proteins and a reduced capacity to degrade them. This suggests that aging SNpc neurons are prone to develop proteolytic stress, which may account for their specific vulnerability in PD. Indeed, mild neuronal loss and Lewy bodies are found in the SNpc in 10%–15% of individuals over the age of 65 years who die without clinical evidence of neurological illness (160,161). It is possible that PD represents an extreme form of age-related proteolytic stress, wherein ongoing compensatory responses to genetic and environmental factors that promote protein accumulation eventually fail, resulting in cell loss sufficient to manifest as clinical disease.

The Ubiquitin-Proteasome System and Other Biochemical Changes in Parkinson's Disease

There are several important biochemical changes that have been detected in the brain in PD subjects. In particular, there is evidence for oxidative stress, mitochondrial damage, inflammation and apoptosis (Table 4.2). There is some evidence to suggest that UPS dysfunction could cause or be linked to these defects. The UPS plays a major role in controlling levels of short-lived regulatory/function proteins that are linked to antioxidant defense mechanisms (162,163), mitochondrial activity (164,165), inflammatory responses (166), and anti-apoptotic pathways (167). Indeed, it has been shown that impairment of proteasomal function causes oxidative stress (168), mitochondrial dysfunction (168), pro-inflammatory reactions (169), and apoptosis (164). Further, there is in vitro evidence that cell damage induced by proteasome inhibitors is synergistically increased by agents that induce oxidative stress or promote protein misfolding (15,137,170,172). Conversely, oxidative stress and mitochondrial dysfunction can induce proteasomal dysfunction, possibly by increasing the protein load to the point that it overwhelms the proteasome system or by impairing ATP production necessary for normal UPS function. Thus, there are reasons to consider that there is a close relationship and interplay between UPS dysfunction and the other biochemical/molecular changes that occur in PD.

SUMMARY

Cells normally maintain a balance between the generation and clearance of unwanted proteins (Fig. 4.3). Proteolytic stress occurs when the levels of unwanted proteins exceed the cell's capacity to clear and degrade them. This results in protein accumulation, aggregation, disruption of critical intracellular processes, and cell death (15,18). A growing body of evidence suggests that altered UPS function and protein mishandling are common features underlying the different familial and sporadic forms of PD. Notably, familial PD has been observed in patients with parkin mutations (which could prevent ubiquitination of target proteins) and UCH-L1 mutations (which could impair deubiquitination of ubiquitinated proteins). Familial PD has also been observed in patients with α-synuclein mutations or duplication/triplication of the wild-type protein. These could result in excess levels of misfolded and aggregated α-synuclein proteins that exceed the degradation capacity of the UPS system and could impair normal proteasomal function. Sporadic PD also has been linked to defects in the UPS and is associated with inhibition of proteasomal enzymatic activity and failed compensatory upregulation of proteasomal activators. Other gene mutations recently described in association with familial PD are less clearly linked to the UPS, although little is currently known about their function or how they might cause cell death leading to PD.

PD is also linked to mutations in several as yet uncharacterized genes, and it will be interesting to determine if these encode proteins that interfere with normal UPS activity. Defects in UPS function could also account for Lewy body formation in PD, the age-related vulnerability of the SNpc, and the other biochemical features of the illness. Further support for this hypothesis is provided by in vitro and in vivo laboratory studies that indicate that proteasome inhibition induces relatively selective degeneration of dopamine neurons coupled with Lewy bodylike inclusions and a progressive model of PD.

Collectively, this information suggests that proteolytic stress secondary to genetic or environmentally based defects in proteins formation or UPS function might be the common factor underlying the different forms of PD. As such, this concept provides novel targets for the development of putative neuroprotective agents for PD, and such approaches are actively being explored. Many unanswered questions remain. First, it has not yet been established that the proteasomal defects and protein accumulation found in cases of sporadic PD are primary events and do not occur secondary to an alternate etiopathogenic process. Indeed, agents that damage mitochondria or cause oxidative stress can induce secondary proteasomal damage. As such, impaired UPS function might still be of extreme importance in promoting the pathogenic cascade, but less so than if it were the inciting event. Second, a relationship between UPS dysfunction and familial cases of PD can only be reasonably proposed for some of the mutations that have been identified to date, and even here there is still much speculation. A better understanding of why individual mutations cause PD is required before we can unequivocally implicate the UPS as a cause of PD in patients with these mutations. Third, the animal model of PD caused by systemic exposure to proteasome inhibitors remains to be replicated. Indeed, several groups have been unable to replicate this model. An understanding is critical of what factors (i.e., source, solubility, absorption of toxin, animal species, housing, etc.) determine why some groups have been able, and others have not, to generate this promising model. Confirmation that systemic exposure to a proteasome inhibitor induces a predictive, reproducible, progressive model of PD that mirrors the biochemical and pathologic changes seen in the disease would provide strong support for the concept that a defect in the capacity of the UPS to clear unwanted proteins is a key factor in the etiopathogenesis of PD.

REFERENCES

1. Hattori N, Mizuno Y. Pathogenetic mechanisms of parkin in Parkinson's disease. *Lancet* 2004;364:722–724.
2. Moore DJ, West AB, Dawson VL, Dawson TM. Molecular pathophysiology of Parkinson's disease. *Ann Rev Neurosci* 2005;25:55–84.
3. McNaught KS, Olanow CW. Proteolytic stress: A unifying concept in the etiopathogenesis of familial and sporadic Parkinson's disease. *Ann Neurol* 2003;53(3 Suppl 1): S73–86.
4. Tanner CM. Is the cause of Parkinson's disease environmental or hereditary? Evidence from twin studies. *Adv Neurol* 2003;91: 133–142.
5. Jenner P. Oxidative stress in Parkinson's disease. *Ann Neurol* 2003;53:S26–36; discussion S36–38.
6. Orth M, Schapira AH. Mitochondrial involvement in Parkinson's disease. *Neurochem Int* 2002;40:533–541.
7. McGeer PL, McGeer EG. Inflammation and neurodegeneration in Parkinson's disease. *Parkinsonism Relat Disord* 2004;10 Suppl 1:S3–7.
8. Beal MF. Excitotoxicity and nitric oxide in Parkinson's disease pathogenesis. *Ann Neurol* 1998;44:S110–114.
9. Tatton WG, Chalmers-Redman R, Brown D, Tatton, N. Apoptosis in Parkinson's disease: signals for neuronal degradation. *Ann Neurol* 2003;53 Suppl 3:S61–70; discussion S70–72.
10. Petrucelli L, Dawson, TM. Mechanism of neurodegenerative disease: role of the ubiquitin proteasome system. *Ann Med* 2004;36:315–320.
11. Goldberg, AL. Protein degradation and protection against misfolded or damaged proteins. *Nature* 2003;426:859–895.
12. Sherman MY, Goldberg, AL. Cellular defenses against unfolded proteins: a cell biologist thinks about neurodegenerative diseases. *Neuron* 2001;29:15–32.
13. Keller JN, et al. Autophagy, proteasomes, lipofuscin, and oxidative stress in the aging brain. *Int J Biochem Cell Biol* 2004;36:2376–2391.
14. Tse DC, McCreery RL, Adams RN. Potential oxidative pathways of brain catecholamines. *J Med Chem* 1976;19:37–40.
15. Bence NF, Sampat RM, Kopito RR. Impairment of the ubiquitin-proteasome system by protein aggregation. *Science* 2001;292: 1552–1555.
16. Kopito RR. Aggresomes, inclusion bodies and protein aggregation. *Trends Cell Biol* 2000;10:524–530.
17. Grune T, Jung T, Merker K, Davies KJ. Decreased proteolysis caused by protein aggregates, inclusion bodies, plaques, lipofuscin, ceroid, and "aggresomes" during oxidative stress, aging, and disease. *Int J Biochem Cell Biol* 2004;36:2519–2530.
18. Bennett EJ, Bence NF, Jayakumar R, Kopito RR. Global impairment of the ubiquitin-proteasome system by nuclear or cytoplasmic protein aggregates precedes inclusion body formation. *Mol Cell* 2005;17:351–365.
19. Pickart CM. Mechanisms underlying ubiquitination. *Annu Rev Biochem* 2001;70:503–533.
20. Pickart CM, Cohen RE. Proteasomes and their kin: proteases in the machine age. *Nat Rev Mol Cell Biol* 2004;5;177–187.
21. Ciechanover A. Proteolysis: from the lysosome to ubiquitin and the proteasome. *Nat Rev Mol Cell Biol* 2005;6:79–87.
22. DiDonato J, et al. Mapping of the inducible IkappaB phosphorylation sites that signal its ubiquitination and degradation. *Mol Cell Biol* 1996;16:1295–1304.
23. Saric T, Graef CI, Goldberg AL. Pathway for degradation of peptides generated by proteasomes: a key role for thimet oligopeptidase and other metallopeptidases. *J Biol Chem* 2004; 279:46,732.
24. Hartl FU, Hayer-Hartl M. Molecular chaperones in the cytosol: from nascent chain to folded protein. *Science* 2004;295:1852–1858.
25. Muchowski PJ, Wacker JL. Modulation of neurodegeneration by molecular chaperones. *Nat Rev Neurosci* 2005;6:11–22.
26. McNaught KS, Shashidharan P, Perl DP, Jenner P, Olanow CW. Aggresome-related biogenesis of Lewy bodies. *Eur J Neurosci* 2004;16:2136–2148.
27. Rajan, RS, Illing ME, Bence NF, Kopito RR. Specificity in intracellular protein aggregation and inclusion body formation. *Proc Natl Acad Sci USA* 2004;98:13,060–13,065.
28. Johnston JA, Illing ME, Kopito RR. Cytoplasmic dynein/dynactin mediates the assembly of aggresomes. *Cell Motil Cytoskeleton* 2002;53:26–38.
29. Johnston JR, Ward CL, Kopito RR. Aggresomes: a cellular response to misfolded proteins. *J Cell Biol* 1998;143:1883–1898.
30. Kawaguchi Y, et al. The deacetylase HDAC6 regulates aggresome formation and cell viability in response to misfolded protein stress. *Cell* 2003;115:727–738.
31. Arrasate M, Mitra S, Schweitzer ES, Segal MR, Finkbeiner S. Inclusion body formation reduces levels of mutant huntington and the risk of neuronal death. *Nature* 2004;431:805–810.

32. Ciechanover A, Brundin P. The ubiquitin proteasome system in neurodegenerative diseases: sometimes the chicken, sometimes the egg. *Neuron* 2003;40:427–446.

33. Olanow CW, Perl DP, DeMartino GN, McNaught KS. Lewy-body formation is an aggresome-related process: a hypothesis. *Lancet Neurol* 2004;3:496–503.

34. Yamamura Y, Sobue I, Ando K, Iida M, Yanagi T. Paralysis agitans of early onset with marked diurnal fluctuation of symptoms. *Neurology* 1973;23:239–244.

35. Lucking CB, and the French Parkinson's Disease Genetics Study Group. Association between early-onset Parkinson's disease and mutations in the parkin gene. *N Engl J Med* 2000;342:1560–1567.

36. Mori H, et al. Pathologic and biochemical studies of juvenile parkinsonism linked to chromosome 6q. *Neurology* 1998;51:890–892.

37. Farrer M, et al. Lewy bodies and parkinsonism in families with parkin mutations. *Ann Neurol* 2001;50:293–300.

38. Matsumine H, et al. Localization of a gene for an autosomal recessive form of juvenile Parkinsonism to chromosome 6q25.2–27. *Am J Hum Genet* 1997;60:588–596.

39. Kitada T, et al. Mutations in the parkin gene cause autosomal recessive juvenile parkinsonism. *Nature* 1998;392:605–608.

40. Mizuno Y, Hattori N, Mori H, Suzuki T, Tanaka K. Parkin and Parkinson's disease. *Curr Opin Neurol* 2001;14:477–482.

41. Horowitz JM, et al. Immunodetection of Parkin protein in vertebrate and invertebrate brains: a comparative study using specific antibodies. *J Chem Neuroanat* 2001;21:75–93.

42. Shimura H, et al. Familial Parkinson disease gene product, parkin, is a ubiquitin-protein ligase. *Nat Genet* 2000;25:302–305.

43. Shimura H, et al. Ubiquitination of a new form of {alpha}-synuclein by parkin from human brain: implications for Parkinson's disease. *Science* 2001;293:263–269.

44. Imai Y, Soda M, Takahashi R. Parkin suppresses unfolded protein stress-induced cell death through its E3 ubiquitin-protein ligase activity. *J Biol Chem* 2000;275:35,661–664.

45. Imai Y, et al. An unfolded putative transmembrane polypeptide, which can lead to endoplasmic reticulum stress, is a substrate of parkin. *Cell* 2001;105:891–902.

46. Zhang Y, et al. Parkin functions as an E2-dependent ubiquitin-protein ligase and promotes the degradation of the synaptic vesicle-associated protein, CDCrel-1. *Proc Natl Acad Sci USA* 2000;97:13,354–359.

47. Sakata E, et al. Parkin binds the Rpn10 subunit of 26S proteasomes through its ubiquitin-like domain. *EMBO Rep* 2003;4:301–306.

48. Imai Y, et al. CHIP is associated with Parkin, a gene responsible for familial Parkinson's disease, and enhances its ubiquitin ligase activity. *Mol Cell* 2002;10:55–67.

49. Cyr DM, Hohfeld J, Patterson C. Protein quality control: U-box-containing E3 ubiquitin ligases join the fold. *Trends Biochem Sci* 2002;27:368–375.

50. Shimura H, et al. Immunohistochemical and subcellular localization of Parkin protein: absence of protein in autosomal recessive juvenile parkinsonism patients. *Ann Neurol* 1999;45:668–672.

51. Yang Y, Nishimura I, Imai Y, Takahashi R, Lu B. Parkin suppresses dopaminergic neuron-selective neurotoxicity induced by Pael-R in Drosophila. *Neuron* 2003;37:911–924.

52. Petrucelli L, et al. Parkin protects against the toxicity associated with mutant alpha-synuclein: proteasome dysfunction selectively affects catecholaminergic neurons. *Neuron* 2002;36:1007–1019.

53. Itier JM, et al. Parkin gene inactivation alters behaviour and dopamine neurotransmission in the mouse. *Hum Mol Genet* 2003;12:2277–2291.

54. Goldberg MS, et al. Parkin-deficient mice exhibit nigrostriatal deficits but not loss of dopaminergic neurons. *J Biol Chem* 2003;278:43,628–635.

55. Von Coelln R, et al. Loss of locus coeruleus neurons and reduced startle in parkin null mice. *Proc Natl Acad Sci USA* 2004;101:10,744–10,749.

56. Perez FA, Palmiter RD. Parkin-deficient mice are not a robust model of parkinsonism. *Proc Natl Acad Sci USA* 2005;102:2174–2179.

57. Lincoln SJ, et al. Parkin variants in North American Parkinson's disease: cases and controls. *Mov Disord* 2003;18:1306–1311.

58. Leroy E, et al. The ubiquitin pathway in Parkinson's disease. *Nature* 1998;395:451–452.

59. Auberger, et al. Is the PARK5 I93M mutation a cause of Parkinson's disease with cognitive deficits and cortical Lewy pathology? (2005). *16th International Congress on Parkinson's Disease and Related Disorders* Berlin, PT042.

60. Wintermeyer P, et al. Mutation analysis and association studies of the UCHL1 gene in German Parkinson's disease patients. *Neuroreport* 2000;11:2079–2082.

61. Maraganore DM, et al. UCHL1 is a Parkinson's disease susceptibility gene. *Ann Neuron* 2004;55:512–521.

62. Solano SM, Miller DW, Augood SJ, Young AB, Penney JB Jr. Expression of alpha-synuclein, parkin, and ubiquitin carboxy-terminal hydrolase L1 mRNA in human brain: genes associated with familial Parkinson's disease. *Ann Neurol* 2000;47:201–210.

63. Wilkinson KD, Deshpande S, Larsen CN. Comparisons of neuronal (PGP 9.5) and non-neuronal ubiquitin C-terminal hydrolases. *Biochem Soc Trans* 1992;20:631–637.

64. Wilkinson KD, et al. The neuron-specific protein PGP 9.5 is a ubiquitin carboxyl-terminal hydrolase. *Science* 1989;246:670–673.

65. Nishikawa K, et al. Alterations of structure and hydrolase activity of parkinsonism-associated human ubiquitin carboxyl-terminal hydrolase L1 variants. *Biochem Biophys Res Commun* 2003;304:176–183.

66. Osaka H, et al. Ubiquitin carboxy-terminal hydrolase L1 binds to and stabilizes monoubiquitin in neuron. *Hum Mol Genet* 2003;12:1945–1958.

67. McNaught KSP, et al. Impairment of the ubiquitin-proteasome system causes dopaminergic cell death and inclusion body formation in ventral mesencephalic cultures. *J Neurochem* 2002;81:301–306.

68. Saigoh K, et al. Intragenic deletion in the gene encoding ubiquitin carboxy-terminal hydrolase in gad mice. *Nat Genet* 1999;23:47–51.

69. Golbe LI, Di Iorio G, Bonavita V, Miller DC, Duvoisin RC. A large kindred with autosomal dominant Parkinson's disease. *Ann Neurol* 1990;27:276–282.

70. Polymeropoulos MH, et al. Mapping of a gene for Parkinson's disease to chromosome 4q21–q23. *Science* 1996;274:1197–1199.

71. Polymeropoulos MH, et al. Mutation in the alpha-synuclein gene identified in families with Parkinson's disease. *Science* 1997;276:2045–2047.

72. Kruger R, et al. Ala30Pro mutation in the gene encoding alpha-synuclein in Parkinson's disease. *Nat Genet* 1998;18:106–108.

73. Zarranz JJ, et al. The new mutation, E46K, of alpha-synuclein causes Parkinson and Lewy body dementia. *Ann Neurol* 2004;55:164–173.

74. Chartier-Harlin MC, et al. Alpha-synuclein locus duplication as a cause of familial Parkinson's disease. *Lancet* 2004;364:1167–1169.

75. Ibanez P, et al. Causal relation between alpha-synuclein gene duplication and familial Parkinson's disease. *Lancet* 2004;364:1169–1171.

76. Singleton AB, et al. alpha-synuclein locus triplication causes Parkinson's disease. *Science* 2003;302:841.

77. Muenter MD, et al. Hereditary form of parkinsonism–dementia. *Ann Neurol* 1998;43:768–781.

78. Miller DW, et al. Alpha-synuclein in blood and brain from familial Parkinson disease with SNCA locus triplication. *Neurology* 2004;62:1835–1838.

79. Farrer M, et al. Comparison of kindreds with parkinsonism and alpha-synuclein genomic multiplications. *Ann Neurol* 2004;55:174–179.

80. Kotzbauer PT, et al. Fibrillization of alpha-synuclein and tau in familial Parkinson's disease caused by the A53T alpha-synuclein mutation. *Exp Neurol* 2004;187:279–288.

81. Duda JE, et al. Concurrence of alpha-synuclein and tau brain pathology in the Contursi kindred. *Acta Neuropathol (Berl)* 2002;104:7–11.

82. Maroteaux L, Campanelli JT, Scheller RH. Synuclein: a neuron-specific protein localized to the nucleus and presynaptic nerve terminal. *J Neurosci* 1988;8:2804–2815.

83. Jakes R, Spillantini MG, Goedert M. Identification of two distinct synucleins from human brain. *FEBS Lett* 1994;345:27–32.

84. Goedert M. Alpha-synuclein and neurodegenerative diseases. *Nat Rev Neurosci* 2001;2:492–501.

85. Abeliovich A, et al. Mice lacking alpha-synuclein display functional deficits in the nigrostriatal dopamine system. *Neuron* 2000;25:239–252.

86. Conway KA, Harper JD, Lansbury PT. Accelerated in vitro fibril formation by a mutant alpha-synuclein linked to early-onset Parkinson disease. *Nat Med* 1998;4:1318–1320.

87. Weinreb PH, Zhen W, Poon AW, Conway KA, Lansbury PT Jr. NACP, a protein implicated in Alzheimer's disease and learning, is natively unfolded. *Biochemistry* 1996;35:13,709–715.

88. Conway KA, et al. Acceleration of oligomerization, not fibrillization, is a shared property of both alpha-synuclein mutations linked to early-onset Parkinson's disease: implications for pathogenesis and therapy. *Proc Natl Acad Sci USA* 2000;97:571–576.

89. Li J, Uversky VN, Fink AL. Effect of familial Parkinson's disease point mutations A30P and A53T on the structural properties, aggregation, and fibrillation of human alpha-synuclein. *Biochemistry* 2001;40:11,604–613.

90. Lashuel HA, et al. Alpha-synuclein, especially the Parkinson's disease-associated mutants, forms pore-like annular and tubular protofibrils. *J Mol Biol* 2002;322:1089–1102.

91. Caughey B, Lansbury PT. Protofibrils, pores, fibrils, and neurodegeneration: separating the responsible protein aggregates from the innocent bystanders. *Annu Rev Neurosci* 2003;26:267–298.

92. Bennett MC, et al. Degradation of alpha-synuclein by proteasome. *J Biol Chem* 1999:274,33,855–858.

93. Tofaris GK, Layfield R, Spillantini MG. Alpha-synuclein metabolism and aggregation is linked to ubiquitin-independent degradation by the proteasome. *FEBS Letters* 2001:25,504;1–5.

94. Liu CW, Corboy MJ, DeMartino GN, Thomas PJ. Endoproteolytic activity of the proteasome. *Science* 2003;299:408–411.

95. Tanaka Y, et al. Inducible expression of mutant alpha-synuclein decreases proteasome activity and increases sensitivity to mitochondria-dependent apoptosis. *Hum Mol Genet* 2001;10:919–926.

96. Stefanis L, Larsen KE, Rideout HJ, Sulzer D, Greene LA. Expression of A53T mutant but not wild-type alpha-synuclein in PC12 cells induces alterations of the ubiquitin-dependent degradation system, loss of dopamine release, and autophagic cell death. *J Neurosci* 2001;21:9549–9560.

97. Snyder H, et al. Aggregated and monomeric alpha-synuclein bind to the S6' proteasomal protein and inhibit proteasomal function. *J Biol Chem* 2003;278:11,753–759.

98. Liu CW, et al. A precipitating role for truncated alpha-synuclein and the proteasome in alpha-synuclein aggregation: implications for pathogenesis of Parkinson's disease. *J Biol Chem* 2005.

99. Fernagut PO, Chesselet MF. Alpha-synuclein and transgenic mouse models. *Neurobiol Dis* 2004;17:123–130.

100. Lee M, Hyun D, Halliwell B, Jenner P. Effect of the overexpression of wild-type or mutant alpha-synuclein on cell susceptibility to insult. *J Neurochem* 200;76:998–1009.

101. Feany MB, Bender WW. A Drosophila model of Parkinson's disease. *Nature* 2000;404:394–398.

102. Kirik D, et al. Nigrostriatal alpha-synucleinopathy induced by viral vector-mediated overexpression of human alpha-synuclein: a new primate model of Parkinson's disease. *Proc Natl Acad Sci USA* 2003;100:2884–2889.

103. Van Duijn CM, et al. Park7: a novel locus for autosomal recessive early-onset parkinsonism, on chromosome 1p36. *Am J Hum Genet* 2001;69:629–634.

104. Bonifati V, et al. Mutations in the DJ-1 gene associated with autosomal recessive early-onset parkinsonism. *Science* 2003;299:256–259.

105. Bonifati V, Oostra BA, Heutink P. Linking DJ-1 to neurodegeneration offers novel insights for understanding the pathogenesis of Parkinson's disease. *J Mol Med* 2004;82:163–174.

106. Nagakubo D, et al. DJ-1, a novel oncogene which transforms mouse NIH3T3 cells in cooperation with rats. *Biochem Biophys Res Commun* 1997;231:509–513.

107. Abou-Sleiman PM, Healy DG, Quinn N, Lees AJ, Wood NW. The role of pathogenic DJ-1 mutations in Parkinson's disease. *Ann Neurol* 2003;54:283–286.

108. Shang H, Lang D, Jean-Marc B, Kaelin-Lang A. Localization of DJ-1 mRNA in the mouse brain. *Neurosci Lett* 2004;367:273–277.

109. Bandopadhyay R, et al. The expression of DJ-1 (PARK 7) in normal human CNS and idiopathic Parkinson's disease. *Brain* 2004;127:420–430.

110. Yokota T, et al. Down regulation of DJ-1 enhances cell death by oxidative stress, ER stress, and proteasome inhibition. *Biochem Biophys Res Commun* 2003;312:1342–1348.

111. Taira T, et al. DJ-1 has a role in antioxidative stress to prevent cell death. *EMBO Rep* 2004;5:213–218.

112. Olzmann JA, et al. Familial Parkinson's disease-associated L166P mutation disrupts DJ-1 protein folding and function. *J Biol Chem* 2004;279:8506–8515.

113. Lee SJ, et al. Crystal structures of human DJ-1 and Escherichia coli Hsp31, which share an evolutionarily conserved domain. *J Biol Chem* 2003;278:44,552–559.

114. Wilson MA, St Amour CV, Collins JL, Ringe D, Petsko GA. The 1.8-A resolution crystal structure of YDR533Cp from Saccharomyces cerevisiae: a member of the DJ-1/ThiJ/PfpI superfamily. *Proc Natl Acad Sci USA* 2004;101:1531–1536.

115. Moore DJ, et al. Association of DJ-1 and parkin mediated by pathogenic DJ-1 mutations and oxidative stress. *Hum Mol Genet* 2005:14,71–84.

116. Moore DJ, Zhang L, Dawson TM, Dawson VL. A missense mutation (L166P) in DJ-1, linked to familial Parkinson's disease, confers reduced protein stability and impairs homo-oligomerization. *J Neurochem* 2003;87:1558–1567.

117. Shendelman S, Jonason A, Martinat C, Leete T, Abeliovich A. DJ-1 is a redox-dependent molecular chaperone that inhibits alpha-synuclein aggregate formation. *PLoS Biol* 2004;2:e362.

118. Goldberg MS, et al. Nigrostriatal dopaminergic deficits and hypokinesia caused by inactivation of the familial parkinsonism-linked gene DJ-1. *Neuron* 2005;45:489–496.

119. Valente EM, et al. Localization of a novel locus for autosomal recessive early-onset parkinsonism, PARK 6, on human chromosome 1p35–p36. *Am J Hum Genet* 2001;68:895–900.

120. Valente EM, et al. PARK 6-linked parkinsonism occurs in several European families. *Ann Neurol* 2002;51:14–18.

121. Valente EM, et al. Hereditary early-onset Parkinson's disease caused by mutations in PINK1. *Science* 2004;304:1158–1160.

122. Healy DG, Abou-Sleiman PM, Wood NW. PINK, PANK, or PARK? A clinicians' guide to familial parkinsonism. *Lancet Neurol* 2004;3:652–662.

123. Rogaeva E, et al. Analysis of the PINK1 gene in a large cohort of cases with Parkinson disease. *Arch Neurol* 2004;61:1898–1904.

124. Funayama M, et al. A new locus for Parkinson's disease (PARK 8) maps to chromosome 12p11.2–q13.1. *Ann Neurol* 2002;51:296–301.

125. Nichols WC, et al. Genetic screening for a single common LRRK2 mutation in familial Parkinson's disease. *Lancet* 2005;365:410–412.

126. Paisan-Ruiz C, et al. Cloning of the gene containing mutations that cause PARK8-linked Parkinson's disease. *Neuron* 2004;44:595–600.

127. Zimprich A, et al. Mutations in LRRK2 cause autosomal-dominant parkinsonism with pleomorphic pathology. *Neuron* 2004;44:601–607.

128. Di Fonzo A, et al. A frequent LRRK2 gene mutation associated with autosomal dominant Parkinson's disease. *Lancet* 2005;365:412–415.

129. Wszolek ZK, et al. Autosomal dominant parkinsonism associated with variable synuclein and tau pathology. *Neurology* 2004;62:1619–1622.

130. McNaught KS, Belizaire R, Isacson O, Jenner P, Olanow CW. Altered proteasomal function in sporadic Parkinson's disease. *Exp Neurol* 2003;179:38–45.

131. McNaught KS, Jenner P. Proteasomal function is impaired in substantia nigra in Parkinson's disease. *Neurosci Lett* 2001;297:191–194.

132. Tofaris GK, Razzaq A, Ghetti B, Lilley K, Spillantini MG. Ubiquitination of alpha-synuclein in Lewy bodies is a pathological event not associated with impairment of proteasome function. *J Biol Chem* 2003;278:44,405–411.

133. Furukawa Y, et al. Brain proteasomal function in sporadic Parkinson's disease and related disorders. *Ann Neurol* 2002;51:779–782.

134. McNaught KSP, Bjorklund LM, Belizaire R, Jenner P, Olanow CW. Proteasome inhibition causes nigral degeneration with inclusion bodies in rats. *NeuroReport* 2002;13:1437–1441.

135. Fornai F, et al. Fine structure and biochemical mechanisms underlying nigrostriatal inclusions and cell death after proteasome inhibition. *J Neurosci* 2003;23;8955–8966.

136. McNaught KSP, Perl DP, Brownell AL, Olanow CW. Systemic exposure to proteasome inhibitors causes a progressive model of Parkinson's disease. *Ann Neurol* 2004;56:149–162.

137. Bulteau AL, et al. Oxidative modification and inactivation of the proteasome during coronary occlusion/reperfusion. *J Biol Chem* 1999;276:30,057–063.

138. Hendil KB, Hartmann-Petersen R, Tanaka K. 26S proteasomes function as stable entities. *J Mol Biol* 2002;315:627–636.

139. Jenner P, Olanow CW. Understanding cell death in Parkinson's disease. *Ann Neurol* 1998;44:S72–S84.

140. Kisselev AF, Goldberg AL. Proteasome inhibitors: from research tools to drug candidates. *Chem Biol* 2001;8:739–758.

141. Fenteany G, Schreiber SL. Lactacystin, proteasome function, and cell fate. *J Biol Chem* 1998;273:8545–8548.

142. Sin N, et al. Total synthesis of the potent proteasome inhibitor epoxomicin: a useful tool for understanding proteasome biology. *Bioorg Med Chem Lett* 1999;9:2283–2288.

143. Koguchi Y, et al. TMC-95A, B, C, and D, novel proteasome inhibitors produced by Apiospora montagnei Sacc. TC 1093: taxonomy, production, isolation, and biological activities. *J Antibiot (Tokyo)* 2000;53:105–109.

144. Nam S, Smith DM, Dou QP. Ester bond-containing tea polyphenols potently inhibit proteasome activity in vitro and in vivo. *J Biol Chem* 2001;276:13,322–330.

145. Kazi A, et al. A natural musaceas plant extract inhibits proteasome activity and induces apoptosis selectively in human tumor and transformed, but not normal and non-transformed, cells. *Int J Mol Med* 2003;12:879–887.

146. Jana NR, Dikshit P, Goswami A, Nukina N. Inhibition of proteasomal function by curcumin induces apoptosis through mitochondrial pathway. *J Biol Chem* 2004;279:11,680–685.

147. Zhou Y, Shie FS, Piccardo P, Montine TJ, Zhang J. Proteasomal inhibition induced by manganese ethylene-bis-dithiocarbamate: relevance to Parkinson's disease. *Neuroscience* 2004;128:281–291.

148. Ensign JC, Normand P, Burden JP, Yallop CA. Physiology of some actinomycete genera. *Res Microbiol* 1993;144:657–660.

149. Cross T. Aquatic actinomycetes: a critical survey of the occurrence, growth and role of actinomycetes in aquatic habitats. *J Appl Bacteriol* 1981;50:397–423.

150. Spillantini MG, Crowther RA, Jakes R, Hasegawa M, Goedert M. Alpha-synuclein in filamentous inclusions of Lewy bodies from Parkinson's disease and dementia with lewy bodies. *Proc Natl Acad Sci USA* 1998;95:6469–6473.

151. Van Duinen SG, Lammers GJ, Maat-Schieman ML, Roos RA. Numerous and widespread alpha-synuclein-negative Lewy bodies in an asymptomatic patient. *Acta Neuropathol (Berl)* 1999;97:533–539.

152. Taylor JP, et al. Aggresomes protect cells by enhancing the degradation of toxic polyglutamine-containing protein. *Hum Mol Genet* 2003;12:749–757.

153. Cummings CJ, et al. Mutation of the E6-AP ubiquitin ligase reduces nuclear inclusion frequency while accelerating polyglutamine-induced pathology in SCA1 mice. *Neuron* 1999;24:879–892.

154. Keller JN, Hanni KB, Markesbery WR. Possible involvement of proteasomeinhibition in aging: implications for oxidative stress. *Mech Ageing Dev* 2000;113:61–70.

155. Zeng BY, Medhurst AD, Jackson M, Rose S, Jenner P. Proteasomal activity in brain differs between species and brain regions and changes with age. *Mech Ageing Dev* 2005;126:760–766.

156. Floor E, Wetzel MG. Increased protein oxidation in human substantia nigra pars compacta in comparison with basal ganglia and prefrontal cortex measured with an improved dinitrophenylhydrazine assay. *J Neurochem* 1998;70:268–275.

157. El-Khodor BF, Kholodilov NG, Yarygina O, Burke RE. The expression of mRNAs for the proteasome complex is developmentally regulated in the rat mesencephalon. *Brain Res Dev Brain Res* 2001;129:47–56.

158. Conway KA, Rochet JC, Bieganski RM, Lansbury PT Jr. Kinetic stabilization of the alpha-synuclein protofibril by a dopamine-alpha-synuclein adduct. *Science* 2001;294:1346–1369.

159. Cappai R, et al. Dopamine promotes alpha-synuclein aggregation into SDS-resistant soluble oligomers via a distinct folding pathway. *Faseb J* 2005;19:1377–1379.

160. Gibb WR, Lees AJ. The relevance of the Lewy body to the pathogenesis of idiopathic Parkinson's disease. *J Neurol Neurosurg Psychiatry* 1988;51:745–752.

161. Braak H, et al. Staging of brain pathology related to sporadic Parkinson's disease. *Neurobiol Aging* 2003;24:197–211.

162. Atlante A, Bobba A, Calissano P, Passarella S, Marra E. The apoptosis/necrosis transition in cerebellar granule cells depends on the mutual relationship of the antioxidant and the proteolytic systems which regulate ROS production and cytochrome c release en route to death. *J Neurochem* 2003;84:960–971.

163. Jha N, Kumar MJ, Boonplueang R, Andersen JK. Glutathione decreases in dopaminergic PC12 cells interfere with the ubiquitin protein degradation pathway: relevance for Parkinson's disease? *J Neurochem* 2002;80:555–561.

164. Hoglinger GU, et al. Dysfunction of mitochondrial complex I and the proteasome: interactions between two biochemical deficits in a cellular model of Parkinson's disease. *J Neurochem* 2003;86:1297–1307.

165. Lee HJ, Shin SY, Choi C, Lee YH, Lee SJ. Formation and removal of alpha-synuclein aggregates in cells exposed to mitochondrial inhibitors. *J Biol Chem* 2001;27:27.

166. Li Z, Jansen M, Pierre SR, Figueiredo-Pereira ME. Neurodegeneration: linking ubiquitin/proteasome pathway impairment with inflammation. *Int J Biochem Cell Biol* 2003;35:547–552.

167. Jesenberger V, Jentsch S. Deadly encounter: ubiquitin meets apoptosis. *Nat Rev Mol Cell Biol* 2003;3:112–121.

168. Kikuchi S, et al. Effect of proteasome inhibitor on cultured mesencephalic dopaminergic neurons. *Brain Res* 2003;964:228–236.

169. Rockwell P, Yuan H, Magnusson R, Figueiredo-Pereira ME. Proteasome inhibition in neuronal cells induces a proinflammatory response manifested by upregulation of cyclooxygenase-2, its accumulation as ubiquitin conjugates, and production of the prostaglandin PGE(2). *Arch Biochem Biophys* 2000;374:325–333.

170. Sitte N, Merker K, von Zglinicki T, Grune T. Protein oxidation and degradation during proliferative senescence of human MRC-5 fibroblasts. *Free Radic Biol Med* 2000;28:701–708.

171. Okada K, et al. 4-hydroxy-2-nonenal-mediated impairment of intracellular proteolysis during oxidative stress: identification of proteasomes as target molecules. *J Biol Chem* 1999;274:23,787–793.

172. Reinheckel T, et al. Comparative resistance of the 20S and 26S proteasome to oxidative stress. *Biochem J* 1998;335:637–642.

173. Goldberg AL, Cascio P, Saric T, Rock KL. The importance of the proteasome and subsequent proteolytic steps in the generation of antigenic peptides. *Mol Immunol* 2002;39:147–164.

174. Lam YA, Lawson TG, Velayutham M, Zweier JL, Pickart CM. A proteasomal ATPase subunit recognizes the polyubiquitin degradation signal. *Nature* 2002;416:763–767.

175. Forno LS. Neuropathology of Parkinson's disease. *J Neuropathol Exp Neurol* 1996;55:259–272.

176. Shamoto-Nagai M, Maruyama W, Kato Y, et al. An inhibitor of mitochondrial complex I, rotenone, inactivates proteasome by oxidative modification and induces aggregation of oxidized proteins in SH-SY5Y cells. *J Neurosci Res* 2003;74:589–597.

177. Sullivan PG, Dragicevic NB, Deng JH, et al. Proteasome inhibition alters neural mitochondrial homeostasis and mitochondria turnover. *J Biol Chem* 2004;279:20,699–707.

178. Schapira AHV, Cooper JM, Dexter D, et al. Mitochondrial complex I deficiency in Parkinson's disease. *J Neurochem* 1990;54:823–827.

179. Hunot S, Hirsch EC. Neuroinflammatory processes in Parkinson's disease. *Ann Neurol* 2003;53 Suppl 3:S49–S58; discussion S58–S60.

180. Hirsch EC, Hunot S, Faucheux B, Agid Y, Mizuno Y, Mochizuki H, Tatton WG, Tatton N, Olanow CW. Dopaminergic neurons

degenerate by apoptosis in Parkinson's disease. *Mov Disord* 1999;14:383–385.

181. Hegde AN, DiAntonio A. Ubiquitin and the synapse. *Nat Rev Neurosci* 2002;3:854–861.

182. Bezard E, Gross CE, Brotchie JM. Presymptomatic compensation in Parkinson's disease is not dopamine-mediated. *Trends Neurosci* 2003;26:215–221.

183. Obeso JA, Rodriguez-Oroz MC, Lanciego JL, Rodriguez Diaz M. How does Parkinson's disease begin? The role of compensatory mechanisms. *Trends Neurosci* 2004;27:125–127; author reply 127–128.

184. Wilkinson KD. Ubiquitin-dependent signaling: the role of ubiquitination in the response of cells to their environment. *J Nutr* 1999;129(11):1933–1936.

185. Albin R, Young A, Penney J. The functional anatomy of basal ganglia disorders. *J Neurosci.* 1989;12:336–374.

186. DeLong MR. Primate models of movement disorders of basal ganglia origin. *TINS* 1990;13:281–285.

187. Aguilar RC, Wendland B. Ubiquitin: not just for proteasomes anymore. *Curr Opin Cell Biol* 2003;15:184–190.

188. Muratani M, Tansey WP. How the ubiquitin-proteasome system controls transcription. *Nat Rev Mol Cell Biol* 2003;4:192–201.

189. Grunblatt E, Mandel S, Jacob-Hirsch J, et al. Gene expression profiling of parkinsonian substantia nigra pars compacta; alterations in ubiquitin-proteasome, heat shock protein, iron and oxidative stress regulated proteins, cell adhesion/cellular matrix and vesicle trafficking genes. *J Neural Transm* 2004;111: 1543–1573.

Epidemiology of Movement Disorders

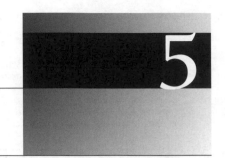

5

Anette Schrag

Epidemiology serves several purposes: It describes the occurrence of disorders, time trends, and geographic differences in their frequency; identifies risk factors that may give clues to the etiology of disorders; provides information for the planning of health care resources; and gives estimates for the prognosis of a disorder. However, epidemiologic studies are usually time-consuming and expensive, so restrictions in resources often limit the methodological rigor that is crucial to the validity of such studies. Differences in the study design, especially case ascertainment methods and inclusion criteria, are important influences on the results of these studies. Epidemiologic studies of movement disorders are particularly complicated by the lack of diagnostic markers that allow an unequivocal diagnosis and by the differences in diagnostic criteria for most movement disorders. As a consequence, variations in diagnostic accuracy are reflected in prevalence rates (number of persons affected at a particular time in a defined population) and incidence rates (number of new cases developing over a defined period of time in a defined population at risk). Furthermore, many epidemiologic studies require large numbers, which will not be easily achieved for some of the rarer disorders. Conclusions from epidemiologic studies should therefore consider the methodology used, particularly in comparisons across studies.

A number of studies have been performed on Parkinson's disease (PD), and great advances in genetic and epidemiologic studies in this disorder have been made in recent years. Few epidemiologic data exist for some of the rarer movement disorders, such as paroxysmal movement disorders. However, there also is increasing knowledge about the epidemiology of other akinetic movement disorders, tremor, dystonia, and other hyperkinetic movement disorders, which are reviewed in this chapter.

PARKINSONISM

Parkinson's Disease

Prevalance

When comparing the results of prevalence studies of PD across geographically and temporally different populations, a number of caveats require consideration to avoid erroneous conclusions. In particular, the method of ascertainment has dramatic influence on the results obtained, as do the choice of diagnostic criteria, the amount of information lost because of nonresponse, the age distribution of the population studied, and survival time. Door-to-door studies, the most time- and cost-intensive of prevalence studies, generally yield higher prevalence rates than studies based on review of medical records and previously made diagnosis, with the percentage of previously undiagnosed cases ranging from 10% to 50%, depending on the health care system in each country (1).

Although the prevalence rates of PD vary between 18 and 418 per 100,000 worldwide (2), the variations are much less marked when the differences between study methodology are considered. Age-adjustment and restriction to studies using similar methodology reduce the variation between prevalence rates to between 102 and 190 per 100,000 population, at least in Western countries. Using unified diagnostic criteria, relative similarity of ascertainment methods, and age adjustment of results, the Euro-parkinson study (1) reported the prevalence rates from 5 European countries within a similar range. However, clusters with a high prevalence of PD have been reported, e.g., in Iceland (2) or on the Faeroe Islands, where prevalence of PD was considerably higher than on the Danish mainland or a neighboring island when the same ascertainment methods were used (3). Similarly, in India and Sicily high prevalence rates of PD have been reported, even when adjustment for differences in age distribution were made (4,5). Conversely, low prevalence rates were reported in other populations, such as in Romanian Gypsies (6) and in northern Africa (7). Although such differences may in large part reflect the sometimes marked differences in methodology, they may also indicate actual differences in the occurrence of PD, which may be due to differences in genetic background or, alternatively, in environmental exposures. This question has been further addressed by a small number of studies comparing prevalence of PD in bi- or multiethnic populations, but the results are conflicting. In a study in New York City over a 4-year period (1988–1991), the age-adjusted prevalence rates were lower for blacks than for whites and Hispanics, although cumulative incidence was higher for blacks, and more deaths occurred among incident black cases, suggesting that in black patients survival with PD is shorter (8). In a door-to-door survey in Cuba, prevalence rates of PD were higher in white than nonwhite subjects (9). Schoenberg et al. conducted two comparative studies with similar case ascertainment methods and identical diagnostic criteria (10). In the biracial population of Copiah County, Mississippi, the prevalence rates of PD in the white and the black population were similar. In Nigeria, on the other hand, the age-adjusted prevalence of PD was 5 times lower (11), suggesting that geographic differences not due to ethnic differences may influence the risk of PD. Along the same lines are the results of prevalence studies in China and Taiwan, populations that share a genetic background but have different levels of industrialization, which have yielded markedly different prevalence rates (14.6 versus 119 per 100,000) (12–14). In addition, the prevalence of PD has been shown to be similar in different ethnic populations (Chinese, Malay, and Indian) in the multiethnic population of Singapore (15). The results of these latter studies taken together suggest that environmental factors play an important role in the occurrence of PD in populations of similar genetic background.

Incidence

A better indicator for the frequency of a chronic disorder in the population than prevalence is the incidence rate, as it is independent of survival, which may vary in temporally or geographically separated populations. However, such studies require larger study populations and/or longer observation times and are therefore much rarer. Reported annual incidence rates of PD range from 4.9 to 26 per 100,000 (16–21). The longitudinal epidemiologic study in Rochester, Minnesota, using review of detailed medical records, reported an annual incidence rate of parkinsonism of 114.7 per 100,000 in the age group 50–99, increasing from 0.8 in the age group 0 to 29 years to 304.8 in the age group 80 to 99 years (19). In an Italian study, the reported annual incidence of PD was 326.3 per 100,000 in those aged 64 to

84 (22). However, the same caveats regarding comparability as for prevalence rates apply.

Association of Sex and Age with Prevalence and Incidence Rates

PD is rare before age 50 years and increases with age to affect approximately 2% in those aged 65 and above (23). Although many record-based studies reported lower prevalence rates in the eldest age group (24), door-to-door studies have not confirmed this drop in prevalence rate in those over 80 (23,25). It appears likely that PD is less frequently diagnosed in older patients, in part due to the difficulties in differentiating features of PD from those of aging, such as postural instability and a small-stepped gait (26,27). Similar ascertainment bias may be responsible in part for the slight male predominance of PD, reported by many record- and clinic-based studies, as few door-to-door studies could confirm this. However, one prospective cohort study in an Italian population aged 65 to 84 also found a 2.13-fold increased risk of PD in men compared with women using screening and personal examination (22). As suggested by Tanner and Aston, a male preponderance, if confirmed in future population-based studies, could suggest an increased X-linked genetic disposition or influence of sex hormones on disease risk or, alternatively, greater exposure to a causative environmental factor in men (28).

Time Trends

Although it has been suggested that PD was rare before the 19th century, recent prevalence data indicate no marked change overall in occurrence over time. However, analysis of mortality and prevalence data suggests that age-specific mortality increased in older and decreased in younger age groups (29). Two recent incidence studies have directly investigated the pattern of PD incidence over time. In Rochester, Minnesota, no significant change in incidence rates from 1976 to 1990 was identified in a well-documented medical record system (30). In contrast, in a Finnish study, Kuopio et al. found an increase in prevalence of PD from 1971 to 1992 from 139 to 166 and in annual incidence of PD from 14.9 to 15.7 per 100,000, which was associated with male predominance and rural living (20). The authors suggested that an increased susceptibility in men and/or a greater exposure to an environmental risk factor in men may account for this increase in the incidence of PD.

Analytic Epidemiology
Genetic Factors

Family history has consistently been reported to be associated with an increased risk of PD compared with controls, particularly in patients with young age of onset, suggesting that genetic factors play a role in the etiology of PD (31–34). The recent discovery of several genes causing parkinsonism, including typical PD, confirms the importance of genetic factors in the etiology of parkinsonism. However, it is uncertain whether this reflects an increased genetic susceptibility in the overall population of patients with PD or pure genetic inheritance in a smaller proportion of cases, with shared familial exposure or biased recall in families of patients with PD accounting for the rest of the increased rate of family history in PD. Twin studies are of particular value to address this question. If genetic factors play an important role in the etiology of a disorder, the concordance rates in monozygotic twins are higher than in dizygotic twins. Most twin studies have not confirmed an overall increased risk of PD in monozygotic twins compared with dizygotic twins (35–37). Tanner et al. conducted the largest of such twin studies in a cohort of World War II veterans in the United States (38). They found no overall difference in concordance rates in monozygotic twins compared with dizygotic twins, arguing for a lack of genetic causation of PD. However, in twins with age of onset below 50 years, the concordance rate in monozygotic twins was significantly increased with 1.0 compared with 0.167 in dizygotic twins. The relative risk was 6.0 (95% confidence interval, 1.69–21.26). These results suggested that genetic factors contribute significantly to the development of PD in those with young onset but do not play a major role in causing typical PD. Positron emission tomography (PET) studies in twins have also been used to assess the genetic contribution to PD. In a PET study in 9 monozygotic twins and 12 dizygotic twins, Vieregge et al. found that the concordance rates in both groups were similar when assessed 8 years apart, arguing against a genetic contribution to PD (39). In contrast, Piccini et al. found that the concordance for subclinical striatal dopaminergic dysfunction was significantly higher in 18 monozygotic than in 16 dizygotic twin pairs. In addition, the asymptomatic monozygotic cotwins all showed progressive loss of dopaminergic function over 7 years and 4 developed clinical PD, whereas none of the dizygotic twin pairs became clinically concordant, arguing for an underlying susceptibility in monozygotic twins of patients with PD (40).

One of the greatest discoveries in the last years in PD research has been the recognition that there are families in whom PD is genetically determined. The first of such mutations was reported in the α-synuclein gene, inherited in an autosomal dominant pattern, which however accounts only for only a small number of cases (41). The autosomal recessively inherited *parkin* gene, on the other hand, appears to account for a substantial minority of cases of sporadic PD, typically of young onset (42). Although the typical phenotype of *parkin*-related parkinsonism differs somewhat from typical PD, the phenotype related to *parkin* mutations is wide and includes typical cases of PD (43). A number of other genes, mainly inherited in an autosomal-recessive fashion, have been reported, particularly in those with young onset parkinsonism. Recently, an autosomal dominant gene, PARK 8 or LRRK2, has been found to account for about 5%–6% of familial and 1%–2% of sporadic cases of PD with a classical late-onset clinical phenotype (44). In addition, known genetic defects have been shown to be linked to a parkinsonian syndrome, including spinocerebellar ataxia

genes and premutations in the fragile-X mental retardation gene (*FMR1;* 45).

These results clearly suggest that genetic factors are important in the etiology of PD, but whether this is a major contribution restricted to a small number of cases or a smaller contribution relevant to the majority of cases at present remains unclear. (For a detailed discussion of the genetics of PD see Chapter 7.)

Environmental Factors

The discovery that 1-methyl-4-phenyl-1,2,3,6-tetrahydropyridine (MPTP), a street drug contaminant, can cause human parkinsonism similar to that in PD lent strong momentum to the hypothesis that PD may be caused by a single environmental toxin. In addition, infectious disease as a cause of PD has been implicated by the endemic encephalitis lethargica leading to postencephalitic parkinsonism. However, the lack of convincing marked geographic or temporal differences in prevalence and incidence rates does not strongly support an environmental exposure as the major cause of PD. Case-control studies in patients with PD, which have attempted to identify potential risk factors for the development of PD, have despite their abundance also not identified strong evidence for a single environmental cause. The most consistent finding in these studies has been the negative association of smoking with the development of PD (46,47), but the exact nature of this relationship is unclear. Possible reasons for this association range from selective survival of nonsmokers (which is unlikely as this negative association is also seen in early-onset cases) to protective effects of smoking to the existence of a common predisposing factor, including personality (24). Other life exposures that have less consistently been found to be associated with PD are working on a farm or having a job that involves head trauma (32), exposure to pesticides (31,48), well-water drinking, and rural living (49). Frequency of bowel movements, coffee drinking, alcohol consumption, head trauma, and hypertension (50–54) have also been reported to be inversely related to PD, independent of smoking history (55). Furthermore, it has been reported that individuals working as teachers or those occupied in health care in Greater Vancouver had a 2- to 2.5-fold risk of PD compared with controls (56). The likelihood that a single environmental factor causes PD is therefore small, and it has been proposed that several environmental causes contribute to the development of PD (57), or that genetic and environmental factors act synergistically to cause PD (32,58). Possible interactions between genes and environment, and of several candidate genes, to produce PD are being investigated. Overall, there are probably several types or causes of PD, with varying contributions from genetic and environmental factors.

Prognosis

Controversy exists with respect to the prognosis of PD. It appears clear that even patients with typical PD may present with considerable variation in phenotype and rate of progression. Some studies have described that presence of gait disturbance is associated with faster disease progression and an increased risk of death (27,59), and other studies have reported that those with older age at onset have a faster rate of progression and a higher incidence of dementia (59–62) but a lower rate of motor complications (62,63). However, with the exception of parkinsonism associated with the mutations described, no pathologic, genetic, or environmental factor has been identified to explain the variation in rate of progression and complications.

Life expectancy is decreased in patients with PD compared with the general population, but reported mortality ratios vary considerably between 1.2 and 3.1 compared with age-matched controls or the general population (5,27,60,64–67). Whether mortality has decreased as a result of dopaminergic treatment remains a matter of controversy. Although few data are available from the pre-levodopa era, mortality data appear to have remained the same, indicating that treatment has not resulted in an improved mortality despite the improvements in quality of life (68). In contrast to control populations, the most common cause of death is pneumonia (5,69).

ATYPICAL PARKINSONISM

Pathologic studies have suggested that up to 35% of patients with a clinical diagnosis of PD coming to autopsy suffered from a different disorder, most commonly progressive supranuclear palsy (PSP), Alzheimer's disease (AD), multiple system atrophy (MSA), and vascular disease (70–72). Until recently, few studies existed on the prevalence and incidence rate of the atypical forms of parkinsonism, including PSP, MSA, and corticobasal degeneration, and these disorders, if differentiated from PD, were often excluded from epidemiologic studies. However, it has become increasingly clear that these disorders are more common than previously thought (73–78).

Progressive Supranuclear Palsy

The first prevalence study of PSP, conducted in New Jersey (79), yielded a prevalence rate of 1.4 per 100,000, approximately 1% of the prevalence of PD. However, the authors emphasized that this was likely to be an underestimate as only diagnosed cases were ascertained and the rate of unrecognized cases was assumed to be high. Since this early study, two population-based studies using standardized diagnostic criteria have reported higher prevalence rates compared with what was previously believed, with 5 to 6 cases of PSP per 100,000, a large proportion of which were undiagnosed prior to the studies (73,74). The incidence of PSP has been reported from 0.3 to 1.1 per 100,000 (80). The most recent study from Olmsted County, Minnesota, which retrospectively analyzed a detailed medical record system and used standardized

diagnostic criteria, reported an incidence rate of 5.3 cases per 100,000 in the ages 50 to 99 (81), which corresponds to the reported prevalence rates in this age group (7). Although few data from different geographic regions are available, PSP has been described in ethnically different populations (82–84), and in the French West Indies atypical parkinsonism and PSP have been reported to be over-represented compared with European and North American populations (85). It has been hypothesized that this high prevalence is due to alimentary causes, such as the consumption of neurotoxic alkaloids contained in herbal teas and tropical fruit (85). It has also been speculated that atypical parkinsonism is more common in individuals of Afro-Caribbean and Indian origin in the PD population in London, England (86), but no epidemiologic data on differential frequency of atypical parkinsonism in these populations are available. Most clinic- and population-based studies reported a slight male preponderance in PSP (81,87,88), but confidence intervals in epidemiologic studies are wide, due to relatively small numbers. The incidence of PSP increases with advancing age (89), with a mean age at onset in the seventh decade. No case of PSP with onset before age 40 has been reported (88,90). Reported mean survival time ranges from 5.3 to 9.7 years (79,81,88,91) with pathologically confirmed survival time up to 18 years (92). Survival appears shorter in those who have early falls, dysphagia, dysarthria, diplopia, and incontinence, and in those who fulfill criteria for probable PSP (93,94). Although the majority of cases with PSP are sporadic, several families with at least two members with PSP have been reported (89). Genetic studies have shown that PSP is associated with inheritance of a specific genotype (H1/H1) in the tau gene. Litvan et al. investigated whether the genotype independently or in conjunction with selected environmental risk factors influences the age at onset, severity, or survival in patients with PSP but found that tau genotyping did not appear to predict the prognosis of PSP (95). Similarly, two other studies did not find any effect of tau genotype on the age of onset of PSP (96,97). Despite the discovery that tau dysfunction is somehow involved in the pathogenesis of PSP, it is also possible that nongenetic factors contribute to neuronal degeneration in PSP. Two case-control studies have been conducted to date that show conflicting results with regard to education and residence in rural areas. Davis et al. (98) conducted a case-control study of 50 cases in New Jersey. The results suggested that rural residence and greater educational attainment but not history of smoking, occupation, exposure to toxins, or hypertension may be significant risk factors for PSP. On the other hand, in a subsequent study of 91 patients, the same authors reported that patients with PSP were found to be less likely to have completed at least 12 years of school. The authors hypothesized that lower level of education may be a proxy for poor early-life nutrition or for occupational or residential exposure to an unknown toxin (99). However, these studies have been criticized for lack of power to detect associations with occupations and exposure to toxins (100). A history of hypertension, which had been postulated to be increased in patients with PSP, has not been found more commonly in autopsy-confirmed cases of PSP, and the previously reported association of PSP and hypertension may have been due to similar presentations of vascular parkinsonism and PSP (101). In addition, no inverse relationship between smoking and PSP has been found, in contrast to PD and MSA, suggesting that smoking habits are associated with different groups of neurodegenerative disorders (102).

Multiple System Atrophy

Multiple system atrophy accounts for 8% to 22% of patients diagnosed with PD coming to pathologic examination (71,72). Although pathologic studies are likely to be biased toward more frequent atypical cases (26), this indicates that MSA is less rare than previously thought. Two epidemiologic studies have found that it affects 4 to 5 people in a population of 100,000 people (73,76), although a recent larger study reported a prevalence of only 2 per 100,000 (78). However, these data are likely to be conservative, as patients not initially presenting with parkinsonism but autonomic failure or ataxia may not have been included in these studies. An incidence study in Olmsted County, Minnesota, using specific criteria, found 9 cases in the years 1976 to 1990 (81), yielding an annual incidence rate of 3.0 per 100,000 for the ages 50 to 99. Given a median survival of 5 to 9 years (103–107), this is comparable to the prevalence rates found in Europe. Symptoms of MSA most commonly begin in the sixth decade with an average age at onset of 54 (104,105,107), but the age of onset ranges between the fourth and eighth decade (104). MSA has been more commonly reported in men, but few population-based data are available to confirm this. A case-control study including 60 MSA patients and 60 controls (108) reported a greater exposure to metal dusts and fumes, plastic monomers and additives, organic solvents, and pesticides in the MSA compared with controls, although this was not confirmed in a more recent study (78). In addition, in the first study symptoms of MSA in relatives were reported by a significantly larger group of patients' relatives than controls (23% vs. 10%). The authors hypothesized that MSA develops as a result of a genetically determined selective vulnerability in the nervous system. However, in contrast to PSP, no case of autopsy-confirmed familial MSA and only one family of clinically probable MSA (109) has been reported, and evidence for an association of genetic factors and MSA is scarce (96,110). More recent case-control studies reported an inverse relationship of MSA and smoking habits, similar to that in PD (102) and an association of farming exposure and MSA, independent of the inverse risk associated with smoking (78).

Distribution of Parkinsonism

The population prevalence of parkinsonism due to vascular disease or use of dopamine receptor–blocking drugs are not well known as these are often excluded from prevalence and incidence studies. They also strongly depend on the frequency of such drug use and the age distribution of the population studied. In the incidence study from Olmsted County, Minnesota, Bower et al. reported that only 42% of all cases of parkinsonism in the years 1976 to 1991 had PD (19). The main differential diagnosis included drug-induced parkinsonism (20%), unspecified parkinsonism (17%), parkinsonism in dementia (14%), and parkinsonism due to other causes (7%). Four percent had PSP, 2% had MSA, and less than 1% (only 1 patient) had a diagnosis of vascular parkinsonism. This is in contrast to the study by Rajput et al. who, using the same hospital record system during the preceding decade, reported that of patients with parkinsonism 86% had PD, 7% had drug-induced parkinsonism, and 1% to 2% had PSP, MSA, and vascular parkinsonism, respectively (17). However, more recent studies from other geographic areas have reported patterns of distribution between the results of the two studies from Olmsted County. A population-based study in elderly people in Spain reported PD in 44%, drug-induced parkinsonism in 32%, parkinsonism with associated features in 1%, unspecified parkinsonism in 7%, and vascular parkinsonism in 4% (18). Baldereschi et al. (22) found that of incident cases of parkinsonism in an elderly population 62% had PD, 10% had drug-induced parkinsonism, 12% had parkinsonism in dementia, 12% had vascular parkinsonism, and 6% had unspecified parkinsonism. Morgante et al. in Sicily reported that 69% had PD, 9% had drug-induced parkinsonism, and 8% had vascular parkinsonism (5), and Schrag et al. (111) found that 66% of all patients with parkinsonism had PD, 18% drug-induced parkinsonism, 7% vascular parkinsonism, 6% atypical parkinsonism, and 2% parkinsonism in dementia (but dementia clearly starting before onset was an exclusion criterion). Postencephalitic parkinsonism, once representing a large proportion of patients with parkinsonism following the worldwide epidemic of encephalitis lethargica between 1916 and 1927, is now rare, as no new epidemics have occurred. However, occasional cases of postencephalitic parkinsonism continue to occur.

HYPERKINETIC MOVEMENT DISORDERS

Essential Tremor

Essential tremor (ET) is probably the most common movement disorder. However, prevalence rates vary widely as epidemiologic studies of ET are hampered by the lack of a biologic marker or a clearly delineated clinical phenotype. It is likely that ET is clinically, pathophysiologically, and genetically a heterogeneous condition (112,113), and phenotypic overlap with other conditions exists. The most difficult differential diagnoses are (a) enhanced physiologic tremor, (b) tremor occurring in association with other conditions, such as dystonia, PD, and peripheral neuropathy, and (c) isolated tremor syndromes, such as voice tremor, which may be either a form fruste of ET or a different condition. A particularly controversial area is the differentiation of ET from tremor in dystonia. Dubinsky et al. found that, although typical ET was found in only 8 of 296 patients in a record review of patients with focal or generalized dystonia (114), a type of tremor was found in 46 (15.5%). Singer et al. reported in a prevalence study of dystonia that tremor occurred in approximately 40% of patients with adult-onset idiopathic focal and segmental dystonia. Eighteen percent had dystonic tremor (tremor in a body part affected by dystonia), and 21% had tremor associated with dystonia (tremor in a different body part) (115). Conversely, in a large study of 678 patients diagnosed with ET, 6.9% also had a coexisting dystonia (116), whereas in another study of 350 patients with ET from a movement disorders clinic, half of all patients (47%) had associated dystonia (117). Electrophysiologic studies reveal differences in some tests between patients with isolated tremor and those with tremor and dystonia (112,118,119). However, a reliable clinical differentiation of individual patients is currently not possible. Some epidemiologic studies therefore excluded patients with dystonia from their analysis, whereas others included them. Another difficulty is the controversy about an association of ET with PD. Some authors contend that ET may predispose to the development of PD (120), whereas others (121) have not been able to confirm an increased association between ET and PD. Various types of neuropathy can be associated with tremor, but the mechanism of this association is poorly understood (122). Finally, an association of tremor with migraine has been demonstrated in familial and sporadic ET (123). Epidemiologic studies of ET are also complicated by the fact that the majority of individuals with tremor have mild symptoms, which may not lead to consultation with a physician or even remain unnoticed by affected subjects and their families. In addition, in many cases there is no positive family history of tremor, even when all family members are examined. Whether these sporadic cases have the same condition or are different from familial ET is unclear, and studies have varied with respect to inclusion of patients without a positive family history of tremor. These difficulties in diagnosis are reflected in the differences between diagnostic criteria that have been employed in epidemiologic studies and the great variability of the results of these studies. Louis et al. demonstrated that the use of different diagnostic criteria results in widely varying prevalence rates (124). Standardization of diagnostic criteria, such as the criteria of the Tremor Research Investigation Group (TRIG), will increase the consistency of findings, but validity will only become evident when a biologic marker becomes

available. Taking into account the limitations of comparability of studies using different ascertainment and diagnostic methods, the prevalence rates ranged from 0.01% to 22% (125). In an analysis of only those studies that provided diagnostic criteria for ET, defined ET as an action tremor, and used community-based rather than service-based designs, Louis et al. (125) reported a narrower range of prevalence rates from 0.4% to 3.9% in the overall population and from 1.3% to 5% in those over the age of 60 years. However, in a recent door-to-door study in Turkey using standardized criteria as opposed to screening instruments, the prevalence of ET was estimated to be 4% with narrow confidence intervals, suggesting that ET may be more common (126). Incidence data are far sparser than prevalence rates, ranging from 8 per 100,000 per year (16) to 23.7 per 100,000 in a longitudinal study in Rochester, Minnesota (127). This study also showed an increase in annual age- and sex-adjusted incidence rate from 5.8 in 1935–1949 to 23.7 in 1964–1979, most likely resulting from underdiagnosis of ET in earlier years. Despite the differences in diagnosis and case ascertainment, which make it difficult to compare incidence and prevalence rates, it is clear that the prevalence of ET increases with age. In one study, the age at onset showed bimodal distribution with peaks in the second and sixth decades (117). In a Finnish study (128), the peak prevalence of ET was 12.6% in the age group 70–79 years, and in a study in Mississippi, there was a tenfold higher prevalence in those aged 70–79 compared with those aged 40–69 (129). In an incidence study from Rochester, Minnesota, incidence rates continuously increased up to the oldest age group with a sharp increase after age 49 (127). However, in a study by Bain et al., which restricted the analysis to family members of index cases with familial ET, all affected family members were symptomatic by the age of 50 with a bimodal age of tremor onset and a median onset age of 15 years (130). Tremor severity and disability, on the other hand, increased with advancing age and tremor duration, possibly in part accounting for the finding of increasing prevalence in cross-sectional studies. Life expectancy of patients with ET is similar to that of the general population, although ET has also been claimed to increase longevity (120,131). Apart from a few studies that found a higher prevalence in women (129) or men (132), ET is largely found to be equally common in women and men, and women appear more likely to develop head tremor (133). Although a slightly higher prevalence of ET in white than black Americans has been reported, this may be related to greater diagnosis than higher prevalence rates (129,132,134).

ET is generally thought to be an autosomal dominantly inherited condition with high but age-dependent penetrance (130). However, the reported percentage of patients with ET with a family history ranges from 17.4% to 100%. This wide range may partly be artifactual and the result of different inclusion criteria, as well as underreporting of a family history, but may also reflect the heterogeneity of this condition. The phenotype of pure autosomal dominantly inherited essential tremor has been well described (130), but it is possible that other phenotypes also exist. Further description of the clinical phenotype will also provide better understanding about the heterogeneity of the condition. Linkage of familial cases of ET with the *DYT 1* gene for childhood-onset generalized dystonia has been excluded (135), but in isolated families linkage of ET to different chromosomes was established. In Iceland a locus on chromosome 3q13 was linked to 16 kindreds with ET fulfilling the TRIG criteria, named *FET1* (136), and linkage has also been reported to a locus on chromosome 2p22-25 (137,138) named *ETM* or *ET2*. Twin studies have confirmed a high concordance rate for ET in monozygotic twins (139). Some studies have reported anticipation in successive generations of families with ET (137), but others could not confirm these findings (130,140), which may have resulted from heightened awareness in the families of such patients. To my knowledge, only one case-control study to assess the influence of nongenetic factors on the occurrence of ET has been reported. Exposures to agricultural chemicals and to domestic animals were suggested as potential risk factors for the occurrence of ET, but this association was not statistically significant in this small study (28 controls and age-matched controls) (141).

Dystonia

Data on the prevalence of dystonia are likely to underestimate the true prevalence of the disorder, as dystonia is commonly underdiagnosed or underreported. In addition to the problems of all epidemiologic studies of movement disorders (lack of a pathologic substrate, reliance on a clinical diagnosis, and a high rate of underdiagnosis), there are also difficulties in the classification (e.g., primary vs. secondary dystonia, generalized vs. focal dystonia) that limit comparability of studies (142). However, since the early descriptions of primary torsion dystonia (PTD) (143), it has been recognized that dystonia is relatively common in Jewish populations, particularly in Jews of Eastern European ancestry (Ashkenazi) (144–147). The initial prevalence rate reported for PTD in Ashkenazi Jews in Israel was 10.8 per million (146), but this was recognized later to be an underestimate due to incomplete case ascertainment in this early survey, and subsequent reassessment of the population resulted in a higher prevalence rate of 43 per million for generalized dystonia (147). Dystonia has also been reported in many other ethnic groups, albeit with varying frequency (12,148–151). In a recent review of all prevalence studies of primary dystonia using record review, Defazio et al. (152) estimated that prevalence studies using the most valid criteria yielded rates of 24–50 per million for primary early-onset dystonia and 101–430 per million for late-onset dystonia. However, even after the exclusion of studies that were flawed, prevalence rates

are likely to be higher due to underdiagnosis in the general population (153). Therefore, population-based studies are of particular relevance, although few have been conducted (12,154). The prevalence rates reported from China (12) and Egypt (154) were comparatively low, with 5 cases of generalized and 3 cases of cervical dystonia per 100,000 in China, and 10 cases of focal dystonia per 100,000 in Egypt. In both studies the only focal dystonia seen was cervical dystonia, and in Egypt no cases with generalized dystonia were found. It has therefore been suggested (155) that case ascertainment was incomplete. A different approach was taken by Risch et al., who calculated the prevalence of early limb-onset generalized dystonia in Ashkenazim in New York from the number of affected individuals on the database from the Dystonia Medical Research Center at the Columbia Presbyterian Medical Center using the number of Ashkenazi Jews from the *American Jewish Yearbook* as the reference population. This resulted in a crude prevalence rate of 50 per million. Assuming a rate of undiagnosed cases of approximately 50% and accounting for those younger than the median age of onset, the prevalence of early limb-onset generalized dystonia was estimated to be as high as 111 per million (156). Although it is likely that the prevalence rate of early limb-onset generalized dystonia in the Ashkenazi population is higher than previously reported, these data need to be interpreted with caution as they are derived indirectly and are based on a number of assumptions.

Among the different types of focal dystonia, the most common type in most studies was cervical dystonia followed by blepharospasm (32%), whereas writer's cramp and spasmodic dysphonia are relatively uncommon. Age-adjusted annual incidence rates in the early epidemiologic study in the Israel population were 0.43 per million in the total Jewish population, 0.98 in European Jews, and 0.11 in Afro-Asians Jews (146). In Rochester, Minnesota, in the years 1950 to 1982, the annual incidence rate of all focal dystonias was reported as 2.4 per 100,000 and of generalized dystonia as 0.2 per 100,000 (142). An incidence study in Britain, relying on referral of all neurologic cases by a number of primary care physicians, obtained an incidence rate of 1 per 100,000 for focal dystonia, but it is likely that underdiagnosis affected the results of this study (16).

With the exception of writer's cramp, focal and segmental dystonia has mostly been reported to be more common in women than men (155,157–159).

A gene for generalized PTD with childhood onset, which contains a three-nucleotide (GAG) deletion and codes for the previously unknown protein torsin A, has been identified on chromosome 9q34 *(DYT1)* (160). It is responsible for most cases of early limb-onset PTD in both Jewish and non-Jewish kindreds (161,162). Transmission mostly follows an autosomal dominant pattern of inheritance with low penetrance. Although there is considerable phenotypic heterogeneity within and between kindreds, the typical clinical features of *DYT1*-associated dystonia are limb onset and spread to the trunk but rare involvement of craniofacial muscles. In contrast, late-onset PTD tends to begin in craniocervical muscles or an arm and rarely becomes generalized. In a minority of cases, late-onset dystonia is associated with a positive family history (163), but it is not usually associated with the *DYT1* gene (164). However, other loci causing PTD have been mapped and other loci are likely to be identified in adult-onset focal dystonias. These findings provide evidence for the genetic heterogeneity of dystonia (for review, see 165). The report of a family, including a pair of monozygotic twins, with variable phenotype (166) also provides evidence for *phenotypic* heterogeneity in adult-onset focal dystonia. It is therefore likely that environmental factors have a role in the expression of genetic predisposition to develop adult-onset PTD. Patients often report trauma or significant viral infection preceding the onset of symptoms (145,158), but epidemiologic evidence regarding the role of such factors is controversial. In a case-control study, Fletcher et al. (167) found that a family history of tremor or stuttering was significantly more common among patients with PTD than control subjects, whereas trauma was not more common in patients with PTD. The authors suggested that if trauma was important in the development of dystonia, it is likely that this is in combination with a preexisting susceptibility. Defazio et al. performed a large case-control study on risk factors for the development of primary adult-onset dystonia in Italy (168). In 202 patients with adult-onset dystonia and 202 age- and sex-matched controls, head or face trauma with loss of consciousness and family history of tremor or dystonia were associated with an increased risk of adult-onset dystonia, whereas hypertension and cigarette smoking exerted a protective effect. There was also a positive association between local injury to a body part and dystonia of that body part. The same group also reported that previous head or face trauma with loss of consciousness, age of onset, and female gender increased the risk of spread in patients with blepharospasm (169).

Age of onset is generally older in patients with blepharospasm and oromandibular dystonia than in patients with other focal dystonias, and younger for generalized dystonia (142,155). However, Nutt et al. reported that any of the focal dystonias could occur later in life (142). Progression of dystonia is more likely in cases with early-onset dystonia, whereas in most cases of adult-onset primary dystonia there is no or minimal spread to contiguous body parts (145). In a study of 115 patients with PTD with onset before age 22 and 472 with onset after age 21, Greene et al. reported that patients with onset in the lower extremities tended to be younger at onset than those with onset in the upper extremities, to have rapid spread of symptoms to other body parts, and to develop generalized dystonia. Patients with onset in the upper extremities were more likely to experience spread of symptoms many years after the disease began. In less than 20% of those with

onset before age 22, symptoms began with torticollis, and in 67% of them there was no spread to other body parts. In adults, dystonic symptoms remained focal in the majority (170). Similarly, in 51 PTD cases identified in Israel the most rapid deterioration occurred in patients with juvenile onset in the lower limbs, particularly in the first 2 years following onset. The rate of evolution was not influenced by gender or familial inheritance but was more rapid in non-Ashkenazi Jews (171). Remissions of dystonia occur in a small minority of patients (145,158).

Tourette's Syndrome

Tourette's syndrome (TS) is a disorder of multiple motor tics and one or more vocal (phonic) tics, which are typically waxing and waning. This variability in symptoms and lack of awareness in many subjects, in addition to the absence of a biologic marker and controversies on diagnostic criteria, pose difficult problems for the conduct of epidemiologic studies. Furthermore, studies in populations of different age groups and different sex distribution are difficult to compare because TS is more common in the male population and symptoms decrease with age. Most epidemiologic studies in adults have yielded prevalence rates of 30 to 50 per 100,000 (172–177). However, surveys in schoolchildren have yielded higher rates. The more recent epidemiologic studies have found that TS affects between 0.1% and 3.0% of schoolchildren (172,178–182), and an even higher percentage have tics not fulfilling *DSM-IV-TR* criteria for TS (which, however, no longer require that the tics cause impairment or are distressing to the individual). It is unclear whether these milder tic disorders represent forme fruste of TS or a separate disorder, and this difficulty in delineation of the phenotype complicates epidemiologic and genetic research. In addition, there are an association and considerable overlap with a number of other disorders, such as attention deficit hyperactivity disorder, obsessive–compulsive disorder, other anxiety disorders, mood disorder, and behaviorial disorders (182,183). The exact relationship of these to TS is unclear as they may reflect the variable expression of a single disorder, a shared underlying etiology, aq selection bias, or a consequence of the social and personal impact of the disorder. Comorbidity with these disorders appears to be more common in males with the exception of obsessive–compulsive behaviors (184–189) and is associated with higher levels of behavioral problems and functional impairment (174,190). The prevalence of TS in children with special educational needs is considerably higher than in regular schoolchildren, and other tic disorders occur in almost 30% of these children (172,191,192). In one study, 65% of children with emotional and behavioral difficulties, 24% of children with learning difficulties, and 6% of "problem children" had tics, most of whom fulfilled criteria for TS, whereas none of the normal children did. Conversely, 46% of 138 children with TS were found to have experienced school-related problems, and the presence of attention deficit hyperactivity disorder was a significant predictor of these (193). Children with autism also have been reported to have an increased rate of TS, with 4.3% fulfilling criteria for TS and an additional 2.2% having probable TS (194). Although many patients with TS even without comorbidity underachieve socially, the condition is found in all socio-economic groups. TS has been described worldwide, and its characteristics are very similar across cultures (195,196), supporting a common genetic basis. Males are probably about four times more commonly affected than females, but the male-to-female ratio ranges from 1.6 to 10.1 (174,175,177,195,197–199).

It has been suggested that there has been an increase in the prevalence of TS over the last decade (200), but this may have been the result of greater recognition of this disorder and higher referral to hospitals (201) because very few of all patients in the community (16%) consult a doctor (202). The incidence of TS has been reported from a study in Rochester, Minnesota (201), which identified individuals seeking medical advice over a 12-year period. Only 3 male individuals were identified, yielding an annual incidence rate of 0.46 per 100,000. However, since many subjects are unaware of their tics or insufficiently disabled to seek medical advice, and since physicians often do not correctly diagnose the disorder, the true incidence is likely to be much higher.

The natural history of TS is relatively well studied. The average onset age of motor tics in TS is 7 years but ranges from 2 to 21 years. Phonic tics usually occur later, with a mean age of onset of 11 years. Tic frequency or severity improve in the majority of TS patients in late adolescence or early adulthood (203,204). In a birth cohort study, Leckman et al. (205) found progressive worsening of tics until the age of 10, with a subsequent improvement of tic severity in the majority of cases. By the age of 18, half of the cohort were virtually tic free.

There is no doubt that genetic factors play an important role in the etiology of TS (206,207). The inheritance mostly follows an autosomal dominant inheritance pattern with variable expression and penetrance (185,208), and several areas have been implicated to be associated with TS (209). There is also growing evidence for bilineal transmission, with the father typically affected by childhood tics and the mother by symptoms of obsessive–compulsive disorder (210–212). Despite enormous research efforts, a gene responsible for TS has not yet been found, although several regions of interest have been identified. A number of reasons for this difficulty have been suggested. The assumed model for inheritance may be wrong; the phenotype may not be accurately delineated or the condition may be genetically heterogeneous; multiple genes may interact to produce TS (213); or environmental factors, such as infection or birth injury, in addition to a genetic vulnerability may determine the manifestation of TS (179,214–217). In particular, the recent description of the

pediatric autoimmune neuropsychiatric disorders associated with streptococcal infections (PANDAS syndrome) (218), which links the occurrence of obsessive–compulsive disorder and/or tic disorder with prepubertal symptom onset to streptococcal infections and neuropsychiatric symptoms, has strengthened the argument for the relevance of infectious factors in the pathogenesis of TS.

Huntington's Disease and Sporadic Chorea

Huntington's disease (HD) is the most common cause of familial chorea, although a number of HD look-alikes have now been described. It is an autosomal dominantly inherited disorder with complete penetrance, which is caused by an expanded sequence of CAG repeats in a gene on chromosome 4p16.3 that codes for the *huntington* protein (219). Nongenetic factors do not appear to influence the disease expression (220). HD occurs worldwide with prevalence rates between 2 and 12 per 100,000 (221), but lower prevalence rates have been reported in black populations, as well as in Finland, Japan, and China. Lower frequency of HD has been associated with smaller CAG repeat lengths and different distribution of CCG alleles in these populations compared with Western European populations, suggesting that, in addition to European emigration, new mutations make a contribution to geographic variation of prevalence rates (222,223). The investigation of clusters, as in Venezuela (224), has significantly advanced genetic research in HD. The incidence rate of HD is approximately 0.02 to 0.65 per 100,000 (225,226). Although it has been suggested that prevalence rates have declined through genetic counseling (227), such a decline in incidence and prevalence rates has not been confirmed by others. Age at onset is mostly in the mid-40s, but ranges from 2 years to more than 80 years. Younger onset is associated with more common presentation of rigidity, tremor, myoclonus, and epilepsy (Westphal variant), but many older patients also become akinetic-rigid and dystonic in the advanced stages. Onset age has been shown to correlate inversely with the length of the CAG repeat segment, particularly if onset is before age 30 years. In addition, paternal transmission is associated with earlier onset, leading to anticipation over several generations when the gene is inherited through the father. However, substantial variability remains, which appears related to both additive genetic and environmental factors (228). Median survival has been reported as long as 16.2 years (229), and many patients survive for more than 20 years, probably depending on the quality of care during the advanced stages. The main causes of death are pneumonia and cardiovascular disease, but the risk of suicide also is increased in patients with HD and in unaffected siblings at risk for HD (230).

No population prevalence data for sporadic chorea are available. However, in tertiary referral centers, vascular disease is the most common cause of sporadic chorea, which often improves over time, but rarer causes also include Huntington's disease (231).

Tardive Dyskinesia

Prolonged treatment with a variety of agents, particularly dopamine receptor–blocking drugs, can cause involuntary hyperkinetic movements or tardive dyskinesia (TD). TD comprises the whole range of abnormal involuntary movements, including chorea, tics, myoclonus, tremor, stereotypies, and dystonia, although tardive dystonia differs from TD with respect to risk factors and prognosis (232). Particularly characteristic are buccolinguomasticatory dyskinesias and involuntary movements of axial muscles, such as body rocking, but TD also may involve any other body part, often with a bizarre appearance. TD also is frequently associated with drug-induced parkinsonism and tardive motor restlessness (akathisia). A background prevalence of dyskinesia in elderly patients has been reported as 3%–4% (233), and the rate of dyskinesia is increased in patients with (untreated) schizophrenia. A meta-analysis of studies in patients with untreated schizophrenia estimated the prevalence of dyskinesia in this patient group from 4% in first-episode schizophrenia to 12% for chronically ill patients younger than 30, 25% for those between 30 and 50, and to 40% for those older than 60 (234). However, the authors acknowledged the limited precision of this estimate because only data from the preneuroleptic era, evaluations of first-episode patients before neuroleptic treatment, and assessment of drug-naive patients in developing countries could be used. A review of 56 prevalence surveys of TD in neuroleptic-treated patients and 19 samples of untreated individuals yielded an average prevalence of 20% in neuroleptic-treated patients and a 5% prevalence of "spontaneous" dyskinesia (235). The prevalence of tardive dyskinesia in patients on dopamine receptor–blocking agents is approximately 20%–40%, but estimates range from 1.5% to 62% (232), reflecting differences in sample characteristics, duration of exposure, and type of medication (236–240). Given the lower incidence of extrapyramidal side effects with atypical neuroleptics, prevalence rates in treated, chronic schizophrenia are likely to fall where these agents are used. Prospective studies, which are likely to more accurately reflect risk than retrospective studies, have yielded a risk of TD after 5 years of treatment with neuroleptics between 20% (241) and 35% (242) in Western populations, with similar rates of 22.3% reported in Japan (236). The annual incidence rate was reported to be much higher in adults older than 45 (30%) than in younger adults (4% to 5%) (237). Overall, increased risk for the development of TD has been found in patients with older age (243), dementia (243), affective disorder (244), or diabetes mellitus (245), and in women (246,247). However, it is unclear whether these risk factors are merely a reflection of populations more likely to have greater exposure to dopamine receptor–blocking drugs or indicate

greater susceptibility in these populations. In addition, it has been reported that those with other extrapyramidal side effects of neuroleptics, such as acute dystonic reaction or drug-induced parkinsonism, are more likely to develop TD, suggesting that an underlying susceptibility to extrapyramidal side effects exists that predisposes some patients to the development of TD on dopamine receptor antagonists. Comparisons across different ethnic groups are hampered by differences in study populations and exposure to dopamine receptor–blocking drugs. Nevertheless, it has been suggested that the risk may be lower in some Asian populations (246,248,249), whereas others have not confirmed this (250) or found a higher risk of TD in nonwhite populations (241).

The prognosis of TD is controversial and depends on a number of factors, including age, cumulative dose, and duration of exposure to the provoking drug. After discontinuation of neuroleptics, many patients improve during the months following withdrawal, especially if they are younger than 60 years. However, cessation of neuroleptic treatment may also be followed by the onset or worsening of TD (in about 40% of previously asymptomatic patients), so-called withdrawal dyskinesia (251), which usually but not always resolves. Other patients will exhibit irreversible dyskinesias even after cessation of treatment. Reports of improvement or cessation have varied in the time of follow-up, cumulative dose, and type of treatment, and studies involving consistent drug exposure are difficult to conduct as treatment usually is dependent on individual patients' requirements of treatment for their underlying disorder. The range of reported partial or complete remission rates has therefore varied widely from 2% (252) to 100% (253). In patients with ongoing neuroleptic treatment, TD tends to plateau, although TD increases in severity in some patients and improves in others (237,242,254,255). Yassa et al. (256) reported that after a 10-year follow-up of 44 patients with TD, 50% had no change in their TD severity, 20% experienced improvement, and 30% experienced a worsening of their TD. In a study from Japan (248), the severity of TD was unchanged in 39%, improved in 18%, fluctuated in 21%, and worsened in only 21%. Fernandez et al. (257) reported resolution of TD symptoms in 62%, improvement in 4%, no change in 15%, and deterioration in 19%. In this study, parkinsonism worsened in 81% despite falling daily drug burden. Reported predictors of improvement have been younger age and affective disorder (258), but not all studies have confirmed this (248). In addition, European American were reported to have better prognosis than African Americans, even after adjustment for age, drug dose, and duration of treatment (259).

Restless Legs Syndrome

Restless legs syndrome (RLS), also known as Ekbom's syndrome, is characterized by an urge to move the legs, usually accompanied or caused by uncomfortable and unpleasant sensations in the legs particularly during periods of rest or inactivity, and worse in the evening or night. Most cases of RLS remain undiagnosed in the community (approximately 90%), and reported prevalence rates in studies using varying criteria have ranged from 3% to 29% (260–266). It has been reported to be uncommon (3%) in those between 18 and 29 years, while affecting 19% of those 80 years and older (262). However, although prevalence increases with age, about one-third of patients reported that their first symptoms started before age 10 (265). Remissions of at least a month occurred in 15% in one study, but severity generally also increases with age (265,267). Severity of RLS appears to be higher in women, and some studies have found a female preponderance of RLS (261,263) (13.9% vs. 6.1%), whereas others did not find a gender difference (262). RLS has been reported worldwide, with similar rates in European, North American, South American, and Japanese samples. However, the prevalence rates reported from some other populations, including India and Singapore, were lower (268,269). There is no doubt that genetic factors are important in RLS, with approximately 60% of affected individuals reporting a positive family history (265), and autosomal dominant inheritance with possible anticipation has been implicated in such families (267). One twin study reported a concordance rate of 83% in identical twins. While linkage to loci on chromosomes 9, 12, and 14 has been reported, these findings have not been replicated in other families. On the other hand, RLS is more common in patients with uremia than in controls (25.9% vs. 13%) (270), and it has been found to be associated with pregnancy, diabetes mellitus, iron deficiency Parkinson's disease with or without anemia, neuropathy and radiculopathy, rheumatoid arthritis, and folate and magnesium deficiencies. Therefore, a distinction between hereditary and nonhereditary RLS has been made, and hereditary cases have been found to be associated with earlier symptom onset and slower progression (271). To assess the validity of this differentiation, Winkelmann et al. assessed the risk factors in 300 patients diagnosed with RLS. In 23%, RLS was associated with uremia (272). Forty-two percent of those with idiopathic RLS and 12% of those with uremic RLS had a definite family history of RLS confirmed by interview with the affected family member. Another 13% of those with idiopathic RLS and 6% of those with uremic RLS had a possible family history of RLS. Age of onset was younger in those with hereditary RLS. However, apart from worsening during pregnancy in those with hereditary RLS, there were no differences in the phenotype between those with hereditary and nonhereditary RLS, indicating that both subgroups of RLS present with a very similar phenotype.

PSYCHOGENIC MOVEMENT DISORDERS

The diagnosis of psychogenic movement disorder (PMD) is conspicuously difficult. As no laboratory test is available to diagnose this condition, the diagnosis depends on clinical judgment and the neurologist's clinical experience with movement disorders. Diagnostic criteria, which are based on the degree of diagnostic certainty, have been developed (273). Factor et al. reported that 3.3% of patients in a movement disorder clinic fulfilled the categories of "documented" and "clinically established" PMD (summarized as "clinically definite") based on those criteria (274). Earlier studies from other movement disorder clinics have also reported similar rates (275,276). Population-based data on the prevalence of PMD are not available, but PMDs are among the most common medically unexplained symptoms; according to some estimates, 25% to 60% of symptoms investigated in primary care do not have a physical explanation (277). As the majority of patients with mild or transient forms of medically unexplained symptoms are not referred to tertiary referral centers, probably only the more persistent or severe forms of PMD are seen in movement disorder clinics. In the study by Factor et al., tremor was the most common PMD (274), followed by dystonia, myoclonus, and parkinsonism. In other centers, psychogenic dystonia was the most common psychogenic movement disorder. Fahn and Williams reported that the majority of patients suffered from multiple types of movement disorders and that only 21% had a single type of movement disorder that remained stable over time (273). In a study that followed patients with PMD seen in a movement disorder clinic for a mean of 3.2 years, outcome was poor, with persistence in abnormal movements in more than 90% of subjects. There was also a high prevalence of mental illness, especially anxiety, depression, and other somatic complaints. Poor outcome was associated with long duration of symptoms, insidious onset of movements, and psychiatric comorbidity (278). This relatively poor outcome was consistent with that reported for somatoform disorders in general (279).

SUMMARY

Epidemiologic studies give important clues to the etiology of disease, provide the basis for health policy and planning, and guide clinicians in giving prognostic advice. Although advances in diagnostic measures, progress in genetic research, and effective treatments that improve the prognosis have become available for many movement disorders, diagnostic difficulties still impede epidemiologic research and comparability among studies. Improved and more standardized diagnostic criteria and ascertainment methods, as well as collaborative cross-cultural and interdisciplinary efforts incorporating genetic, epidemiologic, and diagnostic methods, are required for future studies to advance our knowledge of the epidemiology of movement disorders.

REFERENCES

1. de Rijk MC, Launer LJ, Berger K, et al. Prevalence of Parkinson's disease in Europe: a collaborative study of population-based cohorts—Neurologic Diseases in the Elderly Research Group. *Neurology* 2000;54:S21–S23.
2. Zhang ZX, Roman GC. Worldwide occurrence of Parkinson's disease: an updated review. *Neuroepidemiology* 1993;12:195–208.
3. Wermuth L, Joensen P, Bunger N, et al. High prevalence of Parkinson's disease in the Faroe Islands. *Neurology* 1997;49: 426–432.
4. Bharucha NE, Bharucha EP, Bharucha AE, et al. Prevalence of Parkinson's disease in the Parsi community of Bombay, India. *Arch Neurol* 1988;45:1321–1323.
5. Morgante L, Salemi G, Meneghini F, et al. Parkinson disease survival: a population-based study. *Arch Neurol* 2000;57:507–512.
6. Milanov I, Kmetski TS, Lyons KE, et al. Prevalence of Parkinson's disease in Bulgarian gypsies. *Neuroepidemiology* 2000;19:206–209.
7. Ashok PP, Radhakrishnan K, Sridharan R, et al. Epidemiology of Parkinson's disease in Benghazi, North-East Libya. *Clin Neurol Neurosurg* 1986;88:109–113.
8. Mayeux R, Marder K, Cote LJ, et al. The frequency of idiopathic Parkinson's disease by age, ethnic group, and sex in northern Manhattan, 1988–1993. *Am J Epidemiol* 1995;142:820–827.
9. Giroud Benitez JL, Collado-Mesa F, Esteban EM. Prevalence of Parkinson disease in an urban area of the Ciudad de La Habana province, Cuba: door-to-door population study. *Neurologia* 2000;15:269–273.
10. Schoenberg BS, Anderson DW, Haerer AF. Prevalence of Parkinson's disease in the biracial population of Copiah County, Mississippi. *Neurology* 1985;35:841–845.
11. Schoenberg BS, Osuntokun BO, Adeuja AO, et al. Comparison of the prevalence of Parkinson's disease in black populations in the rural United States and in rural Nigeria: door-to-door community studies. *Neurology* 1988;38:645–646.
12. Li SC, Schoenberg BS, Wang CC, et al. A prevalence survey of Parkinson's disease and other movement disorders in the People's Republic of China. *Arch Neurol* 1985;42:655–657.
13. Wang SJ, Fuh JL, Teng EL, et al. A door-to-door survey of Parkinson's disease in a Chinese population in Kinmen. *Arch Neurol* 1996;53:66–71.
14. Wang YS, Shi YM, Wu ZY, et al. Parkinson's disease in China. Coordinational Group of Neuroepidemiology, PLA. *Chin Med J (Engl)* 1991;104:960–964.
15. Tan LC, Venketasubramanian N, Hong CY, Sahadevan S, Chin JJ, Krishnamoorthy ES, Tan AK, Saw SM. Prevalence of Parkinson disease in Singapore: Chinese vs Malays vs Indians. *Neurology* 2004;62:1999–2004.
16. MacDonald BK, Cockerell OC, Sander JW, et al. The incidence and lifetime prevalence of neurological disorders in a prospective community-based study in the UK. *Brain* 2000;123:665–676.
17. Rajput AH, Offord KP, Beard CM, et al. Epidemiology of parkinsonism: incidence, classification, and mortality. *Ann Neurol* 1984;16:278–282.
18. Benito-Leon J, Bermejo-Pareja F, Morales-Gonzalez JM, Porta-Etessam J, Trincado R, Vega S, Louis ED, for the Neurological Disorders in Central Spain (NEDICES) Study Group. Incidence of Parkinson disease and parkinsonism in three elderly populations of central Spain. *Neurology* 2004;62:734–741.
19. Bower JH, Maraganore DM, McDonnell SK, et al. Incidence and distribution of parkinsonism in Olmsted County, Minnesota, 1976–1990. *Neurology* 1999;52:1214–1220.
20. Kuopio AM, Marttila RJ, Helenius H, et al. Changing epidemiology of Parkinson's disease in southwestern Finland. *Neurology* 1999;52:302–308.
21. Marttila RJ, Rinne UK. Epidemiology of Parkinson's disease in Finland. *Acta Neurol Scand* 1976;53:81–102.
22. Baldereschi M, Di Carlo A, Rocca WA, et al. Parkinson's disease and parkinsonism in a longitudinal study: two-fold higher incidence in men. ILSA Working Group. Italian Longitudinal Study on Aging. *Neurology* 2000;55:1358–1363.
23. de Rijk MC, Tzourio C, Breteler MM, et al. Prevalence of parkinsonism and Parkinson's disease in Europe: the Europarkinson Collaborative Study. European Community Concerted Action on the Epidemiology of Parkinson's disease. *J Neurol Neurosurg Psychiatry* 1997;62:10–15.
24. Ben Shlomo Y. How far are we in understanding the cause of Parkinson's disease? *J Neurol Neurosurg Psychiatry* 1996;61:4–16.
25. Tison F, Dartigues JF, Dubes L, et al. Prevalence of Parkinson's disease in the elderly: a population study in Gironde, France. *Acta Neurol Scand* 1994;90:111–115.
26. Maraganore DM, Anderson DW, Bower JH, et al. Autopsy patterns for Parkinson's disease and related disorders in Olmsted County, Minnesota. *Neurology* 1999;53:1342–1344.
27. Bennett DA, Beckett LA, Murray AM, et al. Prevalence of parkinsonian signs and associated mortality in a community population of older people. *N Engl J Med* 1996;334:71–76.
28. Tanner CM, Aston DA. Epidemiology of Parkinson's disease and akinetic syndromes. *Curr Opin Neurol* 2000;13:427–430.
29. Ben Shlomo Y. The epidemiology of Parkinson's disease. *Baillieres Clin Neurol* 1997;6:55–68.
30. Rocca WA, Bower JH, McDonnell SK, et al. Time trends in the incidence of parkinsonism in Olmsted County, Minnesota. *Neurology* 2001;57:462–467.
31. Tanner CM, Goldman SM. Epidemiology of Parkinson's disease. *Neurol Clin* 1996;14:317–335.
32. Taylor CA, Saint-Hilaire MH, Cupples LA, et al. Environmental, medical, and family history risk factors for Parkinson's disease: a New England–based case control study. *Am J Med Genet* 1999;88:742–749.
33. Rybicki BA, Johnson CC, Peterson EL, et al. A family history of Parkinson's disease and its effect on other PD risk factors. *Neuroepidemiology* 1999;18:270–278.
34. Rocca WA, McDonnell SK, Strain KJ, Bower JH, Ahlskog JE, Elbaz A, Schaid DJ, Maraganore DM. Familial aggregation of Parkinson's disease: The Mayo Clinic family study. *Ann Neurol* 2004;56: 495–502.
35. Duvoisin RC, Eldridge R, Williams A, et al. Twin study of Parkinson disease. *Neurology* 1981;31:77–80.
36. Marttila RJ, Kaprio J, Koskenvuo M, et al. Parkinson's disease in a nationwide twin cohort. *Neurology* 1988;38:1217–1219.
37. Wirdefeldt K, Gatz M, Schalling M, Pedersen NL. No evidence for heritability of Parkinson disease in Swedish twins. *Neurology* 2004;63:305–311.
38. Tanner CM, Ottman R, Goldman SM, et al. Parkinson disease in twins: an etiologic study. *JAMA* 1999;281:341–346.
39. Vieregge P, Hagenah J, Heberlein I, et al. Parkinson's disease in twins: a follow-up study. *Neurology* 1999;53:566–572.
40. Piccini P, Burn DJ, Ceravolo R, et al. The role of inheritance in sporadic Parkinson's disease: evidence from a longitudinal study of dopaminergic function in twins. *Ann Neurol* 1999;45:577–582.
41. Chan DK, Mellick G, Cai H, et al. The alpha-synuclein gene and Parkinson disease in a Chinese population. *Arch Neurol* 2000;57: 501–503.
42. Lucking CB, Durr A, Bonifati V, et al., for the French Parkinson's Disease Genetics Study Group. Association between early-onset Parkinson's disease and mutations in the *parkin* gene. *N Engl J Med* 2000;342:1560–1567.
43. Klein C, Pramstaller PP, Kis B, et al. Parkin deletions in a family with adult-onset, tremor-dominant parkinsonism: expanding the phenotype. *Ann Neurol* 2000;48:65–71.
44. Gilks WP, Abou-Sleiman PM, Gandhi S, et al. A common LRRK2 mutation in idiopathic Parkinson's disease. *Lancet* 2005;365: 415–416.
45. Jacquemont S, Hagerman RJ, Leehey MA, et al. Penetrance of the fragile X-associated tremor/ataxia syndrome in a premutation carrier population. *JAMA* 2004; 291: 460–69, S125–S127.
46. Gorell JM, Rybicki BA, Johnson CC, et al. Smoking and Parkinson's disease: a dose-response relationship. *Neurology* 1999;52:115–119.
47. Hellenbrand W, Seidler A, Robra BP, et al. Smoking and Parkinson's disease: a case-control study in Germany. *Int J Epidemiol* 1997;26:328–339.
48. Seidler A, Hellenbrand W, Robra BP, et al. Possible environmental, occupational, and other etiologic factors for Parkinson's disease: a case-control study in Germany. *Neurology* 1996;46:1275–1284.
49. Kuopio AM, Marttila RJ, Helenius H, et al. Environmental risk factors in Parkinson's disease. *Mov Disord* 1999;14:928–939.

50. Ross GW, Abbott RD, Petrovitch H, et al. Association of coffee and caffeine intake with the risk of Parkinson disease. *JAMA* 2000;283:2674–2679.

51. Hellenbrand W, Seidler A, Boeing H, et al. Diet and Parkinson's disease. I: A possible role for the past intake of specific foods and food groups—results from a self-administered food-frequency questionnaire in a case-control study. *Neurology* 1996;47:636–643.

52. Hellenbrand W, Boeing H, Robra BP, et al. Diet and Parkinson's disease. II: A possible role for the past intake of specific nutrients—results from a self-administered food-frequency questionnaire in a case-control study. *Neurology* 1996;47:644–650.

53. Benedetti MD, Bower JH, Maraganore DM, et al. Smoking, alcohol, and coffee consumption preceding Parkinson's disease: a case-control study. *Neurology* 2000;55:1350–1358.

54. Bower JH, Maraganore DM, Peterson BJ, McDonnell SK, Ahlskog JE, Rocca WA. Head trauma preceding PD: a case-control study. *Neurology* 2003;60:1610–1615.

55. Paganini-Hill A. Risk factors for Parkinson's disease: the leisure world cohort study. *Neuroepidemiology* 2001;20:118–124.

56. Tsui JK, Calne DB, Wang Y, et al. Occupational risk factors in Parkinson's disease. *Can J Public Health* 1999;90:334–337.

57. Marion SA. The epidemiology of Parkinson's disease—current issues. *Adv Neurol* 2001;86:163–172.

58. Elbaz A, Grigoletto F, Baldereschi M, et al, for the Europarkinson Study Group. Familial aggregation of Parkinson's disease: a population-based case-control study in Europe. *Neurology* 1999;52:1876–1882.

59. Jankovic J, Kapadia AS. Functional decline in Parkinson disease. *Arch Neurol* 2001;58:1611–1615.

60. Hely MA, Morris JG, Reid WG, et al. Age at onset: the major determinant of outcome in Parkinson's disease. *Acta Neurol Scand* 1995;92:455–463.

61. Goetz CG, Tanner CM, Stebbins GT, et al. Risk factors for progression in Parkinson's disease. *Neurology* 1988;38:1841–1844.

62. Schrag A, Ben Shlomo Y, Brown R, et al. Young-onset Parkinson's disease revisited—clinical features, natural history, and mortality. *Mov Disord* 1998;13:885–894.

63. Denny AP, Behari M. Motor fluctuations in Parkinson's disease. *J Neurol Sci* 1999;165:18–23.

64. Hely MA, Morris JG, Traficante R, et al. The Sydney multicentre study of Parkinson's disease: progression and mortality at 10 years. *J Neurol Neurosurg Psychiatry* 1999;67:300–307.

65. Montastruc JL, Desboeuf K, Lapeyre-Mestre M, et al. Long-term mortality results of the randomized controlled study comparing bromocriptine to which levodopa was later added with levodopa alone in previously untreated patients with Parkinson's disease. *Mov Disord* 2001;16:511–514.

66. Uitti RJ, Ahlskog JE, Maraganore DM, et al. Levodopa therapy and survival in idiopathic Parkinson's disease: Olmsted County project. *Neurology* 1993;43:1918–1926.

67. Herlofson K, Lie SA, Arsland D, Larsen JP. Mortality and Parkinson disease: a community based study. *Neurology* 2004;62:937–942.

68. Poewe W. The Sydney multicentre study of Parkinson's disease. *J Neurol Neurosurg Psychiatry* 1999;67:280–281.

69. Wermuth L, Stenager EN, Stenager E, et al. Mortality in patients with Parkinson's disease. *Acta Neurol Scand* 1995;92:55–58.

70. Hughes AJ, Daniel SE, Lees AJ. Improved accuracy of clinical diagnosis of Lewy body Parkinson's disease. *Neurology* 2001;57:1497–1499.

71. Hughes AJ, Daniel SE, Kilford L, et al. Accuracy of clinical diagnosis of idiopathic Parkinson's disease: a clinico-pathological study of 100 cases. *J Neurol Neurosurg Psychiatry* 1992;55:181–184.

72. Rajput AH, Rozdilsky B, Rajput A. Accuracy of clinical diagnosis in parkinsonism: a prospective study. *Can J Neurol Sci* 1991;18:275–278.

73. Schrag A, Ben Shlomo Y, Quinn NP. Prevalence of progressive supranuclear palsy and multiple system atrophy: a cross-sectional study. *Lancet* 1999;354:1771–1775.

74. Nath U, Ben Shlomo Y, Thomson RG, et al. The prevalence of progressive supranuclear palsy (Steele-Richardson-Olszewski syndrome) in the UK. *Brain* 2001;124:1438–1449.

75. Trenkwalder C, Schwarz J, Gebhard J, et al. Starnberg trial on epidemiology of Parkinsonism and hypertension in the elderly: prevalence of Parkinson's disease and related disorders assessed by a door-to-door survey of inhabitants older than 65 years. *Arch Neurol* 1995;52:1017–1022.

76. Tison F, Yekhlef F, Chrysostome V, et al. Prevalence of multiple system atrophy. *Lancet* 2000;355:495–496.

77. Vanacore N, Bonifati V, Fabbrini G, et al, for the European Study Group on Atypical Parkinsonisms (ESGAP). Epidemiology of multiple system atrophy. *Neurol Sci* 2001;22:97–99.

78. Chrysostome V, Tison F, Yekhlef F, Sourgen C, Baldi I, Dartigues JF. Epidemiology of multiple system atrophy: a prevalence and pilot risk factor study in Aquitaine, France. *Neuroepidemiology* 2004;23:201–108.

79. Golbe LI, Davis PH, Schoenberg BS, et al. Prevalence and natural history of progressive supranuclear palsy. *Neurology* 1988;38:1031–1034.

80. Vanacore N, Bonifati V, Colosimo C, et al, for the European Study Group on Atypical Parkinsonisms (ESGAP). Epidemiology of progressive supranuclear palsy. *Neurol Sci* 2001;22:101–103.

81. Bower JH, Maraganore DM, McDonnell SK, et al. Incidence of progressive supranuclear palsy and multiple system atrophy in Olmsted County, Minnesota, 1976 to 1990. *Neurology* 1997;49:1284–1288.

82. Iwatsubo T. Japanese clinical statistical data of progressive supranuclear palsy. *Nippon Rinsho* 1992;50(suppl):134–138.

83. Scrimgeour EM. Progressive supranuclear palsy in a Zimbabwean man. *West Afr J Med* 1993;12:175–176.

84. Radhakrishnan K, Thacker AK, Maloo JC, et al. Descriptive epidemiology of some rare neurological diseases in Benghazi, Libya. *Neuroepidemiology* 1988;7:159–164.

85. Caparros-Lefebvre D, Elbaz A, for the Caribbean Parkinsonism Study Group. Possible relation of atypical parkinsonism in the French West Indies with consumption of tropical plants: a case-control study. *Lancet* 1999;354:281–286.

86. Chaudhuri KR, Hu MT, Brooks DJ. Atypical parkinsonism in Afro-Caribbean and Indian origin immigrants to the UK. *Mov Disord* 2000;15:18–23.

87. Santacruz P, Uttl B, Litvan I, et al. Progressive supranuclear palsy: a survey of the disease course. *Neurology* 1998;50:1637–1647.

88. Litvan I, Mangone CA, McKee A, et al. Natural history of progressive supranuclear palsy (Steele-Richardson-Olszewski syndrome) and clinical predictors of survival: a clinicopathological study. *J Neurol Neurosurg Psychiatry* 1996;60:615–620.

89. De Yebenes JG, Sarasa JL, Daniel SE, et al. Familial progressive supranuclear palsy: description of a pedigree and review of the literature. *Brain* 1995;118(Pt 5):1095–1103.

90. Golbe LI. The epidemiology of progressive supranuclear palsy. *Adv Neurol* 1996;69:25–31.

91. Maher ER, Lees AJ. The clinical features and natural history of the Steele-Richardson-Olszewski syndrome (progressive supranuclear palsy). *Neurology* 1986;36:1005–1008.

92. Frasca J, Blumbergs PC, Henschke P, et al. A clinical and pathological study of progressive supranuclear palsy. *Clin Exp Neurol* 1991;28:79–89.

93. Wenning GK, Litvan I, Jankovic J, et al. Natural history and survival of 14 patients with corticobasal degeneration confirmed at postmortem examination. *J Neurol Neurosurg Psychiatry* 1998;64:184–189.

94. Nath U, Ben-Shlomo Y, Thomson RG, Lees AJ, Burn DJ. Clinical features and natural history of progressive supranuclear palsy: a clinical cohort study. *Neurology* 2003;60:910–916.

95. Litvan I, Baker M, Hutton M. Tau genotype: no effect on onset, symptom severity, or survival in progressive supranuclear palsy. *Neurology* 2001;57:138–140.

96. Morris HR, Schrag A, Nath U, et al. Effect of ApoE and tau on age of onset of progressive supranuclear palsy and multiple system atrophy. *Neurosci Lett* 2001;312:118–120.

97. Molinuevo JL, Valldeoriola F, Alegret M, et al. Progressive supranuclear palsy: earlier age of onset in patients with the tau protein A0/A0 genotype. *J Neurol* 2000;247:206–208.

98. Davis PH, Golbe LI, Duvoisin RC, et al. Risk factors for progressive supranuclear palsy. *Neurology* 1988;38:1546–1552.

99. Golbe LI, Rubin RS, Cody RP, et al. Follow-up study of risk factors in progressive supranuclear palsy. *Neurology* 1996;47: 148–154.

100. Litvan I. Update on epidemiological aspects of progressive supranuclear palsy. *Mov Disord* 2003;18(suppl 6): S43–S50.

101. Colosimo C, Osaki Y, Vanacore N, Lees AJ. Lack of association between progressive supranuclear palsy and arterial hypertension: a clinicopathological study. 2003;18:694–697.

102. Vanacore N, Bonifati V, Fabbrini G, et al, for the European Study Group on Atypical Parkinsonisms (ESGAP). Smoking habits in multiple system atrophy and progressive supranuclear palsy. *Neurology* 2000;54:114–119.

103. Ben Shlomo Y, Wenning GK, Tison F, et al. Survival of patients with pathologically proven multiple system atrophy: a meta-analysis. *Neurology* 1997;48:384–393.

104. Wenning GK, Ben Shlomo Y, Magalhaes M, et al. Clinical features and natural history of multiple system atrophy: an analysis of 100 cases. *Brain* 1994;117:835–845.

105. Saito Y, Matsuoka Y, Takahashi A, et al. Survival of patients with multiple system atrophy. *Intern Med* 1994;33:321–325.

106. Testa D, Filippini G, Farinotti M, et al. Survival in multiple system atrophy: a study of prognostic factors in 59 cases. *J Neurol* 1996;243:401–404.

107. Kurisaki H. Prognosis of multiple system atrophy: survival time with or without tracheostomy. *Rinsho Shinkeigaku* 1999;39: 503–507.

108. Nee LE, Gomez MR, Dambrosia J, et al. Environmental-occupational risk factors and familial associations in multiple system atrophy: a preliminary investigation. *Clin Auton Res* 1991;1:9–13.

109. Wullner U, Abele M, Schmitz-Huebsch T, Wilhelm K, Benecke R, Deuschl G, Klockgether T. Probable multiple system atrophy in a German family. *J Neurol Neurosurg Psychiatry* 2004;75: 924–925.

110. Iwahashi K, Miyatake R, Tsuneoka Y, et al. A novel cytochrome P-450IID6 (CYPIID6) mutant gene associated with multiple system atrophy. *J Neurol Neurosurg Psychiatry* 1995;58:263–264.

111. Schrag A, Ben Shlomo Y, Quinn NP. Cross-sectional prevalence survey of idiopathic Parkinson's disease and parkinsonism in London. *BMJ* 2000;321:21–22.

112. Munchau A, Schrag A, Chuang C, et al. Arm tremor in cervical dystonia differs from essential tremor and can be classified by onset age and spread of symptoms. *Brain* 2001;124:1765–1776.

113. Louis ED, Ford B, Barnes LF. Clinical subtypes of essential tremor. *Arch Neurol* 2000;57:1194–1198.

114. Dubinsky RM, Gray CS, Koller WC. Essential tremor and dystonia. *Neurology* 1993;43:2382–2384.

115. Singer MS, Wissel JW, Mueller JM, et al. Prevalence of tremor syndromes in focal and segmental dystonia: a service based epidemiological study in the adult population of Tyrol, Austria. *Mov Disord* 2000;15(suppl 3):155.

116. Koller WC, Busenbark K, Miner K, for the Essential Tremor Study Group. The relationship of essential tremor to other movement disorders: report on 678 patients. *Ann Neurol* 1994;35:717–723.

117. Lou JS, Jankovic J. Essential tremor: clinical correlates in 350 patients. *Neurology* 1991;41:234–238.

118. Jedynak CP, Bonnet AM, Agid Y. Tremor and idiopathic dystonia. *Mov Disord* 1991;6:230–236.

119. Elble RJ, Moody C, Higgins C. Primary writing tremor: a form of focal dystonia? *Mov Disord* 1990;5:118–126.

120. Jankovic J, Beach J, Schwartz K, et al. Tremor and longevity in relatives of patients with Parkinson's disease, essential tremor, and control subjects. *Neurology* 1995;45:645–648.

121. Pahwa R, Koller WC. Is there a relationship between Parkinson's disease and essential tremor? *Clin Neuropharmacol* 1993;16:30–35.

122. Cardoso FE, Jankovic J. Hereditary motor-sensory neuropathy and movement disorders. *Muscle Nerve* 1993;16:904–910.

123. Baloh RW, Foster CA, Yue Q, et al. Familial migraine with vertigo and essential tremor. *Neurology* 1996;46:458–460.

124. Louis ED, Ford B, Lee H, et al. Diagnostic criteria for essential tremor: a population perspective. *Arch Neurol* 1998;55:823–828.

125. Louis ED, Ottman R, Hauser WA. How common is the most common adult movement disorder? Estimates of the prevalence of essential tremor throughout the world. *Mov Disord* 1998;13:5–10.

126. Dogu O, Sevim S, Camdeviren H, et al. Prevalence of essential tremor: door-to-door neurologic exams in Mersin Province, Turkey. *Neurology* 2003 23;61:1804–1806.

127. Rajput AH, Offord KP, Beard CM, et al. Essential tremor in Rochester, Minnesota: a 45-year study. *J Neurol Neurosurg Psychiatry* 1984;47:466–470.

128. Rautakorpi I, Takala J, Marttila RJ, et al. Essential tremor in a Finnish population. *Acta Neurol Scand* 1982;66:58–67.

129. Haerer AF, Anderson DW, Schoenberg BS. Prevalence of essential tremor: results from the Copiah County study. *Arch Neurol* 1982;39:750–751.

130. Bain PG, Findley LJ, Thompson PD, et al. A study of hereditary essential tremor. *Brain* 1994;117(pt 4):805–824.

131. Herskovits E, Figueroa E, Mangone C. Hereditary essential tremor in Buenos Aires (Argentina). *Arq Neuropsiquiatr* 1988;46:238–247.

132. Louis ED, Marder K, Cote L, et al. Differences in the prevalence of essential tremor among elderly African Americans, whites, and Hispanics in northern Manhattan, NY. *Arch Neurol* 1995;52:1201–1205.

133. Hardesty DE, Maraganore DM, Matsumoto JY, Louis ED. Increased risk of head tremor in women with essential tremor: longitudinal data from the Rochester Epidemiology Project. *Mov Disord* 2004;19:529–533.

134. Louis ED, Fried LP, Fitzpatrick AL, Longstreth WT Jr, Newman AB. Regional and racial differences in the prevalence of physician-diagnosed essential tremor in the United States. *Mov Disord* 2003;18:1035–1040.

135. Conway D, Bain PG, Warner TT, et al. Linkage analysis with chromosome 9 markers in hereditary essential tremor. *Mov Disord* 1993;8:374–376.

136. Gulcher JR, Jonsson P, Kong A, et al. Mapping of a familial essential tremor gene, FET1, to chromosome 3q13. *Nat Genet* 1997;17:84–87.

137. Higgins JJ, Pho LT, Nee LE. A gene (ETM) for essential tremor maps to chromosome 2p22–p25. *Mov Disord* 1997;12:859–864.

138. Higgins JJ, Loveless JM, Jankovic J, et al. Evidence that a gene for essential tremor maps to chromosome 2p in four families. *Mov Disord* 1998;13:972–977.

139. Lorenz D, Frederiksen H, Moises H, Kopper F, Deuschl G, Christensen K. High concordance for essential tremor in monozygotic twins of old age. *Neurology* 2004;62:208–211.

140. Mengano A, Di Maio L, Maggio MA, et al. Benign essential tremor: a clinical survey of 82 patients from Campania, a region of southern Italy. *Acta Neurol (Napoli)* 1989;11: 239–246.

141. Salemi G, Aridon P, Calagna G, et al. Population-based case-control study of essential tremor. *Ital J Neurol Sci* 1998;19: 301–305.

142. Nutt JG, Muenter MD, Aronson A, et al. Epidemiology of focal and generalized dystonia in Rochester, Minnesota. *Mov Disord* 1988;3:188–194.

143. Schwalbe W. *Eine eigentuemliche tonische Krampfform mit hysterischen Symptomen.* Berlin: Universitaets-Buchdruckerei von Gustav Schade, 1980.

144. Alter M, Kahana E, Feldman S. Differences in torsion dystonia among Israeli ethnic groups. *Adv Neurol* 1976;14:115–120.

145. Cooper IS, Cullinan T, Riklan M. The natural history of dystonia. *Adv Neurol* 1976;14:157–169.

146. Korczyn AD, Kahana E, Zilber N, et al. Torsion dystonia in Israel. *Ann Neurol* 1980;8:387–391.

147. Zilber N, Korczyn AD, Kahana E, et al. Inheritance of idiopathic torsion dystonia among Jews. *J Med Genet* 1984;21:13–20.

148. Lee LV, Pascasio FM, Fuentes FD, et al. Torsion dystonia in Panay, Philippines. *Adv Neurol* 1976;14:137–151.

149. Gimenez-Roldan S, Lopez-Fraile IP, Esteban A. Dystonia in Spain: study of a Gypsy family and general survey. *Adv Neurol* 1976;14:125–136.

150. Golden GS. Dystonia in the black and Puerto Rican population. *Adv Neurol* 1976;14:121–124.

151. Sempere AP, Duarte C, Coria F, et al. Prevalence of idiopathic focal dystonias in the province of Segovia, Spain. *J Neurol* 1994;241:S124.

152. Defazio G, Abbruzzese G, Livrea P, Berardelli A. Epidemiology of primary dystonia. *Lancet Neurol* 2004;3:673–678.

153. Muller J, Kiechl S, Wenning GK, et al. The prevalence of primary dystonia in the general community. *Neurology* 2002 24;59: 941–943.

154. Kandil MR, Tohamy SA, Fattah MA, et al. Prevalence of chorea, dystonia, and athetosis in Assiut, Egypt: a clinical and epidemiological study. *Neuroepidemiology* 1994;13:202–210.

155. Duffey PO, Butler AG, Hawthorne MR, et al. The epidemiology of the primary dystonias in the north of England. *Adv Neurol* 1998;78:121–125.

156. Risch N, de Leon D, Ozelius L, et al. Genetic analysis of idiopathic torsion dystonia in Ashkenazi Jews and their recent descent from a small founder population. *Nat Genet* 1995;9: 152–159.

157. Soland VL, Bhatia KP, Marsden CD. Sex prevalence of focal dystonias. *J Neurol Neurosurg Psychiatry* 1996;60:204–205.

158. Claypool DW, Duane DD, Ilstrup DM, et al. Epidemiology and outcome of cervical dystonia (spasmodic torticollis) in Rochester, Minnesota. *Mov Disord* 1995;10:608–614.

159. Castelon Konkiewitz ECK, Trender I, Kamm CK, et al. The epidemiology of dystonia in Munich. *Mov Disord* 2000;15(suppl 3): 145.

160. Ozelius LJ, Page CE, Klein C, et al. The *TOR1A (DYT1)* gene family and its role in early onset torsion dystonia. *Genomics* 1999;62:377–384.

161. Klein C, Brin MF, de Leon D, et al. De novo mutations (GAG deletion) in the *DYT1* gene in two non-Jewish patients with early-onset dystonia. *Hum Mol Genet* 1998;7:1133–1136.

162. Warner TT, Fletcher NA, Davis MB, et al. Linkage analysis in British and French families with idiopathic torsion dystonia. *Brain* 1993;116(pt 3):739–744.

163. Stojanovic M, Cvetkovic D, Kostic VS. A genetic study of idiopathic focal dystonias. *J Neurol* 1995;242:508–511.

164. Bressman SB, Heiman GA, Nygaard TG, et al. A study of idiopathic torsion dystonia in a non-Jewish family: evidence for genetic heterogeneity. *Neurology* 1994;44:283–287.

165. Bressman SB. Dystonia: phenotypes and genotypes. *Rev Neurol (Paris)* 2003;159:849–856.

166. Uitti RJ, Maraganore DM. Adult onset familial cervical dystonia: report of a family including monozygotic twins. *Mov Disord* 1993;8:489–494.

167. Fletcher NA, Harding AE, Marsden CD. A case-control study of idiopathic torsion dystonia. *Mov Disord* 1991;6:304–309.

168. Defazio G, Berardelli A, Abbruzzese G, et al. Possible risk factors for primary adult onset dystonia: a case-control investigation by the Italian Movement Disorders Study Group. *J Neurol Neurosurg Psychiatry* 1998;64:25–32.

169. Defazio G, Berardelli A, Abbruzzese G, et al. Risk factors for spread of primary adult onset blepharospasm: a multicentre investigation of the Italian Movement Disorders Study Group. *J Neurol Neurosurg Psychiatry* 1999;67:613–619.

170. Greene P, Kang UJ, Fahn S. Spread of symptoms in idiopathic torsion dystonia. *Mov Disord* 1995;10:143–152.

171. Zilber N, Inzelberg R, Kahana E, et al. Natural course of idiopathic torsion dystonia among Jews. *Neuroepidemiology* 1994;13: 195–201.

172. Comings DE, Himes JA, Comings BG. An epidemiologic study of Tourette's syndrome in a single school district. *J Clin Psychiatry* 1990;51:463–469.

173. Bruun RD. Gilles de la Tourette's syndrome: an overview of clinical experience. *J Am Acad Child Psychiatry* 1984;23:126–133.

174. Caine ED, McBride MC, Chiverton P, et al. Tourette's syndrome in Monroe County school children. *Neurology* 1988;38: 472–475.

175. Burd L, Kerbeshian J, Wikenheiser M, et al. Prevalence of Gilles de la Tourette's syndrome in North Dakota adults. *Am J Psychiatry* 1986;143:787–788.

176. Apter A, Pauls DL, Bleich A, et al. A population-based epidemiological study of Tourette syndrome among adolescents in Israel. *Adv Neurol* 1992;58:61–65.

177. Apter A, Pauls DL, Bleich A, et al. An epidemiologic study of Gilles de la Tourette's syndrome in Israel. *Arch Gen Psychiatry* 1993;50:734–738.

178. Wong CK, Lau JT. Psychiatric morbidity in a Chinese primary school in Hong Kong. *Aust N Z J Psychiatry* 1992;26:459–466.

179. Mason A, Banerjee S, Eapen V, et al. The prevalence of Tourette syndrome in a mainstream school population. *Dev Med Child Neurol* 1998;40:292–296.

180. Zohar AH, Ratzoni G, Pauls DL, et al. An epidemiological study of obsessive-compulsive disorder and related disorders in Israeli adolescents. *J Am Acad Child Adolesc Psychiatry* 1992;31: 1057–1061.

181. Nomoto F, Machiyama Y. An epidemiological study of tics. *Jpn J Psychiatry Neurol* 1990;44:649–655.

182. Kurlan R, Como PG, Miller B, et al. The behavioral spectrum of tic disorders: a community-based study. *Neurology* 2002 13;59: 414–420.

183. Robertson MM. Tourette syndrome: associated conditions and the complexities of treatment. *Brain* 2000;123(pt 3):425–462.

184. Curtis D, Robertson MM, Gurling HM. Autosomal dominant gene transmission in a large kindred with Gilles de la Tourette syndrome. *Br J Psychiatry* 1992;160:845–849.

185. Eapen V, Pauls DL, Robertson MM. Evidence for autosomal dominant transmission in Tourette's syndrome: United Kingdom cohort study. *Br J Psychiatry* 1993;162:593–596.

186. Noshirvani HF, Kasvikis Y, Marks IM, et al. Gender-divergent aetiological factors in obsessive-compulsive disorder. *Br J Psychiatry* 1991;158:260–263.

187. Pauls DL, Raymond CL, Stevenson JM, et al. A family study of Gilles de la Tourette syndrome. *Am J Hum Genet* 1991;48: 154–163.

188. Grados MA, Riddle MA, Samuels JF, et al. The familial phenotype of obsessive-compulsive disorder in relation to tic disorders: the Hopkins OCD family study. *Biol Psychiatry* 2001;50: 559–565.

189. Santangelo SL, Pauls DL, Goldstein JM, et al. Tourette's syndrome: what are the influences of gender and comorbid obsessive-compulsive disorder? *J Am Acad Child Adolesc Psychiatry* 1994;33: 795–804.

190. Freeman RD, Fast DK, Burd L, et al. An international perspective on Tourette syndrome: selected findings from 3,500 individuals in 22 countries. *Dev Med Child Neurol* 2000;42:436–447.

191. Kurlan R, Whitmore D, Irvine C, et al. Tourette's syndrome in a special education population: a pilot study involving a single school district. *Neurology* 1994;44:699–702.

192. Kurlan R, McDermott MP, Deeley C, et al. Prevalence of tics in schoolchildren and association with placement in special education. *Neurology* 2001;57:1383–1388.

193. Eapen V, Robertson MM, Zeitlin H, et al. Gilles de la Tourette's syndrome in special education schools: a United Kingdom study. *J Neurol* 1997;244:378–382.

194. Burd L, Severud R, Klug MG, et al. Prenatal and perinatal risk factors for Tourette disorder. *J Perinat Med* 1999;27:295–302.

195. Staley D, Wand R, Shady G. Tourette disorder: a cross-cultural review. *Compr Psychiatry* 1997;38:6–16.

196. Robertson MM, Trimble MR. Gilles de la Tourette syndrome in the Middle East: report of a cohort and a multiply affected large pedigree. *Br J Psychiatry* 1991;158:416–419.

197. Baron-Cohen S, Scahill VL, Izaguirre J, et al. The prevalence of Gilles de la Tourette syndrome in children and adolescents with autism: a large scale study. *Psychol Med* 1999;29:1151–1159.

198. Robertson MM. The Gilles de la Tourette syndrome: the current status. *Br J Psychiatry* 1989;154:147–169.

199. Tanner CM, Goldman SM. Epidemiology of Tourette syndrome. *Neurol Clin* 1997;15:395–402.

200. Traverse L. Prevalence of Tourette syndrome in a mainstream school population. *Dev Med Child Neurol* 1998;40:847–848.

201. Lucas AR, Beard CM, Rajput AH, et al. Tourette syndrome in Rochester, Minnesota, 1968–1979. *Adv Neurol* 1982;35: 267–269.

202. Baron-Cohen S, Mortimore C, Moriarty J, et al. The prevalence of Gilles de la Tourette's syndrome in children and adolescents with autism. *J Child Psychol Psychiatry* 1999;40:213–218.

203. Bruun RD, Shapiro AK, Shapiro E, et al. A follow-up of 78 patients with Gilles de la Tourette's syndrome. *Am J Psychiatry* 1976;133:944–947.

204. Erenberg G, Cruse RP, Rothner AD. The natural history of Tourette syndrome: a follow-up study. *Ann Neurol* 1987;22: 383–385.

205. Leckman JF, Zhang H, Vitale A, et al. Course of tic severity in Tourette syndrome: the first two decades. *Pediatrics* 1998;102:14–19.
206. Abe K, Oda N. Incidence of tics in the offspring of childhood tiquers: a controlled follow-up study. *Dev Med Child Neurol* 1980;22:649–653.
207. Pauls DL. Update on the genetics of Tourette syndrome. *Adv Neurol* 2001;85:281–293.
208. Pauls DL, Leckman JF. The inheritance of Gilles de la Tourette's syndrome and associated behaviors: evidence for autosomal dominant transmission. *N Engl J Med* 1986;315:993–997.
209. Simonic I, Nyholt DR, Gericke GS, et al. Further evidence for linkage of Gilles de la Tourette syndrome (GTS) susceptibility loci on chromosomes 2p11, 8q22, and 11q23-24 in South African Afrikaners. *Am J Med Genet* 2001;105:163–167.
210. Kurlan R, Eapen V, Stern J, et al. Bilineal transmission in Tourette's syndrome families. *Neurology* 1994;44:2336–2342.
211. McMahon WM, van de Wetering BJ, Filloux F, et al. Bilineal transmission and phenotypic variation of Tourette's disorder in a large pedigree. *J Am Acad Child Adolesc Psychiatry* 1996;35:672–680.
212. Hanna PA, Janjua FN, Contant CF, et al. Bilineal transmission in Tourette syndrome. *Neurology* 1999;53:813–818.
213. Comings DE, Wu S, Chiu C, et al. Polygenic inheritance of Tourette syndrome, stuttering, attention deficit hyperactivity, conduct, and oppositional defiant disorder: the additive and subtractive effect of the three dopaminergic genes—DRD2, D beta H, and DAT1. *Am J Med Genet* 1996;67:264–288.
214. Hasstedt SJ, Leppert M, Filloux F, et al. Intermediate inheritance of Tourette syndrome, assuming assortative mating. *Am J Hum Genet* 1995;57:682–689.
215. Walkup JT, LaBuda MC, Singer HS, et al. Family study and segregation analysis of Tourette syndrome: evidence for a mixed model of inheritance. *Am J Hum Genet* 1996;59:684–693.
216. Lougee L, Perlmutter SJ, Nicolson R, et al. Psychiatric disorders in first-degree relatives of children with pediatric autoimmune neuropsychiatric disorders associated with streptococcal infections (PANDAS). *J Am Acad Child Adolesc Psychiatry* 2000;39:1120–1126.
217. Leckman JF, Dolnansky ES, Hardin MT, et al. Perinatal factors in the expression of Tourette's syndrome: an exploratory study. *J Am Acad Child Adolesc Psychiatry* 1990;29:220–226.
218. Swedo SE, Leonard HL, Mittleman BB, et al. Identification of children with pediatric autoimmune neuropsychiatric disorders associated with streptococcal infections by a marker associated with rheumatic fever. *Am J Psychiatry* 1997;154:110–112.
219. The Huntington's Disease Collaborative Research Group. A novel gene containing a trinucleotide repeat that is expanded and unstable on Huntington's disease chromosomes. *Cell* 1993;72:971–983.
220. Di Maio L, Squitieri F, Napolitano G, et al. Onset symptoms in 510 patients with Huntington's disease. *J Med Genet* 1993;30:289–292.
221. Tanner CM, Goldman SM. Epidemiology of movement disorders. *Curr Opin Neurol* 1994;7:340–345.
222. Squitieri F, Andrew SE, Goldberg YP, et al. DNA haplotype analysis of Huntington disease reveals clues to the origins and mechanisms of CAG expansion and reasons for geographic variations of prevalence. *Hum Mol Genet* 1994;3:2103–2114.
223. Andrew SE, Hayden MR. Origins and evolution of Huntington disease chromosomes. *Neurodegeneration* 1995;4:239–244.
224. Penney JB Jr, Young AB, Shoulson I, et al. Huntington's disease in Venezuela: 7 years of follow-up on symptomatic and asymptomatic individuals. *Mov Disord* 1990;5:93–99.
225. Morrison PJ, Nevin NC. Huntington disease in County Donegal: epidemiological trends over four decades. *Ulster Med J* 1993;62:141–144.
226. Pavoni M, Granieri E, Govoni V, et al. Epidemiologic approach to Huntington's disease in northern Italy (Ferrara area). *Neuroepidemiology* 1990;9:306–314.
227. Harper PS, Tyler A, Smith S, et al. Decline in the predicted incidence of Huntington's chorea associated with systematic genetic counselling and family support. *Lancet* 1981;2:411–413.
228. Wexler NS, Lorimer J, Porter J, et al, for the U.S.–Venezuela Collaborative Research Project. Venezuelan kindreds reveal that genetic and environmental factors modulate Huntington's disease age of onset. *Proc Natl Acad Sci USA* 2004;101:3498–3503.
229. Roos RA, Hermans J, Vegter-van der Vlis M, et al. Duration of illness in Huntington's disease is not related to age at onset. *J Neurol Neurosurg Psychiatry* 1993;56:98–100.
230. Sorensen SA, Fenger K. Causes of death in patients with Huntington's disease and in unaffected first degree relatives. *J Med Genet* 1992;29:911–914.
231. Piccolo I, Defanti CA, Soliveri P, Volonte MA, Cislaghi G, Girotti F. Cause and course in a series of patients with sporadic chorea. *J Neurol* 2003;250:429–435.
232. Gimenez-Roldan S, Mateo D, Bartolome P. Tardive dystonia and severe tardive dyskinesia: a comparison of risk factors and prognosis. *Acta Psychiatr Scand* 1985;71:488–494.
233. Blanchet PJ, Abdillahi O, Beauvais C, Rompre PH, Lavigne GJ. Prevalence of spontaneous oral dyskinesia in the elderly: a reappraisal. *Mov Disord.* 2004;19:892–896.
234. Fenton WS. Prevalence of spontaneous dyskinesia in schizophrenia. *J Clin Psychiatry* 2000;61(suppl 4):10–14.
235. Kane JM, Smith JM. Tardive dyskinesia: prevalence and risk factors, 1959 to 1979. *Arch Gen Psychiatry* 1982;39:473–481.
236. Koshino Y, Madokoro S, Ito T, et al. A survey of tardive dyskinesia in psychiatric inpatients in Japan. *Clin Neuropharmacol* 1992;15:34–43.
237. Jeste DV, Caligiuri MP. Tardive dyskinesia. *Schizophr Bull* 1993;19:303–315.
238. McCreadie RG, Robertson LJ, Wiles DH. The Nithsdale schizophrenia surveys. IX: Akathisia, parkinsonism, tardive dyskinesia and plasma neuroleptic levels. *Br J Psychiatry* 1992;160:793–799.
239. Wojcik JD, Falk WE, Fink JS, et al. A review of 32 cases of tardive dystonia. *Am J Psychiatry* 1991;148:1055–1059.
240. McDermid SA, Hood J, Bockus S, et al. Adolescents on neuroleptic medication: is this population at risk for tardive dyskinesia? *Can J Psychiatry* 1998;43:629–631.
241. Morgenstern H, Glazer WM. Identifying risk factors for tardive dyskinesia among long term outpatients maintained with neuroleptic medications: results of the Yale Tardive Dyskinesia Study. *Arch Gen Psychiatry* 1993;50:723–733.
242. Yassa R, Nastase C, Dupont D, et al. Tardive dyskinesia in elderly psychiatric patients: a 5-year study. *Am J Psychiatry* 1992;149:1206–1211.
243. Krabbendam L, van Harten PN, Picus I, et al. Tardive dyskinesia is associated with impaired retrieval from long-term memory: the Curacao Extrapyramidal Syndromes Study: IV. *Schizophr Res* 2000;42:41–46.
244. O'Hara P, Brugha TS, Lesage A, et al. New findings on tardive dyskinesia in a community sample. *Psychol Med* 1993;23:453–465.
245. Woerner MG, Saltz BL, Kane JM, et al. Diabetes and development of tardive dyskinesia. *Am J Psychiatry* 1993;150:966–968.
246. Yassa R, Jeste DV. Gender differences in tardive dyskinesia: a critical review of the literature. *Schizophr Bull* 1992;18:701–715.
247. Muscettola G, Pampallona S, Barbato G, et al. Persistent tardive dyskinesia: demographic and pharmacological risk factors. *Acta Psychiatr Scand* 1993;87:29–36.
248. Koshino Y, Wada Y, Isaki K, et al. A long-term outcome study of tardive dyskinesia in patients on antipsychotic medication. *Clin Neuropharmacol* 1991;14:537–546.
249. Pi EH, Gutierrez MA, Gray GE. Cross-cultural studies in tardive dyskinesia. *Am J Psychiatry* 1991;150:991.
250. Chong SA, Mahendran R, Machin D, Chua HC, Parker G, Kane J. Tardive dyskinesia among Chinese and Malay patients with schizophrenia. *J Clin Psychopharmacol* 2002;22:26–30.
251. Gardos G, Cole JO, Tarsy D. Withdrawal syndromes associated with antipsychotic drugs. *Am J Psychiatry* 1978;135:1321–1324.
252. Glazer WM, Morgenstern H, Schooler N, et al. Predictors of improvement in tardive dyskinesia following discontinuation of neuroleptic medication. *Br J Psychiatry* 1990;157:585–592.
253. Chiu HF, Leung JY, Lee S. Tardive dystonia in Chinese. *Singapore Med J* 1989;30:441–443.
254. Glazer WM, Morgenstern H. Predictors of occurrence, severity, and course of tardive dyskinesia in an outpatient population. *J Clin Psychopharmacol* 1988;8:10S–16S.

255. Gardos G, Casey DE, Cole JO, et al. Ten-year outcome of tardive dyskinesia. *Am J Psychiatry* 1994;151:836–841.
256. Yassa R, Nair NP. A 10-year follow-up study of tardive dyskinesia. *Acta Psychiatr Scand* 1992;86:262–266.
257. Fernandez HH, Krupp B, Friedman JH. The course of tardive dyskinesia and parkinsonism in psychiatric inpatients: 14-year follow-up. *Neurology* 2001;56:805–807.
258. Glazer WM, Morgenstern H, Doucette JT. Predicting the long-term risk of tardive dyskinesia in outpatients maintained on neuroleptic medications. *J Clin Psychiatry* 1993;54:133–139.
259. Wonodi I, Adami HM, Cassady SL, Sherr JD, Avila MT, Thaker GK. Ethnicity and the course of tardive dyskinesia in outpatients presenting to the motor disorders clinic at the Maryland psychiatric research center. *J Clin Psychopharmacol* 2004;24:592–598.
260. Lavigne GJ, Montplaisir JY. Restless legs syndrome and sleep bruxism: prevalence and association among Canadians. *Sleep* 1994;17:739–743.
261. Rothdach AJ, Trenkwalder C, Haberstock J, et al. Prevalence and risk factors of RLS in an elderly population: the MEMO study. Memory and Morbidity in Augsburg Elderly. *Neurology* 2000;54:1064–1068.
262. Phillips B, Young T, Finn L, et al. Epidemiology of restless legs symptoms in adults. *Arch Intern Med* 2000;160:2137–2141.
263. Rijsman R, Neven AK, Graffelman W, Kemp B, de Weerd A. Epidemiology of restless legs in The Netherlands. *Eur J Neurol* 2004;11:607–611.
264. Hening W, Walters AS, Allen RP, Montplaisir J, Myers A, Ferini-Strambi L. Impact, diagnosis and treatment of restless legs syndrome (RLS) in a primary care population: the REST (RLS epidemiology, symptoms, and treatment) primary care study. *Sleep Med* 2004;5:237–246.
265. Walters AS, Hickey K, Maltzman J, et al. A questionnaire study of 138 patients with restless legs syndrome: the "Night-Walkers" survey. *Neurology* 1996;46:92–95.
266. Gosselin N, Lanfranchi P, Michaud M, et al. Age and gender effects on heart rate activation associated with periodic leg movements in patients with restless legs syndrome. *Clin Neurophysiol* 2003;114:2188–2195.
267. Trenkwalder C, Seidel VC, Gasser T, et al. Clinical symptoms and possible anticipation in a large kindred of familial restless legs syndrome. *Mov Disord* 1996;11:389–394.
268. Tan EK, Seah A, See SJ, et al. Restless legs syndrome in an Asian population: a study in Singapore. *Mov Disord* 2001;16:577–579.
269. Bhowmik D, Bhatia M, Tiwari S, et al. Low prevalence of restless legs syndrome in patients with advanced chronic renal failure in the Indian population: a case controlled study. *Ren Fail* 2004;26:69–72.
270. Miranda M, Araya F, Castillo JL, et al. Restless legs syndrome: a clinical study in adult general population and in uremic patients. *Rev Med Chil* 2001;129:179–186.
271. Ondo W, Jankovic J. Restless legs syndrome: clinico-etiologic correlates. *Neurology* 1996;47:1435–1441.
272. Winkelmann J, Wetter TC, Collado-Seidel V, et al. Clinical characteristics and frequency of the hereditary restless legs syndrome in a population of 300 patients. *Sleep* 2000;23:597–602.
273. Fahn S, Williams DT. Psychogenic dystonia. *Adv Neurol* 1988;50:431–455.
274. Factor SA, Podskalny GD, Molho ES. Psychogenic movement disorders: frequency, clinical profile, and characteristics. *J Neurol Neurosurg Psychiatry* 1995;59:406–412.
275. Marsden CD. Hysteria: a neurologist's view. *Psychol Med* 1986;16:277–288.
276. Lempert T, Dieterich M, Huppert D, et al. Psychogenic disorders in neurology: frequency and clinical spectrum. *Acta Neurol Scand* 1990;82:335–340.
277. Kirkwood CR, Clure HR, Brodsky R, et al. The diagnostic content of family practice: 50 most common diagnoses recorded in the WAMI community practices. *J Fam Pract* 1982;15:485–492.
278. Feinstein A, Stergiopoulos V, Fine J, et al. Psychiatric outcome in patients with a psychogenic movement disorder: a prospective study. *Neuropsychiatry Neuropsychol Behav Neurol* 2001;14:169–176.
279. Hiller W, Rief W, Fichter MM. How disabled are patients with somatoform disorders? *Gen Hosp Psychiatry* 1997;19:432–438.

Nonmotor Symptoms in Parkinson's Disease

6

Werner Poewe

INTRODUCTION

Idiopathic Parkinson's disease (PD) is generally considered a paradigmatic movement disorder, since most patients present with one or more of the cardinal motor features and current treatment strategies focus on dopamine replacement to at least partially correct the disturbances of movement caused by striatal dopamine deficiency. However, it has long been recognized that the neuropathology underlying PD involves many brain areas beyond the dopaminergic nigrostriatal system, including areas that are not directly involved in motor control, such as the locus coeruleus, dorsal vagal nucleus, raphe nuclei of the brainstem, the hypothalamus, the olfactory tubercle, and large parts of the limbic cortex and neocortex (1,2). Pathology also extends into the peripheral autonomic nervous system, involving sympathetic ganglia, cardiac sympathetic efferents, and the myenteric plexus of the gut (2). It is, therefore, not surprising that a majority of, if not all, patients with PD reveal a variety of nonmotor symptoms—either as a spontaneous complaint or upon specific questioning (3,4). In addition, drugs used to treat motor symptoms frequently induce such nonmotor side effects as orthostatic hypotension, hallucinations, somnolence, insomnia, or leg edema, adding to the overall burden of the nonmotor spectrum of parkinsonian morbidity. More recently it has also become clearer that nonmotor dysfunction in PD may actually antedate overt signs and symptoms of motor disturbance (5), and a recent hypothesis about neuropathological stages of PD suggests that Lewy body pathology in the nigrostriatal system only develops after lower brainstem areas and the olfactory system have become affected (1). This has led to clinical studies assessing olfactory dysfunction or REM (rapid eye movement) sleep behavior disorder (RBD) as

potential risk factors for later development of PD in otherwise asymptomatic individuals (6,7).

Independent of their role as early or "preclinical" markers, nonmotor symptoms become increasingly prevalent and obvious over the course of the illness and are a major determinant of quality of life, progression of overall disability, and nursing home placement (8).

Spectrum of Nonmotor Symptoms in Parkinson's Disease

Nonmotor symptoms in PD involve a multitude of functions, including disorders of sleep–wake cycle regulation, cognitive function, regulation of mood and hedonistic tone, autonomic nervous system function, and sensory function and pain perception (see Table 6.1). In their various combinations they may eventually become the chief complaints and therapeutic challenges in advanced stages of PD.

Sensory Symptoms and Pain

Sensory symptoms and, in particular, spontaneous pain had already been recognized as part of PD in the earliest clinical descriptions of the disorder. Parkinson himself noted "rheumatic pain" ipsilateral to the extremity first affected by rest-tremor (9), and Charcot noted it in his famous lectures on cramps, muscular aching, rheumatoid and neuralgic pains experienced by patients with PD (10). More recent series investigating sensory symptoms and pain in parkinsonian patients—excluding secondary pain due to osteoarthritic or rheumatic conditions, neuralgic pain due to neuropathy or root lesions, or other causes of pain commonly observed in elderly populations—have reported such primary sensory symptoms in 40%–50% of patients (11,12,13). Symptoms are described as numbness,

TABLE 6.1

NONMOTOR FEATURES OF PARKINSON'S DISEASE

Neuropsychiatric Dysfunction	Mood disorders Apathy and anhedonia Frontal executive dysfunction Dementia and psychosis
Sleep Disorders	Sleep fragmentation and insomnia REM sleep behavior disorder (RBD) Periodic limb movements in sleep (PLMS) / Restless legs syndrome (RLS) Excessive daytime somnolence
Autonomic Dysfunction	Orthostatic hypotension Urogenital dysfunction Constipation
Sensory Symptoms and Pain	Olfactory dysfunction Abnormal sensations Pain

TABLE 6.2

SENSORY SYMPTOMS IN FLUCTUATING PARKINSON'S DISEASE

Symptom	Frequency (%)	Associated with Off Periods (%)
Tightening sensation	42	76
Tingling sensation	38	95
Diffuse pain	36	89
Neuralgic pain	18	78
Burning sensation	8	75

N = 50
From Witjas et al. (17).

tingling, burning, aching, coldness, heat, and pain. One series found such symptoms in 43 of 101 patients with PD, compared to only 8% of an age-matched control population (11). Pain was the most common sensory complaint in that study and was most often described as an intermittent poorly localized cramplike or aching sensation without accompanying visible cramping or dystonia. Several authors have noted painful sensations as a presenting symptom (11,12,14) and this was true for 9% of patients with primary sensory symptoms in one series (11). Spontaneous limb pain in PD is often reported as proximal and more prominent in the limb first and more severely affected (11,12,14,15,16). Complaints of aching lateral shoulder pain initially affected by rigidity, akinesia, and tremor often lead to unnecessary referrals and investigations and occasionally even shoulder surgery for suspected impingement or lesions to the rotator cuff.

When sensory symptoms and pain were studied in patients with levodopa-related motor fluctuations, they often were found to be linked to "off states" (13,15,16,17) (see Table 6.2). Such primary sensory symptoms and forms of pain related to off periods have to be differentiated from painful dystonic spasms, most commonly affecting the distal lower limb, which have been described as early-morning or off-period dystonia (18,19,20). Quinn et al. have drawn attention to the fact that spontaneous pain in fluctuating PD also can occur rarely as a peak dose phenomenon (16).

The pathophysiology underlying sensory symptoms and pain in PD is poorly understood. Peripheral neuropathies were clinically or neurophysiologically excluded in most series, and one study has also found normal somatosensory-evoked potentials in parkinsonian patients with sensory complaints (12). Studies provide further evidence that pain in PD is probably a result of altered central pain processing as part of the neurodegenerative process. Djaldetti et al. (21) found significantly reduced heat pain thresholds in patients with PD compared to control subjects and further increases in thermal pain sensitivity in those PD patients reporting spontaneous pain compared to those without. In addition, pain thresholds were markedly more reduced on the side more affected by PD in those with unilateral or asymmetric disease. Possible explanations include loss of dopaminergic, pain-inhibiting descending input to dorsal horn synapses resulting from substantia nigra or ventral tregmental dopaminergic cell loss. Alternatively, dopaminergic denervation could potentially induce central hypersensitivity to pain stimuli via basal-ganglia–thalamic connections. Nondopaminergic mechanisms could also be involved— for example, loss of noradrenergic descending pain inhibitory input from the locus coeruleus to the dorsal horn of the spinal cord (22). Finally, it has to be recognized that the widespread cortical Lewy body degeneration also can affect areas of the central pain processing system, including the cingulate gyrus, insular cortex, amygdala, and hypothalamus.

Olfactory Dysfunction

A number of studies have unequivocally established olfactory dysfunction as an early clinical sign in PD that affects some 90% of patients (23). Olfactory dysfunction is a less frequent finding in the parkinsonian variant of Multiple System Atrophy (MSA), is mild in patients with Progressive Supranuclear Palsy (PSP) (23,24), and has not been found in vascular parkinsonism (23). While almost universal in PD, hyposmia does not appear to be a feature of young-onset parkinsonian patients carrying mutations in the PARKIN gene (25), which raises the issue of the specificity of hyposmia to Lewy body disorders or synucleinopathies. A recent study of olfactory function in 361 first-degree relatives of PD patients identified 40 subjects with strictly defined hyposmia based on impaired odor detection, discrimination, and identification. These clinically asymptomatic subjects as well as 38 normosmic controls were followed with clinical examination and dopamine transporter SPECT imaging over 2 years when 10% of the hyposmic subjects with reduced DAT binding at baseline-developed clinical PD. The remaining hyposmic subjects showed a significantly greater decline of DAT transporter binding during follow-up compared to none of the normosmic controls (6). These results highlight the potential of olfactory function testing as a screening tool for persons at risk for PD.

The exact pathophysiology underlying olfactory dysfunction in PD remains obscure. Neuropathological studies of the olfactory bulbs and olfactory tract are sparse and have produced conflicting evidence of both loss and increase of the TH-positive neurons (26), and one study has suggested that relative increase of DA neurones in the olfactory bulbs might cause excessive inhibitory dopaminergic synaptic activity and thus deficient olfactory processing (27). Braak et al. (27a) have identified α-synuclein pathology with Lewy bodies and Lewy neurites in the olfactory system in subjects with clinical signs of PD and without nigral pathology, and they suggested that this type of pathology—together with Lewy pathology in the lower brainstem—could represent the earliest stages of parkinsonian neurodegeneration. Recently, a quantitative voxel-based study using diffusion-weighted magnetic resonance (MR) images and SPM-analysis has found a consistent increase in diffusivity exclusively in the area of the olfactory tracts in PD patients compared to controls (28).

Autonomic Dysfunction

Autonomic dysfunction is an almost universal feature of PD and includes orthostatic hypotension (OH), urinary and sexual dysfunction, and constipation (3).

Orthostatic Hypotension

Retrospective chart reviews in a large series of 135 cases of pathologically proven PD found evidence for symptomatic orthostatic hypotension OH in 30% of cases, bladder dysfunction in 32%, and constipation in 36% (4). Senard et al., when studying 91 patients with idiopathic PD in a cardiovascular laboratory with tilt table examinations, found systolic blood pressure drops of greater than 20 mmHg in 58% of their patients. In 20% of cases, OH was symptomatic and symptomatic OH correlated with dopaminergic medication dose on one hand and duration severity of PD on the other (29). Compared to multiple system atrophy, symptomatic OH is a late feature in PD: Wenning and coworkers in a small series of postmortem-confirmed cases of PD and MSA found mean latencies to symptomatic OH of 24 months in 15 patients with MSA compared to 166 months in 11 patients with PD (30). Mechanisms of OH may differ between MSA and PD: While the central autonomic nervous system bears the brunt of pathology related to autonomic failure, in MSA peripheral sympathetic cardiovascular denervation is

prominent in PD, as shown in multiple studies of cardiac MIBG szintigraphy in both disorders (31).

Autonomic failure is also prominent in patients with pathologically proven dementia with Lewy bodies (DLB) where dysautonomia was found in 28 of 29 patients with pathologically proven DLB (32). A recent study has provided evidence that at least OH is also more pronounced in PD patients with dementia, compared to PD patients without dementia. In a small cardiovascular function study, Peralta et al. found systolic blood pressure drops upon head-up tilt in 50% of patients with PD and dementia compared to only 7% of patients without clinically defined dementia (33). These observations in PD dementia and DLB suggest a potential link between spread of Lewy body pathology to neocortical and limbic structures and parts of the peripheral autonomic nervous system.

Constipation

Lewy body pathology in the peripheral autonomic nervous system in PD also includes the myenteric plexus with subsequent colonic sympathetic denervation (34). Clinically this is associated with a high prevalence of prolonged intestinal transit time and constipation in PD. Several case control studies have reported increased prevalence of constipation in PD of between 28% and 61% compared to control cases (6%–33%) (35,36,37), and one series found either constipation or prolonged intestinal transit time in as many as 80% of patients with PD (38). Importantly, constipation has been reported as a prominent complaint prior to onset of overt motor symptoms in about half the patients in one series (37). In line with such observations, a large prospective follow-up study in 6790 male participants of the Honolulu Heart Programme found evidence for increased relative risk for PD in males with less than one bowel movement per day compared to subjects with one, two, or more than two movements per day in the order of a 2.7- to 4.5-fold increase (39). As for hyposmia, constipation may turn out to be one of the earliest symptoms of Lewy body degeneration in PD.

Urogenital Dysfunction

Urogenital dysfunction in PD includes erectile and ejaculatory failure, urinary frequency and urgency, incomplete bladder emptying, double micturition, and urging continence. Similar to OH, urogenital failure is a late feature of PD with mean latencies of 144 months compared to 12 months in MSA in one postmortem case series (30). The most common abnormality of micturition in PD patients is related to detrusor hyperreflexia, while detrusor hypoactivity seems to be less prominent (40). In addition, paradoxical co-contractions of the urethral sphincter muscle has been described as a correlate of off-period voiding dysfunction in PD (41). Patients with mild detrusor hyperactivity may complain about nocturia with or without urgency during daytime, while urge incontinence is a feature of only advanced PD.

TABLE 6.3

PRACTICAL MANAGEMENT OF AUTONOMIC DYSFUNCTION IN PARKINSON'S DISEASE

Orthostatic Hypotension	Elastic stockings High salt intake Head-up tilt Fludrocortisone 0.1–0.3 mg/d - Midodrine 2.5–10 mg/d - Etilefrine 15–25 mg/d	
Neurogenic Bladder Symptoms	Detrusor Hyperreflexia Retention Nocturnal polyuria	Oxybutynine 5–15 mg/d Tolterodine 2–4 mg/d Trospiumchloride 20–40 mg/d Bethanechol chloride 25–75 mg/d Intermittent self catheterization Desmopressin spray 10–0 mcg/night
Erectile Dysfunction	50 mg sildenafil (CAVE: orthostatic hypotension) 10 mg vardenafil 20 mg tadalafil 3 mg apomorphine sublingual	
Constipation	Stop anticholinergics Ensure adequate fluid Add laxatives (macrogol)	

Urological examination and urodynamic investigations are mandatory to correctly identify the type of dysfunction underlying a parkinsonian patient's bladder problem and initiate appropriate treatment.

Treatment of Autonomic Dysfunction in PD

Management of autonomic failure in PD is largely based on pragmatic recommendations without firm evidence for efficacy from controlled clinical trials (42). Available studies of drugs to treat orthostatic hypotension have been performed in mixed populations of patients with neurogenic hypotension, sometimes including individuals with PD. Results of such trials support the pragmatic recommendation to α-adrenergic agents or mineralocorticoids together with physical measures in the treatment of OH in PD (see Table 6.3).

Similarly, anticholinergic agents to treat neurogenic bladder dysfunction with detrusor hyperreflexia have not been studied specifically in PD but should be tried based on findings in therapeutic trials related to other types of neurogenic bladder symptoms. While oxybutinine and tolterodine cross the blood–brain barrier and may worsen cognitive dysfunction in PD, this is not the case for trospium chloride, which may be preferable in PD dementia (43,44,45). Sildenafil has been found efficacious in one randomized-placebo controlled study in PD patients with erectile dysfunction (46), and pragmatic trials of other phosphodiesterase inhibitors or dopamine agonists like apomorphine may be warranted. The practical management options for common types of autonomic dysfunction in PD are summarized in Table 6.3.

Neuropsychiatric Dysfunction

Contrary to J. Parkinson's orginal descriptions about "the senses and intellect being uninjured," PD is clearly associated with a variety of alterations in mood, initiative, hedonistic tone, and cognitive functioning (see Table 6.4).

Depression

Loss of initiative and assertiveness, as well as anhedonia and anxiety, are common complaints and findings in patients with PD. The reported prevalence of major depression in PD ranges from a low of 4% to a high of 70% with a mean of about 40% (47,48). This figure has been confirmed by more recent studies showing the presence of

TABLE 6.4

NEUROPSYCHIATRIC FEATURES OF PARKINSON'S DISEASE

Mood Disorder	Anhedonia, apathy Anxiety Depression
Cognitive Dysfunction	Dysexecutive syndrome Visuospatial dysfunction Dementia Psychosis

Complex Behavioral Disorders	DA dysregulation syndrome
	   (hedonistic homeostatic
	   dysregulation)
	Punding

depressive symptoms in 36%–50% of patients with PD (49). Depression has a major impact on quality of life in PD (50). It has been suggested that the majority of depressed PD patients satisfy criteria for major depression according to *DSM-IV* (51), whereas more recent series suggest that this percentage may actually be much lower with the majority of patients presenting with symptoms of "minor depression" or "dysthymic disorder" (52). Patients with PD and depressive symptoms generally show less self-blame, guilt, sense of failure, and fewer self-destructive thoughts than patients with primary major depression and also rarely commit suicide (48). On the other hand, features of anxiety and panic attacks are frequently encountered, as are loss of interest and initiative, fatigue, indecisiveness, and anhedonia. Depressive episodes or panic attacks have been found to precede the onset of motor symptoms in up to 30% of patients with PD (5).

While some of the depressive symptoms in PD may actually occur as a reaction at the time of first diagnosis, the general consensus is that PD-specific pathology with multiple transmitter deficiencies in mesocortical monoaminergic systems plays a major role, including the mesocorticolimbic DA projection, as well as the mesocortical noradrenergic and serotonergic projections. Specifically, dopaminergic cell loss in the ventral tegmental area (VTA) with subsequent orbitofrontal dopaminergic denervation may contribute to apathy and anhedonia, which are typical of parkinsonian depression (53). In addition cortico-limbic noradrenergic denervation through cell loss in the locus coeruleus has also been discussed, but the majority of neurochemical correlates of parkinsonian depression relate to serotonergic denervation via serotonergic cell loss in the raphe nucleus (54). Recent PET studies have demonstrated reduction of 5-HT1A receptor binding in the limbic cortex and frontal and temporal cortical areas in depressed PD patients (55). Depression in PD, therefore, is likely multifactorial, with complex pathophysiology likely involving underactivity of orbitofrontal and limbic cortical areas.

In contrast to the frequency and clinical impact of depression in PD, limited data from controlled clinical trials are available to guide treatment decisions in such patients (42). The role of dopaminergic tone is illustrated by clinical anecdotes of off-period related depressive episodes in PD and by studies showing anti-anxiolytic and mood-brightening short-term effects of levodopa infusions in patients with fluctuating PD (56). There have been anecdotal claims of antidepressant efficacy of dopamine agonists, initially related to bromocriptine (57) and more recently also to pergolide and pramipexole in small-scale trials (58). In a study of the effects of selegiline on motor fluctuations, Lees and coworkers (59) failed to detect any significant changes in depression score in a subgroup analysis. However, depression was not the primary target of this trial. In another study, after 6 weeks of therapy, Hamilton Rating Scale for Depression (HAM-D) scores

showed significantly greater improvement in patients receiving combined MAO-A (moclobemide 600 mg/day) plus MAO-B (selegiline 10 mg/day) inhibition compared to treatment with moclobemide alone (60). However, this study was confounded by motor improvement in the combined treatment group.

Antimuscarinic agents are an established treatment modality in major depression. The only randomized placebo-controlled study in PD depression dates back more than 20 years and is related to nortryptiline (titrated from 25 mg/day to a maximum of 150 mg/day) (61), which showed a significant improvement over placebo, on a depression rating scale designed by the author. Although the use of SSRIs in PD-associated depression has been reported as beneficial in numerous small, open-label studies covering a variety of agents (fluoxetine, sertraline, paroxetine) (62), to date only one small double-blind placebo-controlled study of sertraline has assessed this approach. No statistically significant differences in the change of Montgomery Asberg Depression Rating Scale MADRS scores were detected between treatment arms, but the study was not sufficiently powered to allow firm conclusions (63). The two largest uncontrolled trials of SSRIs in the treatment of depression in PD investigated the use of paroxetine in 33 and 65 patients over a period of 3 to 6 months (64,65). In both studies, paroxetine was titrated to 20 mg/day and produced statistically significant improvements over baseline in HAM-D rating scores. There were no changes in United Parkinson's Disease Rating Scale UPDRS motor scores in either study, but in the Ceravolo study (64), one patient reported worsening of tremor, and in the Tesei study (65), two (3%) withdrawals were related to worsened off time or tremor. Avila and coworkers (66) compared nefazodone with fluoxetine. Significant improvements in Beck Depression Inventory (BDI) scores were observed with both treatments.

Reboxetine (67) and venlafaxine (68) have been reported beneficial in PD-associated depression. However, these studies have been small and of short duration.

A recent review identified 21 articles, covering a total of 71 patients with PD receiving electroconvulsive therapy (ECT) to treat concomitant depression (42). These data are insufficient to conclude on the efficacy and safety of ECT to treat depression in PD. Two double-blind studies have assessed repetitive transcranial magnetic stimulation (rTMS) in PD depression. There was no difference between sham and effective stimulation with respect to depression and PD measures (69). A class I study (70) found rTMS as effective as fluoxetine in improving depression at week 2, an effect maintained to week 8. However, interpretation of this study is hampered by lack of a placebo.

In the absence of controlled-trial data, drug treatment of depression in PD should focus on sufficient dopamine-substitution for optimal control of motor symptoms and use add-on antidepressant agents with the choice between antimuscarinic agents, SSRIs, or the newer combined serotonergic–adrenergic agents, depending on patient profile and individual safety and tolerability.

Cognitive Dysfunction and Dementia

Subtle cognitive deficits are almost universally identified even in early PD upon detailed neuropsychological testing (71). They relate to frontal executive dysfunction with impaired problem solving and defective planning and organization of goal-directed behavior, as well as difficulties with set shifting, visuospatial deficits, and some impairment of learning and memory (72). Community-based studies have suggested that some 30%–40% of patients with PD will develop clinically defined dementia. A meta-analysis of prevalence studies on dementia in PD has estimated that 31% of PD patients fullfill diagnostic criteria for dementia and that PD dementia accounts for around 4% of degenerative dementias and may have a population-based prevalence of between 0.2% and 0.5% in those aged older than 65 (73).

The development of dementia has significant impact on the natural history of PD and has been shown to be associated with more rapid progression of disability, increased risk for nursing home placement, and increased mortality (74,75,76). The clinical profile of PD dementia includes aspects of psychomotor-slowing apathy and bradyphrenia, deficits in memory retrieval, impaired set shifting, problem solving, poor visuospatial function, fluctuations in attention and cognition, and prominent mood and personality disorders, hallucinosis, and psychosis while language and praxis remain largely intact (77). Whether or not dementia with Lewy bodies (DLB) is a distinct clinical entity from PD dementia is currently a matter of debate. Several small-scale and one randomized placebo-controlled trial have suggested efficacy of cholinesterase inhibition in improving cognitive function and erratic and psychotic behavior in patients with PD dementia (78,79). The underlying pathology may include Alzheimer's-type changes, cortical Lewy body degeneration, and vascular lesions, but Lewy body degeneration has been suggested to be the major driving factor for the development of dementia in PD (73).

Therapeutic trials in PD dementia for the most part have been small scale and open label. The only controlled trial data relate to the use of cholinesterase inhibitors. The only available large-scale randomized placebo-controlled study was performed with rivastigmine and with mean daily doses of around 9 mg of rivastigmine showed significant improvements of cognitive dysfunction as assessed by the ADAS-cog subscale and caregiver-based interviews of global change (79). Hallucinosis, psychotic symptoms, and erratic behavior also improved at the expense of some increase in tremor in about 10% of patients but without global worsening of parkinsonism as assessed by the UPDRS. Small-scale placebo-controlled studies suggest efficacy also of donepezile (78,80), while galantamine and

tacrine have only been tested in open label studies. Overall, while cognitive improvements may only be modest at group level, individual patients may gain significant profit from cholinesterase inhibition.

Psychosis

Hallucinosis and psychotic episodes are among the most challenging of the parkinsonian nonmotor symptoms. Although there have been few systematic and prospective studies of incidence and risk factors for psychosis in PD, recent drug trials in early PD have found incidences of hallucinosis and psychosis in up to 17% of patients (81), and cross-sectional surveys in outpatient clinic populations have reported a 40% prevalence of hallucinations in PD (82). Psychosis has been identified as a major risk factor for nursing home placement in PD (75), and early psychotic reactions to dopaminergic replacement in PD have been correlated with subsequent development of cognitive decline and dementia (83). Drug-induced psychosis in PD is more common in elderly patients than in those with cognitive impairment. Hallucinosis and psychosis can be triggered by all major classes of antiparkinsonian agents, including dopamine agonists, levodopa, MAO-B inhibitors, amantadine, and anticholinergics. Several randomized controlled studies suggest that dopamine agonists are more likely to induce hallucinosis than levodopa (81,84). The clinical spectrum of psychosis in PD includes visual illusions, visual hallucinations with retained insight, and florid paranoid hallucinatory psychosis and delusions. Visual phenomena are the predominant type of hallucinations in PD, and they are usually well formed, colorful, and rich in detail, while acoustic and tactile hallucinations are less common and, if present, usually occur in association with visual hallucinations (85). Management of psychosis in PD should be based on careful assessment and elimination of contributing or triggering factors in each individual case. This includes reductions of polypharmacy with antiparkinsonian and other centrally active drugs as much as possible, as well as proper treatment of such medical conditions as pneumonia, urinary tract infection, phlebitis, exsiccosis, or electrolyte disturbances. When reducing and simplifying antiparkinsonian combination therapies, drugs with unfavorable risk–benefit ratios regarding cognitive side effects versus antiparkinsonian efficacy should be tapered or removed first—for example anticholinergics or amantadine before tapering dopaminergic drugs. Similarly, dopamine agonists, by virtue of their greater potential to induce psychosis, should be tapered before levodopa. Frequently, however, patients with drug-induced psychosis need adjunct treatment with atypical antipsychotics. Currently clozapine remains the only drug with proven antipsychotic efficacy without motor worsening, as shown by placebo-controlled randomized trials. Altogether, two 4-week randomized controlled trials have documented antipsychotic efficacy without worsening of UPDRS motor scores (86,87), and an open-label extension of one of these studies provided evidence for maintained efficacy over an additional 12 weeks (88). Leucopenia is a rare but serious adverse event with clozapine (0.38% of those exposed according to Honigfeld et al. [89]). Consistently reported side effects even with low-dose clozapine include sedation, dizziness, increased drooling, orthostatic hypotension, and weight gain.

Olanzapine, on the other hand, has failed to show antipsychotic efficacy in 2 randomized controlled trials (90,91), while both studies also found significant motor worsening with olanzapine as was shown before in a prematurely stopped trial versus clozapine (92).

Quetiapine has been used in several open-label trials and was generally associated with improvement in some 80% of patients (93), although with some degree of motor worsening in almost 30%. However, a recent placebo-controlled trial failed to demonstrate significant improvement in psychosis using quetiapine at doses under 100 mg (94). This is in contrast to higher doses used in many of the open-label reports (95,96).

More recently, several open-label studies have claimed antipsychotic efficacy of rivastigmine (97,98) or donepezil (99,100) in PD patients, and hallucinations also have been improved in a placebo-controlled study of rivastigmine in PD dementia (79).

Sleep Disorders

Sleep disorders are among the most frequent nonmotor problems of PD (101). They include difficulties falling asleep, frequent awakenings, nocturnal cramping, painful dystonia, or nocturnal motor symptoms with difficulties turning in bed, motor restlessness, or clear-cut restless legs syndrome (RLS), nighttime incontinence, nocturnal confusion, hallucinosis, and daytime sleepiness. The awareness of the clinical implications of these disturbances has only increased in recent years, prompting new research.

Multiple contributing factors and clinical manifestations are involved. The motor abnormalities of parkinsonism, for example nocturnal tremor, nocturnal akinesia, off-period dystonia, and RLS or periodic limb movements in sleep (PLMS) are possible causes. The neurodegeneration of PD impacts the sleep structure. This induces sleep fragmentation, reduced sleep efficiency, reduced slow-wave sleep, reduced REM sleep and RBD. Respiratory disturbances and autonomic disturbances are other possible mechanisms.

Restless Legs Syndrome

RLS symptoms are often reported in PD, but prevalence studies of RLS in PD are few with inconsistent results. In addition, clinical overlapping between RLS, "wearing-off"-related lower limb discomfort and restlessness, and akathisia complicate the clinical assessments of true RLS in PD. Underlying pathophysiology potentially shared by RLS and PD is mainly suggested by similarities in treatment response. Functional imaging studies in RLS are still inconclusive, although some authors have found subtle deficits in nigrostriatal terminal function. Long-term prospective studies of RLS cohorts will clarify whether or not RLS is associated with an increased risk for development of PD (102).

REM Sleep Behavior Disorder

Of those disturbances of sleep architecture described in PD patients, RBD may be the most closely related to parkinsonian neurodegeneration of brainstem nuclei. RBD has been defined as a loss of REM-sleep muscle atonia with tonic and phasic activity in the chin and extremity EMG associated with jerking or sometimes violent limb and body movements that appeared to be related to dream content (103). A number of studies have assessed the frequency of RBD in PD populations and have found much higher rates than could be accounted for by chance given the low prevalence of idiopathic RBD. Comella et al. (104) in an interview-based study of 61 PD patients identified 9 individuals (15%) who met stringent RBD criteria, another 15% reported sleep-related injuries likely reflecting RBD, with a total of 25% of patients either meeting RBD criteria or reporting sleep-related injuries. In a polysomnographic study of 33 patients, Gangnon et al. (105) found that one-third met polysomnographic criteria for RBD and more than 50% had REM sleep episodes without atonia (RWA). In a similar study, Wetter et al. found 40% of 45 PD patients with either RWA or RBD on polysomnography (106).

Even more intriguing than the relatively high prevalence of RBD in PD populations is the frequent occurence of parkinsonian comorbidity in studies of RBD cohorts. In one study of 53 patients with RBD, Olsen et al. (107) found 47% to be suffering from PD and another 26% from MSA. Several reports have drawn attention to the fact that so-called idiopathic RBD may precede by years the onset of PD, MSA, or dementia with Lewy bodies (108,109). Schenck et al. have reported on a cohort of 29 patients with idiopathic RBD in whom 39% developed overt PD after about 4 years of follow-up, and this figure grew even further to 60% after extended follow-up of 7 years (108,110). There is some evidence for subclinical nigrostriatal presynaptic dysfunction as assessed by 18-F-Dopa PET or dopamine transporter SPECT in idiopathic RBD (111,112), and a recent study has found significant olfactory dysfunction in a group of individuals with idiopathic RBD compared to normal controls, providing further evidence that both hyposmia and RBD could indeed be linked to the earliest stages of neurodegeneration in PD as hypothesized by Braak et al. (1).

Another interesting association is related to RBD in PD and the occurrence of sleep-onset REM episodes and daytime hallucinosis (113).

Daytime Sleepiness

Following the original alert by Frucht et al. about dopamine agonist-induced episodes of irresistible sleep in patients taking pramipexole or ropinirole (114), many studies have investigated the prevalence of excessive daytime sleepiness (EDS) in parkinsonian cohorts. Hobson et al. (115), using a cutoff score of 7 on the Epoworth Sleepiness Scale (ESS), found EDS in half of their nondemented, fully functioning PD patients. Comparative studies versus age-matched controls again identify significantly higher frequencies of EDS in PD (33%–41% versus 11%–19% controls) (116,117). The issue of sudden-onset sleep has also been assessed by several authors, and the two largest series have reported prevalences of 4%–6% of PD patients with this symptom (115,118).

In summary, studies into EDS and sudden-onset sleep in PD have failed to detect significant differences between patients on ergot dopamine agonists compared to nonergot dopamine agonists regarding ESS scores or EDS (115, 117,118), while these have been consistently significant correlations among total dopaminergic drug dose and ESS scores, EDS, and sudden-onset sleep. One study assessed relative frequencies of sudden-onset sleep with different types of treatments and found ESS in 2.9% of those on levodopa monotherapy compared to 5.3% on dopamine agonist monotherapy versus 7.3% on combined treatments with levodopa and dopamine agonists (118).

Management of sleep disorders in PD is complex and has to target underlying mechanisms. Dopamine agonists may be helpful in sleep fragmentation due to nocturnal motor disability or RLS/PLMS. Clonazepam may be considered in RBD, and CPAP in some patients. Atypical neuroleptics or cholinesterase inhibitors may improve sleep in patients with nocturnal episodes of confusion or hallucinosis. Modafinil has some success in patients with EDS. Usually, mechanisms are multiple and treatment multimodal. Overall, sleep problems in PD remain a major therapeutic challenge.

CONCLUSIONS

Nonmotor symptoms are universal features of idiopathic PD and involve dysfunction in the neuropsychiatric, sensory, and autonomic domains. To summarize, they add significantly to overall disability caused by PD and are critical determinants of health-related quality of life of affected patients. In the era of effective symptomatic therapies to treat the motor symptoms of PD, nonmotor dysfunction has developed into a major prognostic factor for overall disease burden and everyday function in PD. In addition, there is increasing evidence that nonmotor dysfunction antedates clinical manifestations of motor symptoms of PD by years or even decades and may thus turn out to be a critical target for early-diagnosis paradigms and identification of at-risk populations. In addition to defining predictive values of certain types of nonmotor dysfunction, including hyposmia, future research on RBD or autonomic dysfunction must focus on the development of effective symptomatic therapies for PD nonmotor symptoms.

REFERENCES

1. Braak H, del Tredici K, Rub U, et al. Staging of brain pathology related to sporadic Parkinson's disease. *Neurobiol Aging* 2003;24: 197–211.
2. Forno LS. Pathology of Parkinson's disease. In: Marsden CD, Fahn S, eds. *Movement Disorders, Neurology 2*. London: Butterworths International Medical Reviews 1982:25–40.
3. Goetz CG, Lutge W, Tanner CM. Autonomic dysfunction in Parkinson's disease. *Neurology* 1986;36:73–75.
4. Magalhaes M, Wenning GK, Daniel SE, Quinn NP. Autonomic dysfunction in pathologically confirmed multiple system atrophy and idiopathic Parkinson's disease: a retrospective comparison. *Acta Neurol Scand* 1995;91:98–102.
5. Santamaria J, Tolosa E, Valles A. Parkinson's disease with depression: a possible subgroup of idiopathic parkinsonism. *Neurology* 1986;36:1130–1133.
6. Ponsen MM, Stoffers D, Booij J, et al. Idiopathic hyposmia as a preclinical sign of Parkinson's disease. *Ann Neurol* 2004;56: 173–181.
7. Stiasny-Kolster K, Magerl W, Oertel WH, Möller JC, Treede RD. Static mechanical hyperalgesia without dynamic tactile allodynia in patients with restless legs syndrome. *Brain* 2004;127:773–782.
8. Hely MA, Morris JG, Reid WG, Trafficante R. Sydney Multicenter study of Parkinson's disease: non-L-Dopa-responsive problems dominate at 15 years. *Mov Disord* 2005;20:190–199.
9. Parkinson J. *An Essay on the Shaking Palsy*. London: Sherwood, Neely and Jones; 1817:47.
10. Charcot JM. *Lectures on Diseases on the Nervous System*. Sigerson S, trans. London: The New Syndenham Society; 1877:1;137.
11. Snider SR, Fahn S, Isgreen W, Cote LJ. Primary sensory symptoms in parkinsonism. *Neurology* 1976;26:423–429.
12. Koller WC. Sensory symptoms in Parkinson's disease. *Neurology* 1984;34:957–959.
13. Goetz CG, Tanner CM, Levy M, Wilson RS, Garron DC. Pain in Parkinson's disease. *Mov Disord* 1986;1:45–49.
14. Schott GD. Pain in Parkinson's disease. *Pain* 1985;22:407–411.
15. Nutt JG, Carter JH. Sensory symptoms in parkinsonism related to central dopaminergic function. *Lancet* 1984;2:456–457.
16. Quinn NP, Koller WC, Lang AE, Marsden CD. Painful Parkinson's disease. *Lancet* 1986;1:1366–1369.
17. Witjas T, Kaphan E, Azulay JP, Blin O, Ceccaldi M, Pouget J, Poncet M, Cherif AA. Nonmotor fluctuations in Parkinson's disease: frequent and disabling. *Neurology* 2002;13:59:408–413.
18. Melamed E. Early-morning dystonia: a late side-effect of long-term levodopa therapy in Parkinson's disease. *Arch Neurol* 1979;36:308–310.
19. Lees AJ, Hardie RJ, Stern GM. Kinesigenic foot dystonia as a presenting feature of Parkinson's disease. *J Neurol Neurosurg Psychiatry* 1984;47:885.
20. Poewe W, Lees AJ, Stern GM. Dystonia in Parkinson's disease: clinical and pharmacological features. *Ann Neurol* 1988;23:73–78.
21. Djaldetti R, Shifrin A, Rogowski Z, et al. Quantitative measurement of pain sensation in patients with Parkinson disease. *Neurology* 2004;62:2171–2175.
22. Buzas B, Max MB. Pain in Parkinson disease. *Neurology* 2004;62: 2156–2167.
23. Katzenschlager R, Zijlmans J, Evans A, Watt H, Lees AJ. Olfactory function distinguishes vascular parkinsonism from Parkinson's disease. *J Neurol Neurosurg Psychiatry* 2004;75:1749–1752.
24. Wenning GK, Shephard B, Hawkes C, Petruckevitch A, Lees A, Quinn N. Olfactory function in atypical parkinsonian syndromes. *Acta Neurol Scand* 1995;91:247–250.
25. Khan NL, Katzenschlager R, Watt H, Bhatia KP, Wood NW, Quinn N, et al. Olfaction differentiates parkin disease from early-onset parkinsonism and Parkinson disease. *Neurology* 2004;62: 1224–1226.
26. Pearce RK, Hawkes CH, Daniel SE. The anterior olfactory nucleus in Parkinson's disease. *Mov Disord* 1995;10:283–287.
27. Huisman E, Uylings HB, Hoogland PV. A 100% increase of dopaminergic cells in the olfactory bulb may explain hyposmia in Parkinson's disease. *Mov Disord* 2004;19:687–692.
27a. Braak H, Del Tredici K, Rub U, et al. Staging of brain pathology related to sporadic Parkinson's disease. *Neurobiol Aging* 2003;24: 197–211.

28. Scherfler C, Schocke MF, Seppi K, et al. Voxel-wise analysis of diffusion weighted imaging reveals disruption of the olfactory tract in Parkinson's disease. *Brain* 2006;129:538–542.

29. Senard JM, Rai S, Lapeyre-Mestre M, et al. Prevalence of orthostatic hypotension in Parkinson's disease. *J Neurol Neurosurg Psychiatry* 1997;63:584–589.

30. Wenning GK, Scherfler C, Granata R, Bosch S, Verny M, Chaudhuri KR, et al. Time course of symptomatic orthostatic hypotension and urinary incontinence in patients with post-mortem confirmed parkinsonian syndromes: a clinicopathological study. *J Neurol Neurosurg Psychiatry* 1999;67:620–623.

31. Braune S, Reinhardt M, Schnitzer R, Riedel A, Lücking CH. Cardiac uptake of [123-I])-MIBG separates Parkinson's disease from multiple system atrophy. *Neurology* 1999;53:1020–1025.

32. Horimoto Y, Matsumoto M, Akatsu H, et al. Autonomic dysfunctions in dementia with Lewy bodies. *J Neurol* 2003;250:530–533.

33. Peralta C, Werner P, Holl B, Kiechl S, Willeit J, Seppi K, et al. Parkinsonism following striatal infarcts: incidence in a prospective stroke unit cohort. *J Neural Transm* 2004;111:1473–1483.

34. Den Hartog Jager WA, Bethlem J. The distribution of Lewy bodies in the central and autonomic nervous system in idiopathic paralysis agitans. *J Neurol Neurosurg Psychiatry* 1960;23:283–290.

35. Edwards LL, Quigley EM, Pfeiffer RF. Gastrointestinal dysfunction in Parkinson's disease: frequency and pathophysiology. *Neurology* 1992;42:726–732.

36. Singer C, Weiner WJ, Sanchez-Ramos JR. Autonomic dysfunction in men with Parkinson's disease. *Eur Neurol* 1992;32:134–140.

37. Korczyn AD. Autonomic nervous system disturbances in Parkinson's disease. *Adv Neurol* 1990;53:463–468.

38. Jost WH. Gastrointestinal motility problems in patients with Parkinson's disease: effects of antiparkinsonian treatment and guidelines for management. *Drugs Aging* 1997;10:249–258.

39. Abbott RD, Petrovitch H, White LR, et al. Frequency of bowel movements and the future risk of Parkinson's disease. *Neurology* 2001;57:456–462.

40. Fowler CJ. Investigation and treatment of bladder and sexual dysfunction in diseases affecting the autonomic nervous system. In: Mathias CJ, Bannister SR, eds. *Autonomic Failure: A Textbook of Clinical Disorders of the Autonomic Nervous System.* 4th ed. London: Oxford; 1999;30:296–303.

41. Christmas TJ, Kampster PA, Chapple CR, et al. Role of subcutaneous apomorphine in parkinsonian voiding dysfunction. *Lancet* 1988;2:1451–1453.

42. Goetz CG, Koller WC, Poewe W, Rascol O, Sampaio C, for the MDS Task Force. Management of Parkinson's disease: an evidence based review. *Mov Disord* 2002;17(suppl 4).

43. Tsao JW, Heilmann KM. Transient memory impairment and hallucinations associated with tolterodine use. *N Engl J Med* 2003;349:2274–2275.

44. Womack KB, Heilmann KM. Toterodine and memory: dry but forgetful. *Arch Neurol* 2003;60:771–773.

45. Todorova A, Vonderheid-Guth B, Dimpfel W. Effects of tolterodine, trospium chloride and oxybutinin on the central nervous system. *J Clin Pharmacol* 2001;41:636–644.

46. Hussain IF, Brady CM, Swinn MJ, et al. Treatment of erectile dysfunction with sildenafil citrate (Viagra) in parkinsonism due to Parkinson's disease or multiple system atrophy with observations on orthostatic hypotension. *J Neurol Neurosurg Psychiatry* 2002;72:681.

47. Cummings JL. Depression and Parkinson's disease: a review. *Am J Psychiatry* 1992;149:443–454.

48. Mayeux R, Denaro J, Hemenegildo N, Marder K, Tang MX, Cote LJ, et al. A population-based investigation of Parkinson's disease with and without dementia. Relationship to age and gender. *Arch Neurol* 1992;49:492–497.

49. Shulman LM, Taback RL, Bean J, Weiner WJ. Comorbidity of the nonmotor symptoms of Parkinson's disease. *Mov Disord* 2001;16:507–510.

50. Schrag A, Jahanshahi M, Quinn N. What contributes to quality of life in patients with Parkinson's disease? *J Neurol Neurosurg Psychiatry* 2000;69:308–312.

51. Starkstein SE, Mayberg HS, Leiguarda R, Preziosi TJ. A prospective longitudinal study of depression, cognitive decline, and physical impairments in patients with Parkinson's disease. *J Neurol Neurosurg Psychiatry* 1992;55:377–382.

52. Tandberg E, Larsen JP, Aarsland D, Cummings JL. The occurrence of depression in Parkinson's disease: a community-based study. *Arch Neurol* 1996;53:175–179.

53. Damier P, Hirsch EC, Agid Y, Graybiel AM. The substantia nigra of the human brain. II. Patterns of loss of dopamine-containing neurons in Parkinson's disease. *Brain* 1999;122:1437–1448.

54. Mayeux R, Stern Y, Sano M, et al. The relationship of serotonin to depression in Parkinson's disease. *Mov Disord* 1988;3:237–244.

55. Doder M, Rabiner EA, Turjanski N, et al. Brain serotonin 1A receptors in Parkinson's disease with and without depression measured by positron emission tomography with 11C-WAY 100635. *Mov Disord* 2000;15:213.

56. Maricle RA, Nutt JG, Carter JH. Mood and anxiety fluctuation in Parkinson's disease associated with levodopa infusion: preliminary findings. *Mov Disord* 1995;10:329–332.

57. Agid Y, Ruberg M, Dubois B, Pillon B, et al. Parkinson's disease and dementia. *Clin Neropharmacol* 1986;9(suppl 2):22–36.

58. Rektorová I, Rector I, Bares M, et al. Pramipexole and pergolide in the treatment of depression in Parkinson's disease: a national multicentre prospective randomized study. *Eur J Neurol* 2003;10: 399–406.

59. Lees AJ, Shaw KM, Kohout LJ, Stern GM. Deprenyl in Parkinson's disease. *Lancet* 1977;15:791–795.

60. Steur EN, Ballering LA. Moclobemide and selegiline in the treatment of depression in Parkinson's disease. *J Neurol Neurosurg Psychiatry* 1997;63:547.

61. Andersen J, Aabro E, Gulmann N, Hjelmsted A, Pedersen HE. Antidepressive treatment in Parkinson's disease: a controlled trial of the effect of nortriptyline in patients with Parkinson's disease treated with L-Dopa. *Acta Neurol Scand* 1980;62:210–219.

62. Weintraub D, Morales KH, Moberg PJ, et al. Antidepressant studies in Parkinson's disease: a review and meta-analysis. *Mov Disord* 2005;20:1161–1169.

63. Leentjens AF, Vreeling FW, Luijeckx GJ, Verhey FR. SSRIs in the treatment of depression in Parkinson's disease. *Int J Geriatr Psychiatry* 2003;18:552–554.

64. Ceravolo R, Nuti A, Piccinni A, Dell'Agnello G, Bellini G, et al. Paroxetine in Parkinson's disease: effects on motor and depressive symptoms. *Neurology* 2000;55:1216–1218.

65. Tesei S, Antonini A, Canesi M, Zecchinelli A, Mariani CB, Pezzoli G. Tolerability of paroxetine in Parkinson's disease: a prospective study. *Mov Disord* 2000;15:986–989.

66. Avila A, Cardona X, Martin-Baranera M, Maho P, Sastre F, Bello J. Does nefazodone improve both depression and Parkinson disease? A pilot randomized trial. *J Clin Psychopharmacol* 2003;23: 509–513.

67. Lemke MR. Effect of reboxetine on depression in Parkinson's disease patients. *J Clin Psychiatry* 2002;63:300–304.

68. Bayulkem K, Torun F. Therapeutic efficiency of venlafaxin in depressive patients with Parkinson's disease. *Mov Disord* 2002;17 (suppl 5):P204.

69. Okabe S, Ugawa Y, Kanazawa I. Effectiveness of rTMS on Parkinson's Disease Study Group: H.2-Hz repetitive transcranial magnetic stimulation has no add-on effects as compared to a realistic sham stimulation in Parkinson's disease. *Mov Disord* 2003;18: 382–388.

70. Fregni F, Santos CM, Myczkowski ML, et al. Repetitive transcranial magnetic stimulation is as effective as fluoxetine in the treatment of depression in patients with Parkinson's disease. *J Neurol Neurosurg Psychiatry* 2004;75:1171–1174.

71. Lees AJ, Smith E. Cognitive deficits in the early stages of Parkinson's disease. *Brain* 1983;106:257–270.

72. Dubois B, Pillon B. Cognitive deficits in Parkinson's disease. *J Neurol* 1997;244:2–8.

73. Aarsland D, Zaccai J, Brayne C. A systematic review of prevalence studies of dementia in Parkinson's disease. *Mov Disord* 2005;20: 1255–1263.

74. Biggins CA, Boyd JL, Harrop FM, et al. A controlled, longitudinal study of dementia in Parkinson's disease. *J Neurol Neurosurg Psychiatry* 1992;55:566–571.

75. Goetz CG, Stebbins GT. Risk factors for nursing home placement in advanced Parkinson's disease. *Neurology* 1993;43: 2227–2229.

76. Marder K, Tang MX, Cote L, Stern Y, Mayeux R. The frequency and associated risk factors for dementia in patients with Parkinson's disease. *Arch Neurol* 1995;52:695–701.

77. Emre M. Dementia associated with Parkinson's disease. *Lancet Neurol* 2003;2:229–237.
78. Aarsland D, Laake K, Larsen JP, Janvin C. Donepezil for cognitive impairment in Parkinson's disease: a randomised controlled study. *J Neurol Neurosurg Psychiatry* 2002;72:708–712.
79. Emre M, Aarsland D, Albanese A, Byrne EJ, Deuschl G, De Deyn PP, et al. Rivastigmine for dementia associated with Parkinson's disease. *N Engl J Med* 2004;351:2509–2518.
80. Leroi I, Brandt J, Reich SG, Lyketsos CG, et al. Randomized placebo-controlled trial of donepezil in cognitive impairment in Parkinson's disease. *Int J Geriatr Psychiatry* 2004;19:1–8.
81. Rascol O, Brooks DJ, Korczyn AD, De Deyn PP, Clarke CE, Lang AE, for the 056 Study Group. A five-year study of the incidence of dyskinesia in patients with Parkinson's disease who were treated with ropinirole or levodopa. *N Engl J Med* 2000;18: 1481–1491.
82. Fenelon G, Mahieux F, Huon R, Ziegler M. Hallucinations in Parkinson's disease: prevalence, phenomenology and risk factors. *Brain* 2000;123:733–745.
83. Goetz CG, Vogel C, Tanner CM, Stebbins GT. Early dopaminergic drug-induced hallucinations in parkinsonian patients. *Neurology* 1998;51:811–814.
84. Parkinson Study Group. Pramipexole vs. levodopa as initial treatment for Parkinson disease: a randomized controlled trial. *JAMA* 2000;284:1931–1938.
85. Poewe W. Psychosis in Parkinson's disease. *Mov Disord* 2003;18 (suppl 6):S80–S87.
86. Parkinson Study Group. Low-dose clozapine for the treatment of drug-induced psychosis in Parkinson's disease. *N Engl J Med* 1999;340:757–763.
87. French Clozapine Parkinson Study Group. Clozapine in drug-induced psychosis in Parkinson's disease. *Lancet* 1999;353:2041.
88. Factor SA, Friedman JH, Lannon MC, Oakes D, Bourgeois K, and the Parkinson Study Group. Clozapine for the treatment of drug-induced psychosis in Parkinson's disease: results of the 12 week open label extension in the PSYCLOPS trial. *Mov Disord* 2001;16: 135–139.
89. Honigfeld G, Arellano F, Sethi J, Bianchini A, Schein J. Reducing clozapine-related morbidity and mortality: 5 years of experience with the Clozaril National Registry. *J Clin Psychiatry* 1998;59:3–7.
90. Ondo W, Levy J, Vuong K, Hunter C, Jankovic J. Olanzapine treatment for dopaminergic-induced hallucinations. *Mov Disord* 2002;17:1031–1035.
91. Breier A, Sutton V, Feldman P, et al. Olanzapine in the treatment of dopaminetic-induced psychosis in patients with Parkinson's disease. *Biol Psychiatry* 2002;52:438–445.
92. Goetz C, Blasucci L, Leurgans S, Pappert E. Olanzapine and clozapine: comparative effects on motor function in hallucinating PD patients. *Neurology* 2000;55:748–749.
93. Fernandez H, Friedman J, Jacques C, and Rosenfeld M. Quetiapine for the treatment of drug-induced psychosis in Parkinson's disease. *Mov Disord* 1999;14:484–487.
94. Ondo WG, Tintner R, Voung KD, Lai D, Ringholz G. Double bind, placebo-controlled, unforced titration parallel trial of quetiapine for dopaminergic-induced hallucinatosis in Parkinson's disease. *Mov Disord* 2005;20:958–963.
95. Fernandez HH, Trieschmann ME, Burke MA, Jacques C, Friedman JH. Long-term outcome of quetiapine use for psychosis among Parkinsonian patients. *Mov Disord* 2003;18:510–514.
96. Juncos JL, Roberts VJ, Evatt ML, Jewart RD, Wood CD, Potter LS, Jou HC, Yeung PP. Quetiapine improves psychotic symptoms and cognition in Parkinson's disease. *Mov Disord* 2004;19: 29–35.
97. Reading P, Luce A, McKeith I. Rivastigmine in the treatment of parkinsonian psychosis and cognitive impairment. *Mov Disord* 2001;16:1171–1174.
98. Bullock R, Cameron A. Rivastigmine for the treatment of dementia and visual hallucinations associated with Parkinson's disease: a case series. *Curr Med Res Opin* 2002;18:258–264.
99. Fabbrini G, Barbanti P, Aurilia C, Pauletti C, Lenzi GL, Meco G. Donepezil in the treatment of hallucinations and delusions in Parkinson's disease. *Neurol Sci* 2002;23:41–43.
100. Bergmann J, Lerner V. Successful use of donepezil for the treatment of psychotic symptoms in patients with Parkinson's disease. *Clin Neuropharmacol* 2002;25:107–110.
101. Tandberg E, Larsen JP, Karlsen K. A community-based study of sleep disorders in patients with Parkinson's disease. *Mov Disord* 1998;13:895–899.
102. Poewe W, Högl B. Akathisia, restless legs and periodic limb movements in sleep in Parkinson's disease. *Neurology* 2004;63 (suppl 3):12–16.
103. Schenck CH, Bundlie SR, Ettinger MG, Mahowald MW. Chronic behavioral disorders of human REM sleep: a new category of parasomnia. *Sleep* 1986;9:293–308.
104. Comella CL, Nardine TM, Diederich NJ, Stebbins GT. Sleep-related violence, injury, and REM sleep behaviour disorder in Parkinson's disease. *Neurology* 1998;51:526–529.
105. Gangnon JF, Bedard MA, Tantini ML, et al. REM sleep behaviour disorder and REM sleep without atonia in Parkinson's disease. *Neurology* 2002;59:585–589.
106. Wetter TC, Trenkwalder C, Gershanik O, Högl B. Polysomnographic measures in Parkinson's disease: a comparison between patients with and without REM sleep disturbances. *Wien Klin Wochenschr* 2001;113:2249–2253.
107. Olson EJ, Boeve BF, Silber MH. Rapid eye movement sleep behaviour disorder: demographic, clinical and laboratory findings in 93 cases. *Brain* 2000;123:331–339.
108. Schenck CH, Bundlie SR, Mahowald MW. Delayed emergence of a parkinsonian disorder in 38% of 29 older men initially diagnosed with idiopathic rapid eye movement sleep behavior disorder. *Neurology* 1996;46:388–393.
109. Boeve BF, Silber MH, Ferman TJ, et al. REM sleep behavior disorder and degenerative dementia: an association likely reflecting Lewy body disease. *Neurology* 1998;51:363–370.
110. Schenck CH, Callies AL, Mahowald MW. Increased percentage of slow-wave sleep in REM sleep behavior disorder (RBD): a reanalysis of previously published data from a controlled study of RBD reported in SLEEP. *Sleep* 2003;26:1066.
111. Albin RL, Koeppe RA, Chervin RD, et al. Decreased striatal dopaminergic innervation in REM sleep behavior disorder. *Neurology* 2000;55:1410–1412.
112. Eisensehr I, Linke R, Noachtar S, et al. Reduced striatal dopamine transporters in idiopathic rapid eye movement sleep behaviour disorder: comparison with Parkinson's disease and controls. *Brain* 2000;123:1155–1160.
113. Arnulf I, Bonnet AM, Damier P, et al. Hallucinations, REM sleep, and Parkinson's disease: a medical hypothesis. *Neurology* 2001;57:1350–1351.
114. Frucht S, Rogers JD, Greene PE, et al. Falling asleep at the wheel: motor vehicle mishaps in persons taking pramipexole and ropinirole. *Neurology* 1999;52:1908–1910.
115. Hobson DE, Lang AE, Martin WR, Razmy A, Rivest J, Fleming J. Excessive daytime sleepiness and sudden-onset sleep in Parkinson's disease: a survey by the Canadian Movement Disorders Group. *JAMA* 2002;287:455–463.
116. Högl B, Saletu M, Brandauer E, Glatzl S, Frauscher B, Seppi K, Ulmer H, Wenning G, Poewe W. Modafinil for the treatment of daytime sleepiness in Parkinson's disease: a double-blind, randomized, crossover, placebo-controlled polygraphic trial. *Sleep* 2002;25:905–909.
117. Brodsky MA, Godbold J, Roth T, Olanow CW. Sleepiness in Parkinson's disease: a controlled study. *Mov Disord* 2003;18: 668–672.
118. Paus S, Brecht HM, Koster J, Seeger G, Klockgether T, Wullner U. Sleep attacks, daytime sleepiness, and dopamine agonists in Parkinson's disease. *Mov Disord* 2003;18:659–667.

7

Etiology and Pathogenesis of Parkinson's Disease

Serge Przedborski

Parkinson's disease (PD) is a common adult-onset neurodegenerative disorder whose disabling cardinal motor signs are mainly engendered by the loss of dopaminergic neurons in the substantia nigra. To date, researchers still have a limited understanding of the key molecular events that provoke neurodegeneration in this disease. A prevalent etiologic hypothesis is that PD may result from a complex interaction between environmental toxic factors, genetic susceptibility traits, and aging. As for its pathogenesis, the discovery of PD genes has led to the hypothesis that misfolding of proteins and dysfunction of the ubiquitin-proteasome pathway may be pivotal in the cascade of deleterious events underlying the demise of dopaminergic neurons. Previously implicated culprits in PD neurodegeneration, such as mitochondrial dysfunction, oxidative stress, and inflammation, may also produce deleterious effects on dopaminergic neurons. This chapter discusses the evidence and the ongoing lines of research relevant to the quest of unraveling the cause and mechanism of neuronal death in PD.

DEFINITION AND DIAGNOSTIC CONSIDERATIONS

Over the past decade, PD has garnered widespread interest, in part because several public figures and celebrities were identified as having this illness. PD is considered to be the second most common degenerative disorder of the aging brain after the dementia of Alzheimer's. In keeping with this, it is estimated that currently more than a million individuals are affected with PD in the United States alone, and, with the aging character of the society, this figure is forecasted to rise dramatically over the coming years. The overall incidence of PD in the United States (which surges upward after the age of 60) is roughly 13.4 per 100,000 people/year (1), and it is approximately twice as frequent in men than in age-matched women (1). Whether PD frequency varies among ethnic groups or geographic location remains an unsettled issue (1).

PD is progressive with a mean age at onset of 55. Although the introduction of effective symptomatic treatment such as levodopa has prolonged survival, PD patients, especially with severe parkinsonism or dementia (2), still exhibit a higher mortality risk compared to healthy controls (3). The mean disease duration of PD, as defined by the period between onset of the clinical manifestations to death, has been estimated to be 10.1 to 12.8 years (4,5). It remains uncertain whether the observed shortened life expectancy of PD patients results from the disease per se or rather from the ensuing motor and cognitive impairments, which increase the odds of fatal accidental falling, aspiration pneumonia, pressure skin ulcers, malnutrition, and dehydration. Relevant to this point is the finding that twice as many PD patients die from pneumonia as in the age-matched control population (4). This is more than a parochial discussion of semantics, as it goes to the heart of how to best care for PD patients.

As illustrated in Figure 7.1, the main neuropathological feature of PD is the loss of neuromelanin-containing dopaminergic neurons of the nigrostriatal pathway (6),

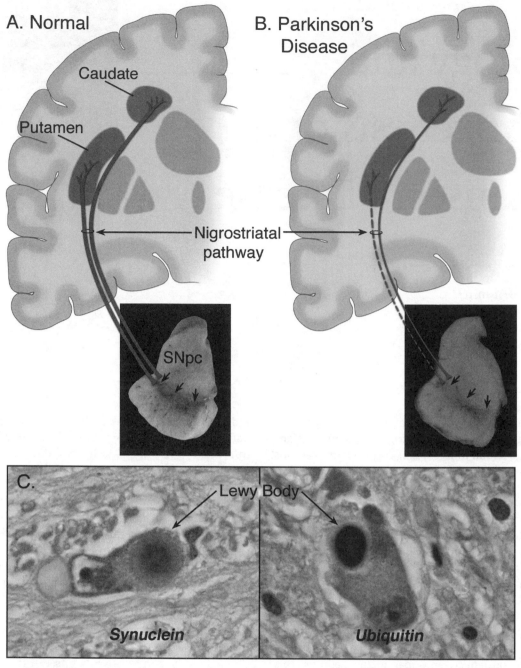

Figure 7.1 Neuropathology of Parkinson's disease (PD). **A:** Schematic representation of the normal nigrostriatal pathway (*in dark grey*). It is composed of dopaminergic neurons whose cell bodies are located in the substantia nigra pars compacta (SNpc; *see arrows*). These neurons project (*thick solid grey lines*) to the basal ganglia and synapse in the striatum (i.e., putamen and caudate nucleus). The photograph demonstrates the normal pigmentation of the SNpc produced by neuromelanin within the dopaminergic neurons. **B:** Schematic representation of the diseased nigrostriatal pathway (*in dark grey*). In PD, the nigrostriatal pathway degenerates. There is a marked loss of dopaminergic neurons that project to the putamen (*dashed line*) and a much more modest loss of those that project to the caudate (*thin grey solid line*). The photograph demonstrates depigmentation (i.e., loss of dark pigment neuromelanin; arrows) of the SNpc due to the marked loss of dopaminergic neurons. **C:** Immunohistochemical labeling of intraneuronal inclusions (Lewy bodies) in an SNpc dopaminergic neuron. Immunostaining with an antibody against alpha-synuclein reveals a Lewy body (*black arrow*) with an intensely immunoreactive central zone surrounded by a faintly immunoreactive peripheral zone (*left photograph*). Conversely, immunostaining with an antibody against ubiquitin yields more diffuse immunoreactivity within the Lewy body (*right photograph*). (Dauer W, Przedborski S. Parkinson's disease: mechanisms and models. *Neuron* 2003; 39:889–909, with permission.)

which, in depleting the brain of dopamine (7), leads to the emergence of motor abnormalities such as tremor at rest, rigidity, slowness of voluntary movement, and postural instability (8). By the time patients become symptomatic, however, ~60% of nigral dopaminergic neurons have been lost and striatal content in dopamine has been reduced by ~80%. It can thus be concluded that disease onset predates the expression of the motor manifestations of PD, which by ^{18}F-fluorodeoxyglucose with positron emission tomography (PET) has been estimated to be about 4.5 years (9). In addition to demonstrating that the presymptomatic period of PD appears to be relatively short, this PET study also documented that the pattern of glucose metabolic alterations in PD is not consistent with the idea that neurodegeneration in this illness is a simple exacerbation of the normal age-related decay of the nigrostriatal dopaminergic system (9). Although the lion's share of attention is consistently paid to the nigrostriatal pathway, it must be remembered that in reality degenerative changes in PD are not restricted to the nigrostriatal pathway and that neuropathological findings can be found in many other dopaminergic and nondopaminergic cell groups, including the locus coeruleus, raphe nuclei, and nucleus basalis of Meynert (10). This is a particularly important notion with respect to the proper management of PD, as some quite disabling features, especially in advanced patients, such as postural instability and cognitive impairment, may not find their pathophysiology in the damage of the dopaminergic system and usually fail to improve with levodopa therapy.

Also important is the fact that more than 30 different neurological syndromes share PD clinical features (Table 7.1). Thus, a definite diagnosis of PD often is achieved only at autopsy and customarily relies not only on finding a loss of nigrostriatal dopaminergic neurons but also on the identification of intraneuronal inclusions, or Lewy bodies, that can be seen in many of the surviving cells of all affected brain regions (Fig. 7.1). Lewy bodies are spherical eosinophilic cytoplasmic aggregates of fibrillary nature that, as illustrated in Figure 7.1, are composed of a variety of proteins, including alpha-synuclein, parkin, ubiquitin, and neurofilaments (11,12). Many authorities, however, question whether identification of Lewy bodies should still be necessary for the diagnosis of PD, in light of the fact that cases of inherited PD linked to parkin mutations typically lack Lewy bodies and are still considered as cases of PD. These facts raise the question as to whether the current nosology of parkinsonian syndromes may not have to be revised to distance itself from the classification typically based on the disease's clinical and neuropathological hallmarks, to evolve toward a classification based on the disease's molecular characteristics. Conceivably, in this novel approach, parkinsonian syndromes that used to belong to distinct categories may become grouped together because of a common molecular defect. Although the usefulness of such a proposed recasting would have to be demonstrated,

TABLE 7.1
PARKINSONIAN SYNDROMES

Primary Parkinsonism
    Parkinson's disease (sporadic, familial)

Secondary Parkinsonism
    Drug-induced: dopamine antagonists and depletors
    Hemiatrophy–hemiparkinsonism
    Hydrocephalus: normal-pressure hydrocephalus
    Hypoxia
    Infectious: postencephalitic
    Metabolic: parathyroid dysfunction
    Toxin: Mn, CO, MPTP, cyanide
    Trauma
    Tumor
    Vascular: multiinfarct state

Parkinson-Plus Syndromes
    Cortical-basal ganglionic degeneration
    Dementia syndromes: Alzheimer's disease, diffuse Lewy-body disease, frontotemporal dementia
    Lytico-Bodig (Guamanian Parkinsonism–dementia–ALS)
    Multiple system atrophy syndromes: striatonigral degeneration, Shy-Drager syndrome, sporadic OPCA, motor neuron disease–parkinsonism
    Progressive pallidal atrophy
    Progressive supranuclear palsy

Familial Neurodegenerative Diseases
    Hallervorden-Spatz disease
    Huntington's disease
    Lubag (X-linked dystonia–parkinsonism)
    Mitochondrial cytopathies with striatal necrosis
    Neuroacanthocytosis
    Wilson's disease

ALS, amyotrophic lateral sclerosis; CO, carbon monoxide; Mn, manganese; MPTP, 1-methyl-4-phenyl-1,2,3,6-tetrahydropyridine; olivopontocerebellar degeneration, OPCA.
Source: From Dauer W, Przedborski S. Parkinson's disease: mechanisms and models. *Neuron* 2003;39:889–909, with permission.

the idea deserves, at the very least, serious consideration as the issue of diagnostic heterogeneity is a well-recognized hurdle for clinical trials geared toward testing neuroprotective agents for PD.

ETIOLOGIC THEORIES OF SPORADIC PARKINSON'S DISEASE

The etiology of almost all occurrences of PD remains unknown. In more than 90% of the cases, PD arises as a sporadic condition, i.e., in the absence of any apparent genetic linkage, but in the remaining instances the disease is unquestionably inherited (Table 7.2). Nonetheless, first-degree relatives of sporadic PD patients are two to three times more likely to have PD than relatives of controls (13). It is therefore not surprising that until now, all of the hypotheses regarding the etiology of sporadic PD have been focused primarily on environmental toxins and genetic factors. As pointed out by Tanner et al. in the previous edition of this chapter (14), the precept about the etiology of PD has for a long time been that a single or, at most, a few genes or environmental factors are sufficient to cause PD in most individuals and that both genetic and environmental risk would operate *independently*. The current school of thought, however, proposes a more multifactorial view of the problem by which diseases such as PD would result from a complex interplay of genetic and environmental factors. Based on this scenario, even in the presence of a known single-gene pathogenic mutation, PD would arise only when both the genetic variant and the deleterious environmental exposure coincide. In this context, a genetic variation would not necessarily cause disease but rather would influence a person's susceptibility to environmental factors. Hence, a person may not inherit the disease state per se but rather a set of susceptibility traits to certain environmental factors placing that person at higher risk of developing PD.

ENVIRONMENTAL TOXINS

According to the *environmental hypothesis*, PD-related neurodegeneration is provoked by exposure to a dopaminergic neurotoxin. The progressive nature of the neurodegeneration of PD would either result from a persistent toxic exposure that causes a sustained insult or from a circumscribed toxic exposure that initiates a self-perpetuating cascade of deleterious events. Relevant to the environmental hypothesis are numerous human epidemiological studies that have implicated consumption of well water, residence in a rural setting, farming and its associated exposure to herbicides and pesticides with an elevated risk for PD. These epidemiological notions have been reviewed comprehensively by Tanner et al. in the previous edition of this chapter (14), and will thus not be rehashed. Instead, only selected and recent epidemiology data will be discussed in the following pages.

From the outset it is stressed that none of the epidemiological studies to date have convincingly linked a specific environmental toxin to the cause of sporadic PD. Nevertheless, cigarette smoking and coffee drinking are inversely associated with PD (15), reinforcing the concept that environmental factors may indeed contribute to PD susceptibility or etiology. It is thus plausible that the lack of compelling evidence incriminating specific environmental factors simply reflects the limitations of our current analytic methodologies. Moreover, there are several known parkinsonian neurotoxins that potentially could be accumulating in our environment. For instance, exposure to 1-methyl-4-phenyl-1,2,3,6-tetrahydropyridine (MPTP), a by-product of 1-methyl-4-phenyl-4-propionoxypiperidine synthesis (16), causes a clinical condition in humans (17) and several other mammalian species almost identical to PD. Although autopsy studies of MPTP-intoxicated individuals with parkinsonism have consistently demonstrated

a profound degeneration of the nigrostriatal dopaminergic pathway, no Lewy body has ever been found in these post-mortem brain samples (18,19). Moreover, despite the impressive resemblance between PD and MPTP intoxication, MPTP has never been recovered from brain tissues or body fluids of PD patients.

Another potential environmental toxin is 1-methyl-4-phenylpyridinium (MPP$^+$), the active metabolite of MPTP, which has been developed as Cyperquat™, an herbicide (never commercialized), and paraquat, both of which are structurally similar (Fig. 7.2). Both MPP$^+$ and paraquat are polar molecules and consequently do not passively cross the blood–brain barrier (BBB). Of these two toxins, only for paraquat was an active transport system at the level of the BBB been identified (20), making it possible at least for the latter to accumulate in the brain and inflict damage. Consistent with this view is the demonstration that systemic administration of paraquat to rodents is associated with the degeneration of nigrostriatal neurons and the formation of Lewy body-like inclusions (21). Chronic exposure to paraquat has also been associated in a case-controlled study in Taiwan with an increased risk of developing PD (22). Interestingly, as noted by Thiruchelvam et al. (23), manganese ethylenebisthiocarbamate shows a striking geographic overlap with paraquat and has been implicated in cases of PD-like syndrome in agricultural workers, and it seems to exacerbate the dopaminergic neurotoxicity of paraquat. If paraquat were to be an environmental toxicant implicated in PD, the latter observation suggests that one should probably not think of the contribution of an environmental insult to the cause of PD in terms of a single toxin but rather in terms of

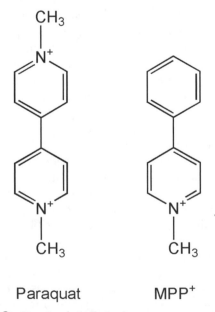

Figure 7.2 Structural similarity between paraquat (*left*) and MPP$^+$ (*right*). The only difference between these two compounds is the second N-methyl-pyridium group that paraquat has instead of the phenyl group seen in MPP$^+$.

a combination of toxic agents such as paraquat, manganese ethylenebisthiocarbamate, and possibly others.

What about rotenone as an environmental culprit? Rotenone is the most potent member of the rotenoids, a family of natural cytotoxic compounds extracted from various parts of *Leguminosa* plants. Like MPP$^+$, rotenone is a mitochondrial poison that is present in the environment and abundantly used around the world as insecticide and piscicide used to kill unwanted lake fish (24). Although rats chronically intoxicated with rotenone display nigrostriatal damage with Lewy body-like inclusions (25), it is unlikely to cause PD because rotenone is unstable, lasting only a few days in the environment (24). Indeed, rotenone breaks down readily by exposure to sunlight. Nearly all the toxicity of the compound is lost in 5 to 6 days of spring sunlight or 2 to 3 days of summer sunlight. Rotenone is also broken down rapidly in soil and in water. Also arguing against an etiologic role of rotenone in PD is the demonstration that chronic ingestion of rotenone for 24 months at doses 30 times greater that used to model PD by systemic infusion (25) failed to cause any behavioral or neuropathological features of the disease in rats (26). Nevertheless, there is one case of fatal rotenone poisoning following its acute ingestion (26). At autopsy, rotenone was found in the blood, liver, and kidney but not in the brain.

Another possibility, which does not, in the strict sense of the word, fall into the environmental category, is that an endogenous toxin may be responsible for PD neurodegeneration. As discussed elsewhere (27), distortions of normal metabolism might create toxic substances because of environmental exposures or inherited differences in metabolic pathways. One obvious source of endogenous toxins may be the metabolism of dopamine, which may generate harmful reactive oxygen species (ROS) (28). Consistent with the endogenous toxin hypothesis is the report that patients harboring specific polymorphisms in the gene encoding for the xenobiotic detoxifying enzyme cytochrome P450 may be at greater risk of developing young-onset PD (29). Further, isoquinoline derivatives and 6-hydroxydopamine, which are both toxic to dopamine neurons, have been recovered respectively from the brain (30) and urine of PD patients (31). Yet the link between polymorphisms in the xenobiotic-metabolizing enzymes and risk of PD remains equivocal, and a comprehensive discussion on this important topic can be found in Paolini et al. (32). From the preceding discussion, it can be concluded that, at this point, the environmental hypothesis of PD remains highly speculative but by no means negligible.

MITOCHONDRIAL GENETICS AND PARKINSON'S DISEASE

For several decades, a mitochondrial defect has been proposed as an etiologic factor in PD, but when one scrutinizes the available evidence it appears that this appealing notion is nothing more than presumptive. For instance, all mitochondrial DNA of a zygote originate from the ovum, thus it is traditionally viewed that diseases linked to mitochondrial mutations are maternally inherited. To date, it is true that some epidemiological evidence supports a maternal inheritance pattern in a subset of PD patients (33,34). Furthermore, polymorphisms in subunits of complex I of the electron transport chain have been proposed as susceptibility genes in subgroups of PD patients (35,36). Although thus far true cases of PD linked to a mitochondrial mutation are still lacking, it should be mentioned that a point mutation (A1555G) in the 12SrRNA gene has been implicated in a maternally inherited deafness associated with levodopa-responsive parkinsonism (37). Subsequently, a distinct heteroplasmic, maternally inherited 12SrRNA point mutation (T1095C) was found in another pedigree with sensorineural deafness, levodopa-responsive parkinsonism, and neuropathy (38). These mutation were not found, however, in 20 cases of sporadic PD, suggesting that the 12SrRNA mutations are not likely to be a common cause of PD. It can thus be concluded that current data supporting the mitochondrial genetic hypothesis of PD etiology are only circumstantial and indirect. That said, mitochondrial alterations may still be instrumental in both the etiology and pathogenesis of PD (see the following) through molecular defects other than a mitochondrial mutation.

PARKINSON'S DISEASE MENDELIAN GENETICS

Since the discovery in 1997 that missense mutations in alpha-synuclein cause a rare form of PD, there has been a resurgence of interest in genetic factors that contribute to the etiology of the disease. Since mutations in parkin, ubiquitin C-terminal hydrolase L1 (UCH-L1), DJ-1, PINK1, and LRRK2/dardarin have also been identified as causes of familial forms of PD (see the following), and linkages for a number of other kindreds have been identified (Table 7.2). In addition to their detection in familial PD, mutations in parkin and LRRK2 were also found in a number of patients without apparent family history for PD (39,40). Moreover, large-scale genetic epidemiological studies have revealed a single-nucleotide polymorphism in tau to be associated with PD susceptibility (41), and both apolipoprotein E and probably more than one gene on chromosome 1p have been reported to influence age at onset for PD (42,43). Heterozygosity for a mutation in the glucocerebrosidase gene may also predispose to PD (44).

Worth noting is the fact that studies of monozygotic twins demonstrated a lack of concordance for PD, and thus this finding has been frequently cited as evidence arguing against a strong genetic contribution to sporadic PD (45). Yet, the interpretation of twin studies in PD is often complicated by the fact that twins may be clinically discordant for PD for up to 20 years (46). Moreover, a study utilizing

TABLE 7.2

GENES AND LOCI LINKED TO FAMILIAL PARKINSON'S DISEASE

Locus	Chromosomal Location	Gene/ Protein	Inheritance	Atypical PD Features	Lewy Bodies
PARK1	4q21	α-synuclein*	AD	Early onset Lower prevalence of tremor	Yes
PARK2	6q25.2–q27	Parkin	AR	Early juvenile onset More frequent dystonia and levodopa-induced dyskinesias Slower disease progression	Mostly negative#
PARK3	2p13	Unknown	AD	Dementia in some patients Rapid progression	Yes
PARK4†	4p15	Unknown	AD	Early onset Rapid progression Dementia Autonomic dysfunction Postural tremor	Yes
PARK5	4p14	UCH-L1	AD	None	Unknown
PARK6	1p36	PINK1	AR	Early onset Slow progression	Unknown
PARK7	1p36	DJ-1	AR	Early onset Psychiatric symptoms Slow progression	Unknown
PARK8	12p11.2–q13.1	LRRK2/dardarin	AD	None	Some
PARK9	1p36	Unknown	AR	Juvenile onset Spasticity Supranuclear gaze paralysis Dementia	Unknown

AD, autosomal dominant; AR, autosomal recessive. * Including mutations and wild-type multiplications. # Lewy bodies reported in one patient with parkin mutations (64). †The initial PARK4 linkage to 4p15 could not be confirmed, and the PD phenotype in this family was subsequently linked to a PARK1 variant, i.e., alpha-synuclein triplication (56).
Source: Vila M, Przedborski S. Genetic clues to the pathogenesis of Parkinson's disease. *Nat Med* 2004;10(suppl):S58–S62, with permission.

[18]F-fluorodopa with PET to investigate the dopaminergic function in twin pairs clinically discordant for PD found significantly greater concordance for monozygotic but not dizygotic twins (47). These observations emphasize the need to utilize functional imaging to identify patients with subclinical disease in such studies and suggest that the actual contribution of genetic factors to the cause of PD may be more significant than thought initially.

α-Synuclein Mutations and Overexpression

Three missense mutations (A53T, A30P, E46K) in the α-synuclein gene are linked to a dominantly inherited PD (48–50). Clinical and pathological features typical of PD have been found in patients with any of the three mutations, although some atypical features have also been noted (49,51). Conversely, α-synuclein mutations have not been found in sporadic PD (52). Therefore, the idea that mutant α-synuclein and sporadic PD share common

pathogenic mechanisms relies predominantly on the observation that alpha-synuclein is a major component of Lewy bodies in sporadic PD (53). Transgenic overexpression of mutant α-synuclein in mice or flies has been generally associated with the development of some of the neuropathological features of PD, such as intraneuronal proteinaceous inclusions (27). These studies, together with the finding that alpha-synuclein ablation in mice does not lead to neurodegeneration (54,55), support the concept that α-synuclein mutations operate by a toxic gain-of-function mechanism.

Remarkably, multiplication of the gene encoding for wild-type α-synuclein can also cause an autosomal dominant PD phenotype (56–58). An important finding that has emerged from these studies is that relatively small alterations in α-synuclein expression can have marked impacts on the disease phenotype. In the study by Chartier-Harlin et al. (57), individuals with alpha-synuclein gene duplication had a mean age of onset of 48 years, with a disease duration of approximately 17 years. Similarly, in the study by Ibáñez and collaborators (58), both patients with the duplication mutation had onsets of the disease at ages 46 and 50. Conversely, in the report by Singleton et al. (56), affected individuals carried four copies of the α-synuclein gene and developed a rapidly progressive (mean duration: 8 years) and young-onset form of PD (mean age: 38 years). It thus seems that the higher the expression level of α-synuclein, the more malignant the PD phenotype. The fact that increased amounts of wild-type α-synuclein can cause PD also advocates for the idea that the cytotoxic function gained by mutant α-synuclein proteins is not a newly acquired property but rather the enhancement of a native property. However, the nature of the gained function is still enigmatic, in part because the normal function of alpha-synuclein is just beginning to be elucidated. The fact that this prevalent presynaptic protein is abundant in Lewy bodies prompted many investigators to believe that its propensity to misfold and form α-synuclein fibrils may be responsible for its neurotoxicity. More can be read about the hypothesized toxic mechanisms of alpha-synuclein in Dauer et al. (27) and Vila et al. (59).

Parkin Mutations

Loss-of-function mutations in the gene encoding parkin cause recessively inherited parkinsonism (60). Although this form of parkinsonism was originally termed *autosomal recessive juvenile parkinsonism*, the clinical phenotype includes a man with onset at age 64 and other older-onset patients. In general, however, parkin mutations are found in PD patients with onset before age 30, particularly those with a family history consistent with recessive inheritance (61). Clinically, parkin mutant patients display the classic signs of parkinsonism but with marked improvement of symptoms with sleep, abnormal dystonic movements, and a striking response to levodopa. Heterozygote mutations in parkin may also lead to dopaminergic dysfunction and later onset of parkinsonism, consistent with a mechanism of haploinsufficiency (62,63). Pathologically, parkin-related PD is characterized by loss of substantia nigra pars compacta (SNpc) dopaminergic neurons, but it is not typically associated with Lewy bodies (61), in that Lewy bodies were definitely identified in only a single patient harboring a parkin mutation (64). Unexpectedly, attempts to recapitulate parkin loss of function in mice and flies have not succeeded in producing a conclusive PD phenotype (65–67). Nevertheless, those engineered animals are not completely normal, as they appear to exhibit mitochondrial defects (66–68), suggestive of those described in sporadic PD (27).

To date, it is uncertain how parkin mutations lead to dopaminergic neuron degeneration, but one clue has emerged from the identification of its normal function, which is E3 ubiquitin ligase (69,70), a component of the ubiquitin-proteasome system. The way E3 ligases work is by conferring target specificity through their capacity

of binding to specific molecules or classes of molecules, thereby facilitating the polyubiquitination necessary for targeting to the proteasome. Since many parkin mutations abolish its E3 ligase activity, it is suggested that the accumulation of misfolded parkin substrates could be responsible for the demise of SNpc dopaminergic neurons in PD. Several investigations highlight the multiplicity of parkin substrates and how these might play a key role in neuronal death (27). However, none of the identified parkin substrates appear specifically enriched in dopaminergic neurons. Also noteworthy is the lack of Lewy bodies in most PD patients carrying parkin null mutations (71), suggesting that parkin E3 ligase activity might be needed for Lewy body formation.

Ubiquitin C-Terminal Hydrolase-L1 Mutation/Polymorphism

This enzyme is ubiquitously expressed in the brain and catalyzes the hydrolysis of C-terminal ubiquityl esters; it is thought to participate in recycling ubiquitin ligated to misfolded proteins after their degradation by the proteasome. A single dominant mutation (I93M) in ubiquitin C-terminal hydrolase-L1 (UCH-L1) has been linked with the development of an inherited form of PD (72). Although this I93M mutation presumably decreases UCH-L1 hydrolase activity, most experts still doubt that a loss of UCH-L1 function could generate a PD phenotype mainly because mice carrying a UCH-L1 null mutation do display dramatic foci of neurodegeneration in the nervous system, but without any evidence of dopaminergic pathology (73). Contrasting with the controversial deleterious role of UCH-L1 193M, several studies have raised the prospect that a polymorphism (S18Y) in UCH-L1 could reduce the risk of developing PD, especially among young individuals (74). However, at this point none of the findings relative to UCH-L1 as either an etiologic or a risk factor in PD have received widespread acceptance, and the current consensus is that much work has to be done to clarify the possible involvement of UCH-L1 in PD.

DJ-1 Mutations

DJ-1 is a homodimeric, multifunctional protein ubiquitously expressed in human tissues, including the brain. Thus far, at least 11 different DJ-1 mutations, including missense, truncating, splice-site mutations and large deletions, have been linked to an autosomal recessive form of PD (75–77). Although DJ-1 mutations account for a small fraction of familial PD, it is now recommended to systematically screen for DJ-1 mutations in all cases of recessively inherited early-onset forms of the disease (78). These mutations are found throughout the four of the seven exons of the DJ-1 gene. Although little is known about the function of DJ-1, it is predicted that many, if not all of the identified mutations, would cause either a lack of DJ-1 expression or the transcription of an unstable and functionally deficient product.

Cells lacking DJ-1 have been reported to be more susceptible to a variety of stresses, including oxidative attack. These findings prompted researchers to propose that DJ-1 protects cells through some kind of antioxidant effect. However, whether this is indeed the case is still a matter of intense investigation. Structural studies also indicate that DJ-1 shares similarities with the bacterial heat shock protein Hsp31 a stress-inducible chaperone (79). In keeping with this observation is the demonstration that wild-type DJ-1 does exhibit chaperone activity (80). However, this Hsp31-like activity is not detectable when DJ-1 is in reducing conditions (which mimics the physiological intracellular environment) but is detectable when in oxidative conditions (which mimics an oxidative stress situation) (80). Furthermore, the PD-associated DJ-1 mutation L166M abolishes this redox-dependent chaperone activity (80). Collectively, these data are consistent with the emerging idea that wild-type DJ-1 functions as a redox-dependent chaperone that in response to intracellular oxidative stress becomes activated to assist the cell in coping with the rising amount of oxidatively damaged, misfolded proteins.

PINK-1 Mutations

Autozygosity mapping of a large consanguineous Sicilian family located the PARK6 locus linked to an autosomal recessive form of PD to chromosome 1p35–36 (81). PARK6 was then linked to an early-onset recessive PD in 8 additional families from 4 different European countries (82). By sequencing candidate genes within the PARK6 region in affected members from each family, two homozygous mutations were found in the PTEN-induced putative kinase 1 (PINK1)/BRPK gene (83). Several additional PINK1 mutations linked to PD have been reported subsequently (84,85). Although most data regarding PINK1 mutations argue for the mutant protein to exert its deleterious effects by a loss of function, reduced striatal ^{18}F flurodopa uptake found by PET in asymptomatic PARK6 heterozygote subjects raises the possibility that PINK1 mutations may in fact operate by haploinsufficiency or by a dominant negative effect (86).

To date, little is known about how mutant PINK1 could kill cells. The rare available data dealing with this question indicate that neuroblastoma cells transiently transfected with either wild-type or mutant PINK1 do not exhibit any impairment in viability (83). However, if neuroblastomas are challenged with a proteasome inhibitor such as MG132, neuroblastomas engineered to express high amounts of wild-type PINK1 resist the cytotoxicity of this drug, whereas neuroblastomas engineered to express high amounts of mutant PINK1 die (83). These results suggest that the loss of PINK1 function may render dopaminergic neurons more vulnerable to injury. In adult mice, PINK1 is ubiquitously expressed among tissues with an apparently high

expression in the brain (87). Both human and mouse PINK1 possess a serine/threonine kinase domain as the sole known functional domain (87,88). Presumably PINK1 also has a mitochondrial targeting motif consistent with the observation that it localizes to the mitochondria in transfected cell lines (83). Of the two initially identified mutations, one is a missense mutation (G309D) in the putative kinase domain, while the second is a nonsense mutation (W437OPA) truncating the last 145 amino acids of the C-terminus of the kinase domain (83). Both of these mutations are expected to impair PINK1 kinase activity or substrate recognition. However, with the subsequently identified PINK1 mutations (84,85), it can now be concluded that most but not all known PD-causing PINK1 mutations are predicted to alter its kinase activity, a fact that casts doubts on a defect in PINK-1-mediated phosphorylation truly being the deleterious mechanism by which this mutant protein provokes neurodegeneration.

LRRK2/Dardarin Mutations

PARK8 locus linked to families with autosomal-dominant, late-onset parkinsonism has been located to chromosome 12p11.2–q13.1 (89). The subsequent sequencing of 29 genes within the PARK8 region revealed 5 missense mutations and 1 putative splice-site mutation in a gene encoding a large, multifunctional protein: leucine-rich repeat kinase 2 (LRRK2) (90) or dardarin (91). LRRK2/dardarin missense mutations were also found in 5 PD families of different origin (91). In both studies, the identified mutations segregated with disease and affected individuals were heterozygous for the mutation. Whether the Japanese Sagamihara kindred, in which the PARK8 linkage was initially identified (89), carries one of the identified LRRK2/dardarin mutations remains to be demonstrated. It has been estimated that LRRK2/dardarin mutations could account for more than 5% of all familial cases of PD (92), and even more remarkable is the finding that out of 482 sporadic PD patients, 8 were heterozygote for the G2019S LRRK2/dardarin mutation (40). As stated by the authors of this fascinating finding, the absence of family history in 5 of the PD patients harboring the LRRK2/dardarin mutation suggests either reduced penetrance or a de novo occurrence. As with the other PD-causing mutations, the function of LRRK2/dardarin in both normal and pathological situations remains unknown. At this point, it is believed that LRRK2/dardarin belongs to a family of multifunctional Ras/GTPase proteins, named *Roc* (for Ras of complex proteins). Moreover, specific motifs in LRRK2/dardarin sequence also suggest that protein–protein interactions play an important role in its function, a view that led to the idea that LRRK2/dardarin may function as a component of a multiprotein complex.

Postmortem examinations of several PD-linked PARK8 cases revealed a remarkable neuropathological heterogeneity. In all 6 patients carrying an LRRK2/dardarin mutation who came to autopsy, there was neuronal loss and gliosis in the substantia nigra. In some cases, the loss of SNpc dopaminergic neurons was not associated with Lewy bodies as in parkin-linked PD, whereas in others, the loss of SNpc dopaminergic neurons was associated with Lewy bodies. In the latter cases, Lewy bodies were restricted to the brainstem as in typical PD, or widespread in brainstem and cortex as in diffuse Lewy body disease. In one case, there were also tau-immunoreactive lesions in both neurons and glial cells, as in progressive supranuclear palsy (PSP). Finally, some patients also showed evidence of anterior horn motor neuron loss with spheroids, reminiscent of amyotrophic lateral sclerosis.

GENE DEFECTS AND MECHANISM OF CELL DEATH

Although genetic forms of PD are rare, the strong impetus for so avidly studying these uncommon occurrences of PD is fueled by the expectation that the phenotypic similarity between familial and sporadic PD indicates that both instances share key neurodegenerative mechanisms. As discussed previously (59), among various plausible mechanistic hypotheses (Fig. 7.3), available data favor impaired protein degradation and accumulation of misfolded proteins as the unifying factor linking genetic alterations to dopaminergic neurodegeneration in familial PD. According to this reasoning, alpha-synuclein and DJ-1 mutations would cause abnormal protein conformations, overwhelming the main cellular protein degradation systems, namely the proteasomal and lysosomal pathways, whereas parkin and UCH-L1 mutations would undermine the cell's ability to detect and degrade misfolded proteins. The common end result of these different perturbations is thus expected to be a cellular buildup of altered proteins that should have been cleared. This scenario fails, however, to explain why an accumulation of "misfolded proteins," which is likely to occur in all cells, would inflict greater damage to dopaminergic neurons in familial PD. Perhaps nigrostriatal dopaminergic neurons are less amenable to coping with "misfolded protein stress" because of a higher basal load of damaged proteins due to dopamine-mediated oxidative events. Also poorly addressed by the preceding scenario is the link between previously identified factors in PD neurodegeneration, such as mitochondrial dysfunction or oxidative stress, which will be discussed in the following section, and the molecular events engendered by the PD-causing mutations. The hypothesized location in mitochondria of DJ-1 and PINK1 and the role in oxidative stress played by DJ-1 may emerge as critical in our effort to reconcile the different aspects of the unified pathogenic cascade of PD. Too little is thus far known about LRRK2/dardarin to speculate how and where this new mutant protein will fit into this proposed scenario (Fig. 7.3).

Pathogenesis of Parkinson's Disease

If etiology refers to the factor that initiates the disease process in PD, pathogenesis refers to the actual mechanisms by which the demise of dopaminergic neurons occur. Although there is no clear boundary between etiology and pathogenesis, this somewhat artificial dichotomy has proved useful from a didactic point of view. To date, there are two major theories regarding the pathogenesis of PD. One hypothesizes that misfolding and aggregation of proteins is key to the neurodegenerative process, whereas the other asserts that mitochondrial dysfunction and related oxidative stress, including toxic oxidized dopamine species, are responsible. Also, inflammatory events are a feature of PD neuropathology, and mounting evidence supports its contribution to neurodegeneration of PD (93). Until recently, most insights into disease pathogenesis have come from human autopsy specimens. Postmortem studies, although useful, also suffer major limitations. For instance, it is usually the case that the cells of main interest—that is, dopaminergic neurons—are greatly depleted in typical autopsy specimens, which usually consist primarily of glial cells and nondopaminergic neurons. Thus, in the absence of experimental models, it is often difficult to reach any reliable mechanistic conclusions, and one is usually left with the intractable dilemma of whether a reported alteration reflects the cause or is simply a consequence of the neurodegenerative process. It should also be mentioned that the pathogenic factors noted previously are not mutually exclusive, and one of the key aims of current PD research is to identify all of the various factors implicated in the death of dopaminergic neurons in PD and to determine in which sequence they intervene in this deleterious cascade. Of great importance for deciphering possible therapies for PD is to determine whether these pathogenic factors eventually converge to engage a common downstream pathway such as apoptosis, or whether they remain divergent until neuronal death.

Misfolding and Aggregation of Proteins

The abnormal deposition of proteinaceous material in the brain in the form of large aggregates detectable by light microscopy is a typical feature of many age-related neurodegenerative diseases, including PD. Even with differences in composition and location of these inclusions, their presence in many diseases of the brain might indicate that these protein aggregations or related events might be toxic to neurons. As previously proposed (27), the observed intraneuronal aggregates, such as Lewy bodies in PD, may cause damage directly, possibly by cell deformation or interference in intracellular trafficking. It also may be that Lewy bodies sequester proteins necessary for cell survival, so depriving the neuron. If so, should there not be a direct correlation between inclusion formation and neurodegeneration? The answer to this question is still ambiguous

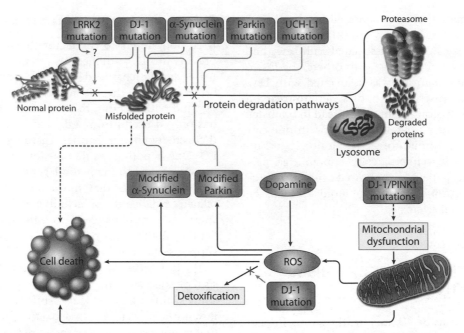

Figure 7.3   Genetic mutations and the pathogenesis of PD. Misfolded proteins may contribute to PD neurodegeneration. Mutant alpha-synuclein and DJ-1 may be misfolded (*blue arrows*), thus overwhelming the ubiquitin (proteasomal) and lysosomal degradation pathways. Other mutant proteins, such as parkin and UCH-L1, may lack their wild-type function. Both of these proteins, which belong to the ubiquitin-proteasome system, upon mutation may no longer exert their ubiquitin ligase activity, thus damaging the ability of the cellular machinery to detect and degrade misfolded proteins (*red arrows*). Mutations in DJ-1 may also alter its supposed chaperone activity, disrupting the refolding of damaged proteins or the targeting and delivery of damaged proteins for degradation (*red arrows*). These different alterations may lead to the accumulation of unwanted proteins, which, by unknown mechanisms (*dashed arrows*) may lead to neurodegeneration. Oxidative stress generated by mitochondrial dysfunction and dopamine metabolism may also promote protein misfolding as a result of post-translational modifications, especially of alpha-synuclein and parkin. Oxidative stress in PD may also originate from a defect in the reduced capacity of DJ-1 to detoxify reactive oxygen species, whereas the mitochondrial dysfunction may, at least in part, derive from defective activity and mislocation of DJ-1 and PINK1. Mitochondrial dysfunction, oxidative stress, and protein mishandling are thus tightly interconnected in this hypothesized pathogenic cascade. LRRK2 function is unknown. Additional possible interactions have been omitted for clarity. (Adapted from Vila M, Przedborski S. Genetic clues to the pathogenesis of Parkinson's disease. *Nat Med* 2004;10 Suppl:S58–62. With permission.) (See color section.)

as studies of Huntington's disease and other polyglutamine diseases (94,95) suggest that there is no straightforward link between the aggregate load and neurodegeneration, whereas studies of amyotrophic lateral sclerosis argue that there might be (96,97). Alternatively, cytoplasmic protein inclusions might not be passively derived from precipitated misfolded proteins but rather from an active process with intent to sequester misfolded proteins from the cellular environment. Accordingly, inclusion formation may be a protective process aimed at removing soluble misfolded proteins (94,98–100).

Aside from insoluble proteinaceous material, soluble misfolded proteins could also be toxic through a variety of mechanisms. For instance, soluble misfolded species seem capable of triggering apoptosis via a c-Jun amino-terminal Kinase (JNK)-dependent mechanism (101). The identification of ubiquitin and chaperones in Lewy bodies (99,102) is further evidence of the presence of soluble misfolded proteins in PD, because chaperones bind specifically to the exposed hydrophobic surface of soluble misfolded

proteins. The ability of chaperones such as Hsp70 to protect against neurodegeneration provoked by disease-related proteins also supports the view that soluble misfolded proteins are neurotoxic. Indeed, Auluck et al. (99) found that overexpression of Hsp70 prevented alpha-synuclein–mediated dopaminergic neuron loss in a *Drosophila* model of PD.

As discussed by Dauer and Przedborski (27), pathogenic mutations in patients with inherited PD are thought to cause disease directly by inducing abnormal and possibly toxic protein conformations or indirectly by interfering with the processes that normally recognize or process misfolded proteins. In sporadic PD, there is similar attention on both direct protein-damaging modifications and dysfunction of chaperones, proteasomes, or autophagy that may indirectly contribute to the accumulation of misfolded proteins. The triggers for dysfunctional protein metabolism in sporadic PD are now beginning to be revealed. One such initiator may be oxidative stress, long thought to play a key role in the pathogenesis of PD through damage caused by ROS. The tissue content of abnormally oxidized proteins (which may misfold) increases with age, and neurons may be especially susceptible because they are postmitotic. In PD, Lewy bodies contain oxidatively modified alpha-synuclein, which in vitro exhibits a greater propensity toward aggregation than does unmodified alpha-synuclein (103). Environmental factors could also initiate protein aggregation in PD as several herbicides and pesticides induce misfolding or aggregation of alpha-synuclein (104–106).

There also appears to be an age-related decline in the ability of cells to handle misfolded proteins (107). Cells respond to misfolded proteins by inducing chaperones, but if not properly refolded they are targeted for proteasomal degradation by polyubiquitination. With aging, the ability of cells to induce a variety of chaperones is impaired. Similarly, there is loss of proteasomal function during aging, with one report of selective loss of the 20S subunit of the proteasome in the postmortem PD brain (108). Furthermore both in vitro (109–111) and in vivo studies (112) suggest that inhibition of proteasomal activity leads to accumulation of alpha-synuclein or the formation of ubiquitinated alpha-synuclein–containing aggregates. Conversely, alpha-synuclein interacts with and may be degraded by the proteasome (113,114) and autophagy (115), and overexpression of alpha-synuclein leads to perturbations in the protein degradation systems (116). Proteasomal and autophagy dysfunctions and the accumulation of misfolded proteins may thus provoke a vicious cycle, with each insult reinforcing the other.

Mitochondrial Dysfunction and Oxidative Stress

The discovery that MPTP blocks the mitochondrial electron transport chain by inhibiting complex I allowed for the possibility that an oxidative phosphorylation defect could play a role in the pathogenesis of PD (117). Consistent with this view is that subsequent studies have identified abnormalities in complex I activity in PD, interestingly, not only in the brains of PD patients (118) but also in platelets (119). Low complex I activity in cybrid cells, which have been generated by the fusion of cells deficient in mitochondrial DNA with patient-derived platelets rich with mitochondrial DNA (120), led to the conclusion either that the observed complex I deficit was inherited from the mitochondrial genome or that some systemic toxicity caused mutations in mitochondrial DNA. However, as mentioned previously, no mitochondrial DNA mutation has been reproducibly identified in PD patients.

Almost all molecular oxygen is consumed by mitochondrial respiration, and such oxidants as superoxide radicals and hydrogen peroxide are continuously produced as byproducts. Inhibition of complex I increases the production of the ROS, which may form secondary oxidants, including hydroxyl radicals and peroxynitrite. All these oxidants may cause cellular damage by reacting with nucleic acids,

proteins, and lipids, and one target of these reactive species may be the electron transport chain itself (121), leading to mitochondrial damage and further production of ROS. Supporting the occurrence of oxidative stress in PD are the demonstrations that several biological markers of oxidative damage are elevated in the SNpc of PD brains (122). Also, the content of the antioxidant glutathione is reduced in the SNpc of PD brains (123), consistent with increased ROS, although this could also indicate a primary reduction of protective mechanisms against ROS.

The presence of ROS would increase the quantity of misfolded proteins, increasing the demand on the ubiquitin-proteasome system to remove them. Dopaminergic neurons may be a particularly fertile environment for the generation of ROS, as the normal metabolism of dopamine by monoamine oxidase (MAO) produces hydrogen peroxide and superoxide radicals, and autooxidation of dopamine produces dopamine quinone (124), a molecule that damages proteins by reacting with cysteine residues. Mitochondria-related energy failure may disrupt vesicular storage of dopamine, causing the free cytosolic concentration of dopamine to rise and allowing harmful dopamine-mediated reactions to damage cellular components. Dopaminergic neurons contain neuromelanin, which can bind ferric iron and reduce it to its reactive ferrous form (125). Midbrain dopaminergic groups differ markedly in the percentage of neuromelanin-pigmented neurons they contain, and PD-related neuron loss is more profound in cell groups that normally contain a greater percentage of neuromelanin-pigmented neurons (6). Further, there is a relative sparing of nonpigmented neurons in PD (6). Postnatal dopaminergic neurons exposed to low doses of levodopa accumulate a black pigment similar to neuromelanin (126), suggesting that the formation of neuromelanin is related to the presence of dopamine. Together, these results suggest that dopamine may be pivotal in rendering SNpc dopaminergic neurons particularly susceptible to oxidative attack.

Despite the large body of literature documenting mitochondrial dysfunction and indices of oxidative damage in autopsy tissue from PD patients, all these reported observations are correlative in nature. There are no data that convincingly link a *primary* abnormality of oxidative phosphorylation or ROS generation with PD; many of these abnormalities could be concomitant to dying cells. Indeed, of the many diseases known to result from mutations directly affecting the oxidative phosphorylation, i.e., mitochondrial cytopathies, parkinsonism is a rare feature and, when encountered, the parkinsonism is almost always accompanied by other symptoms that are not observed in PD.

Inflammation

The loss of dopaminergic neurons in postmortem PD brains is associated with marked microglial and, to a lesser extent, astrocyte activation (127–130). Activated microglial cells are found predominantly in proximity to free neuromelanin in the neuropil, and they sometimes agglomerate onto remaining neurons, producing an image of neuronophagia (127). In PD, inflammation seems to be secondary to neuronal pathology and not a primary pathogenic event. It is thus hypothesized that signals arising from injured neurons stimulate the inflammatory response via subtle alterations in the CNS microenvironment (e.g., ionic imbalances) or rather gross spillage of intraneuronal contents. Also relevant to the initiation of neuroinflammatory response in PD is the demonstration that neurons treated with proteasome inhibitors accumulate ubiquitinated proteins and increase the production of prostaglandins, which can activate glial cells (131).

It is established that both microglia and astrocytes, once activated, acquire phagocytic properties and become capable of producing an array of inflammatory mediators and other deleterious molecules, including ROS and nitric oxide. In keeping with this, in the SNpc of PD patients (but not controls), numerous astrocytes are immunoreactive for inducible nitric oxide synthase (iNOS) (132) while microglia are positive for nicotinamide adenine dinucleotide phosphate (NADPH)-oxidase (133). Enhanced immunostaining for proinflammatory cytokines—such as tumor necrosis factor alpha (TNF-α), interleukin-1β (IL-1β), interferon-γ (IFN-γ), and, for the macrophage cell surface, antigen FcϵR11/CD23—is also observed in the SNpc from PD patients, in both astrocytes and microglial cells (134). These cytokines may act in PD on at least two levels. First, while cytokines are produced by glial cells, they can stimulate other astrocytes and microglia not yet activated, thereby amplifying the inflammatory response and consequently the glial-mediated assault on neighboring neurons. In vitro studies by Hunot et al. (134) found that IFN-γ together with TNF-α and IL-1β not only activates glial cells, but it also stimulates the glial expression of FcϵR11/CD23, which leads to the induction of inducible nitric oxide synthase iNOS and the release of TNF-α. Second, glial-derived cytokines may also act directly on dopaminergic neurons by binding to specific cytokine receptors on the surface of these cells, such as those for TNF (135). Upon activation, these receptors trigger intracellular signaling pathways that may ultimately set off the programmed cell death (PCD) machinery, discussed in the following section. It is thus proposed that neuroinflammation does not initiate PD neurodegeneration but can promote its progression, whereby stimulating the worsening of PD symptoms.

Mode of Cell Death

Regardless of the mechanisms involved in the neurodegenerative process of PD, it may be asked whether a common downstream pathway mediates all PD-related neuronal loss, or whether there is significant heterogeneity in the pathways activated in different compromised neurons in a single patient, or among different patients with PD. The answers to these questions bear upon the development of therapeutic strategies for PD, and bear upon whether PD is a disease or rather a syndrome (i.e., multiple distinct pathological entities with similar phenotype). Over the past decade, PCD has emerged as an inescapable component in the mechanism of cell death in a wide variety of pathological situations, including diseases of the aging brain (136). Although physiological PCD is known to be crucial during normal development and as a homeostatic mechanism in some systems, inappropriate recruitment of this molecular machinery in the mature brain has been proposed as a main contributor to neurodegeneration. Until recently, investigators have explored the possibility that PCD occurs in PD autopsy specimens by searching for neurons that display features of apoptosis, a morphological correlate of PCD. As reviewed by Jellinger, these morphological studies have yielded conflicting results (137). Complicating matters, if apoptosis does occur in PD, it may be difficult to detect those apoptotic cells by morphological means because the rate of neuronal loss in PD may be low (138) and apoptotic cells reportedly disappear in a matter of hours (139). In addition, there may be nonapoptotic forms of PCD (140,141). Accordingly, most recent studies in PD have ascertained the content and status of molecular components of PCD instead of relying on morphological approaches. For example, studies of the PCD Bax molecule demonstrate an increased number of Bax-positive SNpc dopaminergic neurons in PD (142), and, compared to controls, there is an increased neuronal expression of the pro-PCD Bax protein in PD, suggesting that these cells are undergoing early PCD (143). SNpc dopaminergic neurons with increased expression and subcellular redistribution of the anti-PCD protein Bcl-xL and with activated PCD effector protease caspase-3 have also been found in greater proportion in PD (144,145). Remarkably, the Bcl-2 family member BAG5 has emerged as a potential promoter of neurodegeneration in PD by inhibiting both parkin E3 ligase activity and Hsp70-mediated refolding of misfolded proteins (146). Other molecular markers of PCD are altered in PD, including the activation of caspase-8 (147), caspase-9 (148), and the translocation of cytochrome c, an electron carrier and mediator of PCD (M. Vila, personal communication, June, 2000). Studies of PCD in PD remain descriptive in nature, and it is uncertain whether the changes are a primary abnormality of PCD regulation or simply an appropriate "suicide" decision by cells seriously injured by any of the toxic processes reviewed in this section.

SUMMARY

Advances in epidemiologic, genetic, and basic science research are generating plausible hypotheses regarding the cause of PD. These advances, rather than narrowing the focus to a single genetic or environmental cause, have led to an understanding of PD as a complex disorder with multiple etiologies and with a pathogenic cascade made of numerous deleterious factors. Thanks to rare genetic mutations causing familial forms of PD, a better understanding of mechanisms potentially important for the common sporadic form of PD has now been acquired. Alpha-synuclein is an important constituent in Lewy bodies, and environmental and genetic influences may lead to abnormal aggregation of this protein that, in turn, could cause neuronal dysfunction and death. The role of parkin and UCH-L1 in the ubiquitin-proteasomal system suggests that impaired regulation of protein degradation may play a role in PD, and promising insights into dopaminergic neurodegeneration are to be expected from studies on DJ-1, PINK1, and LRRK2/dardarin. Exposure to environmental toxins may interrupt energy production in the mitochondria or cause increased levels of oxidative stress that, in turn, might lead directly to cell injury or death. Here, inflammation and PCD appear respectively as key modulators of the overall extent of the neurodegenerative process and as plausible downstream effectors of neuronal demise. An individual's ability to respond to environmental insults may be determined by genetic polymorphisms that code for metabolic enzymes with reduced or increased ability to metabolize exogenous or endogenous toxins.

Although the numerous potential causes of dopaminergic neuronal degeneration and clinical PD are complex and daunting, they also provide the opportunity for intervention at multiple steps. The development of successful future therapies and preventive measures depends on a sound understanding of the interaction of environmental, molecular, and genetic factors involved in PD.

ACKNOWLEDGMENTS

The author thanks Mr. Matthew Lucas for his assistance in preparing this manuscript and is supported by NIH/ NINDS Grants RO1 NS42269, P50 NS38370, and P01 NS11766-27A2, NIH/NIA RO1 AG21617-01, NIH/NIEHS R21 ES013177, the U.S. Department of Defense Grant DAMD 17-03-1, the Parkinson's Disease Foundation (New York), the Lowenstein Foundation, The Muscular Dystrophy Association/The Wings Over Wall Street.

REFERENCES

1. Van Den Eeden, SK, Tanner, CM, Bernstein, AL, et al. Incidence of Parkinson's disease: variation by age, gender, and race/ethnicity. *Am J Epidemiol* 2003;157:1015–1022.
2. Levy G, Tang MX, Louis ED, et al. The association of incident dementia with mortality in PD. *Neurology* 2002;59:1708–1713.
3. Elbaz A, Bower JH, Peterson BJ, et al. Survival study of Parkinson's disease in Olmsted County, Minnesota. *Arch Neurol* 2003;60:91–96.
4. Beyer MK, Herlofson K, Arsland D, et al. Causes of death in a community-based study of Parkinson's disease. *Acta Neurol Scand* 2001;103:7–11.
5. Fall PA, Saleh A, Fredrickson M, et al. Survival time, mortality, and cause of death in elderly patients with Parkinson's disease: a 9-year follow-up. *Mov Disord* 2003;18:1312–1316.
6. Hirsch E, Graybiel AM, Agid YA. Melanized dopaminergic neurons are differentially susceptible to degeneration in Parkinson's disease. *Nature* 1988;334:345–348.
7. Price KS, Farley IJ, Hornykiewicz O. Neurochemistry of Parkinson's disease: relation between striatal and limbic dopamine. *Adv Biochem Psychopharmacol* 1978;19:293–300.
8. Fahn S, Przedborski S. Parkinsonism. In: Rowland, LP, ed. *Merritt's neurology*. 11th ed. New York: Lippincott Williams & Wilkins, 2006;828–846.
9. Moeller JR, Eidelberg D. Divergent expression of regional metabolic topographies in Parkinson's disease and normal aging. *Brain* 1997;120:2197–2206.
10. Braak H, Braak E, Yilmazer D, et al. Nigral and extranigral pathology in Parkinson's disease. *J Neural Transm Suppl* 1995;46:15–31.
11. Shults CW. Lewy bodies. *Proc Natl Acad Sci* 2006;103:1661–1668.
12. Spillantini MG, Schmidt ML, Lee VMY, et al. α-synuclein in Lewy bodies. *Nature* 1997;388:839–840.
13. Marder K, Levy G, Louis ED, et al. Familial aggregation of early- and late-onset Parkinson's disease. *Ann Neurol* 2003;54:507–513.
14. Tanner C, Goldman SM, and Ross GW. Etiology of Parkinson's disease. In: Jankovic J, Tolosa E, eds. *Parkinson's Disease and Movement Disorders*. 4th ed. Philadelphia: Lippincott Williams & Wilkins, 2002;90–103.
15. Hernan MA, Takkouche B, Caamano-Isorna F, et al. A meta-analysis of coffee drinking, cigarette smoking, and the risk of Parkinson's disease. *Ann Neurol* 2002;52:276–284.
16. Langston JW, Ballard P, Irwin I. Chronic parkinsonism in humans due to a product of meperidine-analog synthesis. *Science* 1983;219:979–980.
17. Ballard P, Tetrud JW, Langston JW. Permanent human parkinsonism due to 1-methyl-4-phenyl-1,2,3,6-tetrahydropyridine (MPTP): 7 cases. *Neurology* 1985;35:949–956.
18. Davis GC, Williams AC, Markey SP, et al. Chronic parkinsonism secondary to intravenous injection of meperidine analogs. *Psychiatry Res* 1979;1:249–254.
19. Langston JW, Forno LS, Tetrud J, et al. Evidence of active nerve cell degeneration in the substantia nigra of humans years after 1-methyl-4-phenyl-1,2,3,6-tetrahydropyridine exposure. *Ann Neurol* 1999;46:598–605.
20. McCormack AL, Di Monte DA. Effects of L-dopa and other amino acids against paraquat-induced nigrostriatal degeneration. *J Neurochem* 2003;85:82–86.
21. Manning-Bog AB, McCormack AL, Purisai MG, et al. Alpha-synuclein overexpression protects against paraquat-induced neurodegeneration. *J Neurosci* 2003;23:3095–3099.
22. Liou HH, Tsai MC, Chen CJ, et al. Environmental risk factors and Parkinson's disease: a case-control study in Taiwan. *Neurology* 1997;48:1583–1588.
23. Thiruchelvam M, Brockel BJ, Richfield EK, et al. Potentiated and preferential effects of combined paraquat and maneb on nigrostriatal dopamine systems: environmental risk factors for Parkinson's disease? *Brain Res* 2000;873:225–234.
24. Hisata J. Final supplemental environmental impact statement. Lake and stream rehabilitation: rotenone use and health risks. Washington Department of Fish and Wildlife, 2002.
25. Betarbet R, Sherer TB, MacKenzie G, et al. Chronic systemic pesticide exposure reproduces features of Parkinson's disease. *Nat Neurosci* 2000;3:1301–1306.
26. Marking L. Oral toxicity of rotenone to mammals. *Investigations in Fish Control* 1988;94.
27. Dauer W, Przedborski S. Parkinson's disease: mechanisms and models. *Neuron* 2003;39:889–909.
28. Cohen G. Oxy-radical toxicity in catecholamine neurons. *Neurotoxicology* 1984;5:77–82.
29. Sandy MS, Armstrong M, Tanner CM, et al. CYP2D6 allelic frequencies in young-onset Parkinson's disease. *Neurology* 1996;47:225–230.
30. Nagatsu T. Isoquinoline neurotoxins in the brain and Parkinson's disease. *Neurosci Res* 1997;29:99–111.

31. Andrew R, Watson DG, Best SA, et al. The determination of hydroxydopamines and other trace amines in the urine of parkinsonian patients and normal controls. *Neurochem Res* 1993;18:1175–1177.

32. Paolini M, Sapone A, Gonzalez FJ. Parkinson's disease, pesticides and individual vulnerability. *Trends Pharmacol Sci* 2004;25:124–129.

33. Wooten GF, Currie LJ, Bennett JP, et al. Maternal inheritance in Parkinson's disease. *Ann Neurol* 1997;41:265–268.

34. Swerdlow RH, Parks JK, Davis JN 2nd, et al. Matrilineal inheritance of complex I dysfunction in a multigenerational Parkinson's disease family. *Ann Neurol* 1998;44:873–881.

35. Kosel S, Grasbon-Frodl EM, Mautsch U, et al. Novel mutations of mitochondrial complex I in pathologically proven Parkinson's disease. *Neurogenetics* 1998;1:197–204.

36. Van der Walt JM, Nicodemus KK, Martin ER, et al. Mitochondrial polymorphisms significantly reduce the risk of Parkinson's disease. *Am J Hum Genet* 2003;72:804–811.

37. Shoffner JM, Brown M, Huoponen K, et al. A mitochondrial DNA (mtDNA) mutation associated with maternally inherited deafness and Parkinson's disease (PD). *Neurology* 1996;46:A331.

38. Thyagarajan D, Bressman S, Bruno C, et al. A novel mitochondrial 12SrRNA point mutation in parkinsonism, deafness, and neuropathy. *Ann Neurol* 2000;48:730–736.

39. Lucking CB, Durr A, Bonifati V, et al, for French Parkinson's Disease Genetics Study Group. Association between early-onset Parkinson's disease and mutations in the parkin gene. *N Engl J Med* 2000;342:1560–1567.

40. Gilks WP, bou-Sleiman PM, Gandhi S, et al. A common LRRK2 mutation in idiopathic Parkinson's disease. *Lancet* 2005;365:415–416.

41. Martin ER, Scott WK, Nance MA, et al. Association of single-nucleotide polymorphisms of the tau gene with late-onset Parkinson's disease. *JAMA* 2001;286:2245–2250.

42. Zareparsi S, Camicioli R, Sexton G, et al. Age at onset of Parkinson's disease and apolipoprotein E genotypes. *Am J Med Genet* 2002;107:156–161.

43. Li YJ, Scott WK, Hedges DJ, et al. Age at onset in two common neurodegenerative diseases is genetically controlled. *Am J Hum Genet* 2002;70:985–993.

44. Aharon-Peretz J, Rosenbaum H, Gershoni-Baruch R. Mutations in the glucocerebrosidase gene and Parkinson's disease in Ashkenazi Jews. *N Engl J Med* 2004;351:1972–1977.

45. Tanner CM, Ottman R, Goldman SM, et al. Parkinson's disease in twins: an etiologic study. *JAMA* 1999;281:341–346.

46. Dickson D, Farrer M, Lincoln S, et al. Pathology of PD in monozygotic twins with a 20-year discordance interval. *Neurology* 2001;56:981–982.

47. Piccini P, Burn DJ, Ceravolo R, et al. The role of inheritance in sporadic Parkinson's disease: evidence from a longitudinal study of dopaminergic function in twins. *Ann Neurol* 1999;45:577–582.

48. Polymeropoulos MH, Lavedan C, Leroy E, et al. Mutation in the alpha-synuclein gene identified in families with Parkinson's disease. *Science* 1997;276:2045–2047.

49. Kruger R, Kuhn W, Muller T, et al. Ala30Pro mutation in the gene encoding alpha-synuclein in Parkinson's disease. *Nat Genet* 1998;18:107–108.

50. Zarranz JJ, Alegre J, Gomez-Esteban JC, et al. The new mutation, E46K, of alpha-synuclein causes Parkinson and Lewy body dementia. *Ann Neurol* 2004;55:164–173.

51. Spira PJ, Sharpe, DM, Halliday G, et al. Clinical and pathological features of a Parkinsonian syndrome in a family with an Ala53Thr alpha-synuclein mutation. *Ann Neurol* 2001;49:313–319.

52. Munoz E, Oliva R, Obach V, et al. Identification of Spanish familial Parkinson's disease and screening for the Ala53Thr mutation of the alpha-synuclein gene in early onset patients. *Neurosci Lett* 1997;235:57–60.

53. Spillantini MG, Crowther RA, Jakes R, et al. α-Synuclein in filamentous inclusions of Lewy bodies from Parkinson's disease and dementia with Lewy bodies. *Proc Natl Acad Sci USA* 1998;95:6469–6473.

54. Abeliovich A, Schmitz Y, Farinas I, et al. Mice lacking alpha-synuclein display functional deficits in the nigrostriatal dopamine system. *Neuron* 2000;25:239–252.

55. Dauer W, Kholodilov N, Vila M, et al. Resistance of alpha-synuclein null mice to the parkinsonian neurotoxin MPTP. *Proc Natl Acad Sci USA* 2002;99:14,524–14,529.

56. Singleton AB, Farrer M, Johnson J, et al. Alpha-synuclein locus triplication causes Parkinson's disease. *Science* 2003;302:841.

57. Chartier-Harlin MC, Kachergus J, Roumier C, et al. Alpha-synuclein locus duplication as a cause of familial Parkinson's disease. *Lancet* 2004;364:1167–1169.

58. Ibáñez P, Bonnet AM, Debarges B, et al. Causal relation between alpha-synuclein gene duplication and familial Parkinson's disease. *Lancet* 2004;364:1169–1171.

59. Vila M, Przedborski S. Genetic clues to the pathogenesis of Parkinson's disease. *Nat Med* 2004;10(suppl):S58–S62.

60. Kitada T, Asakawa S, Hattori N, et al. Mutations in the parkin gene cause autosomal recessive juvenile parkinsonism. *Nature* 1998;392:605–608.

61. Mizuno Y, Hattori N, Mori H, et al. Parkin and Parkinson's disease. *Curr Opin Neurol* 2001;14:477–482.

62. Hilker R, Klein C, Ghaemi M, et al. Positron emission tomographic analysis of the nigrostriatal dopaminergic system in familial parkinsonism associated with mutations in the parkin gene. *Ann Neurol* 2001;49:367–376.

63. Hedrich K, Marder K, Harris J, et al. Evaluation of 50 probands with early-onset Parkinson's disease for Parkin mutations. *Neurology* 2002;58:1239–1246.

64. Farrer M, Chan P, Chen R, et al. Lewy bodies and parkinsonism in families with parkin mutations. *Ann Neurol* 2001;50:293–300.

65. Goldberg MS, Fleming SM, Palacino JJ, et al. Parkin-deficient mice exhibit nigrostriatal deficits but not loss of dopaminergic neurons. *J Biol Chem* 2003;278:43,628–635.

66. Pesah Y, Pham T, Burgess H, et al. *Drosophila* parkin mutants have decreased mass and cell size and increased sensitivity to oxygen radical stress. *Development* 2004;131:2183–2194.

67. Greene JC, Whitworth AJ, Kuo I, et al. Mitochondrial pathology and apoptotic muscle degeneration in *Drosophila* parkin mutants. *Proc Natl Acad Sci USA* 2003;100:4078–4083.

68. Palacino JJ, Sagi D, Goldberg MS, et al. Mitochondrial dysfunction and oxidative damage in parkin-deficient mice. *J Biol Chem* 2004;279:18,614–18,622.

69. Shimura H, Hattori N, Kubo S, et al. Familial Parkinson's disease gene product, parkin, is a ubiquitin-protein ligase. *Nat Genet* 2000;25:302–305.

70. Zhang Y, Gao J, Chung KK, et al. Parkin functions as an E2-dependent ubiquitin-protein ligase and promotes the degradation of the synaptic vesicle-associated protein, CDCrel-1. *Proc Natl Acad Sci USA* 2000;97:13,354–13,359.

71. Hayashi S, Wakabayashi K, Ishikawa A, et al. An autopsy case of autosomal-recessive juvenile parkinsonism with a homozygous exon 4 deletion in the parkin gene. *Mov Disord* 2000;15:884–888.

72. Leroy E, Boyer R, Auburger G, et al. The ubiquitin pathway in Parkinson's disease. *Nature* 1998;395:451–452.

73. Saigoh K, Wang YL, Suh JG, et al. Intragenic deletion in the gene encoding ubiquitin carboxy-terminal hydrolase in gad mice. *Nat Genet* 1999;23:47–51.

74. Maraganore DM, Lesnick TG, Elbaz A, et al. UCHL1 is a Parkinson's disease susceptibility gene. *Ann Neurol* 2004;55:512–521.

75. Bonifati, V, Rizzu P, Van Baren MJ, et al. Mutations in the DJ-1 gene associated with autosomal recessive early-onset parkinsonism. *Science* 2003;299:256–259.

76. Hague S, Rogaeva E, Hernandez D, et al. Early-onset Parkinson's disease caused by a compound heterozygous DJ-1 mutation. *Ann Neurol* 2003;54:271–274.

77. Abou-Sleiman PM, Healy DG, Quinn N, et al. The role of pathogenic DJ-1 mutations in Parkinson's disease. *Ann Neurol* 2003;54:283–286.

78. Hedrich K, Djarmati A, Schafer N, et al. DJ-1 (PARK7) mutations are less frequent than Parkin (PARK2) mutations in early-onset Parkinson's disease. *Neurology* 2004;62:389–394.

79. Quigley PM, Korotkov K, Baneyx F, et al. The 1.6-A crystal structure of the class of chaperones represented by Escherichia coli Hsp31 reveals a putative catalytic triad. *Proc Natl Acad Sci USA* 2003;100:3137–3142.

80. Shendelman S, Jonason A, Martinat C, et al. DJ-1 is a redox-dependent molecular chaperone that inhibits alpha-synuclein aggregate formation. *PLoS Biol* 2004;2:1764–1773.

81. Valente EM, Bentivoglio AR, Dixon PH, et al. Localization of a novel locus for autosomal recessive early-onset parkinsonism,

PARK6, on human chromosome 1p35–p36. *Am J Hum Genet* 2001;68:895–900.

82. Valente EM, Brancati F, Ferraris A, et al. PARK6-linked parkinsonism occurs in several European families. *Ann Neurol* 2002;51:14–18.

83. Valente EM, Abou-Sleiman PM, Caputo V, et al. Hereditary early-onset Parkinson's disease caused by mutations in PINK1. *Science* 2004;304:1158–1160.

84. Rogaeva E, Johnson J, Lang AE, et al. Analysis of the PINK1 gene in a large cohort of cases with Parkinson's disease. *Arch Neurol* 2004;61:1898–1904.

85. Rohe CF, Montagna P, Breedveld G, et al. Homozygous PINK1 C-terminus mutation causing early-onset parkinsonism. *Ann Neurol* 2004;56:427–431.

86. Khan NL, Valente EM, Bentivoglio AR, et al. Clinical and subclinical dopaminergic dysfunction in PARK6-linked parkinsonism: an 18F-dopa PET study. *Ann Neurol* 2002;52:849–853.

87. Nakajima A, Kataoka K, Hong M, et al. BRPK, a novel protein kinase showing increased expression in mouse cancer cell lines with higher metastatic potential. *Cancer Lett* 2003;201:195–201.

88. Unoki M, Nakamura Y. Growth-suppressive effects of BPOZ and EGR2, two genes involved in the PTEN signaling pathway. *Oncogene* 2001;20:4457–4465.

89. Funayama M, Hasegawa K, Kowa H, et al. A new locus for Parkinson's disease (PARK8) maps to chromosome 12p11.2–q13.1. *Ann Neurol* 2002;51:296–301.

90. Zimprich A, Biskup S, Leitner P, et al. Mutations in LRRK2 cause autosomal-dominant parkinsonism with pleomorphic pathology. *Neuron* 2004;44:601–607.

91. Paisan-Ruiz C, Jain S, Evans EW, et al. Cloning of the gene containing mutations that cause PARK8-linked Parkinson's disease. *Neuron* 2004;44:595–600.

92. Nichols WC, Pankratz N, Hernandez D, et al. Genetic screening for a single common LRRK2 mutation in familial Parkinson's disease. *Lancet* 2005;365:410–412.

93. Przedborski S, Goldman JE. Pathogenic role of glial cells in Parkinson's disease. In: Hertz L, ed. *Non-neuronal cells of the nervous system: function and dysfunction* New York: Elsevier, 2004;967–982.

94. Cummings CJ, Reinstein E, Sun Y, et al. Mutation of the E6-AP ubiquitin ligase reduces nuclear inclusion frequency while accelerating polyglutamine-induced pathology in SCA1 mice. *Neuron* 1999;24:879–92.

95. Saudou F, Finkbeiner S, Devys D, et al. Huntington acts in the nucleus to induce apoptosis but death does not correlate with the formation of intranuclear inclusions. *Cell* 1998;95:55–66.

96. Bruijn LI, Becher MW, Lee MK, et al. ALS-linked SOD1 mutant G85R mediated damage to astrocytes and promotes rapidly progressive disease with SOD1-containing inclusions. *Neuron* 1997;18:327–338.

97. Turner BJ, Atkin JD, Farg MA, et al. Impaired extracellular secretion of mutant superoxide dismutase 1 associates with neurotoxicity in familial amyotrophic lateral sclerosis. *J Neurosci* 2005;25:108–117.

98. Cummings CJ, Sun Y, Opal P, et al. Over-expression of inducible HSP70 chaperone suppresses neuropathology and improves motor function in SCA1 mice. *Hum Mol Genet* 2001;10:1511–1518.

99. Auluck PK, Chan HY, Trojanowski JQ, et al. Chaperone suppression of alpha-synuclein toxicity in a *Drosophila* model for Parkinson's disease. *Science* 2002;295:865–868.

100. Warrick JM, Chan HY, Gray-Board GL, et al. Suppression of polyglutamine-mediated neurodegeneration in *Drosophila* by the molecular chaperone HSP70. *Nat Genet* 1999;23:425–428.

101. Gabai VL, Meriin AB, Yaglom JA, et al. Role of Hsp70 in regulation of stress-kinase JNK: implications in apoptosis and aging. *FEBS Lett* 1998;438:1–4.

102. Forno LS, Langston JW. Lewy bodies and aging: relation to Alzheimer's and Parkinson's diseases. *Neurodegeneration* 1993;2:19–24.

103. Giasson BI, Duda JE, Murray IV, et al. Oxidative damage linked to neurodegeneration by selective alpha-synuclein nitration in synucleinopathy lesions. *Science* 2000;290:985–989.

104. Manning-Bog AB, McCormack AL, Li J, et al. The herbicide paraquat causes up-regulation and aggregation of alpha-synuclein in mice: paraquat and alpha-synuclein. *J Biol Chem* 2002;277:1641–1644.

105. Uversky VN, Li J, Fink AL. Pesticides directly accelerate the rate of alpha-synuclein fibril formation: a possible factor in Parkinson's disease. *FEBS Lett* 2001;500:105–108.

106. Lee HJ, Shin SY, Choi C, et al. Formation and removal of alpha-synuclein aggregates in cells exposed to mitochondrial inhibitors. *J Biol Chem* 2002;277:5411–5417.

107. Sherman MY, Goldberg AL. Cellular defenses against unfolded proteins: a cell biologist thinks about neurodegenerative diseases. *Neuron* 2001;29:15–32.

108. McNaught KS, Belizaire R, Jenner P, et al. Selective loss of 20S proteasome alpha-subunits in the substantia nigra pars compacta in Parkinson's disease. *Neurosci Lett* 2002;326:155–158.

109. Rideout HJ, Larsen KE, Sulzer D, et al. Proteasomal inhibition leads to formation of ubiquitin/alpha-synuclein-immunoreactive inclusions in PC12 cells. *J Neurochem* 2001;78:899–908.

110. McNaught KS, Mytilineou C, Jnobaptiste R, et al. Impairment of the ubiquitin-proteasome system causes dopaminergic cell death and inclusion body formation in ventral mesencephalic cultures. *J Neurochem* 2002;81:301–306.

111. Tofaris GK, Layfield R, Spillantini MG. Alpha-synuclein metabolism and aggregation is linked to ubiquitin-independent degradation by the proteasome. *FEBS Lett* 2001;509:22–26.

112. McNaught KS, Bjorklund LM, Belizaire R, et al. Proteasome inhibition causes nigral degeneration with inclusion bodies in rats. *Neuroreport* 2002;13:1437–1441.

113. Ghee M, Fournier A, Mallet J. Rat alpha-synuclein interacts with Tat binding protein 1, a component of the 26S proteasomal complex. *J Neurochem* 2000;75:2221–2224.

114. Bennett MC, Bishop JF, Leng Y, et al. Degradation of alpha-synuclein by proteasome. *J Biol Chem* 1999;274:33,855–33,858.

115. Cuervo AM, Stefanis L, Fredenburg R, et al. Impaired degradation of mutant alpha-synuclein by chaperone-mediated autophagy. *Science* 2004;305:1292–1295.

116. Stefanis L, Larsen KE, Rideout HJ, et al. Expression of A53T mutant but not wild-type alpha-synuclein in PC12 cells induces alterations of the ubiquitin-dependent degradation system, loss of dopamine release, and autophagic cell death. *J Neurosci* 2001;21:9549–9560.

117. Nicklas WJ, Youngster SK, Kindt MV, et al. MPTP, MPP+ and mitochondrial function. *Life Sci* 1987;40:721–729.

118. Schapira AH, Cooper JM, Dexter D, et al. Mitochondrial complex I deficiency in Parkinson's disease. *J Neurochem* 1990;54:823–827.

119. Parker WD Jr, Boyson SJ, Parks JK. Abnormalities of the electron transport chain in idiopathic Parkinson's disease. *Ann Neurol* 1989;26:719–723.

120. Swerdlow RH, Parks JK, Miller SW, et al. Origin and functional consequences of the complex I defect in Parkinson's disease. *Ann Neurol* 1996;40:663–671.

121. Cohen G. Oxidative stress, mitochondrial respiration, and Parkinson's disease. *Ann N Y Acad Sci* 2000;899:112–120.

122. Przedborski S, Jackson-Lewis V. ROS and Parkinson's disease: a view to a kill. In: Poli G, Cadenas E, Packer L, eds. *Free Radicals in Brain Pathophysiology*. New York: Marcel Dekker, Inc., 2000;273–290.

123. Sian J, Dexter DT, Lees AJ, et al. Alterations in glutathione levels in Parkinson's disease and other neurodegenerative disorders affecting basal ganglia. *Ann Neurol* 1994;36:348–355.

124. Graham DG. Oxidative pathways for catecholamines in the genesis of neuromelanin and cytotoxic quinones. *Mol Pharmacol* 1978;14:633–643.

125. Zecca L, Tampellini D, Gerlach M, et al. Substantia nigra neuromelanin: structure, synthesis, and molecular behaviour. *Mol Pathol* 2001;54:414–418.

126. Sulzer D, Bogulavsky J, Larsen KE, et al. Neuromelanin biosynthesis is driven by excess cytosolic catecholamines not accumulated by synaptic vesicles. *Proc Natl Acad Sci USA* 2000;97:11,869–11,874.

127. McGeer PL, Itagaki S, Boyes BE, et al. Reactive microglia are positive for HLA-DR in the substantia nigra of Parkinson's and Alzheimer's disease brains. *Neurology* 1988;38:1285–1291.

128. Forno LS, DeLanney LE, Irwin I, et al. Astrocytes and Parkinson's disease. *Prog Brain Res* 1992;94:429–436.

129. Banati RB, Daniel SE, Blunt SB. Glial pathology but absence of apoptotic nigral neurons in long-standing Parkinson's disease. *Mov Disord* 1998;13:221–227.

130. Mirza B, Hadberg H, Thomsen P, et al. The absence of reactive astrocytosis is indicative of a unique inflammatory process in Parkinson's disease. *Neuroscience* 2000;95:425–432.

131. Rockwell P, Yuan H, Magnusson R, et al. Proteasome inhibition in neuronal cells induces a proinflammatory response manifested by upregulation of cyclooxygenase-2, its accumulation as ubiquitin conjugates, and production of the prostaglandin PGE(2). *Arch Biochem Biophys* 2000;374:325–333.

132. Hunot S, Boissière F, Faucheux B, et al. Nitric oxide synthase and neuronal vulnerability in Parkinson's disease. *Neuroscience* 1996;72:355–363.

133. Wu DC, Teismann P, Tieu K, et al. NADPH oxidase mediates oxidative stress in the 1-methyl-4-phenyl-1,2,3,6-tetrahydropyridine model of Parkinson's disease. *Proc Natl Acad Sci USA* 2003;100:6145–6150.

134. Hunot S, Dugas N, Faucheux B, et al. FceRII/CD23 is expressed in Parkinson's disease and induces, in vitro, production of nitric oxide and tumor necrosis factor-alpha in glial cells. *J Neurosci* 1999;19:3440–3447.

135. Boka G, Anglade P, Wallach D, et al. Immunocytochemical analysis of tumor necrosis factor and its receptors in Parkinson's disease. *Neurosci Lett* 1994;172:151–154.

136. Vila M, Przedborski S. Neurological diseases: targeting programmed cell death in neurodegenerative diseases. *Nat Rev Neurosci* 2003;4:365–375.

137. Jellinger KA. Cell death mechanisms in Parkinson's disease. *J Neural Transm* 2000;107:1–29.

138. McGeer PL, Itagaki S, Akiyama H, et al. Rate of cell death in parkinsonism indicates active neuropathological process. *Ann Neurol* 1988;24:574–576.

139. Raff MC, Barres BA, Burne JF, et al. Programmed cell death and the control of cell survival: lessons from the nervous system. *Science* 1993;262:695–700.

140. Clarke PGH. Apoptosis versus necrosis. In: Koliatsos VE, Ratan RR, eds. *Cell Death and Diseases of the Nervous System.* New Jersey: Humana Press, 1999; 3–28.

141. Sperandio S, de Belle I, Bredesen DE. An alternative, nonapoptotic form of programmed cell death. *Proc Natl Acad Sci USA* 2000;97:14,376–14,381.

142. Hartmann A, Michel PP, Troadec JD, et al. Is Bax a mitochondrial mediator in apoptotic death of dopaminergic neurons in Parkinson's disease? *J Neurochem* 2001;76:1785–1793.

143. Tatton NA. Increased caspase 3 and Bax immunoreactivity accompany nuclear GAPDH translocation and neuronal apoptosis in Parkinson's disease. *Exp Neurol* 2000;166:29–43.

144. Hartmann A, Hunot S, Michel PP, et al. Caspase-3: a vulnerability factor and final effector in apoptotic death of dopaminergic neurons in Parkinson's disease. *Proc Natl Acad Sci USA* 2000;97:2875–2880.

145. Hartmann A, Mouatt-Prigent A, Vila M, et al. Increased expression and redistribution of the antiapoptotic molecule Bcl-xL in Parkinson's disease. *Neurobiol Dis* 2002;10:28–32.

146. Kalia SK, Lee S, Smith PD, et al. BAG5 inhibits parkin and enhances dopaminergic neuron degeneration. *Neuron* 2004;44:931–945.

147. Hartmann A, Troadec JD, Hunot S, et al. Caspase-8 is an effector in apoptotic death of dopaminergic neurons in Parkinson's disease, but pathway inhibition results in neuronal necrosis. *J Neurosci* 2001;21:2247–2255.

148. Viswanath V, Wu Y, Boonplueang R, et al. Caspase-9 activation results in downstream caspase-8 activation and bid cleavage in 1-methyl-4-phenyl-1,2,3,6-tetrahydropyridine-induced Parkinson's disease. *J Neurosci* 2001;21:9519–9528.

Genetics of Parkinson's Disease

8

Thomas Gasser

INTRODUCTION

Over the last few years, several genes for monogenically inherited forms of Parkinson's disease (PD) have been mapped and/or cloned. In a small number of families with autosomal dominant inheritance and typical Lewy body pathology, mutations have been identified in the gene for α-synuclein. Aggregation of this protein in Lewy bodies may be a crucial step in the molecular pathogenesis of familial and sporadic PD. Mutations in the gene for LRRK2 also cause autosomal-dominant PD, with α-synuclein pathology in some but not in all mutation carriers. Mutations in the parkin gene, in DJ-1, and in PINK1 cause autosomal recessive parkinsonism of early onset. Parkin has been implicated in the cellular protein degradation pathways, functioning as a ubiquitin ligase, whereas DJ-1 has been linked to the oxidative stress response, and PINK1 is thought to act in mitochondria.

Evidence is emerging that at least α-synuclein also plays a direct role in the etiology of the common sporadic form of PD. This is so far not the case for other PD genes. However, it is likely that the cellular pathways identified in rare monogenic variants of PD also shed light on the molecular pathogenesis in typical sporadic PD.

Parkinsonism is a clinically defined syndrome, characterized by variable combinations of akinesia, rigidity, tremor, and postural instability, which may occur in the context of a number of different neurodegenerative diseases. The most common cause of parkinsonism is PD. In PD, parkinsonism is caused by a degeneration of dopaminergic neurons of the substantia nigra, leading to a deficiency of dopamine in their striatal projection areas. The Lewy bodies, characteristic eosinophilic inclusions, are found in surviving dopaminergic neurons but also, though less abundantly, in other parts of the brain and have been considered essential for the pathologic diagnosis of PD.

Genetic research of the past 15 years, in particular the mapping and cloning of a number of genes that cause, when mutated, monogenically inherited forms of the disorder, has shown that PD is actually not a disease entity but rather a heterogeneous group of diseases associated with a spectrum of clinical and pathological changes. Although each of the different mutations and loci identified to date appears to be directly responsible in only a relatively small number of families, evidence is accumulating that the molecular pathways identified may be common to more than one genetic form of parkinsonism and may, in one way or another, also play a role in the common sporadic disease. This will—eventually—allow for the development of novel protective and therapeutic strategies.

MONOGENIC FORMS OF PARKINSON'S DISEASE

A minority of patients with the typical clinical picture of PD have a positive family history compatible with a Mendelian (autosomal dominant or autosomal recessive) inheritance. As a rule, age at onset in many (but not all) of these patients is younger than that of patients with sporadic disease, but no other specific clinical signs or symptoms distinguish familial from sporadic cases. Pathologically, all forms have in common a predominant degeneration of dopaminergic neurons of the substantia nigra, although in some forms the pathologic process appears to be more selective (as in parkin-associated parkinsonism, PARK2), whereas in others the degenerative process is more widespread. Some forms demonstrate typical Lewy body

TABLE 8.1

GENETICALLY DEFINED FORMS OF PARKINSON'S DISEASE AND PARKINSONISM

Locus/Gene	Inheritance	Onset	Pathology	Map Position	Gene
PARK1	Dominant	~40	Nigral degeneration with Lewy bodies	4q21	α-synuclein
PARK2	Recessive	20–40	Nigral degeneration without Lewybodies	6q25	parkin
PARK3	Dominant	~60	Nigral degeneration with Lewy bodies Plaques and tangles in some	2p13	?
PARK4	Dominant	30–60	Nigral degeneration with Lewy bodies Vacuoles in neurons of the hippocampus	4q21	α-synuclein duplications and triplications
PARK5	Dominant	~50	No pathology reported	4p14	ubiquitin C-terminal hydrolase L1
PARK6	Recessive	30–40	No pathology reported	1p35–37	PINK1
PARK7	Recessive	30–40	No pathology reported	1p38	DJ-1
PARK8	Dominant	~60	Variable α-synuclein and tau pathology	12cen	LRRK2
PARK10	Dominant (?)	50–60	No pathology reported	1p32	?
PARK11	Dominant (?)	Late	No pathology reported	2q34	?

pathology (PARK1, PARK3), whereas in others the pathology differs from that considered to be typical for PD in some cases but not in others (PARK8). Remarkably, pathology can even vary within single families. These observations indicate that different, and probably interrelated pathogenic pathways, are likely to lead to the process of nigral cell death.

AUTOSOMAL DOMINANT FORMS OF PARKINSONISM

Several genetic loci have been identified by linkage studies to cosegregate with parkinsonism in families with dominant inheritance (Table 8.1). To date, at least two of these genes, α-synuclein (α-SYN) and, recently, leucine-rich repeat kinase 2 (LRRK2) have been identified. The status of the third, ubiquitin C-terminal hydrolase L1 (UCHL1, or PARK5) is still controversial. These discoveries have proven to be extremely fruitful.

PARK1/4: PARKINSON'S DISEASE CAUSED BY MUTATIONS IN, OR MULTIPLICATIONS OF, THE GENE FOR α-SYNUCLEIN

The first PD gene to be recognized was mapped to the long arm of chromosome 4 in a large family with dominant inheritance and relatively early age at onset (mean 44 years), but otherwise typical PD with Lewy body pathology, and identified as the gene for α-synuclein (1). Only three different point mutations have been recognized (1–3), each representing a single mutational event, all in large, multigenerational families. No α-synuclein point mutations have been found in sporadic PD (4).

Although α-synuclein mutations are rare, their identification was extremely important, as it led to the discovery that the encoded protein is the major fibrillar component of the Lewy body (5), the proteinaceous inclusion that has, since Friedrich Lewy's original description in 1917, been considered to be the pathologic hallmark of PD in both familial and sporadic cases.

This finding supports a central role of α-synuclein in the development of PD, and α-synuclein staining has replaced staining for ubiquitin as the most sensitive tool in the detection of Lewy bodies. The currently favored hypothesis states that the amino acid changes in the α-synuclein protein associated with PD may favor the β-pleated sheet conformation, which in turn may lead to an increased tendency to form aggregates (6). However, the precise relationship between the formation of aggregates and cell death is unknown. It has been hypothesized that a failure of proteasomal degradation of α-synuclein and other proteins may lead to an accumulation of toxic compounds, possibly consisting of α-synuclein protofibrils (7), ultimately leading to cell death (8). Another possible mechanism could be a deficient chaperone-mediated lysosomal clearance of α-synuclein (9).

A direct link between α-synuclein and PD is supported by the recent discovery that not only point mutations but also multiplications of the wild-type sequence of the α-synuclein gene (duplications and triplications) cause parkinsonism with or without dementia with α-synuclein inclusions (10,11) in some families. This finding is of mechanistic importance because it indicates that a mere increase in α-synuclein levels, which also can be measured in the blood in cases with triplications (12), can be toxic to neurons. On a population level, dosage mutations of SNCA, the gene encoding α-synuclein are again a rare cause of dominant parkinsonism and are not found in the sporadic disease (13,14).

The clinical picture in the affected subjects from pedigrees with α-synuclein mutations or multiplications ranges from typical idiopathic PD to dementia with Lewy bodies (3), although age at onset is lower (mean of about 35 to 45 years with a wide range), and progression appears to be more rapid than in sporadic cases (15,16).

The recognition of the relevance of α-synuclein expression levels have revitalized studies looking at polymorphisms in SNCA, which might influence expression levels, in the sporadic disease. Earlier results had been controversial. Some but not all studies found a complex polymorphic dinucleotide repeat polymorphism (NACP-Rep1) located about 4 kilobases (kb) upstream of the transcriptional start site of SNCA to be associated with sporadic PD. A recent study confirmed an earlier report (17) on the association of PD with single nucleotide polymorphisms (SNPs) in the SNCA promotor (18). In a more general approach, Müller et al. first defined the haplotype structure of the entire SNCA gene by analyzing more than 50 SNPs across the gene. They found a strong association of a haplotype comprising exons 5 and 6 and the 5′-UTR of the SNCA gene with PD, conferring a relative risk of about 1.4 in heterozygous carriers of the risk haplotype and about 2 in homozygotes (19). It is of course likely that more than one mechanism regulates α-synuclein expression. Specific binding of a nuclear protein—Poly (ADP ribose) polymerase-1 (PARP-1)—to the NACP-Rep1 sequence was discovered (20) and may be responsible, at least in part, for the association of specific alleles of this repeat sequence with PD. If confirmed, pharmacologic manipulation of α-synuclein expression may be a possible therapeutic strategy to prevent PD in susceptible individuals.

A relatively small protein, α-synuclein is abundantly expressed in many parts of the brain and localized mostly to presynaptic nerve terminals. Many aspects of the normal function of α-synuclein are still unknown. The protein has been shown to bind to brain vesicles and other cellular components (21) and may be functionally involved in brain plasticity. However, knockout mice for α-synuclein show only subtle alterations in dopamine release under certain experimental conditions, but no other phenotype (22).

There is still no good explanation for the striking selectivity of neuronal damage, which is prominent in dopaminergic cells whereas α-synuclein is abundantly expressed in many areas of the brain. The identification of proteins that specifically bind α-synuclein, such as synphilin (23), may shed new light on this important question. In addition, several animal models have been described recently. Transgenic mice overexpressing α-synuclein, both the normal and the mutated human sequence, under different promoters (24,25) show accumulation of the protein but do not mimic the full degenerative process in the substantia nigra. A transgenic *Drosophila* model may be more true to the human disease (26). Interestingly, pathology in this model appears to be mediated by mitochondrial dysfunction, at least in muscle tissue (27), and can be partially rescued by coexpression of molecular chaperones (28).

Park3: Parkinson's Disease Linked to Chromosome 2

Another dominant locus has been described (PARK3), located on chromosome 2p13, in a subset of families with autosomal dominant inheritance and typical Lewy body pathology (29). Clinical features resemble relatively closely those of sporadic PD, including a similar mean age of onset (59 years in these families), and the penetrance of the mutation was estimated to be 40%, suggesting that it might also play a role in apparently sporadic cases. To date, however, linkage has not been confirmed in other families and the gene has not been identified, despite screening a relatively large number of candidate genes (30). Interestingly, however, two independent reports implicate the PARK3 locus as a disease-modifying locus influencing age at onset in two independent sib pair cohorts with PD (31,32). Another European sib pair study identified a linkage peak in this region (33). A further study refined this association to a region near the sepiapterine reductase gene (34). Sepiapterine reductase is involved in dopamine synthesis. This finding may indicate that the SPR gene is modifying age of onset of PD.

Park5: Parkinsonism Associated with a Mutation in the Gene for Ubiquitin Hydrolase L1

A missense mutation in the gene for ubiquitin carboxy-terminal hydrolase L1 gene (UCHL1), which is located on chromosome 4p, has been identified in affecteds in one family of German ancestry, (35). To date, no other bona fide pathogenic mutations of this gene have been identified. However, a polymorphism in the UCHL1 gene has been found to be associated with sporadic PD in several studies, including a large meta-analysis (36).

PARK8: Parkinsonism Caused by Mutations in the Gene for Leucine-Rich Repeat Kinase 2

Another locus for a dominant form of PD has been mapped in a large Japanese family to the pericentromeric region of chromosome 12. Affecteds in this family showed typical levodopa-responsive parkinsonism with onset in their fifties. Pathologically, nigral degeneration was found but no Lewy bodies or other distinctive inclusions (37).

Recently, the PARK8 gene has been identified: The disease is caused by point mutations in the gene for leucine-rich repeat kinase 2 (LRRK2) (38,39). The encoded protein has also been called *dardarin* (39). The gene spans a genomic region of 144 kb, with 51 exons encoding 2527 amino acids (Fig. 8.1). The gene is expressed in all brain regions and also in all peripheral tissues examined so far, although at low levels.

LRRK2-associated PD is remarkable for several reasons. First, mutations in the LRRK2 gene appear to be the most

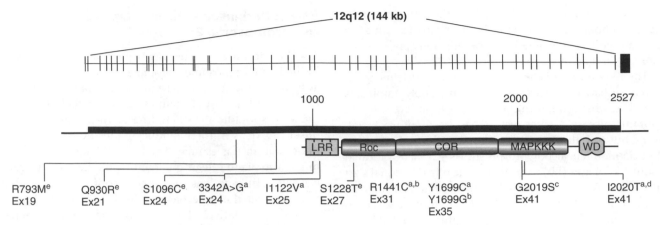

Figure 8.1 Genomic structure and functional domains of LRRK2. The gene spans a genomic distance of 144 kb and contains 51 exons. LRR, leucine rich repeat; Roc, Ras of complex proteins: COR, C-terminal of Roc; MAPKKK, mitogen-activated kinase kinase kinase; WD, Beta-Propeller. Mutations as published in: [a](38); [b](39); [c] (40) (41–43); [d](45); [e]Berg et al.

common cause discovered to date of autosomal-dominant inherited parkinsonism. Four different mutations were detected in 5 of 34 dominant families studied by Zimprich et al. (38). (In two of the families, the same mutation, R1441C, arose independently, based on the analysis of polymorphisms closely surrounding the gene.) The same codon was affected in the group of Basque families studied by Paisan-Ruiz et al. (39), but this mutation resulted in a different amino-acid exchange.

One particularly common mutation, Gly2019Ser, was detected on a founder haplotype across several European populations (40) and in up to 5%–6% of several large cohorts of families with dominant parkinsonism (41,42), and even in 1%–2% of patients with sporadic late-onset disease (43).

Second, clinical signs and symptoms resemble typical sporadic PD in most families. This is true also for age of onset, which is on average in the late fifties and sixties in the families described. Therefore, of the PD genes identified to date, LRRK2 mutations are by far the most common genetic cause of inherited PD and mimic typical sporadic late-onset disease most clearly.

Third, although the clinical picture appears to resemble typical PD, the associated pathology is remarkably variable. Pathologic changes include abnormalities consistent with Lewy body Parkinson's disease, diffuse Lewy body disease, nigral degeneration without distinctive histopathology, and progressive supranuclear palsy (PSP)-like tau aggregation. LRRK2 mutations may therefore be an upstream event in the cascade leading to neurodegeneration with different pathologies.

By sequence homology, LRRK2 can be assigned to the group of recently identified ROCO proteins (44) and contains a protein kinase domain of the MAPKKK class, suggesting a role in intracellular signaling pathways, but its precise function is still undetermined. Mutations appear to be clustered in functionally important regions, which are highly conserved through the species (Fig. 8.1).

AUTOSOMAL RECESSIVE FORMS OF PARKINSONISM

One of the surprising developments of recent years was the recognition of the relatively high proportion of patients with early-onset parkinsonism caused by recessive mutations in several genes (Table 8.1). To date, three have been identified: parkin (PARK2), PINK1 (PARK6), and DJ-1 (PARK7). Again, the study of the function of these genes has provided valuable insight into the molecular mechanisms of dopaminergic degeneration.

PARK2: Autosomal Recessive Juvenile Parkinsonism (AR-JP) Caused by Mutations in the Gene for Parkin

Juvenile cases of parkinsonism with recessive inheritance (families with affected siblings but no transmission from one generation to the next) were first recognized in Japan. The genetic locus for autosomal recessive juvenile parkinsonism (AR-JP) has been mapped to chromosome 6. Mutations were identified in a large gene in that region that was called *parkin* (46). Clinically, these patients suffer from levodopa-responsive parkinsonism and often develop early and severe levodopa-induced motor fluctuations and dyskinesias. Some show diurnal fluctuations, with symptoms becoming worse later in the day. Dystonia at onset of the disease is common.

Parkin mutations turned out to be a common cause of parkinsonism with early onset, particularly in individuals with evidence of recessive inheritance. Nearly 50% of families from a population of sibling pairs collected by Lücking et al. for the European Consortium on Genetic

Susceptibility in PD showed parkin mutations (47). Also, parkin mutations are responsible for the majority of sporadic cases with very early onset (before age 20) and are still common (25%) when onset is between 20 and 35. Prevalence is almost certainly well below 5% in those with onset later than 45.

Several studies have described the clinical spectrum of parkin-associated parkinsonism. Mean age at onset in a European population was 32 years; progression of the disease was usually relatively slow, but levodopa-associated fluctuations and dyskinesias occurred frequently. Dystonia (usually in a lower extremity) at disease onset was found in about 40% of patients, and brisk reflexes of the lower limbs were present in 44% (47). Psychiatric abnormalities have been recognized in PD patients with parkin mutations (48), but there have been no systematic studies to determine whether this is a characteristic feature associated with parkin mutations. Phenotype–genotype studies implicate that the type of mutation may influence the clinical phenotype to a certain degree: Patients with at least one missense mutation showed a faster progression of the disease with a higher United Parkinson's Disease Rating Scale (UPDRS) motor score than carriers of truncating mutations. Missense mutations in functional domains of the parkin gene resulted in earlier onset (49).

The question of whether heterozygous mutations in the parkin gene can cause parkinsonism or can confer an increased susceptibility for typical late-onset PD is still unsettled. There is evidence from imaging studies (50) that heterozygotes may have mildly reduced uptake of fluorodopa in the basal ganglia. Furthermore, families with heterozygous mutation carriers manifesting symptoms of PD been described (51,52). On the other hand, the frequency of heterozygous mutations in the parkin gene was found to be similar in elderly healthy individuals, compared to a cohort with late-onset typical PD (53), and in a large family reported recently, 12 heterozygous carriers of a particular parkin mutation (ex3delta40) were asymptomatic (54). Also, in a group of families with PD showing anticipation (late-onset PD in the parent generation and early-onset PD in the offspring), genotyping results did not support the explanation that the presence of single or compound heterozygous parkin mutations contribute to this phenomenon (55). Therefore, at present the data are still insufficient to confidently judge the role of single heterozygous parkin mutations in the development of PD.

Knowledge of the neuropathology of molecularly confirmed cases of AR-JP is still based on only a few cases. Severe and rather selective degeneration of neurons in the substantia nigra and the locus coeruleus, usually with absence of Lewy bodies, has been described (56). However, a later publication found typical Lewy bodies in a single patient (52). In another case with parkin mutations, tau was found in the inclusions (57), and most recently, another case was reported showing α-synuclein positive inclusions that resemble Lewy bodies in some respects but

differ in some of their staining properties (58). It is still unclear whether these differences may be attributed to differential effects of parkin mutations on the E3-ubiquitin ligase function.

As mutations in parkin cause parkinsonism, in all likelihood by a loss-of-function mechanism, the study of the normal function of parkin should provide insight into the molecular pathogenesis of the disorder. Several groups have now shown that parkin, a protein found in the cytosol but also associated with membranes, functions in the cellular ubiquitination/protein degradation pathway as a ubiquitin ligase (59). It has been hypothesized that the loss of parkin function may lead to the accumulation of a nonubiquitinated substrate that is deleterious to the dopaminergic cell but, due to its nonubiquitinated nature, does not accumulate in typical Lewy bodies. Several proteins have been shown to interact with parkin. However, the putative toxic protein, which has been hypothesized to accumulate due to the lack of parkin in patients (or in knockout animals, for that matter), has not yet been identified.

However, novel functions of parkin are being identified, and it is possible that they may be of equal or even greater relevance to the pathogenesis of PD. For example it has been shown that parkin does not only mediate the well-studied ubiquitinylation via lysin48 (K48), which directs ubiquitinylated proteins for proteasomal degradation, but also via lysin63 (K63), which may play a role in intracellular signalling processes and also in Lewy body formation (60). Additional clues to other possibly relevant functions of parkin have been derived from the proteomic analysis of parkin-/—mice. A recent study revealed a decreased abundance of a number of proteins involved in mitochondrial function or oxidative stress, accompanied by a reduction in respiratory capacity of striatal mitochondria, a decreased serum antioxidant capacity, and increased protein and lipid peroxidation (61). This corresponds well to recent analyses of *Drosophila* parkin[-/-]models. Greene et al. extended an earlier study that had detected mitochondrial pathology, apoptotic muscle degeneration, and locomotor defects in *Drosophila* parkin[-/-]mutants (27) and found that these changes are associated with a profound increase of expression of genes involved in the defense against oxidative stress (62) and that loss-of-function mutations in genes for oxidative stress components enhance the parkin mutant phenotypes. These novel findings indicate that proteasomal dysfunction, although supported by several lines of evidence, may not be the sole mechanism contributing to neurodegeneration in parkin-related disease.

Whatever the mechanism, increasing evidence suggests an important role for parkin in dopamine neuron survival. Overexpression of wild-type rat parkin could protect against the toxicity of mutated human A30P α-synuclein in a rat lentiviral model of PD. The parkin-mediated neuroprotection was associated with an increase in hyperphosphorylated α-synuclein inclusions, suggesting a key role for parkin in the genesis of Lewy bodies (63).

Recessive Early-Onset Parkinsonism Linked to Chromosome 1 (PARK6 and PARK7)

Mutations in the DJ-1 gene (PARK7) are another rare cause of autosomal-recessive parkinsonism (64,65). The clinical picture with early onset and slow progression is similar to the other recessive Parkinson syndromes. Following the initial discovery of two mutations in an Italian and a Dutch family (66), only two additional bona fide pathogenic mutations—one homozygous (67) and one compound heterozygous (68)—have been identified.

The normal function of DJ-1 and its role in dopamine cell degeneration is unknown, but there is evidence that links DJ-1 to oxidative stress response and mitochondrial function. Canet-Aviles et al. have shown that, in the presence of oxidative stress, wild-type DJ-1 translocates to the outer mitochondrial membrane and is associated with neuroprotection (69). Interestingly, DJ-1 is expressed mostly in astrocytes in normal and PD brains, stressing the importance of glial–neuronal interaction in PD (70).

Again, the pathogenic role of several single heterozygous sequence variants detected in cohorts of early-onset PD is unclear (65,68).

Recently, mutations in the PINK1-gene (PARK6) have been identified as another cause for autosomal-recessive early-onset parkinsonism (71). This gene is particularly interesting within the context of the findings linking PD to mitochondrial dysfunction and oxidative stress, as discussed previously, as PINK1 encodes a mitochondrially located kinase. Mutations in the PINK1-gene are much less common than parkin mutations and probably account for only 1%–2% of early-onset cases (72–75). Again the question of the role of single heterozygous mutations is unsettled. In 5 of 100 patients studied by Valente et al. (72), only a single mutation was identified. Age at onset in the heterozygotes was in the fourth to fifth decade (range, 37–47 years). Among healthy control individuals, 2 of 200 also carried one heterozygous missense mutation. Together with previous positron emission tomography studies demonstrating nigrostriatal abnormalities in clinically asymptomatic PARK6 carriers, this observation argues that haploinsufficiency of PINK1 may represent a susceptibility factor toward parkinsonism.

GENETIC CONTRIBUTION TO SPORADIC PARKINSON'S DISEASE

Although molecular genetic analysis has produced significant progress in families with parkinsonian phenotypes with Mendelian inheritance, it must be remembered that in the great majority of cases PD is a sporadic disorder. However, the fact that genetic factors play a role also in families without a clear inheritance pattern is now firmly established. Secondary cases of PD are found more frequently among relatives of patients with PD than in unaffected control populations. Population-based case-control studies indicate that the relative risk for first-degree family members of PD patients is increased in the order of 2 to 3 (76,77), although it should be borne in mind that the genetic contribution is for the largest part contributed by earlier-onset cases. This is supported by a large twin study that indicated that genetic causes may be particularly important in young-onset cases (onset before age 50 years) but appeared low in those with later onset above age 50 (78). It should be mentioned, however, that the strength of the genetic effect and its relative importance in different populations is still under debate. Two studies published in 2004 showed little evidence for an inherited component in Swedish twins (79) or in elderly PD patients with onset after 66 years (77) on the other hand it is clear that LRRK2-mutations account for 1% to 2% of all cases in most series of sporadic PD.

Most attempts to identify the susceptibility genes that are operative in populations of patients with sporadic PD have followed a candidate gene approach. Based on pathologic, pathobiochemical, and epidemiologic findings, hypotheses on the etiology of PD can be generated, and genetic polymorphisms have been examined within—or closely linked to—genes that are thought to be involved in these pathways. Despite a large number of initial positive results, findings have not been confirmed beyond doubt in most cases. Only recently, several positive studies have confirmed initial results for an association of α-synuclein with the sporadic disease (18,19).

A second approach toward the identification of putative genetic risk factors for PD without clear Mendelian inheritance is the genome-wide analysis of a large population of small PD families (affected sib pairs or affected pedigree members) with polymorphic DNA markers. The results of four of these studies have now become available (33,80–82). Several genomic regions with moderately positive lod scores (1–1.5) have been identified in these studies, but only a few regions appeared in more than one study, which did not allow any firm conclusion to be drawn.

Nevertheless, both approaches will be valuable in the future to identify genetic risk factors for PD, because increasing genotyping capacities and improved statistical methods will allow us to greatly expand the data sets and to encompass larger patient populations and/or much denser marker maps across the entire genome.

OTHER GENETIC DISORDERS PRESENTING WITH SIGNS AND SYMPTOMS OF PARKINSONISM

Over time, it has become apparent that a number of inherited neurodegenerative conditions that are, in most cases, neuropathologically and clinically clearly distinct from PD, can present with signs and symptoms of parkinsonism. These disorders may sometimes, at least in the initial stages, mimic idiopathic PD. They include disorders characterized by a predominance of tau-positive inclusions with and without mutations in the MAPTau gene, including the group of frontotemporal dementias with parkinsonism linked to chromosome 17 (FTDP-17) (83) and the related phenotypes of (PSP) and cortico-basal ganglionic degeneration (CBGD). In a small number of patients, a phenotype resembling typical PSP or CBGD is in fact associated with tau gene mutations (84,85). Although no tau mutations can be identified in most patients with PSP or CBGD, there is a clear genetic susceptibility to the disease related to a particular haplotype of DNA markers surrounding the tau gene (86).

The spinocerebellar ataxias (SCAs) are caused by expansions of cytosine–adenine–guanine (CAG) repeat sequences. The core syndrome is usually that of a progressive cerebellar ataxia with or without additional neurologic features. Patients with SCA2 and SCA3 have occasionally been found to present with levodopa-responsive parkinsonism (87,88).

Parkinson's disease has also been described occasionally as occurring in association with Gaucher's disease, a recessive disorder of sphingolipid metabolism caused by mutations in the gene for glucocerebrosidase (GBA). A strong association of PD with (mostly heterozygous) mutations in the GBA gene has been reported in Ashkenazi Jews (89), an ethnic group with a particularly high incidence of Gaucher's. More than 30% of a group of Ashkenazi PD patients had GBA mutations, compared to a general frequency of mutation carriers in this population of about 4%. The relevance of this intriguing finding remains to be determined in large patient cohorts of different ethnic backgrounds.

CONCLUSION

The genetic findings in rare inherited forms of PD have contributed to our understanding of the clinical, neuropathologic, and genetic heterogeneity of PD. The variability of clinical features, such as age at onset, occurrence of dementia, or other associated features found within single families, suggests that a single genetic cause (the pathogenic mutation in a given family) can lead to a spectrum of clinical manifestations. On the other hand, individuals with different genetic defects and different neuropathology may be clinically indistinguishable from each other and fulfill all presently accepted criteria of idiopathic PD. It is therefore apparent that a new genetic classification of PD that is only partially congruent with the classic clinical-pathologic classification is about to emerge.

At present, there is convincing evidence that genetic factors are important in the etiology of at least a subset of patients with PD. Probably only a small percentage of cases with dominant or recessive inheritance can be explained directly by mutations in the genes that have been identified to date, but the molecular pathways also may be important in the sporadic disease. The study of these pathways will provide important insight into the molecular pathogenesis of nigral degeneration. However, it appears that intense efforts are still needed to unravel the full spectrum of etiologic factors leading to the sporadic form of this common neurodegenerative disorder.

REFERENCES

1. Polymeropoulos MH, Lavedan C, Leroy E, et al. Mutation in the α-synuclein gene identified in families with Parkinson's disease. *Science* 1997;276:2045–2047.
2. Krüger R, Kuhn W, Müller T, et al. Ala39Pro mutation in the gene encoding α-synuclein in Parkinson's disease. *Nat Genet* 1998;18: 106–108.
3. Zarranz JJ, Alegre J, Gomez-Esteban JC, et al. The new mutation, E46K, of alpha-synuclein causes Parkinson and Lewy body dementia. *Ann Neurol* 2004;55:164–173.
4. Berg D, Niwar M, Maass S, et al. Alpha-synuclein and Parkinson's disease: implications from the screening of more than 1,900 patients. *Mov Disord* 2005;20:1191–1194.
5. Spillantini MG, Schmidt ML, Lee VM, Trojanowski JQ, Jakes R, Goedert M. Alpha-synuclein in Lewy bodies. *Nature* 1997;388: 839–840.
6. Goedert M, Spillantini MG, Davies SW. Filamentous nerve cell inclusions in neurodegenerative diseases. *Curr Opin Neurobiol* 1998;8:619–632.
7. Goldberg MS, Lansbury Jr PT. Is there a cause-and-effect relationship between alpha-synuclein fibrillization and Parkinson's disease? *Nat Cell Biol* 2000;2:E115–E119.
8. McNaught KS, Olanow CW, Halliwell B, Isacson O, Jenner P. Failure of the ubiquitin-proteasome system in Parkinson's disease. *Nat Rev Neurosci* 2001;2:589–594.
9. Cuervo AM, Stefanis L, Fredenburg R, Lansbury PT, Sulzer D. Impaired degradation of mutant alpha-synuclein by chaperone-mediated autophagy. *Science* 2004;305:1292–1295.
10. Singleton AB, Farrer M, Johnson J, et al. Alpha-synuclein locus triplication causes Parkinson's disease. *Science* 2003;302:841.
11. Ibáñez P, Bonnet AM, Debarges B, et al. Causal relation between alpha-synuclein gene duplication and familial Parkinson's disease. *Lancet* 2004;364:1169–1171.
12. Miller DW, Hague SM, Clarimon J, et al. Alpha-synuclein in blood and brain from familial Parkinson's disease with SNCA locus triplication. *Neurology* 2004;62:1835–1838.
13. Hofer A, Berg D, Asmus F, et al. The role of alpha-synuclein gene multiplications in early-onset Parkinson's disease and dementia with Lewy bodies. *J Neural Transm* 2005;112:1249–1254.
14. Gispert S, Trenkwalder C, Mota-Vieira L, Kostic V, Auburger G. Failure to find alpha-synuclein gene dosage changes in 190 patients with familial Parkinson's disease. *Arch Neurol* 2005;62: 96–98.
15. Golbe LI, Di Iorio G, Bonavita V, Miller DC, Duvoisin RC. A large kindred with autosomal dominant Parkinson's disease. *Ann Neurol* 1990;27:276–282.
16. Spira PJ, Sharpe DM, Halliday G, Cavanagh J, Nicholson GA. Clinical and pathological features of a Parkinsonian syndrome in a family with an Ala53Thr alpha-synuclein mutation. *Ann Neurol* 2001;49:313–319.
17. Farrer M, Maraganore DM, Lockhart P, et al. Alpha-synuclein gene haplotypes are associated with Parkinson's disease. *Hum Mol Genet* 2001;10:1847–1851.
18. Pals P, Lincoln S, Manning J, et al. Alpha-synuclein promoter confers susceptibility to Parkinson's disease. *Ann Neurol* 2004;56: 591–595.
19. Mueller JC, Fuchs J, Hofer A, et al. Multiple regions of alpha synuclein are associated with Parkinson's disease. *Ann Neurol* 2005;57:535–541.
20. Chiba-Falek O, Kowalak JA, Smulson ME, Nussbaum RL. Regulation of alpha-synuclein expression by poly (ADP ribose) polymerase-1 (PARP-1) binding to the NACP-Rep1 polymorphic site upstream of the SNCA gene. *Am J Hum Genet* 2005;76:478–492.

21. Jensen PH, Nielsen MS, Jakes R, Dotti CG, Goedert M. Binding of alpha-synuclein to brain vesicles is abolished by familial Parkinson's disease mutation. *J Biol Chem* 1998;273:26,292–26,294.

22. Abeliovich A, Schmitz Y, Farinas I, et al. Mice lacking alpha-synuclein display functional deficits in the nigrostriatal dopamine system. *Neuron* 2000;25:239–252.

23. Engelender S, Kaminsky Z, Guo X, et al. Synphilin-1 associates with alpha-synuclein and promotes the formation of cytosolic inclusions. *Nat Genet* 1999;22:110–114.

24. Masliah E, Rockenstein E, Veinbergs I, et al. Dopaminergic loss and inclusion body formation in alpha-synuclein mice: implications for neurodegenerative disorders. *Science* 2000;287:1265–1269.

25. Kahle PJ, Neumann M, Ozmen L, et al. Subcellular localization of wild-type and Parkinson's disease-associated mutant alpha-synuclein in human and transgenic mouse brain. *J Neurosci* 2000;20:6365–6373.

26. Feany MB, Bender WW. A *Drosophila* model of Parkinson's disease. *Nature* 2000;404:394–398.

27. Greene JC, Whitworth AJ, Kuo I, Andrews LA, Feany MB, Pallanck LJ. Mitochondrial pathology and apoptotic muscle degeneration in *Drosophila* parkin mutants. *Proc Natl Acad Sci USA* 2003;100:4078–4083.

28. Auluck PK, Chan HY, Trojanowski JQ, Lee VM, Bonini NM. Chaperone suppression of alpha-synuclein toxicity in a *Drosophila* model for Parkinson's disease. *Science* 2002;295:865–868.

29. Gasser T, Müller-Myhsok B, Wszolek ZK, et al. A susceptibility locus for Parkinson's disease maps to chromosome 2p13. *Nat Genet* 1998;18:262–265.

30. West AB, Zimprich A, Lockhart PJ, et al. Refinement of the PARK3 locus on chromosome 2p13 and the analysis of 14 candidate genes. *Eur J Hum Genet* 2001;9:659–666.

31. DeStefano AL, Lew MF, Golbe LI, et al. PARK3 influences age at onset in Parkinson's disease: a genome scan in the GenePD study. *Am J Hum Genet* 2002;70:1089–1095.

32. Pankratz N, Uniacke SK, Halter CA, et al. Genes influencing Parkinson's disease onset: replication of PARK3 and identification of novel loci. *Neurology* 2004;62:1616–1618.

33. Martinez M, Brice A, Vaughan JR, et al. Genome-wide scan linkage analysis for Parkinson's disease: the European genetic study of Parkinson's disease. *J Med Genet* 2004;41:900–907.

34. Karamohamed S, DeStefano AL, Wilk JB, et al. A haplotype at the PARK3 locus influences onset age for Parkinson's disease: the GenePD study. *Neurology* 2003;61:1557–1561.

35. Leroy E, Boyer R, Auburger G, et al. The ubiquitin pathway in Parkinson's disease [letter]. *Nature* 1998;395:451–452.

36. Maraganore DM, Lesnick TG, Elbaz A, et al. UCH-L1is a Parkinson's disease susceptibility gene. *Ann Neurol* 2004;55:512–521.

37. Funayama M, Hasegawa K, Kowa H, Saito M, Tsuji S, Obata F. A new locus for Parkinson's disease (PARK8) maps to chromosome 12p11.2–q13.1. *Ann Neurol* 2002;51:296–301.

38. Zimprich A, Biskup S, Leitner P, et al. Mutations in LRRK2 cause autosomal-dominant parkinsonism with pleomorphic pathology. *Neuron* 2004;44:601–607.

39. Paisan-Ruiz C, Jain S, Evans EW, et al. Cloning of the gene containing mutations that cause PARK8-linked Parkinson's disease. *Neuron* 2004;44:595–600.

40. Kachergus J, Mata IF, Hulihan M, et al. Identification of a novel LRRK2 mutation linked to autosomal dominant parkinsonism: evidence of a common founder across european populations. *Am J Hum Genet* 2005;76:672–680.

41. Nichols WC, Pankratz N, Hernandez D, et al. Genetic screening for a single common LRRK2 mutation in familial Parkinson's disease. *Lancet* 2005;365:410–412.

42. Di Fonzo A, Rohe CF, Ferreira J, et al. A frequent LRRK2 gene mutation associated with autosomal dominant Parkinson's disease. *Lancet* 2005;365:412–415.

43. Gilks WP, Abou-Sleiman PM, Gandhi S, et al. A common LRRK2 mutation in idiopathic Parkinson's disease. *Lancet* 2005;365:415–416.

44. Bosgraaf L, Van Haastert PJ. Roc: a Ras/GTPase domain in complex proteins. *Biochim Biophys Acta* 2003;1643:5–10.

45. Funayama M, Hasegawa K, Ohta E, et al. An LRRK2 mutation as a cause for the parkinsonism in the original PARK8 family. *Ann Neurol* 2005;57:918–921.

46. Kitada T, Asakawa S, Hattori N, et al. Mutations in the parkin gene cause autosomal recessive juvenile parkinsonism. *Nature* 1998;392:605–608.

47. Lücking CB, Dürr A, Bonifati V, et al. Association between early-onset Parkinson's disease and mutations in the parkin gene. *N Engl J Med* 2000;342:1560–1567.

48. Khan NL, Graham E, Critchley P, et al. Parkin disease: a phenotypic study of a large case series. *Brain* 2003;126(Pt 6):1279–1292.

49. Lohmann E, Periquet M, Bonifati V, et al. How much phenotypic variation can be attributed to parkin genotype? *Ann Neurol* 2003;54:176–185.

50. Hilker R, Klein C, Ghaemi M, et al. Positron emission tomographic analysis of the nigrostriatal dopaminergic system in familial parkinsonism associated with mutations in the parkin gene. *Ann Neurol* 2001;49:367–376.

51. Pramstaller PP, Kis B, Eskelson C, et al. Phenotypic variability in a large kindred (family LA) with deletions in the parkin gene. *Mov Disord* 2002;17:424–426.

52. Farrer M, Chan P, Chen R, et al. Lewy bodies and parkinsonism in families with parkin mutations. *Ann Neurol* 2001;50:293–300.

53. Lincoln SJ, Maraganore DM, Lesnick TG, et al. Parkin variants in North American Parkinson's disease: cases and controls. *Mov Disord* 2003;18:1306–1311.

54. Munhoz RP, Sa DS, Rogaeva E, et al. Clinical findings in a large family with a parkin ex3delta40 mutation. *Arch Neurol* 2004;61:701–704.

55. Poorkaj P, Moses L, Montimurro JS, Nutt JG, Schellenberg GD, Payami H. Parkin mutation dosage and the phenomenon of anticipation: a molecular genetic study of familial parkinsonism. *BMC Neurol* 2005;5:4.

56. Mori H, Kondo T, Yokochi M, et al. Pathologic and biochemical studies of juvenile parkinsonism linked to chromosome 6q [see comments]. *Neurology* 1998;51:890–892.

57. Van De Warrenburg BP, Lammens M, Lucking CB, et al. Clinical and pathologic abnormalities in a family with parkinsonism and parkin gene mutations. *Neurology* 2001;56:555–557.

58. Sasaki S, Shirata A, Yamane K, Iwata M. Parkin-positive autosomal recessive juvenile parkinsonism with alpha-synuclein-positive inclusions. *Neurology* 2004;63:678–682.

59. Shimura H, Hattori N, Kubo S, et al. Familial parkinson disease gene product, parkin, is a ubiquitin-protein ligase. *Nat Genet* 2000;25:302–305.

60. Lim KL, Chew KC, Tan JM, et al. Parkin mediates nonclassical, proteasomal-independent ubiquitination of synphilin-1: implications for Lewy body formation. *J Neurosci* 2005;25:2002–2009.

61. Palacino JJ, Sagi D, Goldberg MS, et al. Mitochondrial dysfunction and oxidative damage in parkin-deficient mice. *J Biol Chem* 2004;279:18,614–18,622.

62. Greene JC, Whitworth AJ, Andrews LA, Parker TJ, Pallanck LJ. Genetic and genomic studies of *Drosophila* parkin mutants implicate oxidative stress and innate immune responses in pathogenesis. *Hum Mol Genet* 2005;14:799–811.

63. Lo Bianco C, Schneider BL, Bauer M, et al. Lentiviral vector delivery of parkin prevents dopaminergic degeneration in an alpha-synuclein rat model of Parkinson's disease. *Proc Natl Acad Sci USA* 2004;101:17,510–17,515.

64. Healy DG, Abou-Sleiman PM, Valente EM, et al. DJ-1 mutations in Parkinson's disease. *J Neurol Neurosurg Psychiatry* 2004;75:144–145.

65. Hedrich K, Djarmati A, Schafer N, et al. DJ-1 (PARK7) mutations are less frequent than Parkin (PARK2) mutations in early-onset Parkinson's disease. *Neurology* 2004;62:389–394.

66. Bonifati V, Rizzu P, Van Baren MJ, et al. Mutations in the DJ-1 gene associated with autosomal recessive early-onset parkinsonism. *Science* 2002;299:256–259.

67. Hering R, Strauss KM, Tao X, et al. Novel homozygous p.E64D mutation in DJ1 in early onset Parkinson's disease (PARK7). *Hum Mutat* 2004;24:321–329.

68. Abou-Sleiman PM, Healy DG, Quinn N, Lees AJ, Wood NW. The role of pathogenic DJ-1 mutations in Parkinson's disease. *Ann Neurol* 2003;54:283–286.

69. Canet-Aviles RM, Wilson MA, Miller DW, et al. The Parkinson's disease protein DJ-1 is neuroprotective due to cysteine-sulfinic acid-driven mitochondrial localization. *Proc Natl Acad Sci USA* 2004;101:9103–9108.

70. Bandopadhyay R, Kingsbury AE, Cookson MR, et al. The expression of DJ-1 (PARK7) in normal human CNS and idiopathic Parkinson's disease. *Brain* 2004;127(Pt 2):420–430.

71. Valente EM, Abou-Sleiman PM, Caputo V, et al. Hereditary early-onset Parkinson's disease caused by mutations in PINK1. *Science* 2004;304:1158–1160.

72. Valente EM, Salvi S, Ialongo T, et al. PINK1 mutations are associated with sporadic early-onset parkinsonism. *Ann Neurol* 2004; 56:336–341.

73. Hatano Y, Li Y, Sato K, et al. Novel PINK1 mutations in early-onset parkinsonism. *Ann Neurol* 2004;56:424–427.

74. Rogaeva E, Johnson J, Lang AE, et al. Analysis of the PINK1 gene in a large cohort of cases with Parkinson's disease. *Arch Neurol* 2004;61:1898–1904.

75. Rohe CF, Montagna P, Breedveld G, Cortelli P, Oostra BA, Bonifati V. Homozygous PINK1 C-terminus mutation causing early-onset parkinsonism. *Ann Neurol* 2004;56:427–431.

76. Marder K, Tang MX, Mejia H, et al. Risk of Parkinson's disease among first-degree relatives: a community-based study. *Neurology* 1996;47:155–160.

77. Rocca WA, McDonnell SK, Strain KJ, et al. Familial aggregation of Parkinson's disease: the Mayo Clinic family study. *Ann Neurol* 2004;56:495–502.

78. Tanner CM, Ottman R, Goldman SM, et al. Parkinson's disease in twins: an etiologic study. *JAMA* 1999;281:341–346.

79. Wirdefeldt K, Gatz M, Schalling M, Pedersen NL. No evidence for heritability of Parkinson's disease in Swedish twins. *Neurology* 2004;63:305–311.

80. DeStefano AL, Golbe LI, Mark MH, et al. Genome-wide scan for Parkinson's disease: the GenePD Study. *Neurology* 2001;57: 1124–1126.

81. Scott WK, Nance MA, Watts RL, et al. Complete genomic screen in Parkinson's disease: evidence for multiple genes. *JAMA* 2001;286: 2239–2244.

82. Pankratz N, Nichols WC, Uniacke SK, et al. Genome screen to identify susceptibility genes for Parkinson's disease in a sample without parkin mutations. *Am J Hum Genet* 2002;71:124–135.

83. Reed LA, Wszolek ZK, Hutton M. Phenotypic correlations in FTDP-17. *Neurobiol Aging* 2001;22:89–107.

84. Pastor P, Pastor E, Carnero C, et al. Familial atypical progressive supranuclear palsy associated with homozygosity for the delN296 mutation in the tau gene. *Ann Neurol* 2001;49:263–267.

85. Bugiani O, Murrell JR, Giaccone G, et al. Frontotemporal dementia and corticobasal degeneration in a family with a P301S mutation in tau. *J Neuropathol Exp Neurol* 1999;58:667–677.

86. Baker M, Litvan I, Houlden H, et al. Association of an extended haplotype in the tau gene with progressive supranuclear palsy. *Hum Mol Genet* 1999;8:711–715.

87. Gwinn-Hardy K, Chen JY, Liu HC, et al. Spinocerebellar ataxia type 2 with parkinsonism in ethnic Chinese. *Neurology* 2000;55:800–805.

88. Gwinn-Hardy K, Singleton A, O'Suilleabhain P, et al. Spinocerebellar ataxia type 3 phenotypically resembling Parkinson's disease in a black family. *Arch Neurol* 2001;58:296–299.

89. Aharon-Peretz J, Rosenbaum H, Gershoni-Baruch R. Mutations in the glucocerebrosidase gene and Parkinson's disease in Ashkenazi Jews. *N Engl J Med* 2004;351:1972–1977.

Disease-Modifying Strategies in Parkinson's Disease

9

Cristina Sampaio   *Olivier Rascol*

INTRODUCTION

Problem Statement

The typical course of Parkinson's disease (PD) is one of gradual worsening over a decade or more, corresponding to ongoing neuronal loss affecting cells in the pigmented nuclei of the brainstem, particularly in the substantia nigra. There is a preclinical phase of uncertain duration, probably about 5 years (1), during which loss of dopaminergic neurons progresses until the threshold for clinical symptoms is reached. The estimated neuron loss by the time of diagnosis is about 60% (2). PD progression ultimately leads to important disability, handicap, and death (3). Despite current best standard of care, mortality among PD patients is still higher than the general population one (4). Given this course, there is a growing interest in developing interventions that can change it for the better. It is believed that to obtain an important clinical impact on the natural course of disease, the intervention should have a long-lasting effect that goes beyond the immediate control of signs and symptoms. This is the essence of the disease-modifying concept.

Definitions

There is no consensus on the definition of the term *disease-modifying*. A disease-modifying drug for relapsing–remitting multiple sclerosis is one that can postpone disability in contrast to those that only reduce the frequency of relapses (5). For a neurodegenerative disorder, a disease-modifying drug is usually considered to be one that can reduce the progression rate. To some extent, this intuitively implies an effect in the physiopathologic mechanism of the disease (6). This last, narrow perspective equates with the concept of neuroprotection, which describes a mechanism of action rather than the consequence of an intervention. From the patient perspective, what is relevant, however, is the occurrence of long-lasting changes in disability, regardless and independently of the mechanism. Thus, we believe that a disease-modifying intervention should be defined as one that is able to have a "long-lasting" effect on disability, although we recognize the difficulties in defining the qualifier: "long-lasting."

The Food and Drug Administration (FDA) links disease-modifying effects in a neurodegenerative disorder to an effect in the mechanism of the neurodegenerative process, meaning that it prefers the narrow, mechanistic approach to the concept. The European Medicines Evaluation Agency (EMEA) has not yet expressed a public view on this matter. In fact, two stances can be adopted. One is a disease-centered stance where the dichotomy is treatments that interfere with the mechanisms of the disease versus treatments that only have an effect on the expression of signs and symptoms. The other stance is patient centered. It distinguishes treatments that produce a clinically relevant long-lasting benefit from the ones that produce only transitory effects. In this chapter, we adopt the patient-centered approach in which a disease-modifying intervention is one that prevents/postpones disability. We favor this approach because it is all encompassing and does not overemphasize the importance of preserving neurons to get a relevant benefit. There is a widespread belief that only by protecting or rescuing threatened neurons is it possible to obtain a long-lasting benefit, but this is not necessarily so. The concept of neuroprotection is undoubtedly attractive, but a long-lasting benefit will only be obtained, by this mechanism, if the proportion of neurons that is saved or rescued is significant. Estimates of how large this fraction should be are lacking. It is unlikely that small neuroprotective effects will be clinically relevant. Moreover, most of the preclinical experiments to test potential effects upon neuronal death in PD focus on dopaminergic cells. A number of the most debilitating parkinsonian signs—including dementia, depression, psychosis, falls, orthostatic hypotension, urinary incontinence, constipation, and impotence—are not dependent on dopaminergic denervation. Therefore, it is not expected that they should be sensitive to interventions that would spare dopaminergic neurons alone.

Assuming the broad concept of disease modification, we will argue that levodopa is the best-documented disease-modifying intervention for PD given that it changes the course of the disease by inducing motor fluctuations and dyskinesias (undesirable) and that it has impact on an important milestone: death (desirable)(6).

OUTCOMES OF A DISEASE-MODIFYING STRATEGY IN PARKINSON'S DISEASE

To establish if an intervention has or has not had an effect on prevention/postponement of disability in controlled clinical trials, it is necessary to evaluate clinically relevant endpoints. Outcomes definition is a critical step in the process of establishing if an intervention is disease modifying. For example, the series of trials comparing levodopa to various dopamine agonists (7,8,9,10), which used time to occurrence of dyskinesias or time to motor complications as a primary outcome, has been criticized for not

having used an outcome clearly related with disability (11), which would have made the translation of the results to clinical practice less contentious. These debates are unavoidable because there is a trade-off between the clinical relevance of an outcome and the time frame in which it occurs, with the more relevant outcomes happening later in the disease than the less relevant outcomes, which makes the options for an outcome a matter of feasibility (12,13). A parameter for evaluating the feasibility of an outcome is what we designated by the outcome T30 or T50, which is the time it takes, in months or years, for 30% (T30) or 50% (T50) of a theoretical cohort of early PD patients to reach the defined outcome. Table 9.1 provides examples of values for T30 and T50.

Clinically Relevant Outcomes

Clinically relevant outcomes usually are established by means of consensus expert opinion, although other, more systematic approaches that can reflect patients concerns are available, such as qualitative research methodologies including focus groups (14). Among those outcomes that are consensual, those in Table 9.1 are the most frequently mentioned. However, it is doubtful that postponing death is a goal if disability and handicap are not positively modified. This discussion has never been particularly heated among researchers of PD because the remoteness of this outcome from the moment of diagnosis makes it an unlikely choice. So far only one trial used death as a prespecified outcome (15). Nevertheless, contrary to other opinions (12,13) we consider death inappropriate as an outcome to evaluate a potential disease-modifying intervention in PD because it is not obligatory that delaying death is necessarily associated with delaying disability.

The binary outcomes presented in Table 9.2 should be considered stand-alone outcomes, with a clinical importance of their own, which makes them worth pursuing and distinguishing from surrogate endpoints. Nonetheless, those

---

TABLE 9.1

CRUDE ESTIMATES OF THE TIME NEEDED FOR 30% (T30) OR 50% (T50) OF A COHORT OF EARLY PARKINSON'S DISEASE PATIENTS TO REACH THE DESIGNATED ENDPOINTS

Endpoints	T30 (years)	T50 (years)
Need for dopaminergic therapy[1]	< 1 year	~ 1.5
Occurrence of postural instability (Hoehn & Yahr stage 3)[1]	~ 4	~ 7
Dyskinesias on LD[a2]	~ 3	~ 5
Motor fluctuations on LD[a2]	~ 4	~ 6
Death[1]	> >10	—

[a] The yearly change in annual incidence is probably nonlinear; highest incidence appears in the first year of exposure. 1. Estimates based on data from the DATATOP cohort. 2. Estimates based on data from the PELMOPET cohort.

TABLE 9.2

BINARY OUTCOMES

Disability Milestones	Need for dopaminergic therapy Loss of critical ADLs Occurrence of (disabling) postural instability (Hoehn & Yahr stage 3) Loss of independent ambulation (Hoehn & Yahr stage 4)
Handicap Milestones	Loss of employability Institutionalization
Life Milestones	Death

endpoints are not equal in their clinical relevance. In particular, "need for dopaminergic therapy" calls for the following explanation: Postponing dopaminergic therapy is not a goal in itself. In fact, a recent review of the scientific evidence released most of the fears that levodopa would be neurotoxic (16). Hitherto, "need for dopaminergic therapy" represents a level of disability that is clinically relevant and has been operationalized in different protocols (17,18). It is arguable that this endpoint is too early and any benefit related to it might not be maintained later. The counterargument is that if a patient is kept, *long enough*, in a level of disability below the threshold for needing dopaminergic therapy, it might be worthwhile, even if after reaching that level the disease follows its usual course without change.

In this context and from the patient's perspective, it is important to note that it is not relevant how the listed outcomes are delayed, whether by preserving neuron health or by providing symptomatic control or both. What is relevant is for how long those outcomes are delayed. However, the view that disease modification implies preservation or rescue of neurons pushed investigators to attempt to disentangle what is a strictly symptomatic effect (short-lasting) from a neuroprotective effect (long-lasting) by means of innovative trial designs, like randomized start trials or randomized withdrawal trials (19). There is no room in this context to engage in a detailed discussion of those designs. Nevertheless, it is important for the sake of information to note that none of those designs has been validated for the purpose and their interpretation is fraught by innumerable confounding factors. Designs that include washout periods are confounded by dropouts (patients do not stay for the duration of the washout), nocebo effects, unknown biologic half-life for the drugs that have been washed out, etc. The fancier randomized start trial, partially used in the TEMPO (20) study, where rasagiline was compared with placebo, is far from having been confirmed as useful for disentangling symptomatic from protective effects. Nevertheless, to have an opportunity to achieve that goal, the primary analysis of a randomized start trial must take place at the end of the second period, it should use a repeated measures model instead of a single-point analysis, and the occurrence of differential dropouts must be compensated by an appropriate imputation method. So far no properly analyzed

randomized start trial has been published. When and if it comes up, the further challenge will be to interpret a possible difference in terms of clinical relevance.

Biomarkers and Surrogate Endpoints

As defined by Temple (21), a surrogate endpoint of a clinical trial is a laboratory measurement or a physical sign used as a substitute for a clinically meaningful endpoint that measures directly how a patient feels, functions, or survives. Changes induced on a surrogate endpoint by a therapy are expected to reflect changes in a clinically meaningful endpoint.

A correlate does not a surrogate make. It is a common misconception that if an outcome is a correlate (that is, correlated with the true clinical outcome) it can be used as a valid surrogate endpoint (that is, a replacement for the true clinical outcome). However, proper justification for such replacement requires that the effect of the intervention on the surrogate endpoint predicts the effect on the clinical outcome—a much stronger condition than correlation (22). There are no validated surrogate endpoints in PD.

Biomarker is a characteristic that is objectively measured and evaluated as an indicator of normal biological processes, pathogenic processes, or pharmacologic responses to a therapeutic intervention (23). Several biomarkers have been proposed or used in the context of PD. They were comprehensively reviewed by Mitchell et al. (24). For the discussion of disease-modifying interventions, functional brain imaging is one type of biomarker of special interest.

In 18F-fluorodopa (L-3,4-dihydroxyphenylalanine) positron emission tomography (PET), fluorodopa is injected intravenously and taken up by nigrostriatal neurons in a manner similar to levodopa. It is then decarboxylated to fluorodopamine, which is released and metabolized like dopamine. The level of radioactivity during this process is measured. It is dependent on the number of active neurons.

Another approach to functional imaging is based on visualizing the dopamine transporter located on dopaminergic nerve terminals where it actively pumps dopamine back into neurons. Two radioligands—^{123}I-β-CIT (2β-carboxymethoxy-3β-{4-iodophenyl}tropane) and ^{123}I-FPCIT (N-ω-fluoropropyl-2β-carboxymethoxy-3β-{4-iodophenyl}tropane)—are used to label the presynaptic dopamine transporter for SPECT imaging. The imaging reflects the uptake of the tracer into the striatum, its binding to the dopamine transporter, and its release and metabolism.

Although several trials have used these biomarkers either as primary endpoints—REAL-PET (25)—or secondary endpoints—CALM-PD (8), PELMOPET (10), ELLDOPA (26)—the interpretation of the results is full of hurdles: Some patients classified as PD patients by clinicians have normal scans (these can be 5% to 15% of a given cohort), the treatment used might impact on the image results, and the existence of longitudinal correlation between imaging and clinical status is not yet demonstrated. There also are very important challenges to such correlation. The most striking example comes from the transplantation experiments where a clear survival of the transplant does not translate into any obvious clinical benefit (27,28). Beyond this example, because it can be argued that transplanted cells are exogenous and do not reflect the paradigm of the analysis in cohorts of early PD patients, the fact is that there is no strong evidence: The few studies available are small and show a large intersubject variability, the decrease in signal in imaging techniques does not correlate with the clinical status, and this would be just the first criteria for imaging to achieve the status of a surrogate endpoint (see the preceding). Several factors are to be considered when interpreting imaging data: the effect of the treatment being assessed on the marker—for example, dopamine agonist may downregulate dopamine transporters; this effect being wrongly interpreted as reflecting missing neurons; and the sensitivity and reproducibility of the technique being used.

At present, there are no validated surrogate endpoints for disability in PD. In certain circumstances, the available imaging techniques can be used as biomarkers, but the data generated should be interpreted with caution. Nevertheless, it is desirable to use them as secondary endpoints in clinical trials, which will increase the knowledge database and ultimately lead to a better-informed use.

The community of scientists (academic and industry) interested in developing new treatments for neurodegenerative disorders is struggling not only with the paradigms to prove a clinical relevant effect, as described, but also with paradigms that will allow a quick evaluation of the potential of candidate drugs to avoid the need to start long-term, large-size sample trials in the dark, not knowing which is the optimal dose or if there is a good basis to believe the drug in question is worth testing. To address this issue the National Institutes of Health (NIH) in the United States provided funds to a dedicated program. In the context of this program, four candidate drugs (creatine, coenzyme Q10, minocycline, and neuroimmunophilin) to be tested in clinical trials were selected using systematic criteria. This program also stimulates creative thinking around the topic of how to explore the potential of candidate drugs. This has lead to importation from the field of oncology of the concept of futility studies, which are low-resource trials in which the goal is to declare as failures drugs that do not achieve a predefined success criteria (29).

DISEASE-MODIFYING STRATEGIES IN PARKINSON'S DISEASE

Proven Strategies

Treatment with Levodopa

Levodopa (L-dopa) has an established role as one of the most efficacious antiparkinsonian agents documented by decades of clinical use. The effect size of L-dopa in PD is large and robust and argues against possible biases that

usually affect uncontrolled studies. Therefore, it now seems irrelevant to discuss the evidence basis of L-dopa's well-established efficacy. Nevertheless, this unquestionable efficacy was recently confirmed in a history-making randomized clinical trial known as ELLDOPA (26). The discussion of the remarkable achievement that ELLDOPA represents is beyond our discussion. Yet it is relevant to highlight that ELLDOPA results show a clear dose-response for L-dopa efficacy on PD disability as measured by the United Parkinson's Disease Rating Scale (UPDRS). It also suggests, at a clinical level, that L-dopa may have a "protective" effect while the imaging data suggest the opposite. This is another blow for the attempt to establish imaging as a surrogate endpoint in PD. To the end of supporting that L-dopa is disease modifying, the most relevant argument is that the introduction of L-dopa in the therapeutic armamentarium changed the natural history of the disease by reducing the disability drastically and by having an impact on the time of death, at least in the first 5 years after initiation of treatment, as documented by observational studies (6,30). The most likely mechanism by which this result is achieved is the large symptomatic effect of size on motor symptoms, yet the contribution from other mechanisms cannot be excluded. It is also well-documented that the chronic use of L-dopa does produce long-lasting molecular changes at the level of the basal ganglia, which are associated and probably are an important contributor to the occurrence of motor fluctuations and dyskinesias that were unknown in the pre-levodopa era (31). Such changes do not correspond to a favorable or desirable modification of the disease, but they indisputably change the clinical phenomenology of disease progression.

Promising Strategies

Marketed Medicinal Products
Early Use of Dopamine Agonists
In terms of promising strategies, the crux of the matter is the strategy rather than the drugs, that is, the critical topic is how to start dopaminergic therapy rather than the therapy itself. It is well-known that the five randomized controlled trials (RCTs) (7,8,9,10,32) that compared the strategy of initiating therapy with a dopamine agonist to starting it with levodopa showed consistently that dyskinesias and probably motor fluctuations could be delayed by starting treatment with a dopamine agonist, although this was at the cost of less control of motor symptoms. The imaging data associated with these trials are so far unclear taking in accounting for the confounding factors already mentioned. Despite the clear clinical results obtained in RCTs, there are important doubts regarding the clinical relevance of those results (11) because the lack of clear evidence that disability has been delayed in a clinically meaningful manner remains unclear: When dyskinesias or motor fluctuations first occur, they are not severe enough to be disabling from a clinical perspective. No convincing data are available to show that the early use of a dopamine agonist delays the

occurrence of severe and disabling dyskinesias or on–off fluctuations. Therefore, it is impossible to conclude that starting dopaminergic therapy with a dopamine agonist is a disease-modifying strategy. This inconclusiveness is due mainly to the doubts about the impact on disability, although the difficulties in interpreting the imaging data also contribute.

MAO-B Inhibitors

Selegiline. There are five RCTs, including a megatrial (800 patients)—DATATOP—that have compared selegiline to placebo in the ability to postpone the level of disability associated with the need of dopaminergic therapy. These trials were reviewed in the movement disorders evidence-based review of PD treatments (33). In this regard, all trials were highly consistent in showing that selegiline is effective in postponing for more than 6 months this early level of disability, which may be considered clinically relevant, independently of the mechanism by which it is achieved and remains unknown, despite several attempts to disentangle selegiline symptomatic versus protective effects. It seems that in the early phase of the disease, selegiline does postpone disability but later on there is a catching up, suggested by the data obtained on the follow-up of the DATATOP cohort. Overall, there is no true disease-modifying effect because later-stage disability is not affected.

The fears raised by the UK-PDRG trial that selegiline, when associated with L-dopa, would increase mortality are now put to rest because those findings could never be confirmed (34,35), and it is now accepted that the signal in the UK-PDRG was most likely a chance effect.

Selegiline is, therefore, not considered a disease-modifying drug in PD because its effect seems to be clustered in the early phase of the disease and it is transitory, disappearing in the later stages. Nevertheless, in this early phase, there is an effect that is clinically interesting and can be seen as a benchmark for development of other drugs.

Rasagiline. Like selegiline, rasagiline mesylate is an irreversible MAO inhibitor with high selectivity for the B form of the enzyme. It is more potent than selegiline on a weight basis, such that 0.5—1 mg/day causes total inhibition of platelet MAO-B in humans (36). Unlike selegiline, it is devoid of amphetamine-like metabolites.

Rasagiline proved to be an efficacious antiparkinsonic agent. In monotherapy, its symptomatic effect is modest, but adjunct to levodopa it rivals the effect of entacapone (37). The hypothesis that rasagiline might be disease modifying in the strict sense of having neuroprotective effect has been explored in the TEMPO study (20). This study was a classic drug versus placebo 6-month follow-up study to which an additional 6-month double-blind extension was added, in which patients who had been on placebo in the first period were switched to rasagiline 1 mg. At the end of this extra 6-month period, both groups were compared. The group

that had been exposed to placebo in the initial period of study had higher UPDRS scores than the group started on rasagiline from the beginning. This lead to the interpretation that rasagiline had a long-lasting effect that patients exposed to placebo in the first part of the study missed and could not catch up to with the late introduction of rasagiline.

However, this result is only suggestive of a potential neuroprotective effect: It does not allow concluding that this potential effect has a relevant effect size in the patient's perspective; the caveat remains that if the follow-up had been prolonged (the total follow-up is 1 year), the treated arm might have caught up to the placebo, as happened in the DATATOP cohort.

Coenzyme Q10. Coenzyme Q10 is a commonly used "health supplement" that is being pursued in PD for its ability to augment mitochondrial complex I activity and serve as an antioxidant. Its use targets a metabolic abnormality detected in the PD brain and systemically in a reduction in activity of the first step in the mitochondrial chain of electron transport. Coenzyme Q10 is among the few substances to have a dedicated section in this chapter because some data on it have been obtained in RCTs. The exploratory trial conducted by Schultz et al. (38) revealed some promising positive results. This trial involved 80 otherwise untreated PD subjects receiving oral coenzyme Q10 at up to 1200 mg/day. Over the 16 months of drug administration, there was a worsening of 6.69 points in the 1200 mg/day treatment group while the placebo group deteriorated 11.99 points ($p = 0.04$) in the adjusted mean score for total UPDRS. No improvement was seen at the lower doses of 300 and 600 mg/day. Further analysis indicated that most of the benefit from 1200 mg/day was attributable to fewer declines in activities of daily living rather than to amelioration of clinical signs on examination.

Almost as a déjà vu experience, evocative of the selegiline/DATATOP study, there have been suggestions that coenzyme Q10 might have small, short-term, and therefore symptomatic effects (39).

Nevertheless, given the results available, coenzyme Q10 has been selected by the NIH program to be studied further. In phase II, a futility study is evaluating a dose of 2400 mg/day (40).

Interventions Identified by the National Institutes of Health Task Force

The NIH clinical trials program is currently addressing two important issues in translational research and clinical trials: (1) the identification and prioritization of interventions for testing, and (2) the design and implementation of pilot clinical trials (the already discussed futility studies) that efficiently select agents for further study in comparative efficacy trials (41). NIH believes that even a small neuroprotective effect with a minimally toxic agent would be important to detect. This last assumption might not be true because a small effect in each individual suffering from a neurodegenerative disorder might not have any relevant impact on overall disability. In the field of cerebrovascular disorders, the thinking is different because a small relative reduction of events can have a huge public health impact.

As part of an NIH program to test drugs with the potential to slow the progression of PD, NIH established the Committee to Identify Neuroprotective Agents for Parkinson's (CINAPS) to systematically gather and evaluate information about candidate interventions. CINAPS was composed of clinical pharmacologists, neurologists, clinical trialists, and laboratory-based experts in neurodegeneration. The group established explicit criteria, including mechanism and rationale, efficacy in animal models of PD, safety and tolerability in humans, pharmacokinetics, and preliminary evidence of activity in humans. CINAPS gathered information on 59 different compounds. The published literature on each compound was then used to rate these agents on the prespecified criteria. Twelve compounds with a variety of mechanisms of action were found to be good candidates for phase II–IV clinical trials assessing neuroprotection in PD (42) (Table 9.3). The two ongoing National Institute of Neurological Disorders and Stroke (NINDS)-sponsored trials (each trial tests two compounds against placebo), known as the Neuroprotection Exploratory Trials in PD (NET-PD), are testing four compounds (creatine 10 mg/day, minocycline 1200 mg/day, coenzyme Q10 2400 mg/day, neuroimunophilin ligand—GPI 1485—4000 mg/day) identified by CINAPS.

Creatine is a widely available nutritional supplement. Creatine is converted to phosphocreatine, which in turn can function as an energy buffer by transferring a phosphoryl group to adenosine diphosphate (ADP). It may act as an indirect antioxidant by enhancing energy transduction and may inhibit mitochondrial permeability transition. In doses of 1% to 2% of diet by weight, creatine appears protective in 1-methyl-4-phenyl-1,2,3,6-tetrahydropyridine (MPTP) rodent models and in transgenic Huntington's disease (HD) and amyotrophic lateral sclerosis (ALS) models. There is extensive literature on use and tolerability in athletes at doses up to 20 g/day, and there are some data on safety and tolerability in patients with neurologic disorders at doses up to 10 g/day.

Minocycline is a tetracycline antibiotic with good brain penetration that has been shown to inhibit microglial-related inflammatory events, as well as the apoptotic cascade. Animal studies in ALS and PD models show convincing evidence of neuroprotection, and the compound appears to be safe for chronic administration. Nevertheless, minocycline is also being evaluated in a placebo-controlled randomized trial for multiple systemic atrophy (MSA) in the framework of European Multiple Systemic Atrophy Study Group (EMSA-SG) (43).

Coenzyme Q 10 has already been described.

GPI 1485 is an investigational new drug that belongs to a class of small molecule compounds called *neuroimmunophilin ligands*. In preclinical experiments, neuroimmunophilin ligands have been shown to repair and regenerate damaged nerves without affecting normal, healthy nerves. GPI 1485 has been studied in PD patients in a 6-month clinical trial sponsored by Amgen. Data from the trial are published only as a press release, which indicates that the primary endpoint was negative but the drug was well tolerated.

Other Interventions Undergoing Clinical Trials

This section will be rather incomplete because the public sources of data vary on details. It is possible that several clinical trials are ongoing without having been registered in a public database. Fischer compiled a list of drugs being developed for neurodegenerative diseases as of 2004 (44). In this list, there are 37 products out of a total of 226 quoted to be on study for PD. Many others are intended for neurodegenerative disorders. Among the 37 PD products, 10 (APBPI 124, CEP-1347, ganglioside GM1, iometopane, NS 2330, P 58, rasagiline, safinamide, talampanel, TCH 346) are said to have entered clinical trials to test potential neuroprotective properties. It is not easy to obtained details of these studies. Therefore, the following drugs should be considered to be examples from a longer list.

CEP-1347 (Cephalon Inc./Lundbeck) is a small molecule that acts as an inhibitor of mixed lineage kinase-3, a major component in the transcription factor c-Jun-mediated terminal kinase signaling pathway involved in apoptotic neuron death. With CEP-1347, several pathways leading to experimental loss of neuronal PC12 cells, sympathetic

TABLE 9.3

THE 12 PRODUCTS PRIORITIZED FOR CLINICAL TRIALS TO EVALUATE PUTATIVE NEUROPROTECTION

Product	Mechanism of Action
Caffeine	Adenosine antagonist
Coenzyme Q10	Antioxidant/mitochondrial stabilizer
Creatine	Mitochondrial stabilizer
Estrogen[a]	Undetermined/multiple
GPI 1485	Trophic factor
GM-1 ganglioside	Trophic factor
Minocycline	Anti-inflammatory/anti-apoptotic
Nicotine*	Unknown
Pramipexole	Antioxidant/vesicular trafficking
Ropinirole	Antioxidant
Rasagiline	Antioxidant/anti-apoptotic
Selegiline	Antioxidant/anti-apoptotic

Adapted from Rovinga BM, Fagan SC, Hart RG, et al. Neuroprotective agents for clinical trials in Parkinson's disease: a systematic assessment. *Neurology* 2003;60:1234–1240.
[a] Unlike candidates for clinical trials given the established deleterious effects on outcomes other than neuroprotection.

neurons, and various in vivo models of neurodegeneration can be blocked. In MPTP-induced Parkinsonism, for example, this compound has improved survival of neurons in the substantia nigra. A randomized, placebo-controlled study of CEP-1347 was carried out to demonstrate its safety and tolerability, with 50 mg twice being explored as a potential neuroprotective agent in a clinical trial—the PRECEPT study) (45).

GM1 ganglioside has been shown to stimulate recovery of the damaged dopamine system under a number of different circumstances. In addition to rescue of damaged dopamine neurons, it is claimed that GM1 enhances the synthesis of dopamine in remaining nigrostriatal neurons following MPTP exposure. In 1999, a randomized, placebo-controlled trial was sponsored by NIH. In January 2004, this trial was still ongoing (46).

Deep-Brain Stimulation

Deep-brain stimulation (DBS) can be used in different targets (pallidum, subthalamic nucleus) and in different surgical paradigms. Today, bilateral subthalamic stimulation is being favored by most centers (47). The place to review the benefit–risk relationship of these strategies is elsewhere in this book. They are nevertheless mentioned here because some data suggest that they have the potential to produce large and maintained, beneficial motor effects in advanced PD patients. This potential is yet to be evaluated in long-term, controlled studies measuring global disability outcomes. If those potential beneficial effects prove to be long-lasting, DBS might claim disease-modifying properties in the broad sense mentioned in the early sections of this chapter.

Strategies Known to Have Failed

As for the ongoing trials, it is difficult to retrieve accurately the data on interventions that were tested and failed, because most of these trials never are published, which is regrettable. The following cases should be taken as examples from a larger set.

Vitamin E (VIT E) is an important antioxidant. It was first tested for its potential as a neuroprotectant in the DATATOP trial (17). It failed to show a benefit. Since then VIT E has been tested in several large controlled trials for neurodegenerative and other diseases. It always failed to determine a benefit, and in a couple of instances it was not possible to exclude a deleterious effect (48).

Riluzole has a complex mechanism of action. Among other molecular actions, it blocks the presynaptic release of glutamate. It is currently marketed for slowing progression of amyotrophic lateral sclerosis. A wide range of laboratory studies has highlighted the potential role of glutamatergic excitotoxicity in neurodegenerative diseases, including PD. Studies in animal models of parkinsonism have pointed to the role that might be played by activation of N-methyl-D-aspartate (NMDA) receptors by glutamate. Most compounds with potent glutamatergic blockade have proved to be too toxic for clinical use. A multicenter, randomized, placebo-controlled trial with riluzole was undertaken to test for possible protection against PD progression. The trial in PD was halted because lack of efficacy was determined after an interim analysis (49).

TCH 346 (also designated in laboratory research reports as CGP 3466 or CGP 3466B) is a compound owned by Novartis Pharmaceuticals. It shares some structural similarities with selegiline, but it does not inhibit MAO-B. Its presumed mechanism as a neuroprotective agent is through binding to the gylceraldehyde-3-phosphate dehydrogenase (GAPDH). There is considerable evidence that GAPDH enacts a key step in age-induced neuron apoptosis. The potential neuroprotective effect of TCH 346 was tested for slowing progression of amyotrophic lateral sclerosis and for PD (in large, multicenter, independent, clinical trials). The ALS trial failed to show a benefit, which has only been reported as a communication to the patients association (50). The PD trial is long finished and no public statement on it exists, which makes the presumption that it also failed very likely.

CONCLUSIONS

There are two cultures surrounding the concept of disease-modifying interventions in PD. One is focused on the disease processes. Its most important goal is to find an intervention that can interfere with the mechanism of disease and by doing this to delay disease progression. In this paradigm it is of the utmost importance to disentangle symptomatic from protective effects by means of sophisticated trial design and analysis. Another approach is to work on a patient-centered concept. In this framework, the goal is to achieve a long-lasting delay in disability.

Assuming a disease-centered paradigm, no single intervention has proved to be disease modifying. On a patient-centered paradigm, levodopa—due to its effect in postponing death—can be considered disease modifying. A number of promising strategies were reviewed, but available data are scant. Selegiline is able to postpone early disability, but this advantage is lost later. All other interventions are in the study phase, although some are more advanced (results are likely to appear sooner) than others, for example rasagiline and coenzyme Q10.

REFERENCES

1. Morrish PK, Sawle GV, Brooks DJ. An ^{18}F dopa-PET and clinical study of the rate of progression in Parkinson Disease. *Brain* 1996;119:585–591.
2. Fearnley JM, Lees AJ. Ageing and Parkinson's disease: substantia nigra regional selectivity. *Brain* 1991;114:2283–2301.
3. Poewe WH, Wenning GK. The natural history of Parkinson's disease. *Ann Neurol* 1998;44(suppl 1):S1–S9.
4. Joseph C, Chassan JB, Koch ML. Levodopa in Parkinson disease: a long-term appraisal of mortality. *Ann Neurol* 1978;2:116–118.

5. CPMP note for guidance on clinical investigation of medicinal products for the treatment of mulotiple sclerosis. Available at: http://www.emea.eu.int/pdfs/human/ewp/056198en.pdf. Accessed March 25, 2005.

6. Clarke CE. Does levodopa therapy delay death in Parkinson's disease? a review of the evidence. *Mov Disord* 1995;10:250–256.

7. Rascol O, Brooks DJ, Korczyn AD, De Deyn PP, Clarke CE, Lang AE, for the 056 Study Group. A five-year study of the incidence of dyskinesia in patients with early Parkinson's disease who were treated with ropinirole or levodopa. *N Engl J Med* 2000;342:1484–1491.

8. Holloway RG, Shoulson I, Fahn S, Kieburtz K, et al. Pramipexole vs levodopa as initial treatment for Parkinson disease: a 4-year randomized controlled trial. *Arch Neurol* 2004;61:1044–1053.

9. Bracco F, Battaglia A, Chouza C, Dupont E, Gershanik O, Marti Masso JF, Montastruc JL, for the PKDS009 Study Group. The long-acting dopamine receptor agonist cabergoline in early Parkinson's disease: final results of a 5-year, double-blind, levodopa-controlled study. *CNS Drugs* 2004;18:733–746.

10. Oertel WH, Wolters E, Sampaio C, Gimenez-Roldan S, et al. Pergolide versus L-dopa monotherapy in early Parkinson's disease patients: the PELMOPET* study. *Mov Dis* 2005; in press.

11. Holloway RG, Dick AW. Clinical trial end points: on the road to nowhere? *Neurology* 2002;58:679–686.

12. Kieburtz K. Designing neuroprotection trials in Parkinson's disease. *Ann Neurol* 2003;53(suppl 3):S100–S107.

13. Clarke CE. A "cure" for Parkinson's disease: can neuroprotection be proven with current trial designs? *Mov Disord* 2004;19:491–498.

14. Parsons M, Greenwood J. A guide to the use of focus groups in health care research: part 1. *Contemp Nurse* 2000;9:169–180.

15. Lees AJ, Katzenschlager R, Head J, Ben-Shlomo Y. Ten-year follow-up of three different initial treatments in de-novo PD: a randomized trial. *Neurology* 2001;57:1687–1694.

16. Olanow CW, Agid Y, Mizuno Y, et al. Levodopa in the treatment of Parkinson's disease: current controversies. *Mov Disord* 2004;19: 997–1005.

17. Parkinson Study Group. Effect of deprenyl on the progression of disability in early Parkinson's disease. *N Engl J Med* 1989;321: 1364–1371.

18. LeWitt P, Oakes D, Cui L, for the Parkinson Study Group. The need for levodopa as an end point of Parkinson's disease progression in a clinical trial of selegiline and alpha-tocopherol. *Mov Disord* 1997;12:183–189.

19. Leber P. Observations and suggestions on antidementia drug development. *Alzheimer Dis Assoc Disord* 1996;10(suppl 1):31–35.

20. Parkinson Study Group. A controlled trial of rasagiline in early Parkinson disease: the TEMPO Study. *Arch Neurol* 2002;59: 1937–1943.

21. Temple RJ. A regulatory authority's opinion about surrogate endpoints. In: Nimmo WS, Tucker GT, eds. *Clinical Measurement in Drug Evaluation.* New York: J Wiley; 1995.

22. Fleming TR, DeMets DL. Surrogate end points in clinical trial: are we being misled? *Ann Intern Med* 1996;125:605–613.

23. Biomarkers Definition Working Group. Biomarkers and surrogate endpoints: preferred definitions and conceptual framework. *Clin Pharmacol Ther* 2001;69:89–95.

24. Michell AW, Lewis SJC, Foltynie T, Barker RA. Biomarkers and Parkinson's disease. *Brain* 2004;127:1693–1705.

25. Whone AL, Watts RL, Stoessl AJ, et al. Slower progression of Parkinson's disease with ropinirole versus levodopa: the REAL-PET study. *Ann Neurol* 2003;54:93–101.

26. Fahn S, Oakes D, Shoulson I, et al. Levodopa and the progression of Parkinson's disease. *N Engl J Med* 2004;351:2498–2508.

27. Olanow CW, Goetz CG, Kordower JH, et al. A double-blind controlled trial of bilateral fetal nigral transplantation in Parkinson's disease. *Ann Neurol* 2003;54:403–414.

28. Freed CR, Greene PE, Breeze RE, et al. Transplantation of embryonic dopamine neurons for severe Parkinson's disease. *N Engl J Med* 2001;344:710–719.

29. Elm JJ, Goetz CG, Ravina B, et al. A responsive outcome for Parkinson's disease neuroprotection futility studies. *Ann Neurol* 2005;57:197–203.

30. Uitti RJ, Ahlskog JE, Maraganore DM, et al. Levodopa therapy and survival in idiopathic Parkinson's disease: Olmsted County project. *Neurology* 1993;43:1918–1926.

31. Nutt JG. Motor fluctuations and dyskinesia in Parkinson's disease. *Parkinsonism Relat Disord* 2001;8:101–108.

32. Montastruc JL, Rascol O, Senard JM, Rascol A. A randomised controlled study comparing bromocriptine to which levodopa was later added, with levodopa alone in previously untreated patients with Parkinson's disease: a five year follow up. *J Neurol Neurosurg Psychiatry* 1994;57:1034–1038.

33. Goetz CG, Koller W, Poewe W, Rascol O, Sampaio C. Management of Parkinson's disease: an evidence-based review. *Mov Disord* 2002;17(suppl 4):S1–S166.

34. Ives NJ, Stowe RL, Marro J, et al. Monoamine oxidase type B inhibitors in early Parkinson's disease: meta-analysis of 17 randomised trials involving 3525 patients. *BMJ* 2004;329:593.

35. Olanow CW, Myllyla VV, Sotaniemi KA, Larsen JP, et al. Effect of selegiline on mortality in patients with Parkinson's disease: a meta-analysis. *Neurology* 1998;51:825–830.

36. Sterling J, Veinberg A, Lerner D, et al. R (+) N-propargyl-l-aminoindan (rasagiline) and derivatives: highly selective and potent inhibitors of monoamine-oxidase B. *J Neural Transm Suppl* 1998;52:301–305.

37. Rascol O, Brooks DJ, Melamed E, Oertel W, Poewe W, Stocchi F, Tolosa E, for the LARGO study group. Rasagiline as an adjunct to levodopa in patients with Parkinson's disease and motor fluctuations (LARGO, Lasting effect in Adjunct therapy with Rasagiline Given Once daily, study): a randomised, double-blind, parallel-group trial. *Lancet* 2005:365:947–954.

38. Shults CW, Oakes D, Kieburtz K, et al. Effects of coenzyme Q10 in early Parkinson disease: evidence of slowing of the functional decline. *Arch Neurol* 2002;59:1541–1550.

39. Muller T, Buttner T, Gholipour AF, Kuhn W. Coenzyme Q10 supplementation provides mild symptomatic benefit in patients with Parkinson's disease. *Neurosci Lett* 2003 May 8;341:201–204.

40. Parkinson's disease research agenda. Available at: http://www .ninds.nih.gov/about_ninds/plans/nihparkinsons_agenda.htm. Accessed March 25, 2005.

41. Ravina BM, Janis S, Keleti J, Marler JM. Funding evidence: The National Institute of Neurological Disorders and Stroke clinical trials program. *NeuroRx* 2004;1:317–322.

42. Ravina BM, Fagan SC, Hart RG, et al. Neuroprotective agents for clinical trials in Parkinson's disease: a systematic assessment. *Neurology* 2003;60:1234–1240.

43. The European Multiple System Atrophy Study Group. Available at http://111.emsa.sg.org/index.html. Accessed March 25, 2005.

44. Fischer F, Matthisson M, Herrling P. List of drugs in development for neurodegenerative diseases. *Neurodegenerative Dis* 2004;1:50–70.

45. Parkinson Study Group. The safety and tolerability of a mixed lineage kinase inhibitor (CEP-1347) in PD. *Neurology* 2004 Jan 27;62:330–332.

46. GM1 ganglioside effects on Parkinson's disease. Available at: http://Clinicaltrials.gov. Accessed March 25, 2005.

47. Walter BL, Vitek JL. Surgical treatment for Parkinson's disease. *Lancet Neurol* 2004;3:719–728

48. Miller ER 3rd, Pastor-Barriuso R, Dalal D, et al. Meta-analysis: high-dosage vitamin E supplementation may increase all-cause mortality. *Ann Intern Med* 2005 Jan 4;142:37–46.

49. Rascol O, Olanow CW, Brooks D, et al. A 2-year multicenter placebo-controlled, double blind parallel group study of the effect of riluzole in Parkinson's disease. *Mov Disord* 2002;17:39.

50. Amyotrophic lateral sclerosis. Abstract available at: http://www .focusonals.com/novartis_drug_does_not_slow_als_progression. htm. Accessed March 25, 2005.

Pharmacological Management of Parkinson's Disease

10

Eduardo Tolosa   Regina Katzenschlager

While many aspects of the neurodegenerative process underlying Parkinson's disease (PD) are now understood, treatments with proven disease-modifying effects have not yet reached the stage of clinical applicability. However, since the introduction of the first dopamine-replacing drug, levodopa (L-dopa), considerable further progress has been made with respect to the symptomatic treatment of the parkinsonian motor features, and a wide range of dopaminergic treatments are now available. As the disease advances, motor as well as nonmotor symptoms become more prominent, and the latter can even dominate the clinical picture. It is increasingly recognized that several nondopaminergic neurotransmitter systems are involved in PD, which may give rise to significant clinical problems. These often have more impact on patients' and carers' quality of life than the primary parkinsonian motor signs do and include dementia, depression, behavioral and sleep disturbances, autonomic dysregulation, impaired balance, and falls. In advanced stages, one also increasingly encounters problems related to drug treatment, which may be difficult to distinguish from symptoms related directly to PD.

The clinical features of the motor and nonmotor problems in the early stages of PD are described elsewhere in this book (chapter 6 by Poewe). These are largely related to the cardinal motor symptoms of the disorder. In advanced PD, problems closely linked to the long-term side effects of drugs used for treatment are prominent. An increased risk of motor complications is encountered with the use of L-dopa, while other clinically relevant problems,

such as neuropsychiatric complications or blood pressure drops, are more likely to occur with drugs such as dopamine agonists, amantadine, or anticholinergics (Table 10.1). With this close interaction of disease-related and treatment-related factors in mind, the structure for this chapter was chosen in such a way that the clinical problems encountered in PD are described first and subsequently the various drugs available for their management are presented. In another section, treatment approaches to important nonmotor problems are discussed (with the exception of cognitive dysfunction, which is covered in Chapter 12), and in the last part of this chapter, management recommendations are given for typical situations in early, stable, and advanced PD.

PROBLEMS IN PARKINSON'S DISEASE PREDOMINANTLY ASSOCIATED WITH THE DOPAMINERGIC SYSTEM

In the early stages, motor symptoms that relate to the cardinal manifestation of the disease—mostly tremor and bradykinesia—are those that alarm the patients and their families and bring the patient to medical attention. They reflect progressive degeneration of dopaminergic nigral cells and respond to dopaminergic replacement therapy. Nonmotor symptoms also may occur early, such as anosmia or rapid eye movement (REM) sleep behavior disorder (RBD), but these are less disabling and worrisome to the

TABLE 10.1
COMMON CLINICAL PROBLEMS ENCOUNTERED IN ADVANCED PARKINSON'S DISEASE

Complications related to dopaminergic therapy

- Motor and nonmotor fluctuations
- Dyskinesia
- Neuropsychiatric problems: hallucinosis and behavioural disorders (e.g., dopaminergic dysregulation, punding, hypersexuality)
- Excessive daytime sleepiness
- Leg edema

Disease-related motor complications

- Gait difficulties (freezing)
- Postural imbalance (falls)
- Dysarthria

Disease-related nonmotor symptoms

- Depression,
- Dementia
- Sleep disorders (REM behavior disorders, insomnia)
- Autonomic dysfunction
- Sensory symptoms

TABLE 10.2
FLUCTUATIONS IN MOTOR DISABILITY IN PARKINSON'S DISEASE

Unrelated to drugs

Kinesia paradoxica
Freezing of gait
Sleep benefit (improvement of symptoms after sleep)
Stress-related tremor

Related to L-dopa treatment

Nocturnal and early morning akinesia
Wearing off (end-of-dose deterioration)[a]
Delayed onset effect (delayed *on*)
Dose failure (no *on*)
Super *off*
Unpredictable (random) on–off fluctuations

[a] Can also occur with dopamine agonists

patients who rarely complain about them. Depression or pain may be early manifestations, but usually, the disability inflicted by motor symptoms is what determines the timing and type of medication with which we initiate treatment.

The initiation of antiparkinsonian treatment in early idiopathic PD is followed by a phase of good to excellent symptomatic response in nearly all patients ("honeymoon phase"). A stable response may be sustained in some patients throughout the course of their illness, but the majority will develop motor complications. Motor complications include fluctuations, which are characterized by a shortening of the response to individual L-dopa doses, and dyskinesias or involuntary movements.

Motor Fluctuations

In early PD, the clinical effect following an individual L-dopa dose wanes slowly and may still be detectable after days and up to weeks (long-duration L-dopa response). As the disease progresses, the duration of effect gradually becomes shorter and patients become aware of a missed or delayed dose as their parkinsonian symptoms and signs reemerge. The time when this wearing off at the end of a dose effect first becomes noticeable depends on the dosing intervals in each patient's drug regimen. Eventually, the clinical response closely reflects peripheral L-dopa pharmacokinetics, characterized by a plasma half-life of 1–1.5 hours. At later stages, some patients experience *unpredictable fluctuations*, which occur independently of the timing of medication and which may, therefore, cause

considerable distress. *Delayed on* refers to a prolonged latency to the onset of a noticeable drug effect following intake. *Dose failure*, a complete lack of effect of individual doses, causes distress and carries the additional risk of worsened dyskinesias if patients attempt to compensate for the missed effect by taking additional medication. The various types of fluctuations in motor disability occurring in PD, both disease and drug related, are listed in Table 10.2.

Dyskinesias

Dyskinesias are involuntary, hyperkinetic movements and may occur at any stage during the motor cycle in fluctuating patients (Table 10.3). Dyskinesias tend first to become apparent during the peaks in plasma concentration and clinical effect following each dose of dopaminergic medication, and later on they often are present during the entire duration of drug effect (*peak dose dyskinesia*). At earlier stages, they may go unnoticed by patients while carers and observers are aware of their presence and may be socially embarrassed. While patients themselves may prefer mild or moderate forms of dyskinesias to the immobility and the nonmotor symptoms of off-periods, severe chorea and more complicated patterns such as ballistic, stereotypic, and dystonic dyskinesias pose a considerable burden on patients and may be a major cause of disability in advanced PD. Dyskinesias may be predominant at the onset and end of a dose effect (*diphasic dyskinesia*). These often involve one or both legs and often have stereotypical or ballistic features. *Off-period dyskinesias* are usually dystonic, often affect the lower limbs, and may be painful. Such cramping of feet and toes typically occurs in the early morning hours or upon awaking, when plasma concentrations of drugs are lowest (Poewe 1988). All dyskinesias tend to be more marked on the side of the body or in the limb most affected by parkinsonism.

TABLE 10.3
TYPES OF DRUG-INDUCED DYSKINESIAS

Peak dose dyskinesia (*on* or interdose dyskinesia)

Limbs and trunk: mostly choreic movements
Craniocervical: mostly dystonic movements

Diphasic dyskinesia (beginning-of-dose, end-of-dose dyskinesia)

Occur at begining or end of dose effect
Stereotyped, ballistic and dystonic movements
Sometimes accompanied by profuse sweating, tachycardia, and anxiety
Tremor may worsen with begining-of-dose dyskinesia

Off-period dystonia

Mostly distal in one leg
Frequently painful
Sometimes isolated occurrence early in the morning (early morning dystonia)
Worse when walking

Frequency of Motor Complications

Incidence figures for motor complications vary in the literature. In a meta-analysis of published prospective studies, the risk of dyskinesias as well as fluctuations after 5 years was found to be around 40% (Ahlskog 2001), while a study showed that response fluctuations may be a fairly early phenomenon when subtle and nonmotor signs are also considered (Stacy 2005). Some information on long-term risk is available from prospective treatment trials, which showed a further increase at 10 (Lees 2001) and 15 years (Hely 2005) although motor complications were considered disabling in less than half of the affected patients. Age at onset has an important impact: In young-onset PD, dyskinesias have been reported in up to 94% of patients (Schrag 1998). A population-based study showed a 5-year dyskinesia incidence of 16% in patients with onset after 70 years of age compared with 50% when onset was between 40 and 59 years of age (Kumar 2005).

Pathophysiology of Motor Complications

The exact mechanisms underlying motor fluctuations and dyskinesias are not yet completely understood. While the peripheral pharmacokinetics of L-dopa remain unchanged throughout the course of the illness (Nutt 1996; Fabbrini 1987), presynaptic nigrostriatal nerve terminals gradually lose their ability to store dopamine as the neurodegeneration progresses. Therefore, fluctuations in plasma dopamine levels can no longer be buffered by reuptake into presynaptic terminals. This storage hypothesis is useful for explaining some of the changes that occur in later-stage PD, but ample evidence now exists for a far more complex basis of the development of motor complications.

Although the overall risk of developing dyskinesias has been shown to increase with the duration (Grandas 1999) and dose (Schrag 1998) of L-dopa treatment, the timing of L-dopa initiation as such does not appear to be the primary factor. Rather, current evidence suggests that the degree of nigrostriatal degeneration and the mode of drug administration are of central importance (Olanow 2004). The role of the degree of neuronal loss is supported by the short latency to the occurrence of motor complications in the presence of severe nigrostriatal degeneration: Motor complications develop within days following L-dopa initiation in 1-methyl-4-phenyl-1,2,3,6-tetra-hydropyridine (MPTP)-treated primates, where there is a 90%–95% cell loss (Pearce 1995), and within weeks or months in PD patients in whom treatment was started at an advanced stage (Onofrj 1998) or in MPTP-induced parkinsonism (Langston 1983). Because disease severity determines the timing and doses of symptomatic treatment to a large degree, these factors and their respective roles in the development of motor complications are difficult to disentangle in PD patients.

Age at disease onset is another factor intrinsic to the disease process that is related to the risk of motor complications. As already outlined, younger age of onset is associated with a higher rate of fluctuations and dyskinesias.

As yet, neither the rate of neuronal loss nor the age of onset are amenable to modification. However, treatment-related factors also contribute to the risk of motor complications. As neurodegeneration progresses, the activation of dopamine receptors becomes increasingly dependent on the peripheral availability of exogenous dopaminergic agents. Some of these, such as L-dopa, have a short half-life, and because of reduced striatal buffer capacity, fluctuations in plasma L-dopa concentration may be translated into peaks and troughs in striatal dopamine concentration. The result is intermittent receptor activation, which is in contrast to physiological conditions, where nigrostriatal neurons fire at a relatively constant rate (Delong 1983). Consequently, plastic changes in gene expression and in neuropeptide formation occur within the striatal pathways (Graybiel 2000, Gerfen 1990). These changes lead to alterations in the firing patterns of basal ganglia output neurons, which convey signals to cortical motor regions (Olanow 2000, Filion 1991).

Continuous dopaminergic stimulation has been shown to normalize neuropeptide expression (Hadj 2000). Changes in opioid gene expression and increased internalization of D1 receptors have also been described to be involved in dyskinesia formation and to be associated with intermittent but not continuous drug administration (Morissette 1997, Dumartin 1998).

Evidence supporting the role of continuous receptor stimulation includes the finding in MPTP-treated primates that equally effective doses of L-dopa and short-acting dopamine agonists induce more dyskinesias than long-acting agonists (Bedard 1986, Pearce 1995, Hadj 2000).

In de novo PD, randomized controlled trials have shown that, in comparison with initial L-dopa therapy, patients randomized to long-acting dopamine agonists had a smaller risk of motor complications (Rascol 2000, Parkinson Study Group 2000, Rinne 1998, Lees 2001, Rinne 1998a, Bracco 2004). However, these studies also demonstrate that a delay in the occurrence of motor complications in the agonist arms was achieved at the expense of significantly worse motor scores, which has mainly been attributed to the superior symptomatic effect of L-dopa.

In patients with advanced PD, individual doses of the potent dopamine agonist apomorphine induce the same extent of dyskinesias as L-dopa (Kempster 1990), whereas continuous subcutaneous application can lead to improvement or complete reversal of dyskinesias (Colzi 1998, Katzenschlager 2005, Manson 2001). Similar findings have been demonstrated with the dopamine agonist lisuride (Baronti 1992, Stocchi 2002, Obeso 1986) but also with L-dopa, where intravenous or enteral administration alleviates motor fluctuations and dyskinesias (Quinn 1982, Kurlan 1986, Syed 1998, Sage 1988, Nilsson 2001, Nyholm 2003).

In summary, the currently available evidence supports the concept that the manner of administration of dopaminergic drugs is of central importance, and it argues against a specific detrimental effect of L-dopa.

PROBLEMS IN PARKINSON'S DISEASE PREDOMINANTLY ASSOCIATED WITH NONDOPAMINERGIC SYSTEMS

A number of clinical problems occur in PD that are not, or are only partly, related to the nigrostriatal dopaminergic system and which, therefore, respond poorly to dopamine replacement therapy. This occurs because the neurodegenerative process in PD does not only spread within the dopaminergic system but also involves other neurotransmitters, such as the serotoninergic, noradrenergic, and glutamatergic systems. Additional neuropathological changes may also have a role, such as cerebrovascular disease or Alzheimer's pathology, which are frequently associated with PD pathology in patients with dementia, but the precise mechanism is not yet fully understood for all nondopaminergic problems.

Early signs include olfactory dysfunction, depression, and REM behavior disorder (RBD). Later-stage nondopaminergic complications often have significant clinical relevance and include cognitive decline, hallucinations and psychosis, depression, behavioral and sleep disturbances, dysarthria, dysphagia, impaired balance and falls, freezing while in the on state, and autonomic dysfunction. A recent 15-year follow-up study concluded that factors such as dementia and falls often are more important and more difficult to manage than motor complications in advanced PD (Hely 2005).

In patients with motor fluctuations, nonmotor problems associated with the off periods are much more common than usually recognized, and they may cause significant distress (Witjas 2002, Stacy 2005). The nonmotor off symptoms most frequently reported in one study were anxiety, drenching sweats, slowness of thinking, fatigue, akathisia, irritability, and hallucinations; and in another study, patients reported tiredness most frequently (Stacy 2005). In one study, all patients who had motor fluctuations also experienced at least one nonmotor problem during off phases (Witjas 2002). Dopaminergic mechanisms are important in nonmotor fluctuations, and they can improve with optimization of dopaminergic therapies.

The current pathophysiological concepts and clinical aspects of nonmotor complications are outlined in Chapter 6, and their management is covered at the end of this chapter.

CLASSES OF DRUGS FOR THE SYMPTOMATIC TREATMENT OF MOTOR FUNCTION IN PARKINSON'S DISEASE

The drugs discussed in this section are used for the management of those motor aspects of PD that are related to the dopaminergic deficit in PD, in particular the cardinal motor signs, tremor, bradykinesia, and rigidity. As outlined, severe motor impairment may occur, particularly in later stages of the disease, independently of dopaminergic function, for example, freezing during on phases and loss of balance. Possible management approaches will be discussed in a later section of this chapter, but for these problems, the dopaminergic drugs discussed here typically have a very limited role.

L-dopa

L-dopa, the precursor of dopamine, is an aromatic amino acid that occurs naturally in a number of leguminous plants. The highest concentration is found in the bean plant mucuna pruriens, which has been used in Ayurvedic medicine since 1500 BC, including for conditions resembling parkinsonism (Manyam 1990, Katzenschlager 2004). Synthetic L-dopa was introduced into Western medicine in the early 1960s (Birkmayer 1961, Cotzias 1967) and has since remained the gold standard among antiparkinsonian drugs due to the degree of symptom relief it is capable of providing. L-dopa continues to be the most powerful orally active antiparkinsonian drug; only apomorphine matches its effect on motor function.

L-dopa has a marked symptomatic effect on all components of the cardinal parkinsonian motor signs—bradykinesia, rigidity, and tremor—and in many patients L-dopa therapy initially leads to complete or nearly complete reversal of symptoms. L-dopa increases the duration of time patients remain independent and employable, and

TABLE 10.4
TREATMENT OF PARKINSON'S DISEASE WITH L-DOPA

Advantages of L-dopa Therapy:

- The vast majority of patients who start treatment with L-dopa experience good to excellent functional benefit.
- Tolerability is usually good.
- The antiparkinsonian effect is maintained throughout the course of the illness.
- L-dopa is not toxic to humans.
- There is evidence to show that L-dopa extends life expectancy.
- L-dopa improves quality of life.
- L-dopa is the drug of choice for treatment of elderly patients, and in the presence of neuropsychiatric problems.
- L-dopa today remains the gold standard and the most effective drug for the symptomatic treatment of Parkinson's disease.

Limitations of L-dopa Therapy

- Development of motor and nonmotor fluctuations.
- Dyskinesias.
- Limited or no response of some symptoms (e.g., freezing of gait, dysautonomia, dysarthria).
- Occurrence of nonmotor dopaminergic adverse effects (less frequently than with other drugs): nausea, neuropsychiatric problems including hallucinosis, sleepiness, autonomic problems.

there is evidence to suggest a beneficial effect on life expectancy, although this has not been confirmed in all studies (Rajput 2001, Guttman 2001, Clarke 1995). While a wide range of other symptomatic treatment options is available, which are often used now to delay the use of L-dopa, virtually all patients will at some stage require the more powerful symptomatic effects of L-dopa (Table 10.4).

Basic Pharmacology and Metabolism

L-dopa is absorbed in the gastrointestinal tract at the level of the small intestines, where it uses the large neutral amino acid transport system, competing with protein from food. The same transport system is utilized to cross the blood–brain barrier. The plasma half-life of L-dopa is 1–1.5 hours. In the periphery, it is metabolized to dopamine by aromatic amino acid decarboxylase (AADC), and to 3-O-methyl dopa by catechol-O-methyltransferase (COMT). Due to the high peripheral degradation rate of L-dopa, high doses were required in the early days of L-dopa therapy, which were associated with dopaminergic side effects such as nausea, vomiting, and orthostatic reactions. The introduction of decarboxylase inhibitors greatly facilitated L-dopa treatment and either carbidopa or benserazide are now routinely coadministered with each L-dopa dose. They block peripheral degradation of L-dopa to dopamine, thus increasing plasma concentrations and allowing more L-dopa to cross the

blood–brain barrier. This enables a reduction of exogenous L-dopa by 60%–80%, while dopaminergic side effects occur much less frequently (Rinne 1973, Mars 1973). The gastrointestinal mucosa is also a site for decarboxylation of oral L-dopa (Bergmark 1972), and decarboxylase inhibitors enhance duodenal L-dopa absorption (Pletscher 1971).

The latency to a clinical effect after L-dopa ingestion depends on a number of variables. At all stages of PD, gastric emptying time may have an impact, which is delayed by food and is also slowed by PD itself (Djaldetti 1996), as well as by anticholinergic drugs. Intestinal absorption is influenced by the competition of dietary proteins for the transmucosal transport system. In individual patients, particularly when dyskinesias or acute tolerability are a concern, slowing L-dopa absorption may be helpful, and these patients may prefer to take L-dopa with food. In the majority of cases, however, a reliable and rapid effect is desired and patients should be informed that taking L-dopa with meals may limit its absorption and may delay the clinical response. Although peripheral L-dopa pharmacokinetics remain unchanged throughout the course of the illness, disease severity has been shown to have an impact on the time from ingestion to effect, with a mean delay of 53 minutes in patients at Hoehn & Yahr stages I and II to 28 minutes at stage IV (Sohn 1994).

Limitations of L-dopa Therapy and the Issue of L-dopa Toxicity

While L-dopa continues to be highly effective for many years with respect to the cardinal parkinsonian motor signs, its use is limited by several factors (Table 10.4). Motor fluctuations and dyskinesias develop in the majority of patients; L-dopa has no or little effect on clinically important nondopaminergic problems such as dementia, depression, on-period freezing, autonomic dysfunction, or sleep disturbances; and it does not modify the underlying neurodegenerative process.

Ever since treatment-related motor complications became apparent following the introduction of L-dopa, a potential negative or toxic effect on a cellular level has been discussed. In vitro, either toxic or protective effects on dopaminergic neurons have been demonstrated, depending on the experimental conditions such as L-dopa concentration and the presence or absence of glia cells and ascorbic acid (Michel 1990, Mytilineou 1993, Mena 1999, Han 1996). In vivo, L-dopa induces neither dopaminergic cell death in normal animals (Lyras 2002, Perry 1984), nor additional cell death in lesioned animals (Murer 1998, Datla 2001), and trophic effects were found in some models (Olanow 2004). Similarly, there is no neuropathological evidence of L-dopa–induced neural degeneration in humans without PD who received chronic high-dose L-dopa (Quinn 1986).

In patients with early PD, recent functional neuroimaging studies using position emission tomography (PET) and single-photon emission computed tomography (SPECT) tracer uptake as a surrogate marker of nigrostriatal function have reported a slower decline in tracer uptake on dopamine agonists compared with L-dopa (Marek 2002, Whone 2003). As these studies lacked a placebo arm, it is not clear whether this observation was due to a drug-related pharmacologic response, an agonist-related protective effect, or a direct effect of L-dopa. A recently reported placebo-controlled, double-blind trial (the ELLDOPA study) in untreated PD patients demonstrated that compared with placebo, the three L-dopa arms showed a slower rate of decline in United Parkinson's Disease Rating Scale (UPDRS) motor scores after washout, and, importantly, this was observed in a dose-dependent manner. Conversely, the rate of changes on β-CIT-SPECT was increased (Parkinson Study Group 2004). The significance of these imaging findings remains to be determined. It has been suggested that sufficient proof is as yet lacking that PET and SPECT tracers can be used reliably as surrogate markers of the degree of neurodegeneration (Ravina 2005, Morrish 2003). The clinical results of all these studies argue against any meaningful deleterious effect of L-dopa.

In the light of the cumulative available data, the current consensus is that there is no evidence to indicate that L-dopa is toxic to dopaminergic neurons in PD patients. Ample evidence now exists to suggest that the short half-life of L-dopa and the manner of its administration are much more likely to be related to the development of motor complication than some property of the molecule itself (Olanow/Agid 2004, Chase 2000, Obeso 2000, Nutt 2000).

Practical Use of L-dopa

Based on theoretical concerns and on interpretations of recent comparative trials, where a smaller risk of motor complications was found in the agonist arms, the use of L-dopa in clinical practice has changed over the past few years, at least in those parts of the world where alternative drugs (which are usually more expensive) are available. Many clinicians have advocated initiating therapy with a dopamine agonist in virtually all patients, and L-dopa doses now are often kept at the lower end of the range in an attempt to minimize the risk of later-stage complications. While this approach is indeed useful in the majority of younger patients, it is important to keep in mind that the trials comparing early L-dopa and agonist treatment consistently showed significantly better and longer-lasting motor improvement in the L-dopa arms. The consequences of undertreatment may ultimately hamper employability and may lead to social withdrawal or, at later stages, to complications associated with bradykinesia, such as falls.

For each patient, the best initial dose should be determined individually. In early PD or when first adding L-dopa, daily doses are usually between a minimum of 150 mg and up to 400 mg, or more in some cases. As the disease progresses, adaptations should be made as required and as tolerated. The patient's current needs in terms of symptom control, including employment status, should be weighed against factors, such as age, that have an impact on the individual risk of motor complications. Additional L-dopa also may be required to cover for the discontinuation of other dopaminergic drugs in the course of the illness due to reduced tolerability, for example, in the presence of dementia or psychosis. Eventually, the total daily L-dopa dose may be in the order of 1000–2000 mg/day or higher.

Tolerability

The use of L-dopa is associated with an increased risk of motor complications, as outlined. In contrast, with respect to short-term tolerability, it offers a favorable side-effect profile compared with the other classes of antiparkinsonian agents.

L-dopa, like any dopaminergic drug, can induce typical dopaminergic adverse effects such as orthostatic hypotension, nausea, vomiting, drowsiness, and, rarely, peripheral edema. The addition of decarboxylase inhibitors in routine clinical practice has greatly limited these side effects. Although direct comparative data to support this are lacking in rare cases of persistent lack of L-dopa tolerability, it may be useful to switch to a preparation containing a different decarboxylase inhibitor. However, compared with other drugs used in the treatment of parkinsonism, including dopamine agonists, L-dopa tends to be better tolerated with respect to these dopaminergic effects (Goetz/Koller 2002, Rascol 2000, Lees 2001, Bracco 2004).

Unplanned episodes of sleep during daytime, including while driving a vehicle, were originally described in nonergot dopamine agonists but now also have been shown to be associated with other agonists, and they may occur in L-dopa monotherapy (Ferreira 2001).

L-dopa can be associated with psychosis and confusion, but these problems tend to be less pronounced than with other antiparkinsonian agents, and L-dopa is typically the drug of choice in patients with dementia or hallucinosis (Hubble 2002, Olanow/Agid 2004).

Strategies to Modify L-dopa Administration

There are various manners in which L-dopa can be administered. Once motor complications have occurred, the timing and dosage may be adjusted, for example, by using frequent smaller doses in order to minimize peak-dose complications. In patients without disabling peak-dose dyskinesias, larger L-dopa doses may be helpful to extend the duration of on periods. Other strategies include L-dopa intake with meals to delay its absorption, reduction in concomitant dietary protein in order to avoid competition with other amino acids for absorption, and the use of preparations with different release properties.

Controlled-Release L-dopa

This formulation leads to a longer delay to peak plasma concentrations with prolonged half-life and a slower decline in plasma levels and clinical effect. Controlled-release L-dopa is available with either decarboxylase inhibitor, although different mechanisms are used to achieve delayed absorption: L-dopa/carbidopa is embedded in a slowly dissolving matrix (LeWitt 1989, Yeh 1989), while L-dopa/benserazide floats on the surface of gastric content (Erni 1987).

In patients with motor complications, conflicting results have been reported in the literature: Some (Goetz 1988, Poewe 1986, Wolters 1996, Hutton 1989) but not all (Jankovic 1989) studies showed prolonged daily on time or shorter off duration, while in some cases study design or reported data were insufficient for definite conclusions (Goetz/Koller 2002).

While some patients with wearing off benefit from the longer effect duration of controlled-release L-dopa, the clinical use of these preparations is often hampered by their lower bioavailability. Intestinal absorption is reduced, and it is also less reliable, which may cause delayed on or dose failures and can make it difficult to achieve a constant dose effect. Due to low bioavailability, required dosages are higher than with standard L-dopa, usually by around 30%. To overcome the disadvantage of a longer delay to on, slow-release and standard L-dopa can be administered in combination. Controlled-release L-dopa may be used at bedtime to improve mobility during the night, although a definite benefit of this common approach has not been proven (U.K. Madopar CR Study Group 1989).

In view of its ability to induce fewer peaks and troughs in plasma concentration compared with standard L-dopa, there were hopes that using a controlled-release preparation as initial treatment in early PD might delay motor complications. Two double-blind, controlled 5-year trials failed to demonstrate such a reduction in the risk of motor complications compared with regular L-dopa (Dupont 1996, Block 1997, Koller 1999). In one of these studies, dosing was only twice daily, thus making it unlikely that plasma concentrations and receptor stimulation were more continuous than with standard L-dopa (Block 1997; Koller 1999). The design of this particular study therefore precludes firm conclusions.

Dual-Release L-dopa

This formulation, which is currently available in only a few countries, combines immediate and slow-release properties in one tablet. A single-dose study in fluctuating patients showed a significantly shorter delay to peak L-dopa concentrations with dual-release compared with slow-release L-dopa while plasma half-life was similar. The delay to a clinical effect was 43 minutes with dual-release and 81 minutes with slow-release L-dopa. On-time duration was significantly longer, and no increase in dyskinesias occurred on dual-release L-dopa (Descombes 2001).

Soluble L-dopa Formulations

Soluble L-dopa formulations dissolve and are absorbed quickly, and a clinical effect usually sets in very reliably around 20–30 minutes after ingestion, compared to 30–60 minutes with standard L-dopa. Soluble L-dopa can be useful for delayed morning start-up time or as a rescue medication to provide quick relief from bothersome or disabling off symptoms. However, due to its short half-life, the duration of effect is also shorter and, therefore, chronic or very frequent use should be avoided in view of the pulsatility of its action in the striatum. Although as yet there are no data to prove that soluble L-dopa use is directly associated with increased motor complications, evidence from other short-acting drugs suggests that these should be used sparingly. Moreover, recent data showed an association of dopaminergic rescue medication (of any kind) with behavioral and motor abnormalities including punding, which may be related to receptor sensitization, including in neural systems mediating psychomotor functions (Evans 2004).

L-dopa Infusion

Continuous L-dopa administration via an intravenous route is difficult due to its low solubility in water and its lack of stability at room temperature (Nyholm 2003). The development of a stable water-based gel suspension of L-dopa/carbidopa in methylcellulose has enabled continuous daytime infusion into the duodenum via a transabdominal delivery system. Enteral L-dopa infusion avoids gastric emptying as a factor of delayed or erratic L-dopa absorption. This results in nearly stable plasma profiles and, consequently, in a sustained reduction in motor fluctuations and dyskinesias (Kurlan 1986, 1988; Syed 1998; Sage 1988; Nyholm 2003). L-dopa infusion therapies are currently used mainly in Scandinavian countries and the United States, but a European license has been obtained. While this treatment approach is expensive and invasive and requires special expertise, long-term data are available to show that in patients with refractory fluctuations and dyskinesias, marked and sustained improvements can be achieved (Nilsson 2001).

COMT Inhibitors

L-dopa is metabolized via two main pathways: decarboxylation and O-methylation. Blocking peripheral decarboxylation by adding a decarboxylase (AADC) inhibitor has long been the standard in L-dopa treatment. When AADC is inhibited, methylization of L-dopa to 3-O-methyldopa becomes more prominent. This process is catalyzed by catechol-O-methyltransferase (COMT). By inhibiting COMT, slower degradation of L-dopa and thus prolonged maintenance of plasma levels can be achieved.

Two COMT-inhibiting substances are in clinical use: entacapone and tolcapone. While entacapone acts only on peripheral L-dopa, tolcapone also crosses the blood–brain barrier and inhibits central L-dopa degradation. Moreover, tolcapone has a longer half-life than entacapone. When administered in combination with L-dopa, both drugs lead to prolonged availability of L-dopa in the gastrointestinal tract and to increased plasma half-life, thereby prolonging the clinical effect of L-dopa. Peak L-dopa plasma concentrations are not significantly increased and, importantly, COMT inhibitors do not prolong the delay to peak concentrations (Limousin 1995). This is in contrast to slow-release L-dopa formulations for which the delay to a noticeable clinical effect is longer than with standard preparations. COMT inhibitors can be used in conjunction with slow-release L-dopa, where similar pharmacologic effects have been demonstrated as with standard L-dopa (Stocchi 2004).

Entacapone

Entacapone is rapidly absorbed and has a half-life similar to that of L-dopa (1–1.2 hours). The dose of entacapone that has been shown to offer the best ratio of efficacy and tolerability is 200 mg. Therefore, the standard manner of administration is 200 mg of entacapone together with each L-dopa dose.

A triple-combination tablet is available containing 200 mg entacapone and three different doses of L-dopa/carbidopa (50/12.5 mg, 100/25 mg, and 150/37.5 mg). This combination drug has been shown to be bioequivalent to separate administration while being rated as preferable by patients (Brooks 2005).

Entacapone in Fluctuating Patients

Four large, prospective, randomized, controlled 6-month studies investigated the role of entacapone in patients with motor fluctuations and found a significant increase in daily on time of 1–1.7 hours, with a concomitant reduction in off time. No studies powered for direct comparison are available, but a trial of the MAO-B inhibitor rasagiline used entacapone as an active comparator and found similar results with respect to off time reduction (Rascol 2005). Studies that included total UPDRS and activities of daily living (ADL) subscores found modest but significant improvements (Poewe 2002, Rascol 2005, Reichmann 2005). A 12%–16% reduction in the mean L-dopa dose was reported in most studies, and this occurred mainly in response to increased dyskinesias (Parkinson's Study Group 1997, Rinne/Larsen 1998, Brooks 2005, Poewe 2002).

Entacapone in Patients Without Motor Fluctuations

A small randomized, controlled 6-month study in 41 patients with stable disease found activities of daily living significantly improved and an L-dopa reduction of 40 mg/day (Brooks 2003). A larger 24-week study in 750 stable patients permitted no changes in L-dopa doses (Olanow/Kieburtz 2004). Several quality-of-life scales and clinical global assessments improved significantly, but UPDRS motor scores did not change significantly.

Tolcapone

Tolcapone is rapidly absorbed and has a half-life of 1–4 hours. It is therefore administered 3 times daily at doses of 100 mg or 200 mg, irrespective of the timing of L-dopa doses.

The European Union (EU) license of tolcapone was suspended until recently due to liver toxicity. Its use now will be on condition of close safety monitoring as outlined in the following paragraphs.

Tolcapone in Patients with Motor Fluctuations

Several large randomized, placebo-controlled multicenter studies showed tolcapone to be significantly more effective than placebo (Rajput 1997, Kurth 1997, Myllyla 1997, Baas 1997, Adler 1998). On time was increased and off time reduced by 1–2 hours per day, and L-dopa could be significantly reduced. A randomized, open-label study comparing pergolide and tolcapone as add-on to L-dopa in fluctuating patients found similar efficacy but some evidence of better tolerability on tolcapone (Koller/Lees 2001). Another study used bromocriptine as an active comparator in a randomized, open-label design and found no significant differences in on and off time or UPDRS scores, although there was a significant difference in L-dopa dose reduction in favor of tolcapone (Tolcapone Study Group 1999).

Tolcapone in Patients Without Motor Fluctuations

A 6-month study in stable PD patients (Waters 1997) found small but significant improvements in total UPDRS scores, motor scores, and activities of daily living; L-dopa was decreased slightly. Improved activities of daily living were also found in a smaller 6-week study (Dupont 1997). However, both studies also included patients with mild motor fluctuations, which somewhat limits the conclusions with respect to stable PD.

Summary of Efficacy of COMT Inhibitors

In patients with motor fluctuations, both entacapone and tolcapone reduce off duration and enable a reduction of L-dopa while motor disability during on periods is only modestly improved (Deane 2004a, Deane 2004b). Tolcapone is associated with a larger L-dopa reduction, and a recent study shows that a switch from entacapone to tolcapone can further increase on time duration, without a significant difference in the resulting dyskinesias (Agid 2005).

In patients with stable PD and no or mild fluctuations, significant improvements have been found with respect to activities of daily living and, in one study with entacapone, quality-of-life scores. Motor scores were not significantly improved on entacapone and only mildly improved on tolcapone. These results support a possible role of COMT inhibitors in the symptomatic treatment of patients who have not yet developed motor complications.

Tolerability and Safety of COMT Inhibitors

Hepatotoxicity

The most clinically relevant adverse effect of a COMT inhibitor is the potential for hepatotoxicity associated with tolcapone. Most cases of liver dysfunction occurred 1–6 months after initiation of therapy. Fulminant hepatic failure has been reported, including three fatal cases. The drug license was subsequently suspended in the European Union, although this suspension has now been lifted. Tolcapone can now be prescribed in the EU for patients refractory to or intolerant of entacapone, provided strict regulations with respect to blood testing are adhered to before starting and during the entire duration of treatment (Borges 2005). Similar restrictions exist in the United States. The precise mechanism of tolcapone-associated hepatotoxicity has not been fully elucidated. Hepatotoxicity has not been conclusively demonstrated in entacapone, and hypotheses to explain these differences in safety profiles have included different metabolic pathways in the liver and the finding that tolcapone uncouples mitochondrial oxidative phosphorylation, which is a recognized cause of liver toxicity (Brooks 2004, Nissinen 1997).

Other Adverse Effects

As these drugs enhance the pharmacological effects of L-dopa, dopaminergic side effects may occur or may increase. This includes dyskinesias, which can often be counteracted by reducing L-dopa. Other dopaminergic effects include nausea, orthostatic hypotension, or peripheral edema. Urine discoloration occurs in a large proportion of patients, particularly on entacapone, and is due to the nitrocatechol structure of the drugs and their metabolites. Although this is of no medical relevance, it may be irritating to some patients. Diarrhea, ranging from mild to severe, has been reported in 8%–20% of patients on entacapone but is rarely the cause of stopping treatment. Tolcapone has been shown to lead to more severe forms of diarrhea, and 8%–10% of patients in clinical trials discontinued treatment for this reason. The time of onset is usually between weeks and months after initiation of treatment.

COMT Inhibitors and Prevention of Motor Complications

As outlined, the current concept of the formation of motor complications in PD is essentially based on two main factors: degree of neurodegeneration and pulsatility of drug treatment. Evidence supporting this concept includes the reversal of dyskinesias on continuous subcutaneous apomorphine or enteral L-dopa, and a correlation between the half-life of drugs and the emergence of motor complications in animal models and humans. This has given rise to expectations that prolonging L-dopa half-life by adding a COMT inhibitor early in the disease, before motor complications have developed, might lead to a sufficiently continuous dopaminergic stimulation to reduce this risk. Indeed animal data support this hypothesis: A recent study investigating repeated small L-dopa doses combined with entacapone versus L-dopa alone in untreated MPTP-lesioned primates found, in line with previous rodent data, reduced dyskinesia induction (Smith 2005). However, even though the MPTP primate model has proved to be an excellent predictor of the clinical effect of antiparkinsonian drugs, conclusions from these preclinical data are premature.

Results from an ongoing large trial (STRIDE-PD), which as yet have not been released, address the clinically important question of whether the early combination of L-dopa with a COMT inhibitor may be a useful strategy to avoid motor complications in patients with PD.

Dopamine Agonists

In an attempt to alleviate symptoms of parkinsonism, compounds have been sought that can stimulate dopamine (DA) receptors. These drugs are generally regarded as "dopamine agonists," but most of them do not duplicate the pharmacological properties of dopamine. Besides stimulating DA receptors these compounds, for example, have activity in other neurochemical systems, and some ergot compounds are known to have mixed agonist–antagonist profiles at the DA receptors.

Schwab et al. (Schwab 1951) observed transient improvement of rigidity and tremor in parkinsonian patients after injection of the emetic drug apomorphine. At that time, the dopaminergic properties of this drug were not known. Cotzias et al. (Cotzias 1970) later carried out extensive studies with apomorphine and also tested a congener N-n propyl-norapomorphine. This drug proved effective but was not well-tolerated and was toxic to some patients. In the 1970s, an ergot dopamine agonist bromocriptine (Calne 1974) was tested in PD in an attempt to overcome the limitation of high-dose L-dopa therapy and was shown to be efficacious. Since then bromocriptine and a number of dopamine agonists have been introduced into the market. Proposed advantages of this class of drugs over L-dopa in the management of PD include longer striatal half-life, direct stimulation of receptors bypassing degenerating nigrostriatal neurons, lack of competition for transport in the gut or at the blood–brain barrier, option of alternate routes of administration, and association with reduced incidence of motor complications, their antioxidant effects, and the possibility that they may provide neuroprotection (Tolosa 1997).

Eight different orally administered dopamine agonists are presently approved and marketed for the treatment of PD: bromocriptine, cabergoline, dihydroergocryptine, lisuride, pergolide, piribedil, pramipexole, and ropinirole. Among these agonists, five are ergot derivatives (bromocriptine, cabergoline, dihydroergocryptine, lisuride, and pergolide), while the three others are not (piribedil, pramipexole, and ropinirole). Apomorphine is a nonergot dopamine agonist administered parenterally.

Mechanism of Action

The various dopamine agonists in use have different receptor stimulation profiles and different effects upon non-DA receptors. They also differ in their pharmacokinetic properties (Jankovic 2002). The clinical consequences of such differences remain mostly theoretical and cannot be used to influence a practice based on strong clinical evidence. Among the eight orally active dopamine agonists, all are usually prescribed on a t.i.d. regimen, except cabergoline, which is the only one that is prescribed once (or twice) daily as it has the longest plasma elimination half-life (60 hours) (Watts 1997).

Among the dopamine agonists, intrinsic potency at the D2 receptors can differ by one or more orders of magnitude, but trials have not revealed any major differences in their overall clinical efficacy. Most studies of dopaminergic agonists have concluded that stimulation of D2 receptors accounts for most or all of the benefits exerted against parkinsonian features (Piercey 1995, Jenner 1997). This D2 effect also explains why all dopamine agonists can induce similar peripheral (gastrointestinal: nausea and vomiting; cardiovascular: orthostatic hypotension; central neuropsychiatric: somnolence, psychosis, hallucinations) side effects.

Apart from binding to dopamine and nondopamine receptors, dopamine agonists have in vitro and in vivo properties (free radical scavenging, reduction in dopamine turnover, anti-apoptotic effect) that explain why they have been tested as putative "neuroprotective" agents to reduce the progression of PD (Olanow 1998, Carvey 1997, Zou 1999, Zou 2000, Ogawa 1994).

Efficacy and tolerability in individual patients may vary greatly with different agonists, and switches are therefore advisable if the clinical effect is unsatisfactory or if adverse effects occur on a given agonist.

Dopamine Agonists in Early Stages of Parkinson's Disease: Symptomatic Effect and Prevention of Motor Complications

The benefit of the agonists as monotherapy in mild PD has been shown in large, prospective, randomized, double-blind, placebo-controlled trials. In these trials ropinirole, pramipexole, cabergoline, dihydroergocryptine (Bergamasco 2000) or pergolide (Barone 1999) used as monotherapy provided antiparkinsonian benefits to early PD superior to placebo. These benefits are particularly powerful in patients with Hoehn and Yahr stages I and II (Tolosa 1987, Rascol 1982, Adler 1997, Sethi 1998, Kieburtz 1997, Shannon 1997, Rinne 1997, Rinne 1998). For safety reasons, however (see *Safety*), pergolide is not used anymore as first-line antiparkinsonian medication.

Direct comparison studies of the dopamine agonists as monotherapy are lacking. The clinical relevance of the reported differences—bromocriptine versus ropinirole (Korczyn 1998, Korczyn 1999) and bromocriptine versus pergolide (Mizuno 1995)—if any, remains questionable, especially since the exact dose equivalence between the different agonists remains unknown.

There are no published direct head-to-head comparisons between any agonist given as monotherapy and any other antiparkinsonian medication frequently used in early PD such as the MAO-B inhibitors, amantadine, or the anticholinergics. Changes reported in the UPDRS with most agonists are usually greater than those reported with MAO-B inhibitors, suggesting a possibly greater symptomatic effect of the agonists.

Trials comparing dopamine agonists as monotherapy against L-dopa—ropinirole (Rascol 2000), pramipexole (Parkinson Study Group 2000), cabergoline (Rinne 1998), bromocriptine (Montastruc 1994), and pergolide (Oertel 2005) have been performed. Patients randomized to the agonist arm had less improvement in motor impairments and disability. In terms of tolerability, hallucinations were significantly worse with ropinirole than in the L-dopa arm, and somnolence was worse with pramipexole. Withdrawals because of adverse events were greater with the agonists than with L-dopa. The proportion of patients capable of remaining on an agonist monotherapy falls progressively over years to less than 20% after 5 years of treatment (Montastruc 1994, Parkinson's Disease Research Group of the United Kingdom 1993, Rinne 1998, Parkinson Study Group 2000, Rascol 2000). For this reason, after some years of treatment, most patients who start on an agonist will receive L-dopa as a replacement or an adjunct treatment to keep control of the parkinsonian motor signs.

Several prospective randomized, controlled trials have compared the probability of developing motor complications in patients receiving an agonist versus L-dopa–treated controls. These trials have consistently demonstrated the ability of the early use of an agonist to reduce the incidence of motor complications while at the same time motor improvement was significantly better in the respective L-dopa arms. One study included quality-of-life measures that corroborated better symptomatic improvement on L-dopa (Parkinson Study Group 2000). Such studies, of 2 to 5 years duration, are available for cabergoline (Rinne 1998), pramipexole (Parkinson Study Group 2000 ropirinole), ropinirole (Rascol 2000, Whone 2003), and pergolide (Oertel 2005). Ten-year results of a study comparing bromocriptine and L-dopa similarly showed less risk of motor complications at the expense of less motor improvement in the agonist arm (Lees 2001). Conflicting results have been reported with lisuride (Rinne 1989, Allain 2000), and published controlled data are lacking for other orally active agonists (dihydroergocryptine, piribedil). In two recent clinical trials, chronic treatment with ropinirole or pramipexol (Marek 2002, Whone 2002) was associated with a slower decline of imaged striatal signal, compared to L-dopa monotherapy. The results of these neuroimaging studies, however, could well reflect a pharmacological effect on proteins that interact with the imaging radioligands and the role of neuroimaging as a surrogate marker has been questioned (Albin 2003). In both these studies, patients experienced greater clinical improvement with L-dopa than with a dopamine agonist.

Trials indicating that starting treatment with an agonist reduces the risk of motor complications support a treatment strategy for early PD in which dopamine agonists are used as initial therapy and supplemental L-dopa is added when symptoms cannot be satisfactorily controlled with a dopamine agonist as monotherapy. The clinical importance of the ability of a dopamine agonist to reduce or delay "time to motor complications," however, is tempered by the fact that there is no direct demonstration that this translates into disability and quality-of-life benefit on longer follow-up.

Dopamine Agonists as Adjuncts to L-dopa in Advanced Parkinson's Disease

Several trials have shown that dopamine agonists such as pergolide (Sage 1986, Jankovic 1986, Olanow 1994), pramipexole (Guttman 1997, Lieberman 1997, Wermuth 1998, Pinter 1999, Mizuno 2003), or ropinirole (Rascol et al. 1996, Lieberman 1998) effectively reduce off time in patients with L-dopa–related motor fluctuations. Less convincing evidence exists for bromocriptine (Hoehn 1985, Toyokura 1985, Guttman 1997) and cabergoline (Hutton 1996). There are only open-label or anecdotal data to suggest that other agonists like lisuride or piribedil could improve motor fluctuations.

Reported evidence (bromocriptine vs cabergoline, lisuride vs pergolide) suggest that efficacy is similar among the various agonists. The same was true when comparing bromocriptine (Tolcapone Study Group 1999) and pergolide (Koller 2001) to the COMT inhibitor tolcapone. No other comparisons have been published.

When used as monotherapy or as adjunct to L-dopa therapy, adequate dosing of the agonists is important, depending on individual responsiveness and tolerability. However, the dose ranges vary among these drugs. Licensing details vary among countries, but usual maximum doses are between 4 mg/day and 6 mg/day for pramipexole, cabergoline, pergolide, and lisuride, whereas bromocriptine (20 mg/day) and ropinirole (24 mg/day) have higher dosing ranges. Underdosing is frequently encountered when patients are referred as "refractory" to treatment. As with all dopaminergic drugs, adaptations and increases are required in most patients during the course of their illness.

Safety

Currently available dopamine agonists share a wide range of side effects with L-dopa that are due to peripheral and central dopaminergic stimulation. Both types of adverse effects occur more frequently on agonists than on L-dopa monotherapy. Nausea and vomiting, postural hypotension, dizziness, bradycardia, and other signs of autonomic peripheral stimulation are common peripheral dopaminergic side effects of all dopamine agonists. Erythromelalgia-like reactions have been described with the ergot agonists, and leg edema is also commonly observed with most agonists. The mechanism of such an adverse drug reaction is poorly understood.

Central side effects include confusion, hallucinations and psychosis, and excessive daytime sleepiness (Calne 1984, Tolosa 1997). Insomnia also can occur. Some reports have suggested that nonergot agonists such as pramipexole and ropinirole may induce sleep attacks without warning (Frucht 1999), raising the question of safety of these medications for those who drive. Subsequent reports have described similar problems with other nonergot agonists and even with L-dopa monotherapy (Ferreira 2000, Hobson 2002).

There is no convincing evidence that any agonist is better tolerated than bromocriptine. However, postmarketing surveillance shows that the rare but severe risk of pleuropulmonary/retroperitoneal fibrosis is greater with ergot than with nonergot agonists. Restrictive valvular heart disorders only recently have been recognized as a relevant adverse event associated with dopamine agonists. Although this appears to be more common in ergot agonists, some evidence suggests that the problem may be related to an affinity to serotonin receptor subtypes rather than ergot properties. To date, pergolide has been the most frequently reported drug to cause valvular changes (Van Camp et al. 2004). Pergolide is only used nowadays as a second-line alternative option, when other agonists fail to provide adequate control of symptoms. However, severe restrictive heart valve changes requiring surgery have been described with cabergoline as well (Pinero 2005). At this stage, insufficient data are available to draw conclusions on the magnitude of the problem, and data from larger studies must be awaited to establish the relative safety of individual dopamine agonists.

When added to L-dopa, a dopamine agonist can trigger first-time dyskinesias or more commonly exacerbate existing L-dopa–induced dyskinesias (Tolosa 1993). Both peak dose and diphasic dyskinesias can be aggravated by orally administered agonists. Such an occurrence requires reduction of L-dopa dose for optimal control of the patient's symptoms. The effect of an agonist on L-dopa–induced dyskinesia might be related to the doses of the agonist used, occurring rarely with low doses. In general, worsening of dyskinesias is not a serious consequence of the addition of a dopamine agonist as long as L-dopa dosages are reduced appropriately.

Parenteral Apomorphine

Apomorphine is the oldest and the most potent dopamine agonist in clinical practice, acting on both D1 and D2 receptor subtype families. When given as a single dose, the magnitude of its effect is equivalent to that of oral L-dopa, but it has a considerably faster onset (5–15 minutes) and shorter duration (mean 40 minutes) of effect (Duby 1972). Due to its low bioavailability, it cannot be administered orally, but subcutaneous (SC) injections can be very effective in rapidly resolving off states in patients with motor fluctuations.

Intermittent subcutaneous injection therapy, using an average of 3–4 mg per injection, can be a useful option for quick relief from off periods in selected patients (Ostergaard 1995, Dewey 2001, Hughes 1993, Frankel 1990). Patients suitable for this treatment must have offs despite optimization of their oral drug regimen. They must be able to distinguish their off symptoms from other conditions such as dyskinesias. Patients who suffer from sudden, unexpected offs often benefit from this rescue medication. Pretreatment assessments include an apomorphine challenge test to determine responsiveness and to establish effective doses, and to observe for side effects, such as nausea, postural hypotension, confusion, or somnolence. Patient selection and counseling must be based on the fact that the optimum response that can be expected is equal to the patient's best L-dopa response, and that patients whose on periods are associated by dyskinesias also will likely experience dyskinesias following apomorphine injections. To counteract dopaminergic side effects such as nausea, domperidone at a dose of 20 mg 3 times daily should be initiated at least 3 days before any apomorphine treatment is started.

Apomorphine given via continuous subcutaneous infusion during waking hours leads to large reductions in daily off-time (Colzi 1998, Kanovsky 2002, Manson 2002,

Stocchi 2001, Katzenschlager 2005). Several, but not all, studies have shown marked and sustained antidyskinetic effects in patients on continuous subcutaneous apomorphine therapy (44%–83% reduction in dyskinesia severity compared to baseline). Dyskinesia reduction is significantly more marked in those patients who gradually manage to substantially reduce their oral dopaminergic therapy, or who achieve "apomorphine monotherapy" (i.e., apomorphine pump treatment only during the waking day with complete discontinuation of oral drugs) (Colzi 1998, Manson 2002, Stocchi 2001, Katzenschlager 2005). This is in keeping with the current concept of dyskinesia formation and believed to be due to the replacement of pulsatile with continuous dopamine receptor stimulation. Although randomized-controlled studies are lacking, the magnitude of the antidyskinetic effect of apomorphine encountered in some studies is comparable to that reported with deep brain stimulation of the subthalamic nucleus, and the reduction in oral dopaminergic medication is also similar. The maximum dyskinesia improvement has been observed around 12 months following the initiation of pump treatment, on mean daily doses of around 100 mg (Manson 2002). While the usual daily duration of pump treatment is around 14–16 hours, some patients with severe nocturnal off symptoms benefit from 24-hour administration.

Potential side effects of continuous apomorphine treatment include nausea, orthostatic hypotension, somnolence, and—rarely—hypersexuality or other behavioral disturbances, and skin nodule formation. Hemolytic anemia are rare, but regular checks for full blood count and Coomb's test are recommended. Confusion or hallucinations may occur, although there is increasing evidence that these neuropsychiatric problems may actually improve compared to baseline (Alegret 2004, Morgante 2004, Manson 2002). A positive effect on mood has also been observed (DiRosa et al. 2003).

Transdermal Delivery of Dopamine Agonists

In an attempt to minimize L-dopa–related motor complications, dopaminergic agents with longer half-life than L-dopa have been developed. Routes of delivery alternative to the oral route can produce relatively constant levels of dopaminergic stimulation and can include intravenous or intraintestinal infusions of L-dopa and subcutanous infusions of lisuride or apomorphine. Moreover, currently continuous noninvasive dopaminergic stimulation can be achieved via transdermal drug delivery systems (Pfeiffer 2005). Two such drugs are currently being tested in patients with PD: rotigotine and lisuride.

Rotigotine is a lipid-soluble, nonergoline, selective D2 dopamine receptor agonist with a structure similar to dopamine and apomorphine (Jenner 2005) It has potent antiparkinsonian activity in MPTP monkeys (Belluzzi

1994). Rotigotine cannot be given orally because of extensive GI metabolism, but its high lipid solubility makes it ideal as a transdermal preparation. In the transdermal product, rotigotine is dissolved in a silicone adhesive and then spread across a silicone backing that permits uniform release of the drug at a constant rate, with drug delivery directly proportional to the size of the patch. The system produces a stable drug release and steady-state plasma concentrations over a period of 24 hours when administered once every 24 hours.

Clinical trials have demonstrated both the efficacy and the tolerability of rotigotine administered by the transdermal route. Two randomized placebo-controlled trials have shown rotigotine administered transdermally to be an effective once-daily drug for the treatment of early PD. In one trial by the Parkinson Study Group (Parkinson Study Group 2003) enrolling 242 patients, improvement occurred in combined motor and activities of daily living scores of the UPDRS, and a dose response relationship was evident from 4.5 mg to 13.5 mg. In a second trial (Watts 2004) with a total of 227 patient with early PD, placebo rotigotine significantly reduced UPDRS part 2 and 3 scores compared with placebo. Furthermore, there was a significantly higher proportion of responders at the end of treatment when compared with placebo (48% vs 19%). There was no evidence of tachyphylaxis related to continuous dopaminergic stimulation, and benefits persisted for up to 27 weeks.

Transdermal rotigotine has been tested in patients with motor complications on L-dopa treatment. Preliminary results have been published only in abstract form. Clinically significant reductions in off time were observed in two large trials. A large placebo effect occurred in one trial (Quinn 2001), resulting in nonsignificant differences in off-time reduction between rotigotine and placebo. A more recent study found a significant difference in the reduction in off time between active treatment groups (rotigotine 40 cm^2 and 60 cm^2 patches) and the placebo group at 24 weeks of treatment (LeWitt 2004).

Rotigotine at therapeutic doses displays a good safety profile and is generally well tolerated. Its use was associated with the characteristic adverse reactions to dopamine agonists such as nausea, excessive daytime sleepiness, and dizziness. Application-site reactions are common but usually mild or moderate in nature. These required discontinuation of treatment in 5% of patients. Rotigotine had no clinically relevant effects on laboratory parameters or physical examination.

A transdermal lisuride preparation has also recently been tested as adjunctive treatment in PD (Woitalla 2004). Lisuride is an 8-alpha-aminoergoline compound with a strong affinity for dopamine and serotonin receptors and a rather short plasma half-life of about 2 hours. It is currently used in its oral form and can be given SC as well. In this short trial, 8 patients with advanced disease and motor fluctuations were treated for a brief period of time (up to 8 days of treatment). Improvement in motor fluctuations was noted. Transient skin irritation occurred in half of the patients. Large trials with transdermal lisuride are in progress to assess its efficacy and tolerability in both de novo and fluctuating patients.

MAO-B Inhibitors

MAO-B plays an important role in the biotransformation of dopamine in the human brain. It constitutes about 80% of the total MAO activity in the human brain and is the predominant form of the enzyme in the striatum. Inhibitors of this enzyme block the oxidative deamination of dopamine and increase its half-life in the brain. There are currently two MAO-B inhibitors commercialized for the treatment of PD: selegiline (deprenyl) and rasagiline. Both are irreversible MAO-B inhibitors, which means that the duration of their effect, rather than either drug's plasma half-life, reflects the ability of the body to resynthesize the enzyme.

Mechanism of Action

Selegiline, at the doses commonly used of 10 mg/day, produces a selective and irreversible MAO-B inhibition with only minimal effects upon MAO-A, an enzyme that is involved in the deamination of serotonin and noradrenaline (Mercuri 1997). Selegiline is extensively metabolized in humans mainly in the liver to form desmethylselegiline and methamphetamine, which are further metabolized to amphetamine. These metabolites may contribute to the dopaminergic effect of the drug and can explain some of the stimulating effects of the drug. Blockade of presynaptic dopamine receptors and inhibition of dopamine reuptake from the synapse by selegiline has also been suggested to contribute to the dopaminergic effect of the drug (Knoll 1983, Knoll 1992). Selegiline also has been shown to protect nigral neurons against damage by oxygen free radicals generated during MAO-B activity, to protect against MPP + toxicity in the MPTP model of parkinsonism, and to have an anti-apoptotic effect in vitro and in vivo in experimental animals (Tatton 1998, Ansari 1993, Tatton 1993, Carrillo 1993, Ju 1994).

Rasagiline is a novel second-generation propargylamine that irreversibly and selectively inhibits monoamine oxidase type B (Youdim 2001, Finberg 1998). Unlike the prototype propargylamine selegiline, which is metabolized to amphetamine derivatives, rasagiline is biotransformed to aminoindan, a nonamphetamine compound. Rasagiline is well tolerated with infrequent cardiovascular or psychiatric side effects, and at the recommended therapeutic dose of 1 mg once daily, tyramine restriction is unnecessary. In addition to MAO-B inhibition, the propargylamine chain also confers dose-related antioxidant and antiapoptotic effects, which have been associated with neuroprotection in multiple experimental models (Blandini 2004, Maruyama 2001). Thus, in addition to symptomatic benefits, rasagiline offers the promise of clinically relevant neuroprotection.

Therapeutic Efficacy

Selegiline

Monotherapy with oral selegiline (10 mg/day) reduces symptom severity and, during prolonged therapy, delays the need to start L-dopa in previously untreated patients with early PD (Parkinson Study Group 1989, Parkinson Study Group 1996, Myllyla 1992, Olanow 1995, Palhagen 1998, Teravainen 1990). These symptomatic effects of selegiline are considered modest. In a meta-analysis by Ives et al. (Ives 2004), it has been estimated that the differences versus placebo at 3 months follow-up is about 2.78 points in the total UPDRS score and close to 2 in the motor part of the UPDRS.

The standard oral formulation has been shown to improve PD symptoms in patients with motor fluctuations, but a consistent effect in reducing off time in patients with wearing off has not been shown (Goetz/Koller 2002). A recent study with orally disintegrating tablets of selegiline (Waters 2004) showed that this formulation of selegiline significantly reduces off time when used as adjunctive therapy with L-dopa in patients with motor fluctuations.

Trials with selegiline have looked into the effect of selegiline in preventing or delaying motor complications (Caraceni 2001, Shoulson et al. 2002). It was concluded that selegiline is not efficacious in preventing dyskinesias. In a follow-up trial with the original DATATOP cohort, freezing of gait occurred more commonly in placebo than in selegiline-treated patients (28.9% vs 15.5%; $P = 0.003$) (Shoulson 2002).

Rasagiline

For the management of PD, rasagiline is efficacious across the span of PD stages ranging from monotherapy in early disease to adjunct treatment in patients with advancing disease and motor fluctuations.

In a double-blind randomized trial on monotherapy in early PD (Parkinson Study Group 2002), rasagiline or placebo was given to patients during 26 weeks. Patients receiving rasagiline 1 mg/day or 2 mg/day showed improvement in parkinsonism (UPDRS scores) relative to the placebo group. The outcome for the ADL subscale was also in favor of the rasagiline 2 mg/day group, and the proportion of responders in the rasagiline groups was significantly higher than for placebo recipients. Compared with placebo, patients receiving rasagiline had significantly improved quality-of-life measures during the 26 weeks of the study.

Rasagiline given as a once-daily medication without titrations reduced off time by approximately 1 hour, a reduction of about 20%. Two double-blind, placebo-controlled, randomized clinical trials have assessed the efficacy of rasagiline in patients with Parkinson's disease experiencing L-dopa–related motor fluctuations, the Parkinson's Rasagiline: Efficacy and Safety in the Treatment of "Off" (PRESTO) and the Lasting Effect in Adjunct Therapy with Rasagiline Given Once-Daily trials (LARGO) (Rascol 2005, Parkinson Study Group 2005). Both studies were placebo controlled. The LARGO study also included an active comparator arm, for which patients received entacapone 200 mg administered with each L-dopa dose. Primary efficacy variable in both trials was the change from baseline in daily off time assessed by patient's diaries. A significant reduction in daily off time occurred in both trials in patients receiving rasagiline relative to placebo. Although the LARGO study was not designed to directly compare rasagiline and entacapone, the results demonstrate that the clinical effects on off time were similar with these two compounds.

MAO-B Inhibitors and Neuroprotection

In the hope that selegiline might afford neuroprotection, clinical trials have compared the effect of selegiline with that of placebo on the evolution of disability in de novo patients. One trial compared selegiline with placebo in 54 untreated patients (Tetrud 1989), and the DATATOP study (Parkinson Study Group 1989) investigated both selegiline and vitamin E in a double-blind prospective study of 800 PD patients. Both studies demonstrated that selegiline significantly delayed the development of disability requiring L-dopa therapy. Although a neuroprotective effect of selegiline cannot be ruled out, it is generally considered that these beneficial effects are due to a symptomatic amelioration of PD by selegiline.

Rasagiline has not been studied fully with respect to demonstrating an effect on disease progression. The TVP-1012 in Early Monotherapy for Parkinson's Disease Outpatients (TEMPO) study (Parkinson Study Group 2002) used a delayed-start design, in which one arm initiated active treatment with a 6-month delay. The results of this study suggest that there might be a benefit to starting treatment early. However, data available today are insufficient to draw conclusions on a potential clinically relevant disease-modifying effect and the results of a sufficiently powered, larger trial must be awaited.

Safety and Tolerability of MAO-B Inhibitors

Both selegiline and rasagiline when employed as monotherapy or combined with L-dopa have proven to be well tolerated drugs. Due to their selective MAO-B inhibition, both are devoid of a "cheese effect" (the tyramine increase observed with MAO-A inhibitors) when administered at currently recommended doses.

No major differences with respect to adverse events were detected between the inhibitors and placebo in several clinical trials when given to de novo patients.

The clinical relevance of the amphetamine and metamphetamine metabolites of selegiline is not fully clear, but they are considered to underlie the occurrence or worsening of neuropsychiatric problems and insomnia sometimes observed with selegiline. Insomnia may improve when the drug is administered early in the day.

When administered with L-dopa, both MAO inhibitors may increase dopaminergic effects, which include nausea, orthostatic hypotension, increase in dyskinesias, confusion, and hallucinations. These symptoms are reversible with reduction of L-dopa or the MAO inhibitor. In the LARGO and PRESTO studies, where L-dopa could be adjusted during the first weeks of treatment, dyskinesias were not significantly modified.

Overall, the available MAO-B inhibitors are well tolerated and considered safe. One large prospective study in de novo patients reported increased mortality after 2 and 4 years of treatment with L-dopa plus selegiline compared with L-dopa alone (Parkinson's Disease Research Group of the United Kingdom 1993). Although altered cardiovascular responses have been demonstrated in patients on selegiline and L-dopa (Churchyard 1999), a clinically relevant impact of these findings has not been confirmed in any other trials and the initial finding of increased mortality is generally regarded as a statistical artefact (Olanow 1998, Ives 2004).

Amantadine

Amantadine hydrochloride (ATD) was originally introduced as an antiviral agent effective against A2 Asian influenza (Davies 1964, Dolin 1982) and was fortuitously noted to be useful in relieving clinical symptoms in a patient with PD in 1969 (Schwab 1969). Since then, several clinical trials have established the drug as a useful, well-tolerated agent for the symptomatic treatment of PD. The finding that ATD is a noncompetitive antagonist of the N-methyl-D-aspartate (NMDA) receptor with its implications on the glutamatergic toxic hypothesis on PD and the putative antidyskinetic action of the drug have renewed clinical and theoretical interest in ATD.

The drug is readily absorbed (blood levels peak 1–4 hours after an oral dose of 2.5 mg/kg) and poorly metabolized in humans (more than 90% of an ingested dose can be recovered unchanged in the urine) (Bleidner 1965, Berger 1985, Franz 1975, Ing 1974).

The exact mechanism of action of ATD in PD still remains unclear. Most of the behavioral and neurochemical studies indicate that ATD can interact with catecholamines, especially dopamine. ATD may act presynaptically and postsynaptically. Presynaptically, it enhances the release of stored catecholamines from intact dopaminergic terminals by an amphetamine-like mechanism (Von Voigtlander 1973, Grelak 1970, Farnebo 1971, Stromberg 1971). It also inhibits catecholamine reuptake processes at the presynaptic terminal (Heikkila 1972, Heimans 1972, Bailey 1975).

Postsynaptically, it can activate DA receptors directly (Allen 1981) and can produce changes in the dopamine receptor conformation that fixates the receptor in a high-affinity (agonist-like) configuration (Gianutsos 1985, Allen 1983). Nondopaminergic properties of ATD also have been proposed, including an anticholinergic action (Stone 1977, Nastuck 1976) and an NMDA receptor-blocking effect (Greenamyre 1991). The therapeutic benefit of ATD in PD may be mediated in part by this blockade of glutamate receptors. ATD is able to displace the noncompetitive NMDA receptor antagonist MK-801 from the NMDA receptor complex (Kornhuber 1991). Importantly, this NMDA receptor antagonistic action is exerted at therapeutic levels (Stoof 1992).

ATD was first given to a large group of patients with PD by Schwab et al. (Schwab 1969). In this uncontrolled study, 107 (66%) of 163 patients treated with a maximum daily dosage of 200 mg showed improvement consisting of a reduction in akinesia and rigidity and some lessening of tremor. One-third of the patients who experienced remarkable initial reduction of symptoms, particularly in akinesia and rigidity, showed a slow but steady loss of benefit after 4–8 weeks. In another 58%, benefit was sustained over 3 to 8 months of treatment. In a subsequent publication (Schwab 1972), it was observed that the beneficial effect of ATD usually occurred within the first 24 hours, sometimes following the first 100 mg capsule. When treatment with the drug was stopped, there was a prompt reappearance of symptoms within 24 hours.

Subsequent studies have confirmed the antiparkinsonian properties of ATD. The degree of improvement described in these trials, however, has varied, with open trials giving much more favorable results. In these trials, ATD was compared with placebo either as single therapy or as add-on in patients on anticholinergics. These studies indicated a useful if modest antiparkinsonian effect (Cox 1973, Parkes 1974, Butzer 1975, Fahn 1975).

The effect of ATD on the different elements of the parkinsonian syndrome has been repeatedly described as qualitatively similar to that of L-dopa in that it improves all cardinal manifestations of the illness. A detailed analysis of these studies, however, discloses disparate results. Two studies (Schwab 1969, Parkes 1970) described a modest effect on akinesia and a lesser effect on tremor. Other authors (Gilligan 1970, Bauer 1974, Butzer 1975, Parkes 1970) reported greater effects on tremor than on akinesia. Judging from the studies reported, there are no clear predictors of a positive response to ATD.

Although direct comparative studies are lacking, it can be concluded that the antiparkinsonian potency of ATD is clearly inferior to that of L-dopa but, at least, similar to that of the anticholinergics. The degree of improvement achieved tends to be similar whether or not the patients are taking anticholinergic drugs. Most open-label studies report that the conditions of one-third to two-thirds of patients improve and that the drug causes few side effects. Acceptance by patients was good in most of the trials, and improvement in functional disability was greater than improvement in physical signs. The reverse was true in a few studies.

ATD also has been studied as an adjunctive treatment to L-dopa. In one study in patients without motor complications, ATD was found beneficial when compared with baseline and with placebo, although the follow-up was short (Savery 1971). Improvement was more noticeable in patients on low doses of L-dopa in another trial (Fehling 1973). The effect of ATD on motor fluctuations has been studied in two double-blind randomized clinical trials. In one study a significant decrease in off time versus placebo was described (Verhagen Metman 1998). Another study (Luginger 2000) found no significant differences in hours on or off, but this study included only 11 patients and was powered to detect differences in dyskinesias.

Several clinical trials have shown that ATD has a potent antidyskinetic effect in patients taking L-dopa (Verhagen Metman 1999). The clinical relevance of several of theses studies is limited because they assessed the antidyskinetic effect of acute challenges of ATD (Verhagen Metman 1998, Snow 2000, Del Dotto 2001). In one recent study concerning amantadine use in controlling dyskinesia in advanced PD (Thomas 2004), amantadine increased on time when compared with placebo, whereas off time decreased, although not significantly. Several subjects treated with ATD experienced a rebound in dyskinesia severity after drug discontinuation. ATD was found to decrease dyskinesia scores by 45% compared with placebo. This decrease in dyskinesia, though, was reported to last only from 3 to 8 months.

Safety and Tolerability

Side effects of ATD in patients with PD are usually mild and do not limit treatment. In the original report (Schwab 1969) on a group of 163 patients treated with maximal daily dosages of 200 mg/day, 22% experienced some type of side effect. The most common side effects are livedo reticularis and ankle edema (Shealy et al. 1970), dryness of mouth, and difficulty focusing. Persistent bilateral ankle edema occurred in 22% of patients in one study and tends to occur within 2–8 weeks of starting ATD treatment (Parkes 1970). Livedo reticularis is a common undesirable side effect at therapeutic dosages and is probably related to the vasoconstrictor effect of catecholamines released by ATD (Pearce 1974). It generally appears in the legs and occasionally on the buttocks and arms. Patients usually do not complain about livedo reticularis, and it is generally found on routine inspection of the skin. One report described this in 90% of the patients in the study (Parkes 1970). Occurrence of livedo reticularis does not require discontinuation of the drug.

Dryness of mouth, blurred vision, and, when present, palpitations and jitteriness are considered atropinelike side effects related to the anticholinergic properties of ATD (Sartori 1984). More uncommon but more troublesome are mental aberrations such as confusion, depression, nightmares, insomnia, agitation, visual hallucinations, and psychosis (Shealy 1970). Objective neurologic findings can include ataxia, slurred speech, and, rarely, convulsion.

An evidence-based review of the literature (Goetz 2002) concluded that ATD for PD "has an acceptable risk, without specialized monitoring."

In conclusion, ATD hydrochloride is useful in the treatment of the motor symptoms of PD. It leads to an improvement in all cardinal symptoms. Patients' acceptance is usually good, and the incidence of significant side effects is low when it is administered in the 200–300 mg/day range (Goetz 2002; Editorial 1980). Administered alone or in combination with MAO-B inhibitors (or anticholinergics), ATD has a definite place in the treatment of symptoms in the early, mild stages of PD when it may allow for a delay in the introduction of dopamine agonists or L-dopa. There is some evidence, however, that the therapeutic efficacy of ATD tends to diminish after months of continuous administration, thus adding ATD to optimal L-dopa treatment to improve motor fluctuations in advanced PD is of questionable value but can be tried if additional therapeutic effects are desired.

The results of recent double-blind studies show that ATD is useful in reducing L-dopa–induced dyskinesias in the short term and support the antidyskinetic potential of NMDA antagonism as a possibility of modifying dyskinesias. It remains still to be determined whether this observed antidyskinetic effect is sustained over longer periods of treatment.

Anticholinergic Medications for Parkinson's Disease

Ordenstein (1867), following the observations of his professor Jean-Martin Charcot, first described the beneficial effect of the belladonna alkaloids (mainly containing atropine as active component) on tremor and other Parkinson's disease symptoms. Subsequent investigators, such as Gowers (1888) at the end of the 19th century, agreed that other substances—such as indian hemp (containing *cannabis sativa*), scopolamine (hyoscine), and hyoscyamine (duboisine)—were effective in mitigating tremor and muscular rigidity. In 1945 Feldburg discovered that acetylcholine was also a central neurotransmitter that was abundant in the striatum at the synaptic vesicles of nerve terminals (Feldburg 1945), and he suggested a central effect for anticholinergic drugs. For more than half a century, the belladonna alkaloids formed the mainstay of the medical management of the Parkinson's syndrome. These natural products were substituted in the 1960s by a series of synthetic anticholinergics and antihistaminics (Strang 1965).

Anticholinergics improve symptoms of PD through a central anticholinergic effect exerted in the striatum. Duvoisin showed that cholinesterase inhibitors, which can penetrate the brain, increase the severity of Parkinson's disease symptoms (Duvoisin 1966, Duvoisin 1967), an effect that can be reversed by anticholinergics, such as benzotropine. This observation provides a rationale for the use of anticholinergics in PD and supports the notion that a state of striatal cholinergic preponderance exists in PD (Barbeau 1962). It is thought that the antimuscarinic properties of the anticholinergics mediate their anti-parkinsonian properties (Velasco 1982, Nashold 1959). Another proposed mechanism of action is the inhibition of dopamine reuptake in the striatum (Coyle 1969).

Centrally active anticholinergics (muscarinic receptors antagonists) exert a modest improvement, but the percentage of patients reported to improve with these drugs has varied greatly, from 43% to 77% in open trials (Strang 1965, Corbin 1949) and from 20% to 40% in double-blind studies (Parkes 1974). Studies of trihexyphenidyl (Martin 1974), benzotropine (Tourtellotte 1982), and bornaprine (Cantello 1986) in L-dopa–treated patients indicate that adjunctive anticholinergics have only a minor effect on PD symptoms in patients on L-dopa therapy.

It is frequently stated that anticholinergics are more effective in alleviating resting tremor and rigidity than akinesia and that the major benefit derived from their use is precisely from their tremorolytic effects (Strang 1965, Ebling 1971, Obeso 1987, Doshay 1957, Burns 1964). Reports suggesting that anticholinergics do not have a specific antitremor effect, however, abound in the literature (Marshall 1968, Yahr 1968), and two recent reviews (Goetz 2002, Katzenschlager 2003) indicate that data suggesting such a tremor-specific effect are inconclusive. Therapeutic differences among the various synthetic anticholinergics are probably minor, but some patients may tolerate one better than the other.

Today, the anticholinergics are occasionally used as initial treatment in the early stages of the disease. However, they are no longer used as first-line drugs since they have been replaced gradually by other medications such as the MAO-B inhibitors or the modern dopamine agonists. These latter drugs have shown a reduced incidence of motor complications when compared to L-dopa, with nearly comparable clinical efficacy in the case of dopamine agonists. No such studies have been performed with the anticholinergics. Furthermore, no trials have compared the symptomatic effects of dopamine agonists directly with those of the anticholinergics. Despite a lack of definite data to confirm a special role in the management of tremor, anticholinergics are also recommended in patients in whom other therapies such as the agonists, amantadine, or L-dopa have failed to sufficiently control tremor.

In patients on long-term L-dopa therapy and more advanced disease, e.g., patients with associated motor complications such as fluctuations or dyskinesias, the beneficial effect from adding anticholinergics has been questioned (Martin 1974), but some authors believe that in some instances the addition of anticholinergics may convey some benefit (Parkes 1974, Tourtellote 1982, Yahr 1968).

Development of tolerance to the effects of beneficial effects of anticholinergics is said to occur frequently. Some loss of therapeutic benefit is indeed a common clinical observation after months of treatment but could be attributed, at least in part, to disease progression. Withdrawal of anticholinergics, even in patients in whom it is thought that these drugs are no longer effective, invariably results in worsening of the parkinsonian symptoms, at times to a level worse than the patients' baseline state (Hughes 1971, Horrocks 1973).

Anticholinergic drugs have been reported to alleviate dystonic spasms in PD resulting from chronic L-dopa administration, as is the case of early-morning dystonia (Poewe 1987). Poewe et al. (1988) also reported that a challenge with procyclidine in 9 patients with foot dystonia resulted in abolition of dystonia in 6, amelioration in 1, and no effect in the remaining 2 patients.

Safety and Tolerability

The clinical use of this class of drugs is limited by a considerable spectrum of frequent adverse effects. Peripheral adverse effects include tachycardia, constipation (rarely leading to paralytic ileus), urinary retention, blurred vision, and dry mouth (Ebling 1971, Duvoisin 1965). Gingivitis and caries, rarely leading to loss of teeth, may occur (Lang 1989) and reduced sweating may interfere with body temperature regulation.

These effects are reversible when diminishing or with discontinuation of the drug and can even show some tolerance after prolonged exposure. Rarely, some of these side effects can be beneficial, as is the case for dry mouth, which can be advantageous in patients with prominent drooling. Caution must be exercised in elderly male patients with comorbid prostate hypertrophy, due to a high risk for urinary retention. Blurred vision is a common side effect, attributed to reduced accommodation due to parasympathetic blockade. The occurrence of acute narrow-angle glaucoma is extremely rare and can be precipitated in predisposed patients.

The usefulness of anticholinergics is also limited by central side effects. These include sedation, confusion, and psychiatric disturbances, such as hallucinations and psychosis (Porteous 1956, Koller 1984). Impaired mental function (mainly immediate memory and memory acquisition) is a well-documented central side effect that resolves after drug withdrawal (van Herwaarden 1993). Anticholinergics can lead to an exacerbation of frontal lobe dysfunction in PD patients (Sadeh 1982, Syndulko 1981, Dubois 1987). An impairment of higher cortical functions has been found in nondemented PD subjects with an acute subclinical dose of scopolamine (Bedard 1998), and impaired neuropsychiatric function has been demonstrated even in patients without cognitive impairment (Sadeh 1982, Syndulko 1981). These central effects are more likely to occur with advanced age and in patients with dementia (De Smet 1982). The marked involvement of the cholinergic system (i.e., nucleus basalis of Meynert) in PD pathology (Braak 2000, Forster 1912) is probably the basis of the cognitive changes induced by anticholinergics.

Overall, due to the propensity of anticholinergics to induce adverse effects and due to the wider choice of alternative antiparkinsonian drugs with better tolerability, the importance of these drugs in the management of PD has declined in recent years. If they are prescribed, great caution must be exercised when administering anticholinergics, especially to elderly patients, in order to detect any adverse effects early, in particular with respect to cognition.

PRACTICAL APPROACH TO THE MEDICAL TREATMENT OF DE NOVO AND STABLE PARKINSON'S DISEASE

Until agents with proven disease-modifying effects become available, the choice of initial treatment must be tailored to each patient's requirements. When the signs and symptoms of the illness are beginning to interfere with daily activities or with quality of life, it generally seems prudent to initiate symptomatic treatment. The judgment to initiate symptomatic drug treatment is made in discussions between the patient and the treating physician. Available treatments include amantadine, MAO-B inhibitors, dopamine agonists and L-dopa, and anticholinergics (whose use is often limited by an unfavorable side-effect profile). There is general consensus that in the early stage of PD, when the symptoms are noticed but are not troublesome, treatment with L-dopa is not necessary. As outlined in this chapter, early treatment with L-dopa is associated with good functional improvement but carries a higher risk of eventually leading to the development of motor complications in many patients. This is particularly so in younger patients, and it is therefore reasonable to use an L-dopa sparing strategy in this group of patients (age below 60–70 years).

In mildly affected patients, MAO-B inhibitors, amantadine, and, sometimes, anticholinergics may be sufficient as initial treatment. Although comparative trials are lacking, these drugs are likely to have less symptomatic effect than dopamine agonists. The agonists are used widely as initial therapy because of their symptomatic effect and because they have been shown to reduce the risk of motor complications compared with L-dopa treatment. When treatment is initiated with an agonist, L-dopa can then be added when its superior symptomatic effect becomes necessary to maintain full functioning.

While this initial approach is currently considered to be the most appropriate for the majority of younger PD patients, individual factors must be taken into account. Dopamine agonists have a higher risk of causing hallucinations and orthostatic hypotension, including in early PD. There is no general cutoff age for agonists versus L-dopa as initial treatment: The risk of ever developing motor complications is considerably smaller in patients with older age at onset (Kumar 2005), and concern for these treatment-related complications is therefore less prominent in elderly patients.

Conversely, while younger-onset patients have a higher risk of motor complications, their ability to remain employable or physically active may be an important goal. Dopamine agonists will often be the first choice in these patients, but in certain circumstances L-dopa should be considered early, either as monotherapy or in combination with other drugs. This may be the case when agonists are not well tolerated at the required dose, or when the delay to a full effect is too long because of marked disability. Slow-release L-dopa preparations do not confer any benefit with respect to the risk of motor complications when compared to standard L-dopa. The potential benefits of starting L-dopa therapy in association with a dopa decarboxylase inhibitor plus entecapone is currently being investigated in a large randomized trial.

Among the available agonists, nonergot-derived substances are currently favored as first choice because of evidence suggesting an increased risk of cardiac valvular fibrosis and dysfunction (Pritchett 2002) in at least two of the ergot agonists.

Ongoing Management in Stable Disease

In most patients with PD, initial treament is followed by a period of good response which may last from months to decades. However, even during a stable phase, repeated adjustments of treatment according to tolerability and requirements are necessary as the neurodegenerative process continues.

If a patient has started on an MAO-B inhibitor, amantadine, anticholinergic, or a combination of these drugs, a stage will come when, because of worsening motor symptoms, there is a requirement for adding either L-dopa or a dopamine agonist. As with initial treatment, each patient's individual circumstances and treatment goals must be considered before deciding on changes in dosage or agents used. Again, the patient's age and the desire to avoid late motor complications must be weighed against early tolerability and improved motor disability (both of which are better with L-dopa).

If a patient is on dopamine agonist therapy, it is usually best practice to increase the dopamine agonist dose in accordance with tolerability. However, even when the dopamine agonist dose is increased over time, it cannot control parkinsonian symptoms for more than about 3–5 years of follow-up in most patients, and L-dopa must be added at some stage in nearly all patients.

If a patient is on L-dopa already, the choice whether to increase L-dopa or to add a dopamine agonist will depend on the same deliberations already outlined in this text.

Studies of the COMT inhibitors in nonfluctuating patients have shown significant improvements in secondary outcome measures, including activities of daily living and quality-of-life data. UPDRS motor scores were not significantly improved in all studies, but this may be related to a reduction in L-dopa.

PRACTICAL APPROACH TO THE MEDICAL TREATMENT OF MOTOR FLUCTUATIONS AND DYSKINESIAS

The term *advanced PD* usually refers to patients suffering from the classical motor syndrome of PD along with other motor or nonmotor complications, either disease-related (e.g., freezing) or treatment-related (e.g., fluctuations, dyskinesias or hallucinations).

The goal in management of motor fluctuations is to increase daytime on duration without inducing unacceptable treatment-related side effects. It often requires a determined patient and a doctor with patience to achieve significant improvements.

Wearing Off

In patients with wearing off, optimizing L-dopa treatment is often the first step. This includes adjusting individual dosages according to the patients' needs and shortening the intervals between doses. Increasing the daily doses of L-dopa to more than 3 times a day soon becomes a necessity, and some patients with very short duration of effect of each L-dopa dose may need L-dopa dosing every 2 to 3 hours during the waking day, with additional doses at night. Switching from standard L-dopa to a controlled release (CR) formulation can also improve the wearing off and is not uncommonly used to treat nocturnal or early morning akinesia, although a definite benefit of this common approach has never been proven. It should be kept in mind that the gastrointestinal absorption of slow-release preparations is lower and can be less predictable than with standard L-dopa; if this occurs, switching back

---

TABLE 10.5

OPTIONS AVAILABLE TO IMPROVE WEARING-OFF FLUCTUATIONS

1. Improve L-dopa Absorption and Transport

- Avoid competition for intestinal absorption: avoid L-dopa intake with meals; dietary protein restrictions.
  In selected cases:
  - Enhance gastric motility (domperidone).
  - Soluble L-dopa: as rescue medication when regimen otherwise optimized, e.g., early morning offs.
  - In selected refractory cases: duodenal L-dopa infusions.

2. Stabilize L-dopa Plasma Levels

- Adjust L-dopa dose.
- Adjust intervals between intakes.
- Add COMT inhibitors.
- Use sustained release formulations (for nocturnal akinesia and, in selected cases, during daytime).

3. Enhance Striatal Dopamine Concentrations

- Add MAO-B inhibitor.

4. Add Dopamine Agonists

- Oral dopamine agonist
- Transdermal dopamine agonist.
- Intermittent subcutaneous apomorphine injections; as rescue medication when regimen otherwise optimized
- Continuous apomorphine treatment: when fluctuations and dyskinesias are refractory to oral adjustments.
  In selected cases, for refractory OFFs only.

---

to standard formulations should be considered. (See Table 10.5.)

Response to L-dopa varies with meals. Intake with meals may delay L-dopa absorption and result in a weaker response to it. In many patients, intake of L-dopa 1 hour before meals may enhance absorption and induce a more reliable on. Rarely will competition with other amino acids in the diet interfere with L-dopa efficacy. In such cases, reduction in concomitant dietary protein may provide a more stable response to L-dopa throughout the day.

Soluble L-dopa formulations have a more reliable onset of effect (around 30 minutes) and are particularly useful for delayed morning start-up time or as a rescue medication to provide quick relief from bothersome or disabling off symptoms. With very fast-acting agents, such as soluble L-dopa and apomorphine rescue injections, there is a concern with respect to a further increase in the pulsatility of application and receptor stimulation, and these rescue strategies should be used sparingly and only after the other adjustment options of oral treatment have been fully explored. In addition, it is advisable for the patient to avoid lying down after the ingestion of L-dopa, at least for those patients who notice a quicker effect if they exercise.

Other effective strategies are adding a COMT or an MAO-B inhibitor. On average, both types of drugs reduce off time by 1 to 1.5 hours. However, tolcapone is potentially hepatotoxic and is only recommended in patients for whom all other available medications have failed. Both strategies increase and prolong the presence of dopamine in the striatum and therefore carry a risk of increasing dyskinesias. This is best handled by attempting to reduce L-dopa first. A combined add-on treatment of COMT and MAO-B inhibitors is possible and useful as there is no evidence of a ceiling effect reached when one enzymatic pathway is blocked.

Oral dopamine agonists, which have a longer biological half-life than L-dopa, can also be used in combination with standard or CR L-dopa. They can be added on to COMT and MAO-B inhibitor therapy. Although direct comparisons are lacking, there is strong evidence to suggest that dopamine agonists are the most effective agents when used in combination with L-dopa for the alleviation of off states. If worsening of dyskinesias occurs, it is suggested to first reduce the L-dopa dose. In a small number of patients whose dyskinesias are very sensitive to dopamine replacement treatment with L-dopa, this drug may have to be replaced almost totally by a dopamine agonist. All dopamine agonists are useful in reducing off time. The ergot derivatives are rarely associated with fibrosis, such as the pleura and the heart, and consequently the more recently introduced dopamine agonists such as pramipexol and ropinirole, which do not appear to have this side effect, are used more commonly.

Amantadine was shown to improve motor fluctuations in most, if not all, studies and may be a useful additional strategy.

Complex and Unpredictable Motor Fluctuations

In patients with more complex fluctuations and in whom sudden random offs develop, the same strategies applied for the treatment of wearing off should be considered. Delayed on or dose failure ("no-on") are frequently part of the on–off fluctuations and are likely to be related to poor gastric emptying. In these instances, intake of L-dopa on an empty stomach should be tried.

Most patients with drug-related motor complications will eventually receive a combination of several of these treatments because a single strategy will not provide adequate control of fluctuations. The choice of drugs is mainly based on safety, tolerability, and ease of use.

Should the above-mentioned strategies result in insufficient improvement, other strategies that can be employed include the use of subcutaneous apomorphine either intermittently with a penjet or as continuous subcutaneous infusion through a pump. This can be remarkably useful in alleviating recurrent off periods both during the day and at night. Continuous daytime infusion of L-dopa into the duodenum via a transabdominal delivery system constitutes another alternative. These treatment modalities are options to be considered for patients with complex and unpredictable offs refractory to all oral adjustments, and dyskinesias.

Dyskinesias

Dyskinesias may be mild and even may go unnoticed by the patients requiring no treatment. However, they interfere frequently with voluntary movements of the limbs and with gait, cause fatigue, are socially disabling, and can be painful. Some patients avoid or mininimize L-dopa intake to avoid those symptoms. In the management of dyskinesias, it is important to first establish which pattern of dyskinesia—that is, peak dose, diphasic, or off-period dyskinesia—is predominant. It is also important to understand the nature of associated motor fluctuations since any drug modification to improve dyskinesia will also modify the control of parkinsonism. If the history is not clear and the physician has not observed the dyskinesia described by the patient, it is worthwhile to ask the patient to stay in the clinic through 1 or 2 dose cycles for observation purposes.

Reduction of the L-dopa dose or giving more frequent but smaller doses is usually a first approach to treat dyskinesias. While this frequently improves dyskinesias, the effect of reducing and fractioning the daily dose of L-dopa is often followed by a shorter and less predictable antiparkinsonian effect. Moreover, onset and end of dose (diphasic) dyskinesia may increase in intensity.

Dopamine agonists can induce dyskinesias in patients treated with L-dopa, but they induce much less dykinesia than L-dopa. Addition of a dopamine agonist is frequently accompanied by a reduction in the L-dopa dose and results in less dyskinesia and better control of parkinsonism throughout the day. In some patients with severe dyskinesias, increasing doses of the dopamine agonist allows reduction of L-dopa to a bare minimum. Dopamine agonists administered at night can also alleviate early morning dystonia.

In some instances, it may be necessary to discontinue or reduce an MAO-B or COMT inhibitor to reduce dyskinesias. Sometimes a concomitant dopamine agonist may have to be reduced as well if further reduction in L-dopa is not possible. Changes in these medications are frequently followed by worsening of wearing-off.

Adding amantadine at doses of 200–400 mg per day is a common strategy used to control dyskinesias. It is usually well tolerated, and the reduction in dyskinesias is not accompanied by a concomitant increase in parkinsonism. Some patients treated with amantadine experience a rebound in dyskinesia severity after drug discontinuation. Recently a double-blind, randomized trial comparing amantadine and placebo found that amantadine decreases dyskinesia scores by 45% compared with placebo. This decrease in dyskinesias was found to last only from 3 to 8 months. The question of whether the antidyskinetic effect of amantadine is sustained for longer periods of time will have to be established in further studies.

The atypical antipsychotics clozapine and quetiapine also have been reported to reduce L-dopa–related dyskinesias (Durif 2004, Pierelli 1998, Baron 2003). However, clozapine is associated with such potential serious adverse events as agranulocytosis and myocarditis, which limit its use, while quetiapine may lead to sedation and its antidyskinetic effect remains to be demonstrated in controlled studies.

Continuous apomorphine infusion remains an effective strategy to treat dyskinesias if oral medication fails since it has been shown to improve off time dramatically and at the same time to significantly reduce daytime dyskinesia. This is likely due to its L-dopa sparing effect and to a gradual switch from oral, pulsatile to continuous striatal dopaminergic stimulation. Continuous delivery of L-dopa into the duodenum via an enteral delivery system also can lead to marked reductions in dyskinesias in selected patients.

Dystonic spasms can be a sign of L-dopa overdosage as in peak dose dyskinesias, or it can occur when plasma L-dopa is low, such as early in the morning before the first dose of L-dopa. Off-period dystonia can occur anytime when the patient is off.

TABLE 10.6
PHARMACOLOGICAL MANAGEMENT OF L-DOPA–INDUCED DYSKINESIAS

1. Peak-Dose Dyskinesias

- Adjust L-dopa dose/schedule.
- Adjust dosage of other dopaminergic drugs (MAO-B and COMT inhibitors and dopamine agonists).
- Add amantadine.
- Use continuous drug delivery (subcutaneous apomorphine, duodenal L-dopa).
- Consider atypical neuroleptic (e.g., clozapine).

2. Diphasic Dyskinesias

- Smooth out response oscillations: see options for wearing off.
- Avoid sustained-release L-dopa.
- Add/increase dopamine agonist.
- Use subcutaneous apomorphine bolus injections at selected times.
- Use continuous drug delivery.

3. Early Morning/off-Period Dystonia

- Bedtime L-dopa (sustained-release preparations).
- Bedtime dopamine agonists.
- Add L-dopa dose 1 to 2 hours before getting up from bed.
- Consider baclofen, lithium, diazepam.
- Inject botulinum toxin type A into dystonic muscles.

All strategies used for the management of wearing off can be helpful in alleviating early morning and off-period dystonia. Supplementing L-dopa with a dopamine agonist can be useful, and using CR L-dopa at bedtime might be helpful. In some patients, taking a dose of L-dopa 1 or 2 hours before getting out of bed in the morning can succesfully prevent early morning off and accompanying dystonia.

Some patients respond to lithium or baclofen for relief from off-period dystonia. In selected cases, the injection of botulinum toxin also can result in improvement in off-period dystonia, such as blepharospasm or painful toe extension spasms.

Subcutaneous injections of apomorphine administered via penjet can be used to improve diphasic dyskinesias by injecting the drug immediately before the beginning of the on or off periods. Table 10.6 summarized the pharmacological management of L-dopa induced dyskinesias.

MANAGEMENT OF TREMOR IN PARKINSON'S DISEASE

The management of tremor presenting in the initial stages of PD should not be considered a separate clinical challenge from managing the other cardinal motor problems in PD. The dosage of dopaminergic agents, including L-dopa, dopamine agonists, COMT inhibitors, or amantadine, should be increased according to tolerability and requirement. Only when all dopaminergic options have been explored, should different strategies be recommended, such as adding clozapine or considering stereotactic surgery.

There is no evidence of clinically relevant differences in the anti-tremor effect among the available dopamine agonists. Pramipexole and pergolide have been compard head to head in two small randomized studies. Both agents were found to be significantly superior to placebo in alleviating parkinsonian tremor at comparable doses, without significant differences between the active arms. A higher dropout rate was reported on pergolide due to side effects, in particular nausea (Navan 2003, Navan 2005).

The new MAO-B inhibitor rasagiline has been shown to significantly improve parkinsonian motor signs, including tremor, in early PD (Parkinson Study Group 2002) and advanced PD (Rascol 2005).

Anticholinergics have a long-standing reputation of being valuable in the management of parkinsonian tremor. However, little evidence is available to support a special role in this indication. While a small single-dose challenge study comparing the dopamine agonist pergolide with the anticholinergic benzhexol found a somewhat greater tremor reduction on benzhexol (Schrag 1999), a systematic review by the Cochrane Collaboration found no evidence of a greater response of tremor with anticholinergics compared with the other cardinal motor signs (Katzenschlager 2003). As outlined in the section on anticholinergics, these drugs carry a considerably higher risk of peripheral and cognitive adverse effects. They should, therefore, have a minor role in the routine management of PD but can be used in young and cognitively intact patients, always under monitoring for adverse effects.

Other Medical Treatment Options to Manage Tremor

A Cochrane review looking at the effect of beta-blockers in parkinsonian tremor did not find sufficient evidence to draw conclusions on their efficacy or safety (Crosby 2003). Randomized-controlled studies exist, but they have been small, and problems with design or reporting preclude firm conclusions. Although these studies and anecdotal evidence suggest a role of propanolol in this indication, well-designed studies are required. Beta-blockers are associated with a risk of a drop in heart rate, and cardiac or pulmonary contraindications must be ruled out before considering their use.

Clozapine is an atypical neuroleptic that has been shown to significantly reduce parkinsonian tremor in several randomized-controlled studies. A double-blind crossover trial comparing low-dose clozapine (3 mg/day) and benztropine (39 mg/day) for the treatment of tremor in PD found these two agents to be equally effective (Friedman 1997). An open-label, add-on study of clozapine at a mean dose of 45 mg/day over 15.5 months found a significant improvement from baseline (Bonuccelli 1997). The use of clozapine is limited in practice due to its potential to cause agranulocytosis in 1%–2% of patients.

To date, there is limited evidence suggesting a possible small effect of gabapentin on parkinsonism including tremor. A small placebo-controlled crossover trial showed significant improvement in the UPDRS, although the difference was not significant for individual motor signs (Olson 1997). In another small placebo-controlled study, motor UPDRS scores were significantly improved while all other parameters, including on and off times, remained unchanged (VanBlercom 2004).

Primidone and clonazepam may improve various types of tremor but have been shown to be ineffective in the treatment of parkinsonian tremor in one study (Koller 1987).

In patients for whom tremor is part of motor fluctuations refractory to medical treatment options, either continuous subcutaneous apomorphine therapy or stereotactic surgery should be considered. Surgery for PD is covered in a different chapter of this book (see Chapter 49).

TREATMENT OF NONMOTOR SYMPTOMS

Although disability in PD is generally related to motor problems (e.g., bradykinesia, tremor, gait and balance impairment, speech difficulties, dyskinesias), it is also important for the treating clinician to be aware of the clinical impact of nonmotor symptoms in PD. Nonmotor features may have a considerable impact on patients' quality of life, and not rarely they can represent the most disabling feature of a patient's experience with PD. Nonmotor features should be looked for actively by clinicians as patients may not volunteer these problems or may not be aware of their association with PD. The use of screening questionnaires has been advocated for this purpose (Stacy 2005, Chaudhuri 2005).

Nonmotor symptoms are often still considered to be late-stage complications, whereas they may occur early in the course of the illness and may indeed be present before the onset of noticeable motor symptoms. Nonmotor symptoms occurring as part of end-of-dose wearing off require dopaminergic treatment. Nonmotor features that require specific pharmacological treatment occurring in the early stages mainly include depression and other psychological and mental changes, constipation, hypotension, or sensory symptoms, including pain. Cognitive deterioration is the most severe nonmotor symptom of advanced PD. Detailed descriptions of nonmotor features are described in Chapter 6, and the treatment of dementia is described in Chapter 12.

MEDICAL TREATMENT OF ORTHOSTATIC HYPOTENSION AND URINARY AND SEXUAL DYSFUNCTION IN PARKINSON'S DISEASE

The autonomous nervous system is affected in 70%–80% of PD patients, and this may be the cause of significant morbidity (Zesiewicz 2003). In most cases, this is a late occurrence, but some PD patients have clinically significant autonomic symptoms early into their illnesses. Precise estimates of frequency are hampered by a confounding influence of the drugs used to treat PD, and by some diagnostic uncertainty in the differential diagnosis of PD and multiple systemic atrophy (MSA).

Orthostatic Hypotension

Orthostatic hypotension occurs in at least 20% of PD patients and correlates with disease duration (Zesiewicz 2003). It is believed to be related primarily to peripheral autonomic dysfunction, as shown by the ubiquitous distribution of Lewy bodies and reduced cardiac uptake of the postganglionic tracer meta-iodobenzylguanidine (MIBG) (Courbon 2003). These pathological and pharmacological characteristics clearly differentiate autonomic failure in PD from MSA (Courbon 2003). In addition, dopaminergic therapy can have a negative impact upon orthostatic hypotension (Goetz 2002).

Blood pressure drops on standing do not always cause symptoms. One study found that orthostatic hypotension was symptomatic in only 20% of PD patients (Senard 1997). Pharmacological treatment for orthostatic hypotension should be considered when it is symptomatic and limits activities of daily living. Some of the drugs that potentially may be useful for the treatment of PD-related autonomic dysfunction have been tested in conditions other than PD, in particular in MSA or pure autonomic failure (PAF), or in autonomic dysfunction secondary to peripheral neuropathies. Only very few randomized controlled trials exist of drugs for autonomic dysfunction specifically caused by PD. When considering the use of drugs tested in conditions other than PD, it should be kept in mind that efficacy, as well as safety, of treatments may differ between those conditions and PD. Supine hypertension may be a complication of treating orthostatic hypotension and must be checked.

Midodrine is a peripherally acting alpha-adrenergic drug that acts on both the arterial and the venous system without direct cardiac effects. Two randomized, placebo-controlled studies have been published in mixed patient populations: One study investigated 30 mg/day for up to 4 weeks in 97 patients, 22 of whom had PD, and it found a significant increase in blood pressure. In the PD subgroup, the response rate was 69% (Jankovic 1993). In another study, only 19 out of 162 patients had PD. A significant increase in blood pressure occurred on 30 mg/day of midodrine (Low 97). Adverse events are mostly sympathomimetic and include piloerection, pruritus, paresthesia, and urinary retention or urgency. Supine hypertension was reported in 4%–8% of patients in these studies and may be of clinical importance. Due to its short half-life and good bioavailability, midodrine can be taken intermittently when needed, e.g., before meals at doses of 2.5–10 mg 3 times/day (Wright 1998). As its mechanism of action is strictly peripheral, central effects of sympathic stimulation do not occur.

Fludrocortisone increases renal sodium reabsorption and increases potassium secretion. Increased blood volume and cardiac output are thought to underlie the effect on blood pressure. A small uncontrolled study in 6 PD patients showed improved blood pressure and orthostatic symptoms (Hoehn 1975). Doses are usually started at 0.1 mg/day and titrated upward to 0.3 mg twice daily. Hypokalemia, edema, and supine hypertension may occur. It has been suggested that sleeping in a head-up tilt position may improve orthostatic hypotension in the morning by reducing nocturnal renal sodium loss (Ten Harkel 1992).

Etilefrine is a sympathomimetic agent acting on alpha and beta adrenergic receptors. A single-blind short-term study in 15 PD patients showed increased blood pressure and improved orthostatic hypotension on 15 mg/day. Adverse effects include sympathomimetc reactions and hypertension (Miller 1973).

Indomethacine is a cyclo-oxygenase inhibitor that was shown in a small, uncontrolled short-term trial in 12 PD patients to significantly improve orthostatic blood pressure drop at a dose of 50 mg 3 times/day (Abate 1979). Gastric side effects may occur.

Yohimbine is an alpha-2 adrenergic antagonist that increases catecholamine levels. A controlled study in 17 PD patients failed to demonstrate an effect on orthostatic hypotension (Senard 1993).

L-threo-3,4-dihydroxyphenylserine (L-DOPS) is a noradrenaline precursor that prevents postprandial hypotension (Mathias 1999). In patients with MSA and PAF, a dose-dependent effect on orthostatic hypotension was observed in an uncontrolled study, with 300 mg twice daily showing most effective control (Mathias 2001). A small study in 15 PD patients showed significant improvements in the occurrence of syncope and in orthostatic hypotension on a mean dose of 460 mg/day (Yanagisawa 1998).

Agents that have been shown to be effective in orthostatic hypotension due to various underlying conditions include the somatostatin analog octreotide and the vasopressin analog desmopressin, administered as tablets or as a nasal spray (Mathias 1999), and dihydroergotamine (Lubke 1976). There are no published trials available on the use of these drugs in patients with PD.

In MSA and PAF, the oral ingestion of water has been demonstrated to significantly increase seated and standing blood pressure and to improve orthostatic symptoms without adversely affecting cardiac function parameters (Young 2004). Increasing salt intake (to 120 mmol/day) was shown to significantly improve orthostatic tolerance in a randomized controlled trial in patients with neurally mediated syncope (El-Sayed 1996). There are no published data on the effect of water ingestion or increased salt intake, or of caffeine, specifically in PD-related autonomic dysfunction. Elastic stockings are effective in MSA patients but have not been investigated in PD.

Bilateral subthalamic stimulation for PD has recently been shown to have no significant effect on cardiovascular function, including heart rate variability and postural blood pressure changes (Holmberg 2005).

Urinary Dysfunction

Problems related to urinary function occur in up to 71% of PD patients (Zesiewicz 2003) and can take the form of urinary frequency and urgency, and urge incontinence and urinary retention may occur. Currently, no evidence from controlled trials is available on drug treatment of these problems specifically in PD, but agents that have been investigated for urinary dysfunction in other conditions are commonly used in PD patients.

The approach to urinary dysfunction in PD is similar to those for other elderly patients with these complaints and must include a search for underlying treatable causes, such as infection, prostate hypertrophy, gynecological causes, diabetes, delirium, or drug effects. In PD, a common cause of urinary complaints including incontinence may be reduced mobility due to bradykinesia or imbalance, which may impair the patient's ability to reach the toilet in time. This mechanism should always be considered because of the possibility of specific treatment if the disability is due to dopamine-responsive factors. Nocturia can sometimes be improved by simply reducing fluid intake in the evening. The medical management of urinary problems in PD should usually be carried out in collaboration with a urologist because the choice of treatment depends largely on the type of urodynamic abnormality.

In urinary frequency and urgency, commonly used drugs include the antimuscarinic agents oxybutinine and tolteridone, which relax detrusor muscles and can control detrusor hyperactivity. These may be used only if postmicturition residual volumes are normal. Side effects include dry mouth, constipation, drowsiness, blurred vision, and cognitive dysfunction, including confusion and delirium. Tricyclic antidepressants may also be used in this indication but may be limited by a similar side-effect profile, particularly in elderly patients. All anticholinergics may induce urinary retention.

Stress incontinence due to sphincter dysfunction may be treated with alpha agonists, but the possible emergence of arterial hypertension must be considered.

When distressing nocturia is refractory to all other measures, intranasal desmopressin can be considered at night. This vasopressor analog has a proven effect on nocturia in other conditions, but very limited data are available in patients with PD. Desmopressin may induce hyponatremia and water retention and must, therefore, be used with caution. The smallest effective dose should be determined, and regular blood and urine tests for electrolytes should be performed (Suchowersky 1995).

Intermittent self-catheterization or a permanent suprapubic or transurethral catheter must be considered when other approaches fail, particularly in the presence of refractory urinary retention.

Sexual Dysfunction

Erectile dysfunction may emerge as part of autonomic impairment in the course of PD, and impairment of sexual function also frequently affects women with PD. However, if erectile dysfunction occurs early into the illness, the clinician should be alerted to alternative diagnoses, in particular MSA. The management of erectile dysfunction should include a search for other underlying causes, such as prostate problems or diabetes.

Parkinsonian motor impairment as such may affect sexual functions. If the history reveals hypokinesia or tremor as an important factor, an increase in dopaminergic medication (e.g., as an additional dose when required) may be appropriate. Conversely, dyskinesias may require adjustments in the timing or dosage of medication. Dopaminergic drugs also increase sexual desire.

Antidepressants are frequently used in PD and may interfere with sexual function in both men and women. A switch to different antidepressant agents may be helpful. In patients on antidepressants without PD, adding the phospho-diesterase inhibitor sildenafil has been shown to be effective (Rudkin 2004).

Few clinical trials of treatments for erectile dysfunction have been carried out specifically in PD patients. Sildenafil was investigated in a small randomized, placebo-controlled study in 12 PD and 12 MSA patients. A significant improvement in various parameters for sexual function was found on 50 mg sildenafil. In the PD group, changes in blood pressure were minimal while in some MSA patients, orthostatic hypotension was unmasked (Hussain 2001). Orthostatic hypotension must be considered a potential side effect of phosphor-diesterase inhibitors in parkinsonian patients, and measuring supine and standing blood pressure before prescribing sildenafil has been recommended. No data are available on the use in PD of the other phospho-diesterase inhibitors, tadalafil and vardenafil, but in men without PD, safety profiles have been shown to be similar to sildenafil.

Other treatment strategies that are used despite a lack of data in PD patients include yohimbine (2 mg) and intracavernous injections of vasodilators. Penis implants may be considered in selected cases. A transient erection following sublingual or subcutaneous administration of apomorphine was first noted in PD patients. Although investigations of apomorphine specifically for erectile dysfunction in PD are not available, its effect may not be sustained and reliable enough in many cases. In men without PD, sildenafil recently has been demonstrated to be significantly more effective than apomorphine (Pavone 2004).

Conversely, hypersexuality and abnormal sexual behavior can occur in PD. A relation to higher doses of dopaminergic drug treatment and to self-medication exists, and hypersexual behavior is a typical component of the dopamine dysregulation syndrome (Evans 2004). These problems may improve if dopaminergic doses are reduced or if different agents are chosen. Rarely, apomorphine treatment must be discontinued for this reason.

MEDICATIONS FOR DYSPHAGIA, SIALORRHEA, AND GASTROINTESTINAL PROBLEMS

No drugs are available for the treatment of dysphagia in PD. Anticholinergics can produce improvement (Penner 1942) but also in some cases worsen dysphagia (Bramble 1978). Percutaneous botulinum toxin injections of the cricopharyngeal muscle has been tried successfully to treat dysphagia in four PD patients (Restivo 2002). Drooling is not normally considered an autonomic disorder but rather a consequence of inefficient and infrequent swallowing in PD. In some cases, the use of 1 to 2 mg glycopyrrolate 1 to 4 times per day, or addition of an anticholinergic medication (including tricyclic antidepressants), or the scopolamine patch may be of benefit (Adler 2005).

Intraparotid injections of botulinum toxin A also have been used to treat drooling in PD. In a small study by Pal et al. (Pal 2000), subjective improvement in drooling occurred in 67% of patients. In another small study (Friedman 2001), similar improvements were documented after the application of botulinum A toxin. These favorable results were confirmed in several double-blind studies (Lipp 2002, Mancini 2003, Ondo 2004), and a recent study found significantly greater reduction in saliva production when botulinum toxin injections were guided by ultrasound (Dogu 2004). Side effects reported after intraparotid botulinum toxin injections include dry mouth and dysphagia and facial nerve and artery damage from the injection could also occur.

Constipation is the most familiar gastrointestinal feature of PD. It is thought to reflect an increase in colon transit time. It may occur secondary to the disease itself or may be a side effect of the medications (dopaminergic, anticholinergic) used to treat PD. Constipation causes discomfort, and in some instances intestinal pseudoobstruction or actual obstruction due to volvulus can occur (Eadie 1965, Quigley 1996, Caplan 1965).

Constipation is thought to occur in about 20% to 30% of PD patients (Edwards 1991, Siddiqui 2002). Epidemiological studies suggest that constipation can precede the motor symptoms of PD. In the Honolulu Heart study (Abbott 2001), men who reported having less than one bowel movement daily had a 2.7 times higher risk of developing PD than did men who had daily bowel movements, and a 4 times higher rate than did men who had 2 or more bowel movements a day.

No specific drugs are available to treat constipation in PD. Usual measures are applied when this problem occurs in PD and should include increased water intake, dietary bulk, exercise, stool softeners, laxatives, lactulose, and, in some cases, enemas. Prokinetic agents have also been used in the treatment of slow-transit constipation in PD, but their efficacy is doubtful. Good effects have been found with macrogol, a polyethylene glycol electrolyte solution that works on an osmotic basis (Eichhorn 2001). Cisapride has been reported effective in the short term (Jost 1997), but it is not recommended due to its potential cardiotoxicity. Neurotrophin 3 has been reported to be useful in a small double-blind study (Pfeiffer 2002). There has been an anecdotal report that colchicines can reduce constipation in PD (Sandyk 1984).

Difficulties with defecation also occur in PD. Improvement also has been documented after apomorphine injections (Mathers 1989, Edwards 1993). Botulinumtoxin injections into the puborectalis muscle have been used successfully in the treatment of parkinsonian defecatory dysfunction (Albanese 1997). However, fecal incontinence is a potentially troublesome complication of such an approach.

Difficulties with defecation may be limited to off periods as one of the nonmotor signs of wearing off, and these cases should be managed as outlined elsewhere in this chapter.

MANAGEMENT OF DEPRESSION IN PARKINSON'S DISEASE

Around 40% of patients with PD experience depression during the course of their illness. The importance of this problem is highlighted by the fact that most studies investigating factors contributing to quality of life in PD found depression to have a major impact (Kuopio 2000, Schrag 2000). The precise neurophysiological basis for depression in PD has not been clarified. Current concepts include a decreased serotonergic tone in PD patients; dopamine deficiency in mesolimbic and mesocortical structures; and a neurotransmitter imbalance in combination with psychosocial factors and coping ability. A direct role of the basal ganglia in mood control is suggested by findings in subthalamic stimulation that may produce opposite mood effects depending on the precise location.

Clinically, the manifestations of depression differ somewhat between people with and without PD. While both share features such as lowered mood, anhedonia, and lack of interest, in patients with PD there is less evidence of the feeling of guilt while anxiety and irritability are more prominent (Leentjens 2004). Risk factors for depression in PD do not differ greatly from those in the general population and include female gender, higher age, and family history of depression. Depression may occur several years before the emergence of motor signs and has been considered to be either an early nonmotor sign or a biological risk factor for PD (Oertel 2001).

Even though the major role of depression in PD has now been recognized, there is still a remarkable lack of well-designed, randomized, controlled trials specifically investigating therapeutic options in PD. Mood swings which occur as part of treatment-response fluctuations require optimization of dopaminergic therapy.

Uncontrolled studies and observational reports exist of several antidepressants, usually describing significant changes from baseline. However, a recent systematic review (Ghazi-Noori 2003) identified only two published randomized-controlled trials of antidepressant drugs in PD patients (Andersen 1980, Wermuth 1998). One 16-week crossover study reported better results on nortriptylin (25–150 mg) compared with placebo but failed to state whether this difference was statistically significant (Andersen 1980). Conversely, a 52-week study did not demonstrate a significant difference between citalopram (10–40 mg) and placebo (Wermuth 1998).

In current clinical practice, the management of depression in PD patients reflects the assumption that the underlying pathophysiological processes may be similar or identical to depression in patients without PD, and all classes of antidepressants are used. While clearcut evidence of efficacy is lacking, information on tolerability and safety is available from uncontrolled studies.

Serotonin reuptake inhibitors (SSRIs) are usually considered the drugs of first choice. Possible adverse effects include sexual dysfunction, gastrointestinal symptoms, weight gain, and agitation. A possible worsening of parkinsonian motor function has been discussed but is unlikely to pose a clinically relevant limitation (Tesei 2000). A recent short-term study in 14 PD patients showed that 2 weeks of treatment with paroxetine did not lead to worsening of the motor response to intravenous L-dopa (Chung 2005). Although larger and controlled studies are lacking, a report from the French Pharmacovigilance Database found no significant differences in reported motor worsening between SSRIs and other antidepressants (Gony 2003). There is a small but definite risk of an interaction of SSRIs with the MAO-B inhibitor selegiline: Increased serotonergic tone may lead to the "serotonine syndrome," characterized by confusion, stupor, fever, myoclonus, tremor, sweating or diarrhea, and the combination of these drugs should be avoided.

Tricyclic antidepressants may have a role, particularly where sedation or sleep improvement is desired. However, the risks associated with this class of drugs may be of special relevance in PD patients: Peripheral anticholinergic effects on intraocular pressure, accommodation, saliva secretion, bladder function, and gastrointestinal passage times may be more clinically relevant than in a younger, otherwise healthy patient population. Due to a central anticholinergic mechanism, impairment of cognition and worsening of neuropsychiatric problems are not uncommon, and all PD patients on tricyclic antidepressants must be monitored for the emergence of these adverse effects.

Other antidepressant drugs are routinely used in PD patients: Venlafaxine is a mixed serotonergic and noradrenergic reuptake inhibitor that also may have an anticholinergic component. Venlafaxine has an activating rather than a sedating effect and may, thereby, increase agitation. It should be avoided in hypertensive patients, while a mildly increasing effect on blood pressure may be desirable in some patients with orthostatic hypotension (Okun 2002). Mirtazapine is a presynaptic alpha-2 antagonist that increases central noradrenergic and serotonergic neurotransmission. Due to its histamine receptor blocking effect,

it causes sedation and is best given at bedtime. It improves anxiety and can be used for the treatment of insomnia (Okun 2002).

Monoamino oxidase (MAO)-A inhibitors, such as moclobemide, are of very limited usefulness due to their specific side effects and interactions: These include acute confusional states; serotonergic hyperstimulation, in particular when combined with serotonergic agents; and hypertensive reactions that may occur spontaneously or in response to food containing tyramine, such as some cheeses or red wine. This class of drugs, therefore, has a very limited role in clinical practice.

Antidepressant effects have recently been attributed to dopamine agonists, although this remains to be confirmed in randomized, double-blind trials comparing agonists and antidepressants. An open-label study suggests superior mood enhancement on pramipexole compared with pergolide (Rektoroval 2003), and post-hoc subanalysis of a long-term double-blind study in fluctuating patients showed that, compared with L-dopa alone, add-on pramipexole was associated with improved scores for depression and initiative, as measured on UPDRS/part 1 (Möller 2005).

No controlled studies are available on the role of electroconvulsive therapy or psychotherapy in the management of depression in PD, although open observations and case series suggest a possible role for electroconvulsive therapy in some patients refractory to medical treatment (Moellentine 1998).

BEHAVIORAL ABNORMALITIES ASSOCIATED WITH DOPAMINERGIC TREATMENT IN PARKINSON'S DISEASE

In the course of treatment a substantial number of patients develop psychiatric complications of antiparkinsonian treatment. These complications include vivid dreams, hallucinations, delusions, hypomania, hypersexuality, and the so-called *dopamine dysregulation syndrome*. We describe here in some detail the less common and underecognized dopamine dysregulation syndrome and associated behavioral abnormalities since its recognition is essential for appropriate treatment. The management of drug-related psychosis in PD is summarized in Table 10.7.

Patients with dopamine dysregulation syndrome develop a pattern of compulsive dopaminergic drug use, which includes taking increasing quantities of medication beyond those required to treat motor disabilities and continuing to request more dopaminergic drugs. This occurs despite the emergence of drug-induced motor complications, in particular dyskinesias (Giovannoni 2000, Lawrence 2003). Predisposing factors include young age at disease onset, high dopaminergic drug intake, past drug use, depression, novelty-seeking personality traits, and alcohol intake (Evans/Lawrence 2005).

TABLE 10.7

MANAGEMENT OF HALLUCINOSIS IN PARKINSON'S DISEASE (WITH OR WITHOUT CONCOMITANT DEMENTIA)

A stepwise approach is recommended:

- Eliminate precipitating factors, such as infections, dehydratation, impairment in sensory functions such as vision or hearing.
- Discontinue medication that may be contributing:
    - sedatives, anxiolytics, anticholinergic agents, including many antidepressants and drugs for bladder hyperactivity, and others.
- Discontinue antiparkinsonian drugs with high risk of inducing neuropsychiatric problems, in the following order:
    - anticholinergics
    - amantadine
    - selegiline
    - dopamine agonists
    - L-dopa (+/− COMT inhibitors)
- If these measures are insufficient, options with a specific effect on hallucinations are:
    - Neuroleptics:
      Clozapine: small risk of motor worsening but agranulocytosis
      Quetiapin: available data suggest acceptable risk/benefit ratio
      Risperidone, olanzapin: marked risk of motor worsening
    - Cholinesterase inhibitors: An effect on hallucinosis has been demonstrated with rivastigmine.
- Due to a delayed effect of cholinesterase inhibitors, acute phases may require the use of neuroleptics (in some cases combined with sedatives, e.g., benzodiazepines). Once the acute hallucinatory phase has been controlled, cholinesterase inhibitors may (partly) replace neuroleptics.

A behavioral abnormality that may be associated with high doses of dopaminergic replacement therapy and often with dopamine dysregulation is "punding" (Friedman 1994, Evans 2004, Evans/Katzenschlager 2005). This phenomenon was first described in amphetamine addicts and is a complex stereotyped behavior characterized by an intense fascination with repetitive manipulations of technical equipment; the continual handling, examining, and sorting of objects; grooming; hoarding; or using a computer. These activities are carried out during on phases, and they are often associated with dyskinesias. Initially, the activities are mainly present at night, and if abnormal behavior is suspected, it is important to inquire how patients cope with insomnia, particularly because patients rarely report punding behavior spontaneously. Punding is acknowledged as disruptive and unproductive by the patients, but attempts to interrupt the behavior typically lead to irritability and dysphoria. It is important to note that punding is distinct from both obsessive–compulsive and manic disorder.

It is believed that punding in vulnerable persons results from a process of psychomotor stimulation, mediated by ventral striatal structures, and an increasing inability to control automatic response mechanisms resulting from impaired frontal lobe function. It is closely linked to reward responses and a sensitization process induced by dopaminergic therapy is believed to have a central role. This is supported by the recent finding of an association with frequent use of short-acting rescue medication, such as soluble L-dopa and apomorphine injections (Evans 2004).

Other abnormalities in reward-seeking behavior observed in PD patients on dopaminergic treatment include hypersexuality or excessive gambling (Serrano-Duenas 2002, Molina 2000, Dodd 2005) or binge eating.

These behavioral abnormalities only recently have been described in some detail. Their epidemiology and causal relationships are being explored. Unusually large doses and liberal modifications of drug regimes and demand for higher doses despite being on with severe dyskinesias should alert the treating clinician that dopamine overuse and associated behavioral problems may exist (Schrag 2004). At this stage, while there is evidence to suggest a frequent association with dopamine agonists, no clear conclusions can be drawn as to which agents are more likely to induce behavioral change, and these abnormalities may also occur on L-dopa monotherapy.

Management strategies of dopamine dysregulation and associated behavioral abnormalities include reducing dopaminergic therapy whenever possible, in particular rescue and self-medication, or switching to different agents and symptomatic treatment of any coexisting psychiatric conditions such as depression. Atypical neuroleptics are sometimes but not always helpful (Evans 2004). In severe cases of hypersexuality, anti-androgen treatment with cyproterone has been used successfully (Evans 2004).

REFERENCES

Abate G, Polimeni RM, Cuccurrullo F, Puddu P, Lenzi S. Effects of indomethacine on postural hypotension in Parkinsonism. *Br Med J* 1979;2:1466–1468.

Abbott RD, Petrovitch H, White, LR, et al. Frequency of bowel movements and the future risk of Parkinson's disease, *Neurology* 57 (2001);456–462.

Adler C. Non motor complications in Parkinson's disease. *Mov Disord* 2005;20(suppl 11):S23–S29.

Adler CH, Sethi KD, Hauser RA, et al. Ropinirole for the treatment of early Parkinson's disease. *Neurology* 1997;49:393–399.

Adler CH, Singer G, O'Brien C, et al. Randomized, placebo-controlled study of tolcapone in patients with fluctuation Parkinson's disease treated with levodopa-carbidopa. *Arch Neurol* 1998;55:1089–1095.

Agid Y, Oertel W, Factor S. Entacapone to tolcapone switch study: multicentre double-blind, randomized, active-controlled trial in advanced Parkinson's disease. *Mov Disord* 2005;20(suppl 19):S94.

Ahlskog JE, Muenter MD. Frequency of levodopa-related dyskinesias and motor fluctuations as estimated from the cumulative literature. *Mov Disord* 2001;16:448–458.

Albanese A, Maria G, Bentivoglio A, Brisinda G, Cassetta E, Tonali P. Severe constipation in Parkinson's disease relieved by botulinum toxin, *Mov Disord* 1997;12:764–766.

Albin RL, Frey KA. Initial agonist treatment of Parkinson's disease: a critique. *Neurology* 2003;60:390–394.

Alegret M, Valldeoriola F, Marti M, Pilleri M, Junque C, Rumia J, Tolosa E. Comparative cognitive effects of bilateral subthalamic stimulation and subcutaneous continuous infusion of apomorphine in Parkinson's disease. *Mov Disord* 2004;19. 1463–1469.

Allen RM. Evidence for direct receptor effect of amantadine. *Neurosci Abstr* 1981;7:11.

Andersen J, Aabro E, Gulman N, Hjelmsted A, Pedersen HE. Antidepressive treatment in Parkinson's disease: a controlled trial of the effect of nortriptyline in patients with Parkinson's disease treated with L-dopa. *Acta Neurol Scand* 1980;62:210–219.

Ansari KS, Yu PH, Kruck TP, et al. Rescue of axotomized immature rat facial motoneurons by R(-)-deprenyl: stereospecificity and independence from monoamine oxidase inhibition. *J Neurosci* 1993;13:4042–4053.

Baas H, Beiske AG, Ghika J, et al. Cathechol-O-methyltransferase inhibition with tolcapone reduces the "wearing off" phenomenon and levodopa requirements in fluctuating parkinsonian patients. *J Neurol Neurosurg Psychiatry* 1997;63:421–428.

Bailey EV, Stone TW. The mechanism of action of amantadine in parkinsonism: a review. *Arch Int Pharmacodyn* 1975;216:246–262.

Barbeau A, Sourkes TL, Murphy CF. Les catécholamines dans la maladie de Parkinson's. In: Ajuriaguerra J, ed. *Monoamines et système nerveux central.* Geneva: Georg; 1962:247–262.

Baron MS, Dalton WB. Quetiapine as treatment for dopaminergic-induced dyskinesias in Parkinson's disease. *Mov Disord* 2003; 18:1208–1209.

Barone P, Bravi D, Bernejo-Pareja F, et al. Pergolide monotherapy in the treatment of early PD: a randomized controlled study. *Neurology* 1999;53:573–579.

Baronti F, Mouradian MM, Davis TL, et al. Continuous lisuride effects on central dopaminergic mechanisms in Parkinson's disease. *Ann Neurol* 1992;32:776–781.

Bauer RB, McHenry JT. Comparison of amantadine, placebo, and levodopa in Parkinson's disease. *Neurology* 1974;24:715–720.

Bedard PJ, Di Paolo T, Falardeau P, Boucher R. Chronic treatment with L-DOPA, but not bromocriptine induces dyskinesia in MPTP-parkinsonian monkeys: correlation with [3H]spiperone binding. *Brain Res* 1986;379:294–299.

Bedard MA, Lemay S, Gagnon JF, Masson H, Paquet F. Induction of a transient dysexecutive syndrome in Parkinson's disease using a subclinical dose of scopolamine. *Behav Neurol* 1998; 11: 187–195.

Belluzzi JD, Domino EF, May JM, et al. N-0923, a selective D2 receptor agonist, is efficacious in rat and monkey models of Parkinson's disease. *Mov Disord* 1994;9:147–154.

Bergamasco B, Frattola L, Muratorio A, et al. Alpha-dihydroergocryptine in the treatment of de novo parkinsonian patients: results of a multicentre, randomized, double-blind, placebocontrolled study. *Acta Neurol* 2000;101:372–380.

Berger JR, Weiner WJ. Exacerbation of Parkinson's disease following the withdrawal of amantadine. *Neurology* 1985;35(suppl 1):200.

Bergmark J, Carlsson A, Granerus AK, Jagenburg R, Magrusson T, Svanborg A. Decarboxylation of orally administered L-dopa in the human digestive tract. *Naunyn-Schmied Arch Pharmacol* 1972;272:437.

Birkmayer W and Hornykiewicz O. Der L-3,4 Dioxyphenylalanin (Dopa) Effekt bei der Parkinson-Akinese. *Wien klin Wschr* 1961;73:787–788.

Blandini F, Armentero MT, Fancellu R, et al. Neuroprotective effect of rasagiline in a rodent model of Parkinson's disease. *Exp Neurol* 2004;187:455–459.

Bleidner WE, Harman JB, Hewes WE, Lynes TE, Hermann EC. Absorption, distribution and excretion of amantadine hydrochloride. *J Pharmacol Exp Ther* 1965;150:484–490.

Block G, Liss C, Scott R, Irr J, Nibbelink D. Comparison of immediaterelease and controlled release carbidopa/levodopa in Parkinson's disease: a multicenter 5-year study. *Eur Neurol* 1997;37:23–27.

Bonuccelli U, Ceravolo R, Salvetti S, et al. Clozapine in Parkinson disease tremor: effects of acute and chronic administration. *Neurology* 1997;49:1587–1590.

Borges N. Tolcapone in Parkinsons disease: Liver toxicity and clinical efficacy. *Expert Opin Drug Saf* 2005;4:69–73.

Braak H, Braak E. Pathoanatomy of Parkinson's disease. *J Neurol* 2000 Apr; 247(suppl 2):II3–II10.

Bracco F, Battaglia A, Chouza C, et al, and the PKDS009 Study Group. The long-acting dopamine receptor agonist cabergoline in early Parkinson's disease: final results of a 5-year, double-blind, levodopa-controlled study. *CNS Drugs* 2004; 18:733–746.

Bramble MG, Cunliffe J, Dellipiani AW. Evidence for a change in neurotransmitter affecting oesophageal motility in Parkinson's disease, *J Neurol Neurosurg Psychiatry* 1978; 41:709–712.

Brooks DJ. Safety and tolerability of COMT inhibitors. *Neurology* 2004;62(suppl 1):S39–S46.

Brooks DJ, Agid Y, Eggert K, Widner H, Ostergaard K, Holopainen A, and the TC-INIT Study Group. Treatment of end-of-dose wearing-off in parkinson's disease: stalevo (levodopa/carbidopa/entacapone) and levodopa/DDCI given in combination with Comtess/Comtan (entacapone) provide equivalent improvements in symptom control superior to that of traditional levodopa/DDCI treatment. *Eur Neurol* 2005;53:197–202.

Brooks DJ, Sagar H, and the UK-Irish Entacapone Study Group. Entacapone is beneficial in both fluctuating and non-fluctuating patients with Parkinson's disease: a randomised, placebo controlled, double blind, six month study. *J Neurol Neurosurg Psychiatry* 2003;74:1071–1079.

Burns D, DeJong D, Solis-Quiroga OII. Effects of trihexyphenidyl hydrochloride (Artane) on Parkinson's disease. *Neurology* 1964; 14:13–31.

Butzer JF, Silver DE, Sahs AL. Amantadine in Parkinson's disease a double blind, placebo-controlled cross-over study with long-term follow-up. *Neurology* 1975;25:603–606.

Calne DB, Burton K, Beckman J, Martin WR. Dopamine agonists in Parkinson's disease. *Can J Neurol Sci* 1984;11(suppl 1): 221–224.

Calne DB, Teychenne PF, Claveria LE, Eastman R, Greenacre JK, Petrie A. Bromocriptine in parkinsonism. *Br Med J* 1974;4: 442–444.

Cantello R, Riccio A, Gilli M. Bornaprine vs placebo in Parkinson's disease: double-blind controlled cross-over trial in 30 patients. *Ital J Neurol Sci* 1986;7:139–143.

Caplan LH, Jacobson HG, Rubinstein BM, Rotman MZ. Megacolon and volvulus in Parkinson's disease. *Radiology* 1965;85:73–79.

Caraceni T, Musicco M. Levodopa or dopamine agonists, or deprenyl as initial treatment for Parkinson's disease: a randomized multi-center study. *Parkinsonism Relat Disord* 2001;7:107–114.

Carrillo MC, Kanai S, Sato Y, et al. The optimal dosage of (-) deprenyl for increasing superoxide dismutase activities in several brain regions decreases with age in male Fischer 344 rats. *Life Sci* 1993;52:1925–1934b.

Carvey PM, Pieri S, Ling ZD. Attenuation of levodopa-induced toxicity in mesencephalic cultures by pramipexole. *J Neural Transm* 1997;104:209–228.

Chase TN, Justin DO. Striatal mechanisms and pathogenesis of parkinsonian signs and motor complications. *Ann Neurol* 2000;47(suppl 1):S122–S130.

Chaudhuri KR, Yates L, Martinez-Martin P. The non-motor symptom complex of Parkinson's disease: a comprehensive assessment is essential. *Curr Neurol Neurosci Rep* 2005;5:275–283.

Chung KA, Carlson NE, Nutt JG. Short-term paroxetine treatment does not alter the motor response in PD. *Neurology* 2005; 4:1797–1798.

Churchyard A, Mathias CJ, Lees AJ. Selegiline-induced postural hypotension in Parkinson's disease: a longitudinal study on the effects of drug withdrawal. *Mov Disord* 1999;14:246–251.

Clarke CE. Does levodopa therapy delay death in Parkinson's disease? A review of the evidence. *Mov Disord* 1995;10:250–256.

Colzi A, Turner K, Lees AJ. Continuous subcutaneous waking day apomorphine in the long term treatment of levodopa induced inter-dose dyskinesias in Parkinson's disease. *J Neurol Neurosurg Psychiatry* 1998;64:573–576.

Corbin KB. Trihexyphenidyl: evaluation of a new agent in treatment of parkinsonism. *JAMA* 1949;141:377–382.

Cotzias GC, Papavasiliou PS, Fehling C, Kaufman B, Mena I. Similarities between neurologic effects of L-dopa and of apomorphine. *N Engl J Med* 1970;282:31–33.

Cotzias GC, Van Woert MH, Schiffer LM. Aromatic amino acids and modification of parkinsonism. *N Engl J Med* 1967;276:374–379.

Courbon F, Brefel-Courbon C, Thalamas C, et al. Cardiac MIBG scintigraphy is a sensitive tool for detecting cardiac sympathetic denervation in Parkinson's disease. *Mov Disord* 2003;18:890–897.

Cox B, Danta G, Schnieden H, Yuill GM. Interactions of L-dopa and amantadine in patients with Parkinsonism. *J Neurol Neurosurg Psychiatry* 1973;36:354–361.

Coyle JT, Snyder SH. Antiparkinsonian drugs: inhibition of dopamine uptake in the corpus striatum as a possible mechanism of action. *Science* 1969;166:899–901.

Crosby NJ, Deane KH, Clarke CE. Beta-blocker therapy for tremor in Parkinson's disease. *Cochrane Database Syst Rev* 2003;(1): CD003361.

Datla KP, Blunt SB, Dexter DT. Chronic L-dopa administration is not toxic to the remaining dopaminergic nigrostriatal neurons, but instead may promote their functional recovery, in rats with partial 6-OHDA or FeCl$_3$ nigrostriatal lesions. *Mov Disord* 2001;16:424–434.

Davies WL, Grunert RR, Haff RF, et al. Antiviral activity of 1-adamantamine (amantadine). *Science* 1964;144:862–863.

De Smet Y, Ruberg M, Serdaru M, Dubois B, Lhermitte F, Agid Y. Confusion, dementia, and anticholinergics in Parkinson's disease. *J Neurol Neurosurg Psychiatry* 1982;45:1161–1164.

Deane KHO, Spieker S, Clarke CE. Catechol-O-methyltransferase inhibitors for levodopa-induced complications in Parkinson's disease. The Cochrane Database of Systematic Reviews 2004 a; (4):CD004554.

Deane KHO, Spieker S, Clarke CE. Catechol-O-methyltransferase inhibitors versus active comparators for levodopa-induced complications in Parkinson's disease. The Cochrane Database of Systematic Reviews 2004 b;(4):CD004553.

Del Dotto P, Pavese N, Gambaccini G, et al. Intravenous amantadine improves levodopa-induced dyskinesias: an acute double-blind placebo-controlled study. *Mov Disord* 2001;16:515–520.

DeLong MR, Crutcher MD, Georgopoulos AP. Relations between movement and single cell discharge in the substantia nigra of the behaving monkey. *J Neurosci* 1983;3:1599–1606.

Descombes S, Bonnet AM, Gasser UE, et al. Dual-release formulation, a novel principle in L-dopa treatment of Parkinson's disease. *Neurology* 2001;56:1239–1242.

Dewey RB, Hutton JT, LeWitt PA, Factor SA. A randomized, double-blind, placebo-controlled trial of subcutaneously injected apomorphine for Parkinsonian off-state events. *Arch Neurol* 2001; 58:1385–1392.

Di Rosa AE, Epifanio A, Antonini A, et al. Continuous apomorphine infusion and neuropsychiatric disorders: a controlled study in patients with advanced Parkinson's disease. *Neurol Sci* 2003; 24:174–175.

Djaldetti R, Baron J, Ziv I, Melamed E. Gastric emptying in Parkinson's disease: patients with and without response fluctuations. *Neurology* 1996;46:1051–1054.

Dodd ML, Klos KJ, et al. Pathological gambling caused by drugs used to treat Parkinson disease. *Arch Neurol* 2005;62:1–5.

Dogu O, Apaydin D, Sevim S, Talas DU, Aral M. Ultrasound-guided versus "blind" intraparotid injections of botulinum toxin-A for the treatment of sialorrhoea in patients with Parkinson's disease. *Clin Neurol Neurosurg* 2004;106:93–96.

Dolin R, Reichman RC, Madore HP, Maynard R, Linton PN, Webber-Jones J. A controlled trial of a amantadine and rimantadine in the prophylaxis of influenza A infection. *N Engl J Med* 1982;307: 580–584.

Doshay LJ, Constable K. Treatment of paralysis agitans with orphenadrine (Disipal) hydrochloride. *JAMA* 1957;163: 1352–1357.

Dubois B, Danze F, Pillon B, Cusimano G, Lhermitte F, Agid Y. Cholinergic-dependent cognitive deficits in Parkinson's disease. *Ann Neurol* 1987;22:26–30.

Duby SE, Cotzias GC, Papavasiliou PS, Lawrence WH. Injected apomorphine and orally administered levodopa in parkinsonism. *Arch Neurol* 1972;27:424–480.

Dumartin B, Caille I, Gonon F, Bloch B. Internalization of D1 dopamine receptor in striatal neurons in vivo as evidence of activation by dopamine agonists. *J Neurosci* 1998;18: 1650–1661.

Dupont E, Anderson A, Boqs J, et al. Sustained-release Madopar HBS compared with standard Madopar in the long-term treatment of de novo parkinsonian patients. *Acta Neurol Scan* 1996;93:14–20.

Dupont E, Burgunder JM, Findley LJ, Olsson JE, Dorflinger E, for the Tolcapone in Parkinson's Disease Study Group II (TIPS II). Tolcapone added to levodopa in stable parkinsonian patients: a double-blind placebo-controlled study. *Mov Disord* 1997;12: 928–934.

Durif F, Debilly B, Galitzky M, et al. Clozapine improves dyskinesias in Parkinson's disease: a double-blind, placebo-controlled study. *Neurology* 2004;62:381–388.

Duvoisin RC. A review of drug therapy in parkinsonism. *Bull NY Acad Med* 1965;41:898–910.

Duvoisin RC. The mutual antagonism of cholinergic and anticholinergic agents in parkinsonism. *Trans Am Neurol Assoc* 1966;91: 73–79.

Duvoisin RC. Cholinergic–anticholinergic antagonism in parkinsonism. *Arch Neurol* 1967;17:124–136.

Eadie MJ and Tyrer JH. Alimentary disorder in parkinsonism, *Aust Ann Med* 14 (1965), pp. 13–22.

Ebling P. The medical management of Parkinson's disease before the introduction of L-dopa. *Aust NZ J Med* 1971;1(suppl):35–38.

Editorial. The posology of amantadine: A note of caution. *JAMA* 1980;243:844–845.

Edwards LL, Pfeiffer RF, Quigley EM, Hofman R, Balluff M. Gastrointestinal symptoms in Parkinson's disease. *Mov Disord* 1991;6:151–156.

Edwards LL, Quigley EMM, Harned RK, Hofman R, Pfeiffer RF. Defecatory function in Parkinson's disease: response to apomorphine. *Ann Neurol* 1993;33:490–493.

Eichhorn TE, Oertel WH. Macrogol 3350/electrolyte improves constipation in Parkinson's disease and multiple system atrophy. *Mov Disord* 2001;16:1176–1177.

El-Sayed H, Hainsworth R. Salt supplement increases plasma volume and orthostatic tolerance in patients with unexplained syncope. *Heart* 1996;75:134–140.

Erni W, Held K. The hydrondynamically balanced system: a novel principle of controlled drug release. *Eur Neurol* 1987; 27(suppl 1):21–27.

Evans AH, Katzenschlager R, Paviour D, et al. Punding in Parkinson's disease: its relation to the dopamine dysregulation syndrome. *Mov Disord* 2004;19:397–405.

Evans AH, Lawrence AD, Potts J, Appel S, Lees AJ. Factors influencing susceptibility to compulsive dopaminergic drug use in Parkinson's disease. Neurology. 2005 Nov 22;65(10):1570–1574.

Fabbrini G, Juncos J, Mouradian MM, Serrati C, Chase TN. Levodopa pharmacokinetic mechanisms and motor fluctuations in Parkinson's disease. *Ann Neurol* 1987;21:370–376.

Fahn S, Isgreen WP. Long term evaluation of amantadine and levo-dopa combination in parkinsonism by double-blind cross-over analyses. *Neurology* 1975;25:695–700.

Farnebo LO, Fuxe K, Goldstein M, Hamberger B, Ungerstedt U. Dopamine and noradrenaline releasing action of amantadine in the central and peripheral nervous system: a possible mode of action in Parkinson's disease. *Eur J Pharmacol* 1971;16: 27–38.

Fehling C. The effect of adding amantadine to optimum L-dopa dosage in Parkinson's syndrome. *Acta Neurol Scand* 1973;49: 245–251.

Feldburg W. Present views on the mode of action of acetylcholine in the central nervous system. *Physiol Rev* 1945;25:596–642.

Ferreira JJ, Galitzky M, Brefel-Courbon C, et al. "Sleep attacks" as an adverse drug reaction of levodopa monotherapy. *Mov Disord* 2000;15(suppl 3):P661.

Ferreira JJ, Thalamas C, Montastruc JL, Castro-Caldas A, Rascol O. Levodopa monotherapy can induce "sleep attacks" in Parkinson's disease patients. *J Neurol* 2001;248:426–427.

Filion M, Tremblay L. Abnormal spontaneous activity of globus pallidus neurons in monkeys with MPTP-induced parkinsonism. *Brain Res* 1991;547:142–151.

Finberg JP, Wang J, Bankiewicz K, et al. Increased striatal dopamine production from L-DOPA following selective inhibition of monoamine oxidase B by R(+)-N-propargyl-1-aminoindan (rasagiline) in the monkey. *J Neural Transm Suppl* 1998;52: 279–285.

Forster E, Lewy FH. Paralysis agitans. In: Lewandowsky, M, ed. *Pathologische Anantomie: Handbuch der Neurologie*. Berlin: Springer Verlag; 1912:920–933.

Frankel JP, Lees AJ, Kempster PA, et al. Subcutaneous apomorphine in the treatment of Parkinson's disease. *J Neurol Neurosurg Psychiatry* 1990;53:96–101.

Franz DN. Drugs for Parkinson's disease. In: Goodmann LS, Gilman A, eds. *The Pharmacological Basis of Therapeutics*. New York: Macmillan, 1975.

Friedman A, Potulska A. Quantitative assessment of parkinsonian sialorrhea and results of treatment with botulinum toxin. *Parkinsonism Relat Disord* 2001;7:329–332.

Friedman JH, Koller WC, Lannon MC, et al. Benztropine versus clozapine for the treatment of tremor in Parkinson's disease. *Neurology* 1997;48:1077–1081.

Friedman JH. Punding on levodopa. *Biol Psychiatry* 1994;36:350–351.

Frucht S, Rogers JD, Green PD, Gordon MF, Fahn S. Falling asleep at the wheel: motor vehicle mishaps in persons taking pramipexole and ropinirole. *Neurology* 1999;52:1908–1910.

Gerfen CR, Engber TM, Mahan LC, et al. D1 and D2 dopamine receptor-regulated gene expression of striatonigral and striatopallidal neurons. *Science* 1990;250:1429–1432.

Ghazi-Noori S, Chung TH, Deane KHO, Richards H, Clarke CE. Therapies for depression in Parkinson's disease. *The Cochrane Database of Systematic Reviews*. 2003;10:59–65.

Gianutsos G, Chute S, Dunn JP. Pharmacological changes in dopaminergic systems induced by long-term administration of amantadine. *Eur J Pharmacol* 1985;110:357–361.

Gilligan BS, Veale J, Wodak J. Amantadine hydrochloride in the treatment of Parkinson's disease. *Med J Aust* 1970;2:634–637.

Giovannoni G, O'Sullivan JD, Turner K, Manson AJ, Lees AJ. Hedonistic homeostatic dysregulation in patients with Parkinson's disease on dopamine replacement therapies. *J Neurol Neurosurg Psychiatry* 2000;68:423–428.

Goetz CG, Koller WC, Poewe W, et al, Movement Disorders Society Task Force. Management of Parkinson's disease: an evidence-based review. *Mov Disord* 2002;17(suppl 4).

Goetz CG, Koller WC, Poewe W, Rascol O, Sampaio C. Amantadine and other antiglutamate agents. *Mov Disord* 2002;17(Suppl 4): S13–S22.

Goetz CG, Tanner CM, Shannon KM, Carroll VS, Klawans HL. Controlled-release long-acting levodopa/carbidopa combination in Parkinson's disease patients with and without motor fluctuations. *Neurology* 1988;38:1143–1145.

Gony M, Lapeyre-Mestre M, Montastruc JL, and the French Network of Regional Pharmacovigilance Centres. *Clin Neuropharmacol* 2003;26:142–145.

Gowers WR. A manual of disease of the nervous system. Philadelphia: P. Blakiston, Son and Company, 1888.

Grandas F, Galiano ML, Tabernero C. Risk factors for levodopa-induced dyskinesias in Parkinson's disease. *J Neurol* 1999;246: 1127–1133.

Graybiel AM, Canales JJ, Capper-Loup C. Levodopa-induced dyskinesias and dopamine-dependent stereotypies: a new hypothesis. *Trends Neurosci* 2000;23(suppl 10):S71–S77.

Greenamyre JT, O'Brien CF. N-methyl-D-aspartate antagonists in the treatment of Parkinson's disease. *Arch Neurol* 1991;48: 977–981.

Grelak RP, Clarek R, Stump JM, Vernier VG. Amantadine-dopamine interaction: possible mode of action in parkinsonism. *Science* 1970;169:203–204.

Guttman M, The International Pramipexole-Bromocriptine Study Group. Double-blind comparison of pramipexole and bromocriptine treatment with placebo in advanced Parkinson's disease. *Neurology* 1997;49:1060–1065.

Guttman M, Slaughter PM, Theriault ME, DeBoer DP, Naylor CD. Parkinsonism in Ontario: increased mortality compared with controls in a large cohort study. *Neurology* 2001;57: 2278–2282.

Hadj Tahar A, Gregoire L, Bangassoro E, Bedard PJ. Sustained cabergoline treatment reverses levodopa-induced dyskinesias in parkinsonian monkeys. *Clin Neuropharmacol* 2000;23: 195–202.

Han SK, Mytilineou C, Cohen G. L-DOPA up-regulates glutathione and protects mesencephalic cultures against oxidative stress. *J Neurochem* 1996;66:501–510.

Heikkila RE, Cohen G. Evaluation of amantadine as a releasing agent or uptake blocker for 3H-dopamine in rat brain slices. *Eur J Pharmacol* 1972;20:156–160.

Heimans RL, Rand MJ, Fennesy MR. Effects of amantadine on uptake and release of dopamine by a particulate fraction of rat basal ganglia. *J Pharm Pharmacol* 1972;24:875–879.

Hely MA, Morris JGL, Reid WGJ, Trafficante R. Sydney multicenter study of Parkinson's disease: Non-L-dopa-responsive problems dominate at 15 years. *Mov Disord* 2005;20:190–199.

Hobson DE, Lang AE, Martin WR, Razmy A, Rivest J, Fleming J. Excessive daytime sleepiness and sudden-onset sleep in Parkinson's disease: a survey by the Canadian Movement Disorders Group. *JAMA* 2002;287:455–463.

Hoehn MM. Levodopa-induced postural hypotension: treatment with fludrocortisone. *Arch Neurol* 1975;32:50–51.

Hoehn MM, Elton RL. Low dosages of bromocriptine added to levodopa in Parkinson's disease. *Neurology* 1985;35:199–206.

Holmberg B, Corneliusson O, Elam M. Bilateral stimulation of nucleus subthalamicus in advanced Parkinson's disease: no effects on, and of, autonomic dysfunction. *Mov Disord* 2005; 20:976–981.

Horrocks PM, Vicary DJ, Rees JE, Parkes JD, Marsden CD. Anticholinergic withdrawal and benzhexol treatment in Parkinson's disease. *J Neurol Neurosurg Psychiatry* 1973;36: 936–941.

Hubble JP. Long-term studies of dopamine agonists. *Neurology* 2002;58(suppl 1):S42–S50.

Hughes AJ, Bishop S, Kleedorfer B, et al. Subcutaneous apomorphine in Parkinson's disease: response to chronic administration for up to 5 years. *Mov Disord* 1993;8:165–170.

Hughes RC, Polgar JG, Weightman D, Walton JN. Levodopa in Parkinsonism: the effects of withdrawal of anticholinergic drugs. *Br Med J* 1971;2:487–491.

Hussain IF, Brady CM, Swinn MJ, Mathias CJ, Fowler CJ. Treatment of erectile dysfunction with sildenafil citrate (Viagra) in parkinsonism due to Parkinson's disease or multiple system atrophy with observations on orthostatic hypotension. *J Neurol Neurosurg Psychiatry* 2001;71:371–374.

Hutton JT, Koller WC, Ahlskog JE, et al. Multicenter, placebo-controlled trial of cabergoline taken once daily in the treatment of Parkinson's disease. *Neurology* 1996;46:1062–1065.

Hutton JT, Morris JL, Bush DF, Smith ME, Liss CL, Reines S. Multicenter controlled study of Sinemet CR vs Sinemet (25/100) in advanced Parkinson's disease. *Neurology* 1989;39(suppl 2): 67–72.

Ing TS, Rahn AC, Armbruster KFS, Oyama JH, Klawans HL. Accumulation of amantadine hydrochloride in renal insufficiency. *N Engl J Med* 1974;291:1257.

Ives NJ, Stowe RL, Marro J, et al. Monoamine oxidase type B inhibitors in early Parkinson's disease: meta-analysis of 17 randomised trials involving 3525 patients. *BMJ* 2004;329:593.

Jankovic J. Therapeutic strategies in Parkinson's disease. In: Jankovic J, Tolosa E. eds. *Parkinson's Disease and Movement Disorders*. Philadelphia: Lippincott Williams & Wilkins, 2002: 116–152.

Jankovic J, Gilden JL, Hiner BC, et al. Neurogenic orthostatic hypotension: a double-blind, placebo controlled study with midodrine. *Am J Med* 1993;95:38–48.

Jankovic J, Orman J. Parallel double-blind study of pergolide in Parkinson's disease. *Adv Neurol* 1986;45:551–553.

Jankovic J, Schwartz K, Vander Linden C. Comparison of Sinemet CR4 and standard Sinemet: double blind and long-term open trial in parkinsonian patients with fluctuations. *Mov Disord* 1989; 4:303–309.

Jenner P. Is stimulation of D-1 and D-2 dopamine receptors important for optimal motor functioning in Parkinson's disease? *Eur J Neurol* 1997;4(suppl 3):S3–S11.

Jenner P. A novel dopamine agonist for the transdermal treatment of Parkinson's disease. *Neurology* 2005;65(suppl 1):S3–S5.

Jost WH, Schimrigk K. Long-term results with cisapride in Parkinson's disease. *Mov Disord* 1997;12:423–425.

Ju WYH, Hollan DP, Tatton WG. (-)-Deprenyl alters the time course of death of axotomized facial motoneurons and the hypertrophy of neighboring astrocytes in immature rats. *Exp Neurol* 1994;126:1–14.

Kalir HH, Mytilineou C. Ascorbic acid in mesencephalic cultures: effects on dopaminergic neuron development. *J Neurochem* 1991;57:458–464.

Kanovsky P, Kubova D, Bares M, et al. Levodopa-induced dyskinesias and continuous subcutaneous infusions of apomorphine: results of a two-year, prospective follow-up. *Mov Disord* 2002;17:188–191.

Katzenschlager R, Evans A, Manson A, et al. Mucuna pruriens in Parkinson's disease: a double-blind clinical and pharmacological study. *J Neurol Neurosurg Psychiatry* 2004;75:1672–1677.

Katzenschlager R, Hughes A, Evans A, et al. Continuous subcutaneous apomorphine therapy improves dyskinesias in Parkinson's disease: a prospective study using single-dose challenges. *Mov Disord* 2005;20:151–157.

Katzenschlager R, Sampaio C, Costa J, Lees AJ. Anticholinergics for symptomatic management of Parkinson's disease (Cochrane Review). *Cochrane Database Syst Rev* 2003;(2):CD003735.

Kaufmann H, Nahm K, Purohit D, Wolfe D. Autonomic failure as the initial presentation of Parkinson's disease and dementia with Lewy bodies. *Neurology* 2004;63:1093–1095.

Kempster PA, Frankel JP, Stern GM, et al. Comparison of motor response to apomorphine and levodopa in Parkinson's disease. *J Neurol Neurosurg Psychiatry* 1990;53:1004–1007.

Kieburtz K, Shoulson I, McDermontt M, et al. Safety and efficacy of pramipexole, in early Parkinson's disease: a randomized dose-ranging study. *JAMA* 1997;278:125–130.

Knoll J. Deprenyl (selegiline): the history of its development and pharmacological action. *Acta Neurol Scand* 1983;95:57–80.

Knoll J. The pharmacological profile of (-) deprenyl (selegiline) and its relevance for humans: a personal view. *Pharmacol Toxicol* 1992;70:317–321.

Koller W, Lees A, Doder M, Hely M, and the Tolcapone/Pergolide Study Group. Randomized trial of tolcapone versus pergolide as add-on to levodopa therapy in Parkinson's disease patients with motor fluctuations. *Mov Disord* 2001;16:858–866.

Koller WC. Disturbance of recent memory functions in parkinsonian patients on anticholinergic therapy. *Cortex* 1984;20: 307–311.

Koller WC, Herbster G. Adjuvant therapy of parkinsonian tremor. *Arch Neurol* 1987;44:921–923.

Koller WC, Hutton JT, Tolosa E, et al. Immediate-release and controlled-release carbidopa/levodopa in PD: a 5-year randomized multicenter study. *Neurology* 1999;53:1012–1019.

Korczyn AD, Brooks DJ, Brunt ER, Poewe WH, Rascol O, Stocchi F. Ropinirole versus bromocriptine in the treatment of early Parkinson's disease:a 6-month interim report of a 3-year study. 053 Study Group. *Mov Disord* 1998:13:46–51.

Korczyn AD, Brunt ER, Larsen JP, Nagy Z, Poewe WH, Ruggieri S. A 3-year randomized trial of ropinirole and bromocriptine in early Parkinson's disease. The 053 Study Group. *Neurology* 1999;53:364–370.

Kornhuber J, Bormann J, Hubers M, Rusche K, Riederer P. Effects of the 1-amino-adamantanes at the MK-801-binding site of the NMDA-receptor-gated ion channel: a human postmortem brain study. *Eur J Pharmacol* 1991;206:297–300.

Kumar N, Van Gerpen JA, Bower JH, Ahlskog JE. Levodopa-dyskinesia by age of Parkinson's disease onset. *Mov Disord* 2005;20:342–344.

Kuopio AM, Marttila RJ, Helenius H, Toivonen M, Rinne UK. The quality of life in Parkinson's disease. *Mov Disord* 2000;15:216–223.

Kurlan R, Rothfield KP, Woodward WR, et al. Erratic gastric emptying of levodopa may cause random fluctuations of parkinsonian mobility. *Neurology* 1988;38:419–421.

Kurlan R, Rubin AJ, Miller C, et al. Duodenal delivery of levodopa for on-off fluctuations in parkinsonism: preliminary observations. *Ann Neurol* 1986;20:262–265.

Kurth MC, Adler CH, St. Hilaire M, et al, and the Tolcapone Fluctuator Study Group. Tolcapone improves motor function and reduces levodopa requirement in patients with Parkinson's disease experiencing motor fluctuations: a multicenter, double-blind, randomized, placebo-controlled trial. *Neurology* 1997;48:81–87.

Lang AE, Blair RDG. Anticholinergic drugs and amantadine in the treatment of Parkinson's disease. In: Calne DB, ed. *Handbook of Experimental Pharmacology*, Vol. 88. Berlin, Heidelberg: Springer Verlag, 1989.

Langston JW, Ballard P, Tetrud JW, Irwin I. Chronic Parkinsonism in humans due to a product of meperidine-analog synthesis. *Science* 1983;219:979–980.

Lawrence AD, Evans AH, Lees AJ. Compulsive use of dopamine replacement therapy in Parkinson's disease: reward systems gone awry? *Lancet Neurol* 2003;2:595–604.

Lees AJ, Katzenschlager R, Head J, Ben-Shlomo Y, on behalf of the Parkinson's disease research group on the United Kingdom. Ten-year follow-up of three different initial treatments in de-novo PD: a randomized trial. *Neurology* 2001;57:1687–1694.

Leentjens, AF. Depression in Parkinson's disease: conceptual issues and clinical challenges. *J Geriatr Psychiatry Neurol* 2004;17:120–126.

LeWitt PA, Chang F-L, Fazzini E, et al. Rotigotine CDS patch in advanced stage, idiopathic Parkinson's disease: a parallel group, open label, dose escalation trial. *Neurology* 2004;62(suppl 5): A399.

LeWitt PA, Nelson MV, Berchou RC, et al. Controlled-release carbidopa/levodopa (Sinemet 50/200 CR4): clinical and pharmacokinetic studies. *Neurology* 1989;39(suppl 2):45–53.

Lieberman A, Olanow CW, Sethi K, et al. A multi-center, double-blind, placebo-controlled trial of ropinirole as an adjunct to L-dopa in the treatment of Parkinson's disease patients with motor fluctuations. *Neurology* 1998;51:1057–1062.

Lieberman A, Ranhosky A, Korts D. Clinical evaluation of pramipexole in advanced Parkinson's disease: results of a double-blind, placebo-controlled, parallel—group study. *Neurology* 1997;49: 162–168.

Limousin P, Pollak P, Pfefen JP, Tournier-Gervason CL, Dubuis R, Perret JE. Acute administration of levodopa-benserazide and tolcapone, a COMT inhibitor, in Parkinson's disease. *Clin Neuropharm* 1995;18:258–265.

Lipp A, Trottenberg T, Beyer D, Kupsch A, Arnold G. Treatment of drooling in Parkinson's disease and motorneuron disease with botulinum toxin A. *Naunyn Schmiedebergs Arch Pharmacol* 2002:365(suppl 2):R38.

Low PA, Gilden JL, Freeman R, Sheng KN, McElligott MA. Efficacy of midodrine vs. placebo in neurogenic orthostatic hypotension: randomized, double-blind multicenter study. *JAMA* 1997;277:1046–1051.

Lubke KO. A controlled study with dihydroergot in patients with orthostatic dysregulation. *Cardiology* 1976;61(suppl 1):333–341.

Luginger E, Wenning GK, Bosch S, Poewe W. Beneficial effects of amantadine on L-dopa-induced dyskinesias in Parkinson's disease. *Mov Disord* 2000;15:873–878.

Lyras L, Zeng BY, McKenzie G, Pearce RK, Halliwell B, Jenner P. Chronic levodopa does not increase oxidative damage or impair the function of the nigro-striatal pathway in normal cynomologus monkeys. *J Neural Transm* 2002;109:53–67.

Mancini F, Zangaglia R, Cristina S, et al. Double blind, placebo-controlled study to evaluate the efficacy and safety of botulinum toxin type A in the treatment of drooling in parkinsonism. *Mov Disord* 2003;18:685–688.

Manson AJ, Hanagasi H, Turner K, et al. Intravenous apomorphine therapy in Parkinson's disease: clinical and pharmacokinetic observations. *Brain* 2001;124:331–340.

Manson AJ, Turner K, Lees AJ. Apomorphine monotherapy in the treatment of refractory motor complications of Parkinson's disease: long-term follow-up study of 64 patients. *Mov Disord* 2002;17:1235–1241.

Manyam B. Paralysis agitans and levodopa in "Ayurveda": ancient Indian medical treatise. *Mov Disord* 1990;5:47–48.

Marek K, Seybl J, Shoulson I, et al, for the Parkinson Study Group. Dopamine transporter brain imaging to assess the effects of pramipexole vs levodopa on Parkinson's disease progression. *JAMA* 2002;287:1653–1661.

Mars H. Modification of levodopa effect by systemic decarboxylase inhibition. *Arch Neurol* 1973;28:91–95.

Marshall J. Tremor. In: Vinken PJ, Bruyn GW, eds. *Handbook of Clinical Neurology: Diseases of Basal Ganglia.* Amsterdam: Elsevier North-Holland; 1968:809–825.

Martin WE, Lowenson RB, Resch JA, Baker AB. A controlled study comparing trihexyphenidyl hydrochloride plus levodopa with placebo plus levodopa in patients with Parkinson's disease. *Neurology* 1974;24:912–919.

Maruyama W, Youdim MB, Naoi M. Antiapoptotic properties of rasagiline, N-propargylamine-1(R)-aminoindan, and its optical (S)-isomer, TV1022. *Ann N Y Acad Sci* 2001;939:320–329.

Mathers SE, Kempster PA, Law P, et al. Anal sphincter dysfunction in Parkinson's disease. *Arch Neurol* 1989;46:1061–1064.

Mathias CJ, Kimber JR. Postural hypotension: causes, clinical features, investigation, and management. *Annu Rev Med* 1999;50:317–336.

Mathias CJ, Senard JM, Braune S, et al. L-threo-dihydroxyphenylserine (L-threo-DOPS; droxidopa) in the management of neurogenic orthostatic hypotension: a multi-national, multi-center, dose-ranging study in multiple system atrophy and pure autonomic failure. *Clin Autonom Res* 2001;11:235–242.

Mena MA, Casarejos MJ, Yebenes JG. Neurotoxic and neurotrophic effects of L-dopa on dopamine neurons. *Recent Res Devel Neurochem* 1999;2:91–97.

Mercuri NB, Scarponi M, Bonci A, et al. Monoamine oxidase inhibition causes a long-term prolongation of the dopamine-induced responses in rat midbrain dopaminergic cells. *J Neurosci* 1997;17:2267–2272.

Michel PP, Hefti F. Toxicity of 6-hydroxydopamine and dopamine for dopaminergic neurons in culture. *J Neurosci Res* 1990;26:428–435.

Miller E, Wiener L, Bloomfield D. Etilefrine in the treatment of levodopa-induced orthostatic hypotension. *Arch Neurol* 1973;29:99–103.

Mizuno Y, Kondo T, Narabayashi H. Pergolide in the treatment of Parkinson's disease. *Neurology* 1995;45(suppl 31):S13–S21.

Mizuno Y, Yanagisawa N, Kuno S, et al. Randomized, double-blind study of pramipexole with placebo and bromocriptine in advanced Parkinson's disease. *Mov Disord* 2003;18:1149–1156.

Moellentine C, Rummans T, Ahlskog JE, et al. Effectiveness of ECT in patients with parkinsonism. *J Neuropsychiatry Clin Neurosci* 1998;10:187–193.

Molina JA, Sainz-Artiga MJ, Fraile A, et al. Pathologic gambling in Parkinson's disease: a behavioral manifestation of pharmacologic treatment? *Mov Disord* 2000;15869–872.

Möller JC, Oertel WH, Köster J, Pezzoli G, Provinciali L. Long-term efficacy and safety of pramipexole in advanced Parkinson's disease: results from a European multicenter trial. *Mov Disord* 2005;20:602–610.

Montastruc JL, Rascol O, Senard JM, Rascol A. A randomised controlled study comparing bromocriptine to which levodopa was later added, with levodopa alone in previously untreated patients with Parkinson's disease: a five-year follow-up. *J Neurol Neurosurg Psychiatry* 1994;57:1034–1038.

Morgante L, Basile G, Epifanio A, et al. Continuous apomorphine infusion (CAI) and neuropsychiatric disorders in patients with advanced Parkinson's disease: a follow-up of two years. *Arch Gerontol Geriatr Suppl* 2004;9:291–296.

Morissette M, Goulet M, Soghomonian JJ, Bedord PJ, Di Paolo T. Preproenkephalin mRNA expression in the caudate-putamen of MPTP monkeys after chronic treatment with the D2 agonist U91356A in continuous or intermittent mode of administration: comparison with L-DOPA therapy. *Brain Res Mol Brain Res* 1999;49:55–62.

Morrish PK. How valid is dopamine transporter imaging as a surrogate marker in research trials in Parkinson's disease? *Mov Disord* 2003;18(suppl 7):S63–70.

Murer MG, Dziewczapolski G, Menalled LB, et al. Chronic levodopa is not toxic for remaining dopamine neurons, but instead promotes their recovery, in rats with moderate nigrostriatal lesions. *Ann Neurol* 1998;43:561–575.

Myllyla VV, Jackson M, Larsen JP, Baas H. Efficacy and safety of tolcapone in levodopa-treated Parkinson's disease patients with "wearing-off" phenomenon: a multicenter, double-blind, randomized, placebo-controlled trial. *Eur J Neurol* 1997;4:333–341.

Myllyla VV, Sotaniemic KA, Vuorinen JA, Heinonen EA. Selegiline as initial treatment in de novo parkinsonian patients. *Neurology* 1992;42:339–343.

Mytilineou C, Han S-K, Cohen G. Toxic and protective effects of L-DOPA on mesencephalic cell cultures. *J Neurochem* 1993;61:1470–1478.

Nashold BS. Cholinergic stimulation of globus pallidus in man. *Prc Soc Exp Biol Med* 1959;101:68–69.

Nastuck WC, Su PC, Doubilet P. Anticholinergic and membrane activities of amantadine in neuromuscular transmission. *Nature* 1976;264:76–79.

Navan P, Findley LJ, Jeffs JA, Pearce RK, Bain PG. Randomized, double-blind, 3-month parallel study of the effects of pramipexole, pergolide, and placebo on Parkinsonian tremor. *Mov Disord* 2003;18:1324–1331.

Navan P, Findley LJ, Undy MB, Pearce RK, Bain PG. A randomly assigned double-blind cross-over study examining the relative anti-parkinsonian tremor effects of pramipexole and pergolide. *Eur J Neurol* 2005;12:1–8.

Nilsson D, Nyholm D, Aquilonius SM. Duodenal levodopa infusion in Parkinson's disease long-term experience. *Acta Neurol Scand* 2001;104:343–348.

Nissinen E, Kaheinen P, Penttila KE, Kaivola J, Lindin IB. Entacapone, a novel catechol-O-methyltransferase inhibitor for Parkinson's disease, does not impair mitochondrial energy production. *Eur J Neurol* 1997;340:287–294.

Nutt JG. Pharmacodynamics of levodopa in Parkinson's disease. *Clin Exp Pharmacol Physiol* 1995;22:837–840.

Nutt JG, Obeso JA, Stocchi F. Continuous dopamine-receptor stimulation in advanced Parkinson's disease. *Trends Neurosci* 2000;23(suppl):S109–S115.

Nyholm D, Askmark H, Gomes-Trolin C, et al. Optimizing levodopa pharmacokinetics: intestinal infusion versus oral sustained-release tablets. *Clin Neuropharm* 2003;26:156–163.

Obeso JA, Luquin MR, Martinez-Lage JM. Lisuride infusion pump: a device for the treatment of motor fluctuations in Parkinson's disease. *Lancet* 1986;i:467–470.

Obeso JA, Martínez-Lage M. Anticholinergics and amantadine. In: Koller W, ed. *Handbook of Parkinson's Disease.* New York: Marcel Dekker; 1987:309–316.

Oertel WH, Höglinger GU, Ceracheni T, et al. Depression in Parkinson's disease: an update. *Adv Neurol* 2001;86:373–383.

Oertel WH, Wolters E, Sampaio C, et al. Pergolide versus levodopa monotherapy in early Parkinson's disease patients: the PELMOPET study. *Mov Disord* 2006;21:343–353.

Ogawa N, Tanaka K, Asanuma M, et al. Bromocriptine protects mice against 6-hydroxydopamine and scavenges hydroxyl free radicals in vitro. *Brain Res* 1994;657:207–213.

Okun MS, Watts RL. Depression associated with Parkinson's disease. *Neurology* 2002;58(suppl):S63–S70.

Olanow CW, Agid Y, Mizuno Y, et al. Levodopa in the treatment of Parkinson's disease: current controversies. *Mov Disord* 2004;19:997–1005.

Olanow CW, Alberts MJ. Double-blind controlled study of pergolide mesylate as an adjunct to Sinemet in the treatment of Parkinson's disease. *Adv Neurol* 1987;45:555–560.

Olanow CW, Fahn S, Muenter M. A multicenter double-blind placebo-controlled trial of pergolide as an adjunct to Sinemet in Parkinson's disease. *Mov Disord* 1994;9:40–47.

Olanow CW, Hauser RA, Gauger L, et al. The effect of deprenyl and levodopa on the progression of Parkinson's disease. *Ann Neurol* 1995;38:771–777.

Olanow CW, Jenner P, Brooks D. Dopamine agonists and neuroprotection in Parkinson's disease. *Ann Neurol* 1998;44:167–174.

Olanow CW, Kieburtz K, Stern M, et al, for the US01 Study Team. Double-blind, placebo-controlled study of entacapone in levodopa-treated patients with stable Parkinson's disease. *Arch Neurol* 2004;61:1563–1568.

Olanow CW, Myllyla VV, Sotaniemi KA, et al. Effect of selegiline on mortality in patients with Parkinson's disease: a meta-analysis. *Neurology* 1998; 51: 825–830.

Olanow CW, Schapira AHV, Rascol O. Continuous dopamine-receptor stimulation in early Parkinson's disease. *Trends Neurosci* 2000;23(suppl):S117–S126.

Olson WL, Gruenthal M, Mueller ME, Olson WH. Gabapentin for parkinsonism: a double-blind, placebo-controlled, crossover trial. *Am J Med* 1997;102:60–66.

Ondo WG, Hunter C, Moore W. A double-blind placebo-controlled trial of botulinum toxin B for sialorrhea in Parkinson's disease. *Neurology* 2004;62:37–40.

Onofrj M, Paci C, Thomas A. Sudden appearance of invalidating dyskinesia-dystonia and off fluctuations after the introduction of levodopa in two dopaminomimetic drug naïve patients with stage IV Parkinson's disease. *J Neurol Neurosurg Psychiatry* 1998;65:605–606.

Ordenstein L. Sur la paralysie et la sclerose en plaque generalisé. Paris: Martinet, 1867.

Ostergaard L, Werdelin L, Odin P, et al. Pen injected apomorphine against off phenomena in late Parkinson's disease: a double blind, placebo controlled study. *J Neurol Neurosurg Psychiatry* 1995;58:681–687.

Pal PK, Calne DB, Calne S, Tsui JKC. Botulinum toxin A as a treatment for drooling saliva in PD. *Neurology* 2000;54:244–247.

Palhagen S, Heinonan EH, Hagglund J, et al, for the Swedish Parkinson Study Group. Selegiline delays the onset of disability in de novo parkinsonian patients. *Neurology* 1998;51:520–525.

Parkes JD, Baxter RCH, Curzon G, et al. Treatment of Parkinson's disease with amantadine and levodopa. *Lancet* 1970;1:1083–1087.

Parkes JD, Baxter RC, Marsden CD, Rees JE. Comparative trial of benzhexol, amantadine and levodopa in the treatment of Parkinson's disease. *J Neurol Neurosurg Psychiatry* 1974;37:422–426.

Parkinson Study Group. Effect of deprenyl on the progression of disability in early Parkinson's disease. *N Engl J Med* 1989;321:1364–1371.

Parkinson Study Group. Impact of deprenyl and tocopherol treatment on Parkinson's disease in DATATOP subjects not requiring levodopa. *Ann Neurol* 1996;39:29–36.

Parkinson Study Group. Entacapone improves motor fluctuations in levodopa-treated Parkinson's disease patients. *Ann Neurol* 1997;42:747–755.

Parkinson Study Group. Pramipexole vs levodopa as initial treatment for Parkinson's disease: a randomized controlled trial. *JAMA* 2000;284:1931–1938.

Parkinson Study Group. A controlled trial of rasagiline in early (rasagiline mesylate) Parkinson's disease: the TEMPO study. *Arch Neurol* 2002;59:1937–1943.

Parkinson Study Group. A controlled trial of rotigotine monotherapy in early Parkinson's disease. *Arch Neurol* 2003;60:1721–1728.

Parkinson Study Group. A randomized placebo-controlled trial of rasagiline in levodopa-treated patients with Parkinson's disease and motor fluctuations: the PRESTO Study. *Arch Neurol* 2005;62:241–248.

Parkinson Study Group. Levodopa and the progression of Parkinson's disease. *New Engl J Med* 2004;351:2498–2508.

Parkinson's Disease Research Group of the United Kingdom. Comparisons of therapeutic effects of levodopa, levodopa and selegiline, and bromocriptine in patients with early, mild Parkinson's disease: three years interim report. *BMJ* 1993;307:469–472.

Pavone C, Curto F, Anello G, Serretta V, Almasio PL, Pavone-Macaluso M. Prospective, randomized, crossover comparison of sublingual apomorphine (3 mg) with oral sildenafil (50 mg) for male erectile dysfunction. *J Urol* 2004;172:2347–2349.

Pearce LA, Waterbury LD, Green HD. Amantadine hydrochloride: alteration in peripheral circulation. *Neurology* 1974;24:468.

Pearce RK, Jackson M, Smith L, Jenner P, Marsden CD. Chronic L-DOPA administration induces dyskinesias in the 1-methyl-4-phenyl-1,2,3,6-tetrahydropyridine-treated common marmoset (Callithrix Jacchus). *Mov Disord* 1995;10:731–740.

Pearce RKB, Jenner P, Marsden CD. De novo administration of ropinirole and bromocriptine induces less dyskinesia than L-dopa in the MPTP-treated marmoset. *Mov Disord* 1998;13:234–241.

Penner A, Druckerman LJ. Segmental spasms of the esophagus and their relation to parkinsonism, *Am J Dig Dis* 1942;9:282–286.

Perry TL, Yong VW, Ito M, et al. Nigrostriatal dopaminergic neurons remain undamaged in rats given high doses of L-dopa and carbidopa chronically. *J Neurochem* 1984;43:990–993.

Pfeiffer, RF. A promising new technology for Parkinson's disease. *Neurology* 2005;65:S6–S10.

Pfeiffer RF, Markopoulou K, Quigley EM, Stambler N, Cedarbaum JM. Effect of NT-3 on bowel function in Parkinson's disease. *Mov Disord* 220;17:223–224.

Piercey MF, Camacho-Ochoa M, Smith MW. Functional roles for dopamine receptor subtypes. *Clin Neuropharmacol* 1995;18(suppl):S34–S42.

Pierelli F, Adipietro A, Soldati G, Fattapposta F, Pozzessere G, Scoppetta C. Low dosage clozapine effects on L-dopa induced dyskinesias in parkinsonian patients. *Acta Neurol Scand* 1998;97:295–299.

Pinero A, Marcos-Alberca P, Fortes J. Cabergoline-related severe restrictive mitral regurgitation. *N Engl J Med* 2005;353:1976–1977.

Pinter MM, Pogarell O, Oertel WH. Efficacy, safety, and tolerance of the nonergoline dopamine agonist pramipexole in the treatment of advanced Parkinson's disease: a double-blind, placebo controlled, randomized, multicentre study. *J Neurol Neurosurg Psychiatry* 1999;66:436–441.

Pletscher A, Bartholini G. Selective rise in brain dopamine by inhibition of extracerebral levodopa decarboxylation. *Clin Pharm Ther* 1971;12:117–131.

Poewe W, Lees AJ, Steiger D, Stern GM. Foot dystonia in Parkinson's disease: clinical phenomenology and neuropharmacology. *Adv Neurol* 1987;45:357–360.

Poewe W, Lees AJ, Stern GM. Dystonia in Parkinson's disease: Clinical and pharmacological features. *Ann Neurol* 1988;235:73–78.

Poewe WH, Deuschl G, Gordin A, Kultalahti ER, Leinonen M, and the Celomen Study Group. Efficacy and safety of entacapone in Parkinson's disease patients with suboptimal Levodopa response: a 6-month randomized placebo-controlled double-blind study in Germany and Austria (Celomen study). *Acta Neurol Scand* 2002;105:245–255.

Poewe WH, Lees AJ, Stern GM. Treatment of motor fluctuations in Parkinson's disease with an oral sustained-release preparation of

L-dopa: clinical and pharmacological observations. *Clin Neuropharmacol* 1986;9:430–439.

Porteous HB, Ross DDN. Mental symptoms in parkinsonism following benzhexol hydrochloride therapy. *Br Med J* 1956;2: 138–140.

Pritchett AM, Morrison JF, Edwards WD, Schaff HV, Connolly HM, Espinosa RE. Valvular heart disease in patients taking pergolide. *Mayo Clin Proc* 2002;77:1280–1286.

Quigley EMM. Gastrointestinal dysfunction in Parkinson's disease, *Semin Neurol* 1996;16:245–250.

Quinn N, for the SP 511 Investigators. Rotigotine transdermal delivery system (TDS) (SPM 962): a multicenter, double-blind, randomized, placebo controlled trial to assess the safety and efficacy of rotigotine TDS in patients with advanced Parkinson's disease. *Parkinsonism Relat Disord* 2001;7(suppl 1):S66.

Quinn N, Marsden CD, Parkes JD. Complicated response fluctuations in Parkinson's disease: response to intravenous infusion of levodopa. *Lancet* 1982;ii:412–415.

Quinn N, Parkes D, Janota I, et al. Preservation of the substantia nigra and locus ceruleus in a patient receiving levodopa (2kg) plus decarboxylase inhibitor over a four-year period. *Mov Disord* 1986;1:65–68.

Rajput AH. Levodopa prolongs life expectancy and is non-toxic to substantia nigra. *Parkinsonism Relat Disord* 2001;8:95–100.

Rajput AH, Martin W, Saint-Hilaire MH, Dorflinger E, Pedder S. Tolcapone improves motor function in parkinsonian patients with the wearing-off phenomenon: a double-blind, placebo-controlled, multicenter trial. *Neurology* 1997;49:1066–1071.

Rascol A, Montastruc JL, Guirard-Chaumeil B, Clanet M. Bromocriptine as first treatment of Parkinson's disease: long-term results. *Rev Neurol* 1982;138:402–408.

Rascol O, Brooks DJ, Korczyn AD, De Deyn PP, Clarke CE, Lang AE. A five-year study of the incidence of dyskinesia in patients with early Parkinson's disease who were treated with ropinirole or levodopa. *N Eng J Med* 2000;342:1484–1491.

Rascol O, Brooks DJ, Melamed E, Poewe W, Stocchi F, Tolosa E, for the LARGO study group. Rasagiline as an adjunct to levodopa in patients with Parkinson's disease and motor fluctuations (LARGO, Lasting Effect in Adjunct Therapy with Rasagiline Given Once Daily study): a randomised, double-blind, parallel group trial. *Lancet* 2005;365:947–954.

Rascol O, Lees AJ, Senard JM, et al. Ropinirole in the treatment of levodopa-induced motor fluctuations in patients with Parkinson's disease. *Clin Neuropharmacol* 1996;19:234–245.

Ravina B, Eidelberg D, Ahlskog JE, et al. The role of radiotracer imaging in Parkinson's disease. *Neurology* 2005;64:208–215.

Reichmann H, Boas J, Macmahon D, Myllyla V, Hakala A, Reinikainen K, for the ComQol Study Group. Efficacy of combining levodopa with entacapone on quality of life and activities of daily living in patients experiencing wearing-off type fluctuations. *Acta Neurol Scand* 2005;111:21–28.

Rektorova I, Rektor I, Bares M, et al. Promipexole and pergolide in the treatment of depression in Parkinson's disease: a national multicentre prospective randomized study. *Eur J Neurol* 2003;10: 399–406.

Restivo DA, Palmeri A, Marchese-Ragona R. Botulinum toxin for cricopharyngeal dysfunction in Parkinson's disease, *N Engl J Med* 2002;346:1174–1175.

Rinne UK. Lisuride, a dopamine agonist in the treatment of early Parkinson's disease. *Neurology* 1989;39:336–339.

Rinne UK, Bracco F, Chouza C, Dupont E, Gershanik O, Marti Masso JF, Montastruc JL, Marsden CD, and the PKDS 009 Study Group. Early treatment of Parkinson's disease with cabergoline delays the onset of motor complications. results of a double-blind levodopa controlled trial. *Drugs* 1998;55(suppl 1): 23–30.

Rinne UK, Bracco F, Chouza C, et al. Cabergoline in the treatment of early Parkinson's disease: results of the first year of treatment in a double-blind comparison of cabergoline and levodopa. *Neurology* 1997;48:363–368.

Rinne UK, Larsen JP, Siden A, Worm-Petersen J, and the Nomecomt Study Group. Entacapone enhances the reponse to levodopa in parkinsonian patients with motor fluctuations. *Neurology* 1998;51:1309–1314.

Rinne UK, Sonninen V, Sirtola T. Plasma concentration of levodopa in patients with Parkinson's disease. *Eur Neurol* 1973;10: 301–310.

Rudkin L, Taylor MJ, Hawton K. Strategies for managing sexual dysfunction induced by antidepressant medication. *Cochrane Database Syst Rev* 2004 Oct 18;(4):CD003382.

Sadeh M, Braham J, Modan M. Effects of anticholinergic drugs on memory in Parkinson's disease. *Arch Neurol* 1982;39: 666–667.

Sage JI, Duvoisin RC. Long-term efficacy of pergolide in patients with Parkinson's disease. *Clin Neuropharmacol* 1986;9:160–164.

Sage JI, Schuh L, Heikkila RE, et al. Continuous duodenal infusions of levodopa: plasma concentrations and motor fluctuations in Parkinson's disease. *Clin Neuropharmacol* 1988;11:36–44.

Sandyk R, Gillman MA. Colchicine ameliorates constipation in Parkinson's disease. *J R Soc Med* 1984;77:1066.

Sartori M, Pratt CM, Yound JB. Torsade de pointe. Malignant cardiac arrhythmia induced by amantadine poisoning. *Am J Med* 1984;77:388–391.

Savery F. Amantadine and a fixed combination of levodopa and carbidopa in the treatment of Parkinson's disease. *Dis Nerv System* 1971;38:605–608.

Schrag A. Psychiatric aspects of Parkinson's disease: an update. *J Neurol* 2004;251:795–804.

Schrag A, Ben-Shlomo Y, Brown R, Marsden CD, Quinn N. Young-onset Parkinson's disease revisited: clinical features, natural history, and mortality. *Mov Disord* 1998;13:885–894.

Schrag A, Jahanshahi M, Quinn N. What contributes to quality of life in patients with Parkinson's disease? *J Neurol Neurosurg Psychiatry* 2000;69:308–312.

Schrag A, Schelosky L, Scholz U, Poewe W. Reduction of parkinsonian signs in patients with Parkinson's disease by dopaminergic versus anticholinergic single-dose challenges. *Mov Disord* 1999;14: 252–255.

Schwab RS, Amador LV, Lettvin JY. Apomorphine in Parkinson's disease. *Trans Am Neurol Assoc* 1951;76:251–253.

Schwab RS, England AC, Poskanzer DC, Young RR. Amantadine in the treatment of Parkinson's disease. *JAMA* 1969;208: 1168–1170.

Schwab RS, Poskanzer DC, England AC, Young RR. Amantadine in Parkinson's disease: review of more than two years of experience. *JAMA* 1972;222:792–795.

Senard JM, Rai S, Lapeyre-Mestre M, et al. Prevalence of orthostatic hypotension in Parkinson's disease. *J Neurol Neurosurg Psychiatry* 1997;63:584–589.

Senard JM, Rascol O, Rascol A, Montastruc JL. Lack of yohimbine effect on ambulatory blood pressure recording: a double blind cross-over trial in parkinsonians with orthostatic hypotension. *Fundam Clin Pharmacol* 1993;7:465–470.

Serrano-Duenas M. Chronic dopamimetic drug addiction and pathologic gambling in patients with Parkinson's disease: presentation of four cases. *Ger J Psychiatry* 2002;5:62–66.

Sethi KD, O'Brien CF, Hammerstad JP, et al. Ropinirole for the treatment of early Parkinson's disease: a 12-month experience. *Arch Neurol* 1998;55:1211–1216.

Shannon KM, Bennett JP Jr, Friedman JH. Efficacy of pramipexole, a novel dopamine agonist, as monotherapy in mild to moderate Parkinson's disease. *Neurology* 1997;49:724–728.

Shealy CN, Weath JB, Mercier DA. Livedo reticularis in patients with Parkinson's receiving amantadine. *JAMA* 1970;212:1522–1523.

Shoulson I, Oakes D, Fahn S, et al. Impact of sustained deprenyl (selegiline) in levodopa-treated Parkinson's disease: a randomized placebo-controlled extension of the deprenyl and tocopherol antioxidant therapy of parkinsonism trial. *Ann Neurol* 2002;51:604–612.

Siddiqui MF, Rast S, Lynn MJ, Auchus AP, Pfeiffer RF. Autonomic dysfunction in Parkinson's disease: a comprehensive symptom survey, *Parkinsonism Relat Disord* 2002;8:277–284.

Smith LA, Jackson MJ, Al-Barghouthy G, et al. Multiple small doses of levodopa plus entacapone produce continuous dopaminergic stimulation and reduce dyskinesia induction in MPTP-treated drug-naive primates. *Mov Disord* 2005;20:306–314.

Snow BJ, Macdonald L, Mcauley D, Wallis W. The effect of amantadine on levodopa-induced dyskinesias in Parkinson's disease: a double-blind, placebo-controlled study. *Clin Neuropharmacol* 2000;23:82–85.

Sohn YH, Verhagen Metman L, Bravi D, et al. Levodopa peak response time reflects severity of dopamine neuron loss in Parkinson's disease. *Neurology* 1994;44:755–757.

Stacy M, Bowron A, Guttman M, et al. Identification of motor and nonmotor wearing-off in Parkinson's disease: comparison of a patient questionnaire versus a clinician assessment. *Mov Disord* 2005;20:726–733.

Stocchi F, Barbato L, Nordera G, Bolner A, Caraceni T. Entacapone improves the pharmacokinetic and therapeutic response of controlled release levodopa/carbidopa in Parkinson's patients. *J Neural Transm* 2004;111:173–180.

Stocchi F, Ruggieri S, Vacca L, Olanow CW. Prospective randomized trial of lisuride infusion versus oral levodopa in PD patients. *Brain* 2002;125:2058–2066.

Stocchi F, Vacca L, De Pandis MF, Barbato L, Valente M, Ruggieri S. Subcutaneous continuous apomorphine infusion in fluctuating patients with Parkinson's disease: long-term results. *Neurol Sci* 2001;22:93–94.

Stone TW. Evidence for a nondopaminergic action of amantadine. *Neurosci Lett* 1977;4:343–346.

Stoof JC, Booij J, Drukarch B. Amantadine as N-methyl-D-aspartic acid receptor antagonist: new possibilities for therapeutic applications? *Clin Neurol Neurosurg* 1992;94(suppl):S4–S6.

Strang RR. Orphenadrine ("Disipal") in the treatment of parkinsonism: a two-year study of 150 patients. *Med J Aust* 1965;2:448–450.

Stromberg U, Svensson TH. Further studies on the mode of action of amantadine. *Acta Pharmacol Toxicol* 1971;30:161–171.

Suchowersky O, Furtado S, Rohs G. Beneficial effect of intranasal desmopressin for nocturnal polyuria in Parkinson's disease. *Mov Disord* 1995;10:337–340.

Syed N, Murphy J, Zimmerman T Jr, Mark MH, Sage JI. Ten years' experience with enteral levodopa infusions for motor fluctuations in Parkinson's disease. *Mov Disord* 1998;13:336–368.

Syndulko K, Gilden ER, Hansch EC, Potvin AR, Tourtelotte WW, Povin JH. Decreased verbal memory associated with anticholinergic treatment in Parkinson's disease patients. *Int J Neurosci* 1981;14:61–66.

Tatton WG. Selegiline can mediate neuronal rescue rather than neuronal protection. *Mov Disord* 1993;8:S20–S30.

Tatton WG, Chalmers-Redman RME. Mitochondria in neurodegenerative apoptosis: an opportunity for therapy? *Ann Neurol* 1998;44(suppl 1):S134–S141.

Ten Harkel AD, Van Lieshout JJ, Wieling W. Treatment of orthostatic hypotension with sleeping in the head-up tilt position, alone and in combination with fludrocortisone. *J Intern Med* 1992;232:139–145.

Teravainen H. Selegiline in Parkinson's disease. *Acta Neurol Scand* 1990;81:333–336.

Tesei S, Antonini A, Canesi M, Zecchinelli A, Mariani CB, Pessoli G. Tolerability of paroxetine in Parkinson's disease: a prospective study. *Mov Disord* 2000;15:986–989.

Tetrud JW, Langston JW. The effect of deprenyl (selegiline) in the natural history of Parkinson's disease. *Science* 1989;245:519–522.

Thomas A, Iacono D, Luciano AL, Armellino K, Di Iorio A, Onofrj M. Duration of amantadine benefit on dyskinesia of severe Parkinson's disease. *J Neurol Neurosurg Psychiatry* 2004;75(1):141–143.

Tolcapone Study Group. Efficacy and tolerability of tolcapone compared with bromocriptine in levodopa-treated parkinsonian patients. *Mov Disord* 1999;14:38–44.

Tolosa E, Alom J, Martí MJ. Drug-induced dyskinesias. In: Jankovic J, Tolosa E, eds. *Parkinson's Disease and Movement Disorders.* Baltimore: Williams & Wilkins, 1993:375–398.

Tolosa E, Blesa R, Bayes A, Forcadell F. Low dose bromocriptine in the early phases of Parkinson's disease. *Clin Neuropharmacol* 1987;10:168–174.

Tolosa E, Marin C. Dopamine agonists in Parkinson's disease: a clinical review. In: Olanow WC, Obeso JA, eds. Beyond the Decade of the Brain. Vol 2. Dopamine agonists in early Parkinson's disease. 1997:143–161.

Tourtellotte WW, Potvin AR, Syndulko K, et al. Parkinson's disease: Congentin with Sinemet, a better response. *Prog Neuropsychopharmacol Biol Psychiatry* 1982;6:51–55.

Toyokura Y, Mizuno Y, Kase M, et al. Effects of bromocriptine on parkinsonism: a nation-wide collaborative double-blind study. *Acta Neurol Scand* 1985;72:157–170.

U.K. Madopar CR Study Group. A comparison of Madopar CR and standard Madopar in the treatment of nocturnal and early-morning disability in Parkinson's disease. *Clin Neuropharmacol* 1989;12:498–505.

Van Blercom N, Lasa A, Verger K, Masramon X, Sastre VM, Linazasoro G. Effects of gabapentin on the motor response to levodopa: a double-blind, placebo-controlled, crossover study in patients with complicated Parkinson's disease. *Clin Neuropharmacol* 2004;27:124–128.

Van Camp G, Flamez A, Cosyns B, et al. Treatment of Parkinson's disease with pergolide and relation to restrictive valvular heart disease. *Lancet* 2004;363:1179–1183.

Van Herwaarden G, Berger HJ, Horstink MW. Short-term memory in Parkinson's disease after withdrawal of long-term anticholinergic therapy. *Clin Neuropharmacol* 1993; 16:438–443.

Velasco F, Velasco M, Romo R. Effect of carbachol and atropine perfusions in the mesencephalic tegmentum and caudate nucleus of experimental tremor in monkeys. *Exp Neurol* 1982;78:450–460.

Verhagen Metman L, Del Dotto P, van den Munckhof P, et al. Amantadine as treatment for dyskinesias and motor fluctuations in Parkinson's disease. *Neurology* 1998;50:1323–1326.

Verhagen Metman LV, Del Dotto P, LePoole K, Konitsiotis S, Fang J, Chase TN. Amantadine for levodopa-induced dyskinesias: a 1-year follow-up study. *Arch Neurol* 1999;56:1383–1386.

Von Voigtlander PF, Moore KE. Dopamine release from the brain in vivo by amantadine. *Science* 1973;174:408–410.

Waters CH, Kurth M, Bailey P, et al. and the Tolcapone Stable Study Group. Tolcapone in stable Parkinson's disease: efficacy and safety of long-term treatment. *Neurology* 1997;49:665–671.

Waters CH, Sethi KD, Hauser RA, Molho E, Bertoni JM, for the Zydis Selegiline Study Group. Zydis selegiline reduces off time in Parkinson's disease patients with motor fluctuations: a 3-month, randomized, placebo-controlled study. *Mov Disord* 2004;19:426–432.

Watts R. The role of dopamine agonists in early Parkinson's disease. *Neurology* 1997;49(suppl 1):S34–S48.

Watts RL, Wendt RL, Nausied B, et al. Efficacy, safety, and tolerability of the rotigotine transdermal patch in patients with early-stage, idiopathic Parkinson's disease: a multicenter, multinational, randomized, double-blind, placebo-controlled trial. *Mov Disord* 2004;19(suppl 9):S258.

Wermuth L, The Danish Pramipexole Study Group. A double-blind, placebo-controlled, randomized, multi-center study of pramipexole in advanced Parkinson's disease. *Eur J Neurol* 1998;5:235–242.

Wermuth L, Sorensen PS, Timm B, et al. Depression in idiopathic Parkinson's disease treated with citalopram: a placebo-controlled trial. *Nordic J Psychiatry* 1998;52:163–169.

Whone AL, Watts RL, Stoessl AJ, et al. Slower progression of Parkinson's disease with ropinirole versus levodopa: the REAL-PET study. *Ann Neurol* 2003;54:93–101.

Whone AL, Renny P, Davis MR, et al. The REAL-PET study: slower progression in early Parkinson's disease treated with ropinirole compared with L-dopa. *Neurology* 2002;58:A82–A83.

Witjas T, Kaphan E, Azulay JP, et al. Nonmotor fluctuations in Parkinson's disease. *Neurology* 2002;59:408–413.

Woitalla D, Muller T, Benz S, Horowski R, Przuntek H. Transdermal lisuride delivery in the treatment of Parkinson's disease. *J Neural Transm Suppl* 2004;68:89–95.

Wolters EC, Tesselaar HJ. International (NL–UK) double-blind study of Sinemet CR and standard Sinemet (25/100) in 170 patients with fluctuating Parkinson's disease. *J Neurol* 1996;243:235–240.

Wright RA, Kaufmann HC, Perera R, et al. A double-blind, dose-response study of midodrine in neurogenic orthostatic hypotension. *Neurology* 1998;51:120–124.

Yahr M, Duvoisin RC. Medical therapy of parkinsonism. In: Vinken PJ, Bruyn GW, eds. *Handbook of Clinical Neurology: Diseases of Basal Ganglia*. Amsterdam: Elsevier North-Holland; 1968: 283–300.

Yanagisawa N, Ikeda S, Hashimoto T, et al. Effect of L-threo-dops on orthostatic hypotension in Parkinson's disease. *No To Shinkei* 1998;50:157–163.

Yeh KC, August TF, Bush TF, et al. Pharmacokinetics and bioavailability of Sinemet CR: a summary of human studies. *Neurology* 1989;39:25–38.

Youdim MBH, Gross A, Finberg JPM. Rasagiline [N-propargyl-1R(+)-aminoindan], a selective and potent inhibitor of mitochondrial monoamine oxidase B. *Br J Pharmacol* 2001;132: 500–506.

Young TM, Mathias CJ. The effects of water ingestion on orthostatic hypotension in two groups of chronic autonomic failure: multiple system atrophy and pure autonomic failure. *J Neurol Neurosurg Psychiatry* 2004;75:1737–1741.

Zesiewicz TA, Baker MJ, Wahba M, Hauser RA. Autonomic nervous system dysfunction in Parkinson's disease. *Curr Treatm Op Neurol* 2003;5:149–160.

Zou L, Jankovic J, Rowe DB, et al. Neuroprotection by pramipexole against dopamine and levodopa-induced cytotoxicity. *Life Sci* 1999;64:1275–1285.

Zou L, Xu J, Jankovic J, et al. Pramipexole inhibits lipid peroxidation and reduces injury in the substantia nigra induced by the dopaminergic neurotoxin 1-methyl-4-phenyl-1,2,3,6-tetrahydropyridine in C57BL/6 mice. *Neurosci Lett* 2000;281:167–170.

11

Experimental Therapeutics of Parkinson's Disease and the Development of New Symptomatic Medicines for Parkinson's Disease

Olivier Rascol   *Cristina Sampaio*

Since the discovery nearly 40 years ago of levodopa's extraordinary antiparkinsonian properties, nearly all antiparkinsonian drugs marketed today (with the exception of two "old" medicinal products: the anticholinergic trihexyphenidyl and other related compounds, and the antiglutaminergic amantadine whose action mechanism was long unknown) share a common pharmacodynamic mechanism: correction of the striatal dopamine deficiency that is characteristic of Parkinson's disease (PD). These include various dopamine agonists (apomorphine, bromocriptine, cabergoline, dihydroergocriptine, lisuride, pergolide, piribedil, pramipexole, and ropinirole), monoamine oxidase B inhibitors (selegiline and rasagiline) and C-O-methyltransferase inhibitors (entacapone and tolcapone) (1). No one would deny the significant therapeutic advances that these medicinal products have brought to the daily management of symptomatic treatment for PD. As monotherapies or in combination, they significantly improve, to varying degrees, the three cardinal signs of the motor disorders in PD: tremor, akinesia, and rigidity.

Despite these advances, we cannot forget, however, that PD treatment still faces major shortcomings: the mortality of patients remains abnormally high (2) and quality of life is still deeply affected (3). Use of the current dopaminergics just about suffices to control the main signs of the disease during the first years of its development, but after that new symptoms appear and aggravate the clinical picture (Fig. 11.1). Some remain linked, directly or indirectly, with the striatal dopamine deficiency. This is the case with on/off motor fluctuations and dyskinetic involuntary movements, estimated to be suffered by nearly 80% of patients after 10 years of the disease and L-dopa therapy. Apart from the motor complications of L-dopa, patients and doctors are confronted with the challenges of other,

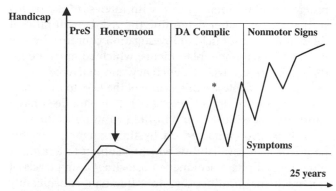

Figure 11.1 Schematic Representation of the Clinical Progression of Parkinson's Disease **PreS**, presymptomatic phase. Its duration remains unknown (perhaps 5–10 years). This corresponds to the period of time when dopaminergic neurons start to die but remain sufficiently numerous (>50% of normal) to allow the brain to compensate for this loss, due to adaptive mechanisms. **Honeymoon**, period of time when the usual symptomatic medications (initiated at the level of the arrow) including L-dopa and DA agonists, alone or in combination, are sufficiently efficacious to control the symptoms in a way that allows the patients to behave without significant difficulties. This period lasts usually 3–6 years. **DA Complic**, period of the disease when the motor complications related to chronic L-dopa therapy (motor fluctuations like on/off and dyskinesias) occurs. During this period, the addition of dopamine (DA) agonists and/or MAO-B inhibitors and/or COMT-inhibitors helps to a certain extent in controlling fluctuations. Amantadine also helps to a certain extent in controlling dyskinesias. Once such medications become insufficient to provide an acceptable result, subthalamic nucleus deep brain stimulation (DBS) is usually considered (*asterisk*). **Nonmotor Signs**, last period of evolution of the disease. This is when most nonmotor signs occur (dementia, psychosis, dysarthria, falls, dysautonomia, etc.). This stage usually occurs after 10 years of evolution, and most of these symptoms are resistant, if not worsened, by dopaminergic treatments and DBS.

even more disabling symptoms, which, if not aggravated by dopamine treatment, are generally resistant to it: cognitive disorders and dementia (4), dysautonomia (orthostatic hypotension, urinary disorders, constipation, impotence, etc.) (5), balance and walking difficulties, with the risk of falling that these entail (6), sleep and waking disorders (7), speech disorders (8), mental and hallucinatory disorders (9), pain (10), etc. Little is still known about the exact prevalence of these symptoms, but they are far from rare: It is estimated that about one-third of Parkinson's patients may experience all of them at one time or another during the course of the disease. Their incidence increases over the years as the disease progresses, threatening the prognosis in the most advanced stages. Most of these admittedly nonmotor symptoms have the characteristic of not "responding" to dopaminergic treatments (nor to functional stereotaxic surgery by deep-brain stimulation of the subthalamic nuclei). This clinical feature common to all these symptoms explains why their physiopathology is often attributed to mechanisms other than striatal dopaminergic lesions, and it also explains why they are easily associated with abnormalities affecting other neurotransmitters (11). PD can no longer be viewed as a simple mobility disease secondary to striatal dopamine deficiency. Based on this

clinical, pathological, and pharmacological assessment, the oversimplified model of striatal dopamine deficiency can be extended so that this disease is considered a more complex neuropsychiatric disease, including not only the subcortical motor circuits but also the central nervous system, borne out by the existence of real peripheral orthosympathetic lesions in the PD patient. It has therefore been recognized that PD is a result of multiple functional and lesional abnormalities, involving a long list of neurotransmitters (acetylcholine, noradrenaline, serotonin, glutamate, peptides, etc.), which contribute, along with dopamine, to the creation of a complete clinical picture of this disease (12). These ideas suggest that focusing our efforts on repairing dopaminergic transmission, as we have done for years, is too restrictive, and at least partly explains the current therapeutic dearth of medical resources available to us.

Armed with these new principles, therapeutic research has for several years already been moving in three different directions:

1. The hope to further improve dopaminergic drugs has not been completely abandoned since further refinements can reasonably be expected in the field, although the solution to all problems faced by PD patients is no longer to be expected from such medications.
2. There are plans to develop so-called "neuroprotective" drugs, which would block or at least slow the degenerative process responsible for neuron death. Better still, there are attempts to take "restorative" steps that would allow us to regain lost ground and find a source of neurons compatible with normal brain function. The road is arduous, on a par with what is at stake therapeutically.
3. A third step, less ambitious but perhaps more pragmatic and accessible to short-term clinical therapeutic applications, consists of researching new symptomatic medicinal products that act on neurotransmitters other than dopamine, at targets in the brain other than the striatum, to relieve symptoms other than just shaking, akinesia, and hypertonia.

The intention of this short review is not to discuss in detail the challenges of research on neuroprotective medicines or neurorestorative treatments for PD; many review articles have been published on this subject (13–16). This strategy, if proven effective by well-designed clinical trials, will revolutionize the treatment not only of PD but also of other neurodegenerative diseases. "Neuroprotection," if successful, should therefore resolve most of the problems experienced by patients by preventing the disease from progressing to a stage where the disability exceeds the symptomatic therapeutic possibilities. In an ideal world, we can dream about controlling neuron death to the point of preventing the patient from reaching the fateful threshold of symptomatic lesion expression, thus maintaining the patient in a permanent "subclinical" state. But the obstacles remain considerable, both from a conceptual point of view (we are far from fully understanding the physiopathological mechanisms of neuron death and the therapeutic targets that result from them) and in terms of application (we are far from knowing how to demonstrate clinically in patients the long-term efficacy and innocuousness of treatments that are potentially neuroprotective). Despite the efforts already made, the clinical results are still poor. Examples include the disappointing results of embryonic mesencephalic neuron transplants (17) and the unanswered questions raised by clinical trials carried out with dopamine agonists intended to document their hypothetical effects as neuroprotectors (18,19). Without being too pessimistic, we can ascertain the obstacles better this way, especially since the neuroprotective or neurorestorative "miracle" must not be restricted to just dopaminergic neurons. Otherwise, without being too naïve, how can we expect the most effective dopaminergic cell or gene therapy to correct or prevent the onset of disabling symptoms not caused by dopamine deficiency, such as dementia disorders or balancing or walking difficulties?

NOVEL DOPAMINERGIC, SYMPTOMATIC ANTIPARKINSONIAN DRUGS

Nigrostriatal dopaminergic synapse deficiency should not, whatever is said, be dismissed out of hand as an "old" hypothesis to be forgotten. It must be admitted that research into dopamine agonists, increasingly selective for various receptor subtypes, has not yet led to the advances that were expected initially when this class of drugs was first introduced. The recent development of dopamine agonists selective for D2–D3 receptors (ropinirole, pramipexole), stripped of most of the serotoninergic and adrenergic effects characteristic of the "old" ergot-derived agonists (bromocriptine, lisuride, and pergolide), has not greatly improved the therapeutic profile of this pharmacological class in terms of efficacy or undesirable effects, except perhaps the much lower risk of fibrosis (20). The few clinical trials carried out with agonists said to be selective for D1 receptors have shown effects differing little from those of nonselective substances, such as L-dopa (21–23). However, these studies remain too few and too fragmented to come to a definitive conclusion, and much work remains to be done before we understand the potential impact of such products on the motor and nonmotor disorders of PD. It is therefore not unreasonable to still hope for further innovations through the development of new dopamine agonists, whether they be fully or partially selective or nonselective (24).

Another area of research with dopamine, on which there have been practically no clinical trials yet, involves the dopamine reuptake site. The leading dopamine reuptake inhibitor is cocaine. The well-known addictive effects of this substance prevent its use in PD, but other drugs in this pharmacological class, such as brasofensine, have been shown to be effective against parkinsonism in various experimental models (25). The first clinical trials are in progress, and we look forward with interest to the results so that we can better determine the risk/benefit ratio of these drugs. A third field of investigation concerns the way in which dopamine replacements, which compensate for the endogenous striatal deficiency, are delivered to the brain. Some people see this as one of the keys to the motor complications of dopatherapy (26). L-dopa indeed has a short plasma elimination half-life (90 minutes on average). It is also characterized by the extremely variable nature of its bioavailability, which is subject to a number of peripheral pharmacokinetic obstacles. Plasma levels of this medicinal product therefore fluctuate considerably from one moment to the next in the same patient, and these "antiphysiological" dopamine fluctuations probably have repercussions on the brain. From an experimental point of view, in primates whose brains have been denervated of dopaminergic neurons by the toxic effect of 1-methyl-4-phenyl-1,2,3,6-tetrahydropyridine (MPTP), it was observed that repeated administration of L-dopa deregulates at a molecular, cellular, and functional level the series of dopaminergic and nondopaminergic mechanisms controlling the motor programs within and below the striatum (27,28). All these deregulations together would lead to the onset of fluctuations and dyskinesia. Indeed, a more constant method of stimulation reduces the experimental and clinical incidence of such disorders (26,29,30). It is perhaps for this reason that the use of dopamine agonists, with longer half-lives than that of L-dopa, reduces the incidence of motor disorders in the early stages of the disease in patients compared with L-dopa therapy (31). In the same vein, MPTP-intoxicated primates undergoing early treatment with L-dopa and the catechol-O-methyltransferase (COMT) inhibitor entacapone (which prolongs the elimination half-life of L-dopa and would thus reduce its variability) are at a lower risk of developing dyskinesia than when treated with L-dopa alone (29). The potential preventive benefit of the early use of this combination is currently undergoing clinical evaluation, showing that new experimental findings can lead to the reevaluation of the therapeutic role of a drug even after it has been marketed (entacapone is in fact officially marketed only for advanced stages of the disease, to treat motor fluctuations *after* they have already been caused by L-dopa). In the same vein, the concept of "constant dopamine stimulation" is now leading to the study of new ways of administering dopaminergics, such as the transdermal route, because this gives particularly stable plasma levels (32).

NOVEL SYMPTOMATIC NONDOPAMINERGIC ANTIPARKINSONIAN DRUGS

Apart from this research on dopaminergics, based on the classic idea of correcting the nigrostriatal dopaminergic deficit, increasing attention is being paid to the antiparkinsonian potential of substances that act through other neurotransmitter systems. We have already emphasized that not all of the abnormalities of PD are associated with dopamine deficiency. Furthermore, the antiparkinsonian properties of alkaloids contained in belladonna were identified in the 19th century, long before the discovery of dopamine and L-dopa. These alkaloids have no dopaminergic effects but do block muscarinic cholinergic receptors. In the Parkinson's patient, many regions of the brain, both striatal and nonstriatal, are deficient in noradrenaline, serotonin, acetylcholine, and a number of other neurotransmitters, peptides, or amino acids (11,12). These abnormalities can generally be explained in two ways: either by a direct mechanism, as a result of the extension of the lesional process beyond the nigrostriatal pathway, or by an indirect mechanism, resulting from the functional imbalances caused by dopaminergic denervation. It is expected that at least partial correction of these abnormalities, using suitable agonists or antagonists, will one day add to or even replace the arsenal of traditional, dopaminergic treatments (33,34).

It is beyond the scope of this chapter to discuss all non-dopaminergic strategies, but glutamatergic receptor antagonists, such as amantadine (for a review, see 35), are increasingly used as antidyskinetic drugs. Amantadine is an old antiviral drug whose antiparkinsonian properties were found by chance in the 1960s, when it happened to be used to treat some Parkinson's patients with influenza. For more than two decades, this medicine enjoyed only marginal interest, given the low level of its symptomatic antiparkinsonian effect and the lack of understanding about its pharmacological action. The concept behind the beneficial effects of the glutamatergic drugs in the treatment of levodopa-related dyskinesias is based on the central role of glutaminergic receptors on the cortico-striatal pathway and dopamine receptors in the nigrostriatal pathway at the efferent GABAergic neurons of the corpus striatum (36). Using the model of motor disorders caused by L-dopa in 6-OH-dopamine-intoxicated rodents, researchers established the link between these abnormalities, the abnormal variability of the dopaminergic stimulation delivered to the animals, and the behavioral expression of their motor disorders. They then showed in vivo that blocking N-methyl-D-aspartate (NMDA) receptors attenuated the clinical expression of this abnormal motor syndrome, both in rodents and in primates (37). They then sought a suitable NMDA receptor antagonist for clinical application of the results of their research. The task was not easy because previous attempts to use NMDA antagonists to treat humans had shown that the use of the leading one, MK-801, was unfortunately accompanied by unacceptable adverse effects, irredeemably compromising its use for therapeutic purposes. The fact that amantadine is not as powerful an NMDA antagonist perhaps explains why it is better tolerated by patients than MK-801, although the drug clearly has antidyskinetic properties, without compromising at the same time the antiparkinsonian response to L-dopa (38).

Studies of interactions between glutamate and dopamine, utilizing animal models, such as MPTP-intoxicated monkeys, promise to provide new leads to potentially effective antidyskinetic drugs (for a review see 39,33). The MPTP primate model also has been used to study a novel class of drugs, the adenosine A2 receptor antagonists, which have been shown to exert an antiparkinsonian effect when administered alone or in combination with L-dopa, with less dyskinesia than that caused by classic dopaminergics (40). One substance in this group, istradefylline, is currently undergoing phase III development for this indication, based on the encouraging results of the initial phase II studies (41). Serotoninergic substances such as sarizotan, a 5-HT1A receptor agonist, exert interesting antidyskinetic effects in primates (42) that seem to have been repeated in the first pilot studies carried out in humans (43). In the same way, it has been shown that alpha 2-adrenergic receptor antagonists, such as idazoxan or fipamezole, have an original pharmacological profile in monkeys, amplifying the antiparkinsonian properties of L-dopa while reducing its dyskinetic effects (44,45). The first studies conducted in patients have turned out to be contradictory at times but are no less stimulating (21,46). Other examples of novel approaches, currently under development in the treatment of PD and levodopa-related complications include agonists and antagonists of opiate receptors (47), cannabinoid receptors (48), serotonin receptors (49), histamine receptors, and others.

While little is known about Parkinson dementia, the use of anticholinesterases for this indication does not necessarily seem illogical when one remembers that cholinergic markers are as low, if not lower, in the cerebral cortex in Parkinson dementia than in Alzheimer's disease. This again takes us away from the classic nigrostriatal motor model, and also from the formerly widespread (but simplistic and outdated) notion of a functional striatal balance between dopamine and acetylcholine, so that our hypotheses are focused on new ideas involving the cortex. The low level of symptomatic therapeutic efficacy of anticholinesterases in Alzheimer's disease is no secret. Despite this, several clinical trials have shown that acetylcholinesterase inhibitors significantly improve the cognitive deficit symptoms of Parkinson dementia (50). Without knowing exactly why, this effect seems at least as significant as in Alzheimer's disease, and mainly happens without appreciable aggravation of the patient's motor signs. Both practice and clinical trials also show that anticholinesterases have a notable antihallucinatory effect in Parkinson patients. Some Parkinson hallucinations correspond to abnormal behavior during rapid eye movement (REM) sleep (51). Since cholinergic nuclei of the brainstem, such as the nucleus subcoeruleus, are involved in the control of the wake/sleep cycle, and these nuclei may be involved in PD, it is possible that the acetylcholinesterase inhibitors act not only at the cortex but also at the brainstem. It is also of interest to develop alpha-1 adrenergic agonists to counteract the postganglionic

TABLE 11.1
CURRENT AND FUTURE TREATMENT FOR PARKINSON'S DISEASE

Current Symptomatic Medications for Parkinson's Disease	Putative Future Symptomatic Medications for Parkinson's Disease
Dopaminergic medications L-dopa + dopadecarboxylase-inhibitors (benzerazide, carbidopa) Dopamine agonists (apomorphine, bromocriptine, cabergoline, dihydroergocriptine, lisuride, pergolide, piribedil, pramipexole, ropinirole) MAO-B inhibitors (selegiline, rasagiline) COMT inhibitors (entacapone, tolcapone)	**Dopaminergic medications** DA agonists (e.g., rotigotine, SLV 308) DA transporter blockers (e.g., brasofensine)
Nondopaminergic medications Anticholinergics (trihexyphenidyl) NMDA glutamate antagonists (amantadine)	**Nondopaminergic medications** Adenosine antagonists (e.g., istradefylline) Glutamate antagonists (NMDA, AMPA, e.g., E2007) Kappa or delta opiate agonists/antagonists Cannabinoid antagonists/agonists Alpha 2 antagonists (e.g., idazoxan, fipamezole) Alpha 1 agonists 5HT1A agonists (e.g., sarizotan) 5HT2 A antagonists (e.g., quetiapine) Cholinesterase inhibitors (e.g., rivastigmine, donepezil) H3 histamine agonists

orthosympathetic deficit at the origin of severe orthostatic hypotension in dysautonomic PD (52). As another example of focusing on nonstriatal targets, clozapine, an "old" atypical neuroleptic, has a surprising antipsychotic effect, attenuating the hallucinations of delirious Parkinson patients without aggravating the motor disorders (53,54).

So little is yet understood about the physiopathology of walking difficulties associated with PD, such as shuffling and hesitation when starting to walk ("freezing"), the loss of postural reflexes, and the risk of falls that the latter entails, that it has proved almost impossible to imagine future new therapeutic opportunities, in the short or medium term, whether they be of a pharmaceutical nature or not. The same is true for other symptoms, such as dysarthria. The absence of suitable experimental models and the vertical bipedal gait and speech specific to humans may partly explain the shortcomings and failures. Moreover, for clinical research, in the absence of validated outcome criteria, it is also difficult to design reliable trials to assess a putative benefit related to any therapeutic intervention in these domains.

REFERENCES

1. Rascol O, Goetz C, Koller W, Poewe W, Sampaio C. Treatment interventions for Parkinson's disease: an evidence based assessment. *Lancet* 2002;359:1589–1598.
2. Lees AJ, Katzenschlager R, Head J, Ben-Shlomo Y. Ten-year follow-up of three different initial treatments in de-novo PD: a randomized trial. *Neurology* 2001;57:1687–1694.
3. Gage H, Hendricks A, Zhang S, Kazis L. The relative health related quality of life of veterans with Parkinson's disease. *J Neurol Neurosurg Psychiatry* 2003;74:163–169.
4. Brown RG, Marsden CD. Cognitive function in Parkinson's disease: from description to theory. *Trends Neurosci* 1990;13:21–29.
5. Senard JM, Brefel-Courbon C, Rascol O, Montastruc JL. Orthostatic hypotension in patients with Parkinson's disease: pathophysiology and management. *Drugs Aging* 2001;18:495–505.
6. Bloem BR, Hausdorff JM, Visser JE, Giladi N. Falls and freezing of gait in Parkinson's disease: a review of two interconnected, episodic phenomena. *Mov Disord* 2004;19:871–84.
7. Brotini S, Gigli GL. Epidemiology and clinical features of sleep disorders in extrapyramidal disease. *Sleep Med* 2004;5:169–179.
8. Pinto S, Ozsancak C, Tripoliti E, Thobois S, Limousin-Dowsey P, Auzou P. Treatments for dysarthria in Parkinson's disease. *Lancet Neurol* 2004;3:547–556.
9. Wint DP, Okun MS, Fernandez HH. Psychosis in Parkinson's disease. *J Geriatr Psychiatry Neurol* 2004;17:127–136.
10. Goetz CG, Tanner CM, Levy M, Wilson RS, Garron DC. Pain in Parkinson's disease. *Mov Disord* 1986;1:45–49.
11. Agid Y. Parkinson's disease: pathophysiology. *Lancet* 1991;337:1321–1324.
12. Lang AE, Obeso JA. Challenges in Parkinson's disease: restoration of the nigrostriatal dopamine system is not enough. *Lancet Neurol* 2004;3:309–316.
13. Mandel S, Grunblatt E, Riederer P, Gerlach M, Levites Y, Youdim MB. Neuroprotective strategies in Parkinson's disease: an update on progress. *CNS Drugs* 2003;17:729–762.
14. Schapira AH, Olanow CW. Neuroprotection in Parkinson disease: mysteries, myths, and misconceptions. *JAMA* 2004;291:358–364.
15. Koller WC, Cersosimo MG. Neuroprotection in Parkinson's disease: an elusive goal. *Curr Neurol Neurosci Rep* 2004;4:277–283.
16. Walter BL, Vitek JL. Surgical treatment for Parkinson's disease. *Lancet Neurol* 2004;3:719–728.
17. Freed CR, Greene PE, Breeze RE, Tsai WY, DuMouchel W, Kao R, Dillon S, Winfield H, Culver S, Trojanowski JQ, Eidelberg D, Fahn S. Transplantation of embryonic dopamine neurons for severe Parkinson's disease. *N Engl J Med* 2001;344:710–719.
18. Whone AL, Watts RL, Stoessl AJ, Davis M, Reske S, Nahmias C, Lang AE, Rascol O, Ribeiro MJ, Remy P, Poewe WH, Hauser RA, Brooks DJ, REAL-PET Study Group. Slower progression of Parkinson's disease with ropinirole versus levodopa: the REAL-PET study. *Ann Neurol* 2003;54:93–101.

19. Clarke CE. A "cure" for Parkinson's disease: can neuroprotection be proven with current trial designs? *Mov Disord* 2004;19:491–498.
20. Rascol O, Pathak A, Bagheri H, Montastruc JL. New concerns about old drugs: valvular heart disease on ergot derivative dopamine agonists as an exemplary situation of pharmacovigilance. *Mov Disord* 2004;19:611–613.
21. Rascol O, Blin O, Thalamas C, Descombes S, Soubrouillard C, Azulay P, Fabre N, Viallet F, Lafnitzegger K, Wright S, Carter JH, Nutt JG. ABT-431, a D1 receptor agonist prodrug, has efficacy in Parkinson's disease. *Ann Neurol* 1999;46:736–741.
22. Rascol O, Nutt JG, Blin O, Goetz CG, Trugman JM, Soubrouillard C, Carter JH, Currie LJ, Fabre N, Thalamas C, Giardina WW, Wright S. Induction by dopamine D1 receptor agonist ABT-431 of dyskinesia similar to levodopa in patients with Parkinson disease. *Arch Neurol* 2001;58:249–254.
23. Rascol O, Arnulf I, Peyro-Saint Paul H, Brefel-Courbon C, Vidailhet M, Thalamas C, Bonnet AM, Descombes S, Bejjani B, Fabre N, Montastruc JL, Agid Y. Idazoxan, an alpha-2 antagonist, and L-DOPA-induced dyskinesias in patients with Parkinson's disease. *Mov Disord* 2001;16:708–713.
24. Bezard E, Ferry S, Mach U, Stark H, Leriche L, Boraud T, Gross C, Sokoloff P. Attenuation of levodopa-induced dyskinesia by normalizing dopamine D3 receptor function. *Nat Med* 2003;9:762–767.
25. Pearce RK, Smith LA, Jackson MJ, Banerji T, Scheel-Kruger J, Jenner P. The monoamine reuptake blocker brasofensine reverses akinesia without dyskinesia in MPTP-treated and levodopa-primed common marmosets. *Mov Disord* 2002;17:877–886.
26. Olanow W, Schapira AH, Rascol O. Continuous dopamine-receptor stimulation in early Parkinson's disease. *Trends Neurosci* 2000;23:S117–S126.
27. Chase TN. The significance of continuous dopaminergic stimulation in the treatment of Parkinson's disease. *Drugs* 1998;55(suppl 1):1–9.
28. Gerfen CR. Dopamine-mediated gene regulation in models of Parkinson's disease. *Ann Neurol* 2000;47(4 suppl 1):S42–S50.
29. Jenner P. Avoidance of dyskinesia: preclinical evidence for continuous dopaminergic stimulation. *Neurology* 2004;62:S47–S55.
30. Stocchi F, Ruggieri S, Vacca L, Olanow CW. Prospective randomized trial of lisuride infusion versus oral levodopa patients with Parkinson's disease. *Brain* 2002;125:2058–2066.
31. Rascol O, Brooks DJ, Korczyn AD, De Deyn PP, Clarke CE, Lang AE, for the 056 Study Group. A five-year study of the incidence of dyskinesia in patients with early Parkinson's disease who were treated with ropinirole or levodopa. *N Engl J Med* 2000;342:1484–1491.
32. The Parkinson Study Group. A controlled trial of rotigotine monotherapy in early Parkinson's disease. *Arch Neurol* 2003;60:1721–1728.
33. Bezard E, Brotchie JM, Gross CE. Pathophysiology of levodopa-induced dyskinesia: potential for new therapies. *Nat Rev Neurosci* 2001;2:577–588.
34. Johnston TH, Brotchie JM. Drugs in development for Parkinson's disease. *Curr Opin Investig Drugs* 2004;5:720–726.
35. Chase TN, Oh JD, Konitsiotis S. Antiparkinsonian and antidyskinetic activity of drugs targeting central glutamatergic mechanisms. *J Neurol* 2000;247(suppl 2):II36–II42.
36. Chase TN. Levodopa therapy: consequences of the nonphysiologic replacement of dopamine. *Neurology* 1998;50(suppl 5):S17–S25.
37. Blanchet PJ, Konitsiotis S, Chase TN. Amantadine reduces levodopa-induced dyskinesias in parkinsonian monkeys. *Mov Disord* 1998;13:798–802.
38. Verhagen Metman L, Del Dotto P, van den Munckhof P, Fang J, Mouradian MM, Chase TN. Amantadine as treatment for dyskinesias and motor fluctuations in Parkinson's disease. *Neurology* 1998;50:1323–1326.
39. Brotchie JM. Adjuncts to dopamine replacement: a pragmatic approach to reducing the problem of dyskinesia in Parkinson's disease. *Mov Disord* 1998;13:871–876.
40. Grondin R, Bedard PJ, Hadj Tahar A, Gregoire L, Mori A, Kase H. Antiparkinsonian effect of a new selective adenosine A2A receptor antagonist in MPTP-treated monkeys. *Neurology* 1999;52:1673–1677.
41. Hauser RA, Hubble JP, Truong DD, Istradefylline US-001 Study Group. Randomized trial of the adenosine A (2A) receptor antagonist istradefylline in advanced PD. *Neurology* 2003;61:297–303.
42. Bibbiani F, Oh JD, Chase TN. Serotonin 5-HT1A agonist improves motor complications in rodent and primate parkinsonian models. *Neurology* 2001;57:1829–1834.
43. Olanow CW, Damier P, Goetz CG, Mueller T, Nutt J, Rascol O, Serbanescu A, Deckers F, Russ H. Multicenter, open-label, trial of sarizotan in Parkinson disease patients with levodopa-induced dyskinesias (the SPLENDID Study). *Clin Neuropharmacol* 2004;27:58–62.
44. Grondin R, Hadj Tahar A, Doan VD, Ladure P, Bedard PJ. Noradrenoceptor antagonism with idazoxan improves L-dopa-induced dyskinesias in MPTP monkeys. *Naunyn Schmiedebergs Arch Pharmacol* 2000;361:181–186.
45. Savola JM, Hill M, Engstrom M, Merivuori H, Wurster S, McGuire SG, Fox SH, Crossman AR, Brotchie JM. Fipamezole (JP-1730) is a potent alpha2 adrenergic receptor antagonist that reduces levodopa-induced dyskinesia in the MPTP-lesioned primate model of Parkinson's disease. *Mov Disord* 2003;18:872–883.
46. Manson AJ, Iakovidou E, Lees AJ. Idazoxan is ineffective for levodopa-induced dyskinesias in Parkinson's disease. *Mov Disord* 2000;15:336–337.
47. Fox S, Silverdale M, Kellett M, Davies R, Steiger M, Fletcher N, Crossman A, Brotchie J. Non-subtype-selective opioid receptor antagonism in treatment of levodopa-induced motor complications in Parkinson's disease. *Mov Disord* 2004;19:554–560.
48. Brotchie JM. CB1 cannabinoid receptor signalling in Parkinson's disease. *Curr Opin Pharmacol* 2003;3:54–61.
49. Nicholson SL, Brotchie JM. 5-hydroxytryptamine (5-HT, serotonin) and Parkinson's disease: opportunities for novel therapeutics to reduce the problems of levodopa therapy. *Eur J Neurol* 2002;9(suppl 3):1–6.
50. Emre M, Aarsland D, Albanese A, Byrne EJ, Deuschl G, De Deyn PP, Durif F, Kulisevsky J, van Laar T, Lees A, Poewe W, Robillard A, Rosa MM, Wolters E, Quarg P, Tekin S, Lane R. Rivastigmine for dementia associated with Parkinson's disease. *N Engl J Med* 2004;351:2547–2549.
51. Arnulf I, Bonnet AM, Damier P, Bejjani BP, Seilhean D, Derenne JP, Agid Y. Hallucinations, REM sleep, and Parkinson's disease: a medical hypothesis. *Neurology* 2000;55:281–288.
52. Pathak A, Senard JM. Pharmacology of orthostatic hypotension in Parkinson's disease: from pathophysiology to management. *Expert Rev Cardiovasc Ther* 2004;2:393–403.
53. Pollak P, Tison F, Rascol O, Destee A, Pere JJ, Senard JM, Durif F, Bourdeix I, on behalf of the French Clozapine Parkinson Study Group. Clozapine in drug induced psychosis in Parkinson's disease: a randomised, placebo controlled study with open follow up. *J Neurol Neurosurg Psychiatry* 2004:75:689–695.
54. Goetz CG, Blasucci LM, Leurgans S, Pappert EJ. Olanzapine and clozapine: comparative effects on motor function in hallucinating PD patients. *Neurology* 2000;55:789–794.

Dementia Associated with Parkinson's Disease: Features and Management

12

Murat Emre

INTRODUCTION

Cognitive aspects of Parkinson's disease (PD) have been largely ignored for many years. This is partly because of the original description that the senses and intellect remain intact, and also because of the short survival time of patients with PD in the past. Thanks to modern treatment, patients with PD have substantially prolonged survival times, with life expectancies close to their healthy peers, and we now understand that cognitive changes, especially dementia, are largely age-dependent phenomena. Thus, in the last few decades dementia associated with PD (PD-D) has been increasingly recognized and better understood. This chapter is devoted to description of epidemiological features, clinical characteristics, underlying neurochemical and neuropathological abnormalities, diagnosis, and treatment of dementia associated with PD.

EPIDEMIOLOGY

Both the prevalence and the incidence of dementia are substantially higher in patients with PD compared to age-matched controls. The *prevalence* figures for PD-D vary substantially across different studies, probably due to differences in study populations, assessment methods, diagnostic tools, and definition of dementia. A meta-analysis of 27 studies suggested a prevalence rate of 40% (1). Several large, cross-sectional, population-based studies have revealed comparable figures, ranging from 41% (2) to 28% (3). *Incidence* figures usually provide a more reliable estimate of frequency for chronic conditions, as they are relatively free of survival bias. The incidence rate of dementia among patients with PD was reported to be six times higher than in controls in a study with 5-year follow-up (4). The cumulative incidence of dementia in patients with PD was assessed in several prospective studies with a sizeable number of patients and lengthy follow-up times. In the majority of these studies, patients free of dementia at baseline were included and the occurrence of newly emerging dementia was assessed after a variable length of time. During 5-year follow-up, dementia was diagnosed in 62% of patients with PD, who were free of this condition at baseline, compared to 17% of controls (5). In a similar study, the cumulative incidence of dementia was 53% after 14 years (6). Finally, prospective follow-up of patients over 8 years, of whom 26% already had dementia at baseline, revealed a cumulative incidence of 78% (7).

A number of *risk factors* have been associated with PD-D, both in cross-sectional studies as associated features and in prospective studies as baseline characteristics predictive of incident dementia. An overview of these risk factors has been provided in a review (8). They include age at onset of PD and at entry to the study, severity of the motor disability, cognitive scores at baseline, confusion or psychosis while being treated with levodopa, early occurrence of drug-related hallucinations, symmetrical disease presentation, axial involvement such as speech impairment and postural imbalance, early occurrence of autonomic failure, unsatisfactory response to dopaminergic treatment, presence of depression, smoking, and excessive daytime sleepiness. Among cognitive features, poor verbal fluency at baseline was found to be significantly and independently associated with incident dementia. Similarly, the presence of subtle involvement of executive functions at baseline and poor performance on verbal memory were reported to predict dementia.

The role of age deserves special attention as it emerges as one of the most significant risk factors, both in cross-sectional and prospective studies: In a population-based study, the prevalence was zero in patients below the age of 50, but 69% above the age of 80 (2). Similarly in a group of patients entered in a prospective observational study, the prevalence after 5 years was 62% and 17% in patients whose disease had begun after or before the age of 70, respectively (5). The combination of old age and severe disease seems to be a particularly detrimental combination: Older patients with a high severity of motor symptoms at baseline had a 9.7 times increased risk of incident dementia, compared to younger patients with lower motor-symptom severity (9). Rapid eye movement (REM) sleep behavior disorder is frequently seen in patients with PD, and this may be even more the case in patients who eventually develop dementia. A close correlation between α-synuclein pathology and REM sleep behavior disorder (RBD) has been described, and a striking observation was that RBD preceded dementia or parkinsonism by a median of 10 years (10).

CLINICAL FEATURES

Theoretically, patients with PD can be afflicted by all types of etiologies that can cause dementia in the population at large, including other degenerative dementias such as Alzheimer's disease (AD). The clinical profile of dementia in such cases will be compatible with the underlying etiology. PD is, however, associated with a highly significant increase in the prevalence and incidence of dementia. This close association strongly suggests that the disease process itself also underlies the dementia syndrome accompanying PD, which has characteristic clinical features. These features can be best summarized as a dysexecutive syndrome with prominent impairment of attention, visuospatial functions, and accompanying behavioral symptoms (Table 12.1). Impairments in individual cognitive domains have been explored in a number of studies, and the extensive literature

TABLE 12.1
CLINICAL FEATURES OF DEMENTIA ASSOCIATED WITH PARKINSON'S DISEASE

Cognitive Features
  Attention: prominent impairment with fluctuations
  Memory: moderate impairment, retrieval deficits with relatively spared storage
  Executive functions: severely impaired
  Visuospatial functions: early and substantial impairment
  Language: impaired word finding and verbal fluency

Behavioral Features
  Apathy
  Hallucinations
  Delusions
  Depressive symptoms

Motor Features
  Symmetrical involvement
  Prominent postural instability and gait disorder
  Tremor dominance less frequent

can be found in two reviews (8,11). Several recent studies compared cognitive profiles in patients with PD-D, dementia with Lewy bodies (DLB) and AD. The results confirmed the similarities between PD-D and DLB, and differences between these two and AD (12–15). These features are summarized in the following paragraphs.

Impairment in *attentional functions* is an early and prominent feature of patients with PD-D. Similar to those with DLB, patients with PD-D have prominent fluctuations in attention and impairment in vigilance, compared to those with AD. Cognitive slowing (bradyphrenia) is more prominent in PD-D patients as compared to patients with AD, and patients with PD-D have longer response durations both in measures of simple and choice reaction time, suggesting that their central processing time is prolonged.

Deficits in *executive functions* (defined as the ability to plan, organize, and perform goal-directed behavior) is the core feature of dementia syndrome associated with PD. These deficits involve tasks requiring concept formation, rule finding, planning, problem solving, set elaboration, set shifting, and set maintenance. Patients have more difficulties with internally cued behavior, that is, when they have to develop their own internal strategies; their performance improves substantially when external cues are provided. Abnormalities in executive functions occur early in the course of PD-D and are prominent throughout the course.

All types of *memory* are impaired in PD-D, including working memory, explicit memory (both verbal and visual) and implicit memory, such as procedural learning. The severity and the profile of impairment, however, differ from the amnesia seen in AD. Patients with PD-D have been reported to have deficits in learning new information; however, these deficits are less severe than those seen in patients with AD. PD-D patients have impaired free recall, but their recognition is significantly better, implying that new information was stored but not readily accessed. Accordingly, when structured cues or multiple choices are provided, retrieval is facilitated. In fact memory scores in patients with PD-D were found to be correlated with executive function test scores, and it was suggested that the memory impairment may be due to difficulties in accessing of memory traces, reflecting a deficiency in internally cued search strategies, or impairment in the ability to generate encoding and retrieval strategies, both due to the dysexecutive syndrome. This is in contrast to the limbic-type memory disorder with abnormalities of storage and consequent deficits of recall, as well as recognition as the key neuropsychological feature in AD.

Early and prominent deficits in *visuospatial* function is another characteristic feature of PD-D. Tasks that require visuospatial analysis and orientation were found to be the most affected, suggesting that impairment in visual perception may be the core of the problem. Visuospatial abstraction and reasoning were found to be more impaired in patients with PD-D compared to patients with AD, whereas visuospatial memory tasks were substantially worse in patients with AD. Impairment becomes especially evident in more complex tasks that require planning and sequencing of response or self-generation of strategies so that deficits in visuomotor tasks may be due partly to problems in sequential organization of behavior and thus to deficits in executive functions.

Language, especially core language functions, were found to be less impaired in patients with PD-D compared to those with AD. Impaired verbal fluency is the main feature, and it was found to be more severe than that seen in patients with AD. Mild anomia (naming or word-finding difficulties) is frequent in the more advanced phases of PD-D, and other deficits include decreased information content of spontaneous speech and impaired comprehension of complex sentences, but these occur to a significantly lesser extent than that seen in patients with AD. The anomia typically progresses to a transcortical-type aphasia with disease progression. In contrast, aphasic-type language abnormalities are prominent early in AD and increase throughout the course of the illness. It was suggested that most of the language deficits, such as impaired verbal fluency and word finding difficulties, may not reflect a true involvement of language functions, but rather may be related to the dysexecutive syndrome, such as impairment of self-generated search strategies.

PD-D is associated with prominent *behavioral symptoms* and changes in personality. The most common neuropsychiatric symptoms are depression, hallucinations, delusions, apathy, and anxiety. Hallucinations and delusions commonly follow treatment with dopaminergic agents, and occur disproportionately frequently in patients with dementia. Visual hallucinations are common, and when minor forms such as feeling of presence were included, they were found in 70% of patients with PD as compared to 25% of those with AD (16). Likewise depressive features were found to be more common in patients with PD than in those with AD. A comparison of patients with PD-D and AD revealed that 83% of those with PD-D, compared to 95% with AD, had at least one psychiatric symptom: Hallucinations were more severe in PD-D, whereas increased psychomotor activity such as aberrant motor behavior, agitation, disinhibition, and irritability were more common in AD. In PD-D apathy was more common in mild stages, while delusions increased with more severe motor and cognitive dysfunction (17).

The *motor features* associated with PD-D were characterized by more symmetrical involvement. Bradykinesia, rigidity, and postural instability have been correlated with more rapid cognitive decline and dementia, whereas tremor dominance has been associated with relative preservation of mental status (18). In a cross-sectional study of motor features in PD, it was found that the postural instability gait disorder (PIGD) subtype was overrepresented in PD-D in contrast to nondemented PD patients (19). It was suggested that L-dopa responsiveness diminishes as cognitive impairment emerges and that proposed mechanisms for L-dopa refractoriness in patients with PD-D include intrinsic striatal α-synuclein pathology, loss of dopamine D2 and D3 receptors, or the emergence of more nondopaminergic features, such as postural instability (19).

NEUROCHEMICAL DEFICITS

The predominant neurochemical impairment in PD, nigrostriatal dopaminergic deficit, was initially assumed also to underlie the cognitive impairment. However, many with PD, especially young patients, may not show any cognitive impairment despite considerable motor dysfunction. In addition, clinical experience demonstrates that dementia does not improve with levodopa treatment, and levodopa may worsen behavioral and cognitive functions, especially in demented patients. These observations suggest that dopaminergic deficit is unlikely to play a major role in PD-D. It was proposed that some cognitive deficits may be due to dopaminergic dysfunction, especially early in the disease process, whereas dopaminergic stimulation may be detrimental in later stages (20). Several experimental findings support this hypothesis. For example, reduced 18F-fluorodopa uptake in the caudate nucleus and frontal cortex correlated with impairment in neuropsychological tests measuring verbal fluency, working memory, and attention, indicating that ascending dopaminergic projections may be involved in mediating some of the cognitive dysfunction in PD (21). Similarly, using fluorodopa and positron emission tomography (PET), a bilateral decline in the anterior cingulate area and ventral striatum, as well as in the right caudate nucleus was shown in PD patients with dementia, as compared to those without dementia, and an impaired mesolimbic and caudate dopaminergic function was suggested to be associated with PD-D (22). In another study, dopamine levels in neocortical areas were found to be decreased to a greater level in demented than in nondemented PD patients (23), suggesting some role for the degeneration of the mesocortical dopaminergic system in dementia.

Involvement of other ascending monoaminergic systems, namely noradrenergic and serotoninergic pathways, was also suggested to underlie cognitive impairment. Locus ceruleus is severely damaged in patients with PD, and both neuronal loss and noradrenaline depletion in locus ceruleus were found to be significantly more severe in demented PD patients (24). In addition, concentration of noradrenaline was reduced in the cerebral neocortex and hippocampus. Nevertheless, there was no difference between demented and nondemented patients (23). Likewise, neuronal loss in raphe nuclei and reduced serotonin concentrations in the striato-pallidal complex and in various cortical areas, notably in the hippocampus and the frontal cortex, were also described; there was, however, no difference between demented and nondemented PD patients (23).

There is substantial evidence that cholinergic deficits due to degeneration of the ascending cholinergic pathways may significantly contribute to cognitive impairment and dementia in patients with PD. Loss of cholinergic neurons in the nucleus basalis of Meynert (nbM) was described in PD-D, shortly after they were reported in AD (25). The extent of neuronal loss in the nbM was reported to be greater in patients with PD than in those with AD (26), and this loss was not associated with AD-type pathology in the cerebral cortex (27). In parallel to these morphological findings, biochemical deficits in the nbM and in the cerebral cortex were also described: Cholinacetyltransferase (ChAT) activity was found to be decreased in the frontal cortex and the nbM of patients with PD, and the decrease was greater in the frontal cortex of PD patients with dementia (28). Extensive reductions of ChAT and acetylcholinesterase (AChE) in all examined cortical areas were described, and ChAT reductions in the temporal neocortex were correlated with the degree of mental impairment, but not with the extent of plaque or tangle formation. In addition in PD, but not in AD, the decrease in neocortical ChAT correlated with the number of neurons in the nbM suggesting that primary degeneration of these cholinergic neurons may be related to declining cognitive function in PD (29). Reductions in ChAT activity were found to be more extensive in the neocortical (especially temporal) region than in the archicortical region. In a comparative study of various pathological and chemical indices, only presynaptic cholinergic markers (including the number of neurons in the nbM) were related to dementia in PD (30). In a comparative study of patients with AD, DLB and PD mean midfrontal ChAT activity was found to be markedly reduced in PD and DLB, compared to normal controls and AD: The activity was reduced to almost 20% of controls in

DLB and PD, whereas in AD it was reduced to 50% of the activity in normals (31). Imaging studies of cortical cholinergic function using PET revealed similar findings: Compared with controls, mean cortical AChE activity was lowest in patients with PD-D (–20%), followed by patients with PD without dementia (–13%) and patients with AD (–9%) (32). These and other studies indicate that the severity of cholinergic deficiency is greater in PD-D than in AD and that these deficits may occur earlier in the clinical course of PD-D. In addition PD-D is associated with neuronal loss also in the pedinculopontine cholinergic pathways that project to structures such as the thalamus (33). Another important finding is that nicotinic receptor binding was found to be reduced in striatum in patients with PD, suggesting a reduced risk of parkinsonism with cholinergic treatment through stimulation of striatal cholinergic receptors (34).

Although the strongest evidence indicates that cholinergic deficits are associated with dementia, it was suggested that impairment in other neurotransmitter systems can also contribute to behavioral and cognitive symptoms. Thus, dopaminergic deficits may partly be responsible for dysexecutive syndrome, cholinergic deficits for impairments in memory, attention and frontal dysfunction, whereas noradrenergic deficits may contribute to impaired attention and serotoninergic deficits to depressive mood (11).

NEUROPATHOLOGY

The site and the type of pathology underlying dementia associated with PD have been somewhat controversial. Three types of pathologies have been suggested, including pathology in subcortical structures, notably dopaminergic cell loss in the medial substantia nigra (SN), co-incident Alzheimer-type pathology and Lewy body (LB) type pathology in limbic and cortical areas.

Dopaminergic cell loss was suggested to underlie dementia in PD by several groups (35,36), which found that cellular loss in the medial part of the SN correlated with dementia, and this correlation was still significant after accounting for amyloid burden (35). A comparison of neuronal loss in the SN of demented and nondemented patients, by others, however, showed no difference and no correlation with dementia (37). Recently, another subcortical structure was proposed as a potential site of pathology. Components of thalamus assigned to the limbic loop were found to be most severely affected by PD-related pathology (LBs and Lewy neurites), compared to a mild pathology in other thalamic nuclei, and it was suggested that damage to the thalamic components of the limbic loop nuclei may also contribute to cognitive, emotional, and autonomic symptoms in patients with PD (33).

Alzheimer-type pathology has been suggested as either the cause of or associated with dementia in PD in a number of studies from the early 1980s onward (38). These studies have been extensively reviewed in two articles (39,40). In fact, senile plaques seem to be present in most cases with advanced dementia and demonstrate high specificity, but they are absent in many cases with cognitive impairment and have low sensitivity (41). An interesting finding is the significant correlation between neocortical LB counts and senile plaques, as well as neurofibrillary tangles, suggesting either common origins for these pathologies or that one may trigger the other (39).

The contribution of AD-type pathology to dementia in PD has been challenged by recent studies in which both AD-type and LB-type pathology have been evaluated in parallel. As a result of these studies, cortical and/or limbic LB-type degeneration has been suggested increasingly to be the main pathology underlying dementia in PD, as first proposed by Kosaka et al. (42). The growing body of evidence supporting this suggestion was provided by studies using α-synuclein antibodies to identify LBs, a more sensitive method than the conventional ubiquitin staining. In four studies using this method, and assessing both AD-type and LB-type pathology, a similar conclusion was reached in all: α-Synuclein-positive neocortical or limbic LBs were found to be associated with cognitive impairment, independent of AD-type pathology (39,41,43,44), and the presence of LBs in the cortex or limbic areas showed the highest correlation with the occurrence of dementia. Another strong evidence that LB-type pathology alone can induce dementia was provided by recent genetic studies. Patients with familial PD with a triplication of the α-synuclein gene seem to develop dementia, whereas those with duplication do not, or do so rarely (45–48). Thus, the type and the severity of the neurodegenerative phenotype may be related to the dose of the α-synuclein gene and consequent quantitative variation in the levels of the α-synuclein protein, the main component of LBs. The presence of limbic or cortical LBs, however, may not always be associated with dementia in patients with PD (49). Therefore, not only the presence but also the topography and burden of LBs may be crucial for the development of dementia.

It was suggested recently that pathological changes in PD follow an ascending order, sequentially involving cerebral structures as the disease advances. This temporospatial pattern may provide a plausible explanation for the late emergence of dementia in the course of PD (50). It is described that the initial lesions in PD occur in certain, susceptible brainstem and anterior olfactory nuclei, less vulnerable nuclear grays, and cortical areas gradually become affected thereafter. The disease process in the brainstem seems to pursue an ascending course, ensuing cortical involvement beginning with the anteromedial temporal mesocortex and then spreading to the neocortex, commencing with high-order sensory association and prefrontal areas, structures that are involved in cognitive functions. This ascending order of pathological changes from brainstem to limbic and neocortical areas may explain why dementia usually develops relatively late in classical PD.

In summary, and on the basis of recent studies, the main pathological change underlying dementia in PD is suggested to be the LB-type degeneration in the cerebral cortex and limbic structures. AD-type pathology seems to be present frequently, but correlates less well with dementia.

GENETIC ASPECTS

There are rare forms of familial PD with dementia. Altered expression of or missense mutations in the α-synuclein gene have been linked to early-onset familial PD, sometimes associated with dementia. As described, the likelihood of dementia was found to be associated with an increase in the additional copies of the gene: Dementia has not been reported in families with duplication of the gene, whereas triplication has been associated with dementia (45–48). The additional copies of the α-synuclein gene result in an excess of the wild-type protein, indicating that the magnitude of increase in the expression of α-synuclein, the major component of Lewy bodies, is important for the development of dementia.

The ApoE4 genotype has been associated with an increased risk of AD. A systematic review and meta-analysis of results from case-control studies reporting ApoE genotype frequencies in PD revealed that, unlike AD, for which the ApoE4 allele increases the prevalence and the ApoE2 allele is protective, the ApoE2 allele, but not the ApoE4 allele, was found to be positively associated with sporadic PD (51). The ApoE2 allele also seems to increase the likelihood of dementia in patients with PD; the risk of dementia for ApoE4 carriers was not any different for persons with or without PD (52).

NEUROIMAGING

Structural and functional imaging studies suggested several features associated with PD-D. None of these features, however, has been specific or sensitive enough to be relied on in routine clinical practice.

In *structural imaging* studies, the presence of dementia in patients with PD was not found to be associated with any specific pattern of structural MRI abnormalities (53). Recently, however, it was suggested that in MRI, temporal lobe atrophy including the hippocampus and the parahippocampal gyrus is more severe in AD patients, whereas there is more severe atrophy of the thalamus and occipital lobe in PD-D (54).

Functional imaging studies have been performed using different methods. Perfusion deficits in single-photon emission computed tomography (SPECT) have been consistently reported in patients with PD-D. Although the reports have been variable, the most consistent findings were temporoparietal perfusion deficits in patients with

PD-D, as compared to those without dementia, in some studies also involving frontal and occipital areas. In a review of SPECT studies performed in PD patients, Bissessur and coworkers (55) reached a similar conclusion: in PD-D, rCBF assessments often demonstrate frontal hypoperfusion or bilateral temporoparietal deficits. Recently, perfusion deficits in precuneus and inferior lateral parietal regions, areas associated with visual processing, were described in patients with PD-D, whereas patients with AD showed a perfusion deficit in the midline parietal region, in a more anterior and inferior location (56). More severe abnormalities in temporoparietal regions of demented PD patients, compared to those without dementia, were also observed with fluorodeoxyglucose PET (FDG-PET) studies, in some studies also including frontal association cortices, the posterior cingulate cortex, or the visual cortex (57).

Using a marker of dopamine transport (which is located on presynaptic dopaminergic terminals), FP-CIT and SPECT, patients with PD, PD-D, and DLB were found to have significant reductions in FP-CIT binding in the caudate and the anterior and posterior putamens compared to patients with AD and controls. Transporter loss in DLB was of similar magnitude to that seen in PD, and the greatest loss in all three areas was seen in patients with PD-D (58). This method can be useful to differentiate patients with PD-D from those with AD, when there is doubt on clinical grounds.

Iodine-123 meta-iodobenzylguanidine (^{123}I-MIBG) is an analog of noradrenaline and may be used in conjunction with SPECT imaging to quantify postganglionic sympathetic cardiac innervation. The heart-to-mediastinum ratio (H/M ratio) is lower in PD than in other akinetic-rigid syndromes and normal controls. In complex cases cardiac ^{123}I-MIBG can be used to distinguish between DLB, PD-D, and AD; patients with PD or DLB have reduced H/M ratios, whereas in AD tracer uptake is normal (59).

DIAGNOSIS OF PD-D

The diagnostic process in patients with PD and suspected dementia can be subsumed into two main steps: first, the diagnosis of the dementia syndrome itself, i.e., differentiating it from conditions mimicking dementia; second, the differential diagnosis as to the etiology of dementia, i.e., if the dementia is due to the neurodegenerative process associated with PD or if it involves other etiologies such as vascular disease (Table 12.2).

The diagnosis of dementia in patients with PD may be confounded by several factors. First, the apparent impairment in certain cognitive domains, such as language, may be difficult to differentiate from the consequences of motor dysfunction. Second, it may be difficult to decide if impairment in activities of daily living, a necessary criteria for the diagnosis of dementia, is due to cognitive or motor dysfunction. Adverse effects of drugs can also complicate the

TABLE 12.2
DIAGNOSTIC PROCESS IN DEMENTIA ASSOCIATED WITH PARKINSON'S DISEASE

Diagnosis of Dementia Syndrome
    Exclude co-morbid depression
    Exclude confusion (systemic, metabolic disorders)
    Exclude adverse effects of drugs

Differential Diagnosis
    Other degenerative diseases presenting with
        parkinsonism and dementia
    Co-incident degenerative dementias, such as AD
    Symptomatic dementias
        Intracranial causes, such as vascular dementia,
            tumors, normal pressure hydrocephalus (NPH)
        Extracranial systemic disorders, such as thyroid
            disease

diagnostic process. Along with a detailed history, especially elucidating the onset, course, pattern, and chronology of the cognitive and behavioral symptoms, it is important to administer appropriate neuropsychological and neuropsychiatric test batteries, which include tests sensitive to executive dysfunction and which can also differentiate the types of deficits in certain cognitive domains, e.g., storage versus retrieval deficit in memory performance.

The differential diagnosis of dementia syndrome includes cognitive impairments associated with the disease but not extensive and severe enough to qualify for dementia, co-morbid depression, confusional states secondary to systemic or metabolic disorders, and adverse effects of drugs. Once a dementia syndrome is diagnosed, the differential diagnosis with regard to the etiology includes other primary degenerative dementing disorders associated with extrapyramidal features (such as progressive supranuclear palsy, corticobasal degeneration, dementia with Lewy bodies), other co-incident neurodegenerative dementias such as AD, and symptomatic forms of dementia due either to intracranial pathologies (e.g., cerebrovascular disease, tumors, normal pressure hydrocephalus) or to extracranial systemic disorders, including reversible dementias, e.g., thyroid dysfunction.

TREATMENT

Based on substantial deficits in cholinergic markers in PD-D, cholinesterase inhibitors (ChE-I) have been investigated in this patient population. There was an initial hesitation to use these drugs in PD-D because of the fear that motor functions may worsen. Following a small, open study with tacrine that described improvement in cognition and no worsening in motor functions in patients with PD and cognitive impairment, a number of studies have been reported with all commercially available ChE-I. These include 2 open studies with tacrine, 7 studies (1 case series, 3 open, and 3 double-blind, placebo-controlled studies) with donepezil, 1 open study with galantamine, and 3 open and 1 large randomized, placebo-controlled study with rivastigmine. These studies, except for the latter, were summarized in a review (60). Although the majority of them were open and all of them were small, involving fewer than 30 patients, the conclusions were similar. There was an improvement in cognition in almost all studies, behavioral symptoms improved in most where they were measured, and motor symptoms did not worsen except in a few patients with worsening tremor under galantamine and worsening of motor functions in some patients under donepezil during long-term treatment. It was also suggested that an abrupt withdrawal of ChE-I in patients with PD-D or DLB should be avoided, which may produce acute cognitive and behavioral decline.

Recently, the first large, randomized, controlled, multi-center study ever conducted with a ChE-I in PD-D was published (61). In this study, which included 541 patients, both primary efficacy endpoints (ADAS-cog as a composite scale of cognition, and CGIC as a scale of change in overall status) showed statistically significant improvements in favor of rivastigmine. Likewise, on all secondary efficacy parameters, there were statistically significant differences in favor of rivastigmine: Neuropsychiatric symptoms as measured with the Neuropsychiatric Inventory showed an improvement on rivastigmine and no change from baseline on placebo, power of attention improved on rivastigmine and worsened on placebo, improvement from baseline was also seen on the Ten Point Clock Drawing test, verbal fluency test, and MMSE on rivastigmine, whereas patients receiving placebo worsened on these scales as compared to the baseline. On the Activities of Daily Living (ADL) scale, patients on rivastigmine showed a minimal worsening, whereas those on placebo had significantly more deterioration. The main adverse events were cholinergic in nature, with nausea and vomiting being the most frequent. Worsening of parkinsonian symptoms was more frequently reported as an adverse event on rivastigmine (27.3% vs 15.6% on placebo), mainly driven by worsening of tremor (10.2% on rivastigmine vs 3.9% on placebo), which was rarely severe: 1.7% of patients discontinued treatment because of worsening tremor. The objective measures of motor symptoms, on the other hand, as assessed by the United Parkinson's Disease Rating Scale (UPDRS), part III, did not reveal any significant differences or trends between the two treatments.

PD-D is frequently associated with psychotic symptoms. These symptoms may improve under treatment with ChE-I, but at times they may necessitate treatment with neuroleptics. Classical neuroleptics are contraindicated, as they may worsen motor function. There have been attempts to treat psychosis in PD with atypical neuroleptics. Randomized, placebo-controlled studies showing significant improvement of psychosis without worsening motor symptoms exist only for clozapine (62,63). Placebo-controlled, randomized trials with olanzapine revealed that it did not significantly improve psychosis but significantly worsened motor function (64). Although not investigated in placebo-controlled trials, risperidone also worsens motor function in patients with PD (65). Large, randomized, controlled studies are lacking for quetiapine; a comparative trial against clozapine suggested that quetiapine may improve psychosis in patients with PD without worsening parkinsonism (66). Thus, on the basis of current data, clozapine and possibly quetiapine should be given the priority in treating psychosis in patients with PD-D.

CONCLUSIONS

PD is frequently associated with dementia, affecting up to 40% of patients in cross-sectional studies and up to 78% in longitudinal studies. The main risk factors are advanced age, severe motor symptoms, and presence of mild cognitive deficits, such as reduced verbal fluency. The clinical presentation can be summarized as a dysexecutive syndrome, and the main features are impaired attention with fluctuations, impairment of executive functions, retrieval-type memory impairment and deficits in visuospatial functions with largely preserved language, except for reduced verbal fluency. Behavioral symptoms such as apathy, hallucinations, and delusions are frequent. The most prominent neurochemical deficit seems to be cholinergic. Dementia correlates best with LB pathology in limbic and cortical areas. There is strong evidence that ChE-I can be beneficial in the treatment of patients with PD-D.

REFERENCES

1. Cummings JL. Intellectual impairment in Parkinson's disease: clinical, pathologic, and biochemical correlates. *J Geriatr Psychiatry Neurol* 1988;1:24–36.
2. Mayeux R, Denaro J, Hemenegildo N, et al. A population-based investigation of Parkinson's disease with and without dementia: relationship to age and gender. *Arch Neurol* 1992;49:492–497.
3. Aarsland D, Tandberg E, Larsen JP, Cummings JL. Frequency of dementia in Parkinson disease. *Arch Neurol* 1996;53:538–542.
4. Aarsland D, Andersen K, Larsen JP, Lolk A, Nielsen H, Kragh-Sorensen P. Risk of dementia in Parkinson's disease: a community-based, prospective study. *Neurology* 2001;56:730–736.
5. Reid WG, Hely MA, Morris JG, et al. A longitudinal study of Parkinson's disease: clinical and neuropsychological correlates of dementia. *J Clin Neurosci* 1996;3:327–333.
6. Read N, Hughes TA, Dunn EM, et al. Dementia in Parkinson's disease: incidence and associated factors at 14 years of follow up. *Parkinsonism and Related Disorders* 2001;7(suppl):S109.
7. Aarsland D, Andersen K, Larsen JP, et al. Prevalence and characteristics of dementia in Parkinson disease: an 8-year prospective study. *Arch Neurol* 2003; 60:387–392.
8. Emre M. Dementia associated with Parkinson's disease. *Lancet Neurology* 2003;2:229–237.
9. Levy G, Schupf N, Tang MX, et al. Combined effect of age and severity on the risk of dementia in Parkinson's disease. *Ann Neurol* 2002;51:722–729.

10. Boeve BF, Silber MH, Parisi JE, et al. Synucleinopathy pathology and REM sleep behavior disorder plus dementia or parkinsonism. *Neurology* 2003;61:40–45.

11. Pillon B, Boller F, Levy R, Dubois B. Cognitive deficits and dementia in Parkinson's disease. In: Boller F, Cappa S, eds. *Handbook of Neuropsychology.* 2nd ed. Amsterdam: Elsevier Sciences B.V.; 2001:311–371.

12. Cahn-Weiner DA, Grace J, Ott BR, et al. Cognitive and behavioral features discriminate between Alzheimer's and Parkinson's disease. *Neuropsychiatry Neuropsychol Behav Neurol* 2002;15:79–87.

13. Aarsland D, Litvan I, Salmon D, et al. Performance on the dementia rating scale in Parkinson's disease with dementia and dementia with Lewy bodies: comparison with progressive supranuclear palsy and Alzheimer's disease. *J Neurol Neurosurg Psychiatry* 2003;74:1215–1220.

14. Noe E, Marder K, Bell KL, et al. Comparison of dementia with Lewy bodies to Alzheimer's disease and Parkinson's disease with dementia. *Mov Disord* 2004;19:60–67.

15. Mosimann UP, Mather G, Wesnes KA, et al. Visual perception in Parkinson's disease dementia and dementia with Lewy bodies. *Neurology* 2004; 63:2091–2096.

16. Fenelon G, Mahieux F, Huon R, Ziegler M. Hallucinations in Parkinson's disease: prevalence, phenomenology and risk factors. *Brain* 2000;123:733–745.

17. Aarsland D, Cummings JL, Larsen JP. Neuropsychiatric differences between Parkinson's disease with dementia and Alzheimer's disease. *Int J Geriatr Psychiatry* 2001;16:184–191.

18. Foltynie T, Brayne C, Barker RA. The heterogeneity of idiopathic Parkinson's disease. *J Neurol* 2002;249:138–145.

19. Burn DJ, Rowan EN, Minett T, et al. Extrapyramidal features in Parkinson's disease with and without dementia and dementia with Lewy bodies: a cross-sectional comparative study. *Mov Disord* 2003;18:884–889.

20. Kulisevsky J. Role of dopamine in learning and memory: implications for the treatment of cognitive dysfunction in patients with Parkinson's disease. *Drugs Aging* 2000;16:365–379.

21. Rinne JO, Portin R, Ruottinen H, et al. Cognitive impairment and the brain dopaminergic system in Parkinson disease: 18F-fluorodopa positron emission tomographic study. *Arch Neurol* 2000;57:470–475.

22. Ito K, Nagano-Saito A, Kato T, et al. Striatal and extrastriatal dysfunction in Parkinson's disease with dementia: a 6-[18 F] fluoro-L-dopa PET study. *Brain* 2002;125:1358–1365.

23. Scatton B, Javoy-Agid F, Rouquier L, et al. Reduction of cortical dopamine, noradrenaline, serotonin and their metabolites in Parkinson's disease. *Brain Res* 1983;275:321–328.

24. Cash R, Dennis T, L'Heureux R, et al. Parkinson's disease and dementia: norepinephrine and dopamine in locus ceruleus. *Neurology* 1987;37:42–46.

25. Whitehouse PJ, Hedreen JC, White CL III, Price DL. Basal forebrain neurons in the dementia of Parkinson disease. *Ann Neurol* 1983;13:243–248.

26. Candy JM, Perry RH, Perry EK, et al. Pathological changes in the nucleus of Meynert in Alzheimer's and Parkinson's diseases. *J Neurol Sci* 1983;59:277–289.

27. Nakano I, Hirano A. Parkinson's disease: neuron loss in the nucleus basalis without concomitant Alzheimer's disease. *Ann Neurol* 1984;15:415–418.

28. Dubois B, Ruberg M, Javoy-Agid F, et al. A subcortico-cortical cholinergic system is affected in Parkinson's disease. *Brain Res* 1983;288:213–218.

29. Perry EK, Curtis M, Dick DJ, et al. Cholinergic correlates of cognitive impairment in Parkinson's disease: comparisons with Alzheimer's disease. *J Neurol Neurosurg Psychiatry* 1985;48:413 421.

30. Perry RH, Perry EK, Smith CJ, et al. Cortical neuropathological and neurochemical substrates of Alzheimer's and Parkinson's diseases. *J Neural Transm Suppl* 1987;24:131–136.

31. Tiraboschi P, Hansen LA, Alford M, et al. Cholinergic dysfunction in diseases with Lewy bodies. *Neurology* 2000;54:407–411.

32. Bohnen NI, Kaufer DI, Ivanco LS, et al. Cortical cholinergic function is more severely affected in parkinsonian dementia than in Alzheimer disease: an in vivo positron emission tomographic study. *Arch Neurol* 2003;60:1745–1748.

33. Rub U, Del Tredici K, Schultz C, et al. Parkinson's disease: the thalamic components of the limbic loop are severely impaired by alpha-synuclein immunopositive inclusion body pathology. *Neurobiol Aging* 2002;23:245–254.

34. Pimlott SL, Piggott M, Owens J, et al. Nicotinic acetylcholine receptor distribution in Alzheimer's disease, dementia with Lewy bodies, Parkinson's disease, and vascular dementia: in vitro binding study using 5-[(125)i]-a-85380. *Neuropsychopharmacology* 2004;29:108–116.

35. Rinne JO, Rummukainen J, Paljarvi L, Rinne UK. Dementia in Parkinson's disease is related to neuronal loss in the medial substantia nigra. *Ann Neurol* 1989;26:47–50.

36. Jellinger KA, Paulus W. Clinico-pathological correlations in Parkinson's disease. *Clin Neurol Neurosurg* 1992;94(suppl): S86–S88.

37. Gaspar P, Gray F. Dementia in idiopathic Parkinson's disease. A neuropathological study of 32 cases. *Acta Neuropathol* (Berl) 1984;64:43–52.

38. Boller F, Mizutani T, Roessmann U, Gambetti P. Parkinson disease, dementia, and Alzheimer disease: clinicopathological correlations. *Ann Neurol* 1980;7:329–335.

39. Apaydin H, Ahlskog JE, Parisi JE, et al. Parkinson disease neuropathology: later-developing dementia and loss of the levodopa response. *Arch Neurol* 2002;59:102–112.

40. Emre M. What causes mental dysfunction in Parkinson's disease? *Mov Disord* 2003;18(suppl 6):S63–S71.

41. Hurtig HI, Trojanowski JQ, Galvin J, et al. Alpha-synuclein cortical Lewy bodies correlate with dementia in Parkinson's disease. *Neurology* 2000;54:1916–1921.

42. Kosaka K, Tsuchiya K, Yoshimura M. Lewy body disease with and without dementia: a clinicopathological study of 35 cases. *Clin Neuropathol* 1988;7:299–305.

43. Mattila PM, Rinne JO, Helenius H, et al. Alpha-synuclein-immunoreactive cortical Lewy bodies are associated with cognitive impairment in Parkinson's disease. *Acta Neuropathol (Berl)* 2000;100:285–290.

44. Kovari E, Gold G, Herrmann FR, et al. Lewy body densities in the entorhinal and anterior cingulate cortex predict cognitive deficits in Parkinson's disease. *Acta Neuropathol (Berl)*. 2003;106:83–88.

45. Singleton AB, Farrer M, Johnson J, et al. Alpha-synuclein locus triplication causes Parkinson's disease. *Science* 2003;302:841.

46. Chartier-Harlin MC, Kachergus J, Roumier C, et al. Alpha-synuclein locus duplication as a cause of familial Parkinson's disease. *Lancet* 2004;364:1167–1169.

47. Farrer M, Kachergus J, Forno L, et al. Comparison of kindreds with parkinsonism and alpha-synuclein genomic multiplications. *Ann Neurol* 2004;55:174–179.

48. Ibáñez P, Bonnet AM, Debarges B, et al. Causal relation between alpha-synuclein gene duplication and familial Parkinson's disease. *Lancet* 2004;364:1169–1171.

49. Colosimo C, Hughes AJ, Kilford L, Lees AJ. Lewy body cortical involvement may not always predict dementia in Parkinson's disease. *J Neurol Neurosurg Psychiatry* 2003;74:852–856.

50. Braak H, Del Tredici K, Rub U, et al. Staging of brain pathology related to sporadic Parkinson's disease. *Neurobiol Aging* 2003;24: 197–211.

51. Huang X, Chen PC, Poole C. APOE-epsilon2 allele associated with higher prevalence of sporadic Parkinson disease. *Neurology* 2004;62:2198–2202.

52. Harhangi BS, de Rijk MC, van Duijn CM, et al. APOE and the risk of PD with or without dementia in a population-based study. *Neurology* 2000;54:1272–1276.

53. Huber SJ, Shuttleworth EC, Christy JA, et al. Magnetic resonance imaging in dementia of Parkinson's disease. *J Neurol Neurosurg Psychiatry* 1989;52:1221–1227.

54. Burton EJ, McKeith IG, Burn DJ, et al. Cerebral atrophy in Parkinson's disease with and without dementia: a comparison with Alzheimer's disease, dementia with Lewy bodies and controls. *Brain* 2004;127:791–800.

55. Bissessur S, Tissingh G, Wolters EC, Scheltens P. rCBF SPECT in Parkinson's disease patients with mental dysfunction. *J Neural Transm Suppl* 1997;50:25–30.

56. Firbank MJ, Colloby SJ, Burn DJ, et al. Regional cerebral blood flow in Parkinson's disease with and without dementia. *Neuroimage* 2003;20:1309–1319.

57. Vander Borght T, Minoshima S, Giordani B, et al. Cerebral metabolic differences in Parkinson's and Alzheimer's diseases matched for dementia severity. *J Nucl Med* 1997;38:797–802.

58. O'Brien JT, Colloby S, Fenwick J, et al. Dopamine transporter loss visualized with FP-CIT SPECT in the differential diagnosis of dementia with Lewy bodies. *Arch Neurol* 2004; 61:919–925.

59. Yoshita M, Taki J, Yamada M. A clinical role for [(123)I]MIBG myocardial scintigraphy in the distinction between dementia of the Alzheimer's type and dementia with Lewy bodies. *J Neurol Neurosurg Psychiatry* 2001;71:583–588.

60. Aarsland D, Mosimann UP, McKeith IG. Role of cholinesterase inhibitors in Parkinson's disease and Dementia with Lewy bodies. *J Geriatr Psychiatry Neurol* 2004;17:164–171.

61. Emre M, Aarsland D, Albanese A, et al. Rivastigmine for dementia associated with Parkinson's disease. *N Engl J Med* 2004;351: 2509–2518.

62. The Parkinson Study Group. Low-dose clozapine for the treatment of drug-induced psychosis in Parkinson's disease. *N Engl J Med* 1999;340:757–763.

63. The French Clozapine Parkinson Study Group. Clozapine in drug-induced psychosis in Parkinson's disease. *Lancet* 1999;353: 2041–2042.

64. Ondo WG, Levy JK, Vuong KD, Hunter C, Jankovic J. Olanzapine treatment for dopaminergic-induced hallucinations. *Mov Disord* 2002;17:1031–1035.

65. Friedman JH, Fernandez HH. Atypical antipsychotics in Parkinson-sensitive populations. *J Geriatr Psychiatry Neurol* 2002;15:156–70.

66. Morgante L, Epifanio A, Spina E, et al. Quetiapine and clozapine in parkinsonian patients with dopaminergic psychosis. *Clin Neuropharmacol* 2004;27:153–156.

Progressive Supranuclear Palsy

13

Lawrence I. Golbe

INTRODUCTION

Until recently, clinical recognition and scientific understanding of progressive supranuclear palsy (PSP) were hindered by the rarity of the condition, its frequent clinical misdiagnosis as Parkinson's disease (PD) and its frequent pathologic misdiagnosis as postencephalitic parkinsonism. Patients lacked useful prognostic and management advice and research was slowed by an insufficiency of accurately diagnosed subjects. Now, six decades after its defining clinicopathologic description (1), these constraints have largely yielded to improvements in clinical recognition and scientific understanding of PSP. The results are that international lay advocacy and support organizations have formed, brain banks have collected hundreds of diagnostically confirmed specimens for the use of researchers, genetic clues to etiology have emerged, and multiple animal models have been developed.

CLINICAL PHENOMENOLOGY

Motor Features

In its early phases, PSP shares bradykinesia, lead-pipe rigidity, facial hypomimia, hypophonia, and postural instability with the other parkinsonian disorders. However, by the time PSP reaches its fully developed, middle stages, its distinctive features will not elude the experienced clinician. At this point, PSP is unique in its combination of severe vertical gaze limitation, hypometric saccades, poor visual fixation with square-wave jerks, tonic contraction of facial muscles with deep nasolabial folds, spastic and/or ataxic dysarthria, prominent pharyngeal dysphagia, postural

instability disproportionate to other parkinsonian signs, and nuchal rigidity disproportionate to limb rigidity, often with erect or retroflexed posture. Other important points that help the clinician distinguish PSP from PD but not from most of the other parkinsonian disorders are its minimal response to dopaminergic medication, near absence of rest tremor, and relatively symmetric motor picture (Table 13.1). Examples of the typical PSP appear in Figure 13.1.

Recognizing the early, subtle, or atypical patient with PSP is more challenging. A helpful clue is postural instability with falls unrelated to obstacles as the initial manifestation. This occurs as the first symptom in approximately 60% of patients in most series (2). The initial or only gait abnormality may be severe gait "freezing" or "apraxia" (3) with no rigidity. By the time of diagnosis, which occurs a mean of approximately 4 years after symptom onset, postural instability is present in nearly all patients (4). In PD, gait disturbance is present in only 11% of patients at presentation, and falls at that point are rare.

The next most common symptoms at PSP presentation are dysarthria and behavioral changes. The former usually begins as nonspecific hypophonia, as in PD, but soon acquires spastic and/or ataxic qualities (5) (Table 13.2). Dysphagia, a major cause of morbidity and mortality in PSP, typically develops later and is present in only 18% of patients within the first 2 years (2). The first behavioral changes tend toward social withdrawal and apathy but also may include irritability and may later expand into the frontal dementia typical of advanced PSP (6). The characteristic downgaze paresis appears relatively late in the course, but for all too many clinicians it is the first clue to the diagnosis.

Rest tremor occurs in 5%–10% of patients, usually early in the course (7). Action or postural tremor occurs in about 25%. The limb rigidity and distal bradykinesia are mild

TABLE 13.1

CLINICAL FEATURES DIFFERENTIATING PROGRESSIVE SUPRANUCLEAR PALSY FROM OTHER MAJOR PARKINSONIAN DISORDERS

	PSP	PD	MSA-P	CBD	MIP
Motor symmetry	+++	+	+++	-	+/-
Axial rigidity	+++	++	++	++	-
Limb dystonia	+	+	+	+++	+/-
Pyramidal signs	+	-	++	+++	++
Apraxia	+	-	-	+++	+
Postural instability	+++	++	++	+	++
Vertical supranuclear gaze restriction	+++	+	++	++	+
Frontal behavior	+++	+	+	++	+
Dysautonomia	-	+	++	-	-
Levodopa response early in course	+	+++	+		-
Levodopa response late in course	-	++	+	-	-
Asymmetric cortical atrophy on MRI	-	-	-	++	+/-

PD, Parkinson's disease; MSA-P, multiple system atrophy of the parkinsonian type; CBD, corticobasal degeneration; MIP, multi-infarct parkinsonism; MRI, magnetic resonance imaging; -, absent or rare; +, occasional, mild, or late; ++, usual, moderate; +++; usual, severe, or early.

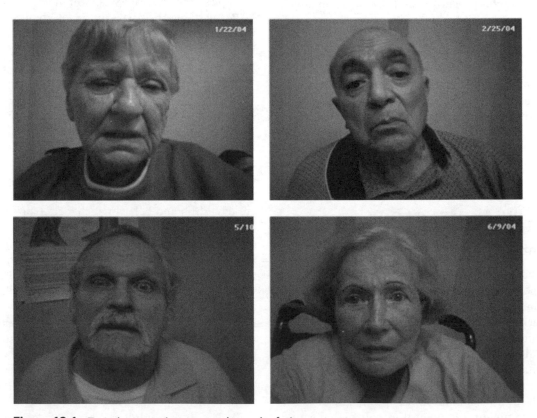

Figure 13.1 Typical progressive supranuclear palsy facies.

TABLE 13.2
COMPONENTS OF DYSARTHRIA IN PROGRESSIVE SUPRANUCLEAR PALSY AND SOME RELATED CONDITIONS

	Hypokinesia	Ataxia	Spasticity
PSP	++	+	+++
PD	+++	-	-
MSA-P	+++	++	+
MSA-C	+	+++	++

PD, Parkinson's disease; MSA-P, multiple system atrophy of the parkinsonian type; MSA-C, multiple system atrophy of the cerebellar type; -, absent or rare; +, occasional, mild, or late; ++; usual, moderate; +++, usual, severe, or early.

relative to axial rigidity. Apraxia and limb dystonia occur in a minority of patients and are milder and less asymmetric than in corticobasal degeneration (CBD) (8).

Eye Movements

The loss of range of downgaze, while relatively specific for PSP, is frequently absent until late in the course and is, in fact, often exceeded by the loss of upgaze. Voluntary gaze without a specific target (i.e., "look down") is usually more difficult than command gaze to a target, which is more difficult than pursuit versions, and reflex gaze is the least and last affected (Table 13.3).

Before gaze amplitude is affected, subtle clues in the ocular examination without the aid of specialized equipment will often suggest a diagnosis of early PSP. These signs include delay in saccade initiation, slowing of vertical saccades (9), saccadic pursuit, breakdown of opticokinetic nystagmus in the vertical plane, disordered Bell's phenomenon, poor convergence, and subtle square-wave jerks (SWJs) evident only during fixation on a distant penlight in a dark room (10,12). The last finding has close to 100% sensitivity (12,13) but low specificity, as SWJs occur commonly in multiple systemic atrophy (MSA) and other cerebellar conditions, and occasionally in PD (13).

The frontal defect impairs the antisaccade task, where the patient is instructed to direct his or her gaze quickly to the examiner's hand that does *not* wave. An altitudinal visual attentional deficit (14) arising from damaged tectal centers may contribute to overloading the fork, poor aim of the urinary stream, poor attention to dress, and apathy for the severity of postural instability.

Another sensitive but nonspecific eye sign is loss of the ability to suppress voluntarily the nystagmus caused by the vestibulo-ocular reflex (VOR) (15). This may be tested in a patient seated in a swivel chair with hands clasped and arms extended, attempting to maintain fixation on one extended thumb as the examiner slowly rotates the chair and patient as a unit.

Eyelid levator inhibition, lid closure inhibition, or blepharospasm occur in about one-third of patients and can cause functional blindness (7,16). The slow blink rate of PSP, often less than 5 per minute, can allow conjunctival drying with annoying reactive inflammation and lacrimation. The electrical blink reflex is severely impaired, unlike in PD, CBD, or MSA (17), which is testament to the profound brainstem pathology in PSP.

TABLE 13.3
EYE MOVEMENT ABNORMALITIES IN PROGRESSIVE SUPRANUCLEAR PALSY BY DISEASE STAGE

Usually precede frank gaze restriction	Hypometric saccades, particularly downward
	Disordered opticokinetic nystagmus, particularly downward
	Slowing of downward saccades (especially when starting at upgaze)
	Square-wave jerks
	Inability to voluntarily suppress the vestibulo-ocular reflex
	Hesitancy (apraxia) on command downgaze
Middle-stage progressive supranuclear palsy	Restriction of range of voluntary downgaze
	Impaired convergence
	Disordered Bell's phenomenon
	Visual grasping
	Lid retraction with reduced blink rate
	Apraxia of lid opening or closing
Late-stage progressive supranuclear palsy	Restriction of range of voluntary horizontal gaze
	Loss of oculocephalic reflex
	Disconjugate gaze
	Disabling blepharospasm

Behavioral Abnormalities

Clinical frontal lobe dysfunction in PSP is often the most disabling area of cognitive loss and can progress rapidly. Behavioral changes were the initial symptom of PSP in 22% of patients in one series (18) and eventually produced disability in at least 80% (7). The dementia of PSP differs from the amnestic, visuospatial, and aphasic dementia of Alzheimer's disease (AD). In PSP, apathy, intellectual slowing, and impairment of executive functions are the consistent findings (19). The executive dysfunction comprises difficulty with shifting mental set, sorting, problem solving, abstract thinking, motor inhibition, and lexical fluency (20). A brief but formal frontal assessment battery is useful for bedside quantification of these deficits (6).

Pseudobulbar laughter, crying, or both are common in PSP, even as a presenting symptom. A nearly constant growling phonation is common in PSP, possibly a function of pseudobulbar emotion and incomplete glottic closure.

Dysautonomia

PSP features little or no dysautonomia, in contrast to MSA, which can otherwise mimic it closely. Orthostatic hypotension is not part of the disorder and the growth hormone response to clonidine is normal (21). The ventilatory arrhythmias and thermoregulatory deficits of MSA have not been described in PSP. However, urinary incontinence, constipation, and erectile dysfunction are common in PSP, possibly because of degeneration of the nucleus of Onuf, a parasympathetic center in the sacral spinal cord (22).

CLINICAL SUBTYPES

Two clinical subtypes of PSP have been described (23). The principal form, called "Steele-Richardson-Olszewski" because of its fidelity to Richardson's original description of PSP, comprises approximately half of all cases of autopsy-confirmed PSP (24). It features early onset of falls, vertical gaze paresis, and cognitive loss. The other form, "PSP-parkinsonism," comprises about one-third of the cases of PSP and features asymmetry, tremor, and a clear but transient levodopa response. The remaining one-sixth of cases conform well to neither syndrome. Biochemical and genetic differences between the two major types are described below and suggest that two etiologically distinct disorders may produce the same pathological phenotype.

Descriptive Epidemiology

The median interval from symptom onset to diagnosis of PSP averages slightly less than 4 years, and survival after that is usually between 2 and 6 years (2,4), depending on aggressiveness of supportive care. One survey found total median survival to be only 5.3 years (24). Survival tends to be shorter for patients with older onset, falls, dysarthria, or diplopia in the first year, or dysphagia within the first 2 years (25).

The prevalence of diagnosed PSP is approximately 1–2 cases per 100,000 population (2,25). But surveys using full, painstaking ascertainment by experienced clinicians who considered a diagnosis of PSP in every person whose symptoms suggested it yield a prevalence of 5–6 cases per 100,000 (24,26), about 3%–5% of the prevalence of PD. This means that three-quarters of persons seeking medical care for symptoms of PSP receive an incorrect or no diagnosis. More practically, it means that the population of patients who could use the services of PSP organizations, support PSP research, and benefit from neuroprotective treatments under development would increase threefold if clinicians had a higher index of suspicion and maximal familiarity with the disease.

The median age at symptom onset is remarkably uniform across most series at 62–63 years (2,4,7). In fact, the variance in age of onset with a typical standard deviation (SD) of 5–6 years (27) is less than in PD, with a typical SD of 11–12 years. This suggests that a relatively unitary, perhaps more easily elucidated, etiology and pathogenesis exist for PSP.

Analytic Epidemiology

Few studies have examined PSP risk factors in controlled fashion. The one finding to emerge has been that subjects with PSP were only 35% as likely to have completed high school as controls (28). This may be interpreted as evidence for the "synaptic reserve" hypothesis, also advanced as a factor in AD, where education creates neural complexity that buffers the effects of a degenerative illness. Alternatively, lesser educational attainment may correlate with greater occupational or residential toxin exposure.

No geographic clusters of PSP have been found, but two PSP-like illnesses occur on remote islands. The Parkinson-dementia complex of Guam is, like PSP, a tauopathy with parkinsonism, subcortical dementia, and prominent vertical eye movement paresis. Genetic factors, dietary toxins, and even parasitic infestation have been suspected but not proven. The dramatically declining incidence of this disorder during the decades over which the island's culture has become Westernized suggests a traditional indigenous dietary practice as the cause (29).

On Guadeloupe, there is a high prevalence of PSP and other dopa-unresponsive, dementing, nontremorous parkinsonian disorders. The few autopsies to date reveal a tauopathy with a pathological signature identical to that of PSP (30). A questionnaire survey implicated the tropical fruits sweetsop and soursop, extracts of which, as will be described, reproduce many features of PSP in laboratory animals (31).

Attempts to transmit PSP to primates (32) and a search for prion protein (33) have been unsuccessful.

Differential Diagnosis

No other disorder reproduces the fully developed picture of PSP, but fragments of this syndrome can be caused by other disorders. The most common of these is PD, but this is true only in the early stages of PSP. Another common disorder that can occasionally be mistaken for PSP is a multi-infarct state (34). It features asymmetry, prominence of pyramidal signs, and vascular lesions on magnetic resonance imaging (MRI). The clinical course rarely displays stepwise progression.

A more difficult differential diagnostic consideration for the clinician is MSA of the parkinsonian type, formerly called *striatonigral degeneration*. MSA, however, usually includes dysautonomic and cerebellar findings, and the eye movement abnormality is not as pronounced as in PSP. Another helpful, if inconstant, clue is antecollis in MSA and retrocollis in PSP.

In the same category is CBD, which can be distinguished from PSP by its marked asymmetry and prominence of asymmetric apraxia and cortical sensory findings. Myoclonus and prominent pyramidal findings are other common features of CBD that are rare in PSP. MSA and CBD share with PSP a 5- to 10-year survival, poor medication response, and nonfamilial incidence. For that reason, differentiating among them given present treatment options is not of critical importance from a purely clinical standpoint.

Dementia with Lewy bodies (DLB) is a common disorder that may be confused with PSP, but it typically includes more prominent psychosis and depression. The rigidity and bradykinesia of DLB respond to levodopa.

Entities that can occasionally resemble PSP but are readily treatable include Wilson's disease, hepatocerebral degeneration, normal-pressure hydrocephalus, myasthenia gravis, Whipple's disease, and tumors of the dorsal brainstem. Creutzfeldt-Jakob disease can mimic PSP and is poorly treatable but requires anti-infectious measures.

Other poorly treatable conditions that can be confused with PSP but require genetic investigation and, possibly, genetic counseling include rigid Huntington's disease, spinocerebellar ataxia type 3, Niemann-Pick disease type C, and rare cases of Gaucher's disease and mitochondrial encephalomyopathy. Those without genetic tests or treatment at present include the various pallidal degenerations, dementia with Lewy bodies, AD with parkinsonism, Pick's disease, progressive subcortical gliosis, postencephalitic parkinsonism, and dementia pugilistica.

The previously described differential diagnosis is more relevant for evaluation of early than for advanced cases, but even at the time of death, PSP is often misdiagnosed. Patients who carry an incorrect diagnosis of PSP at the time of death (if the collection of the PSP Brain Bank at the Mayo Clinic in Jacksonville, Florida, is representative) comprise 24% of the total. In most of these, MSA, DLB, or CBD was the correct diagnosis (35). The retrospective nature of this series makes it difficult to say whether the full PSP clinical syndrome was present in all cases.

DIAGNOSTIC WORKUP

MRI

Unless there is specific reason to suspect one of the unusual disorders in the differential diagnosis, the workup of a patient in whom PSP is suspected after a history and neurological exam consists only of an MRI without contrast. MRI features that help differentiate PSP from the leading competing diagnostic considerations appear in Table 13.4, and MRI images appear in Figure 13.2.

The MRI findings in PSP, which are often absent in the early stages when they would be most useful, are atrophy of the midbrain, particularly its dorsal portion; dilation of the third ventricle, particularly its posterior portion; signal change in the periaqueductal gray matter indicative of gliosis; and, occasionally, an "eye of the tiger" sign in which low signal indicative of iron deposition occurs in a V shape whose arms are the medial and lateral portions of the putamen, leaving a normal central portion (36). This sign also occurs in neurodegeneration with brain iron accumulation type 1 (Hallervorden-Spatz disease) and MSA. Atrophy of the superior cerebellar peduncle has been reported to occur in PSP but not in MSA, a welcome radiographic aid in differentiating these conditions (37).

Functional Imaging

The commonly available functional imaging techniques that may be useful in the diagnosis of PSP are single-photon emission computed tomography (SPECT) using hexamethylpropyleneamine oxime (HMPAO) or another nonspecific metabolic/blood flow tracer and 3H magnetic resonance spectroscopy (MRS). SPECT with HMPAO shows relatively symmetric superior frontal hypoperfusion and variable changes in the basal ganglia (38). MRS shows a reduced n-acetyl aspartate/creatine ratio in the pallidum in PSP and MSA but not in PD (39).

The less widely available positron emission tomography (PET) with 18F-fluorodeoxyglucose gives results similar to HMPAO SPECT but with greater resolution. PET using 18F-fluorodopa reveals loss of tracer uptake to a similar degree in caudate and putamen, while in PD there is greater loss in putamen.

None of these has been shown to differentiate with validity from its competitors early, diagnostically equivocal, PSP. Their utility is merely to provide one more point in an array of diagnostic information.

TABLE 13.4

DIAGNOSTIC CRITERIA FOR PROGRESSIVE SUPRANUCLEAR PALSY AS PROPOSED BY GOLBE ET AL.

Criteria for Progressive Supranuclear Palsy	Criteria for Vertical Supranuclear Gaze Palsy
All 4 of these: Onset at age 40 or later Progressive course Bradykinesia Vertical supranuclear gaze palsy, *per criteria at right*	*Either both of these:* Voluntary downgaze less than 15 degrees (tested by instructing patient to look down without presenting a specific target; accept the best result after several attempts) Preserved horizontal oculocephalic reflexes (except in very advanced stages)
Plus any 3 of these 5: Dysarthria or dysphagia Neck rigidity (to flexion/extension) greater than limb rigidity Neck in a posture of extension Minimal or absent tremor Frequent falls or gait disturbance early in course	*Or all 3 of these:* Slowed downward saccades (defined as slow enough for the examiner to perceive the movement itself) Impaired opticokinetic nystagmus with the stimulus moving downward Poor voluntary suppression of vertical vestibulo-ocular reflex
Without any of these: Early or prominent cerebellar signs Unexplained polyneuropathy Prominent noniatrogenic dysautonomia other than isolated postural hypotension	

Proposed by Golbe et al. (2).

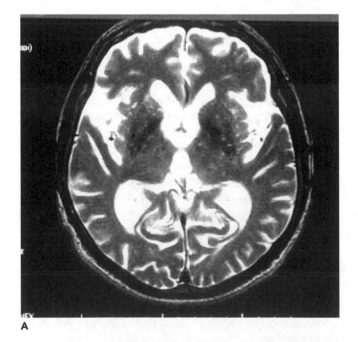
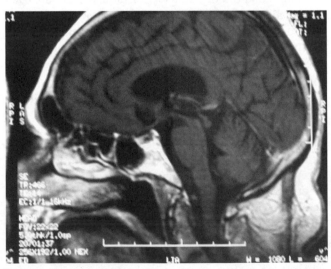

Figure 13.2 MRI signs in progressive supranuclear palsy. **A:** Iron deposition in both lateral and medial putamen with intervening high signal, the "eye of the tiger" sign. **B:** Atrophy of the dorsal midbrain in advanced progressive supranuclear palsy.

TABLE 13.5

DIAGNOSTIC CRITERIA FOR PROGRESSIVE SUPRANUCLEAR PALSY AS PROPOSED BY LITVAN ET AL.

"Possible" Progressive Supranuclear Palsy	"Probable" Progressive Supranuclear Palsy
All 3 of these: Gradually progressive disorder Onset at age 40 or later No evidence for competing diagnostic possibilities *Plus either of these:* Vertical gaze palsy Slowing of vertical saccades *and* prominent postural instability with falls in the first year	*All 5 of these:* Gradually progressive disorder Onset at age 40 or later No evidence for competing diagnostic possibilities Vertical gaze palsy Slowing of vertical saccades *and* prominent postural instability with falls in the first year

Criteria That Would Exclude Progressive Supranuclear Palsy from Consideration:

Recent encephalitis
Alien limb syndrome, cortical sensory defects or temporoparietal atrophy
Psychosis unrelated to dopaminergic treatment
Important cerebellar signs
Important unexplained dysautonomia
Severe, asymmetric parkinsonian signs
Relevant structural abnormality of basal ganglia on neuroimaging
Whipple's disease on cerebrospinal fluid polymerase chain reaction (CSF PCR), if indicated

Proposed by Litvan et al. (40).

Diagnostic Criteria

A set of diagnostic criteria (2) has been formulated for use in settings that permit detailed examination of patients (Table 13.5). Its specificity is 96% (40). Another set (40) includes "probable" clinical criteria with the high specificity necessary to a treatment trial and "possible" criteria sufficiently sensitive for use in a prevalence study (Table 13.6). Although neither set significantly augments diagnostic accuracy for an experienced subspecialist (41) both offer useful guides for most physicians and for research studies requiring a uniform diagnostic definition.

CELLULAR PATHOLOGY

Neurofibrillary Tangles

Neurofibrillary tangles (NFTs), the pathologic hallmark of PSP, are composed of unpaired straight filaments 15–18 nm in diameter. These are composed of at least six protofilaments 2–5 nm in diameter, which, in turn, are composed of aggregated tau protein (42,43). The filaments in PSP occasionally display paired helical filaments of the type seen in AD, particularly in cortical areas (44). The tangles of PSP tend to be globose rather than the flame-shaped tangles of AD. Anti-tau staining also reveals neuropil threads, or curly fibers, in the same neurons that include NFTs and in oligodendroglia of white matter tracts connecting affected areas of gray matter (45).

The antigenic and ultrastructural properties of the filaments of PSP tangles are nearly identical to those of CBD (46). However, the white matter tangles of CBD occur in oligodendroglia rather than in astrocytes, as in most cases of PSP (47).

Cortical NFTs of PSP appear to be antigenically identical to those of AD, most notably with regard to the presence of abnormally phosphorylated tau protein (48). PSP tau exhibits bands on the Western blot test of 64 and 69 kD, whereas AD and Down syndrome tau exhibits those two bands plus one of 55 kD (49). The NFTs of PSP stain weakly or not at all for ubiquitin (50).

Other Changes

Abnormally regenerated synaptic terminal material of Purkinje cells, called *grumose degeneration*, occurs in some cases with PSP, particularly in the cerebellar dentate nucleus (51). Granulovacuolar degeneration, a hallmark of AD, does occur to a mild extent in PSP, but amyloid and senile plaques do not. The swollen, achromatic neurons characteristic of CBD or Pick's disease occur in a few cases of otherwise typical PSP, generally in tegmental and inferior temporal areas (52).

Microglial activation, another pathologic change that occurs in some neurodegenerative disorders, has recently been found in PSP (53). In the brainstem in PSP, microglial activation does not correlate well with the presence of NFTs. This suggests that neither is the direct cause of the other and that microglia may help produce the neuronal loss of PSP.

TABLE 13.6

PRINCIPAL CLINICOPATHOLOGICAL CORRELATES IN PROGRESSIVE SUPRANUCLEAR PALSY

Region	Area	Severity (+ to ++++)	Prominent Clinical Correlate
Cerebrum	Frontal cortex	++	Frontal behavior
	Precentral cortex	++	Frontal motor phenomena
Limbic system	Amygdala	+	Depression
	Hippocampus	++	Memory disorder
Basal ganglia	Caudate	+++	
	Putamen	+++	
	Globus pallidus	++	Bradykinesia, dysarthria, dystonia, postural instability
	Subthalamic nucleus	++++	
	Thalamus (interlaminar nuclei)	+	
Basal forebrain	Nucleus basalis of Meynert	+++	Dementia
	Hypothalamus	+	Dysautonomia
Dorsal midbrain	Superior colliculus	++++	Coordination of head movement with gaze
	Rostral interstitial nucleus of the medial longitudinal fasciculus	+++	
			Vertical gaze palsy
	Periaqueductal gray	++++	
	Oculomotor nucleus	++	
	Interstitial nucleus of Cajal	++	Nuchal rigidity, postural instability
Midbrain tegmentum	Substantia nigra zona compacta	+++	Bradykinesia
	SN zona reticulata	++	Bradykinesia
	Ventral tegmental area	++	Frontal behavior
	Red nucleus	+++	Motor deficit?
	Pedunculopontine nucleus	+++	Postural instability, dementia, sleep disorder
Pons	Locus ceruleus	++	Gait disorder, dementia, depression, sleep disorder
	Nucleus of the dorsal raphe	+++	Frontal behavior, depression, sleep disorder
	Nuclei basis pontis	++	Horizontal saccadic disorder
Medulla	Vestibular nuclei	++	Dysequilibrium, abnormal gaze
Cerebellum	Dentate nucleus	++	Dysarthria, postural instability?
Spinal cord	Nucleus of Onuf	++	Dysautonomia
	Intermediolateral column	++	

ANIMAL MODELS

Over recent years, multiple animal models of tauopathy have been developed. As most of them are transgenic models using mutant versions of tau found in FTD and not in PSP, the fidelity of these models to PSP at the molecular level is not ideal. However, the pathology at the cellular level offers useful clues to the pathogenesis of human PSP and may provide a means of testing treatment. Two mouse models (54,55) feature glial rather than neuronal pathology, rendering them particularly relevant to PSP, and models in *Drosophila* (56,57) and *Caenorhabditis elegans* (58) offer opportunity for high-throughput drug testing. A rat model model (31) using intravenous annonacin,

a mitochondrial toxin occurring in the roots of fruit plants implicated in Guadeloupean atypical parkinsonism, may prove to be more relevant to PSP than a model based on a tau mutation.

ANATOMIC AND NEUROCHEMICAL PATHOLOGY

Overview

The complexity of the anatomical and neurochemical pathology of PSP is one reason for its continuing resistance to pathophysiologic understanding and pharmacologic intervention

TABLE 13.7

MRI FEATURES OF PROGRESSIVE SUPRANUCLEAR PALSY AND SOME OTHER CONDITIONS

	PSP	PD	MSA (OPCA)	MSA (SND)	CBGD	AD
Cortical atrophy	++	+	+/−	+	++/−	++
Putaminal atrophy	−	−	−	++	−	−
Pontine atrophy	+	−	+++	−	+/−	−
Midbrain atrophy	++	−	+	−	+/−	−
Cerebellar atrophy	−	−	++/−	−	−	−
High putaminal iron	−	−	+/−	+/−	−	−

PSP, progressive supranuclear palsy; PD, Parkinson's disease; MSA (OPCA), multiple system atrophy/sporadic olivoponto-cerebellar atrophy; MSA (SND), multiple system atrophy/striatonigral degeneration; CBGD, corticobasal degeneration; AD, Alzheimer's disease; -, absent or rare; +, occasional, mild, or late; ++, usual, moderate; +++, usual, severe, or early.

(59). An overview of the areas of anatomical involvement and their clinical correlates appears in Table 13.7.

The primary involvement in PSP can be classified into four major areas: the cerebral cortex, producing cognitive and behavioral changes; the nigrostriatopallidal area, producing rigidity, bradykinesia, and postural instability; the cholinergic pontomesencephalic area, producing gaze palsies, sleep disturbances and axial motor abnormalities; and the hindbrain area, producing dysarthria and dysphagia (60).

From the standpoint of neurotransmitters involved, dopaminergic damage in the nigrostriatal pathway and cholinergic damage in many areas are the most consistent, severe neurotransmitter-related changes in PSP (61,62). The loss of adrenoceptors is widespread (63), reflecting the wide projections of the severely damaged locus ceruleus. GABA-ergic function of the basal ganglia (in striatum and GPi and GPe) is moderately but widely impaired (64). Unlike in PD, the peptidergic systems and both the mesolimbic and mesocortical dopaminergic systems are intact. Serotonergic receptor sites are reduced in the cortex, but unlike in PD, are normal in basal ganglia (65).

Distribution of Pathology

The area of the brain most consistently involved in PSP is the population of pigmented neurons of the zona compacta of the substantia nigra (66). The damage is relatively uniform, unlike in PD, where the dorsal and extreme lateral portions are minimally affected. The dorsal portion projects principally to the caudate, the ventral to the putamen. This probably explains the relative sparing of presynaptic caudate dopamine reuptake in PD and its involvement in PSP, as measured by 18F-fluorodopa PET (67).

The cholinergic pedunculopontine nucleus (PPN) is severely affected in PSP (68). Experimental lesions of that nucleus can cause severe postural instability (69). Other areas severely and constantly affected in PSP are the external pallidum and to a lesser extent, the internal pallidum (70).

There is little striatal neuronal loss and correspondingly little or no loss of postsynaptic dopamine D1 and D2 receptors (71). In the striatum, the few neurons lost tend to be cholinergic interneurons (72). However, there is an important loss of astrocytes, which display "tufts" of tau-positive material and neuropil threads similar to those in affected neurons (60). Such astrocytic pathology may be unique to PSP and appears to be a primary site of pathology rather than a function of neuronal damage (73).

Brainstem pathology is also important in PSP, with the rostral midbrain most intensely involved. Damage to the nucleus of Darkschewitsch, the rostral interstitial nucleus of the medial longitudinal fasciculus, and the mesencephalic reticular formation may all contribute to the vertical gaze palsy, but their individual contributions have not been sorted out (58).

Variable damage of the substantia nigra pars reticulata (74), a ventral area projecting to the superior colliculus, may also contribute. The ventral tegmental area, red nucleus, and locus ceruleus are also involved (51), but their specific contributions to the clinical deficits are unclear.

The horizontal gaze palsy that appears eventually in most cases is attributable to degeneration of nuclei of the potine base (75). The ocular motor cranial nerve nuclei are the sole examples of cholinergic nuclei to escape important, consistent involvement in PSP.

CLINICAL GENETICS

Familial Clusters

A case-control study (76) elicited reports of "Parkinson's disease" among relatives 5 times as frequently from patients with PSP as from controls. Another study found that 39% of 23 asymptomatic first-degree relatives of patients with PSP, but none of 23 controls, had abnormal scores on a test battery designed to screen for PD (77).

Despite this indirect evidence for subtle familial clustering of PSP, fewer than 1% of patients with PSP have had relatives with that diagnosis. Eight reports of families with more than one member with proven PSP, usually with autosomal dominant transmission and no purely maternal transmission, offer hope of a clue to the cause of sporadic PSP. It is intriguing that some of these families, including a Spanish family that is by far the largest, include additional members with reports of typical PD or essential tremor (78,79).

Molecular Pathology

In the NFTs of PSP, the ratio of human brain tau isoforms is at least 3:1 in favor of 4-repeat tau (49). Disordered regulation of exon 10 splicing may therefore explain tau aggregation into NFTs in PSP and other tauopathies.

Several mutations in and near the 5′ splice site downstream of exon 10 have been described in families with hereditary frontotemporal dementia linked to chromosome 17 (FTD-17), another 4-repeat tauopathy, but not in typical PSP (80,81). These probably disrupt a stem-loop structure in the RNA transcribed at the downstream end of exon 10. This stem loop regulates splicing of the exon 10 transcript, the inappropriate inclusion of which produces an excess of 4-repeat tau. The cause then, of PSP and other sporadic tauopathies, may be dysfunction of the same RNA stem loop but from a different cause.

The H1 haplotype, spanning the tau gene on chromosome 17q21, is present in homozygous form in approximately 90% of patients with PSP but also in approximately 60% of controls (82,83). The pathogenic locus itself is not known and may even lie well outside tau itself, in one of several nearby candidate genes that contribute to the H1 haplotype. Variants of the H1 haplotype are overrepresented in corticobasal degeneration and PD. Efforts are underway to further refine an H1 haplotype variant specific to PSP in hopes of identifying a very small genomic interval harboring the pathogenic sequence (84).

Patients with PSP who carry the H1 haplotype or the H1:H1 genotype do not differ from the others with regard to age of onset, clinical progression (85), anatomical distribution of degeneration, or biochemical features of the abnormal tau protein (86). However, H1 overrepresentation is greater in the recently proposed "Steele-Richardson-Olszewski syndrome" PSP variant than in the "PSP-parkinsonism" variant (23).

A second genomic locus, at chromosome 1q31.1, has been found by linkage analysis to be associated with autosomal dominant PSP in one Spanish family with at least nine affected members (87). The specific causative gene and mutation are not known.

An area of inquiry is the role of transglutaminases in PSP (88). Enzymes normally important in stabilizing protein structure, they are aberrantly activated in PSP and other neurodegenerative disorders by oxidative stress. The resulting cross-linking of tau protein could help explain the formation of NFTs or the dysfunction of other proteins and offers a promising site of action for neuroprotective therapy.

Mitochondrial or Oxidative Mechanisms

Skeletal muscle mitochondrial respiratory function is reduced by about 30% in PSP. Evidence for oxidative stress in brain tissue is marked increases in levels of superoxide dismutase 1 and/or dismutase 2 activity, malondialdehyde, and lipid peroxidation products specifically in areas that degenerate in PSP (89). The cause of this deficiency, as for that in PD, is unclear, but may, again as in PD, be of mitochondrial genetic origin. In both PD and PSP, there is a deficiency of mitochondrial Complex I activity that is of mitochondrial genetic origin. The principal evidence for this is the poor Complex I function of "cybrids," cultured neuronal cells in which mitochondria from patients with PSP (or PD) have been substituted for native mitochondria (90).

PHARMACOTHERAPY

As is the case for most other degenerative disorders, neurotransmitter replacement or receptor stimulation in PSP encounters little or none of the success it has with PD (91,92).

Dopaminergics

The extent and nature of the benefit of levodopa in PSP have not been adequately studied in double-blind fashion, but any benefit is nearly always mild and/or brief (91,93). A double-blind trial of the dopamine receptor agonist pramipexole showed no efficacy and more toxicity than typically observed with levodopa (94). Only the rigidity and bradykinesia, including those components of dysarthria and dysphagia attributable to them, may respond more than would be expected from placebo. At best, only about half of patients with PSP respond usefully to levodopa (93). These patients may mostly comprise the "PSP-parkinsonism" subtype recently described (23).

Hyperkinetic and behavioral side effects of levodopa are rare in PSP (91). This prompts the use of approximately twice the levodopa/carbidopa dosages used for PD with the equivalent degree of parkinsonism. For patients with PSP whose rigidity or bradykinesia impair daily activities, titrating levodopa to 1500 mg/day in three doses (with car-bidopa) should be attempted.

Cholinergics and Anticholinergics

The anticholinergic drug amantadine, which has dopamin-ergic and antiglutamatergic properties as well, is a close second to levodopa in risk/benefit ratio for PSP (91). A trial of amantadine starting at 100 mg daily and increas-ing to a maximum of 100 mg twice daily is worthwhile for most patients with PSP. It should be tapered and discon-tinued if symptomatic benefit is not apparent within a month or if cognitive adverse effects occur.

Trials of cholinergics have been inspired by the severe and widespread degeneration of acetylcholinergic systems in PSP, but donepezil, a commercially available cholinesterase inhibitor minimally effective in AD, has no benefit against PSP (95). Informal experience suggests that the other avail-able cholinesterase inhibitors fare no better and that the antiglutamatergic drug memantine, slightly effective in AD, produces somnolence or confusion in PSP with no cognitive benefit.

Antidepressants

Amitriptyline improved gait and rigidity in 3 of 4 patients in a small, double-blind trial (96). In a retrospective series (91), amitriptyline gave a risk/benefit ratio that was slightly less favorable than those of levodopa and amantadine. Amitriptyline is generally started at 10 mg at bedtime, increasing by that amount each week, given in two divided doses. If 20 mg twice daily proves ineffective, higher dosages are unlikely to do otherwise. Amitriptyline occa-sionally produces a paradoxic worsening of postural insta-bility in PSP. Other classes of antidepressants have not been found to help the motor deficits in PSP but may be useful against depression in those patients. Formal studies, how-ever, are lacking.

Botulinum Toxin

Orbital muscle injection of botulinum is typically highly successful against blepharospasm and apraxia of lid open-ing in PSP (97). Torticollis or retrocollis in PSP may also respond, but caution is dictated by the possibility of ante-rior neck muscle botulinum injections exacerbating the dysphagia of PSP with resulting aspiration. Botulinum toxin may also be useful in focal limb dystonia of PSP (98).

Other Pharmacotherapeutics

The secretions of PSP and the urinary urgency or inconti-nence can be mitigated by a peripherally acting anticholin-ergic. The asymmetric dystonia may respond to baclofen. The sleep disorder may respond to a mild sedative or a tri-cyclic antidepressant at bedtime.

NONPHARMACOLOGIC THERAPY

Gaze and Lid Pareses

Prisms are not usually useful against the vertical gaze pare-sis of PSP but may help diplopia related to dysconjugate gaze. Some patients can overcome the voluntary downgaze palsy by following the fork or other target down to the object of gaze. Low-lying obstacles, such as coffee tables, loose rugs, and children's toys, should be removed from the patient's environment. The chronic conjunctivitis and reac-tive lacrimation caused by the low blink rate may be treated by instillation of lubricants.

Physical, Speech, and Swallowing Therapy

Physical therapy seems to be of little or no benefit against the postural instability of PSP, but regular exercise has a clear psychological benefit (99). Similarly, speech therapy is of little benefit, but the speech pathologist may be able to arrange adjunctive means of communication such as electronic typing devices or simple pointing boards if the visual function permits.

Reducing the risk of aspiration may be the most effective means of prolonging the life of a patient with PSP. Dysphagia in PSP is unlikely to respond to retraining therapy, but the caregivers may be instructed in the preparation of foods of proper consistency, using a blender and cornstarch-based thickeners as necessary. The speech pathologist can teach the patient safer swallowing techniques, such as neck flexion during swallowing and multiple swallows per mouth-ful. A modified barium-swallow radiograph using boluses of varying consistency will guide this advice and should be ordered at the first sign of coughing or choking on fluids.

Placement of a percutaneous feeding gastrostomy pre-sents an ethical dilemma in PSP, where prolongation of life by this means may not be desirable in the advanced stages of the illness. Some indications for the procedure are an episode of aspiration pneumonia, coughing on each mouthful, and excessive time required for feeding. The decision may be guided by the cognitive state of the patient at the time the need for gastrostomy occurs. Experience shows that many patients who declare at the onset of their illness that they would not opt for a gastrostomy feel dif-ferently when the time comes. In practice, patients with PSP who remain communicative are rarely denied the option of a gastrostomy by their family or physician.

Surgical Implants

Deep-brain stimulation that has proven efficacious in PD, tremor disorders, and dystonia is unlikely to benefit PSP but has not been attempted. The involvement in PSP of the downstream nuclei of the basal ganglia, such as the subthalamic nucleus and pallidum, suggest that downregulating those areas would only exacerbate the motor deficit. For similar reasons, implantation of dopamine-producing tissue into the striatum would not help, and a small trial of adrenal medullary autografts in PSP confirms this prediction (100).

Patient Counseling and Resources

Until specific symptomatic or neuroprotective treatment for PSP is available, the most valuable services that health professionals can offer patients are a prompt and accurate diagnosis to avoid unnecessary diagnostic testing and useless treatments and prognostic advice to permit planning of finances, assistive services, and home alterations. Perhaps even more important is to offer hope that research against PSP is proceeding apace and may bring useful treatment while the patient remains able to benefit from it.

Patients and their families derive comfort and information from interacting with others who share this rare illness and are dedicated to the fight against it. The Society for Progressive Supranuclear Palsy (http://www.psp.org) is headquartered in Maryland and serves North America. The Progressive Supranuclear Palsy Association (Europe) (http://www.pspeur.org) is based in the United Kingdom and serves all of Europe. Both organizations offer support meetings and lay-language information to patients and their families. They also offer research funding to scientists internationally and sponsor research symposia.

REFERENCES

1. Steele JC, Richardson JC, Olszewski J. PSP: a heterogeneous degeneration involving the brain stem, basal ganglia and cerebellum, with vertical gaze and pseudobulbar palsy, nuchal dystonia and dementia. *Arch Neurol* 1964;10:333–359.
2. Golbe LI, Davis PH, Schoenberg BS, Duvoisin RC. Prevalence and natural history of progressive supranuclear palsy. *Neurology* 1988;38:1031–1034.
3. Imai H, Nakamura T, Kondo T, Narabayashi H. Dopa-unresponsive pure akinesia or freezing: a condition with a wide spectrum of progressive supranuclear palsy? *Adv Neurol* 1993;60:622–625.
4. Maher ER, Lees AJ. The clinical features and natural history of the Steele-Richardson-Olszewski syndrome (progressive supranuclear palsy). *Neurology* 1986;36:1005–1008.
5. Kluin KJ, Foster NL, Berent S, Gilman S. Perceptual analysis of speech disorders in progressive supranuclear palsy. *Neurology* 1993;43:563–566.
6. Dubois B, Slachevsky A, Litvan I, Pillon B. The FAB: a Frontal Assessment Battery at bedside. *Neurology* 2000;55:1621–1626.
7. Jankovic J, Van der Linden C. Progressive supranuclear palsy (Steele-Richardson-Olszewski syndrome). In: Chokroverty S, ed. *Movement Disorders*. New York: PMA Publishing; 1990:267–286.
8. Bergeron C, Pollanen MS, Weyer L, Lang AE. Cortical degeneration in progressive supranuclear palsy: a comparison with cortical-basal ganglionic degeneration. *J Neuropath Exp Neurol* 1977;56:726–734.
9. Leigh RJ, Riley DE. Eye movements in parkinsonism: it's saccadic speed that counts. *Neurology* 2000;54:1018–1019.
10. Pfaffenbach DD, Layton DD, Kearns TP. Ocular manifestations in progressive supranuclear palsy. *Am J Ophthalmol* 1972;74:1179–1184.
11. Chu FC, Reingold DB, Cogan DG, Williams AC. The eye movement disorders of progressive supranuclear palsy. *Ophthalmology* 1979;86:422–428.
12. Troost BT, Daroff RB. The ocular motor defects in progressive supranuclear palsy. *Ann Neurol* 1977;2:397–403.
13. Rascol O, Sabatini U, Simonetta-Moreau M, Montastruc JL, Rascol A, Clanet M. Square wave jerks in parkinsonian syndromes. *J Neurol Neurosurg Psychiatry* 1991;54:599–602.
14. Rafal RD, Posner MI, Friedman JH, Inhoff AW, Bernstein E. Orienting of visual attention in progressive supranuclear palsy. *Brain* 1988;111:267–280.
15. Rascol O, Clanet M, Senard JM, Montastruc JL, Rascol A. Vestibulo-ocular reflex in Parkinson's disease and multiple system atrophy. *Adv Neurol* 1993;60:395–397.
16. Golbe LI, Davis PH, Lepore FE. Eyelid movement abnormalities in progressive supranuclear palsy. *Mov Disord* 1989;4:297–302.
17. Valls-Solé J, Valldeoriola F, Tolosa E, Marti MJ. Distinctive abnormalities of facial reflexes in patients with progressive supranuclear palsy. *Brain* 1997;120:1877–1883.
18. Birdi S, Rajput AH, Fenton M, et al. Progressive supranuclear palsy diagnosis and confounding features: report on 16 autopsied cases. *Mov Disord* 2002;17:1255–1267.
19. Litvan I, Phipps M, Pharr VL, Hallett M, Grafman J, Salazar A. Randomized placebo-controlled trial of donepezil in patients with progressive supranuclear palsy. *Neurology* 2001;57:467–473.
20. Pillon B, Dubois B, Lhermitte F, Agid Y. Heterogeneity of cognitive impairment in progressive supranuclear palsy, Parkinson's disease, and Alzheimer's disease. *Neurology* 1986;36:1179–1185.
21. Kimber J, Mathias CJ, Lees AJ, et al. Physiological, pharmacological and neurohormonal assessment of autonomic function in progressive supranuclear palsy. *Brain* 2000;123:1422–1430.
22. Scaravilli T, Pramstaller PP, Salerno A, et al. Neuronal loss in Onuf's nucleus in three patients with progressive supranuclear palsy. *Ann Neurol* 2000;48:97–101.
23. Williams DR, de Silva R, Paviour DC, et al. Characteristics of two distinct clinical phenotypes in pathologically proven progressive supranuclear palsy: Richardson's syndrome and progressive supranuclear palsy-parkinsonism. *Brain* 2005;128:1247–1258.
24. Nath U, Ben-Shlomo Y, Thomson RG, Lees AJ, Burn DJ. Clinical features and natural history of progressive supranuclear palsy: a clinical cohort study. *Neurology* 2003;60:910–916.
25. Schrag A, Ben-Shlomo Y, Quinn NP. Prevalence of progressive supranuclear palsy and multiple system atrophy: a cross-sectional study. *Lancet* 1999;354:1771–1775.
26. Bower JH, Maraganore DM, McDonnell SK, Rocca WA. Incidence of progressive supranuclear palsy and multiple system atrophy in Olmsted County, Minnesota, 1976 to 1990. *Neurology* 1997;49:1284–1288.
27. Molinuevo JL, Valldeoriola F, Alegret M, Oliva R, Tolosa E. Progressive supranuclear palsy: earlier age of onset in patients with the tau protein A0/A0 genotype. *J Neurol* 2000;247:206–208.
28. Golbe LI, Rubin RS, Cody RP, et al. Follow-up study of risk factors in progressive supranuclear palsy. *Neurology* 1996;47:148–154.
29. Caparros-Lefebvre D, Elbaz A. Possible relation of atypical parkinsonism in the French West Indies with consumption of tropical plants: a case-control study. *Lancet* 1999;354:281–286.
30. Caparros-Lefebvre D, Sergeant N, Lees A, et al. Guadeloupean parkinsonism: a cluster of progressive supranuclear palsy-like tauopathy. *Brain* 2002;125:801–811.
31. Champy P, Hoglinger GU, Feger J, et al. Annonacin, a lipophilic inhibitor of mitochondrial complex I, induces nigral and striatal neurodegeneration in rats: possible relevance for atypical parkinsonism in Guadeloupe. *J Neurochem* 2004;88:63–69.
32. Brown P, Gibbs CJ, Rodgers-Johnson P, et al. Human spongiform encephalopathy: the National Institutes of Health series of 300 cases of experimentally transmitted disease. *Ann Neurol* 1994; 35:513–529.
33. Jendroska K, Hoffmann O, Schelosky L, Lees AJ, Poewe W, Daniel S. Absence of disease related prion protein in neurodegenerative disorders presenting with Parkinson's syndrome. *J Neurol Neurosurg Psychiatry* 1994;57:1249–1251.
34. Josephs KA, Ishizawa T, Tsuboi Y, Cookson N, Dickson DW. A clinicopathological study of vascular progressive supranuclear palsy: a multi-infarct disorder presenting as progressive supranuclear palsy. *Arch Neurol* 2002;59:1597–1601.
35. Josephs KA, Dickson DW. Diagnostic accuracy of progressive supranuclear palsy in the Society for Progressive Supranuclear Palsy brain bank. *Mov Disord* 2003;18:1018–1026.

36. Savoiardo M, Girotti F, Strada L, Ciceri E. Magnetic resonance imaging in progressive supranuclear palsy and other parkinsonian disorders. *J Neural Transm Suppl* 1994;42:93–110.

37. Paviour DC, Price SL, Stevens JM, Lees AJ, Fox NC. Quantitative MRI measurement of superior cerebellar peduncle in progressive supranuclear palsy. *Neurology* 2005;64:675–679.

38. Habert MO, Spampinato U, Mas JL, et al. A comparative technetium 99m hexamethylpropylene amine oxime SPECT study in different types of dementia. *Eur J Nucl Med* 1991;18:3–11.

39. Federico F, Simone IL, Lucivero V, et al. Usefulness of proton magnetic resonance spectroscopy in differentiating parkinsonian syndromes. *Ital J Neurol Sci* 1999;20:223–229.

40. Litvan I, Agid Y, Calne D, et al. Clinical research criteria for the diagnosis of progressive supranuclear palsy (Steele-Richardson-Olszewski syndrome): report of the NINDS-progressive supranuclear palsy international workshop. *Neurology* 1996;47:1–9.

41. Osaki Y, Ben-Shlomo Y, Lees AJ, Daniel SE, Colosimo C, Wenning G, Quinn N. Accuracy of clinical diagnosis of progressive supranuclear palsy. *Mov Disord* 2004;19:181–189.

42. Powell HC, London GW, Lampert PW. Neurofibrillary tangles in progressive supranuclear palsy. *J Neuropath Exp Neurol* 1974;33:98–106.

43. Tellez-Nagel I, Wisniewski HM. Ultrastructure of neurofibrillary tangles in Steele-Richardson-Olszewski syndrome. *Arch Neurol* 1973;29:324–327.

44. Ghatak NR, Nochlin D, Hadfield MG. Neurofibrillary pathology in progressive supranuclear palsy. *Acta Neuropathol (Berl)* 1980;52:73–76.

45. Probst A, Langui D, Lautenschlager C, Ulrich J, Brion JP, Anderton BH. Progressive supranuclear palsy: extensive neuropil threads in addition to neurofibrillary tangles. *Acta Neuropathol (Berl)* 1988;77:61–68.

46. Ikeda K, Akiyama H, Haga C, Kondo H, Arima K, Oda T. Argyrophilic thread-like structure in corticobasal degeneration and supranuclear palsy. *Neurosci Lett* 1994;174:157–159.

47. Wakabayashi K, Oyanagi K, Makifuchi T, et al. Corticobasal degeneration: etiopathological significance of the cytoskeletal alterations. *Acta Neuropathologica* 1994;87:545–553.

48. Pollock NJ, Mirra SS, Binder LI, Hansen LA, Wood JG. Filamentous aggregates in Pick's disease, progressive supranuclear palsy, and Alzheimer's disease share antigenic determinants with microtubule-associated protein, tau. *Lancet* 1986;2:1211.

49. Flament S, Delacourte A, Verny M, Hauw J-J, Javoy-Agid F. Abnormal tau proteins in progressive supranuclear palsy. *Acta Neuropathol (Berl)* 1991;81:591–596.

50. Lennox G, Lowe J, Morrell K, Landon M, Mayer RJ. Ubiquitin is a component of neurofibrillary tangles in a variety of neurodegenerative diseases. *Neurosci Lett* 1988;94:211–217.

51. Olszewski J, Steele J, Richardson JC. Pathological report on six cases of heterogeneous system degeneration. *J Neuropathol Exp Neurol* 1963;23:187–188.

52. Giaccone G, Tagliavini F, Street JS, Ghetti B, Bugiani O. Progressive supranuclear palsy with hypertrophy of the olives: an immunohistochemical study of argyrophilic neurons. *Acta Neuropathol (Berl)* 1988;77:14–20.

53. Ishizawa K, Dickson DW. Microglial activation parallels system degeneration in progressive supranuclear palsy and corticobasal degeneration. *J Neuropathol Exp Neurol* 2001;60:647–657.

54. Higuchi M, Ishihara T, Zhang B, Hong M, Andreadis A, Trojanowski J, Lee VM. Transgenic mouse model of tauopathies with glial pathology and nervous system degeneration. *Neuron* 2002;35:433–446.

55. Lewis J, McGowan E, Rockwood J, et al. Neurofibrillary tangles, amyotrophy and progressive motor disturbance in mice expressing mutant (P301L) tau protein. *Nat Genet* 2000;25:402–405.

56. Wittmann CW, Wszolek MF, Shulman JM, Salvaterra PM, Lewis J, Hutton M, Feany MB. Tauopathy in Drosophila: neurodegeneration without neurofibrillary tangles. *Science* 2001;293:711–714.

57. Jackson GR, Wiedau-Pazos M, Sang TK, Wagle N, Brown CA, Massachi S, Geschwind DH. Human wild-type tau interacts with wingless pathway components and produces neurofibrillary pathology in Drosophila. *Neuron* 2002;34:509–519.

58. Kraemer BC, Zhang B, Leverenz JB, Thomas JH, Trojanowski JQ, Schellenberg GD. Neurodegeneration and defective neurotrans-

59. mission in a Caenorhabditis elegans model of tauopathy. *Proc Natl Acad Sci USA* 2003;100:9980–9985.

59. Jellinger KA, Bancher C. Neuropathology. In: Litvan I, Agid Y, eds. *Progressive Supranuclear Palsy: Clinical and Research Approaches.* New York: Oxford; 1992:44–88.

60. Hauw J-J, Daniel SE, Dickson D, et al. Preliminary NINDS neuropathologic criteria for Steele-Richardson-Olszewski syndrome (progressive supranuclear palsy). *Neurology* 1994;44:2015–2019.

61. Ruberg M, Javoy-Agid F, Hirsch E, Scatton B, et al. Dopaminergic and cholinergic lesions in progressive supranuclear palsy. *Ann Neurol* 1985;18:523–529.

62. Warren NM, Piggott MA, Perry EK, Burn DJ. Cholinergic systems in progressive supranuclear palsy. *Brain* 2005;128:239–249.

63. Levy R, Ruberg M, Herrero MT, et al. Alterations of GABAergic neurons in the basal ganglia of patients with progressive supranuclear palsy: an in situ hybridization study of GAD_{67} messenger RNA. *Neurology* 1995;45:127–134.

64. Pascual J, Berciano J, Gonzalez AM, Grijalba B, Figols J, Pazos A. Autoradiographic demonstration of loss of alpha-2-adrenoceptors in progressive supranuclear palsy: preliminary report. *J Neurol Sci* 1993;114:165–169.

65. Landwehrmeyer B, Palacios JM. Neurotransmitter receptors in progressive supranuclear palsy. *J Neural Transm* 1994;42(suppl):229–246.

66. Fearnley JM, Lees AJ. Ageing and Parkinson's disease: substantia nigra regional selectivity. *Brain* 1991;114:2283–2301.

67. Brooks DJ, Ibáñez V, Sawle GV, et al. Differing patterns of striatal ^{18}F-dopa uptake in Parkinson's disease, multiple system atrophy, and progressive supranuclear palsy. *Ann Neurol* 1990;28:547–555.

68. Zweig RM, Whitehouse PJ, Casanova MF, et al. Loss of pedunculopontine neurons in progressive supranuclear palsy. *Ann Neurol* 1987;22:18–25.

69. Masdeu JC, Alampur U, Cavaliere R, Tavoulareas G. Astasia and gait failure with damage of the pontomesencephalic locomotor region. *Ann Neurol* 1994;35:619–621.

70. Hardman CD, Halliday GM. The external globus pallidus in patients with Parkinson's disease and progressive supranuclear palsy. *Mov Disord* 1999;14:626–633.

71. Brooks DJ, IbáñezV, Sawle GV, et al. Striatal D_2 receptor status in patients with Parkinson's disease, striatonigral degeneration, and progressive supranuclear palsy, measured with ^{11}C-raclopride and positron emission tomography. *Ann Neurol* 1992;31:184–192.

72. Togo T, Dickson DW. Tau accumulation in astrocytes in progressive supranuclear palsy is a degenerative rather than a reactive process. *Acta Neuropathol (Berl)* 2002;104:398–402.

73. Jackson GR, Wiedau-Pazos M, Sang TK, Wagle N, Brown CA, Massachi S, Geschwind DH. Human wild-type tau interacts with wingless pathway components and produces neurofibrillary pathology in Drosophila. *Neuron* 2002;34:509–519.

74. Halliday GM, Hardman CD, Cordato NJ, Hely MA, Morris JG. A role for the substantia nigra pars reticulata in the gaze palsy of progressive supranuclear palsy. *Brain* 2000;123:724–732.

75. Malessa S, Gaymard B, Rivaud S, et al. Role of pontine nuclei damage in smooth pursuit impairment of progressive supranuclear palsy: a clinical-pathologic study. *Neurology* 1994;44: 716–721.

76. Davis PH, Golbe LI, Duvoisin RC, Schoenberg BS. Risk factors for progressive supranuclear palsy. *Neurology* 1988;38:1546–1552.

77. Baker KB, Montgomery EB Jr. Performance on the PD test battery by relatives of patients with progressive supranuclear palsy. *Neurology* 2001;56:25–30.

78. Rojo A, Pernaute S, Fontán A, et al. Clinical genetics of familial progressive supranuclear palsy. *Brain* 1999;122:1233–1245.

79. Piccini P, de Yebenes J, Lees AJ, et al. Familial progressive supranuclear palsy: detection of subclinical cases using 18F-dopa and 18-fluorodeoxyglucose positron emission tomography. *Arch Neurol* 2001;58:1846–1851.

80. Hutton M, Lendon CL, Rizzu P, et al. Association of missense and 5'-splice-site mutation in tau with the inherited dementia FTDP-17. *Nature* 1998;393:702–705.

81. Spillantini MG, Murrell JR, Goedert M, Farlow MR, Klug A, Ghetti B. Mutation in the tau gene in familial multiple system tauopathy with presenile dementia. *Proc Natl Acad Sci USA* 1998;95:7737–7741.

82. Conrad C, Andreadis A, Trojanowski JQ, et al. Genetic evidence for the involvement of tau in progressive supranuclear palsy. *Ann Neurol* 1997;41:277–281.

83. Pittman AM, Myers AJ, Abou-Sleiman P, et al. Linkage disequilibrium fine-mapping and haplotype association analysis of the tau gene in progressive supranuclear palsy and corticobasal degeneration. *J Med Genet* 2005;42:837–846.

84. Morris HR, Schrag A, Nath U, et al. Effect of ApoE and tau on age of onset of progressive supranuclear palsy and multiple system atrophy. *Neurosci Lett* 2001;312:118–120.

85. Litvan I, Baker M, Hutton M. Tau genotype: no effect on onset, symptom severity, or survival in progressive supranuclear palsy. *Neurology* 2001;57:138–140.

86. Liu WK, Le TV, Adamson J, et al. Relationship of the extended tau haplotype to tau biochemistry and neuropathology in progressive supranuclear palsy. *Ann Neurol* 2001;50:494–502.

87. Ros R, Gomez Garre P, Hirano M, et al. Genetic linkage of autosomal dominant progressive supranuclear palsy to 1q31.1. *Ann Neurol* 2005;57:634–641.

88. Kim SY, Jeiter TM, Steinert PM. Transglutaminases in disease. *Neurochem International* 2002;40:85–103.

89. Albers DS, Augood SJ, Martin DM, Standaert DG, Vonsattel JPG, Beal MF. Evidence for oxidative stress in the subthalamic nucleus in progressive supranuclear palsy. *J Neurochem* 1999;73:881–884.

90. Swerdlow RH, Golbe LI, Parks JK, et al. Mitochondrial dysfunction in cybrid lines expressing mitochondrial genes from patients with progressive supranuclear palsy. *J Neurochem* 2000;75:1681–1684.

91. Nieforth KA, Golbe LI. Retrospective study of drug response in 87 patients with progressive supranuclear palsy. *Clin Neuropharmacol* 1993;16:338–346.

92. Kompoliti K, Goetz CG, Litvan I, Jellinger K, Verny M. Pharmacological therapy in progressive supranuclear palsy. *Arch Neurol* 1998;55:1099–1102.

93. Jankovic J. Controlled trial of pergolide mesylate in Parkinson's disease and progressive supranuclear palsy. *Neurology* 1983;33:505–507.

94. Weiner WJ, Minagar A, Shulman LM. Pramipexole in progressive supranuclear palsy. *Neurology* 1999;52:873–874.

95. Litvan I, Baker M, Hutton M. Tau genotype: no effect on onset, symptom severity, or survival in progressive supranuclear palsy. *Neurology* 2001;57:38–140.

96. Newman GC. Treatment of progressive supranuclear palsy with tricyclic antidepressants. *Neurology* 1985;35:1189–1193.

97. Piccione F, Mancini E, Tonin P, Bizzarini M. Botulinum toxin treatment of apraxia of eyelid opening in progressive supranuclear palsy: report of two cases. *Arch Phys Med Rehab* 1997;78:525–529.

98. Polo KB, Jabbari B. Botulinum toxin-A improves the rigidity of progressive supranuclear palsy. *Ann Neurol* 1994;35:237–239.

99. Sosner J, Wall GC, Sznajder J. Progressive supranuclear palsy: clinical presentation and rehabilitation of two patients. *Arch Phys Med Rehabil* 1993;74:537–539.

100. Koller WC, Morantz R, Vetere-Overfield B, Waxman M. Autologous adrenal medullary transplant in progressive supranuclear palsy. *Neurology* 1989;39:1066–1068.

Multiple System Atrophy

14

Gregor K. Wenning   Felix Geser

INTRODUCTION

Multiple system atrophy (MSA) is a sporadic neurodegenerative disorder characterized clinically by various combinations of parkinsonian, autonomic, cerebellar, or pyramidal symptoms or signs and pathologically by cell loss, gliosis, and glial cytoplasmic inclusions (GCIs) in several brain and spinal cord structures. The term *multiple system atrophy* was introduced in 1969; however, cases of MSA were previously reported under the rubrics of striatonigral degeneration (SND), olivopontocerebellar atrophy (OPCA), Shy-Drager syndrome (SDS), and idiopathic orthostatic hypotension (1). In 1989, GCIs were first described in the brains of patients with MSA, regardless of clinical presentation (2). GCIs were not present in a large series of patients with other neurodegenerative disorders. The abundant presence of GCIs in all clinical subtypes of MSA led to the recognition of SDS, SND, and sporadic OPCA as one disease entity characterized by neuronal multisystem degeneration with unique oligodendroglial inclusion pathology. In the late nineties, α-synuclein immunostaining was recognized as a sensitive marker of inclusion pathology in MSA (Fig. 14.1) (3,4), and MSA is now classified among the "synucleinopathies" along with Parkinson's disease (PD) and dementia with Lewy bodies (DLB). In parallel, clinical recognition greatly improved following the introduction of diagnostic criteria. Quinn was the first to propose a list of criteria (5), and—due to a number of associated pitfalls—new consensus criteria were developed in 1998 (6). Although the diagnosis of MSA is largely based on clinical expertise, several investigations have been proposed to help in the differential diagnosis of this disease.

EPIDEMIOLOGY

Bower et al. reported the incidence of MSA over a 14-year period in Olmsted County, Minnesota. Nine incident cases of MSA were identified, none of which had an onset before the age of 50 years. The reported crude incidence rate was 0.6 cases per 100,000 population per year; when the age band under 50 years was examined, the estimate rose to 3 cases per 100,000 population (7). Estimates of the prevalence of MSA (per 100,000 in the population) in four studies ranged from 1.9–4.9 (8,9,10,11). Whereas many studies report a possible role of environmental toxins in PD, such a role is even more likely in MSA, as this is a sporadic disease. However, only four studies have addressed environmental risk factors in MSA to date (12,13,14). So far no single environmental factor has been established (15), clearly as conferring increased or reduced risks to develop MSA.

PATHOLOGY

In MSA-P (parkinsonian phenotype), the striatonigral system is the main site of pathology, but less severe degeneration can be widespread and usually includes the olivopontocerebellar system. The putamen is shrunken with gray-green discoloration (Fig. 14.2). When putaminal pathology is severe, there may be a cribriform appearance. In early stages, the putaminal lesion shows a distinct topographical distribution with a predilection for the caudal and dorsolateral regions. Degeneration of pigmented nerve cells occurs in the substantia nigra pars compacta, while cells of the substantia nigra pars reticulata are reported as normal.

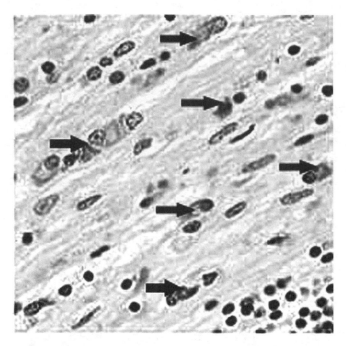

Figure 14.1 α-synuclein immunostaining reveals glial cytoplasmic inclusions in subcortical white matter. Reproduced with permission from: Wenning GK, Colosimo C, Geser F, Poewe, W. Multiple System Atrophy. *Lancet Neurol* 2004;3(2):93–103.

The topographical patterns of neurodegeneration involving the motor neostriatum, efferent pathways, and nigral neurons reflect their anatomical relationship and suggest a common denominator or "linked" degeneration (1).

In MSA-C, the brunt of pathology is in the olivopontocerebellar system, while the involvement of the striatum and substantia nigra is less severe. The basis pontis is atrophic, with loss of pontine neurons and transverse pontocerebellar fibers. In sections stained for myelin, the intact

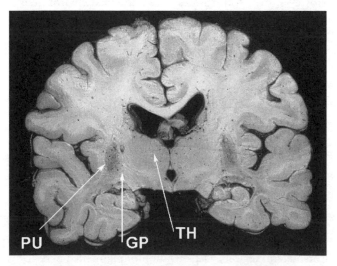

Figure 14.2 Coronal slice of cerebrum. The putamena are symmetrically shrunken. Pallida are atrophic. PU, putamen; GP, globus pallidus; TH, thalamus. Reproduced with permission from: Wenning GK, Geser F, Poewe, W. The 'risus sardonicus' of Multiple System Atrophy. *Mov Disord* 2003;18(10):1211.

descending corticospinal tracts stand out against the degenerated transverse fibers and the atrophic middle cerebellar peduncles. There is a disproportionate depletion of fibers from the middle cerebellar peduncles, compared with the loss of pontine neurons, an observation consistent with a "dying back" process (1).

A supraspinal contribution to the autonomic failure of MSA is now well-established. Sites of cell loss include the dorsal motor nucleus of the vagus, locus ceruleus, and the catecholaminergic neurons of ventrolateral medulla (1). Papp and Lantos (16) have shown marked involvement of pontomedullary reticular formation, providing a supraspinal histological counterpart for impaired visceral function. Disordered bladder, rectal, and sexual function in MSA also have been associated with cell loss in parasympathetic preganglionic nuclei of the spinal cord. These neurons are localized rostrally in Onuf's nucleus between sacral segments S2 and S3 and more caudally in the inferior intermediolateral nucleus, chiefly in the S3 to S4 segments (17). Degeneration of sympathetic preganglionic neurons in the intermediolateral column of the spinal cord is considered contributory to orthostatic hypotension (OH). However, it is noteworthy that there is not always a strong correlation between nerve cell depletion and the clinical degree of autonomic failure (18).

A variety of other neuronal populations are noted to show cell depletion and gliosis with considerable differences in vulnerability from case to case. Various degrees of abnormalities in the cerebral hemisphere, including Betz cell loss, were detected in pathologically proven MSA cases (18,19). Furthermore, anterior horn cells may show some depletion but rarely to the same extent as that occurring in motor neuron disease (20).

PATHOGENESIS

The discovery of GCIs in MSA brains highlighted the unique glial pathology as a biological hallmark of this disorder (2). GCIs are argyrophilic and half moon, oval, or conical in shape and are composed of 20- to 30-nm multilayered tubular filaments (21). Although inclusions have been described in different cellular sites (22), GCIs are most ubiquitous and appear to represent the subcellular hallmark lesion of MSA (21). Their distribution selectively involves basal ganglia, supplementary and primary motor cortex, reticular formation, and the pontocerebellar system (16). Recent data suggest that GCI represent the primary change in MSA and the neuronal pathology develops secondary to the glial pathology (23). GCIs contain classical cytoskeletal antigens, including ubiquitin and tau (21,22). More recently, α-synuclein, a presynaptic protein that is affected by point mutations in familiar PD and that is present in Lewy bodies (LBs), also has been observed in both neuronal and glial cytoplasmic inclusions in brains of patients with MSA (3,4,24). The accumulation of α-synuclein into filamentous inclusions appears to play a key role not only in MSA but also in other α-synucleinopathies such as PD and DLB. The α-synuclein accumulation in GCIs, as well as in neuronal inclusions associated with MSA, precedes their ubiquitination (25). Importantly, α-synuclein, but not ubiquitin, antibodies also reveal numerous degenerating neurites in the white matter of MSA cases (25). This suggests that an as yet unrecognized degree of pathology may be present in the axons of MSA cases, although whether or not neuronal/axonal α-synuclein pathology precedes glial α-synuclein pathology has not been examined.

Alpha-synuclein is exclusively expressed in the soluble fraction of the neuronal cytoplasm in normal humans, while in MSA brains α-synuclein forms insoluble aggregates. Whether the α-synuclein aggregation is induced by some other factor(s) or is the primary trigger of MSA pathology is unknown. Impairment in the ability of oligodendrocytes to degrade α-synuclein, which they may normally produce at low levels, may promote abnormal subcellular aggregation in MSA. Alternatively, selective upregulated or ectopic expression of α-synuclein in glial cells could occur in response to certain pathologic conditions resulting in GCIs. This scenario is supported by experimental studies demonstrating GCI-like inclusion pathology in transgenic mice overexpressing oligodendroglial α-synuclein (26). However, expression levels of α-synuclein mRNA in MSA brains are similar to those of control subjects (27). These results suggest that the transcriptional regulation of the α-synuclein gene is unlikely to be affected in MSA. Similarly, oligodendroglia that were identified by the presence of the transcript for proteolipid protein had negligible levels of α-synuclein mRNA relative to the abundance of this transcript detected in nigral dopamine neurons (28). Nevertheless, overexpression of α-synuclein mRNA may play a role in GCI formation as in cases with MSA-C. α-synuclein mRNA was elevated in GCIs positive oligodendroglia relative to nearby GCI negative oligodendroglia (28). Furthermore, in vitro models of α-synuclein-positive glial aggregations mimic the morphology of GCIs reported in MSA and could be suitable models for studying their role in the pathogenesis of this disease. Indeed, to investigate the consequence of α-synuclein overexpression in glia, Stefanova et al. (29) transfected U373 astrocytoma cells with vectors encoding wild-type human α-synuclein or C-terminally truncated synuclein fused to red fluorescent protein. Alpha-synuclein immunocytochemistry of transfected astroglial cells revealed diffuse cytoplasmic labeling associated with discrete inclusions within both cell bodies and processes. Susceptibility to oxidative stress was increased in astroglial cells overexpressing α-synuclein, particularly in the presence of cytoplasmic inclusions. Furthermore, overexpression of α-synuclein induced apoptotic death of astroglial cells as shown by TUNEL staining. Further morphological studies of the inclusions using immunoelectronmicroscopy (30) revealed an amorphous dense core and a predominantly filamentous halo. Mainly filamentous structures at the border area between the halo and the core are α-synuclein-immunoreactive.

Alpha-synuclein is post-translationally modified by phosphorylation and/or glycosylation. In transfected cells, α synuclein is constitutively phosphorylated at serine residues 87 and 129, with residue 129 being the predominant site (31). Fujiwara et al. also demonstrated that serine 129 of α-synuclein is selectively and extensively phosphorylated in synucleinopathy lesions, and that this phosphorylation promotes fibril formation in vitro (32). Alpha-synuclein is also modified by glycosylation (33). Whether soluble, O-glycosylated αSP22 (a new 22-kilodalton glycosylated form of α-synuclein) mediates specific physiological functions (as found for other O-glycosylated cytoplasmic proteins) and/or has neurotoxic effects in PD or other synucleinopathies remains to be established (33). Using antibodies to specific nitrated tyrosine residues in α-synuclein, Giasson et al. (34) demonstrated extensive and widespread accumulations of nitrated α-synuclein in the signature inclusions of PD, DLB, and MSA brains. The widespread presence of nitrated α-synuclein in diverse intracellular inclusions suggests that oxidation/nitration is involved in the onset and/or progression of these neurodegenerative diseases. Souza et al. (35) showed that exposure of human recombinant α-synuclein to nitrating agents (peroxynitrite/CO_2 or myeloperoxidase/H_2O_2/nitrite) induces formation of nitrated α-synuclein oligomers that are highly stabilized due to covalent cross-linking via the oxidation of tyrosine to form o,o′-dityrosine. Gomez-Tortosa et al. (36) investigated the distribution and relationships of α-synuclein inclusions and 3-nitrotyrosine (3-NT), a marker of protein nitration through oxidative mechanisms, in brains diagnosed with Lewy body diseases or MSA and control brains using double immunohistochemical techniques. Their data showed that protein nitration in Lewy body diseases and MSA cases has a widespread distribution and is associated not only with the α-synuclein deposits. The presence of α-synuclein-positive deposits lacking 3-NT immunoreactivity suggests that nitration is not a prerequisite for α-synuclein deposition.

Accumulation of α-synuclein may require additional proteins as pathologic chaperones. If chaperones are involved, their nature is likely to be unique to MSA because the morphology and array of immunoreactive components in GCIs and neuronal cytoplasmic inclusions NCIs differ from those characterizing Lewy bodies (4). Engelender et al. (37) identified an α-synuclein-associated novel protein, synphilin-1, and reported that co-transfection of both α-synuclein and synphilin-1 in mammalian cells yielded eosinophilic cytoplasmic inclusions resembling LBs. More recently, Wakabayashi et al. (38) showed that synphilin-1 immunoreactivity is present in LBs, as well as in GCIs. Various neuronal and glial inclusions in neurodegenerative disorders other than LB disease and MSA were synphilin-1 negative. Therefore, abnormal accumulation of synphilin-1 appears to be specific for brain lesions in which α-synuclein is a major component. Recent evidence suggests that 14-3-3 proteins also may be linked to the formation of GCIs (39).

CLINICAL PRESENTATION

MSA affects both men and women, usually starts in the sixth decade, and relentlessly progresses with a mean survival of 6–9 years (40,41,42). In some instances, there is considerable variation of disease progression with survival of more than 15 years.

Clinically, cardinal features include autonomic failure, parkinsonism, cerebellar ataxia, and pyramidal signs in any combination. Previous studies suggest that 29%–33% of patients with isolated late-onset cerebellar ataxia and 8% of patients presenting with parkinsonism will eventually develop MSA (43,44,45). Two major motor presentations can be distinguished clinically. Parkinsonian features predominate in 80% of patients (MSA-P subtype), and cerebellar ataxia is the major motor feature in 20% of patients (MSA-C subtype) (6,42). Importantly, both motor presentations of MSA are associated with similar survival times (41). However, MSA-P patients have a more rapid functional deterioration than do MSA-C patients (40).

MSA-P associated parkinsonism is characterized by progressive akinesia and rigidity. Jerky postural tremor and, less commonly, tremor at rest may be superimposed.

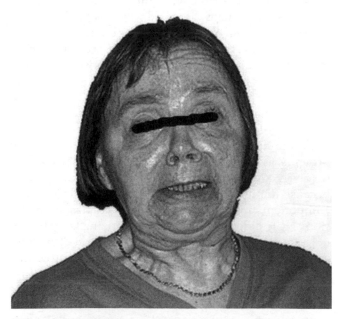

Figure 14.3 A patient with MSA with hypomimia, asymmetric orofacial dystonia, and cervical dystonia affecting the platysma. The patient had a very distinctive quivering, strangled, high-pitched dysarthria, as is seen in 80% of MSA patients. Reproduced with permission from: Wenning GK, Colosimo C, Geser F, Poewe, W. Multiple System Atrophy. *Lancet Neurol* 2004;3(2):93–103.

Frequently, patients exhibit orofacial or craniocervical dystonia (Fig. 14.3) associated with a characteristic quivering, high-pitched dysarthria. Postural stability is compromised early on; however, recurrent falls at disease onset are unusual in contrast to progressive supranuclear palsy (PSP). Differential diagnosis of MSA-P and PD may be exceedingly difficult in the early stages due to a number of overlapping features, such as rest tremor or asymmetrical akinesia and rigidity. Furthermore, L-dopa–induced improvement of parkinsonism may be seen in 30% of MSA-P patients. However, the benefit is transient in most of these subjects, leaving 90% of the MSA-P patients L-dopa unresponsive in the long term. L-dopa–induced dyskinesia affecting orofacial and neck muscles occurs in 50% of MSA-P patients, sometimes in the absence of motor benefit (46). In most instances, a fully developed clinical picture of MSA-P evolves within 5 years of disease onset, allowing a clinical diagnosis during follow-up.

The cerebellar disorder of MSA-C comprises gait ataxia, limb kinetic ataxia, and scanning dysarthria, as well as cerebellar oculomotor disturbances. Patients with MSA-C usually develop additional noncerebellar symptoms and signs, but before doing so may be indistinguishable from other patients with idiopathic late-onset cerebellar ataxia, many of whom have a disease restricted clinically to cerebellar signs and pathologically to degeneration of the cerebellum and olives (43).

Dysautonomia is characteristic of both MSA motor presentations, primarily comprising urogenital and orthostatic dysfunction. Early impotence (erectile dysfunction) is virtually universal in men with MSA, and urinary incontinence or retention, often early in the course or as presenting symptoms, are frequent (42). Disorders of micturition in MSA are due to changes in the complex peripheral and central innervation of the bladder (47) and generally occur more commonly, earlier, and to a more severe degree than in PD. In contrast, constipation occurs equally in PD and MSA. Symptomatic OH is present in 68% of clinically diagnosed patients, but recurrent syncopes emerge in only 15% (42). L-dopa or dopamine agonists may provoke or worsen OH.

CLINICAL DIAGNOSTIC CRITERIA

Clinical diagnostic criteria for MSA were first proposed by Quinn (5,48), who classified patients as either SND- or OPCA-type MSA, depending on the predominance of parkinsonism or cerebellar ataxia. These criteria define two levels of clinical diagnostic certainty (possible, probable) and reserve a definite diagnosis to neuropathological confirmation.

Clinicopathological studies have shown good specificity but poor sensitivity (49) of the Quinn criteria, and more recently operationalized criteria have been proposed by an International Consensus Conference (6) (Table 14.1). The consensus criteria have since been

TABLE 14.1 A
MULTIPLE SYSTEM ATROPHY CONSENSUS CRITERIA

Nomenclature of clinical domains, features (disease characteristics), and criteria (defining features or composite of features) used in the diagnosis of MSA

Domain	Criterion	Feature
Autonomic and urinary dysfunction	Orthostatic fall in blood pressure by 30 mmHg systolic or 15 mmHg diastolic) *or* persistent urinary incontinence with erectile dysfunction in men *or both*	Orthostatic hypotension (by 20 mmHg systolic or 10 mmHg diastolic) Urinary incontinence or incomplete bladder emptying
Parkinsonism	Bradykinesia *plus* rigidity *or* postural instability *or* tremor	Bradykinesia (progressive reduction in speed and amplitude of voluntary movements during repetitive actions) Rigidity Postural instability (loss of primary postural reflexes) Tremor (postural, resting or both)
Cerebellar dysfunction	Gait ataxia *plus* ataxic dysarthria *or* limb ataxia *or* sustained gaze-evoked nystagmus	Gait ataxia (wide-based stance with irregular steps) Ataxic dysarthria Limb ataxia Sustained gaze-evoked nystagmus
Corticospinal tract dysfunction	No defining features	Extensor plantar responses with hyperreflexia

Modified from Gilman S, Low PA, Quinn N, Albanese A, Ben Shlomo Y, Fowler CJ, et al. Consensus statement on the diagnosis of multiple system atrophy. *J Auton Nerv Syst* 1998;74:189–192. Reproduced with permission from: Wenning GK, Geser F. Diagnosis and Treatment of Multiple System Atrophy: An Update. Advances in Clinical Neuroscience and Rehabilitation 2004;3:5–10.

TABLE 14.1 B
MULTIPLE SYSTEM ATROPHY CONSENSUS CRITERIA

Diagnostic categories of MSA

Possible MSA-P	Criterion for parkinsonism, plus two features from separate other domains. A poor L-dopa response qualifies as one feature, hence only one additional feature is required.
Possible MSA-C	Criterion for cerebellar dysfunction, plus two features from separate other domains.
Probable MSA-P	Criterion for autonomic failure/urinary dysfunction, plus poorly L-dopa–responsive parkinsonism.
Probable MSA-C	Criterion for autonomic failure/urinary dysfunction, plus cerebellar dysfunction.
Definite MSA	Pathological confirmation: high density of α-synuclein–positive glial cytoplasmic inclusions associated with degenerative changes in the nigrostriatal (striatonigral degeneration) and olivopontocerebellar pathways (olivopontocerebellar atrophy).

Modified from Gilman S, Low PA, Quinn N, Albanese A, Ben Shlomo Y, Fowler CJ, et al. Consensus statement on the diagnosis of multiple system atrophy. *J Auton Nerv Syst* 1998;74:189–192. Reproduced with permission from: Wenning GK, Geser F. Diagnosis and Treatment of Multiple System Atrophy: An Update. Advances in Clinical Neuroscience and Rehabilitation 2004;3:5–10.

TABLE 14.1 C
MULTIPLE SYSTEM ATROPHY CONSENSUS CRITERIA

Exclusion criteria for the diagnosis of MSA

I. History

Symptomatic onset under 30 years of age
Family history of a similar disorder
Systemic disease or other identifiable causes for features listed in Table 14.1A
Hallucinations unrelated to medication

II. Physical Examination

Criteria for dementia according to the Diagnostic and Statistical Manual of Mental Disorders, fourth edition
Prominent slowing of vertical saccades or vertical supranuclear gaze palsy[a]
Evidence of focal cortical dysfunction, such as aphasia, alien limb syndrome, and parietal dysfunction

III. Laboratory Investigation

Metabolic, molecular genetic, and imaging evidence of an alternative cause of features listed in Table 14.1A

[a] In practice, MSA is most frequently confused with Parkinson's disease or progressive supranuclear palsy (PSP). Mild limitation of upward gaze alone is nonspecific, whereas a prominent (>50%) limitation of upward gaze or any limitation of downward gaze suggests PSP. Before the onset of vertical gaze limitation, a clinically obvious slowing of voluntary vertical saccades is usually easily detectable in PSP and assists in the early differentiation of these two disorders. Reproduced with permission from: Gilman S, Low PA, Quinn N, Albanese A, Ben Shlomo Y, Fowler CJ, Kaufmann H, Klockgether T, Lang AE, Lantos PL, Litvan I, Mathias CJ, Oliver E, Robertson D, Schatz I, Wenning GK. Consensus statement on the diagnosis of multiple system atrophy. *J Auton Nerv Syst* 1998;74:189–192.

widely established in the research community and in movement disorders clinics. They define three diagnostic categories of increasing certainty: possible, probable, and definite. The diagnoses of possible and probable MSA are based on the presence of specific clinical features (Table 14.1A and 14.1B). In addition, exclusion criteria have to be considered (Table 14.1C). A definite diagnosis requires a typical neuropathological lesion pattern with α-synuclein-positive GCIs.

A recent retrospective evaluation of the consensus criteria on pathologically proven cases showed excellent positive predictive values for both possible and probable MSA; however, sensitivity for probable MSA was poor (50). Interestingly, the consensus criteria and Quinn's criteria had similar positive predictive values. Although such formal diagnostic criteria are important for certain types of clinical research, they add little to the problem of detecting early cases, and improved screening instruments are certainly needed.

Besides the poor response to L-dopa, and the additional presence of pyramidal or cerebellar signs or autonomic failure as major diagnostic clues, certain other features ("red flags"), such as orofacial dystonia, stridor, or rapid eye movement sleep behavior disorder (RBD), may raise suspicion of MSA (5,51) (Table 14.2). MSA patients may present with isolated RBD (52). RBD and other sleep disorders matched for disease duration are more common in patients with MSA than in those with PD, reflecting both a profound striatal monoaminergic deficit (53) and diffuse subcortical and brainstem disease in MSA (54).

INVESTIGATIONS

The diagnosis of MSA still rests on the clinical history and neurological examination. Attempts have been made, however, to improve diagnostic accuracy through analysis of cerebrospinal fluid and serum biomarkers, autonomic function tests, structural and functional neuroimaging, and neurophysiological techniques. Typical results that may be obtained using these various investigational tools are summarized in Table 14.3. According to the Consensus Conference on the diagnosis of multiple system atrophy (6), additional investigations, such as autonomic function tests, sphincter electromyography, or neuroimaging, may be used to support the diagnosis or to exclude other conditions. The abnormalities shown in Table 14.3 have been observed in patients with advanced rather than early disease. In the early stages, the investigations may give equivocal results. Therefore, the Consensus Conference considered it premature to incorporate the results of laboratory investigations into the diagnostic guidelines that were established.

TREATMENT

Autonomic Failure

Unfortunately, currently there is no curative therapy for autonomic dysfunction, and so the therapeutic strategy is symptomatic and determined by the extent of impairment of the quality of life in these patients. In all cases it is important to remember that the progressive course of MSA

TABLE 14.2
WARNING FEATURES (RED FLAGS) OF MULTIPLE SYSTEM ASTROPHY*

Motor Red Flags	Definition
Orofacial dystonia	Atypical spontaneous or L-dopa–induced dystonia predominantly affecting orofacial muscles, occasionally resembling *risus sardonicus* of cephalic tetanus.
Pisa syndrome	Subacute axial dystonia with a severe tonic lateral flexion of the trunk, head, and neck (contracted and hypertrophic paravertebral muscles may be present).
Disproportionate antecollis	Chin-on-chest, neck can only with difficulty be passively and forcibly extended to its normal position. Despite severe chronic neck flexion, flexion elsewhere is minor.
Jerky tremor	Irregular (jerky) postural or action tremor of the hands and/or fingers.
Dysarthria	Atypical quivering, irregular, severely hypophonic or slurring high-pitched dysarthria, which tends to develop earlier, be more severe, and be associated with more marked dysphagia compared to PD.
Nonmotor Red Flags	
Abnormal respiration	Nocturnal (harsh or strained, high-pitched inspiratory sounds) or diurnal inspiratory stridor, involuntary deep inspiratory sighs/gasps, sleep apnea (arrest of breathing for ≥10 seconds), and excessive snoring (increase from premorbid level or newly arising).
REM sleep behavior disorder	Intermittent loss of muscle atonia and appearance of elaborate motor activity (striking out with arms in sleep often with talking/shouting) associated with dream mentation.
Cold hands/feet	Coldness and color change (purple/blue) of extremities not due to drugs, with blanching on pressure and poor circulatory return.
Raynaud's phenomenon	Painful "white finger," which may be provoked by ergot drugs.
Emotional incontinence	Crying inappropriately without sadness or laughing inappropriately without mirth.

* Excluding cardinal diagnostic features of MSA, such as orthostatic hypotension, urinary incontinence/retention, L-dopa–unresponsive parkinsonism, cerebellar (ataxia), and pyramidal signs. Also excluding nonspecific features suggesting atypical parkinsonism, such as rapid progression or early instability and falls. Reproduced with permission from: Wenning GK, Geser F, Stampfer-Kountchev M, Tison F. Multiple System Atrophy: An Update. *Mov Disord* 2003;18:534–542.

TABLE 14.3
ADDITIONAL INVESTIGATIONS IN MULTIPLE SYSTEM ATROPHY

Investigation	Typical Results
Cardiovascular autonomic function tests	Orthostatic hypotension (≥20/10 mmHg systolic/diastolic blood pressure drop upon standing) Impaired reflex tachycardia Impaired heart rate variability Impaired Valsalva maneuver Impaired rise of plasma noradrenaline upon standing
Clonidine challenge test	Impaired release of growth hormone (controversial)
Thermoregulatory sweat test, quantitative sudomotor axon reflex test	Sudomotor dysfunction (an-/hypohidrosis) due to pre- and postganglionic sympathetic failure
Sympathetic skin response	Abnormal or absent
Cerebrospinal fluid	Increased neurofilament protein level
External anal sphincter EMG	Denervation (nonspecific)
Cerebral computed tomography	Unhelpful
MRI (1.5 Tesla)	Basal ganglia abnormalities (putaminal atrophy/hyperintense putaminal rim/putaminal hypointensity, infratentorial signal change— hot cross bun sign), cerebellar and/or brain stem atrophy
MRI (diffusion-weighted imaging)	Increase in putaminal diffusion properties (posterior > anterior)
[123I] iodobenzamide single photon emission computed tomography	Reduced striatal dopamine D2 receptor binding
[(123)I] Metaiodobenzylguanidine single photon emission computed tomography	Reduced striatal, frontal, and infratentorial metabolism
No reduction in myocardial metaiodobenzylguanidine uptake [(18)F]-fluorodeoxyglucose positron emission tomography	

Reproduced and modified with permission from: Wenning GK, Geser F. Diagnosis and Treatment of Multiple System Atrophy: An Update. Advances in Clinical Neuroscience and Rehabilitation 2004;3:5–10.

means that a regular review of the treatment is mandatory to adjust measures according to clinical needs.

The rationale in treating the symptoms of OH is based on increasing the intravascular volume with a reduction of volume shift to lower body parts when changing to an upright position. The selection and combination of therapies depends on the severity of symptoms in the individual patient, rather than the extent of blood pressure drop during a tilt test.

The simplest nonpharmacological options include sufficient fluid intake, a high salt diet, an increase in frequency along with smaller meals to reduce postprandial hypotension (by spreading the total carbohydrate intake), and custom-made elastic body garments. During night, head-up tilt increases the intravascular volume by up to 1 liter within a week, which is particularly helpful in improving early morning hypotension. This approach is especially successful in combination with fludrocortisone, which further supports sodium retention.

The next group of drugs to consider are the sympathomimetics. These include ephedrine (with both direct and indirect effects), although at higher doses side effects develop, including tremulousness, loss of appetite, and urinary retention in men.

Among the large number of vasoactive agents that have been evaluated in MSA, only one—the directly acting α-adrenergic agonist midodrine—meets the criteria of evidence-based medicine (55,56,57). Side effects usually are mild and only rarely lead to discontinuation of treatment because of urinary retention or pruritus, predominantly on the scalp.

Another promising drug appears to be the norepinephrine precursor L-threo-3,4-dihydroxyphenylserine (L-DOPS), which has been used for this indication in Japan for years and for which efficacy has now been shown by a recent open, dose-finding trial (58).

If the drugs previously mentioned do not produce the desired effects, selective targeting is needed. The somatostatin analog, octreotide, is often beneficial in postprandial hypotension, presumably because it inhibits release of vasodilatory gastrointestinal peptides and, importantly, it does not enhance nocturnal hypertension.

The vasopressin analog, desmopressin, which acts on renal tubular vasopressin-2 receptors, reduces nocturnal polyuria and improves morning postural hypotension.

The peptide erythropoietin may be beneficial in some patients by raising red cell mass, secondarily improving cerebral oxygenation.

A broad range of drugs (Table 14.4) has been tried in the treatment of postural hypotension, but the value and side effects of many of these have not been adequately determined in MSA patients using appropriate endpoints.

In the management of neurogenic bladder (including measurements of residual urine volumes), clean intermittent catheterization 3–4 times per day is a widely accepted approach to prevent the secondary consequences of poor

TABLE 14.4
PRACTICAL MANAGEMENT OF MULTIPLE SYSTEM ATROPHY

A. Pharmacotherapy

I. For akinesia-rigidity
- L-dopa up to 1000 mg/day, if tolerated
- Dopamine agonists as second-line antiparkinsonian drugs (dosing as for PD patients)
- Amantadine as third-line drug, 100 mg up to 3 times daily

II. For focal dystonia
- Botulinum toxin A

III. For orthostatic hypotension
- Head-up tilt of bed at night
- Elastic stockings or tights
- Increased salt intake
- Fludrocortisone 0.1–0.3 mg/day
- Ephedrine 15–45 mg t.i.d.
- L-threo-DOPS 300 mg b.i.d.
- Midodrine 2.5—10 mg t.i.d.

IV. For postprandial hypotension
- Octreotide 25–50 mcg s.c. 30 minutes before a meal

V. For nocturnal polyuria
- Desmopressin (spray: 10–40 mcg/night; tablet: 100–400 mcg/night)

VI. For bladder symptoms
- Oxybutynin for detrusor hyperreflexia 2.5–5 mg b.i.d–t.i.d.
- Intermittent self-catheterization for retention or residual volume >100 ml

B. Other therapies

- Physiotherapy
- Speech therapy
- Occupational therapy
- Percutaneous endoscopic gastrostomy (PEG) (rarely needed in late stage)
- Provision of wheelchair
- Continuous positive air pressure (CPAP; rarely tracheostomy) for inspiratory stridor

Reproduced with permission from: Wenning GK, Geser F, Stampfer-Kountchev M, Tison F. Multiple System Atrophy: An Update. *Mov Disord* 2003;18:534–542.

micturition (59). It may be necessary, in some cases, to provide the patient with a permanent transcutaneous suprapubic catheter if mechanical obstruction in the urethra or motor symptoms of MSA prevent uncomplicated catheterization.

Pharmacological options with cholinergic agonists or antagonists or alpha-adrenergic substances are usually not successful in reducing post-void residual volume in MSA, but anticholinergic agents such as oxybutynin can improve symptoms of detrusor hyperreflexia or sphincter–detrusor dyssynergy in the early course of the disease. Furthermore, alpha-adrenergic receptor antagonists (prazosin and moxisylyte) have been shown to improve voiding with reduction of residual volumes in MSA patients (60). Urological surgery must be avoided in these patients because postoperative worsening of bladder control is common.

The necessity of a specific treatment for sexual dysfunction must be evaluated individually in each MSA patient. Male impotence can be partially circumvented with the use of intracavernosal papaverine, prostaglandin E1, or penile implants. Preliminary evidence in PD patients (61) suggests that sildenafil also may be successful in treating erectile failure in MSA. Indeed, a trial confirmed the efficacy of this compound in MSA but also suggested caution because of the frequent cardiovascular side effects (62). Erectile failure in MSA also may be improved by oral yohimbine.

Constipation can be relieved by increasing the intraluminal volume, which may be achieved by using macrogol–water solution.

Inspiratory stridor develops in about 30% of patients. Continuous positive airway pressure (CPAP) may be helpful in some of these patients (63). In only about 4%, a tracheostomy is needed and performed.

Motor Disorder

General Approach

Because the results of drug treatment for the motor disorder of MSA are generally poor, other therapies are all the more important. Physiotherapy helps maintain mobility and prevent contractures, and speech therapy can improve speech and swallowing and provide communication aids. Dysphagia may require feeding via a nasogastric tube or even percutaneous endoscopic gastrostomy. Occupational therapy helps to limit the handicap resulting from the patient's disabilities and should include a home visit. Provision of a wheelchair is usually dictated by the liability to falls because of postural instability and gait ataxia but not by akinesia and rigidity per se. Psychological support for patients and partners must be stressed.

Parkinsonism

Parkinsonism is the predominant motor disorder in MSA and, therefore, represents a major target for therapeutic intervention. Although less effective than in PD and despite the lack of randomized controlled trials, L-dopa replacement represents the mainstay of antiparkinsonian therapy in MSA. Open-label studies suggest that 30%–40% of MSA patients may derive benefit from L-dopa at least transiently (42,64). Occasionally, a beneficial effect is evident only when seemingly unresponsive patients deteriorate after L-dopa withdrawal. Preexisting OH is often unmasked or exacerbated in L-dopa–treated MSA patients associated with autonomic failure whereas, in contrast, psychiatric or toxic confusional states appear to be less common than in PD. Results with dopamine agonists have been even more disappointing. Wenning et al. (42) reported a response to oral dopamine agonists only in 4 of 41 patients, and none of 30 patients improved upon receiving bromocriptine, but

3 of 10 who received pergolide had some benefit. Of the L-dopa responders, 22% had a good or excellent response to at least one additional orally active dopamine agonist. Antiparkinsonian effects were noted in 4 of 26 MSA patients treated with amantadine (42), but there was no significant improvement in an open study of nine patients with atypical parkinsonism, including five subjects with MSA (65).

Blepharospasm, as well as limb dystonia, but not antecollis, may respond well to local injections of botulinum toxin A.

Ablative neurosurgical procedures such as medial pallidotomy fail to improve parkinsonian motor disturbance in MSA. However, Visser-Vandewalle et al. report a beneficial effect of bilateral high-frequency subthalamic stimulation in four patients with MSA-P, both in the short term and long term (66).

Cerebellar Ataxia

There is no effective therapy for the progressive ataxia of MSA-C. Occasional successes have been reported with cholinergic drugs, amantadine, 5-hydroxytryptophan, isoniazid, baclofen, and propanolol. For the large majority of MSA-C patients, these drugs proved ineffective. One intriguing observation is the apparent temporary exacerbation of ataxia by cigarette smoking. Nicotine is known to increase the release of acetylcholine in many areas of the brain and probably also releases noradrenaline, dopamine, 5-hydroxytryptophan, and other neurotransmitters. Nicotinic systems may, therefore, play a role in cerebellar function, and trials of nicotinic antagonists such as dihydrobetaerythroidine might be worthwhile in MSA-C.

Practical Therapy

Because of the small number of randomized controlled trials, the practical management of MSA is largely based on empirical evidence ($\leftrightarrow$) or single randomized studies ($\uparrow$), except for three randomized controlled studies of midodrine ($\uparrow\uparrow$). The present recommendations are summarized in Table 14.4.

Future Therapeutic Approaches

Two European research initiatives—European MSA-Study Group (EMSA-SG) and Natural History and Neuroprotection and Parkinson Plus Syndromes (NIPPS)—are presently conducting multicenter intervention trials in MSA. These trials will radically change our approach to MSA. For the first time, prospective data concerning disease progression will become available, allowing us to identify reliably the predictors of survival.

The need for prospective natural history studies has led the EMSA-SG to develop the Unified MSA Rating Scale (UMSARS), including a video teaching tape to standardize severity assessments in specialized clinics and research programs (67). This novel scale also will be useful in the planning and implementation of future multicenter intervention trials. Importantly, accurate data on UMSARS rates of decline as established recently enable sample size calculations (68).

Furthermore, surrogate markers of the disease process will be identified by the EMSA-SG and NNIPPS trials using structural and functional neuroimaging. These markers will allow planning future phase III intervention trials more effectively.

Research into the etiopathogenesis and neuropathology of MSA is being conducted by EMSA-SG, NNIPPS, and the North American MSA-Study Group (NAMSA-SG). A number of animal models have become available as testbeds for preclinical intervention studies (69). This work will lead to a multitude of neuroprotective candidate agents ready to be tested during the next decade.

CONCLUSION

Since the early 1990s, there have been major advances in our understanding of the cellular pathology of MSA. Despite these advances in the pathogenesis of MSA, more work is required to elucidate the cascade of cell death in MSA and to determine exogenous and genetic susceptibility factors, both of which are likely to drive the disease process in this disorder. At the same time, the first multicenter intervention trials have been launched in Europe. Although therapeutic options are limited at present, there is a real hope for a radical change of our approach to this devastating illness.

REFERENCES

1. Geser F, Colosimo C, Wenning G. Multiple system atrophy (MSA). In: Beal F, Lang A, Ludolph A, eds. *Neurodegenerative Diseases: Neurobiology, Pathogenesis and Therapeutics.* Cambridge: Cambridge University Press; 2005;623–662.
2. Papp M, Kahn JE, Lantos PL. Glial cytoplasmic inclusions in the CNS of patients with multiple system atrophy (striatonigral degeneration, olivopontocerebellar atrophy and Shy-Drager syndrome). *J Neurol Sci* 1989;94:79–100.
3. Wakabayashi K, Yoshimoto M, Tsuji S, Takahashi H. Alpha-synuclein immunoreactivity in glial cytoplasmic inclusions in multiple system atrophy. *Neurosci Lett* 1998;249:180–182.
4. Spillantini MG, Crowther RA, Jakes R, Cairns NJ, Lantos PL, Goedert M. Filamentous alpha-synuclein inclusions link multiple system atrophy with Parkinson's disease and dementia with Lewy bodies. *Neurosci Lett* 1998;251:205–208.
5. Quinn N. Multiple system atrophy—the nature of the beast. *J Neurol Neurosurg Psychiatry* 1989;52(suppl):78–89.
6. Gilman S, Low PA, Quinn N, et al. Consensus statement on the diagnosis of multiple system atrophy. *J Auton Nerv Syst*1998;74: 189–192.
7. Bower J, Maraganore D, McDonnell S, Rocca W. Incidence of progressive supranuclear palsy and multiple system atrophy in Olmsted County, Minnesota, 1976 to 1990. *Neurology* 1997;49: 1284–1288.
8. Tison F, Yekhlef F, Chrysostome V, Sourgen C. Prevalence of multiple system atrophy. *Lancet* 2000;355:495–496.
9. Schrag A, Ben-Shlomo Y, Quinn NP. Prevalence of progressive supranuclear palsy and multiple system atrophy: a cross-sectional study. *Lancet* 1999;354:1771–1775.
10. Wermuth L, Joensen P, Bunger N, Jeune B. High prevalence of Parkinson's disease in the Faroe Islands. *Neurology* 1997;49: 426–432.
11. Chio A, Magnani C, Schiffer D. Prevalence of Parkinson's disease in Northwestern Italy: comparison of tracer methodology and clinical ascertainment of cases. *Mov Disord* 1998;13:400–405.
12. Nee LE, Gomez MR, Dambrosia J, Bale S, Eldridge R, Polinsky RJ. Environmental-occupational risk factors and familial associations in multiple system atrophy: a preliminary investigation. *Clin Auton Res* 1991;1:9–13.
13. Vanacore N, Bonifati V, Fabbrini G, et al. Smoking habits in multiple system atrophy and progressive supranuclear palsy. *Neurology* 2000;54:114–119.
14. Hanna P, Jankovic J, Kirkpatrick JB. Multiple system atrophy: The putative causative role of environmental toxins. *Arch Neurol* 1999;56:90–94.
15. Vanacore N, Bonifati V, Fabbrini G, et al. Case-control study of multiple system atrophy. *Mov Disord* 2005;20(2):158–163.
16. Papp M, Lantos PL. The distribution of oligodendroglial inclusions in multiple system atrophy and its relevance to clinical symptomatology. *Brain* 1994;117:235–243.
17. Konno H, Yamamoto T, Iwasaki Y, Iizuka H. Shy-Drager syndrome and amyotrophic lateral sclerosis: cytoarchitectonic and morphometric studies of sacral autonomic neurons. *J Neurol Sci* 1986;73:193–204.
18. Daniel S. The neuropathology and neurochemistry of multiple system atrophy. In: Mathias C, Bannister R, eds. *Autonomic Failure: A Textbook of Clinical Disorders of the Autonomic Nervous System.* Oxford: Oxford University Press; 1999:321–328.
19. Wenning G, Tison F, Ben-Shlomo Y, Daniel SE, Quinn NP. Multiple system atrophy: a review of 203 pathologically proven cases. *Mov Disord* 1997;12:133–147.
20. Sima A, Caplan M, D'Amato CJ, Pevzner M, Furlong JW. Fulminant multiple system atrophy in a young adult presenting as motor neuron disease. *Neurology* 1993;43:2031–2035.
21. Lantos PL. The definition of multiple system atrophy: a review of recent developments. *J Neuropathol Exp Neurol* 1998;57: 1099–1111.
22. Papp M, Lantos PI. Accumulation of tubular structures in oligodendroglial and neuronal cells as the basic alteration in multiple system atrophy. *J Neurog Sci* 1992;107:172–182.
23. Armstrong RA, Cairns NJ, Lantos PL. Multiple system atrophy (MSA): Topographic distribution of the alpha-synuclein-associated pathological changes. *Parkinsonism Relat Disord* 2006, in press.
24. Wakabayashi K, Hayashi S, Kakita A, et al. Accumulation of alpha-synuclein/NACP is a cytopathological feature common to Lewy body disease and multiple system atrophy. *Acta Neuropathol* 1998;96:445–452.
25. Gai WP, Power JH, Blumbergs PC, Blessing WW. Multiple-system atrophy: a new alpha-synuclein disease? *Lancet* 1998;352:547–548.
26. Kahle PJ, Neumann M, Ozmen L, et al. Hyperphosphorylation and insolubility of alpha-synuclein in transgenic mouse oligodendrocytes. EMBO Rep. 2002;3:583–588.
27. Ozawa T, Okuizumi K, Ikeuchi T, Wakabayashi K, Takahashi H, Tsuji S. Analysis of the expression level of alpha-synuclein mRNA using postmortem brain samples from pathologically confirmed cases of multiple system atrophy. *Acta Neuropathol (Berl)* 2001; 102:188–190.
28. Miller DW, Johnson JM, Solano SM, Standaert DG, Young, AB. Expression of alpha-synuclein mRNA in multiple system atrophy. *Funct Neurol* 2004;19:145–146.
29. Stefanova N, Klimaschewski L, Poewe W, Wenning GK, Reindl M. Glial cell death induced by overexpression of alpha-synuclein. *J Neurosci Res* 2001;65:432–438.
30. Stefanova N, Emgard M, Klimaschewski L, Wenning GK, Reindl M. Ultrastructure of alpha-synuclein-positive aggregations in U373 astrocytoma and rat primary glial cells. *Neurosci Lett* 2002;323:37–40.
31. Okochi M, Walter J, Koyama A, et al. Constitutive phosphorylation of the Parkinson's disease associated alpha-synuclein. *J Biol Chem* 2000;275:390–397.
32. Fujiwara H, Hasegawa M, Dohmae N, et al. Alpha-synuclein is phosphorylated in synucleinopathy lesions. *Nat Cell Biol* 2002;4:160–164.
33. Shimura H, Schlossmacher MG, Hattori N, et al. Ubiquitination of a new form of alpha-synuclein by parkin from human brain: implications for Parkinson's disease. *Science* 2001;293:263–269.

34. Giasson BI, Duda JE, Murray IV, et al. Oxidative damage linked to neurodegeneration by selective alpha-synuclein nitration in synucleinopathy lesions. *Science* 2000;290:985–989.

35. Souza JM, Giasson BI, Chen Q, Lee VM, Ischiropoulos H. Dityrosine cross-linking promotes formation of stable alpha-synuclein polymers. Implication of nitrative and oxidative stress in the pathogenesis of neurodegenerative synucleinopathies. *J Biol Chem* 2000;275:18,344–18,349.

36. Gomez-Tortosa E, Gonzalo I, Newell K, Garcia YJ, Vonsattel P, Hyman BT. Patterns of protein nitration in dementia with Lewy bodies and striatonigral degeneration. *Acta Neuropathol (Berl)* 2002;103:495–500.

37. Engelender S, Kaminsky Z, Guo X, et al. Synphilin-1 associates with alpha-synuclein and promotes the formation of cytosolic inclusions. *Nat Genet* 1999;22:110–114.

38. Wakabayashi K, Engelender S, Yoshimoto M, Tsuji S, Ross C, Takahashi H. Synphilin-I is present in Lewy bodies in Parkinson's disease. *Ann Neurol* 2000;47:521–523.

39. Kawamoto Y, Akiguchi I, Nakamura S, Budka H. Accumulation of 14-3-3 proteins in glial cytoplasmic inclusions in multiple system atrophy. *Ann Neurol* 2002;52:722–731.

40. Watanabe H, Saito Y, Terao S, Ando T, Kachi T, Mukai E. Progression and prognosis in multiple system atrophy: an analysis of 230 Japanese patients. *Brain* 2002;125:1070–1083.

41. Ben-Shlomo Y, Wenning G, Tison F, Quinn N. Survival of patients with pathologically proven multiple system atrophy: a meta-analysis. *Neurology* 1997;48:384–393.

42. Wenning GK, Ben Shlomo Y, Magalhaes M, Daniel SE, Quinn NP. Clinical features and natural history of multiple system atrophy. An analysis of 100 cases. *Brain* 1994;117(pt 4):835–845.

43. Abele M, Burk K, Schols L, et al. The aetiology of sporadic adult-onset ataxia. *Brain* 2002;125(pt 5):961–968.

44. Gilman S, Little R, Johanns J, et al. Evolution of sporadic olivopontocerebellar atrophy into multiple system atrophy. *Neurology* 2000;55:527–532.

45. Schwarz J, Tatsch K, Gasser T, et al. 123I-IBZM binding compared with long-term clinical follow up in patients with de novo parkinsonism. *Mov Disord* 1998;13:16–19.

46. Boesch SM, Wenning GK, Ransmayr G, Poewe W. Dystonia in multiple system atrophy. *J Neurol Neurosurg Psychiatry* 2002;72: 300–303.

47. Beck R, Betts C, Fowler C. Genitourinary dysfunction in multiple system atrophy: clinical features and treatment in 62 cases. *J Urol* 1994;151:1336–1341.

48. Quinn N. Multiple system atrophy. In: Marsden CD, Fahn S, eds. *Movement Disorders 3*. London: Butterworth-Heinemann; 1994:262–281.

49. Litvan I, Booth V, Wenning GK, et al. Retrospective application of a set of clinical diagnostic criteria for the diagnosis of multiple system atrophy. *J Neural Transm* 1998;105:217–227.

50. Osaki Y, Wenning GK, Daniel SE, et al. Do published criteria improve clinical diagnostic accuracy in multiple system atrophy? *Neurology* 2002;59:1486–1491.

51. Gouider-Khouja N, Vidailhet M, Bonnet AM, Pichon J, Agid Y. "Pure" striatonigral degeneration and Parkinson's disease: a comparative clinical study. *Mov Disord* 1995;10:288–294.

52. Tison F, Wenning GK, Quinn NP, Smith SJ. REM sleep behaviour disorder as the presenting symptom of multiple system atrophy. *J Neurol Neurosurg Psychiatry* 1995;58:379–380.

53. Gilman S, Koeppe RA, Chervin RD, et al. REM sleep behavior disorder is related to striatal monoaminergic deficit in MSA. *Neurology* 2003;61:29–34.

54. Ghorayeb I, Yekhlef F, Chrysostome V, Balestre E, Bioulac B, Tison F. Sleep disorders and their determinants in multiple system atrophy. *J Neurol Neurosurg Psychiatry* 2002;72:798–800.

55. Jankovic J, Gilden JL, Hiner BC, et al. Neurogenic orthostatic hypotension: a double-blind, placebo-controlled study with midodrine. *Am J Med* 1993;95:38–48.

56. Low PA, Gilden JL, Freeman R, Sheng KN, McElligott MA, for the Midodrine Study Group. Efficacy of midodrine vs placebo in neurogenic orthostatic hypotension: a randomized, double-blind multicenter study. *JAMA* 1997;277:1046–1051.

57. Wright RA, Kaufmann HC, Perera R, et al. A double-blind, dose-response study of midodrine in neurogenic orthostatic hypotension. *Neurology* 1998;51:120–124.

58. Mathias CJ, Senard JM, Braune S, et al. L-threo-dihydroxyphenylserine (L-threo-DOPS; droxidopa) in the management of neurogenic orthostatic hypotension: a multi-national, multi-center, dose-ranging study in multiple system atrophy and pure autonomic failure. *Clin Auton Res* 2001;11:235–242.

59. Ito T, Sakakibara R, Yasuda K, et al. Incomplete emptying and urinary retention in multiple-system atrophy: when does it occur and how do we manage it? *Mov Disord* 2006;21(6):816–823.

60. Sakakibara R, Hattori T, Uchiyama T, et al. Are alpha-blockers involved in lower urinary tract dysfunction in multiple system atrophy? A comparison of prazosin and moxisylyte. *J Auton Nerv Syst* 2000;79:191–195.

61. Zesiewicz TA, Helal M, Hauser RA. Sildenafil citrate (Viagra) for the treatment of erectile dysfunction in men with Parkinson's disease. *Mov Disord* 2000;15:305–308.

62. Hussain IF, Brady CM, Swinn MJ, Mathias CJ, Fowler CJ. Treatment of erectile dysfunction with sildenafil citrate (Viagra) in parkinsonism due to Parkinson's disease or multiple system atrophy with observations on orthostatic hypotension. *J Neurol Neurosurg Psychiatry* 2001;71:371–374.

63. Iranzo A, Santamaria J, Tolosa E, Barcelona Multiple System Atrophy Study Group. Continuous positive air pressure eliminates nocturnal stridor in multiple system atrophy. *Lancet* 2000;356:1329–3130.

64. Parati E, Fetoni V, Geminiani C, et al. Response to L-dopa in multiple system atrophy. *Clin Neuropharmacol* 1993;16:139–144.

65. Colosimo C, Merello M, Pontieri F. Amantadine in parkinsonian patients unresponsive to levodopa: a pilot study. *J Neurol* 1996;243:422–425.

66. Visser-Vandewalle V, Temel Y, Colle H, van der Linden C. Bilateral high-frequency stimulation of the subthalamic nucleus in patients with multiple system atrophy—parkinsonism. Report of four cases. *J Neurosurg* 2003;98:882–887.

67. Wenning GK, Tison F, Seppi K, et al. Development and validation of the Unified Multiple System Atrophy Rating Scale (UMSARS). *Mov Disord* 2004;19:1391–1402.

68. Geser F, Wenning GK, Seppi K, et al. Progression of multiple system atrophy (MSA): a prospective natural history study by the European MSA Study Group (EMSA SG) *Mov Disord* 2006;21(2):179–186.

69. Wenning GK, Geser F, Stampfer Kountchev M, Tison F. Multiple system atrophy: an update. *Mov Disord* 2003;18(suppl 6): 834–842.

Corticobasal Degeneration

15

Anthony E. Lang   *Bradley F. Boeve*   *Catherine Bergeron*

Corticobasal degeneration (CBD) was first described by Rebeiz et al. in their 1968 paper entitled "Cortico-dentatonigral degeneration with neuronal achromasia" (1). Greater than one hundred cases have since been described in the literature, often under such essentially synonymous terms as "cortical basal ganglionic degeneration" and "corti-conigral degeneration with neuronal achromasia" (2,3,4). Although originally described as a late adult-onset, progressive neurodegenerative disorder presenting as a distinctive asymmetric akinetic-rigid syndrome with associated involuntary movements and signs of cortical dysfunction, a wider spectrum of clinical phenotypes has been recognized recently, including presentations with focal cognitive syndromes and altered behavior dependent on the topography of the predominant lesion. Furthermore, a variety of alternative pathologies (or "mimickers") have been reported to occasionally cause the prototypical syndrome (Fig. 15.1). Comparative studies with other neurodegenerative diseases utilizing new immunochemical techniques and electron microscopy have lead to the recognition of substantial similarities [particularly with progressive supranuclear palsy (PSP), Pick's disease, and frontotemporal dementia and parkinsonism linked to chromosome 17 (FTDP-17)], and possibly unique morphologic and biochemical features. The hypothesis that fundamental abnormalities in tau processing may underlie these disorders has been supported by genetic linkage studies. Each of these issues in the clinical and pathologic diagnosis of CBD and its overlap with other neurodegenerative diseases is emphasized.

CLASSICAL CLINICAL FEATURES AND NATURAL HISTORY

Classically, CBD presents in the sixth, seventh, or eighth decade of life with a varied combination of symptoms including stiffness, clumsiness, jerking, and sensory impairment affecting an arm or, less frequently, a leg (Table 15.1) (4,5). Over the next 2–7 years, symptoms and accompanying disability progress as additional limbs are affected—usually the unaffected ipsilateral limb before the contralateral limbs. Mean survival is 7 years after symptom onset with death secondary to a complication of generalized immobility (6,7). Early bilateral bradykinesia or a frontal syndrome (including early dementia, memory or attention disturbances) is predictive of a shorter survival (7). Recent clinicopathologic correlation has cast considerable doubt on the specificity of the classical clinical syndrome for the pathological diagnosis of CBD (8,9,10). Despite several reports of such patients with alternative pathologic findings at postmortem (including PSP, Pick's disease, FTDP-17, nonspecific cortical degeneration with status spongiosus—otherwise termed *frontotemporal lobar degeneration*, Alzheimer's disease, vascular disease, Creutzfeldt-Jacob disease, neurofilament inclusion body disease, sudanophilic leukodystrophy), the typical pathologic features of CBD seem to most commonly accompany this constellation of clinical features (11).

On examination at presentation, most patients demonstrate rigidity, bradykinesia, and apraxia of the affected

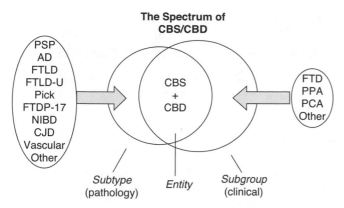

The Spectrum of CBS/CBD

PSP
AD
FTLD
FTLD-U
Pick
FTDP-17
NIBD
CJD
Vascular
Other

CBS
+
CBD

FTD
PPA
PCA
Other

Subtype
(pathology)

Entity

Subgroup
(clinical)

Figure 15.1 Clinicopathologic overlap between the corticobasal syndrome (CBS) and corticobasal degeneration (CBD). The larger of the two circles represents the pathology of CBD, the smaller the multiple pathologies listed to the left. The sizes of the circles and their overlap are not representative of relative frequencies. AD, Alzheimer's disease; CJD, Creatzfeldt-Jakob disease; FTD, frontotemporal dementia; FTLD, frontotemporal lobar degeneration; FTLD-U, frontotemporal lobar degeneration with ubiquitin-positive inclusions; FTDP-17, frontotemporal dementia and parkinsonism linked to chromosome 17; NIBD, neurofilament inclusion body disease; PCA, posterior cortical atrophy; Pick, Pick's disease; PPA, primary progressive aphasia; PSP, progressive supranuclear palsy.

limbs without significant global intellectual impairment or dysphasia. Little or no L-dopa response of parkinsonism is noted. Pronounced asymmetry of limb involvement is a hallmark of the classical disorder. In our experience, buccofacial apraxia at presentation is uncommon, but when present, can significantly impair speech (12). Limb-kinetic apraxia (LKA) is probably the most common form of apraxia seen in CBD, and studies done within the last 10 years have emphasized its characteristics (13,14). However, it is sometimes difficult to distinguish LKA from the clumsiness caused by accompanying bradykinesia, rigidity, and dystonia. It is important not to overdiagnose the presence of apraxia when these motor disturbances are prominent; this has been a common source of misdiagnosis in our experience. Ideomotor limb apraxia is almost universal during the course of CBD (5). Heilman proposed that the dominant parietal lobe stores representations of learned skilled movements (known as praxicons) that are converted into motor programs by anterior premotor regions (especially the supplementary motor area [SMA]) upon verbal command or other external or internal signal (15). Two forms of ideomotor apraxia may result: (a) lesions of the dominant parietal lobe damage the praxicons and result in a bilateral deficit in the performance of skilled movements, in addition to difficulty comprehending and discriminating between well and poorly pantomimed actions; (b) dominant SMA lesions (or subcortical lesions that disconnect the dominant parietal lobe from the SMA) cause a contralateral performance deficit without a discrimination deficit. Leiguarda et al. found ideomotor apraxia without a discrimination deficit to be most frequent in patients with clinically diagnosed CBD lacking

ideational apraxia and significant cognitive impairment, thus suggesting predominant SMA cortical pathology early in the course of classical CBD with recent fluordeoxyglucose positron emission tomography (FDG-PET) findings congruent with this pathologic localization (16). The presence of ideational apraxia in three patients correlated with more severe global cognitive impairment, and all such patients had ideomotor apraxia with a discrimination deficit. This is consistent with dominant parietal and, possibly, more diffuse cortical involvement developing with disease progression.

A rigid, dystonically postured arm with some fingers extended and others forcibly flexed into the palm causing skin maceration characteristically develops early in the course of the illness in a substantial minority (5,17). Jerking of the affected limb due to action-induced and stimulus-sensitive focal reflex myoclonus commonly precedes or accompanies the development of such dystonic postures and, if rhythmic, may mimic tremor (18). However, a classical Parkinsonian resting tremor is not a feature of CBD. Application of light touch or pinprick stimuli usually elicits multiple flexion jerks that, although initially distal, with disease progression may affect the entire limb almost synchronously. Spontaneous myoclonus may also occur but is always superimposed on a background of muscle activity (18). With time, combinations of apraxia, dystonia, rigidity, akinesia, and myoclonus make a limb functionally useless. In those with initial leg involvement, the early development of apraxia may interfere with walking, resulting in a frontal gait disorder with shuffling, start hesitation, and freezing (5). However, isolated gait ignition failure is not a feature of CBD. With disease progression, dysequilibrium becomes a common feature in all patients and postural instability with falls becomes frequent.

At presentation, oculomotor function may be normal or, alternatively, may be abnormal with saccadic pursuit and increased latency of pursuit onset, with increased saccade latency, and difficulty initiating voluntary saccades to command when spontaneous saccades in the same directions are successfully performed (sometimes referred to as apraxia of eye movement) (19). Patients may use head thrusts to improve horizontal saccades (head–eye synergy). Although a true supranuclear gaze palsy may develop later in the clinical course once marked generalized disability is present, an early vertical supranuclear gaze palsy raises the diagnostic possibility of PSP with atypical features due to accompanying cortical degeneration (see the following) (5,19,20). Furthermore, in CBD there is often equally severe vertical and horizontal gaze palsy.

New clinical features develop and preexisting symptoms and signs worsen as the disease progresses with pathological involvement of additional cortical and subcortical areas. Alien limb phenomena (ALP) develop in approximately 50% of patients (21). Classification schemes and definitions for ALP have been proposed. Feinberg et al.

TABLE 15.1

THE NATURAL HISTORY OF THE CLASSICAL SYNDROME OF CBD COMPARED TO PROGRESSIVE SUPRANUCLEAR PALSY AND STRIATONIGRAL DEGENERATION (SND)

Clinical Features	CBD	PSP	SND
Movement Disorders			
Akinesia, rigidity	At presentation—frequent; develops universally	Universal	Universal
Limb dystonia	At presentation—uncommon; develops in ~60%–70%	At presentation—rare; develops occasionally (~25%); may be L-dopa-induced	Uncommon but develops commonly with L-dopa therapy (facial may be an early clue to diagnosis)
Focal reflex myoclonus[a]	At presentation— occasional; develops in ~60%–70%	Uncommon	Frequent
Postural and action tremor	At presentation—occasional; develops in ~50%	Rare	At presentation—occasional; develops frequently
Postural instability, falls, or dysequilibrium	Rare at presentation (though abnormal gait is common in those with leg onset symptoms); develops late in course frequently (~70%–80%)	At presentation—frequent; develops universally	At presentation—occasional; develops frequently
Other dyskinesias (especially athetosis or pseudoathetosis)	At presentation—rare; develops occasionally	Rare	Rare
Cerebral Cortical Features			
Cortical sensory loss	At presentation—uncommon; develops in ~50%	Rare	Rare
Apraxia	At presentation—frequent; develops universally	At presentation—uncommon; develops commonly	Rare
Alien limb	At presentation—rare; develops in ~50%	Rare, although levitation may occur in the presence of marked cortical degeneration	Rare
Frontal release signs, including grasp	At presentation—uncommon; develops in ~50%	At presentation—common; develops frequently	At presentation—rare; develops occasionally
Dementia	At presentation—rare; develops in ~25%[b]	At presentation—uncommon; develops frequently	Rare
Dysphasia	At presentation—rare; develops uncommonly (~15%)[b]	Rare	Rare
Other Features	**CBD**	**PSP**	**SND**
Corticospinal tract signs	At presentation—occasional; develops frequently (~70%)	At presentation—uncommon; develops frequently	At presentation—uncommon; develops frequently
Oculomotor dysfunction	At presentation—occasional (predominantly saccadic pursuit and hypometric saccades); develops frequently (~60%–70%) (true supranuclear gaze palsy remains uncommon throughout course)	At presentation—frequent (may be just impairment of saccades and generation of opticokinetic nystagmus); vertical supranuclear gaze palsy develops in most patients (>90%)	At presentation—rare; develops ataxic eye movements occasionally

(Continued)

TABLE 15.1 CONTINUED			
Other Features	**CBD**	**PSP**	**SND**
Eyelid motor dysfunction	At presentation—uncommon (usually only decreased blink rate or speed); develops frequently with apraxia of lid opening (~20%) or blepharospasm occasionally	At presentation—uncommon; develops frequently with apraxia of lid opening or blepharospasm	At presentation—rare; develops uncommonly
Dysarthria	At presentation—rare; develops frequently (~50%–60%) (often pseudobulbar in character) sometimes due to apraxia	At presentation—common; develops frequently (often pseudobulbar in character)	At presentation—uncommon; develops frequently
Dysphagia	At presentation—rare; develops frequently	At presentation—rare; develops frequently	At presentation—rare; develops frequently
Autonomic Failure	At presentation—rare; incontinence develops frequently	At presentation—rare; incontinence develops frequently	At presentation—occasional (often impotence is first symptom, incontinence or orthostasis may also be present); severe orthostasis and incontinence develop frequently
Cerebellar Signs	Rare	Rare	At presentation—uncommon; develops frequently

[a]See text for discussion of unique physiologic characteristics of myoclonus in CBGD.
[b]These features, especially dementia, may be much more common than generally appreciated in patients who do no present with the "classical" CBD phenotype (see text for details).
Approximate percentage frequencies provided in addition to descriptors where adequate data exists. Rare = 10%; uncommon = 10%–20%; occasional = 20%–30%; common = 30%–50%; frequent = >50%; universal = >90%. Adapted in part, with modifications according to our personal experience, from the following: (1) Rinne JO, Lee MS, Thompson PD, Marsden CD. Corticobasal degeneration: a clinical study of 36 cases. *Brain* 1994;117:1183–1196. (2) Wenning GK, Ben Shlomo Y, Magalhaes M, Daniel SE, Quinn NP. Clinical features and natural history of multiple system atrophy: an analysis of 100 cases. *Brain* 1994;117:835–845. (3) Litvan I, Mangone CA, McKee A, et al. Natural history of progressive supranuclear palsy (Steele-Richardson-Olszewski syndrome) and clinical predictors of survival: a clinicopathological study. *J Neurol Neurosurg Psychiatry* 1996;60:615–620.

have proposed that ALP be divided into frontal and callosal types (22). Frontal ALP occurs in the dominant hand, is characterized by a strong grasp reflex and an uncontrollable tendency to reach for and manipulate objects, and is due to a lesion involving the dominant medial prefrontal cortex, SMA, anterior cingulate gyrus, and anterior corpus callosum. Callosal ALP results from an anterior or midbody corpus callosum lesion with the nondominant hand demonstrating intermanual conflict and diagonistic dyspraxia (acting at cross-purposes in tasks requiring both hands). In CBD patients with ALP, transcranial magnetic stimulation studies indicate an enhanced excitability, or reduced inhibition, of the motor area of the hemisphere contralateral to the ALP, and ipsilateral responses are noted compatible with a disinhibited transcallosal input (23). Levitation consists of relatively simple, nonpurposeful movements of a limb caused by a contralateral parietal lobe lesion, is much less specific for CBD, and may result in misdiagnosis. We would agree with other authorities in

requiring more complex behavior to fulfill criteria for true ALP. In our experience the commonest semipurposeful movement found in CBD that could be characterized as an ALP is utilization behavior with groping and manipulation. It should be borne in mind that among neurodegenerations, ALP is not specific for CBD and complex forms of ALP may be present in Alzheimer's (AD) and Creutzgeldt-Jacob disease (CJD) (21).

Cortical sensory deficits such as sensory extinction, astereognosis, agraphesthesia, and impaired 2-point discrimination account for some patients' complaints of numbness or paresthesiae, but are initially present in only a minority of patients. Later, severe sensory dysfunction may result in pseudoathetotic movements or wandering of the limb without patient awareness. Visual inattention may also develop. Similarly, frontal release signs (e.g., grasp), signs of corticospinal tract dysfunction (including extensor plantar responses and exaggerated deep tendon reflexes), and bulbar dysfunction are uncommon at presentation but become very common later in the disease course. Pseudobulbar palsy with emotional lability or inappropriate jocularity may also be observed (24). Hypokinetic and mixed-type dysarthria frequently impairs communication, and dysphagia with resulting aspiration pneumonia becomes a common source of morbidity and mortality (25). In contrast, severe dysphasia and global dementia remain uncommon (in the classical CBD phenotype) even when mobility is severely compromised, probably due to the topographically restricted predisposition for frontoparietal/pericentral cortical involvement. Yet some degree of dysarthria and dysphasia is present in most cases (26). Extensive neuropsychological testing has revealed mild to moderate global deficits and some specific similarities to PSP (and differences from AD), including a frontal dysexecutive syndrome, explicit learning deficits without retention difficulties easily compensated for by the use of semantic cues for encoding and retrieval, and disorders of dynamic motor execution (temporal organization, bimanual coordination, control, and inhibition) (27). As in AD, however, patients with CBD display prominent deficits on tests of sustained attention/mental control and verbal fluency, and mild deficits on confrontation naming (28). Psychomotor depression is more common and severe than in AD, possibly because of underlying basal ganglia pathology or psychological reaction to debilitating motor deficits with greater preservation of insight (28). Similarly, both depression and irritability are more common than in PSP, in which apathy predominates (29). Unlike both AD and PSP, patients with CBD have asymmetric praxis disorders (27). In reviewing the results of these neuropsychological reports, it is important to emphasize that the patients studied presented with the classical syndrome. It is likely that other neuropsychological patterns would be found in those presenting with alternative features (see the following).

DIFFERENTIAL DIAGNOSIS

CBD may be difficult at times to differentiate from other parkinsonian syndromes, such as multiple system atrophy (MSA) and PSP (Table 15.1). Misdiagnosis has resulted from misinterpretation of poor performance on manual tasks as due to apraxia when, in fact, severe bradykinesia, rigidity, or dystonia was causative. Stimulus-sensitive myoclonus in MSA and PSP may also encourage a misdiagnosis of CBD. PSP may share clinical features more commonly associated with CBD including apraxia, asymmetrical dystonia, and arm levitation. When the supranuclear gaze palsy is mild or absent, as it can sometimes be early on, and these features are present, the differentiation between PSP and CBD becomes most difficult. Leiguarda et al. also found bilateral ideomotor

apraxia for transitive and intransitive movements in 67% and 33%, respectively, of patients with PSP (30). Severity of apraxia correlated with cognitive deficit measured by mini-mental state examination. Although 2 of 12 patients performed abnormally on multiple-step tasks, no patients with PSP failed to comprehend pantomimed tasks or to discriminate between well and poorly performed pantomimes. Although blepharospasm has been well-recognized in PSP, the presence of other forms of dystonia has not been emphasized. Barclay and Lang found that 45% of PSP patients seen at one center manifested some form of dystonia (31). Limb dystonia was common and developed spontaneously in 20 patients (24%) and was L-dopa–induced in two patients. We have also observed arm levitation in pathologically proven PSP (20). These "unusual" clinical features may be more common in the presence of coexistent cortical degeneration. Severe autonomic dysfunction or delusions or hallucinations unrelated to L-dopa therapy have never been reported in pathologically proven CBD. MSA may cause the former, and dementia with Lewy bodies (DLB) may cause both of these problems. AD and nonspecific cortical degeneration (which more often presents as frontotemporal dementia) may present with an asymmetrical motor syndrome (especially progressive apraxia) that is initially indistinguishable from CBD (8,11). Clues that CBD is not the causative pathology include the absence of limb dystonia, milder parkinsonism, and usually more severe cognitive dysfunction. Parietal predominant Pick's disease may be clinically indistinguishable from CBD. Multiple infarcts and CJD also may mimic CBD. A stepwise or rapid progression, respectively, should be the important clue to these alternative diagnoses. Also, magnetic resonance imaging—particularly using fluid attenuation inversion recovery (FLAIR) and diffusion-weighted imaging (DWI)—typically shows increased signal in the basal ganglia and/or cortical ribbon (32). Another diagnostic consideration in younger patients (average age 45) demonstrating a more rapidly progressive course (2.5–4 years) is neurofilament inclusion body disease (NIBD) (33). A further diagnostic consideration in patients demonstrating a somehat more rapid progression is motor neuron inclusion body dementia (34) or frontotemporal lobar degeneration with ubiquitin-positive inclusions. Lastly, FTDP-17 should also be considered in patients with any family history or parkinsonism or dementia. The role of functional neuroimaging and electrophysiologic studies (see the following) in distinguishing these disorders from CBD remains uncertain (with the exception of imaging for multiple infarcts and CJD). The preceding comments apply to the differential diagnosis of the classical syndrome of CBD outlined in the previous section. However, as will be emphasized, the fact that the pathology of CBD may result in alternative clinical presentations broadens the differential diagnosis problem considerably.

ALTERNATIVE CLINICAL PRESENTATIONS

It has become increasingly clear that CBD may present with any of a variety of asymmetric cortical degeneration syndromes (ACDS) more commonly associated with other neurodegenerative diseases (Table 15.2) (35). These syndromes include primary progressive aphasia, frontotemporal dementia, posterior cortical atrophy, progressive hemiparesis, progressive apraxia, and more (10,11, 35,36). From pathologic studies, it is apparent that CBD commonly presents with the dysexecutive/behavioral subtype of frontotemporal dementia, especially when the cortical degeneration predominantly involves the frontal lobes (37,38). CBD should be suspected when patients present with a dementia phenotype characterized by executive dysfunction, poor attention/concentration, behavioral changes, dysphasia, and later development of bilateral motor signs (including non-L-dopa–responsive parkinsonism and pyramidal signs) and urinary incontinence (37). Similarly, when the superior temporal gyrus is the site of early cortical degeneration, presentation with the syndrome of primary progressive aphasia (aka the temporal variant of frontotemporal dementia [FTD]) may result (10). When

the frontal operculum and/or insula in the dominant hemisphere is affected early, nonverbal oral apraxia, apraxia of speech, nonfluent aphasia, or some combination of these may present long before other features develop (12). The broad clinical phenotype of ACDS seems to reflect the predominant area of pathological cortical degeneration and is not specific for any one disease. This situation makes accurate antemortem diagnosis in the absence of a sensitive and specific clinical or laboratory marker very difficult.

Attempts have been made to assess the accuracy of neurologists' clinical diagnosis of CBD. Litvan et al. have assessed the accuracy of neurologists' clinical diagnosis of CBD: Mean sensitivity for CBD was low (35%), but specificity was near perfect (99.6%) (9). Boeve et al. developed diagnostic criteria based on previously published pathologically proven cases and then prospectively applied these criteria (8). At postmortem, only 7 in 13 cases defined, using their criteria, as either clinically definite, probable, or possible had the classical pathology of CBD while the remainder demonstrated alternative findings. Hughes et al. published a study assessing the accuracy of clinical diagnoses made by movement disorders experts at Queen's Square in 143 patients with a parkinsonian

TABLE 15.2
COMMON ALTERNATIVE CLINICAL PRESENTATIONS OF CORTICOBASAL DEGENERATION

Clinical Syndrome	Main Clinical Features[a]	Other Pathologies
Primary Progressive Aphasia	Progressive nonfluent and/or fluent aphasia without global dementia or significant anterograde amnesia, often presenting initially with anomia, frequent paraphasic errors, and loss of speech fluency. Occasionally orofacial apraxia.	Pick's disease FTDP-17 AD PSP FTLD FTLD with ubiquitin-positive inclusions CJD NIBD
Frontotemporal Dementia	Progressive loss of judgment with disinhibition (including distractibility, impulsiveness, compulsiveness, or perseveration), social misconduct, or social withdrawal out of proportion to the degree of anterograde amnesia. Psychometric testing abnormalities on trailmaking, verbal fluency, mazes, or categorization.	Pick's disease FTDP-17 AD PSP FTLD
	Affective symptoms including depression, anxiety, emotional unconcern, or abulia. Early primitive reflexes and incontinence.	FTLD with ubiquitin-positive inclusions CJD NIBD AD
Posterior Cortical Atrophy	Progressive visuospatial/visuoperceptual impairment, Balint's syndrome, Gerstmann's syndrome, relatively preserved memory and insight	Nonspecific neurode-generative changes[b] Creutzfeldt-Jacob disease

[a] Predominant clinical features at presentation and in the early clinical course; thereafter, additional signs commonly develop.
[b] The current nomenclature for nonspecific neurodegenerative changes in the setting of frontotemporal dementia or progressive aphasia is frontotemporal lobar degeneration. This latter term is not appropriate for those with posterior cortical atrophy as the topography is parieto-occipital cortex.
FTDP-17, frontotemporal dementia and parkinsonism linked to chromosome 17; AD, Alzheimer's disease; PSP, progressive supranuclear palsy; FTLD, frontotemporal lobar degeneration; CJD, Creutzfeldt-Jacob disease; NIBD, neurofilament inclusion body disease.

TABLE 15.3

PROPOSED RESEARCH CRITERIA FOR THE DIAGNOSIS OF THE CLINICAL SYNDROME USUALLY ACCOMPANIED BY THE PATHOLOGY OF CORTICOBASAL DEGENERATION

I. Chronic progressive course
II. Asymmetric at onset (includes speech dyspraxia, dysphasia)
III. Presence of:
    1. Higher cortical dysfunction
    and
    2. Movement disorders

1. Higher Cortical Dysfunction	2. Movement Disorder
a. Apraxia	a. *Rigid*/akinetic syndrome
or	resistant to L-dopa
b. Cortical sensory loss	*and*
or	i. Dystonic limb posturing
c. Alien limb	ii. Spontaneous and reflex focal myoclonus

Qualifications of Clinical Features

- Rigidity: must be easily detectable without reinforcement.
- Apraxia: must be more than simple use of limb as object; absence of cognitive/motor abnormalities sufficient to account for the disturbance must be clear.
- Cortical sensory loss: must be able to demonstrate preserved primary sensation and be highly asymmetrical to verify the patient understands the test assignment.
- Alien limb phenomenon: must be more than simple levitation.
- Dystonia: must affect a limb and be present at rest from the outset (i.e., not purely action induced).
- Myoclonus: must spread beyond the digits when provoked by external stimuli.

Exclusion Criteria

- Presentation with cognitive disturbances other than apraxias or speech or language disorders.[a]
- Presence of moderate to severe global dementia while the patient remains ambulatory.[a]
- Presence of L-dopa responsivity (other than mild worsening on withdrawal).
- Presence of down-gaze palsy (including absence of fast component of opticokinetic nystagmus) while patient is still ambulatory.[a]
- Presence of typical parkinsonian rest tremor.
- Presence of severe autonomic disturbances, including symptomatic postural hypotension, urinary or bowel incontinence, and constipation to the point of repeated impaction.
- Presence of sufficient and appropriately located lesions on imaging studies to account for the clinical disturbances.

[a]May exclude cases of classical pathology but more often excludes alternative pathologies (i.e., reduces sensitivity but increases specificity even more).
Adapted from Kumar R, Bergeron C, Pollanen M, Lang AE. Cortical-basal Ganglionic Degeneration. In: Jankovic J, Tolosa E, eds. *Parkinson's Disease & Movement Disorders*. 3rd Edition. Baltimore, MD: Williams & Wilkins, 1998; 297–316.

syndrome coming to autopsy. Only 1 of 3 patients diagnosed with CBD in life had this pathology, and in only 1 of the 4 patients with this pathology had the diagnosis of CBD been made in life (39). These studies mandate the development of validated diagnostic criteria but also raise concerns that this goal may be exceedingly difficult, if not impossible.

Several sets of criteria have been proposed (Table 15.3 and Table 15.4). Given that the classical syndrome seems to correlate best with the pathology of CBD, the research diagnostic criteria outlined in Table 15.3 may offer the best specificity, acknowledging that these rigid clinical criteria are likely to exclude large numbers of patients, especially those with "atypical" or alternative presentations. The features consistent with the corticobasal syndrome (Table 15.4) may be more sensitive but possibly less specific. No consensus has been reached on what set of criteria is most appropriate. Prospective clinicopathologic studies are clearly necessary to refine the criteria and determine the best balance of sensitivity and specificity.

TABLE 15.4
PROPOSED CRITERIA FOR THE DIAGNOSIS OF THE CORTICOBASAL SYNDROME

Core Features

- Insidious onset and progressive course
- No identifiable cause (e.g., tumor, infarct)
- Cortical dysfunction as reflected by at least one of the following:
  - Focal or asymmetric ideomotor apraxia
  - Alien limb phenomenon
  - Cortical sensory loss
  - Visual or sensory hemineglect
  - Constructional apraxia
  - Focal or asymmetric myoclonus
  - Apraxia of speech/nonfluent aphasia
- Extrapyramidal dysfunction as reflected by at least one of the following:
  - Focal or asymmetric appendicular rigidity lacking prominent and sustained L-dopa response
  - Focal or asymmetric appendicular dystonia

Supportive Investigations

- Variable degrees of focal or lateralized cognitive dysfunction, with relative preservation of learning and memory, on neuropsychometric testing
- Focal or asymmetric atrophy on CT or MRI, typically maximal in parietofrontal cortex
- Focal or asymmetric hypoperfusion on SPECT and hypometabolism on PET, typically maximal in parietofrontal cortex +/- basal ganglia +/- thalamus

Adapted from Boeve BF, Lang AE, Litvan I. Corticobasal degeneration and its relationship to progressive supranuclear palsy and frontotemporal dementia. *Ann Neurol* 2003;54:S15–S19. CT, computed tomography; MRI, magnetic resonance imaging; SPECT, single-photon emission computed tomography; PET, positron emission tomography.

TABLE 15.5
FUNCTIONAL IMAGING IN NEURODEGENERATIVE DISEASES

Pathology	FDG-PET or HMPAO-SPECT Scanning	F-DOPA PET Scanning
CBD	Asymmetric hypometabolism/ hypoperfusion in striatum, thalamus, posterior frontal, inferior parietal, and lateral temporal cortex	Reduced uptake equally in caudate and putamen (may be asymmetric)
PSP	Bilateral medial frontal, thalamus, and midbrain hypometabolism/ hypoperfusion	Same as CBD, but symmetric
AD	Hypometabolism/ hypoperfusion in parieto-temporal and frontal association cortex (occasionally asymmetric)	Usually normal
Parkinson's disease with dementia	Parietal +/- occipital and frontal hypometabolism/ hypoperfusion	Uptake reduced in putamen much greater than caudate (usually asymmetric)

AD, Alzheimer's disease; CBD, corticobasal degeneration; FDG-PET, fluorodeoxyglucose positron emission tomography; HMPAO-SPECT, technetium TC-99m-hexamethyl propyleneamine oxime single photon emission computed tomography; F-DOPA PET, 18F-fluoro-L-Dopa PET; PSP, progressive supranuclear palsy.

TABLE 15.6
OFFICE OF RARE DISEASES NEUROPATHOLOGIC CRITERIA FOR THE DIAGNOSIS OF CORTICOBASAL DEGENERATION

Core Features

- Focal cortical neuronal loss, most often in frontal, parietal, and/or temporal regions
- Substantia nigra neuronal loss
- Gallyas/tau-positive neuronal and glial lesions, especially astrocytic plaques and threads, in both white matter and gray matter, most often in superior frontal gyrus, superior parietal gyrus, pre- and post-central gyri, and striatum

Supportive Features

- Cortical atrophy, often with superficial spongiosis
- Ballooned neurons, usually numerous in atrophic cortices
- Tau-positive oligodendroglial coiled bodies

Adapted from Dickson DW, Bergeron C, Chin SS, et al. Office of Rare Diseases neuropathologic criteria for corticobasal degeneration. *J Neuro Pathol Exp Neurol* 2002;61:935–946.

EPIDEMIOLOGY

Although CBD has become a more widely recognized entity, it remains a rare disease of unknown incidence and prevalence. No gender predilection has been identified, and there are equal proportions of patients with left- and right-predominant features. Furthermore, it is not clear what proportion of all patients harboring CBD pathology present in the classical fashion versus an alternative ACDS because current data are largely based on biased samples derived from small autopsy series with cases originating from either movement disorder or dementia clinics. In a population-based assessment of parkinsonism in Olmsted County, Minnesota, no cases of CBD were identified (40); since this series was published, a case with a dementia phenotype and a case with the CBD phenotype have been identified in that county (Boeve BF, personal observation). It is seen considerably less commonly than PSP, which accounts for approximately 5% of cases of parkinsonism seen in specialized movement disorder clinics. CBD constituted 0.9% of patients seen in one large movement disorders clinic. Based on this estimate and corrections for underdiagnosis, Togasaki et al. estimated that the total number of people who will develop CBD in the population is about 4%–6% of the number of those with parkinsonism (41). Based on the incidence of Parkinson's disease, they estimated that the CBD incidence rate would be 0.62–0.92/100,000 per year. Based on a mean survival of 7.9 years, they estimated a prevalence rate of 4.9–7.3/100,000. In considering these estimates, one must keep in mind that overestimation is likely because patients with CBD are more likely to be referred to specialized clinics; however,

these estimates may be low since they consider only the classic lateralized movement disorder presentation and not the dementia phenotype. The cause and risk factors for the development of CBD are currently unknown.

NEUROIMAGING AND NEUROPHYSIOLOGY

Structural and functional imaging and electrophysiologic techniques have been used in an attempt to provide useful adjunctive information in the diagnosis of CBD and information about the pathophysiology of various clinical signs. Except for the study of Josephs et al. described below (43), systematic studies have been carried out only in patients diagnosed with the classical clinical syndrome. Recognizing the clinical heterogeneity of CBD and the variability of pathologic conditions causing the clinical syndrome, it must be acknowledged that it is uncertain how sensitive and specific the defined imaging and physiologic abnormalities are for the pathology of CBD, compared to a specific topographic distribution that may be affected by multiple pathologic entities.

Magnetic resonance imaging (MRI) may demonstrate asymmetric pericentral cortical atrophy in approximately 50%–96% of cases (42); however, Caselli and Jack have suggested that three-dimensional surface-rendered MRI scanning may be considerably more sensitive in detecting subtle cortical atrophy (35). Computerized quantitation and detection of accelerated regional or generalized cerebral atrophy using serial MRI scans, as in patients with AD, might also be applicable in CBD and other ACDS. Hyperintensity of the atrophic cortex and the underlying white matter may be seen on FLAIR images in some cases (42). Hypointensity in the putamen and globus pallidus may also be evident on T_2-weighted images, although we have not been impressed with the presence of these abnormalities and they certainly do not reach the degree seen in striatonigral degeneration or neurodegeneration with brain iron accumulation type 1 (Hallervorden–Spatz syndrome) (42). In a study of MRI features among patients with the CBD phenotype and CBD pathology compared to those with the CBD phenotype and non-CBD pathologies, no MRI finding was identified that differentiated CBD from the CBD mimickers in patients presenting with the CBD clinical phenotype (43). Compared to controls, proton magnetic resonance spectroscopic imaging demonstrates significantly reduced N-acetylaspartate/creatine-phosphocreatine ratio in the centrum semiovale and reduced N-acetylaspartate/choline ratio in the lentiform nucleus and parietal cortex (predominantly contralateral to the worst affected side) (44). Functional imaging studies may help differentiate between CBD and other neurodegenerative diseases (Table 15.5), especially when 18F-fluorodeoxyglucose (FDG) and 18F-fluoro-L-DOPA (F-DOPA) positron emission tomography (PET) are both utilized in a single patient (45). Widespread abnormalities may be revealed even when structural imaging studies appear normal or only minimally abnormal. Areas of cortical hypometabolism or reduced blood flow may reflect a combination of local neuronal loss and deafferentation from adjacent cortical and subcortical regions. Typically FDG or oxygen scans show asymmetrical medial frontal, inferior parietal, and temporal cortical hypometabolism, as well as hypometabolism in the lenticular nucleus and thalamus. Eidelberg et al. (45a) has also suggested that the severity of apraxia and dystonia correlate with severity of cortical and basal ganglia hypometabolism respectively in individual patients. Assessment of the presynaptic dopamine system shows severe, asymmetric reduction in striatal F-DOPA uptake, which is equal in putamen and caudate. There is also reduced basal ganglia IBZM binding on single-photon emission computed tomography (SPECT) examination of postsynaptic D2 receptors. These findings are congruent with widespread substantia nigra neuron loss and similar, though less severe, striatal degeneration (45). Recent studies have also demonstrated differences between PSP and Parkinson's disease with respect to muscarinic and opioid receptor binding; further discrimination of CBD might also be possible using these ligands (45). PET using [C-11]PK 11195 demonstrates evidence for microglial activation in the pathogenesis of CBD (46). Finally, it has been reported that transcranial sonography demonstrates marked hyperechogenicity in the substantia nigra in patients with CBD, a finding similar to that described in idiopathic Parkinson's disease, whereas this is not present in patients with PSP (47). Further studies are required to define the reproducibility and reliability of this observation.

Conventional electrophysiologic studies are generally nonspecifically abnormal or unrevealing (18), although upper limb somatosensory-evoked potentials may be delayed in early CBD in an apraxic upper limb compared to the normal arm. Action and spontaneous myoclonus consists of 25–50 ms bursts of agonist and antagonist muscle co-contraction with a proximal to distal pattern of activation. Stimulus-sensitive and action myoclonus is often repetitive with 60–80 ms interburst intervals. Clinically apparent spontaneous myoclonus occurs on a background of ongoing muscle activity (often dystonic) and subsides if muscle relaxation (as recorded by surface electromyogram [EMG]) can be achieved (18). Unlike typical cortical reflex myoclonus (e.g., as seen in progressive myoclonus epilepsy/ataxia), EEG back averaging rarely provides evidence of a preceding cortical discharge (18). Studies with magnetoencephalography (MEG) may provide further insights into the nature of the cortical mechanisms of myoclonus in CBD; cortical activation on back-averaged MEG preceding myoclonus in CBD has been detected that was not evident on electroencephalogram (EEG) (18). On the other hand, the absence of corticomuscular coherence (EEG–EMG) has been used to argue against a cortical origin of the myoclonus (48). Cortical somatosensory evoked

potentials (SEPs) are usually not enlarged. Later components of the parietal SEPs are poorly formed and dominated by a broad positive wave with a peak latency of approximately 45 ms possibly due to abnormal processing in the sensory cortex (18). Cutaneous reflex latencies in CBD (mean 50 ms) are considerably shorter than in patients with MSA or dementia plus Parkinson's disease (mean 63.5 ms) (18). To the best of our knowledge, no other pathologic entity has been reported to result in myoclonus with these physiologic characteristics, thus this feature may help differentiate CBD from pathologic mimickers that otherwise clinically appear typical of CBD (Fig. 15.2). Further evaluation of this technique in pathologically verified cases is necessary to confirm its sensitivity and specificity. The latency of typical cortical reflex myoclonus is approximately 8 ms longer than that of CBD and is thought to involve abnormal relays through the sensory cortex to motor cortex. Thompson et al. have suggested that a direct sensory input from ventrolateral

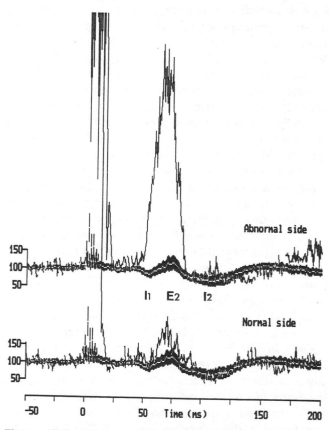

Figure 15.2 Effect of stimulating the middle finger (5 pulses at 500 Hz at twice perception threshold given at time zero) on electromyogram (EMG) of the first dorsal interosseous (FDI) muscle during a 30% maximum contraction (50 sweeps rectified and averaged). The darkened zone represents the mean +/- 2 SE from normal subjects. On the abnormal side of patient 2 (*top trace*), digital nerve stimulation resulted in a strong facilitation of the FDI EMG with a latency of 46 ms replacing the normal inhibitory period "I1." This was not seen on the normal side (*bottom trace*) for patient 1. The mean value of the prestimulus EMG has been normalized to 100%. (Courtesy of Dr. P. Ashby.)

thalamic nuclei to the motor cortex (bypassing the primary sensory cortex) may be the basis for the very short latency reflex myoclonus in CBD, which is only 1–2 ms longer than the sum of the afferent and efferent times to and from the cortex (18). Intra-cortical or thalamo-cortical neuronal inhibition may also be reduced in CBD. This is supported by studies using transcranial magnetic stimulation (TMS) that demonstrate reduced inhibition of voluntary EMG activity with subthreshold stimuli while single suprathreshold stimuli frequently result in repetitive muscle facilitation that has been attributed to repetitive cortical activation. In addition, paired pulse stimulation at short inter-stimulus intervals demonstrates evidence for motor cortex disinhibition (49). Furthermore, a shorter silent period following TMS on the affected side of the brain may be found (18), as well as evidence of impaired transcallosal inhibition (50).

PATHOLOGY

Recently, several advances have been made in the pathologic characterization of CBD, coupled with recognition of features overlapping with other neurodegenerative diseases. As a result, controversy exists with respect to its differentiation from PSP and Pick's disease. Indeed, Kertesz et al. have argued for use of the term *Pick Complex* to lump together a variety of diagnoses, both clinically and pathologically (10). Nevertheless, we believe that CBD is a pathologically distinct disorder with unique histologic and biochemical features. On gross examination, frontoparietal cortical atrophy is usually present but may be mild. Frontotemporal dementia and primary progressive aphasia presentations are associated with additional involvement of the frontal and temporal lobes. Asymmetry is often less obvious pathologically than clinically. A variable degree of ventricular dilatation may be seen. The substantia nigra is severely depigmented in most cases, but this may be much less evident in patients with severe early cognitive symptoms. Routine histological examination of the cortex reveals neuronal loss and gliosis most prominent in the superficial layers; in the most severely involved areas, status spongiosus may be observed. These changes are most evident in grossly atrophic areas but can be seen to a milder degree in less overtly atrophic cortex. Gliosis is usually observed in the subcortical white matter and parallels the degree of cortical degeneration. Neuronal gloss, gliosis, and corticobasal inclusions (see the following) are invariably found in the substantia nigra (3). There is variable involvement of other deep gray structures, including lateral thalamic nuclei, subthalamic nucleus, globus pallidus, striatum, amygdala, nucleus basalis, deep cerebellar nuclei, and other brainstem nuclei.

Ballooned neurons (BNs) (Fig. 15.3A) are characterized by perikaryal swelling, dispersion of Nissl substance, an eccentrically located nucleus, loss of typical cytoplasmic staining (achromasia), and occasional cytoplasmic vacuolation. BNs stain variably with antibodies to ubiquitin and tau but are consistently stained with antibodies to phosphorylated neurofilament epitopes and B-crystallin (38). Among neurodegenerative diseases, the presence of BNs was previously thought characteristic of Pick's disease (so called *Pick cells*) and CBD. However, they have been increasingly recognized in some cases of PSP and less commonly in AD, frontotemporal dementia and parkinsonism motor neuron disease, and CJD (38). Thus, the presence of swollen neurons does not discriminate between different diseases, although their quantity and distribution are of diagnostic relevance.

The occasional presence of frank cortical degeneration—predominantly confined to the premotor and motor cortex with neuronal loss, gliosis, and occasional BNs in PSP—blurs its distinction from CBD (20). Unusual clinical features may be associated with such cases, including limb apraxia, focal dystonia, arm levitation, and absence of supranuclear gaze palsy. Despite these features, CBD can be differentiated on the basis of other pathologic findings, as discussed in the following.

Sensitive immunohistochemical methods, have been used to study the cytoskeletal abnormalities and the neuropathologic overlap between CBD, Pick's disease, and PSP (38). All these disorders have numerous tau-immunoreactive neuronal and glial inclusions in cortical

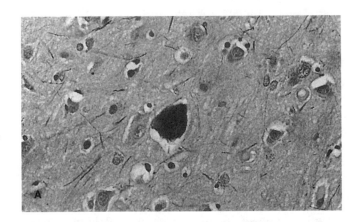

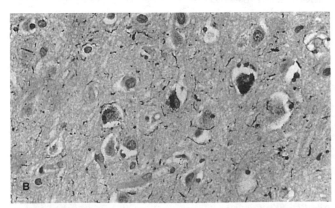

Figure 15.3 Ballooned neuron **(A)** and tau immunoreactive neuronal deposits **(B)** in the neocortex. Thin tau immunoreactive profiles are scattered in the neuropil **(B)**. Neurofilament **(A)** and tau **(B)** immunostains, original magnification x60.

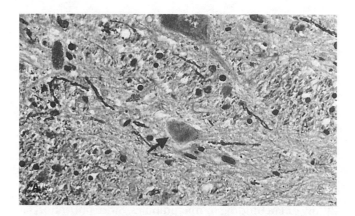

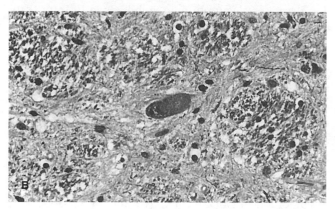

Figure 15.4 Corticobasal inclusions vary in their appearance. They include coarse fibrillary tangles **(A)** and more homogeneous basophilic inclusions **(B)**. Hematoxylin-eosin/luxol fast blue. Original magnification x60.

and subcortical regions. Pathologic diagnostic separation can be achieved by identifying the characteristic *distribution* of neuronal and glial lesions. Cortical tau+ neuronal inclusions in CBD are found in pyramidal and nonpyramidal neurons and may have a distinctive perinuclear, coiled filamentous appearance, but in general they vary greatly in appearance (Fig. 15.3B). Weakly basophilic nigral neuronal inclusions were first described by Gibb et al. and were initially thought to be specific for CBD (corticobasal inclusions); however, examination of additional cases has revealed considerable morphologic heterogeneity ranging from slightly fibrillar to frankly filamentous (Figs. 15.4A and 15.4B) (3). As a result, these inclusions are not reliably distinguishable from tau+ neurofibrillary tangles (NFTs) commonly associated with PSP. Thus, the morphology of neuronal tau+ inclusions is often not sufficiently distinctive to allow differentiation between different diseases. In CBD, cortical tau+ neuronal inclusions are considerably more common than in PSP; in contrast, in PSP the neuronal inclusions are more abundant than in CBD in the deep gray matter and brainstem.

Diagnostic confusion between Pick's disease and CBD has resulted from old classifications describing three subtypes of Pick's disease, recognition that CBD may present with a frontal-lobe dementia syndrome, and recent studies

describing cytoskeletal abnormalities similar to those seen in CBD and other conditions. Pick bodies (PBs) are spherical cortical intraneuronal inclusions seen predominantly in the hippocampal dentate gyrus and frontotemporal cortex that are argyrophilic and ubiquitin and tau immunoreactive. The light microscopic appearance of an individual PB is nonspecific, and both PSP and CBD may contain tau+ structures that appear similar to PBs (38). Nevertheless, when present in sufficient quantity and appropriate distribution, they confirm the diagnosis of Pick's disease. Furthermore, PBs and the Pick-like bodies of CBD have distinct staining characteristics. PBs are strongly argentophilic with Bodian and Bielschowsky stains but negative with the Gallyas stain. The converse is true in CBD. Their tau immunoreactivity is also different: Typical PBs fail to stain with the anti-tau antibody 12E8, which detects phosphorylation at SER 262/356 whereas the CBD inclusions are recognized by 12E8 (51,52).

Astrocytic plaques are distinctive annular clusters of thick, short tau+ deposits within distal processes of cortical astrocytes specific for CBD (53)(Fig. 15.5A). These plaques are not associated with β-amyloid. Astrocytic plaques must be distinguished from thorn-shaped astrocytes, which are not disease specific, and tufted astrocytes most commonly seen in PSP (38). Thorn-shaped astrocytes have their tau

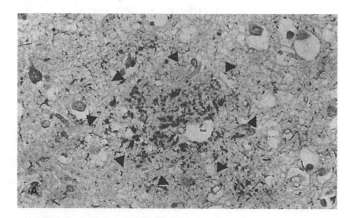

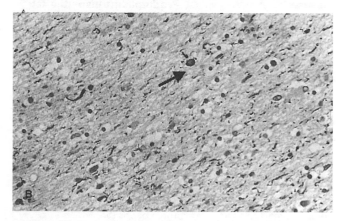

Figure 15.5 A: Tau-immunoreactive astrocytic plaque in the neocortex. **B:** In the white matter, tau immunoreactive profiles and coils (*arrow*) are common. Tau immunostain, original magnification x60.

immunoreactivity localized mainly to perikaryal cytoplasm with extension into the proximal portions of cell processes, whereas the abnormal inclusions of tufted astrocytes are mainly within distal and proximal processes and radiate from the periphery of the astrocytic perikaryon. In CBD, astrocytic inclusions are more common in cortex than in deep gray matter or the brainstem. In each disease, abnormal tau accumulates preferentially in specific subcellular regions of astrocytes. This differential distribution may reflect distinctive pathogenetic mechanisms.

Coiled bodies are oligodendroglial inclusions that appear as a fine bundle of filaments coiled around a nucleus and extending into the proximal part of the cell process (Fig. 15.5B). These ubiquitin-negative, tau-immunoreactive inclusions are morphologically and antigenically distinct from the glial cytoplasmic inclusions seen in multiple system atrophy and, though nonspecific, are most common in cortical and subcortical regions of CBD (38). Thin tau-immunoreactive threads of neuronal and glial origin are seen throughout the gray and white matter (Fig. 15.5B). Although also found in Pick's disease, they are particularly numerous in CBD and PSP.

Table 15.6 outlines the current consensus criteria for the neuropathological diagnosis of CBD.

MOLECULAR NEUROPATHOLOGY

Unique antigenic, biochemical, and ultrastructural characteristics serve to differentiate CBD from other neurodegenerative diseases. Aberrant phosphatase activity has been implicated in the production of abnormal tau protein, and pathological accumulation of hyperphosphorylated tau comprises the abnormal inclusions in neurons and glia. The tau gene is localized to chromosome 17 and has 13 exons. Variable splicing of exons 2, 3, and 10 results in 6 tau isoforms that are variably phosphorylated at specific serine and threonine residues (38,53). Three of these isoforms carry the segment specified by exon 10 and 4 repeats of a microtubule-binding domain (4R tau); the other 3 isoforms lack this fourth domain (3R tau). Normally, 3R tau and 4R tau are in equal concentration. Phosphorylation and differential exon splicing alter the affinity of tau binding to microtubules. Since phosphorylation decreases electrophoretic mobility, tau isoforms cannot be precisely differentiated by electrophoresis alone. Studies using antibodies to exon-specific epitopes allow further differentiation. Differences in the morphology and distribution of tau-immunoreactivity suggest that different isoforms may be implicated in different neurodegenerative diseases (Table 15.7). Immunochemical analysis of cortex in AD, CBD, and Pick's disease and basal ganglia in PSP reveals electrophoretic patterns confirming that the glial and neuronal inclusions in each disease are composed of a distinct complement of phosphorylated tau variants (Table 15.7) (38). There is similarity of the electrophoretic profile of tau in CBD and PSP (68 and 64 kD doublets); however, application of antibodies to exon 3 tau-specific epitopes confirms that in contrast to PSP, inclusions in CBD lack exon 3 sequences. Immunoblot analysis in CBD and PSP shows distinctive patterns of tau fragments, suggesting differing intracellular proteolytic processing of

TABLE 15.7
COMPARATIVE MOLECULAR PATHOLOGY OF SELECT NEURODEGENERATIVE DISEASES

Neurodegenerative Disease	Western Blot of Predominant Insoluble Tau	Tau Exon 10 Expression (4 repeat tau)	Ultrastructure of Abnormal Filaments
CBD	Two bands (64 and 68 kD)	Present	15 nm straight filaments and wide twisted double-stranded form
Pick's disease	Two bands (55 and 64 kD)	Absent (3 repeat tau)	15 nm straight filaments and wide twisted double-stranded form
Progressive supranuclear palsy	Two bands (64 and 68 kD)	Present	15 nm straight filaments
Chromosome-17 linked dementia (Select exon 10 and splice site mutations)	Two bands (64 and 68 kD)	Present (overproduction of 4 repeat tau)	15 nm straight filaments and wide twisted double-stranded form
Chromosome-17 linked dementia (select nonexon 10 mutations)	Three bands (55, 64, and 68 kD as in Alzheimer's disease)	Present	22 nm paired helical filaments (Alzheimer's-like)

Adapted from Dickson DW, Liu WK, Ksiezak-Reding H, Yen SH. Neuropathologic and molecular considerations. *Adv Neurol* 2000;82:9–27.

aggregated tau in these two diseases despite an identical composition of tau isoforms (54). Immunoblots from AD cerebrospinal fluid (CSF) reveal a triplet identical to that found in AD brain homogenate. Increased total CSF tau protein has also been reported in patients with CBD compared to normal controls and patients with PSP (55). Therefore, an antemortem diagnostic test for CBD and other neurodegenerative diseases might be developed if disease-specific electrophoretic profiles of tau protein in CSF are the same as those from postmortem brain homogenates.

The tau in CBD forms paired helical filaments (PHFs) that differ from those in AD by having a longer periodicity of the helical twist and being wider, more polymorphic, and unstable. Scanning transmission electron microscopy, demonstrates that PHFs in CBD exist in a less abundant double-stranded form (with a maximal width of 29 nm and a mass per unit length of 133 kD/nm), which may separate into more abundant single-stranded filaments (which are 15 nm wide and have a mass per unit length of 62 kD/nm) (38). Although 15 nm abnormal straight filaments are also seen in PSP and Pick's disease, paired wide twisted ribbons are seen only in Pick's disease (Table 15.7) (38). Heterogeneity of tau isoforms, differential packing of the tau protein, phosphorylation state, and possibly other posttranslational modifications may contribute to the unique ultrastructure and instability of the abnormal filaments in CBD.

ETIOLOGY

Reports of familial cases of CBD suggest that genetic predisposition may be important. Brown et al. have described a frontal-lobe dementia syndrome in multiple members of two families in a pattern consistent with autosomal dominant inheritance (56). One member of each family underwent pathologic study with findings most consistent with CBD. Furthermore, two other pathologically proven cases have had a first-degree relative with dementia (57). Vérin et al. have reported two brothers with clinical, radiological, and metabolic imaging features of CBD, though pathological confirmation was lacking (58). Boeve et al. reported on a kindred with nonspecific histopathology in which the proband exhibited the CBD phenotype while his brother had typical FTD features (59), again underscoring the heterogeneity of the clinical and pathologic findings and the need to obtain confirmatory neuropathology before accepting familial cases as evidence of a genetic origin in CBD. Caselli et al. have reported two clinically discordant monozygotic twins in which the proband had clinical and imaging evidence suggestive of CBD; neuropsychologic testing in the clinically unaffected twin suggested mild left hemispheric dysfunction and FDG-PET scanning revealed mild global hypometabolism, though MRI scanning was normal (60). Despite the absence of pathologic confirmation, these findings suggest that the second twin might

have presymptomatic CBD. The role of nongenetic factors is unclear but might account for the interval between the twins' symptom onset. If presymptomatic detection becomes possible, trials of neuroprotective therapy might be instituted. Schneider et al. found increased ε4 allele frequency (0.32) of ApoE in their 11 cases of CBD and suggested that ApoE genotype might be important in CBD pathophysiology (24). These results require confirmation in a larger study as three of their cases had concomitant AD, and in 5 of 7 cases, Aβ immunoreactive plaques were identified with at least one ε4 allele, whereas none of the remaining 4 cases with a 3/3 genotype demonstrated any Aβ deposition.

The clinical and pathologic overlap of CBD with PSP (including the presence of widespread tau-immunoreactive pathology), combined with the recent identification of an association between homozygosity for the tau H1 haplotype in PSP, encouraged similar studies in CBD. Using pathologically confirmed cases (to avoid diagnostic errors) an identical association with the H1 haplotype as in PSP has been demonstrated for CBD (61). This has lead to speculation that underlying abnormalities in the tau gene (on chromosome 17q) may be responsible for both CBD and PSP. Further support for this comes from a recent report of a consanguinous family with 2 siblings who demonstrated a CBS one with the pathology of CBD and the other with pathological features of PSP. Both had the H1/H1 haplotype. Three other siblings had clinical features of PSP and 2 of these had the H1/H1 haplotype (61a). This raises an important question regarding the relationship between CBD and a number of disorders linked to chromosome 17q 21–22 (FTDP-17or the so-called *tauopathies*). Recent molecular genetic studies have confirmed that autosomal dominantly inherited FTDP-17 is due to a wide variety of mutations in the tau gene that reduce the ability of tau to bind to microtubules and to promote microtubule assembly (53). Some cases with certain mutations located in exon 10 or the 5'-exon splice site of exon 10 have a pathologic phenotype that is similar to CBD, whereas those with tau mutations outside the microtubule binding domain show tau+ abnormalities but not those typical of CBD (38). Furthermore, Western blots of detergent-soluble tau and ultrastructural studies in these groups of mutations demonstrate additional similarities to CBD and PSP respectively (Table 15.7). Most of the intron splice-site mutations and certain exon 10 mutations result in an increase in the production of 4R tau isoforms, which may form toxic filaments and cause neuron dysfunction and death. Other exon mutations are associated with decreased microtubule binding and assembly, disrupt the neuronal cytoskeleton, and alter fast axonal transport, resulting in neuronal dysfunction. Either a change in the ratio of 3R to 4R tau or mutations in tau can lead to abnormal tau deposition within neurons and glia. This concept has been validated in transgenic mice with overexpression of either wild-type 4R tau or mutant 3R/4R tau, causing neurodegeneration and intracellular accumulation of fibrillar deposits of tau (62). Mutations leading to increased 4R tau cause an accumulation of straight filaments, while 3R tau accumulation leads to PHFs (like AD) (38). Straight filaments do not stain with silver, while PHFs are argyrophilic. Further complicating the situation, familial forms of Pick's disease with tau mutations have recently been reported (63).

FTDP-17 has an age of onset less than 65 years (often in the fourth or fifth decade) and demonstrates selective frontotemporal and basal ganglia involvement. Clinical features are highly variable even within a single family, which suggests that additional genetic or epigenetic factors influence the phenotypic manifestations of neurodegenerative tauopathies. The clinical overlap between CBD and FTDP-17 may be substantial. Bugiani et al. have described a family with a tau mutation in which the father presented with frontotemporal dementia and the son with the classic syndrome of CBD (64). As described, CBD cases with predominantly frontal and/or temporal involvement may be difficult to distinguish from classic frontotemporal dementia, and many experts now consider CBD, Primary Progressive Aphasia (PPA), and FTD within the same spectrum of disorders (10). Pallidopontonigral degeneration (PPND), familial progressive subcortical gliosis (PSG), disinhibition-dementia-parkinsonism-amyotrophy complex (DDPAC), and a family with FTDP-17 resembling PSP have been reported with pathologic findings that include neuronal loss and gliosis, BNs, and tau + neuronal and glial inclusions (53). As a result, only the presence of astrocytic plaques and distinctive isoforms of tau clearly justify considering CBD a completely separate pathologic entity. Indeed, it is possible that PSP, CBD, and FTDP-17 represent the same disorder differing only in underlying additional biological and genetic factors. Additional molecular genetic studies of large numbers of patients with CBD will be necessary to determine if specific abnormalities in the tau gene or genes that control tau processing might be responsible for producing such a wide range of clinical and pathologic phenotypes.

TREATMENT

Unfortunately, there is no treatment that prevents or delays progression in CBD and symptomatic therapy is usually ineffective. Kompoliti et al. retrospectively reviewed the open-label treatment of 147 patients with a variety of drugs at 8 movement disorder centers (65). Parkinsonism was present in 100% of patients, and 24% of patients treated with dopaminergic agents (predominantly L-dopa) showed modest improvement in parkinsonian signs, but none responded dramatically. Poor response to L-dopa, despite universal involvement of nigrostriatal dopaminergic neurons, is probably due to the presence of pathology farther "downstream" in the basal ganglia, thalamus, and SMA. Clonazepam reduced myoclonus in 23% of treated patients, and botulinum toxin injections improved limb dystonia or pain in 6 of 9 patients. Other medications,

such as baclofen, anticonvulsants, steroids, and anticholinergics, were not significantly useful, and central and peripheral side effects were common. Our experience is generally consistent with these results. We have observed apraxia of eyelid opening and closing and abnormal limb movements in two separate CBD patients taking L-dopa, which resolved with drug withdrawal. Therefore, an effort should be made to discontinue L-dopa, especially if a clinical response has been absent or unclear. The only drug that has resulted in some consistent benefit in our hands has been the use of clonazepam for myoclonus, while valproic acid has been ineffective. In contrast to these results, we have had rather unfavorable results with botulinum toxin injections, although others have found that EMG-guided injections of the small muscles of the hand (especially the lumbricals) can be useful for the dystonic fisted posture. There are no data that any form of currently available surgical therapy would be helpful. In addition to drug therapies, intervention by allied health professionals may be helpful. Physical therapists for gait training and use of weighted walkers may help prevent falls. Occupational therapists may devise strategies to accommodate for patients' specific disabilities. Constraint-induced movement therapy (CIMT), in which the patient wears a cumbersome mitten over the less affected hand and is required thereby to use only the more affected limb, can be beneficial to some. However, this is an ardous therapeutic program to follow and any benefit initially obtained is lost as the disease progresses. Speech therapy for dysarthria, dietary manipulation for dysphagia, and advice regarding the timing of the use of percutaneous endoscopic gastrostomy (PEG) are all useful. Clearly, new experimental therapies are necessary to halt the underlying neurodegeneration and provide symptomatic relief to our patients.

FUTURE DIRECTIONS

Although considerable advances have been made in the recognition of the pathologic characteristics of CBD, additional work is necessary to define universally accepted pathological diagnostic criteria based on the presence of specific markers (e.g., tau protein electrophoretic profile). Further studies are needed to define the relationship between CBD, PSP, and the other tauopathies. The current difficulties with clinical diagnosis and clinicopathologic correlation mandate the establishment of a registry of patients who fulfill stringent diagnostic criteria, such as those proposed in this chapter (41). This will permit epidemiological case-control studies and allow the identification of possible risk factors and the development of hypotheses that can be tested in clinical or laboratory settings. However, if the pathology of CBD results in other clinical presentations (e.g., frontotemporal dementia) more often than the classical syndrome, epidemiological studies will be greatly compromised. On the other hand, a homogeneous patient group might allow biochemical and genetic studies and the validation of an antemortem diagnostic marker (e.g., in CSF), which could then be applied to other clinical populations and subsequently permit more definitive epidemiological evaluations. Furthermore, establishing a homogeneous patient group with this rare disorder would allow more successful evaluation of new treatments in the form of multi-institutional pharmacologic therapeutic trials. Some centers are following patients longitudinally with periodic clinical evaluations, functional assessments, neuropsychiatric and neuropsychological measures, and quantitative neuroimaging studies to determine the course of changes based on currently available agents; such data may form the foundation for developing future therapeutic drug trials. As a result of this newly gained knowledge, we might be better able to alleviate the suffering experienced by these unfortunate patients.

ACKNOWLEDGMENTS

Supported in part by the National Parkinson Foundation, and AG16574 from the National Institute on Aging.

REFERENCES

1. Rebeiz JJ, Kolodny EH, Richardson EP. Corticodentatonigral degeneration with neuronal achromasia. *Arch Neurol* 1968;18:20–33.
2. Lippa CF, Smith TW, Fontneau N. Corticonigral degeneration with neuronal achromasia. *J Neurol Sci* 1990;98:301–310.
3. Gibb WRG, Luthert PJ, Marsden CD. Corticobasal degeneration. *Brain* 1989;112:1171–1192.
4. Riley DE, Lang AE, Lewis A, et al. Cortical-basal ganglionic degeneration. *Neurology* 1990;40:1203–1212.
5. Rinne JO, Lee MS, Thompson PD, Marsden CD. Corticobasal degeneration: a clinical study of 36 cases. *Brain* 1994;117:1183–1196.
6. Litvan I, Grimes DA, Lang AE. Phenotypes and prognosis: clinicopathologic studies of corticobasal degeneration. *Adv Neurol* 2000;82:183–196.
7. Wenning GK, Litvan I, Jankovic J, et al. Natural history and survival of 14 patients with corticobasal degeneration confirmed at postmortem examination. *J Neurol Neurosurg Psychiatry* 1998;64:184–189.
8. Boeve BF, Maraganore DM, et al. Pathologic heterogeneity in clinically diagnosed corticobasal degeneration. *Neurology* 1999;53:795–800.
9. Litvan I, Agid Y, Goetz C, et al. Accuracy of the clinical diagnosis of corticobasal degeneration: a clinicopathologic study. *Neurology* 1997;48:119–125.
10. Kertesz A, Martinez-Lage P, Davidson W, Munoz DG. The corticobasal degeneration syndrome overlaps progressive aphasia and frontotemporal dementia. *Neurology* 2000;55:1368–1375.
11. Bhatia KP, Lee MS, Rinne JO, et al. Corticobasal degeneration look-alikes. *Adv Neurol* 2000;82:169–182.
12. Lang AE. Cortical-basal ganglionic degeneration presenting with "progressive loss of speech output and orofacial dyspraxia." *J Neurol Neurosurg Psychiatry* 1992;55:1101.
13. Denes G, Mantovan MC, Gallana A, Cappelletti JY. Limb-kinetic apraxia. *Mov Disord* 1998;13:468–476.
14. Leiguarda RC, Merello M, Nouzeilles MI, Balej J, Rivero A, Nogués M. Limb-kinetic apraxia in corticobasal degeneration: clinical and kinematic features. *Mov Disord* 2003;18:49–59.
15. Heilman KM. The apraxia of CBGD. *Mov Disord* 1996;11:348.
16. Leiguarda R, Lees AJ, Merello M, Starkstein S, Marsden CD. The nature of apraxia in corticobasal degeneration. *J Neurol Neurosurg Psychiatry* 1994;57:455–459.
17. Riley DE, Lang AE, Lewis A, et al. Cortical-basal ganglionic degeneration. *Neurology* 1990;40:1203–1212.
18. Thompson PD, Shibasaki H. Myoclonus in corticobasal degeneration and other neurodegenerations. *Adv Neurol* 2000;82:69–81.
19. Rivaud-Péchoux S, Vidailhet M, Gallouedec G, Litvan I, Gaymard B, Pierrot-Deseilligny C. Longitudinal ocular motor study in corticobasal degeneration and progressive supranuclear palsy. *Neurology* 2000;54:1029–1032.
20. Bergeron C, Pollanen MS, Weyer L, Lang AE. Cortical degeneration in progressive supranuclear palsy: a comparison with cortical-basal ganglionic degeneration. *J Neuro Pathol Exp Neurol* 1997;56:726–734.
21. Hanna PA, Doody RS. Alien limb sign. *Adv Neurol* 2000;82:135–145.
22. Feinberg TE, Schindler RJ, Flanagan NG, Haber LD. Two alien hand syndromes. *Neurology* 1992;42:19–24.
23. Valls-Solé J, Tolosa E, Marti MJ, et al. Examination of motor output pathways in patients with corticobasal ganglionic degeneration using transcranial magnetic stimulation. *Brain* 2001;124:1131–1137.
24. Schneider JA, Watts RL, Gearing M, Brewer RP, Mirra SS. Corticobasal degeneration: neuropathologic and clinical heterogeneity. *Neurology* 1997;48:959–969.
25. Frattali CM, Sonies BC. Speech and swallowing disturbances in corticobasal degeneration. *Adv Neurol* 2000;82:153–160.
26. Graham NL, Bak T, Patterson K, Hodges JR. Language function and dysfunction in corticobasal degeneration. *Neurology* 2003;61:493–499.
27. Pillon B, Blin J, Vidailhet M, et al. The neuropsychological pattern of corticobasal degeneration: comparison with progressive supranuclear palsy and Alzheimer's disease. *Neurology* 1995;45:1477–1483.
28. Massman PJ, Kreiter KT, Jankovic J, Doody RS. Neuropsychological functioning in cortical-basal ganglionic degeneration: differentiation from Alzheimer's disease. *Neurology* 1996;46:720–726.
29. Litvan I, Cummings JL, Mega M. Neuropsychiatric features of corticobasal degeneration. *J Neurol Neurosurg Psychiatry* 1998;65:717–721.
30. Leiguarda RC, Pramstaller PP, Merello M, Starkstein S, Lees AJ, Marsden CD. Apraxia in Parkinson's disease, progressive supranuclear palsy, multiple system atrophy and neuroleptic-induced parkinsonism. *Brain* 1997;120:75–90.
31. Barclay CL, Lang AE. Dystonia in progressive supranuclear palsy. *J Neurol Neurosurg Psychiatry* 1997;62:352–356.
32. Meissner B, Kortner K, Bartl M, et al. Sporadic Creutzfeldt-Jakob disease: magnetic resonance imaging and clinical findings. *Neurology* 2004;63:450–456.
33. Josephs KA, Holton JL, Rossor MN, et al. Neurofilament inclusion body disease: a new proteinopathy? *Brain* 2003;126(pt 10):2291–2303.
34. Grimes DA, Bergeron C, Lang AE. Motor neuron disease-inclusion dementia presenting as cortical-basal ganglionic degeneration. *Mov Disord* 1999;14:674–680.
35. Caselli RJ, Jack CR. Asymmetric cortical degeneration syndromes: a proposed clinical classification. *Arch Neurol* 1992;49:770–780.
36. Tang-Wai DF, Graff-Radford NR, Boeve BF, et al. Clinical, genetic, and neuropathologic characteristics of posterior cortical atrophy. *Neurology* 2004;63:1168–1174.
37. Grimes DA, Lang AE, Bergeron CB. Dementia as the most common presentation of cortical-basal ganglionic degeneration. *Neurology* 1999;53:1969–1974.
38. Dickson DW, Liu WK, Ksiezak-Reding H, Yen SH. Neuropathologic and molecular considerations. *Adv Neurol* 2000;82:9–27.
39. Hughes AJ, Daniel SE, Ben Shlomo Y, Lees AJ. The accuracy of diagnosis of parkinsonian syndromes in a specialist movement disorder service. *Brain* 2002;125:861–870.
40. Bower JH, Dickson DW, Taylor L, Maraganore DM, Rocca WA. Clinical correlates of the pathology underlying parkinsonism: a population perspective. *Mov Disord* 2002;17:910–916.
41. Togasaki DM, Tanner CM. Epidemiologic aspects. *Adv Neurol* 2000;82:53–59.
42. Savoiardo M, Grisoli M, Girotti F. Magnetic resonance imaging in CBD, related atypical parkinsonian disorders, and dementias. *Adv Neurol* 2000;82:197–208.
43. Josephs KA, Tang-Wai DF, Edland SD, et al. Correlation between antemortem magnetic resonance imaging findings and

pathologically confirmed corticobasal degeneration. *Arch Neurol* 2004; 61:1881–1884.

44. Tedeschi G, Litvan I, Bonavita S, et al. Proton magnetic resonance spectroscopic imaging in progressive supranuclear palsy, Parkinson's disease and corticobasal degeneration. *Brain* 1997;120:1541–1552.

45. Brooks DJ. Functional imaging studies in corticobasal degeneration. *Adv Neurol* 2000;82:209–215.

45a. Eidelberg D, Dhawan V, Moeller JR, et al. The metabolic landscape of cortico-basal ganglionic degeneration: regional asymmetries studied with positron emission tomography. *J Neurol Neurosurg Psychiatry* 1991;54:856–862.

46. Henkel K, Karitzky J, Schmid M, et al. Imaging of activated microglia with PET and [^{11}C]PK 11195 in corticobasal degeneration. *Mov Disord* 2004;19:817–821.

47. Walter U, Dressler D, Wolters A, Probst T, Grossmann A, Benecke R. Sonographic discrimination of corticobasal degeneration vs progressive supranuclear palsy. *Neurology* 2004;63:504–509.

48. Grosse P, Kühn A, Cordivari C, Brown P. Coherence analysis in the myoclonus of corticobasal degeneration. *Mov Disord* 2003;18:1345–1350.

49. Frasson E, Bertolasi L, Bertasi V, et al. Paired transcranial magnetic stimulation for the early diagnosis of corticobasal degeneration. *Clin Neurophysiol* 2003;114:272–278.

50. Trompetto C, Buccolieri A, Marchese R, Marinelli L, Michelozzi G, Abbruzzese G. Impairment of transcallosal inhibition in patients with corticobasal degeneration. *Clin Neurophysiol* 2003;114: 2181–2187.

51. Probst A, Tolnay M, Langui D, Goedert M, Spillantini MG. Pick's disease: hyperphosphorylated tau protein segregates to the somatoaxonal compartment. *Acta Neuropathol (Berl)* 1996;92:588–596.

52. Bell K, Cairns NJ, Lantos PL, Rossor MN. Immunohistochemistry distinguishes between Pick's disease and corticobasal degeneration. *J Neurol Neurosurg Psychiatry* 2000;69:835–836.

53. Lee VM, Goedert M, Trojanowski JQ. Neurodegenerative tauopathies. *Annu Rev Neurosci* 2001;24:1121–1159.

54. Arai T, Ikeda K, Akiyama H, et al. Identification of amino-terminally cleaved tau fragments that distinguish progressive supranuclear palsy from corticobasal degeneration. *Ann Neurol* 2004;55:72–79.

55. Urakami K, Wada K, Arai H, et al. Diagnostic significance of tau protein in cerebrospinal fluid from patients with corticobasal degeneration or progressive supranuclear palsy. *J Neurol Sci* 2001;183:95–98.

56. Brown J, Lantos PL, Roques P, Fidani L, Rossor MN. Familial dementia with swollen achromatic neurons and corticobasal inclusion bodies: a clinical and pathological study. *J Neurol Sci* 1996;135:21–30.

57. Mitsuyama Y, Masuda K, Inoue T, Koono M, Koga S, Nakamura J. Primary progressive dementia with swollen chromatolytic neurons. *Dementia* 1992;3:223–231.

58. Verin M, Rancurel G, DeMarco O, Edan G. First familial cases of corticobasal degeneration. *Mov Disord* 1997;12(suppl1):55.

59. Boeve BF, Maraganore DM, Parisi JE, et al. Corticobasal degeneration and frontotemporal dementia presentations in a kindred with nonspecific histopathology. *Dement Geriatr Cogn Disord* 2002;13:80–90.

60. Caselli RJ, Reiman EM, Timmann D, et al. Progressive apraxia in clinically discordant monozygotic twins. *Arch Neurol* 1995;52:1004–1010.

61. Houlden H, Baker M, Morris HR, et al. Corticobasal degeneration and progressive supranuclear palsy share a common tau haplotype. *Neurology* 2001;56:1702–1706.

61a. Tuite PJ, Clark HB, Bergeron C, et al. Clinical and pathologic evidence of corticobasal degeneration and progressive supranuclear palsy in familial tauopathy. *Arch Neurol* 2005;62: 1453–1457.

62. Lewis J, McGowan E, Rockwood J, et al. Neurofibrillary tangles, amyotrophy and progressive motor disturbance in mice expressing mutant (P301L) tau protein. *Nat Genet* 2000;25: 402–405.

63. Neumann M, Schulz-Schaeffer W, Crowther RA, et al. Pick's disease associated with the novel *Tau* gene mutation K369I. *Ann Neurol* 2001;50:503–513.

64. Bugiani O, Murrell JR, Giaccone G, et al. Frontotemporal dementia and corticobasal degeneration in a family with a P301S mutation in *tau*. *J Neuro Pathol Exp Neurol* 1999;58:667–677.

65. Kompoliti K, Goetz CG, Boeve BF, et al. Clinical presentation and pharmacological therapy in corticobasal degeneration. *Arch Neurol* 1998;55:957–961.

Inherited and Sporadic Tauopathies

16

Maria Grazia Spillantini   *Michel Goedert*

INTRODUCTION

Over the past 20 years, a basic understanding of some of the most common neurodegenerative diseases has emerged from the coming together of two independent lines of research. First, the molecular study of the neuropathological lesions that define these diseases led to the identification of their major components. Second, the study of rare, inherited forms of disease resulted in the discovery of gene defects that cause inherited variants of the different diseases. In most cases, the defective genes were found to encode the major components of the neuropathological lesions, or factors that increase their expression. It follows that the basis of the inherited forms of these diseases is a toxic property of the proteins that make up the filamentous lesions. A corollary insight is that a similar toxic property also may underlie the much more common sporadic forms of disease.

Alzheimer's disease (AD) is the most common neurodegenerative disease. Neuropathologically, AD is defined by the presence of abundant extracellular neuritic plaques made largely of the β-amyloid peptide and intraneuronal neurofibrillary lesions composed of the microtubule-associated protein tau (1). Similar tau deposits, in the absence of extracellular deposits, are also the defining characteristic of a number of other neurodegenerative diseases, including progressive supranuclear palsy (PSP), corticobasal degeneration (CBD), Pick's disease (PiD), and argyrophilic grain disease (AGD) (2). For many years, there was no genetic evidence implicating tau protein in the neurodegenerative process. This changed with the discovery of tau gene mutations in the inherited frontotemporal dementia and parkinsonism linked to chromosome 17 (FTDP-17) (3,4,5).

TAU ISOFORMS IN HUMAN BRAIN AND THEIR INTERACTIONS WITH MICROTUBULES

Tau is a natively unfolded microtubule binding protein that is believed to be important for the assembly and stabilization of microtubules. In nerve cells, tau is normally found in axons, but in the tau diseases it is redistributed to the cell body and dendrites. In the normal adult human brain, there are six isoforms of tau, produced from a single gene by alternative mRNA splicing (Fig. 16.1) (6). They differ from one another by the presence or absence of a 29- and 58-amino acid insert in the amino-terminal half of the protein and by the inclusion, or not, of a 31-amino acid repeat, encoded by exon 10 of tau, in the carboxy-terminal half of the protein. The exclusion of exon 10 leads to the production of three isoforms, each containing three repeats, and its inclusion leads to another three isoforms, each containing four repeats. The repeats constitute the microtubule-binding region of tau protein. In normal adult human cerebral cortex, there are similar levels of 3-repeat and 4-repeat isoforms. In developing human brain, only the shortest tau isoform (three repeats and no amino-terminal inserts) is expressed.

The tau molecule can be subdivided into an amino-terminal domain that projects from the microtubule surface and a carboxy-terminal microtubule-binding domain. High- resolution nuclear magnetic resonance (NMR) spec troscopy was used to identify residual structure in a fragment of tau with three microtubule-binding repeats (7). Three regions exhibited a preference for helical conformation, suggesting that these regions may adopt a helical structure when bound to microtubules. Structural work also has begun to shed light in a more

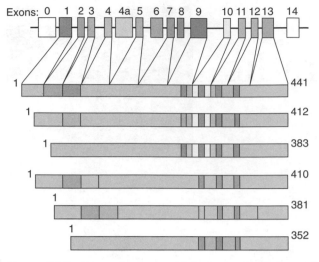

Figure 16.1   Schematic diagram of the human tau gene and the 6 tau isoforms (352 to 441 amino acids) that are generated in the brain through alternative mRNA splicing. The human tau gene consists of 16 exons (E) and extends over approximately 140 kb. E0, which forms part of the promoter, and E14 are noncoding (*in white*). Alternative splicing of E2 (*in red*), E3 (*in green*), and E10 (*in yellow*) gives rise to the 6 tau isoforms. The constitutively spliced exons (E1, E4, E5, E7, E9, E11, E12, E13) are indicated in blue. E6 and E8 (*in violet*) are not transcribed in the human brain. E4a (*in orange*) is only expressed in the peripheral nervous system, where its presence gives rise to the tau isoform known as *big tau*. *Black bars* indicate the microtubule-binding repeats, with three isoforms having three repeats each and three isoforms having four repeats each. The exons and introns are not drawn to scale. (See color section.)

direct manner on the way that tau and microtubules interact. Microtubules were assembled with tubulin and tau in the absence of taxol and in the presence of the natural osmolyte trimethylamine N-oxide (8). One of the repeats in tau had been labeled with nanogold and was localized by three-dimensional analysis of electron micrographs. The tau repeats were found to bind to the inner surface of the microtubule, in a region that overlapped with the taxol-binding site on β-tubulin. Taxol binds to a site in β-tubulin, where β-tubulin has a conserved loop of eight amino acids (TVVPGGDL). Interestingly, part of the tau repeat motif (THVPGGN) resembles this sequence. Since tubulin cannot have evolved to bind taxol, these findings may answer the question of what natural substrate binds in this pocket of β-tubulin. In this model, part of the proline-rich region of tau must provide the link between the amino-terminal projection domain on the outside of the microtubule and the repeat motifs on the inside surface. It could thread through one of the holes between protofilaments. Another model has been derived from experiments in which gold-labeled tau was bound to preassembled, taxolstabilized microtubules (9). Tau was found to bind only to the outer surface of the microtubule, where it localized along the outer ridges of the protofilaments.

TAU FILAMENTS AS NERVE CELL AMYLOID

In human diseases with tau pathology, the normally soluble tau protein is present in an abnormal filamentous form (2). It is also hyperphosphorylated. In AD, tau filaments consist primarily of paired helical filaments (PHFs), with straight filaments (SFs) being a minority species. Electron micrographs of negatively stained isolated filaments show images in which the width of the filament varies between about 8 nm and 20 nm, with a spacing between crossovers of about 80 nm. Although the filament morphologies and their tau isoform composition vary between diseases, it is the repeat region that forms the core of the filament, with the amino- and carboxy-terminal regions forming a fuzzy coat around the filament. During the course of the disease, the fuzzy coat is frequently proteolysed, such that filaments comprise only the repeat region of tau. However, it is the full-length protein that first assembles into filaments.

Incubation of bacterially expressed human tau with sulphated glycosaminoglycans leads to bulk assembly of full-length tau into filaments (10,11). By immunoelectron microscopy, these filaments can be decorated by antibodies directed against the N- and C-terminal regions of tau, but not by an antibody against the microtubule-binding repeat region, exactly like the tau filaments from AD. The assembly is a nucleation-dependent phenomenon and a short amino acid sequence (VQIVYK) in the third microtubule-binding repeat was found to be essential for heparin-induced filament assembly (12). By NMR spectroscopy of three tau repeats, this region showed a marked preference for extended or β-strandlike conformation (7). A separate NMR study on four tau repeats detected additional β-strandlike conformation in the second and fourth repeats (13). In addition to sulphated GAGs, RNA and arachidonic acid have been shown to induce the bulk assembly of full-length tau into filaments. This work provided robust methods for the assembly of full-length tau into filaments. It also made it possible to obtain structural information and to identify compounds that inhibit tau filament formation.

Filaments assembled from either 3- or 4-repeat tau showed cross β-structure by selected area diffraction, X-ray diffraction from macroscopic fibers, and Fourier transform infrared spectroscopy (14). This work was extended to PHFs and SFs extracted from diseased human brain. There had been controversy in the literature with regard to the internal molecular fine structure of these filaments. The difficulty had been to prepare from human brain pure preparations of filaments for analysis. This problem was circumvented by using selected area diffraction from small groups of filaments of defined morphology. Using this approach, PHFs and SFs had a clear cross β-structure, which is the defining feature of amyloid fibers. They share this structure with the extracellular deposits present in systemic and organ-specific amyloid diseases. It is, therefore, appropriate to consider the tauopathies as a form of brain amyloidosis.

Small molecule inhibitors of arachidonic acid- and heparin-induced filament formation of full-length tau have been identified (15,16,17). Prominent among these figure a number of phenothiazines, polyphenols, and porphyrins, which inhibit tau filament formation with IC_{50} values in the low micromolar range and are believed to stabilize soluble oligomeric tau species. The continued identification of inhibitory compounds may pave the way for the development of mechanism-based therapies for the tauopathies.

MUTATIONS IN TAU

Frontotemporal dementias occur as familial forms and, more commonly, as sporadic diseases. They are characterized by a remarkably circumscribed atrophy of the frontal and temporal lobes of the cerebral cortex, often with additional, subcortical changes. In 1994, an autosomal dominantly inherited form of frontotemporal dementia with parkinsonism was linked to chromosome 17q21.2 (18). Subsequently, other forms of frontotemporal dementia were found to be linked to this region, resulting in the denomination *frontotemporal dementia and parkinsonism linked to chromosome 17* (FTDP-17) for this class of disease. All cases of FTDP-17 have so far shown a filamentous pathology made of hyperphosphorylated tau protein (Fig. 16.2). In June 1998, the first mutations in tau in FTDP-17 were reported (3–5). Currently, 37 different mutations have been described in over 100 families with FTDP-17 (Fig. 16.3). Tau mutations are either missense, deletion, or silent mutations in the coding region, or they are intronic mutations located close to the splice-donor site of the intron following the alternatively spliced exon 10.

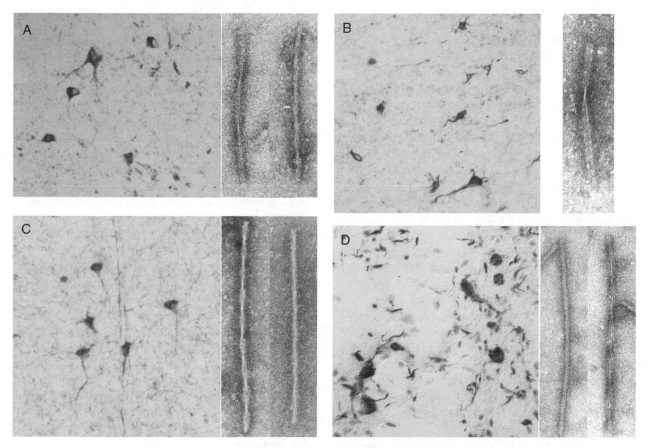

Figure 16.2 Pathologies of frontotemporal dementia and parkinsonism linked to chromosome 17 (FTDP-17), as revealed by immunohistochemistry for hyperphosphorylated tau protein and the presence of tau filaments. **A:** The P301L mutation in exon 10 gives rise to a neuronal and glial tau pathology. Filaments consist of narrow twisted ribbons (*left*) as the majority species and ropelike filaments (*right*) as the minority species. **B:** Mutations in the intron following exon 10 give rise to a neuronal and glial tau pathology. Filaments consist of wide twisted ribbons. **C:** The V337M mutation in exon 12 gives rise to a neuronal tau pathology. Filaments consist of paired helical filaments (*left*) and straight filaments (*right*), like the tau filaments of Alzheimer's disease. **D:** The G389R mutation in exon 13 gives rise to a neuronal tau pathology. Filaments consist of straight filaments (*left*) as the majority species and twisted filaments (*right*) as the minority species. The tau pathology resembles that of Pick's disease.

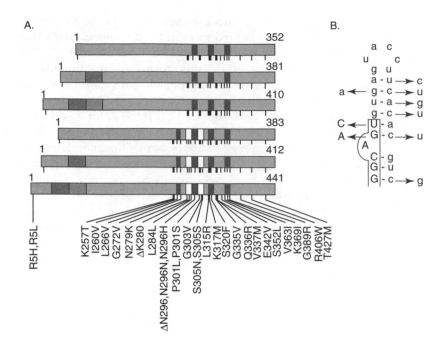

Figure 16.3 Mutations in the tau gene in FTDP-17. **A:** Schematic diagram of the six tau isoforms (352 to 441 amino acids) that are expressed in adult human brain, with mutations in the coding region indicated using the numbering of the 441 amino acid isoform. Twenty-six missense mutations, two deletion mutations, and three silent mutations are shown. **B:** Stem-loop structure in the pre-mRNA at the boundary between exon 10 and the intron following exon 10. Nine mutations are shown, two of which (S305N and S305S) are located in exon 10. Exon sequences are boxed and shown in capital letters, with intron sequences shown in lowercase letters. (See color section.)

FUNCTIONAL EFFECTS OF TAU MUTATIONS

Tau mutations fall into two largely nonoverlapping categories: those that influence the alternative splicing of tau pre-mRNA and those with the primary effect at the protein level (19). Several mutations in exon 10 of tau, such as ΔK280, ΔN296, and N296H, have effects at both RNA and protein levels. In accordance with their location in the microtubule-binding region of tau, most missense mutations reduce the ability of tau to interact with microtubules, as reflected by a reduction in the ability of mutant tau to promote microtubule assembly (20,21). Mutations S305N and Q336R are exceptions, since they slightly increase the ability of tau to promote microtubule assembly, besides having additional effects that may be pathogenic. A reduction in microtubule function is observed when mutant tau is expressed in a number of cell types. Expression of tau with a variety of mutations caused varying degrees of reduced microtubule binding and stability, as well as disorganized microtubule morphology.

A number of mutations in tau may cause FTDP-17, at least in part, by promoting the aggregation of tau protein (22,23). Several studies have demonstrated that some of these mutations, including R5L, K257T, I260V, G272V, ΔK280, P301L, P301S, G335V, Q336R, V337M, and R406W, promote heparin- or arachidonic acid-induced filament formation of tau in vitro relative to wild-type tau. This effect is particularly marked for mutations P301L and P301S. Furthermore, the assembly of mutant tau into filaments following conditional expression in neuroglioma cells has been reported (24). Additional mechanisms may play a role in the case of some coding region mutations. For example, protein phosphatase 2A is known to be the major

tau phosphatase in the brain and to bind to the tandem repeats in tau. Accordingly, several mutant tau proteins have shown reduced binding to protein phosphatase 2A.

Intronic mutations and most coding region mutations in exon 10 (N279K, L284L, ΔN296, N296N, N296H, G303V, S305N, and S305S) increase the splicing of exon 10, thus changing the ratio of 3- and 4-repeat isoforms, resulting in the overproduction of 4-repeat tau (4,5,19,25). Mutation ΔK280 in exon 10 is an apparent exception, since it decreases the splicing of exon 10 in transfection experiments (25). However, it remains to be seen whether this mutation leads to an overproduction of 3-repeat tau in human brain. It is one of the few mutations with effects at both RNA and protein levels. Approximately half of the known tau mutations have their primary effect at the RNA level. Thus, to a significant degree, FTDP-17 is a disease of the alternative mRNA splicing of exon 10 of the tau gene. It follows that a correct ratio of 3-repeat to 4-repeat tau isoforms is essential for preventing neurodegeneration and dementia in midlife. This is all the more surprising, since tau isoform ratios in the adult brain are not conserved between species. Thus, in rodents, only 4-repeat isoforms are expressed, whereas in chicken brain 3-, 4-, and 5-repeat isoforms are present.

The regulation of the alternative splicing of exon 10 is an area of great current interest. It is known to involve multiple cis-acting regulatory elements that either enhance or inhibit utilization of the 5′-splice site of exon 10 (26). These elements are located in exon 10 itself and in the intron following exon 10. Splicing regulatory elements within exon 10 include 2 exon splicing enhancers (ESEs) separated by an exon splicing silencer (ESS). Sequences located at the end of exon 10 and at the beginning of the intron following exon 10 inhibit the splicing of exon 10, probably because of the presence of a stem-loop structure that limits access of the splicing machinery to the 5′-splice site. The determination of the three-dimensional structure of a 25-nucleotide-long RNA from the exon 10-5′-intron junction has shown that this sequence forms a stable, folded stem-loop structure (Fig. 16.3) (27). The stem consists of a single G-C base pair that is separated from a double helix of 6 base pairs by an unpaired adenine. As is often the case with single nucleotide purine bulges, the unpaired adenine at position -2 does not extrude into solution but intercalates into the double helix. The apical loop consists of six nucleotides that adopt multiple conformations in rapid exchange. Downstream of this intron splicing silencer (ISS), an intron splicing modulator has been described. It mitigates exon 10 expression by the ISS.

Pathogenic mutations in the tau gene may alter exon 10 splicing by affecting several of the regulatory elements described in the preceding text. Thus, the intronic mutations (+3, +11, +12, +13, +14, and +16) destabilize the inhibitory stem-loop structure. The S305N mutation and the +3 intronic mutation also may enhance exon 10 splicing by increasing the strength of the 5′-splice site through improved binding of U1snRNA. However, the finding that the S305S mutation, which causes reduced binding of U1snRNA, leads to a predominance of 4-repeat tau, argues against this as the primary effect of the mutations. The N279K mutation may improve the function of the first ESE, thus enhancing exon 10 splicing. Mutation L284L, which enhances exon 10 splicing, may do so by disrupting a potential ESS or by lengthening the first ESE. The effects of the three mutations at codon 296 (ΔN296, N296N, and N296H) are probably through disruption of the ESS.

The high fidelity of splice-site selection is believed to result from the cooperative binding of transacting factors to cis-acting sequences (28). Heterogenous nuclear ribonucleoproteins (hnRNPs) and serine-arginine rich (SR) proteins are involved in splice-site selection. The SR domain-containing proteins Tra2, SF2/ASF, and SRp30c have been found to interact with the first ESE in exon 10 and to function as activators of the alternative splicing of exon 10. In transfection experiments, several other SR proteins, such as SRp20, have been shown to promote the exclusion of exon 10. Moreover, phosphorylation of SR proteins by CDC2-like kinases also has been found to result in the skipping of exon 10.

NEUROPATHOLOGY OF FTDP-17

To a significant degree, the morphologies of tau filaments and their isoform compositions are determined by whether tau mutations affect mRNA splicing of exon 10, or whether they are missense mutations located inside or outside exon 10 (29). The latter give rise to a number of different pathologies.

Mutations in tau resulting in increased splicing of exon 10 lead to the formation of wide twisted ribbon-like filaments that consist only of 4-repeat tau isoforms (Fig. 16.2). Where examined, the tau pathology was widespread and present in both nerve cells and glial cells. This has been shown for the intronic mutations and for mutations N279K, L284L, S305N, S305S, ΔN296, N296N, and N296H in exon 10. Mutation P301L in exon 10, which does not affect alternative mRNA splicing, leads to the formation of narrow twisted ribbons that contain 4-repeat tau isoforms. Biochemical studies have demonstrated that filaments extracted from the brains of patients with the P301L mutation contain predominantly mutant tau. Tau pathology is widespread and present in both nerve cells and glial cells. Compared with mutations that affect the splicing of exon 10, the glial component is less pronounced.

Most coding region mutations located outside exon 10 lead to neuronal tau pathology, without a significant glial component (Fig. 16.2). However, tau deposits in both nerve cells and glial cells have been described for mutations R5H and R5L in exon 1, I260V and L266V in exon 9, and L315R and K317M in exon 11. Two mutations, V337M in exon 12 and R406W in exon 13, lead to the formation of PHFs that contain all 6 tau isoforms, like the tau filaments of AD. Using an antibody specific for tau protein with the R406W mutation, both wild-type and mutant proteins were detected in the abnormal filaments. Mutations K257T, L266V, G272V, L315R, S320F, Q336R, E342V, K369I, and G389R lead to a tau pathology similar or identical to that of PiD. These findings indicate that, depending on the positions of tau mutations in exons 9–13 and the nature of these mutations, a filamentous tau pathology ensues that resembles that of either PSP, CBD, AD, or PiD.

PATHOGENESIS OF FTDP-17

The pathway leading from a mutation in tau to neurodegeneration is unknown. The likely primary effect of most missense mutations is a change in conformation that results in a reduced ability of tau protein to interact with microtubules. It can be overcome by natural osmolytes, such as trimethylamine N-oxide, probably through the promotion of tubulin-induced folding of tau. The primary effect of these mutations may be equivalent to a partial loss of function, with resultant microtubule destabilization and deleterious effects on cellular processes, such as rapid axonal transport. However, in the case of mutations whose primary effect is at the RNA level, this appears unlikely. The net effect of these mutations is a simple overproduction of tau isoforms with four repeats, which are known to interact more strongly with microtubules than do isoforms with three repeats. It is, therefore, possible that in cases of FTDP-17 with intronic mutations and those coding region mutations whose primary effect is at the RNA level, microtubules are more stable than in brain from control individuals. Moreover, some mutations, such as P301L and P301S in exon 10, will only affect

20%–25% of tau molecules, with 75%–80% of tau being wild type, arguing against a simple loss of function of tau as a decisive mechanism. Mice without tau protein are largely normal and exhibit no signs of neurodegeneration (30).

A correct ratio of wild-type 3-repeat to 4-repeat tau may be essential for the normal function of tau in human brain. However, the fact that the tau isoform composition is not conserved in humans, rodents, and chickens argues against this possibility. An alternative hypothesis is that a partial loss of function of tau is necessary for setting in motion the gain of toxic function mechanism that will lead to neurodegeneration. This hypothesis requires that an overproduction of tau isoforms with four repeats results in an excess of tau over available binding sites on microtubules, resulting in the cytoplasmic accumulation of unbound 4-repeat tau. It would probably necessitate the existence of different binding sites on microtubules for 3-repeat and 4-repeat tau. Validation of this hypothesis will require structural information at the atomic level.

From the preceding, a reduced ability of tau to interact with microtubules emerges as the most likely primary effect of the FTDP-17 mutations. It will lead to the accumulation of tau in the cytoplasm of brain cells and will result in its hyperphosphorylation. Over time, hyperphosphorylated tau protein will assemble into abnormal filaments. It is at present unknown whether the filaments themselves cause nerve cell loss, or whether nonassembled, conformationally altered tau is toxic.

RELEVANCE OF TAU MUTATIONS FOR THE SPORADIC TAUOPATHIES

The study of FTDP-17 has established that dysfunction of tau protein can cause neurodegeneration and dementia. It follows that tau dysfunction is most probably also of central importance for the pathogenesis of sporadic diseases with a filamentous tau pathology, such as AD, PSP, CBD, AGD, and PiD. This is further emphasized by the fact that the aforementioned diseases are partially or completely phenocopied by cases of FTDP-17 (19,29).

Nine missense mutations in tau have been shown to give rise to a clinical and neuropathological phenotype reminiscent of PiD. The finding that overproduction of 4-repeat tau causes disease and leads to the assembly of tau with 4 repeats in nerve cells and glial cells may shed light on the pathogenesis of PSP, CBD, and AGD. Neuropathologically, all three diseases are characterized by a neuronal and glial pathology, with the filaments comprising predominantly 4-repeat tau. PSP and CBD can be phenocopied by some tau mutations. Thus, individuals with mutations R5L, N279K, ΔN296, G303V, S305S, and the +16 intronic mutation have presented with a clinical picture similar to PSP, whereas some individuals with mutations N296N, P301S, and K317M suffered from a disease resembling CBD. Intronic mutation +14 and missense mutation K317M can give rise

to cases of FTDP-17 with motor neuron disease, extending the phenotypic spectrum even further.

An association between PSP and a dinucleotide repeat polymorphism in the intron between exons 9 and 10 of tau was described in 1997 (31). Subsequently, a similar genetic association was found for CBD (32). The alleles at this locus carry 11–15 repeats. The A0 allele, with 11 repeats, has a frequency of over 90% in patients with PSP and about 70% in controls. Following from this work, two common tau haplotypes, named H1 (allele frequency of 80%) and H2 (allele frequency of 20%), were identified in populations of European descent (33). Both alleles differ in nucleotide sequence and intron size but are identical at the amino acid level. A recent study has shown that a genomic inversion polymorphism underlies the H1 and H2 haplotypes, explaining the extended linkage disequilibrium in this region and the suppressed H1/H2 recombination (34). It extends over a 900 kb region that encompasses the tau gene along with several other genes. H1 shows considerable diversity and has a normal pattern of linkage disequilibrium, except with H2, whereas H2 appears to be an unrecombining haplotype.

Several subhaplotypes of H1 have been identified. One of these (H1B, also known as H1c) has been linked to PSP and CBD (35,36). A recent study also has reported an association between this subhaplotype and sporadic, late-onset AD (37). The H1B risk has been localized to a 22 kb regulatory region in the large intron preceding coding exon 1 of tau and could be explained by a single nucleotide polymorphism creating a binding site for transcription factor CP2 (erythrocyte factor related to *Drosophila* Elf1 [LBP-1c; LSF]) (36). In addition, several groups have described a significant, but relatively weak, association between the H1 haplotype and idiopathic Parkinson's disease (PD), a disease lacking significant tau pathology (38). The functional consequences resulting from the presence of the H1 or H2 haplotype are incompletely understood. It has been reported that H1 is more effective than H2 at driving expression of a reporter gene in transfected cells, suggesting that tau expression from the H1 haplotype may be higher than from the H2 haplotype (39). Furthermore, the H2 haplotype has been found to be associated with an earlier age of onset in sporadic cases of frontotemporal dementia lacking tau pathology (40). The intron between exons 9 and 10 of tau also contains the putative intronless gene Saitohin, which encodes a predicted protein of 128 amino acids that is poorly conserved. It remains to be seen whether Saitohin exists as a bona fide protein and, if so, what its physiological function may be.

ANIMAL MODELS OF THE TAUOPATHIES

The identification of mutations in tau in FTDP-17 is rapidly leading to the production of transgenic mouse lines that reproduce the essential molecular and cellular features of the human tauopathies (Figs. 16.4 and 16.5). They represent an improvement over earlier lines that

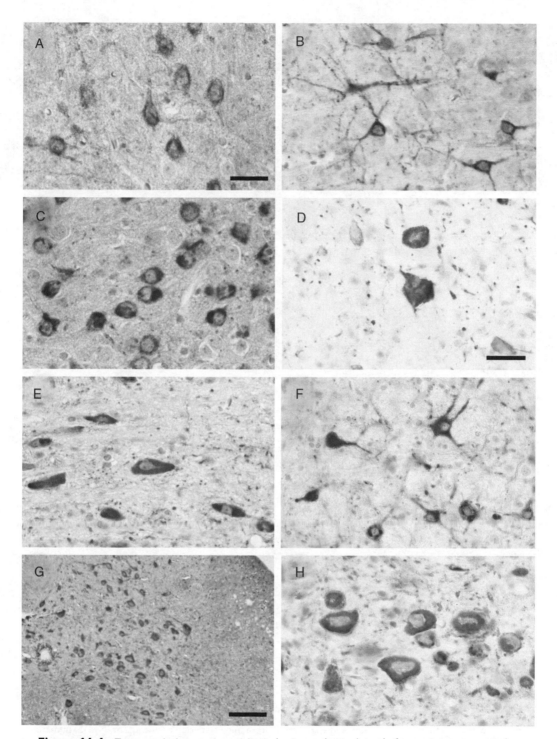

Figure 16.4 Tau protein immunoreactivity in brains and spinal cords from mice transgenic for mutant (P301S) human tau protein. **A, B:** Cerebral cortex. **C:** Amygdala. **D:** Dentate nucleus of the cerebellum. **E, F:** Brainstem. **G, H:** Spinal cord. Scale bars: (A–C,E,F), 40 μm (in A); (D,H), 60 μm (in D); (G), 250 μm.

expressed wild-type human tau in nerve cells and showed signs of axonopathy and amyotrophy but failed to develop abundant tau filaments and nerve cell death.

Mouse lines expressing human tau with mutations P301L, G272V, V337M, R406W, P301S, and the triple mutation G272V, P301L, and V337M in nerve cells or glial cells have

been published. Abundant tau filaments in nerve cells were found in lines expressing 4-repeat P301L or R406W human tau under the control of the murine prion protein promoter and 4-repeat P301S human tau under the control of the murine Thy1 promoter (41,42,43). Filamentous tau protein was hyperphosphorylated in a way similar to the human

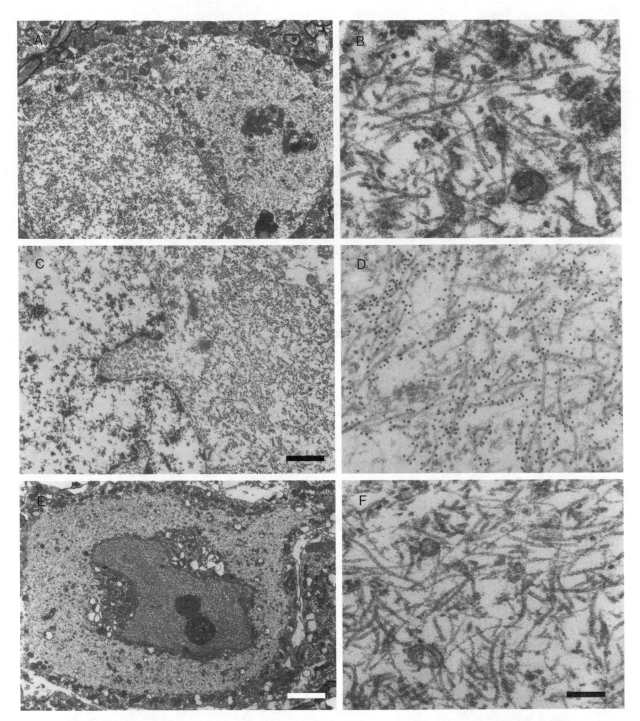

Figure 16.5   Tau filaments in brains and spinal cords from mice transgenic for mutant (P301S) human tau protein. **A, B:** Cerebral cortex. **C, D:** Brainstem. **E, F:** Spinal cord. **B, D, F:** Higher magnification of parts of the cytoplasmic regions from **(A, C, E)**. The electron micrographs in **(C, D)** show immunogold labeling of filaments using a phosphorylation-dependent anti-tau antibody. Scale bars: **C:** 1.5 μm. **A, E:** 5.5 μm (in **E**); **B, D, F:** 300 nm (in **F**).

diseases, and hyperphosphorylation at most sites appeared to precede the assembly of tau into filaments. Moreover, an increase in the phosphorylation of soluble tau resulted in increased filament formation, suggesting that phosphorylation can drive filament assembly (44). In lines transgenic for P301L and P301S tau, nonapoptotic nerve cell loss and a pronounced inflammatory reaction were detected in the spinal cord (42,45,46). The mice suffered from a severe paraparesis and showed signs of neurogenic muscle atrophy.

In a mouse line expressing P301L tau in oligodendrocytes, coexpression of mutant human α-synuclein resulted in the appearance of thioflavin S-positive staining that was not observed in the single transgenic lines (47). Moreover, in vitro experiments have shown that α-synuclein can induce the formation of tau filaments, giving a possible explanation for the co-occurrence of tau and α-synuclein in some neurodegenerative diseases. In mouse lines expressing P301L tau in nerve cells, coexpression of mutant human amyloid precursor protein (APP) or the intracerebral injection of β-amyloid fibrils resulted in an increase in the number of tangle-bearing cells (48,49). In a mouse line triple transgenic for mutant APP, presenilin-1, and P301L tau, the intracerebral injection of anti-Aβ antibodies or of a γ-secretase inhibitor resulted in the disappearance of somatodendritic staining in younger, but not in older, animals (50). It thus appears that extracellular β-amyloid deposits can exacerbate the intraneuronal pathology caused by the expression of mutant human tau protein. However, one must bear in mind that these experiments are artificial to the extent that mutant APP and mutant tau have not been encountered together in human diseases. So far, β-amyloid deposition has not been found to induce the formation of filamentous tau deposits in transgenic mice.

Filamentous tau deposits made of wild-type human tau were observed in a mouse line expressing all 6 human brain tau isoforms in the absence of endogenous mouse tau (51). The observed imbalance between levels of 3- and 4-repeat isoforms may have caused tau pathology in this line, where nerve cells with and without tau inclusions were reported to die. A closer correspondence was observed between cell death and an abnormal reexpression of cell cycle markers, suggesting a possible cause and effect relationship. However, this contrasts with a line transgenic for P301S tau, where cell cycle markers were not reexpressed (52). Endogenous mouse tau has been reported to assemble into filaments in a neurodegenerative condition caused by inactivation of the gene encoding the prolyl isomerase Pin1 (53).

Taken together, the experimental mouse models of human tauopathy reaffirm the notion derived from studies of human diseases that a pathological pathway leading from soluble, monomeric to insoluble, filamentous tau causes neurodegeneration. What is unclear, however, is the precise molecular nature of the offending tau species. Assembly of tau into filaments is a complex process that is likely to involve a number of poorly defined intermediates of varying solubility and, perhaps, toxicity. An apparent dissociation between inclusion formation and neurodegeneration was reported in a model based on the inducible expression of human P301L tau to high levels (54).

Mouse models of the human tauopathies differ from invertebrate models to the extent that overexpression of wild-type and mutant human tau in *C. elegans* and *D. melanogaster* resulted in nerve cell degeneration, in the absence of filament formation (55,56). Phosphorylation of tau was more extensive in the fly than in the worm. In *Drosophila*, phosphorylation of S262 and S356 in tau by PAR-1 kinase, the fly homologue of MARK, appeared to be necessary for the subsequent phosphorylation at other sites, indicating the existence of a hierarchical and temporally ordered phosphorylation process (57). Coexpression of human tau with the fly homologue of GSK3- resulted in accelerated neurodegeneration and formation of tau-immunoreactive inclusions. In contrast to what has been described in FTDP-17, tau-induced neurodegeneration involved programmed cell death. All in all, it thus appears that conformationally altered nonfilamentous human tau protein is neurotoxic in invertebrates. The future will tell whether or not this is also true in mice and men.

REFERENCES

1. St George-Hyslop PH, Farrer LA, Goedert M. Alzheimer disease and frontotemporal dementias: diseases with cerebral deposition of fibrillar proteins. In: Scriver CR, Beaudet AL, Sly WS, Vallee D, eds. *The Metabolic and Molecular Bases of Inherited Disease.* McGraw-Hill, 2001;5875–5899.
2. Lee VMY, Goedert M, Trojanowski JQ. Neurodegenerative tauopathies. *Annu Rev Neurosci* 2001;24:1121–1159.
3. Poorkaj P, Bird TD, Wijsman E, et al. Tau is a candidate gene for chromosome 17 frontotemporal dementia. *Ann Neurol* 1998;43: 815–825.
4. Hutton M, Lendon CL, Rizzu P, et al. Association of missense and 5′-splice-site mutations in tau with the inherited dementia FTDP-17. *Nature* 1998;393:702–706.
5. Spillantini MG, Murrell JR, Goedert M, et al. Mutation in the tau gene in familial multiple system tauopathy with presenile dementia. *Proc Natl Acad Sci USA* 1998;95:7737–7741.
6. Goedert M, Spillantini MG, Jakes R, et al. Multiple isoforms of human microtubule-associated protein tau: sequences and localization in neurofibrillary tangles of Alzheimer's disease. *Neuron* 1989;3:519–526.
7. Eliezer D, Barré P, Kobaslija M, et al. Residual structure in the repeat domain of tau: echoes of microtubule binding and paired helical filament formation. *Biochemistry* 2005;44:1026–1036.
8. Kar S, Fan J, Smith MJ, et al. Repeat motifs of tau bind to the insides of microtubules in the absence of taxol. *EMBO J* 2003;22: 70–77.
9. Al-Bassam J, Ozer RS, Safer D, et al. MAP2 and tau bind longitudinally along the outer ridges of microtubules and protofilaments. *J Cell Biol* 2002;157:1187–1196.
10. Goedert M, Jakes R, Spillantini MG, et al. Assembly of microtubule-associated protein tau into Alzheimer-like filaments induced by sulfated glycosaminoglycans. *Nature* 1996;383: 550–553.
11. Pérez M, Valpuesta JM, Medine M, et al. Polymerization of tau into filaments in the presence of heparin: the minimal sequence requirement for tau-tau interactions. *J Neurochem* 1996;67: 1183–1190.
12. Von Bergen M, Friedhoff P, Biernat J, et al. Assembly of tau protein into Alzheimer paired helical filaments depends on a local sequence motif (306)VQIVYK(311) forming beta structure. *Proc Natl Acad Sci USA* 2000;97:5129–5134.
13. Mukrasch MD, Biernat J, von Bergen M, et al. Sites of tau important for aggregation populate β-structure and bind to microtubules and polyanions. *J Biol Chem* 2005;280:24,978–24,986.
14. Berriman J, Serpell LC, Oberg KA, et al. Tau filaments from human brain and from in vitro assembly of recombinant protein show cross β-structure. *Proc Natl Acad Sci USA* 2003;100: 9034–9038.
15. Chirita C, Necula M, Kuret J. Ligand-dependent inhibition and reversal of tau filament formation. *Biochemistry* 2004;43: 2879–2887.
16. Pickhardt M, Gazova S, von Bergen M, et al. Anthraquinones inhibit tau aggregation and dissolve Alzheimer's paired helical filaments in vitro and in cells. *J Biol Chem* 2005;280:3628–3635.
17. Taniguchi S, Suzuki N, Masuda M, et al. Inhibition of heparin-induced tau filament formation by phenothiazines, polyphenols, and porphyrins. *J Biol Chem* 2005;280:7614–7623.
18. Wilhelmsen KC, Lynch T, Pavlou E, et al. Localization of disinhibition-dementia-parkinsonism-amyotrophy complex to 17q21-22. *Am J Hum Genet* 1994;55:1159–1165.

19. Goedert M, Jakes R. Mutations causing neurodegenerative tauopathies. *Biochim Biophys Acta* 2005;1739:240–250.

20. Hasegawa M, Smith MJ, Goedert M. Tau proteins with FTDP-17 mutations have a reduced ability to promote microtubule assembly. *FEBS Lett* 1998;437:207–210.

21. Hong M, Zhukareva V, Vogelsberg-Ragaglia V, et al. Mutation-specific functional impairments in distinct tau isoforms of hereditary FTDP-17. *Science* 1998;282:1914–1917.

22. Nacharaju P, Lewis C, Easson C, et al. Accelerated filament formation from tau protein with specific FTDP-17 missense mutations. *FEBS Lett* 1999;447:195–199.

23. Goedert M, Jakes R, Crowther RA. Effects of frontotemporal dementia FTDP-17 mutations on heparin-induced assembly of tau filaments. *FEBS Lett* 1999;450:306–311.

24. De Ture M, Ko LW, Easson SH, et al. Tau assembly in inducible transfectants expressing wild-type or FTDP-17 tau. *Am J Pathol* 2002;161:1711–1722.

25. D'Souza I, Poorkaj P, Hong M, et al. Missense and silent tau gene mutations cause frontotemporal dementia with parkinsonism-chromosome 17 type, by affecting multiple alternative RNA splicing regulatory elements. *Proc Natl Acad Sci USA* 1999;96:5598–5603.

26. D'Souza I, Schellenberg GD. Tau exon 10 expression involves a bipartite intron 10 regulatory sequence and weak 5′ and 3′ sites. *J Biol Chem* 2000;277:26,587–26,599.

27. Varani L, Hasegawa M, Spillantini MG, et al. Structure of tau exon 10 splicing regulatory element RNA and destabilization by mutations of frontotemporal dementia and parkinsonism linked to chromosome 17. *Proc Natl Acad Sci USA* 1999;96:8229–8234.

28. Faustino NA, Cooper TA. Pre-mRNA splicing and human disease. *Genes Dev* 2003;17:419–437.

29. Yancopoulou, D, Spillantini MG. Tau protein in familial and sporadic diseases. *Neuromol Med* 2003;4:37–48.

30. Harada A, Oguchi K, Okabe S, et al. Altered microtubule organization in small-calibre axons of mice lacking tau protein. *Nature* 1994;369:488–491.

31. Conrad C, Andreadis A, Trojanowski JQ, et al. Genetic evidence for the involvement of tau in progressive supranuclear palsy. *Ann Neurol* 1997;41:277–281.

32. Di Maria E, Tabaton M, Vigo G, et al. Corticobasal degeneration shares a common genetic background with progressive supranuclear palsy. *Ann Neurol* 2000;47:374–377.

33. Baker M, Litvan I, Houlden H, et al. Association of an extended haplotype in the tau gene with progressive supranuclear palsy. *Hum Mol Genet* 1999;8:711–715.

34. Stefansson H, Helgason A, Thorleifsson G, et al. A common inversion under selection in Europeans. *Nature Genet* 2005;37:129–137.

35. Pastor P, Ezquerra M, Perez JC, et al. Novel haplotypes in 17q21 are associated with progressive supranuclear palsy. *Ann Neurol* 2004;56:249–258.

36. Rademakers R, Melquist S, Cruts M, et al. High-density SNP haplotyping suggests altered regulation of tau gene expression in progressive supranuclear palsy. *Hum Mol Genet* 2005;14:3281–3292.

37. Myers AJ, Kaleem M, Malowe, L, et al. The H1c haplotype at the MAPT locus is associated with Alzheimer's disease. *Hum Mol Genet* 2005;14:2399–2404.

38. Pastor P, Ezquerra M, Munoz E, et al. Significant association between the tau gene A0/A0 genotype and Parkinson's disease. *Ann Neurol* 2000;47:242–245.

39. Kwok JBJ, Teber ET, Loy C, et al. Tau haplotypes regulate transcription and are associated with Parkinson's disease. *Ann Neurol* 2004;55:329–334.

40. Borroni B, Yancopoulou D, Tsutsui M, et al. Association between tau H2 haplotype and age at onset in frontotemporal dementia. *Arch Neurol* 2005;62:1419–1422.

41. Lewis J, McGowan E, Rockwood, J., et al. Neurofibrillary tangles, amyotrophy and progressive motor disturbance in mice expressing mutant (P301L) tau protein. *Nature Genet* 2000;25:402–405.

42. Allen B, Ingram E, Takao M, et al. Abundant tau filaments and nonapoptotic neurodegeneration in transgenic mice expressing human P301S tau protein. *J Neurosci* 2002;22:9340–9351.

43. Zhang B, Higuchi M, Yoshiyama Y, et al. Retarded axonal transport of R406W mutant tau in transgenic mice with a neurodegenerative tauopathy. *J Neurosci* 2004;24:4657–4667.

44. Noble W, Olm V, Takata K, et al. Cdk5 is a key factor in tau aggregation and tangle formation in vivo. *Neuron* 2003;38:555–565.

45. Zehr C, Lewis J, McGowan E, et al. Apoptosis in oligodendrocytes is associated with axonal degeneration in P301L tau mice. *Neurobiol Dis* 2004;15:553–562.

46. Belluci A, Westwood AJ, Ingram E, et al. Induction of inflammatory mediators and microglial activation in mice transgenic for mutant human P301S tau protein. *Am J Pathol* 2004;165:1643–1652.

47. Giasson BI, Forman MS, Higuchi M, et al. Initiation and synergistic fibrillization of tau and alpha-synuclein. *Science* 2003;300:636–640.

48. Lewis J, Dickson DW, Lin WL, et al. Enhanced neurofibrillary degeneration in transgenic mice expressing mutant tau and APP. *Science* 2001;293:1487–1491.

49. Götz J, Chen J, van Dorpe RM, et al. Formation of neurofibrillary tangles in P301L tau transgenic mice by A 42 fibrils. *Science* 2001;293:1491–1495.

50. Oddo S, Billings L, Kesslak JP, et al. A β immunotherapy leads to clearance of early, but not late, hyperphosphorylated tau aggregates via the proteasome. *Neuron* 2004;43:321–332.

51. Andorfer C, Acker CM, Kress Y, et al. Cell-cycle reentry and cell death in transgenic mice expressing nonmutant human tau isoforms. *J Neurosci* 2005;25:5446–5454.

52. Delobel P, Lavenir I, Ghetti B, et al. Cell cycle markers in a transgenic mouse model of human tauopathy: increased levels of cyclin-dependent kinase inhibitors p21Cip1 and p27Kip1. *Am J Pathol.* 2006;168:878–887.

53. Liou YC, Sun A, Ryo XZ, et al. Role of the prolyl isomerase Pin1 in protecting against age-dependent neurodegeneration. *Nature* 2003;424:556–561.

54. SantaCruz K, Lewis J, Spires T, et al. Tau suppression in a neurodegenerative mouse model improves memory function. *Science* 2005;309:476–481.

55. Wittmann CW, Wszolek MF, Shulman JM, et al. Tauopathy in *Drosophila*: neurodegeneration without neurofibrillary tangles. *Science* 2001;293:711–714.

56. Kraemer BC, Zhang B, Leverenz JB, et al. Neurodegeneration and defective neurotransmission in a *Caenorhabditis elegans* model of tauopathy. *Proc Natl Acad Sci USA* 2003;100:9980–9985.

57. Nishimura I, Yang Y, Lu B. PAR-1 kinase plays an initiator role in a temporally ordered phosphorylation process that confers tau toxicity in *Drosophila. Cell* 2004;116:671–682.

Secondary Parkinson's Syndrome

17

Andrew J. Lees

Secondary causes of Parkinsonism continue to influence our thinking on the possible etiology of Parkinson's disease (PD) and, as a consequence, assume an importance far greater than their incidence in neurological practice. A number of monogenetic causes of L-dopa–responsive parkinsonism have been identified in the last 5 years, and together these now comprise about 5% of all cases currently included under the umbrella of PD. The clinical picture associated with each mutation is beginning to be characterized, and it seems probable that the autosomal recessive disorders linked with mutations of the parkin, PINK-1, or more rare DJ-1 protein will be reliably distinguishable on clinical grounds from PD. In addition to α-synuclein and the much more common dardarin mutations (LRRK-2), it is now recognized that a number of other autosomal dominantly inherited trinucleotide repeat disorders, particularly Huntington's disease (see Chapter 18) and SCA2 and 3 (see Chapter 32), can present with parkinsonism rather than chorea or ataxia. The identified genes responsible for familial parkinsonism are covered elsewhere in this book (see Chapter 8), so I have left this important cause of secondary parkinsonism to one side. In previous editions of this textbook, Riley's chapters on secondary parkinsonism embraced the atypical Parkinson's syndromes, which constitute a group of diverse, relatively uncommon and obscure neurodegenerative disorders that may masquerade as PD. Strictly, the term *secondary parkinsonism* should be restricted to bradykinetic syndromes in which a specific cause is known. As separate chapters are devoted to progressive supranuclear palsy (PSP) (Chapter 13), multisystem atrophy (Chapter 14), corticobasal degeneration (Chapter 15), and neurodegeneration with iron accumulation (Chapter 20), these also will not be covered in this chapter. I also have elected arbitrarily to exclude a myriad of rare and esoteric secondary causes in which parkinsonism occurs as part of a more widespread multisystem degeneration and which are only rarely confused with PD. I also have omitted several single case reports linking infectious diseases, drugs, toxins, and inborn errors of metabolism where cause and effect would benefit from further corroborative reports. Despite these restrictions, the number of secondary causes presenting with PD continues to grow, and space will permit only fragmentary accounts of many of the now well-established secondary causes. In addition to the traditional and mandatory divisions relating to cause, I have tried to balance the length of each clinical description to the relative frequency of the causative agent, its contemporaneous interest, the therapeutic opportunity, and the likelihood of achieving accurate diagnosis premortem. For those exotica relegated to tables, the bibliography will provide a stepping stone for additional reading.

IATROGENIC PARKINSONISM

A reversible Parkinson's syndrome caused by the prescription of antipsychotic dopaminergic antagonist drugs or the dopamine-depleting antihypertensive reserpine has been recognized for half a century, and it has proven to be an important piece in the jigsaw paving the way for the "dopamine miracle" of PD therapy (Degkwitz, 1960). Early descriptions seemed to suggest that neuroleptic-provoked Parkinson's syndrome was distinguishable from PD by its symmetry and predominantly bradykinetic-rigid presentation, as well as a tendency to involve the arms more than the legs (Hassin-Baer, 2001). Many patients also developed coexisting neuroleptic-provoked dyskinesias, including akathisia and bucco-linguo-masticatory syndromes. However, other studies, particularly in the elderly, have indicated that the clinical picture may be indistinguishable from PD with marked asymmetry and prominent rest tremor (Hardie, 1988). A number of these patients have an associated moderate to high-frequency postural tremor with an additional kinetic component, and a few also present with a strikingly slow 4–6 Hz perioral tremor that responds to anticholinergic drugs ("the rabbit syndrome") (Villeneuve, 1972). In a Department of Elderly Medicine in Scotland study, 51% of 95 elderly new referrals with parkinsonism seen over a 2-year period were found to be receiving neuroleptics (especially prochlorperazine and thioridazine) (Stephen, 1984). In a further study in a hospital neurology clinic, 24% of 298 patients were taking drugs implicated in causing parkinsonism (the most common being cinnarizine and sulpiride) (Marti Masso, 1993). Inappropriate prescribing is responsible for a large number of iatrogenic cases, and careful and repeated enquiry about concurrent drug use may be needed to identify an offending medication.

Signs of parkinsonism may start within the first few days of dopaminergic blockade, and the majority of cases are present within 3 months of sustained therapy. Occasionally, severe parkinsonism may occur after sudden concurrent antipsychotic and anticholinergic drug withdrawal, possibly due to cholinergic rebound in the face of persisting dopamine receptor blockade. In general practice, the antiemetic metoclopramide and prochlorperazine prescribed as a vestibular sedative are common and frequently overlooked causes. There are also reports of generic medications adulterated with neuroleptics causing parkinsonism (Cosentino, 2000). Anticholinergic drugs are of some symptomatic value when the underlying psychiatric illness precludes neuroleptic discontinuation, but they must be used with great caution in the elderly because of the risk of delirium and amnesia. L-dopa, on the other hand, is ineffective due to striatal D2 receptor blockade (Hardie, 1988). Parkinsonism due to drugs that deplete presynaptic dopamine, such as the antidyskinetic therapy tetrabenazene, may be on the other hand amenable to treatment with L-dopa (Jankovic, 1997). If it is possible to stop the offending antipsychotic, recovery usually occurs over several weeks. Occasionally, after depot phenothiazines, recovery may be delayed for many months. There are also reports of spontaneous improvement of neuroleptic-provoked parkinsonism over time despite continuation of the antipsychotic drug, presumably due to the gradual development of striatal dopamine receptor supersensitivity. However, a few elderly patients fail to recover at all, even after permanent neuroleptic withdrawal when it is usually assumed that PD has been unmasked by pharmacological dopaminergic blockade. In favor of this is the clinical observation that in some patients iatrogenic parkinsonism may recover, only to be followed a few months later by the emergence of idiopathic PD (Rajput, 1982). In patients on long-term neuroleptics who develop parkinsonian symptoms, it is often impossible to distinguish between iatrogenic parkinsonism and emerging PD. SPECT scanning using a dopamine transporter ligand has shown early promise in helping to resolve this diagnostic uncertainty (Tolosa, 2003). In PD, a presynaptic nigrostriatal dopamine deficit will be demonstrated. Clozapine and quetiapine are the only widely prescribed antipsychotic drugs that have not been associated with parkinsonism and offer a therapeutic option for schizophrenic patients who develop disabling movement disorders with other antipsychotic drugs. Great care should be taken with antipsychotic therapy, especially in patients over 50. The need for continuing treatment should also be reviewed periodically, and the dose and duration of antipsychotic drug therapy should be kept to the minimum needed to effectively control psychiatric symptoms. In elderly patients, the routine coadministration of anticholinergic drugs is inadvisable.

Many patients on long-term antipsychotic drugs manifest subtle parkinsonian signs, but these are usually found on routine examination and do not interfere markedly with psychological rehabilitation. It has been estimated that about 10%–15% of patients receiving antipsychotics will develop symptomatic parkinsonism, but accurate epidemiological data are lacking. Dose and duration of therapy, however, do not seem to be definite risk factors, and even the relevance of increasing age as a predisposing factor is by no means certain (Moleman, 1986). Nevertheless, no evidence exists that individuals with a preexisting postural tremor of the hands are at increased risk (Gimenez-Roldan, 1991). Patients with neuroleptic-induced parkinsonism do not appear to have a higher incidence of affected first-degree relatives with PD than do age-matched controls (Myrianthopoulos, 1962), but it has been reported that patients with increased echogenicity on transcranial sonography may be at greater risk (Berg, 2001). Patients with dementia with Lewy bodies (DLB) also have been reported to exhibit extreme neuroleptic sensitivity compared with Alzheimer's disease, leading to the unmasking of cryptic parkinsonism and the potentially fatal neuroleptic malignant syndrome (McKeith, 1992).

Although there is a long list of other drugs reported to cause parkinsonism, the mechanisms for most of these are poorly understood, and many are single-case reports. The calcium channel blockers, particularly flunarizine and high-dose cinnarizine, are common causes in some parts of the world (Micheli, 1987; Marti-Masso, 1998), where they are used as vestibular sedatives and cerebral vasodilators in elderly arteriopaths; dopamine receptor antagonism is believed to be the likely mechanism of causation. Kava kava, a western Pacific herbal sedative widely used in the West until recent scares of hepatotoxicity, can, rarely, lead to parkinsonism and dystonia (Meseguer, 2002). Sodium valproate is a common cause of postural tremor, but a number of convincing cases of reversible Parkinson's syndrome following chronic administration have now been described. Some of these patients have normal dopamine transporter SPECT imaging, suggesting that the cause is unlikely to be presynaptic nigrostriatal dopamine depletion, or the unmasking of PD; some have associated hearing and cognitive deficits (Armon, 1996; Easterford, 2004). Although chorea and dystonia are more common side effects with high-dose phenytoin, a few cases of parkinsonism also have been reported. A number of anticancer chemotherapy drugs, including cyclophosphamide, busulphan, cytosine arabinoside, and 5-fluorouracil, have been implicated in cases of parkinsonism, but the mechanisms underlying these reports remain obscure (Boranic, 1979; Kulkantrakorn, 1996). Cyclo-sporin also has been linked with severe akinetic syndromes (Kim, 2002). Minor concern also continues that benzodiazepines and bupropion, serotonin reuptake inhibitors, central cholinesterase inhibitors, and lithium may aggravate PD. (See Table 17.1.)

TABLE 17.1
DRUG-INDUCED CAUSES OF PARKINSONISM

- Dopamine receptor blocking drugs (neuroleptics, metoclopramide, prochlorperazine, adulterated generics) (Hardie, 1988)
- Dopamine-depleting antichoreic drugs (tetrabenazene) (Jankovic, 1997)
- Calcium channel blockers (flunarizine, cinarrizine, diltiazem, perhexiline, nifedipine, verapamil) (Teive, 2004; Micheli, 1987; Dick, 1989; Gordon, 1981; Garcia-Albea, 1993; Sempere, 1995)
- Antiarrhythmic drugs (amiodarone, procaine) (Gjerris, 1971; Werner, 1989)
- Buspirone, diazepam (Suranyi-Cadotte, 1985)
- Herbal causes, e.g., kava kava, betel nuts (arecoline) (Meseguer, 2002; Deahl, 1989)
- Anticonvulsants sodium valproate, phenytoin (Armon, 1996; Easterford, 2004; Goni, 1985)
- Immunosuppressants (cyclosporin, busulphan, cytosine arabinoside, vincristine, adriamycin) (Boranic, 1979; Kim, 2002; Chuang, 2003; Kulkantrakorn, 1996; Wasserstein, 1996)
- Lithium (Holroyd, 1995; Dallocchio, 2002)
- Alpha-methyldopa
- Cephaloridine (Mintz, 1971)
- Chloroquine (Parmar, 2000)

VASCULAR PARKINSONISM

Classical "lower-half" Parkinson's syndrome, associated with confluent subcortical white matter ischemia and lacunar infarcts, is clinically distinct from PD and presents with start hesitation, motor blocking, a broad-based shuffling gait, and falls (FitzGerald, 1989). The speech may be slurred and some super-added swallowing difficulties, mild arm rigidity, and bradykinesia with slight hypomimia also may occur. Some patients have additional cognitive deficits, pseudobulbar palsy, and pyramidal signs. This clinical syndrome is common in the elderly, and the diagnosis can be supported by magnetic resonance (MR) scanning, as well as a past history of strokes and vascular risk factors. Dopamine transporter SPECT imaging is usually normal (Gerschlager, 2002) and the response to L-dopa variable, but a trial of this up to 1000 mg daily for at least 6 weeks should always be given. Patients with macroscopic basal ganglia lacunar infarcts, lacunae caused by enlarged perivascular spaces, or neuronal nigral loss are more likely to respond favorably to dopaminergic drugs.

A more uncommon and less well-recognized vascular syndrome may follow an acute striatal infarct with limb hemiparesis (Tolosa, 1984; Peralta, 2004). As the corticospinal tract signs resolve, a bradykinetic-rigid syndrome emerges on the same side. Dopamine transporter SPECT may reveal complete absence of uptake on the side of the infarct with complete preservation on the other side (Fig. 17.1). A rest tremor may be present, and the parkinsonism may spread to the other side. A modest response to L-dopa is not uncommon (Zijlmans, 2004).

A recent clinicopathological investigation was conducted in which 17 highly selected patients presented with parkinsonism for which no alternative pathological cause could be found were compared with age-matched controls with comparable vascular risk factors. These cases were identified from an archival pathology collection of more than 600 parkinsonian brains. Microscopic small-vessel disease was more severe in the presumed vascular Parkinson cases. The

majority presented with a "lower-half" Parkinson syndrome but four presented acutely with a hemiparesis and then developed delayed-onset parkinsonism over the following year. These "acute" cases were distinguished pathologically by macroscopically visible lacunar infarcts in regions that could result in reduced thalamocortical drive; intriguingly, four of the patients had additional nigral loss without inclusions. On the basis of this study, operational criteria for the clinical diagnosis of vascular parkinsonism (VP) have been proposed (Ziljmans, 2004) (see Table 17.2). The use of the University of Pennsylvania Smell Test (UPSIT) also may be a helpful discriminator as olfaction appears to be preserved in VP, whereas 80% of patients with PD are hyposmic (Katzenschlager, 2004).

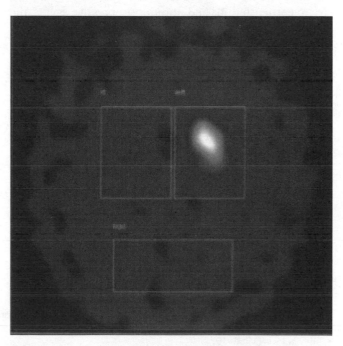

Figure 17.1 Dopamine transporter (DAT scan) SPECT showing unilateral loss of dopamine transporter uptake in a patient with vascular parkinsonism following a strio-capsular infarct.

TABLE 17.2
POSSIBLE CRITERIA FOR THE CLINICAL DIAGNOSIS OF VASCULAR PARKINSONISM

a. Parkinsonism: bradykinesia (slowness of initiation of voluntary movement with progressive reduction in speed and amplitude of repetitive actions in either upper limb or lower limb, including the presence of reduced step length) and at least one of the following: rest tremor, muscular rigidity, or postural instability not caused by primary visual, vestibular, cerebellar, or proprioceptive dysfunction.
b. Cerebrovascular disease, defined by evidence of relevant cerebrovascular disease by brain imaging (CT or MRI) or the presence of focal signs or symptoms that are consistent with stroke.
c. A relationship between the two preceding disorders. In practice: (1) An acute or delayed progressive onset with infarcts in or near areas that can increase the basal ganglia motor output (globus pallidus pars externa or substantia nigra pars compacta) or can decrease the thalamocortical drive directly (ventral lateral nucleus of the thalamus, large frontal lobe infarct). The parkinsonism at onset consists of a contralateral bradykinetic rigid syndrome or shuffling gait, within 1 year after a stroke (vascular parkinsonism). (2) An insidious onset of parkinsonism with extensive subcortical white matter lesions, bilateral symptoms at onset, and the presence of early shuffling gait or early cognitive dysfunction.

Exclusion criteria for vascular parkinsonism: history of repeated head injury, definite encephalitis, neuroleptic treatment at onset of symptoms, presence of cerebral tumor or communicating hydrocephalus on CT or MRI scan, or other alternative explanation for parkinsonism. (Zijlmans, 2004a; Zijlmans, 2004b)

In everyday clinical practice, difficulties surround the relevance in an individual case of extensive subcortical white matter ischemia demonstrated on MR in determining the cause of the parkinsonian syndrome. If the patient responds well and in a sustained fashion to L-dopa (Zijlmans, 2004), is hyposmic, and has an abnormal bilateral reduction in dopamine transporter uptake on SPECT, then PD is probable. However, even here, the subcortical ischemic burden may contribute to the phenomenology, e.g., presence of severe and disproportionate gait, bulbar and cognitive impairments.

Rare cases of Parkinson's syndrome also have been reported in association with systemic lupus erythematosus causing cerebral vasculitis, which is variably responsive to corticosteroids and immunosuppressive agents, the antiphospholipid syndrome, and moyamoya disease (Chacon, 1999).

INFECTIOUS CAUSES

There is copious literature on viral and bacterial causes of parkinsonism stretching back to the celebrated midbrain tuberculomatous "noisette" that invaded the midbrain (Marinesco, 1893) and led Edouard Brissaud to propose that the substantia nigra might be the principal lesion responsible for parkinsonism. Since then, large numbers of infectious agents have been linked occasionally with an acute transient or reversible parkinsonism (see Table 17.3). When the symptoms of parkinsonism develop

TABLE 17.3
INFECTIOUS CAUSES OF PARKINSONISM

- Japanese B encephalitis (Duvoisin, 1965; Pradhan, 1999)
- HIV encephalopathy (Nath, 1993; Hersh, 2001)
- Encephalitis lethargica (von Economo's disease) (Howard, 1987; Dale, 2004)
- Coxsackie B virus (Poser, 1969)
- Measles/SSPE post-vaccinial (Meyer, 1943; Alves, 1992; Sawaishi, 1999)
- Poliomyelitis (Nielsen, 2002)
- St. Louis encephalitis (Wasay, 2000)
- Western equine encephalitis (Schultz, 1977)
- West Nile virus (Robinson, 2003)
- Epstein-Barr virus (Hsieh, 2002)
- Mycoplasma pneumoniae (Kim, 1995; Smith, 2000; Zambrino, 2000)
- Syphilis (Neill, 1953)
- Borreliosis (Lyme disease) (Cassarino, 2003)
- Opportunistic infections causing basal ganglia abscesses (toxoplasma, cryptococcus, mucormycosis) (Bouffard, 2003)
- Neurocysticercosis (Sa, 2005)
- Tuberculosis (Mital, 1974)
- Malaria (Lipton, 1954)

in the acute or convalescent phase of a febrile illness, an infection is often and reasonably the first etiology to be considered. Blood and cerebrospinal fluid should be acquired for culture and virological study; serum for acute and convalescent titres may be extremely helpful in some situations, e.g., if mycoplasma is suspected and (PCR) can be diagnostic. Nevertheless, it is common for no transmissible agent to be identified, and the scarcity of reports for some common viral or bacterial pathogens render their association with parkinsonism far from convincing, e.g., measles and mumps (Meyer, 1943). The underlying pathological mechanisms linking infection with parkinsonism are also unclear in many instances: They may occur as a direct effect of bacterial or viral infection on dopaminergic function, or as a para-infectious autoimmune process.

Japanese B encephalitis is common in Southeast Asia and affects about 50,000 people a year, and movement disorders are relatively frequent and disabling sequelae. Parkinsonism is usually first noted in the early weeks of the illness as consciousness is regained. Distinctive hypodense abnormalities on T2 weighted MR involving the nigra striatum, pallidum, thalamus, and, sometimes, other brain regions have been described. Prognosis for full recovery must be guarded, and residual disability is relatively common (Duvoisin, 1965; Pradhan, 1999).

Epidemic encephalitis lethargica (von Economo's disease) is believed to be caused by an as yet unidentified transmissible agent. During the 1919–1926 pandemic, millions of people died, and, of the survivors, thousands more developed an acute parkinsonism, often indistinguishable from PD. The long-term survivors with postencephalitic parkinsonism were, half a century later, found to be exquisitely responsive to low doses of L-dopa but developed severe chorea, respiratory dyskinesias, motor fluctuations, and psychotoxicity in the first few weeks of treatment, causing the drug to be discontinued in most cases.

Oculogyric crises are a common accompaniment to postencephalitic parkinsonism, and many patients also have associated neurobehavioral disturbances including obsessive–compulsive behavior. The disorder is nonprogressive until old age when some modest deterioration may occur (Calne, 1988). Although the original survivors of the pandemic have almost all died now, sporadic cases of mesencephalitis indistinguishable clinically and pathologically from von Economo's disease continue to be seen: onset is with drowsiness, delirium, and pyrexia with progression to stupor, sleep inversion, central respiratory disturbances, and coma (Howard, 1987). Persistent local synthesis of immunoglobulin G in the cerebrospinal fluid and HLA histocompatibility antigen risk profiles (Lees, 1982) have been reported. Speculation that influenza was the underlying causative agent continues, but recently a postinfectious immunological disorder akin to Sydenham's chorea has been proposed as an alternative explanation (Dale, 2004). Recently MR lesions restricted to the substantia nigra have been demonstrated in acute transient postencephalitic

parkinsonism with improvement of bradykinesia correlating with disappearance of the MR lesion (Savant, 2003).

Cases of parkinsonism have been reported recently in association with West Nile virus, which usually presents neurologically with a meningo-encephalitis or an acute flaccid paralysis (Robinson, 2003). Mycoplasma pneumoniae is occasionally associated with parkinsonism, which emerges usually as the chest infection is resolving (Kim, 1995; Smith, 2000). A few cases of parkinsonism associated with poliomyelitis have been reported (Nielsen, 2002), and I also have seen several patients with chronic polio who have developed PD in middle age.

Human immunodeficiency virus (HIV) can cause Parkinson's syndrome, either as a result of direct viral damage in HIV encephalopathy (Reyes, 1991) or through an opportunistic infection (e.g., toxoplasma or cryptococcal abscess in the basal ganglia) (Nath, 1993; Mirsattari, 1998). A case of pure parkinsonism as the sole manifestation of HIV in an adult has been reported with clear improvement on anti-retroviral medication, and mild benefit from L-dopa (Hersh, 2001). In a recent series of more than 2000 HIV-positive cases from South America, 28 had movement disorders and 14 of these had parkinsonism. In 12, direct HIV infection involving the nigra was believed to be responsible (Mattos, 2002). Subacute sclerosing panencephalitis (SSPE) rarely causes parkinsonism, presenting classically with behavioral disturbances, periodic myoclonus, and cognitive deficits. In one case, serial MRI revealed migratory basal ganglia lesions, suggesting axonal spread. The patient improved initially with L-dopa (Sawaishi, 1999). Diagnosis of SSPE hinges on cerebrospinal fluid (CSF) measles antibody titres, oligoclonal CSF banding, reverse transcription PCR, and a distinctive EEG appearance (Ball, 2003).

TOXIC CAUSES

Manganese toxicity played an indirect but important role in the introduction of L-dopa therapy into clinical practice. Cotzias, working at the Brookhaven Laboratories, studied manganese turnover in Chilean miners who had inhaled ore dust. Most had developed behavioral disturbances after a year or so of exposure to this, with forgetfulness, anxiety, hallucinations, and compulsive behavior, followed months later by parkinsonism and dystonia (Mena, 1967). Manganese was found to accumulate in melanin granules in the substantia nigra, and as a result Cotzias started to explore ways of augmenting neuromelanin in the nigra, including the use of high-dose neat racemic dopa. Manganese-induced parkinsonism is classically symmetrical in onset with early gait problems, postural tremor, and associated dystonia (Wang, 1989). In addition to miners, it has been reported in factory workers making dry batteries (Emara, 1971) and incriminated as the toxin in the fungicide maneb (Ferraz, 1988). It has also recently been described in Ukrainian and Russian drug addicts using a cocktail including potassium permanganate. The response to L-dopa is variable but in general is less than that seen in PD. High signal intensities are seen in the striatum, substantia nigra, and globus pallidus on T1 weighted MRI, and functional imaging of the striatal dopamine system suggests integrity of the nigrostriatal dopamine bundle (Huang, 1989). Pathological studies have revealed significant globus pallidus and nigra zona reticulata damage, and there is also some evidence that slow progression of the extrapyramidal symptoms may occur even after exposure has ceased (Pal, 1999).

Parkinsonism was reported in 11 out of 51 consecutive patients with severe cirrhosis who were hospitalized to assess their eligibility for hepatic transplantation. Presentation was insidious but rapidly progressive, with maximum disability occurring within a year of onset in most cases with early gait disorder and falls and a symmetrical L-dopa–responsive bradykinetic-rigid syndrome. Associated focal dystonia was common, but there was no flapping tremor or dementia and Kayser-Fleischer rings were absent. Blood and spinal fluid manganese levels were elevated to the same level as those found in occupational manganese exposure, and the occurrence of parkinsonism seemed more related to the degree of liver failure than its underlying cause; it also appeared independently of any hepatic encephalopathic episodes. Striking hyperintensity was found in the pallidum and nigra on T1 weighted MRI, identical to changes reported in chronic manganese poisoning. Liver transplantation was able to reverse the pallidal MR hyperintensities and restore manganese levels to normal (Burkhard, 2003). Patients who die in hepatic coma have a seven-fold increase in pallidal manganese levels, which lends support to the role of elevated brain manganese as the cause of parkinsonism in the chronic hepatocerebral syndrome. Children on long-term parenteral nutrition, particularly in association with cholestasis, also have been reported to develop hypermanganesemia with parkinsonism and MR basal ganglia signal abnormalities (Fell, 1996). Recently, it has been claimed that chronic low-level exposure to manganese from welding rods increases the risk of parkinsonism, but further research is needed before any definitive conclusions can be drawn (Sadek, 2003); there also has been concern over the presence of manganese in high-octane fuels (Kaiser, 2003). The exact mechanisms by which manganese neurotoxicity occurs remain to be determined, but increased oxidative stress in vulnerable brain regions as a consequence of mitochondrial toxicity, and auto-oxidation of dopamine, may be important.

It is now more than 20 years since the reports of 1-methyl-4-phenyl–1,2,3,6 tetrahydropyridine (MPTP) induced irreversible L-dopa–responsive parkinsonism. The seven cases originally described by Tetrud and Langston were clinically indistinguishable from PD except for their acute onset and subsequent lack of disease progression (Ballard, 1985; Tetrud, personal communication). All these cases occurred in drug addicts in California who bought from a kitchen chemist a sloppily prepared supply of the meperidine-related designer narcotic MPPP. It became clear subsequently that MPTP had hit the main distribution line of the northern California drug market and that more than 200 individuals had been exposed. Scrupulous investigation over several years led to the identification of a further 22 cases with very soft extrapyramidal signs (Tetrud, 1989). None of these individuals have presented for subsequent follow-up (Tetrud, personal communication), so the possibility that some may have developed parkinsonism cannot be absolutely excluded. It is interesting to speculate whether the seven index cases received a greater hit of MPTP or whether they were genetically predisposed in some way to the toxin. Three of the patients subsequently underwent fetal mesencephalic implants in Lund, Sweden, but despite marked improvement on F-dopa positron emission tomography (PET) imaging, clinical benefit has in the long term been modest (Snow, 2000). Another patient who is now serving a prison sentence has recently had deep brain subthalamic nucleus stimulation with a good initial response. Four of the patients became psychotic, and most have continued to abuse drugs, raising the possibility that cross-sensitization to addictive drugs may have been a predisposing factor in the high frequency of psychiatric complications. Freezing, unresponsiveness to dopa, and early development of dyskinesias, motor fluctuations, and visual hallucinations were reported in most of the patients. Frontal lobe cognitive deficits have been noted on detailed neuropsychological testing, but dementia has not occurred (Tetrud, personal communication). Three cases have come to autopsy (including two of Langston and Tetrud's original seven and a later isolated case who also had been independently exposed to MPTP after synthesising designer drugs). All three had marked nigral neuronal loss, and findings suggestive of an ongoing active pathological process were noted in two, more than a decade after initial exposure (Langston, 1999). No Lewy bodies or neurofibrillary tangles were identified, and—in contrast to PD—there were no extra-nigral lesions. A case was reported of a 38-year-old woman in whom reversible parkinsonism was caused by inhalation of heroin pyrolysate ("chasing the dragon"); over 2 months the woman recovered fully from severe bradykinesia, rigidity, truncal unsteadiness, limited upgaze, and confusion that were associated with severe tetrahydrobiopterin deficiency in the cerebrospinal fluid (Heales, 2004).

An influential report claiming that the serotoninergic spree drug ecstasy (MDMA; 3,4-methylenedioxymethamphetamine) could cause severe dopamine neurotoxicity in monkeys prompted intense but short-lived concern, in addition to existing worries about chronic depression. This was supported by the common "street" observation that ravers developed transient twitching and tremors (Parrott, 2003) and by one or two isolated reports linking parkinsonism to ecstasy use (Kish 2003; Kuniyoshi, 2003; O'Suilleabhain, 2003). However, fear was allayed when the authors retracted their results, having discovered that all but one of their animals had received erroneously (+) methamphetamine (Mithoefer, 2003). Ironically, shortly before this scare and following a highly publicized

TABLE 17.4

TOXIC CAUSES OF PARKINSONISM

- Manganese (miners, welders, MMT in petrol) (Mena, 1967; Emara, 1971; Sadek, 2003; Olanow, 2004)
- Street drugs of addiction: MPTP, heroin pyrolysate, solvent inhalation (toluene), ecstasy (Ballard, 1985; Heales, 2004; Kuniyoshi, 2003; Uitti, 1994)
- Organophosphates (Muller-Vahl, 1999; Arima, 2003)
- Aliphatic hydrocarbons (n-hexane and halogens) (Pezzoli, 1995; Pezzoli, 2000; Tetrud, 1994)
- Methanol/alcohol (Davis, 1999; Carlen, 1987; LeWitt, 1988; Shandling, 1990; Finkelstein, 2002)
- Glyphosate herbicide (glycine derivate) (Barbosa, 2001)
- Carbon disulphide fumigant (Peters, 1988)
- Mercury poisoning (Eto, 2000)
- Cyanide poisoning (Carella, 1988; Rachinger, 2002)

British television documentary in which a young stuntman with PD was shown to benefit strikingly from self-medication with ecstasy, global media interest had spurred some interest in ecstasy as a treatment for PD.

A number of industrial toxins also have been linked occasionally with parkinsonism, but the causative mechanisms are largely poorly understood (see Table 17.4). Carbon disulphide has been implicated for 150 years as a possible cause of parkinsonism, first in the rubber industry and more recently in silo workers exposed to carbon disulfide fumigant vapors (Peters, 1988). Mercury poisoning is most commonly associated with postural tremor (hatters' shakes) and psychotoxicity, but parkinsonism can also occur. Of the victims of Minamata disease (methyl mercury intoxication), 8% had parkinsonism, as well as ataxia, neuropathies, and hearing and visual disturbances (Eto, 2000). A few cases of cyanide-induced parkinsonism have been reported (Carella, 1988; Rosenow, 1995): For example, a 46-year-old geologist who took 1500 mg of potassium cyanide in a suicide bid became comatose after 15 minutes but was treated promptly with sodium thiosulphate, sodium nitrate, and hyperbaric oxygen. He recovered after 3 days, but over the next 3 weeks he developed parkinsonism with a shuffling gait, marked bradykinesia, hypomimia, and mild tremor and rigidity, which responded modestly to L-dopa. Neuroimaging showed striatal lesions and that PET fluorodopa reduced dopa uptake (Rosenberg, 1989). Although the natural pesticide rotenone leads to nigrostriatal damage in animal models, no clinical cases have been described.

METABOLIC AND ENDOCRINOLOGICAL CAUSES

Carbon monoxide poisoning leads not uncommonly to delayed onset postanoxic parkinsonism, which appears usually within 4 weeks but occasionally with delays as long as 6 months after resolution of the acute encephalopathy (Fig. 17.2) (Ringel, 1972). After its appearance, some progressive deterioration may then occur over the next few weeks. Delirium and amnesia are usual in the acute stages, and urinary incontinence is common. Gait disturbances,

dysarthria, and mutism are the most frequently described accompaniments, but dystonia and tremor also may occur. Neuroimaging reveals confluent symmetrical white matter abnormalities involving the centrum semiovale and the corpus callosum and striking low-intensity lesions in the pallidum and to a lesser degree the thalamus and putamen (Lee, 1994). Dopamine transporter SPECT imaging is usually normal as the nigra is spared and the predominant lesion is in the anterior and superior parts of the globus pallidus interna where hemorrhagic necrosis occurs (Sohn, 2000). As a consequence, most cases are unresponsive to L-dopa, but a therapeutic trial always should be carried out. Despite this, the prognosis for substantial gradual improvement over the ensuing months is reasonably good. A delayed-onset postanoxic parkinsonism also may occur following cardiorespiratory arrest, severe prolonged hypotension, or

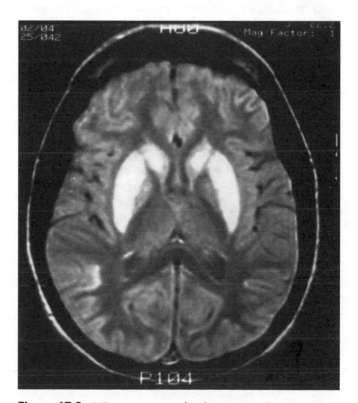

Figure 17.2 MR appearances of carbon monoxide poisoning.

cyanide poisoning (Bhatt, 1993; Rachinger, 2002; Uitti, 1985) with basal ganglia infarction. Despite significant evidence of subcortical damage on imaging, full recovery—especially in children—can occur (Straussberg, 1993).

Uremia, in association with diabetic ketoacidosis, recently has been acknowledged as a not-infrequent cause of acute, potentially reversible parkinsonism, often in association with disturbed consciousness, unsteadiness of gait, slurred speech, and hyperkinetic movement disorders. Altered signal in the basal ganglia is seen on MR, but it remains unclear whether this is a primary metabolic or vascular disturbance (Wang, 2003). A parkinsonian syndrome also has been reported in children undergoing allogenic bone marrow transplantation and under treatment with amphotericin B for pulmonary aspergillosis. All were encephalopathic and also had received cytosine arabinoside, cyclophosphamide, and whole body irradiation (Mott, 1995; Pirker, 1999).

Central pontine myelinolysis results from the rapid correction of hyponatremia or, rarely, from extreme serum hyperosmolality. It usually presents with a tetraparesis and pseudobulbar palsy that, when severe, leads to a locked-in syndrome. Lesions outside the pons occur in 10% of cases, particularly in the basal ganglia, cerebellum, and lateral geniculate body. Parkinsonism may occur and is usually responsive to L-dopa, suggesting the potentially reversible nigrostriatal neuronal demyelination has occurred. Isolated increased signal occurs in the corpus striatum on T2 weighted images.

Myxoedema may be misdiagnosed as early PD, and PD may mask the subsequent development of hypothyroidism. However, there is no proven association between PD and thyroid disease, although both poorly controlled concomitant hyper- or hypothyroidism may lead to marked and abrupt deterioration in motor disability in PD. Hypoparathyroidism has been linked occasionally with parkinsonism. A 35-year-old Indian woman presenting with neuropsychiatric disturbances, increased skin pigmentation, anorexia, weight loss, and severe apathy followed by rapidly worsening bradykinesia, rigidity, and a shuffling gait was confirmed as Addison's disease with plasma cortisols and a synacthen test, and the woman fully recovered after 3 months with corticosteroid supplementation. Following discontinuation for a month of her treatment, all her symptoms returned, but they disappeared again following resumption of cortisol replacement. She has remained asymptomatic for 3 years (Wali, 2003).

PARKINSONIAN SYNDROMES IN WHICH NEUROIMAGING MAY BE HELPFUL

Although some of the other secondary causes of parkinsonism considered in this chapter may have neuroimaging abnormalities (e.g., vascular parkinsonism, Wilson's disease, extrapontine myelinolysis), there are a few rare causes of secondary parkinsonism where neuroimaging may provide a definitive diagnosis. Exclusion of these is often used as an erroneous justification for the systematic MR scanning of all patients presenting with a Parkinson's syndrome. Most of the following conditions will have unusual clinical features or additional physical signs that suggest a diagnosis other than PD and justify neuroimaging.

Hydrocephalus

Communicating hydrocephalus usually presents with rapidly progressive dementia, gait apraxia/ataxia, and urinary incontinence. Furthermore, it may present rarely with an L-dopa responsive parkinsonism, including a pill-rolling tremor (Curran, 1994). There are also a few reports of parkinsonism and a Parinaud's syndrome occurring in association with obstructive hydrocephalus secondary to idiopathic aqueduct stenosis (Zeidler, 1998). If hydrocephalus or evidence of shunt malfunction is found on neuroimaging, then shunt replacement is the treatment of choice; if these are not present, however, then treatment should be initially with L-dopa (Jankovic, 1986). Possible mechanisms of causation include basal ganglia and midbrain compression either by direct pressure or more chronically by impairment of blood flow.

Cerebral Tumors

Cerebral tumors are an uncommon but easily overlooked and potentially curable cause of parkinsonism. Supratentorial tumors, particularly frontoparietal meningiomas, have been described most often, and it may not be until the eventual emergence of other symptoms—such as seizures, cognitive decline, or upper motor neuron signs—that a secondary cause is suspected (Krauss, 1995). Tumors compressing or invading the basal ganglia (Yoshimura, 2002) including astrocytomas (Krauss, 1992) and arteriovenous malformations (Lobo-Antunes, 1974) are also uncommon causes. Secondary hydrocephalus and the delayed effects of craniospinal radiotherapy are other causes linking tumors to parkinsonism.

Head Trauma

Parkinson's syndrome, as a component of posttraumatic encephalopathy in professional boxers and National Hunt steeplechase jockeys is well recognized, and a *striatal variant* of dementia pugilistica is also acknowledged. These patients may closely resemble PD, but speech, gait, and balance problems appear early, the response to dopaminergic drugs is usually poor, and functional imaging (Turjanski, 1997) and MR spectroscopic differences (Davie, 1995) have been described. Most of these cases also have a large cavum septum pellucidum on MRI (Jordan, 2000). However, very few convincing cases of posttraumatic parkinsonism after a single, severe, closed head injury have been described (Bhatt, 2000), although the apallic syndrome with akinetic mutism is well-recognized and a delayed onset Holmes tremor, with demonstrable nigrostriatal damage on dopamine transporter SPECT, is also seen occasionally (Zijlmans, 2002).

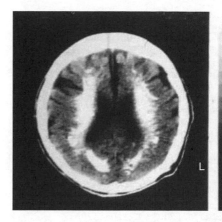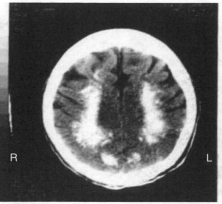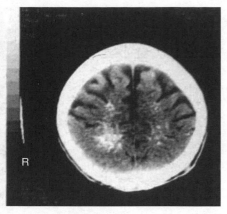

Figure 17.3 CAT scan of familial idiopathic basal ganglia calcification in a 52-year-old patient presenting with parkinsonism.

Chronic extradural and subdural hematomata occasionally present with parkinsonism (Turjanski, 1997) and may be L-dopa responsive. Recently a patient was described who had sustained a life-threatening subdural hematoma and was noted to have a contralateral midbrain peduncular lesion as reported in patients with a Kernohan's notch. Parkinsonism developed, and it was suggested that the supratentorial mass had compressed the upper brain stem thrusting the opposite cerebral peduncle against the rigid edge of the tentorium and producing nigrostriatal damage (Evans, 2004). A 36-year-old man who sustained a severe closed head injury leading to unconsciousness for 24 hours is reported as developing a progressive predominantly right-sided brady-kinetic rigid parkinsonism 6 weeks later, with marked abulia, and had a cerebral infarction due to trauma involving the left caudate and lenticular nucleus. Bilateral, but markedly asymmetrical deficits were found on F-dopa PET, the response to L-dopa was modest and disease progression was very slow (Doder, 1999). Other mechanisms that may be relevant to the development of Parkinson's syndrome after acute head injury include tearing of small brainstem vessels by shearing forces and direct trauma to blood vessels leading to secondary thrombosis.

Hemiparkinsonism/Hemiatrophy

Hemiparkinsonism/hemiatrophy is often associated with dystonia and may occur rarely as a delayed complication of body hemiatrophy or facial hemiatrophy (Parry-Romberg syndrome); contralateral brain atrophy or hypoplasia is apparent on neuroimaging. From the available clinical literature, this disorder seems to be heterogeneous in both its course and response to dopaminergic treatment (Klawans, 1981; Buchman, 1988).

Familial Idiopathic Basal Ganglia Calcification

A small degree of intracerebral calcification is a common incidental finding here: rarely patients may present with parkinsonism where the whole corpus striatum and pallidum appear to be replaced with aggregations of calcium. The dentate also is often calcified and there may be white matter abnormalities. A case of isolated extensive nigral calcification presenting with an akinetic-rigid syndrome also has been described (Fig. 17.3) (Moskowitz, 1971; Kobari, 1997) Some of these cases are familial, and linkage to chromosome 14(IBG1) has been found in some families (Oliveira, 2004). Presentation may be with L-dopa unresponsive parkinsonism, dystonia, dementia, or cerebellar ataxia (Brodaty, 2002). Nasu-Hakola disease is another disorder in which basal ganglia calcification may occur. It is a rare autosomal recessive disorder caused by at least two genes encoding subunits of a cell-membrane–associated receptor complex: TREM 2 and DAP 12. It usually presents in young adults with pain and swelling in the ankles and feet, followed by bone fractures due to polycystic lipomembranous osteodysplasia and is then followed in the fourth decade by a frontal dementia culminating in death in the sixth decade. Although parkinsonism is not a feature of most reports, the basal ganglia radiological abnormalities suggest it may well be a clinical feature in some cases (Klunemann, 2005).

OTHER UNUSUAL CAUSES OF SECONDARY PARKINSONISM

An intention or Holmes' tremor are the commonest movement disorder linked with multiple sclerosis and the distinction between multiple sclerosis and PD exercised the 19th-century neurologists to a degree that seems surprising now. Paroxysmal dyskinesias, palatal tremor, hemiballismus, and dystonia all have been occasionally noted. A number of cases of parkinsonism associated with central nervous system demyelination have been reported, but in some of these a chance association is probable as neither MR anatomical correlation or response of the parkinsonism to corticosteroids can be demonstrated. In only eight reports are central demyelinating lesions seen on neuroimaging linked closely to parkinsonian signs. In these, corticosteroids have, on occasion, been of great benefit,

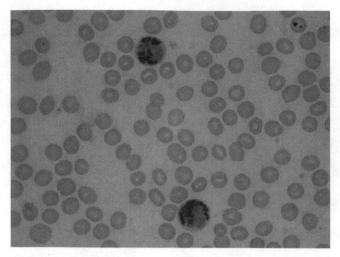

Figure 17.4 Light micrograph of two neutrophils containing numerous giant granules in the cytoplasm markedly stained with peroxidase in peripheral blood smear of a patient with Chédiak-Higashi syndrome. (Photo courtesy of Dr. L. Silveira-Moriyama and Dr T. Gabbi.)

whereas dopaminergic therapy has proved disappointing (Folger et al., 2003). Chediak-Higashi syndrome occasionally presents with parkinsonism and another variety (Silveira-Moriyama, 2004). Neuronal Intranuclear Inclusion body disease should be considered in juvenile cases where a full thickness rectal biopsy may give no diagnosis (O'Sullivan, 2000).

REFERENCES

Alves RS, Barbosa ER, Scaff M. Postvaccinal parkinsonism. *Mov Disord* 1992;7:178–180.

Arima H, Sobue K, So M, et al. Transient and reversible parkinsonism after acute organophosphate poisoning. *J Toxicol Clin Toxicol* 2003;41:67–70.

Armon C, Shin C, Miller P, et al. Reversible parkinsonism and cognitive impairment with chronic valproate use. *Neurology* 1996;47:626–635.

Ball MJ. Unexplained sudden amnesia, postencephalitic Parkinson disease, subacute sclerosing panencephalitis, and Alzheimer disease: does viral synergy produce neurofibrillary tangles? *Arch Neurol* 2003;60:641–642.

Ballard PA, Tetrud JW, Langston JW. Permanent human parkinsonism due to 1-methyl-4-phenyl-1,2,3,6-tetrahydropyridine (MPTP): seven cases. *Neurology* 1985;35:949–956.

Barbosa ER, Lerios de Costa MD, Bacheschi LA, et al. Parkinsonism after glycine-derivate exposure. *Mov Disord* 2001;16:565–568.

Berg D, Siefker C, Becker G. Echogenicity of the substantia nigra in Parkinson's disease and its relation to clinical findings. *J Neurol* 2001;248:684–689.

Bhatt M, Desai J, Mankodi A, et al. Posttraumatic akinetic-rigid syndrome resembling Parkinson's disease: a report on three patients. *Mov Disord* 2000;15:313–317.

Bhatt MH, Obeso JA, Marsden CD. Time course of postanoxic akinetic-rigid and dystonic syndromes. *Neurology* 1993;43:314–317.

Boranic M, Raci F. A Parkinson-like syndrome as side effect of chemotherapy with vincristine and adriamycin in a child with acute leukaemia. *Biomedicine* 1979;31:124–125.

Bouffard JP, Mena H, Ripple M, et al. Mesencephalic cryptococcal abscesses presenting with parkinsonism as an initial manifestation of AIDS. *Mov Disord* 2003;18:1354–1357.

Brodaty H, Mitchell P, Luscombe G, et al. Familial idiopathic basal ganglia calcification (Fahr's disease) without neurological,

cognitive and psychiatric symptoms is not linked to the IBGC1 locus on chromosome 14q. *Hum Genet* 2002;110:8–14.

Buchman AS, Goetz CG, Klawans HL. Hemiparkinsonism with hemiatrophy. *Neurology* 1998;38:527–530.

Burkhard PR, Delavelle J, DuPasquier R, et al. Chronic parkinsonism associated with cirrhosis: a distinct subset of acquired hepatocerebral degeneration. *Arch Neurol* 2003;60:521–528.

Calne DB, Lees AJ. Late progression of post-encephalitic Parkinson's syndrome. *Can J Neurol Sci* 1988;15:135–138.

Carella F, Grassi MP, Savoiardo M, et al. Dystonic-Parkinsonian syndrome after cyanide poisoning: clinical and MRI findings. *J Neurol Neurosurg Psychiatry* 1988;51:1345–1348.

Carlen PL, Wilkinson DA. Reversibility of alcohol-related brain damage: clinical and experimental observations. *Acta Med Scand Suppl* 1987;717:19–26.

Cassarino DS, Quezado MM, Ghatak NR, et al. Lyme-associated parkinsonism: a neuropathologic case study and review of the literature. *Arch Pathol Lab Med* 2003;127:1204–1206.

Chacon J, Garcia-Moreno JM, Valencia J, et al. Parkinson disease of juvenile onset with systemic lupus erythematosus in a presymptomatic stage. *Rev Neurol* 1999;29:725–727.

Chuang C, Constantino A, Balmaceda C, et al. Chemotherapy-induced parkinsonism responsive to levodopa: an underrecognized entity. *Mov Disord* 2003;18:328–331.

Cosentino C, Torres L, Scorticati MC, et al. Movement disorders secondary to adulterated medication. *Neurology* 2000;55:598–599.

Curran T, Lang AE. Parkinsonian syndromes associated with hydrocephalus: case reports, a review of the literature, and pathophysiological hypotheses. *Mov Disord* 1994;9:508–520.

Dale RC, Church AJ, Surtees RA, et al. Encephalitis lethargica syndrome: 20 new cases and evidence of basal ganglia autoimmunity. *Brain* 2004;127(pt 1):21–33.

Dallocchio C, Mazzarello P. A case of Parkinsonism due to lithium intoxication: treatment with Pramipexole. *J Clin Neurosci* 2002;9:310–311.

Davie CA, Pirtosek Z, Barker GJ, et al. Magnetic resonance spectroscopic study of parkinsonism related to boxing. *J Neurol Neurosurg Psychiatry* 1995;58:688–891.

Davis LE, Adair JC. Parkinsonism from methanol poisoning: benefit from treatment with anti-Parkinson drugs. *Mov Disord* 1999;14:520–522.

Deahl M. Betel nut-induced extrapyramidal syndrome: an unusual drug interaction. *Mov Disord* 1989;4:330–332.

Degkwitz R, Frowein R, Kulenkampff C, et al. On the effects of L-dopa in man and their modification by reserpine, chlorpromazine, iproniazid and vitamin B6. *Klin Wochenschr* 1960;38:120–123.

Dick RS, Barold SS. Diltiazem-induced parkinsonism. *Am J Med* 1989;87:95–96.

Doder M, Jahanshahi M, Turjanski N, et al. Parkinson's syndrome after closed head injury: a single case report. *J Neurol Neurosurg Psychiatry* 1999;66:380–385.

Duvoisin RC, Yahr MD. Encephalitis and parkinsonism. *Arch Neurol* 1965;12:227–239.

Easterford K, Clough P, Kellett M, et al. Reversible parkinsonism with normal beta-CIT-SPECT in patients exposed to sodium valproate. *Neurology* 2004;62:1435–1437.

Emara AM, erl-Ghawabi SH, Madkour OI, et al. Chronic manganese poisoning in the dry battery industry. *Br J Ind Med* 1971;28:78–82.

Eto K. Minamata disease. *Neuropathology* 2000;20(suppl):S14–S19.

Evans AH, Gacinovic S, Costa DC, et al. Parkinsonism due to Kernohan notch: clinical, structural, and functional imaging correlates. *Neurology* 2004;62:2333–2334.

Fell JM, Reynolds AP, Meadows N, et al. Manganese toxicity in children receiving long-term parenteral nutrition. *Lancet* 1996;347:1218–1221.

Ferraz HB, Bertolucci PH, Pereira JS, et al. Chronic exposure to the fungicide maneb may produce symptoms and signs of CNS manganese intoxication. *Neurology* 1988;38:550–553.

Finkelstein Y, Vardi J. Progressive parkinsonism in a young experimental physicist following long-term exposure to methanol. *Neurotoxicology* 2002;23:521–525.

FitzGerald PM, Jankovic J. Lower body parkinsonism: evidence for vascular etiology. *Mov Disord* 1989;4:249–260.

Folger S, et al. Parkinsonism as a manifestation of multiple sclerosis. *Mov Disord.* 2003;18(1):108–110.

Garcia-Albea E, Cabrera F, Tejeiro J, et al. Parkinsonism unmasked by verapamil. *Clin Neuropharmacol* 1993;16:263–265.

Gerschlager W, Bencsits G, Pirker W, et al. [123I]beta-CIT SPECT distinguishes vascular parkinsonism from Parkinson's disease. *Mov Disord* 2002;17:518–523.

Gimenez-Roldan S, Mateo D. Cinnarizine-induced parkinsonism: susceptibility related to aging and essential tremor. *Clin Neuropharmacol* 1991;14:156–164.

Gjerris F. Transitory procaine-induced Parkinsonism. *J Neurol Neurosurg Psychiatry* 1971;34:20–22.

Goni M, Jimenez M, Feijoo M. Parkinsonism induced by phenytoin. *Clin Neuropharmacol* 1985;8:383–384.

Gordon M, Gordon AS. Perhexiline maleate as a cause of reversible parkinsonism and peripheral neuropathy. *J Am Geriatr Soc* 1981;29:259–262.

Hardie RJ, Lees AJ. Neuroleptic-induced Parkinson's syndrome: clinical features and results of treatment with levodopa. *J Neurol Neurosurg Psychiatry* 1988;51:850–854.

Hassin-Baer S, Sirota P, Korczyn AD, et al. Clinical characteristics of neuroleptic-induced parkinsonism. *J Neural Transm* 2001;108(11):1299–1308.

Heales S, Crawley F, Rudge P. Reversible parkinsonism following heroin pyrolysate inhalation is associated with tetrahydrobiopterin deficiency. *Mov Disord* 2004;19:1248–1251.

Hersh BP, Rajendran PR, Battinelli D. Parkinsonism as the presenting manifestation of HIV infection: improvement on HAART. *Neurology* 2001;56:278–279.

Holroyd S, Smith D. Disabling parkinsonism due to lithium: a case report. *J Geriatr Psychiatry Neurol* 1995;8:118–119.

Howard RS, Lees AJ. Encephalitis lethargica: a report of four recent cases. *Brain* 1987;110(pt 1):19–33.

Hsieh JC, Lue KH, Lee YL. Parkinson-like syndrome as the major presenting symptom of Epstein-Barr virus encephalitis. *Arch Dis Child* 2002;87:358.

Huang CC, Chu NS, Lu CS, et al. Chronic manganese intoxication. *Arch Neurol* 1989;46:1104–1106.

Jankovic J, Beach J. Long-term effects of tetrabenazine in hyperkinetic movement disorders. *Neurology* 1997;48:358–362.

Jankovic J, Newmark M, Peter P. Parkinsonism and acquired hydrocephalus. *Mov Disord* 1986;1:59–64.

Jordan BD. Chronic traumatic brain injury associated with boxing. *Semin Neurol* 2000;20:179–185.

Kaiser J. Manganese: a high-octane dispute. *Science* 2003;300:926–928.

Katzenschlager R, Zijlmans J, Evans A, et al. Olfactory function distinguishes vascular parkinsonism from Parkinson's disease. *J Neurol Neurosurg Psychiatry* 2004;75:1749–1752.

Kim HC, Han SY, Park SB, et al. Parkinsonism during cyclosporine treatment in renal transplantation. *Nephrol Dial Transplant* 2002;17:319–321.

Kim JS, Choi IS, Lee MC. Reversible parkinsonism and dystonia following probable mycoplasma pneumoniae infection. *Mov Disord* 1995;10:510–512.

Kish SJ. What is the evidence that Ecstasy (MDMA) can cause Parkinson's disease? *Mov Disord* 2003;18:1219–1223.

Klawans HL. Hemiparkinsonism as a late complication of hemiatrophy: a new syndrome. *Neurology* 1981;31:625–628.

Klunemann HH, Ridha BH, Magy L, et al. The genetic causes of basal ganglia calcification, dementia, and bone cysts DAP12 and TREM2. *Neurology* 2005;64:1502–1507.

Kobari M, Nogawa S, Sugimoto Y, et al. Familial idiopathic brain calcification with autosomal dominant inheritance. *Neurology* 1997;48:645–649.

Krauss JK, Nobbe F, Wakhloo AK, et al. Movement disorders in astrocytomas of the basal ganglia and the thalamus. *J Neurol Neurosurg Psychiatry* 1992;55:1162–1167.

Krauss JK, Paduch T, Mundinger F, et al. Parkinsonism and rest tremor secondary to supratentorial tumours sparing the basal ganglia. *Acta Neurochir (Wien)* 1995;133:22–2s9.

Kulkantrakorn K, Selhorst JB, Petruska PJ. Cytosine arabinoside and amphotericin B-induced parkinsonism. *Ann Neurol* 1996;39:413–414.

Kuniyoshi SM, Jankovic J. MDMA and Parkinsonism. *N Engl J Med* 2003;349:96–97.

Langston JW, Forno LS, Tetrud J, et al. Evidence of Active Nerve Cell Degeneration in the Substantia Nigra of Humans Years after 1-Methyl-4-Phenyl-1,2,3,6-Tetrahydropyridine Exposure. *Annals of Neurology* 1999;46:598–605.

Lee MS, Marsden CD. Neurological sequelae following carbon monoxide poisoning clinical course and outcome according to the clinical types and brain computed tomography scan findings. *Mov Disord* 1994;9:550–558.

Lees AJ, Stern GM, Compston DA. Histocompatibility antigens and post-encephalitic Parkinsonism. *J Neurol Neurosurg Psychiatry* 1982;45:1060–1061.

LeWitt PA, Martin SD. Dystonia and hypokinesis with putaminal necrosis after methanol intoxication. *Clin Neuropharmacol* 1988;11:161–167.

Lipton EL. Can malaria cause parkinsonism? Report of a case. *Dis Nerv Syst* 1954;15:184–188.

Lobo-Antunes J, Yahr MD, Hilal SK. Extrapyramidal dysfunction with cerebral arteriovenous malformations. *J Neurol Neurosurg Psychiatry* 1974;37:259–268.

Marinesco B. Sur un cas de tremblement Parkinsonien, hemiplegique symptomatique d'une tumeur du pedoncule cerebral. *Soc de Biol* 1983;27:5.

Marti Masso JF, Carrera N, Urtasun M. Drug-induced parkinsonism: a growing list. *Mov Disord* 1993;8:125.

Marti-Masso JF, Poza JJ. Cinnarizine-induced parkinsonism: ten years later. *Mov Disord* 1998;13:453–456.

Mattos JP, Rosso AL, Correa RB, et al. Movement disorders in 28 HIV-infected patients. *Arq Neuropsiquiatr* 2002;60:525–530.

McKeith I, Fairbarin A, Perry R, et al. Neuroleptic sensitivity in patients with senile dementia of Lewy body type. *BMJ* 1992;305:673–678.

Mena I, Marin O, Fuenzalida S, et al. Chronic manganese poisoning. Clinical picture and manganese turnover. *Neurology* 1967;17:128–136.

Meseguer E, Taboada R, Sanchez V, et al. Life-threatening parkinsonism induced by kava-kava. *Mov Disord* 2002;17:195–196.

Meyer B. Encephalitis after measles with severe parkinsonian rigidity: recovery. *BMJ* 1943;1:508.

Micheli F, Pardal MF, Gatto M, et al. Flunarizine- and cinnarizine-induced extrapyramidal reactions. *Neurology* 1987;37:881–884.

Mintz U, Liberman UA, de Vries A. Parkinsonism syndrome due to cephaloridine. *JAMA* 1971;216:1200.

Mirsattari SM, Power C, Nath A. Parkinsonism with HIV infection. *Mov Disord* 1998;13:684–689.

Mital OP, Sarkari NB, Singh RP. Parkinsonian symptoms in T.B.M. (a case report). *J Assoc Physicians India* 1974;22:629–631.

Mithoefer M, Jerome L, Doblin R.. MDMA ("ecstasy") and neurotoxicity. *Science* 2003;300:1504–1505; author reply, 1504–1505.

Moleman P, Janzen G, von Bargen BA, et al. Relationship between age and incidence of parkinsonism in psychiatric patients treated with haloperidol. *Am J Psychiatry* 1986;143:232–234.

Moskowitz MA, Winickoff RN, Heinz ER. Familial calcification of the basal ganglions: a metabolic and genetic study. *N Engl J Med* 1971;285:72–77.

Mott SH, Packer RJ, Vezina LG, et al. Encephalopathy with parkinsonian features in children following bone marrow transplantations and high-dose amphotericin B. *Ann Neurol* 1995;37:810–814.

Muller-Vahl KR, Kolbe H, Dengler R. Transient severe parkinsonism after acute organophosphate poisoning. *J Neurol Neurosurg Psychiatry* 1999;66:253–254.

Myrianthopoulos NC, Kurland AA, Kurland LT. Hereditary predisposition in drug-induced parkinsonism. *Arch Neurol* 1962;6:5–9.

Nath A, Hobson DE, Russell A. Movement disorders with cerebral toxoplasmosis and AIDS. *Mov Disord* 1993;8:107–112.

Neill KG. An unusual case of syphilitic parkinsonism. *Br Med J* 1953;2:320–322.

Nielsen NM, Rostgaard K, Hjalgrim H, et al. Poliomyelitis and Parkinson disease. *JAMA* 2002;287:1650–1651.

O'Suilleabhain P, Giller C. Rapidly progressive parkinsonism in a self-reported user of ecstasy and other drugs. *Mov Disord* 2003;18:1378–1381.

O'Sullivan JD, Hanagasi HA, Daniel SE, Tidswell P, Davies SW, Lees AJ. Neuronal intranuclear inclusion disease and juvenile parkinsonism. *Mov Disord* 2000;15:990–995.

Olanow CW. Manganese-induced parkinsonism and Parkinson's disease. *Ann N Y Acad Sci* 2004;1012:209–223.

Oliveira JR, Spiteri E, Sobrido MJ, et al. Genetic heterogeneity in familial idiopathic basal ganglia calcification (Fahr disease). *Neurology* 2004;63:2165–2167.

Pal PK, Samii A, Calne DB. Manganese neurotoxicity: a review of clinical features, imaging and pathology. *Neurotoxicology* 1999;20: 227–238.

Parmar RC, Valvi CV, Kamat JR, et al. Chloroquine induced parkinsonism. *J Postgrad Med* 2000;46:29–30.

Parrott AC, Buchanan T, Heffernan TM, et al. Parkinson's disorder, psychomotor problems and dopaminergic neurotoxicity in recreational ecstasy/MDMA users. *Psychopharmacology (Berl)* 2003;167:449–450.

Peralta C, Werner P, Holl B, et al. Parkinsonism following striatal infarcts: incidence in a prospective stroke unit cohort. *J Neural Transm* 2004;111:1473–1483.

Peters HA, Levine RL, Matthews CG, et al. Extrapyramidal and other neurologic manifestations associated with carbon disulfide fumigant exposure. *Arch Neurol* 1988;45:537–540.

Pezzoli G, Antonini A, Barbieri S, et al. n-Hexane-induced parkinsonism: pathogenetic hypotheses. *Mov Disord* 1995;10:279–282.

Pezzoli G, Canesi M, Antonini A, et al. Hydrocarbon exposure and Parkinson's disease. *Neurology* 2000;55:667–673.

Pirker W, Baumgartner C, Brugger S, et al. Severe akinetic syndrome resulting from a bilateral basal ganglia lesion following bone marrow transplantation. *Mov Disord* 1999;14:525–528.

Poser CM, Huntley CJ, Poland JD. Para-encephalitic parkinsonism. Report of an acute case due to coxsackie virus type B 2 and re-examination of the etiologic concepts of postencephalitic parkinsonism. *Acta Neurol Scand* 1969;45:199–215.

Pradhan S, Ogata A, Tashiro K. Parkinsonism due to predominant involvement of substantia nigra in Japanese encephalitis. *Neurology* 1999;53:1781–1786.

Rachinger J, Fellner FA, Stieglbauer K, et al. MR changes after acute cyanide intoxication. *AJNR Am J Neuroradiol* 2002;23: 1398–1401.

Rajput AH, Rozdilsky B, Hornykiewicz, et al. Reversible drug-induced parkinsonism: clinicopathologic study of two cases. *Arch Neurol* 1982;39:644–646.

Reyes MG, Feraldi F, Senseng CS, et al. Nigral degeneration in acquired immune deficiency syndrome (AIDS). *Acta Neuropathol (Berl)* 1991;82:39–44.

Ringel SP, Klawans SP Jr. Carbon monoxide-induced Parkinsonism. *J Neurol Sci* 1972;16:245–251.

Robinson RL, Shahida S, Madan N, et al. Transient parkinsonism in West Nile virus encephalitis. *Am J Med* 2003;115:252–253.

Rosenberg NL, Myers JA, Martin WR. Cyanide-induced parkinsonism: clinical, MRI, and 6-fluorodopa PET studies. *Neurology* 1989;39: 142–144.

Rosenow F, Herholz K, Lanfermann H, et al. Neurological sequelae of cyanide intoxication: the patterns of clinical, magnetic resonance imaging, and positron emission tomography findings. *Ann Neurol* 1995;38:825–828.

Sa DS, Teive HA, Troiano AR, et al. Parkinsonism associated with neurocysticercosis. *Parkinsonism Relat Disord* 2005;11:69–72.

Sadek AH, Rauch R, Schulz PE. Parkinsonism due to manganism in a welder. *Int J Toxicol* 2003;22:393–401.

Savant CS, Singhal BS, Jankovic J, et al. Substantia nigra lesions in viral encephalitis. *Mov Disord* 2003;18:213–216.

Sawaishi Y, Yano T, Watanabe Y, et al. Migratory basal ganglia lesions in subacute sclerosing panencephalitis (SSPE): clinical implications of axonal spread. *J Neurol Sci* 1999;168:137–140.

Schultz DR, Barthal JS, Garrett G. Western equine encephalitis with rapid onset of parkinsonism. *Neurology* 1977;27:1095–1096.

Sempere AP, Duarte J, Cabezas C, et al. Parkinsonism induced by amlodipine. *Mov Disord* 1995;10:115–116.

Shandling M, Carlen PL, Lang AE. Parkinsonism in alcohol withdrawal: a follow-up study. *Mov Disord* 1990;5:36–39.

Silveira-Moriyama L, Moriyama TS, Gabbi TV, Ranvard R, Barbosa ER. Chediak-Higashi syndrome with parkinsonism. *Mov Disord* 2004;19:472–475.

Smith R, Eviatar L. Neurologic manifestations of Mycoplasma pneumoniae infections: diverse spectrum of diseases. A report of six cases and review of the literature. *Clin Pediatr (Phila)* 2000; 39:195–201.

Snow BJ, Vingerhoets FJ, Langston JW, et al. Pattern of dopaminergic loss in the striatum of humans with MPTP induced parkinsonism. *J Neurol Neurosurg Psychiatry* 2000;68:313–316.

Sohn YH, Jeong Y, Kim HS, et al. The brain lesion responsible for parkinsonism after carbon monoxide poisoning. *Arch Neurol* 2000;57:1214–1218.

Stephen PJ, Williamson J. Drug-induced parkinsonism in the elderly. *Lancet* 1984;2:1082–1083.

Straussberg R, Shahar E, Gat R, et al. Delayed parkinsonism associated with hypotension in a child undergoing open-heart surgery. *Dev Med Child Neurol* 1993;35:1011–1014.

Suranyi-Cadotte BE, Nestoros JN, Nair NP, et al. Parkinsonism induced by high doses of diazepam. *Biol Psychiatry* 1985;20: 455–457.

Teive HA, Troiano AR, Germiniani FM, et al. Flunarizine and cinnarizine-induced parkinsonism: a historical and clinical analysis. *Parkinsonism Relat Disord* 2004;10:243–245.

Tetrud JW, Langston JW, Garbe PL, et al. Mild parkinsonism in persons exposed to 1-methyl-4-phenyl-1,2,3,6-tetrahydropyridine (MPTP). *Neurology* 1989;39:1483–1487.

Tetrud JW, Langston JW, Irwin I, et al. Parkinsonism caused by petroleum waste ingestion. *Neurology* 1994;44:1051–1054.

Tolosa E, Coelho M, Gallardo M. DAT imaging in drug-induced and psychogenic parkinsonism. *Mov Disord* 2003;18(suppl 7):S28–S33.

Turjanski N, Lees AJ, Brooks DJ. Dopaminergic function in patients with posttraumatic parkinsonism: an 18F-dopa PET study. *Neurology* 1997a;49:183–189.

Turjanski N, Pentland B, Lees AJ, et al. Parkinsonism associated with acute intracranial hematomas: an [18F]dopa positron-emission tomography study. *Mov Disord* 1997b;12:1035–1038.

Uitti RJ, Rajput AH, Ashenhurst EM, et al. Cyanide-induced parkinsonism: a clinicopathologic report. *Neurology* 1985;35: 921–925.

Uitti RJ, Snow BJ, Shinotoh H, et al. Parkinsonism induced by solvent abuse. *Ann Neurol* 1994;35:616–619.

Villeneuve, A. The rabbit syndrome: a peculiar extrapyramidal reaction. *Can Psychiatr Assoc J* 1972;17(suppl 2):SS69.

Wali GM. Parkinsonism associated with Addison's disease. *Mov Disord* 2003;18:340–342.

Wang HC, Cheng SJ. The syndrome of acute bilateral basal ganglia lesions in diabetic uremic patients. *J Neurol* 2003;250: 948–955.

Wang JD, Huang OC, Hwang YH, et al. Manganese induced parkinsonism: an outbreak due to an unrepaired ventilation control system in a ferromanganese smelter. *Br J Ind Med* 1989;46:856–859.

Wasay M, Diaz-Arrastia R, Suss RA, et al. St Louis encephalitis: a review of 11 cases in a 1995 Dallas, Tex, epidemic. *Arch Neurol* 2000;57:114–118.

Wasserstein PH, Honig LS. Parkinsonism during cyclosporine treatment. *Bone Marrow Transplant* 1996;18:649–650.

Werner EG, Olanow CW. Parkinsonism and amiodarone therapy. *Ann Neurol* 1989;25:630–632.

Yoshimura M, Yamamoto T, Iso-o N, et al. Hemiparkinsonism associated with a mesencephalic tumor. *J Neurol Sci* 2002; 197:89–92.

Zambrino CA, Zorzi G, Lanzi G, et al. Bilateral striatal necrosis associated with Mycoplasma pneumoniae infection in an adolescent: clinical and neuroradiologic follow up. *Mov Disord* 2000;15: 1023–1026.

Zeidler M, Dorman PJ, Ferguson IT, et al. Parkinsonism associated with obstructive hydrocephalus due to idiopathic aqueductal stenosis. *J Neurol Neurosurg Psychiatry* 1998;64:657–659.

Zijlmans J, Booij J, Valk J, et al. Posttraumatic tremor without parkinsonism in a patient with complete contralateral loss of the nigrostriatal pathway. *Mov Disord* 2002;17:1086–1088.

Zijlmans JC, Katzenschlager R, Daniel SE, et al. The L-dopa response in vascular parkinsonism. *J Neurol Neurosurg Psychiatry* 2004a; 75:545–547.

Zijlmans JC, Daniel SE, Hughes AJ, et al. Clinicopathological investigation of vascular parkinsonism, including clinical criteria for diagnosis. *Mov Disord* 2004b;19:630–640.

Huntington's Disease

18

Alexandra Durr

INTRODUCTION

Huntington's disease (HD) is a neurodegenerative disorder transmitted as an autosomal dominant trait. Selective neuronal loss in the striatum leads to chorea and cognitive impairment. It is a progressive disease with onset in midlife, which chronically evolves over many years and for which no curative treatment is available today. The discovery of the underlying gene defect helped to explain some of the clinical variability, especially the variability in age at onset and, to a lesser extent, the disease severity.

For a long time, HD was the prototype of a genetically homogeneous disorder with a single responsible gene, IT15 or HD gene on chromosome 4p, and one single type of mutation, a coding CAG repeat expansion. It is a fact that this mutation is responsible for the vast majority of HD, but today genetic heterogeneity is proven, with the identification of the Junctophilin 3 gene (HDL2) as responsible for a typical HD phenotype in small subgroup of patients. The physiopathology is still not fully understood, but many promising results are expected from the analysis of interacting proteins and animal models. HD was the first adult-onset disease in which predictive testing became possible, which changed medical practice and showed the important role of multistep and multidisciplinary caretaking of at-risk persons.

DIAGNOSIS

Clinical Characteristics

HD can be well recognized on clinical grounds in the presence of (a) behavior, (b) affective and cognitive changes associated with progressive motor dysfunction, and (c) family history consistent with autosomal dominant transmission. The diagnosis is made on clinical examination, and the stereotypical presentation of patients allows a skilled clinician to make the diagnosis on the basis of clinical observation in 90% of the cases (Folstein, 1986).

Early signs of the disease are general restlessness, hygienic neglect, sleep disturbances, behavioral changes, anxiety, and depression. Motor signs follow or are the sign at onset and include involuntary movements that can be suppressed by the patient but not for long. There are typical facial movements and postures with the characteristic raising of the eyebrows and the special facial expression of an astonished look. Examination can show early clumsiness in finger tapping or rapid alternating hand movements. There are uncontrolled finger and truncal movements. The chorea worsens during walking, concentration, and stress, and the clinical examination takes advantage of that by putting the patient in situations in which he or she has to concentrate (i.e., "give the months of the year starting from December backward"). Interestingly, patients often are not aware of their difficulties and do not feel sick or impaired when they are questioned. In general, individuals are more aware of their mood swings than of their movement disorders.

With disease evolution chorea gets worse and impairs gait balance and voluntary movements. Bradykinesia and rigidity are frequent in late stages of the disease or in juvenile cases where chorea can be absent. In an advanced stage, the patient can be positively parkinsonian, often due to antichoreic treatment (Racette, 1998; Reuter, 2000). Dystonic postures of the trunk, neck, and limbs are frequent. Motor speed and gait are affected with increasing risk of falls. Furthermore, the ability to maintain head and trunk posture is lost. In some instances there is clear cerebellar clumsiness and gait. Eye movements are always abnormal (Leigh, 1983). Patients have difficulty initiating saccades, and decreased saccades velocity is evident later on clinical examination. Excessive distractibility does not allow the patient to suppress head movements during examination. These abnormalities are recordable in an early as well as in a presymptomatic stage of the disease (Kirkwood, 2000). The motor score of the Unified Huntington's Disease Rating Scale (UHDRS) includes all motor systems affected and is a useful tool to assess patients and disease progression (Huntington Study Group, 1996; Siesling, 1998).

Hyperreflexia is constant but rarely with extensor plantar reflexes. Dysarthria is common, and speech disturbance is often mixed, sometimes cerebellar. Weight loss is always present, but until now no metabolic cause has been identified in patients with HD that could explain it. Sleep disturbances are frequent, even in an early stage of the disease, with inversion of the day–night rhythm (Hansotia, 1985; Morton, 2005).

Atrophy of the caudate nucleus on cerebral magnetic resonance imaging (MRI) supports the diagnosis, but MRI is used more often to determine whether other conditions are contributing to the neurological dysfunction. Nevertheless, the striatal atrophy may already exist in a preclinical stage (Aylward, 2004). Pathologic studies demonstrate progressive and severe atrophy of the caudate and putamen (Vonsattel, 1985). The proteins with the elongated polyglutamine tracts aggregate and form intraneuronal inclusions. These are found in affected but also nonaffected brain regions. They may precede clinical onset.

In late stages, behavior disturbances are gradually less prominent, motor disability becomes severe, and the patient is dependent, mute, and can be incontinent. The median survival time after onset ranges from 5 years up to more than 25 years.

Psychiatric Features

A wide range of disorders of mental function and behavior occur at any time during the disease (Cummings, 1995). These help to differentiate HD from other choreas that are often without behavioral problems. The most frequent feature is major anxiety and loss of flexibility of the mind (fixed ideas). The anxiety can be disabling and is often associated with depression. In an early phase of the disease, patients show dysphoric, low mood; change in self-esteem with feelings of hopelessness; and loss of interest, energy, and appetite. The premorbid personality becomes less differentiated, and irritability and aggressive and violent behavior result from untreated anxieties. In rare instances and only in young adults, schizophrenic psychosis may occur. In these cases, diagnosis of HD may be delayed because of the absence of chorea due to antipsychotic treatment. The suicidal risk is heightened, ranging

from 9% to 23%, especially when suicidal behavior already exists in the family. The first critical period is immediately before receiving a genetic diagnosis of Huntington's disease, and the second is in a more advanced stage of the disease, when autonomy diminishes (Paulsen, 2005). In general, treatment decisions and care options taken together with a psychiatric team are most helpful for many patients. The psychiatric manifestations respond well to appropriate pharmacological treatment, and patients feel greatly relieved when anxiety is treated early.

Cognitive Deficits

Cognitive changes are always present and can be present early in the disease. They can be the first signs and can precede depression and motor signs (Diamond, 1992; Hahn-Barma, 1998; Paulsen, 2001; Lemiere, 2002; Lemiere, 2004; Ho, 2003; Reading, 2004). One-quarter of mutation carriers without motor impairment show such early cognitive signs as an impaired working memory, slowness of execution, memory dysfunction, and reduced mental flexibility. The losses of mental flexibility and of mental planning and organization of sequential activities interfere greatly with daily life. As for motor disturbances, there is lack of awareness of one's own difficulties (anosognosia). There is no apparent relationship between the onset of cognitive impairment and the CAG repeat expansion (Brandt, 2002). The pattern includes abnormal attention capacities, memory deficit, global inertia defined as subcortical dementia (Mayeux, 1986; Pillon, 1991; Harper, 2002). The neuropsychological profile is that observed in frontal lesions and demonstrates the close relationship between basal ganglia and the prefrontal cortex, individualized as striatofrontal circuits. Lesions of the caudate nucleus disconnect or deactivate the frontal cortex and are responsible for impaired executive functions. Functional MRI studies reveal the early hyperactive frontal cortex (Paulsen, 2004). Early diagnosis can stimulate the patient to undergo cognitive training to avoid intellectual and social isolation.

Juvenile Cases

Juvenile HD (JHD), defined by onset before age 21, accounts for approximately 10% of all HD patients (Harper, 2002; van Dijk, 1986). Transmission of the disease is paternal in 90% of cases, and the number of CAG repeats in the HD gene is larger than 60, usually in the range of 80 to 100 (Duyao, 1993; Telenius, 1993). However, some authors reported maternal transmissions of unusually large expansions (Nance, 1999). The clinical features at onset and during the course of the disease may differ between JHD and adult-onset HD. JHD patients show prominent rigidity, dystonia, seizures, and often minimal chorea (Siesling, 1997; Rasmussen, 2000;

Nance & Myers, 2001). Infant onset can manifest itself as psychomotor regression (Seneca, 2004) and a decline in school performance (Ribai, in press). Epileptic seizures are more common in JHD (Gambardella, 2001). Psychiatric features, depression, or psychosis are also frequent at onset and during the disease (Nance, 2001). Atypical presentation without chorea may cause misdiagnosis or a delayed diagnosis, particularly when the family history is unclear.

OCCURRENCE AND FREQUENCY

HD is rare but exists worldwide, with cases in Europe, North America, South America, and Australia, mostly in Caucasian populations. It has the highest prevalence rates in the region of Lake Maracaibo in Venezuela and the Moray Firth region of Scotland, and it is relatively rare in African blacks and almost absent in Asia (Harper, 2002; Hayden, 1980). Throughout Europe, the prevalence ranges from 5 to 10 per 100,000 (Harper, 2002). Genetic heterogeneity was suspected in a very small proportion of clinical HD cases, 5% to 10%. The HD gene involved in the disease is responsible for more than 90% of HD in Caucasian populations, and another gene (JPH3 or HDL2) is responsible for 40% of clinical HD in South Africa (Table 18.1) In Japan HD is very rare, with 0.11 and 0.45 per 100,000. It is believed that the mutation for HD arose independently in

multiple locations and that its uneven distribution is due to founder effects (Kremer, 1994; Squitieri, 1994; Almqvist, 1995; Watkins, 1995).

CLINICAL GENETICS

Genetic Counseling

The HD gene is the major gene associated with Huntington's disease. A translated trinucleotide CAG repeat expansion is the only mutation observed in the HD gene. There are other more rare genes associated with clinical HD, with a very similar phenotype, especially in the case of HDL2 (Table 18.1).

Prior genetic counseling is needed before DNA analysis confirms the diagnosis. It is important to inform patients and their relatives of the potential implications before blood sampling for DNA testing.

The Huntington's Disease Gene on Chromosome 4P

HD was the first inherited disorder whose defect was mapped to a chromosomal region using linkage studies with DNA markers. The successful positional-cloning strategy finally allowed the identification of the IT15 or HD gene located on chromosome 4p16.3 and its mutation (Huntington's Disease Collaborative Research Group, 1993). The HD gene contains a CAG trinucleotide repeat

TABLE 18.1
GENES AND THEIR MUTATIONS INVOLVED IN HUNTINGTON'S DISEASE

Gene	HD (IT15)	HDL1/PRNP	HDL2	TBP/SCA17
Location	4p16.3	20p12	16q24.3	6q27
OMIM	143100	176640	605268	600075 (TBP) 607136 (SCA17)
Protein	*Huntingtin*	*Prp (Prion protein)*	*JPH3 (Junctophilin3)*	*TBP (Tata-binding protein)*
Mutation	CAG repeat expansion (Normal 9–30 Pathological >36)	192bp insertion	CAG-CTG repeat expansion (Normal 6–35 Pathological 44–59)	CAG repeat (Normal: 27–43 Pathological 44–63)
Frequency among HD phenotype	Europe: frequent >90%	1 family	Europe: none South Africa: >35% North Africa: 3% African Americans: 1%	Several families
Associated clinical features in addition to chorea	Juvenile forms with epileptic features, and pure psychiatric forms	Epileptic seizures, cerebral atrophy on MRI	None	Cerebellar ataxia, cerebellar atrophy on MRI
Selected references	Harper, 2002	Moore, 2001; Xiang, 1998	Holmes, 2001 Margolis, 2004 Stevanin, 2002 Krause, 2002 (abstract)	Stevanin, 2003 Bauer, 2004

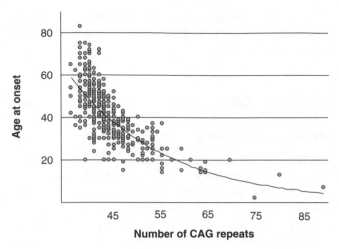

Figure 18.1 Correlation between the size of the CAG repeat expansion in the Huntington's disease gene and the age at onset in 392 patients. r=0.7, which indicates that about 50% of the age at onset is determined by the CAG repeat size. Among the most frequent expansions encountered (41 and 45 CAG repeats), the effect of the CAG repeat explains only 31% of the variance of the age at onset.

in its first exon, which is expanded above the threshold of 36 in a heterozygous state in patients (Fig. 18.1). The mutation is called "unstable" because the expansion may vary in size upon transmission. Although contractions or stable transmission may occur, in most instances the size of the expansion further increases during transmission, resulting in a mean increase of the expansion size in successive generations. There are, however, differences according to the sex of the transmitting parent, paternal transmissions being associated with the greatest instability, and tendency to increase in size.

Repeats not associated with the disease are polymorphic in the normal population and most commonly contain between 15 and 20 CAG repeats. Therefore, normal sizes are 26 or fewer repeats. There are intermediate sizes of repeats ranging from 27 to 35. These alleles are not associated with the disease but are occasionally prone to expansion, even if the risk has been estimated as very rare. Intermediate alleles may show instability during paternal transmissions (Goldberg, 1993; Goldberg, 1995). This means that offsprings of male intermediate allele carriers risk the inheritance of an larger allele associated with an HD phenotype. No expansion of intermediate alleles has been observed through mothers (Chong, 1997). Only 1 case of a 27 CAG repeat that underwent a further expansion during paternal transmission has been reported (Kelly, 1999). Strictly speaking, de novo expansions do not exist since expansions always occur on already intermediate alleles. Factors known to favor the new expansions are paternal transmission and repeats larger than 29 (Goldberg, 1995; Leeflang, 1995).

The pathological repeat size ranges from 36 up to 200 units, but alleles with 40 to 45 repeats account for the majority of patients affected with HD (Snell, 1993; Duyao,

1993; Rubinsztein, 1996; Kremer, 1994). There is an age-dependent reduced penetrance associated with repeat sizes between 36 and 39 repeats (McNeil, 1998). Nevertheless, 39 repeats have been associated with the disease in nearly all cases, and cases with 36, 37, and 38 repeats are rare.

The diagnosis of sporadic HD is a difficult counseling issue because the sudden discovery of a dominant disease frightens. However, the absence of a positive family history with no known cases in the elder generations is due more often to censured family histories, such as early death, adoption, or false paternity (Durr, 1995). The discovery of the mutation in apparently isolated cases has important consequences for all family members since they were not aware of an inherited disorder until the genetic testing. This has to be taken into account and explained to the sporadic HD patient and to relatives before blood sampling and testing.

Presymptomatic and Prenatal Predictive Testing

Genetic testing can be performed in three distinct situations: (a) molecular confirmation of the disease in an affected person, allowing establishment of an already clear clinical diagnosis; (b) revelation of the presence or the absence of the mutation in an asymptomatic at-risk person; and (c) prenatal and preimplantation diagnosis for couples when either partner is a carrier or is at risk for HD.

Predictive testing for an at-risk person allows an unaffected individual to know if he or she is a carrier or not. If preventive and curative treatment would be available, testing could be the ideal situation. Unfortunately, the possibilities of prevention and treatment to date are not good enough to counsel in favor of genetic testing. This means that the discussions and decision making in favor of or against testing will be organized according to individual needs. The predictive value of the genetic test is not strong, since there is no possibility to determine the exact individual age at onset or the severity of the disease progression. The test makes it possible to determine a genotype but not the details of the associated phenotype.

International guidelines have been provided to give a structured predictive testing procedure. This includes pretest counseling and interviews, as well as posttest follow-ups. After 15 years of predictive testing for HD, today most of the difficulties encountered relate to the counseling and to the human aspects of the test. Testing must be a process, which takes place over time (Fig. 18.2). The informed choice should include counseling with caretakers, including geneticist, neurologist, psychologist, and social worker. The teams should be able to deal with untreatable disorders, with uncertain outcome, and with offering support during several years.

Predictive testing requires informed consent. Autonomous decision making is important to avoid regret

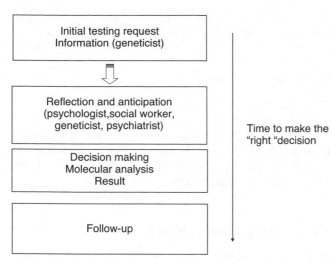

Figure 18.2 Multistep and multidisciplinary testing procedure for presymptomatic testing in individuals at risk for Huntington's disease.

after testing. Reasons for testing includes desire to end uncertainty about the genetic status, to obtain control over the future, to inform already existing children, to conduct prenatal testing, and to be included in future research protocols. However, the fear of not being able to cope with an unfavorable result and the absence of available treatment and prevention explain why only about 20% of at risk persons wish to be tested (Craufurd, 1989; Goizet, 2002). Not all those who start the testing procedure wish to be sampled. In fact, a large proportion of candidates choose not to continue with the test (van der Steenstraten, 1994; Decruyenaere, 1995; Goizet, 2002). However, suicidal reactions after the test have been reported only occasionally (Almqvist, 1999).

Prenatal diagnosis means genetic testing of the fetus with earliest sampling between 12 and 14 weeks of amenorrhea. In Europe, a minority of those at risk for HD have chosen to prevent transmission of the disease by the use of such diagnosis (Simpson, 2002; Lesca, 2002). This is partly explained by the late onset of the disease but also by the 50% risk to undergo pregnancy termination. The fear of exposing the future child to an affected parent is a further concern. Prenatal testing is not a direct consequence of presymptomatic testing, and even ongoing pregnancies do not always precipitate presymptomatic testing. (Simpson, 2002; Harper, 2002; Lesca, 2002; for review see Evers-Kiebooms, 2002b).

Preimplantation diagnosis means genetic testing of embryo prior to transfer. This implies ovarian hyperstimulation, in vitro fertilization, and single-cell DNA analysis. Problems are the low success rate of in vitro fertilization, usually with less than a 30% baby take-home rate, and the fact that single-cell DNA analysis can lead to misdiagnosis. Until today the major indications are nonacceptance of pregnancy termination and decreased fertility (Geraedts, 2002). Another reason for choosing preimplantation diagnosis is the difficulty of not wanting to transmit the disease

but at the same time refusing knowledge of one's own genetic status (Moutou, 2004).

GENOTYPE–PHENOTYPE CORRELATIONS

Age at Onset Variability

Age at onset in HD is determined for about 50% by the CAG repeat expansion in the HD gene (Fig. 18.2). A significant correlation between the number of CAG repeats and the age at onset has been demonstrated (Andrew, 1993; Norremolle, 1995; Snell, 1993; Duyao, 1993) (Fig. 18.2). The relationship between the CAG repeat size and the disease progression is less clear (Kieburtz, 1994; Illarioshkin, 1994). Age at onset is difficult to assess in chronically progressive disorders. This is especially true for HD since the patient is barely aware of his or her own changes and does not complain of motor disturbances, even when they are obvious to the family. Age at onset relies on retrospective event assessment by the spouse or another family member. In most studies, age at onset is defined as the onset of motor signs (chorea), but in the vast majority of these patients, mood and behavior abnormalities precede motor signs. Expansion sizes between 41 and 45 CAG repeats are most frequently encountered, and they explain only 30% of the age at-onset-variance. Family members and individuals with the same length of CAG repeats may have markedly different ages at onset (Fig. 18.2). The overall distribution of age at onset is shaped as a normal distribution with a large majority of patients starting their disease between 30 and 50 years of age, the early-onset cases, as well as the late-onset cases, being rarer. Interestingly, the mean ages at onset vary according to the population's origin: Venezuela: 34 ± 10 years (Wexler, 2004); Canada: 40 ± 13 years (Rosenblatt, 2001); Americans: 37 ± 13 yrs (Rosenblatt, 2001); France: 40 ± 13 yrs . It is, therefore, difficult to predict age at onset in gene carriers, and such information should be handled with care.

Anticipation of age at onset, a well-known phenomenon in HD families, means that age at onset tends to be earlier from one generation to another. This is due partly to an observation bias since there is a tendency to make the diagnosis earlier in the following generations. However, part of the anticipation is due to the instability of the CAG repeat during transmission, more pronounced through fathers than mothers. However, only one-third of fathers transmit a CAG repeat expansion with marked increase in size. Paternal instability is accounted for by the existence of mosaicism of the expansion in the sperm (Duyao, 1993; Telenius, 1993).

Not all the variability of age at onset is explained by the length of the expansion. HD expression may be modulated by other genes (Farrer, 1993; Li, 2003). Several modifiers have been identified, but they each account only for a small additional variance of the age at onset. The polymorphic normal allele was shown to have a moderate effect but only for large expansions ranging from 47 to 83 repeats (Djoussé, 2003). There are (a) a noncoding TAA repeat polymorphism in the GluR6 subunit gene of the kainate receptor, with increasing size associated with younger age at onset (MacDonald, 1999; Rubinsztein, 1997; Chattopadhyay, 2003); (b) a transcription factor, CA150, a human homologue of a *C. elegans* protein interacting with the *huntingtin* protein (Holbert, 2001); (c) 2 polymorphisms in a N-methyl-D-aspartate receptor subset of glutamate receptors NR2B *(GRIN2B)* (Arning, 2005); (d) the UCHL1 (ubiquitin carboxyl-terminal hydrolase L1) S18Y polymorphism (Naze, 2002). In addition, several loci containing potential modifying genes have been found in a large multicenter study (HD maps), but these genes are not yet identified (Li, 2003). Not only hae genetic modifiers been shown to have an effect on age at onset but also environmental factors. Additive genetic factors account for 38%, but environmental factors (familial or general) account for 62% of the age-at-onset variance (Wexler, 2004; van Dellen, 2004). This goes along with the observation that environmental enrichment ameliorates motor symptoms and prevents loss of body weight in transgenic mice (R6/1model) (Spires, 2004). It is also interesting that age at onset can be discordant in monozygotic twins, further supporting the role of environmental factors (Friedman, 2005).

DIFFERENTIAL DIAGNOSIS

Differential diagnosis has to be considered either in isolated cases of HD-like phenotypes or in familial ones. The most common cause of isolated chorea is tardive dyskinesias due to the use of neuroleptics but also due to L-dopa–induced dyskinesias in patients with Parkinson's disease, noradrenergic drugs such as cocaine, or oral contraceptives. Other causes includes thyreotoxicosis, cerebrovascular disease, lupus erythematosus, and polycythemia rubra vera. HIV infection is also a cause of chorea, and AIDS-related disease should be considered in young patients presenting without a family history of movement disorders (Piccolo, 2003). None of those resemble HD closely enough because of the absence of behavior and cognitive changes. The only exception is Sydenham's chorea, which is associated with prominent psychiatric changes, occurs in children, and is known as an autoimmune disorder associated with streptococcal infections. Several autosomal recessive diseases, such as cerebellar ataxia with ocular apraxia type 1, also can exhibit chorea as an associated feature (Le Ber, 2004), Wilson disease, or choreoacanthocytosis. The latter is characterized by chorea, parkinsonism, dystonia, distal myopathy, and acanthocytes of red blood cells. ChAc is the associated responsible gene (Rubio, 1997; Rampoldi, 2001).

The following diseases can be considered as a differential diagnosis in familial HD-like phenotypes.

HDL1 with Epilepsy

The HDL1 locus was identified using linkage analysis in a single family with an HD-like phenotype, including 4 out of 6 patients with chorea and 3 with epileptic features (Xiang, 1998). Consecutively, a 192bp insertion in the octapeptide-coding region in the PRPN gene encoding the *Prion* protein was found (Moore, 2001).

HDL2 Gene, Junctophilin 3

HD was thought to be monogenetic par excellence with one responsible gene and one single mutation in the HD gene. Nevertheless, the involvement of HDL2 or Junctophilin 3 located on chromosome 16q proved genetic heterogeneity (Table 18.1). The responsible mutation is an expanded CTG/CAG repeat. The pathological repeat ranges from 44 to 57 CTG/CAG repeats. Several studies have showed that the HDL2 gene is rarely involved (Margolis, 2001; Margolis, 2004; Stevanin, 2002). The frequencies reported are 1% (6/538) in North America (Margolis, 2004), and 0% (0/44) in Japan (Margolis, 2004), 3% (2/60) in France (Stevanin, 2002), but 35% (7/20) in South Africa (Krause, 2002). Interestingly, this indicates that HDL2 might be frequent in populations from black African ancestry.

Dentatorubro-Pallidoluysian Atrophy

Chorea is part of the clinical spectrum of dentatorubro-pallidoluysian atrophy (DRPLA) (Ikeuchi, 1995). DRPLA is included in the classification of autosomal dominant cerebellar ataxias (SCA) because cerebellar ataxia is often the prominent sign. It is more frequent among Japanese patients (Le Ber, 2003; Ikeuchi, 1995). As in HD and other SCA subtypes (SCA1, 2, 3, 6, 7, 17), the causal mutation is an expanded CAG repeat in the coding region. The phenotype is an association of cerebellar signs, movement disorders, and cognitive impairments. In cases with predominant dystonic and choreic features, the phenotype may be similar to HD.

SCA 17 Spinocerebellar Ataxia 17

Dementia and movement disorders, including chorea, are observed in patients with spinocerebellar ataxia 17 (SCA17), due to a CAG repeat expansions in the Tata-binding protein gene (Fujigasaki, 2001). The occurrence of HD phenotypes due to TBP/SCA17 expansions highlights the clinical overlap between HD and some forms of spinocerebellar ataxias (Stevanin, 2003).

MANAGEMENT

Coordinated interaction between neurologists, geneticists, and psychiatrists/psychologists, social workers, physical therapists, and speech therapists is essential. A management proposal according to early and later stages of the disease is shown in Table 18.2. The Total Functional Capacity (TFC) scale (Shoulson, 1979; Shoulson, 1981), with a maximal score (best) of 13, is useful for assessing the abilities of individuals to work, manage money, perform activities of daily living and household chores, and live at home or in supervised care. Patients lose approximately 0.6 to 0.7 points every year (Feigin, 1995; Marder, 2000).

Treatment

Even if there are no effective therapies to slow the progression or delay the onset of HD, symptoms such as chorea, depression, and anxiety can and must be treated. Difficulties lie not in the choice of medications but in the acceptance and compliance of patients for medications. Atypical antipsychotics—such as clozapine, quetiapine, and olanzapine without sedation—and neuroleptics are the best accepted. They should be introduced at the beginning of the disease to allow better compliance since anxiety will be reduced effectively without sedation. The control of chorea is possible with neuroleptics, but since patients often are not aware of chorea, treatment will be necessary only if gait is impaired. In addition, antichoreic therapy has adverse effects. Dopaminergic blocks with haloperidol are not well tolerated since they produce such side effects as slowing down and speech difficulties and may result in increased clumsiness. The presynaptic monoamine-depleting agent tetrabenazine improves chorea; however, depression is a problematic side effect (Marshall, 2004). There is some evidence that L-dopa improves akinesia and rigidity and helps improve patients' ability for voluntary movements (Racette, 1998; Reuter, 2000). Physical therapy with balance exercises also is helpful. Speech therapy combined with intellectual stimulation and exercise can enhance fluency, strategies for attention deficits, and impaired planification.

Even in the absence of double-blind studies, it is known that selective serotonin reuptake inhibitors are well tolerated

TABLE 18.2
CARE PROPOSAL IN HUNTINGTON'S DISEASE ACCORDING TO DISEASE STAGE

Stage of the Disease	Symptoms	Pharmacological Treatment Proposal	Care
Earlier stage	Chorea: slight and no functional significance	None	Proposal of gymnastics, physical therapy, motivation for doing physical activities Taking care of family members (genetic counseling and psychological care)
	Anxiety and difficulties in concentration and planning strategies	Atypical neuroleptics, SSRI in low doses, anxiolytics Atypical neuroleptics	Psychological support+++ Genetic counseling and information for the family+++ Social support Day-to-day strategies (notebooks, planning charts)
	Sleep disorder Depression	SSRI of other antidepressive agents+++	Psychiatric care+++
	Weight loss Social isolation		Dietary follow-up Social support
Advanced stage	Chorea Hypokinesia, rigidity Anxiety Obsessive behavior Depression Dysphagia, dysarthria Gait difficulties and falls	Neuroleptics Sometimes L-dopa Benzodiazepines Neuroleptics Antidepressant (SSRI+++)	Physical therapy+++ Physical therapy+++ Psychiatric care Support of family and spouse Speech therapy+++ Physical therapy+++ NMDA receptor antagonist
	Weight loss	Protein-complementary diet	Dietary advice Dietary supplementation+++

SSRI: Selective serotonin reuptake inhibitor.

and effective on both depression and anxiety in HD patients. Also, obsessive–compulsive symptoms may respond to treatment with the latter but will respond better to atypical neuroleptics.

Apathy is a common manifestation of HD, but its treatment has not been systematically evaluated. The removal of medications, such as typical antipsychotics (haloperidol and tiapridal) that may contribute to apathy should be considered.

Experimental Therapies

Several double-blinded and placebo-controlled pharmacological trials were carried out between 1999 and 2006. Small effects on chorea scores and motor scores of the UHDRS scale were obtained with riluzole (Huntington Study Group, 1996), amantadine (Verhagen, 2002), tetrabenazine (Marshall, 2004), and unsaturated fatty acids (Vaddadi, 2002). No effects were demonstrated using lamotrigine (Kremer, 1999), creatine (Verbessem, 2003; Tabrizi, 2003), ethyl EPA (Puri, 2005), and coenzyme Q10 (Huntington Study Group, 2005). Until now, none of the pharmacological trials has provided a definite answer for the usefulness of the employed drugs.

The evaluation of neuronal grafting of embryonic neurons is underway in a large series (for review, see Peschanski, 2004). Other strategies for therapeutic approaches are imagined today: (a) directly blocking the mutated gene, as with the use of RNA interference (Xia, 2002); (b) interfering with the apoptotic pathway by inhibiting downstream toxic products of the cascade (Friedlander, 2003); (c) protecting the cells form oxidative stress; and (d) directly replacing the neurons in the striatum by grafting embryonic neurons or stem cells. Several other avenues have to be explored, such as the targeting of energy metabolism (Walker, 2004).

CONCLUSION

HD is a devastating neurodegenerative disorder. Particular care should be given to appropriate genetic counseling of patients and their relatives, especially when there is an apparently sporadic case or when there is a request for predictive testing. Pluridisciplinary care and patient follow-up are important in these situations. The current absence of efficient neuroprotective drugs should lead practitioners to take advantage of all possibilities for symptomatic treatments and for physiotherapy for severe disorders that evolve over decades.

REFERENCES

Almqvist E, Spence N, Nichol K, et al. Ancestral differences in the distribution of the delta 2642 glutamic acid polymorphism is associated with varying CAG repeat lengths on normal chromosomes: insights into the genetic evolution of Huntington disease. *Hum Mol Genet* 1995;4:207–214.

Almqvist EW, Bloch M, Brinkman R, Craufurd D, Hayden MR. A worldwide assessment of the frequency of suicide, suicide attempts, or psychiatric hospitalization after predictive testing for Huntington disease. *Am J Hum Genet* 1999;64: 1293–1304.

Ambrose CM, Duyao MP, Barnes G, Bates GP, Lin CS, Srinidhi J, Baxendale S, Hummerich H, Lehrach H, Altherr M, et al. Structure and expression of the Huntington's disease gene: evidence against simple inactivation due to an expanded CAG repeat. *Somat Cell Mol Genet* 1994;20:27–38.

Andrew SE, Goldberg YP, Kremer B, et al. The relationship between trinucleotide (CAG) repeat length and clinical features of Huntington's disease *Nat Genet* 1993;4:398–340.

Arning L, Kraus PH, Valentin S, et al. NR2A and NR2B receptor gene variations modify age at onset in Huntington disease. *Neurogenetics* 2005;6:25–28.

Aylward EH, Sparks BF, Field KM, et al. Onset and rate of striatal atrophy in preclinical Huntington disease. *Neurology* 2004;63: 66–72.

Bates G, Harper PS. *Huntington's Disease.* London: W.B. Saunders, 2002.

Bauer P, Laccone F, Rolfs A, et al. Trinucleotide repeat expansion in SCA17/TBP in white patients with Huntington's disease-like phenotype. *J Med Genet* 2004;41:230–232.

Brandt J, Shpritz B, Codori AM, Margolis R, Rosenblatt A. Neuropsychological manifestations of the genetic mutation for Huntington's disease in presymptomatic individuals. *J Int Neuropsychol Soc* 2002;8:918–924.

Chattopadhyay B, Ghosh S, Gangopadhyay PK, et al. Modulation of age at onset in Huntington's disease and spinocerebellar ataxia type 2 patients originated from eastern India. *Neurosci Lett* 2003;345:93–96.

Chong SS, Almqvist E, Telenius H, et al. Contribution of DNA sequence and CAG size to mutation frequencies of intermediate alleles for Huntington disease: evidence from single sperm analyses. *Hum Mol Genet* 1997;6:301–309.

Craufurd D, Dodge A, Kerzin-Storrar L, Harris R. Uptake of presymptomatic predictive testing for Huntington's disease. *Lancet* 1989;2:603–605.

Cummings JL. Behavioral and psychiatric symptoms associated with Huntington's disease. *Adv Neurol* 1995;65:179–186.

de Boo GM, Tibben A, Lanser JB, Jennekens-Schinkel A, Hermans J, Maat-Kievit A, Roos RA. Early cognitive and motor symptoms in identified carriers of the gene for Huntington disease. *Arch Neurol* 1997;54:1353–1357.

Decruyenaere M, Evers-Kiebooms G, Boogaerts A, et al. Predictive testing for Huntington's disease: risk perception, reasons for testing and psychological profile of test applicants. *Genet Couns* 1995;6:1–13.

Diamond R, White RF, Myers RH, et al. Evidence of presymptomatic cognitive decline in Huntington's disease. *J Clin Exp Neuropsychol* 1992;14:961–975.

DiFiglia M, Sapp E, Chase KO, Davies SW, Bates GP, Vonsattel JP, Aronin N. Aggregation of huntingtin in neuronal intranuclear inclusions and dystrophic neurites in brain. *Science* 1997;277: 1990–1993.

Di Maio L, Squitieri F, Napolitano G, Campanella G, Trofatter JA, Conneally PM. Suicide risk in Huntington's disease. *J Med Genet* 1993;30:293–295.

Djoussé L, Knowlton B, Hayden M, et al. Interaction of normal and expanded CAG repeat sizes influences age at onset of Huntington disease. *Am J Med Genet A* 2003;119:279–282.

Djousse L, Knowlton B, Hayden MR, et al. Evidence for a modifier of onset age in Huntington disease linked to the HD gene in 4p16. *Neurogenetics* 2004;5:109.

Durr A, Dode C, Hahn V, et al. Diagnosis of "sporadic" Huntington's disease. *J Neurol Sci* 1995;129:51–55.

Duyao M, Ambrose C, Myers R, et al. Trinucleotide repeat length instability and age of onset in Huntington's disease. *Nat Genet* 1993;4:387–392.

Evers-Kiebooms G, Nys K, Harper P, Zoeteweij M, Durr A, Jacopini G, Yapijakis C, Simpson S. Predictive DNA-testing for Huntington's disease and reproductive decision making: a European collaborative study. *Eur J Hum Genet* 2002a;10: 167–176.

Evers-Kiebooms G, Zoeteweiij M, Harper P (eds). Prenatal testing for late onset neurogenetic disorders. BIOS Scientific Publishers Ltd, Oxford, UK, 2002b.

Farrer LA, Cupples LA, Wiater P, Conneally PM, Gusella JF, Myers RH. The normal Huntington disease (HD) allele, or a closely linked gene, influences age at onset of HD. *Am J Hum Genet* 1993;53:125–130.

Feigin A, Kieburtz K, Bordwell K, et al. Functional decline in Huntington's disease. *Mov Disord* 1995;10:211–214.

Folstein SE, Leigh RJ, Parhad IM, Folstein MF. The diagnosis of Huntington's disease. *Neurology* 1986;36:1279–1283.

Friedlander RM. Apoptosis and caspases in neurodegenerative diseases. *N Engl J Med* 2003;348:1365–1375.

Friedman JH, Trieschmann ME, Myers RH, Fernandez HH. Monozygotic twins discordant for Huntington disease after 7 years. *Arch Neurol* 2005;62:995–997.

Fujigasaki H, Martin JJ, De Deyn PP, et al. CAG repeat expansion in the TATA box-binding protein gene causes autosomal dominant cerebellar ataxia. *Brain* 2001;124(pt 10):1939–1947.

Gambardella A, Muglia M, Labate A, et al. Juvenile Huntington's disease presenting as progressive myoclonic epilepsy. *Neurology* 2001;57:708–711.

Geraedts J, Liebaers I. Preimplantation genetic diagnosis for Huntington disease. In: Evers-Kiebooms G, Zoeteweiij M, Harper P, eds. *Prenatal Testing for Late Onset Neurogenetic Disorders.* Oxford, England: BIOS Scientific Publishers Ltd; 2002.

Goizet C, Lesca G, Durr A, and the French Group for Presymptomatic Testing in Neurogenetic Disorders. Presymptomatic testing in Huntington's disease and autosomal dominant cerebellar ataxias. *Neurology* 2002;59:1330–1336.

Goldberg YP, Kremer B, Andrew SE, et al. Molecular analysis of new mutations for Huntington's disease: intermediate alleles and sex of origin effects. *Nat Genet* 1993;5:174–179.

Goldberg YP, McMurray CT, Zeisler J, et al. Increased instability of intermediate alleles in families with sporadic Huntington disease compared to similar sized intermediate alleles in the general population. *Hum Mol Genet* 1993;4:1911–1918.

Hahn-Barma V, Deweer B, Durr A, et al. Are cognitive changes the first symptoms of Huntington's disease? A study of gene carriers. *J Neurol Neurosurg Psychiatry* 1998;64:172–177.

Hansotia P, Wall R, Berendes J. Sleep disturbances and severity of Huntington's disease. *Neurology* 1985;35:1672–1674.

Harper PS, Bates G, Jones L. Oxford Monographs on Medical Genetics Huntington's Disease.

Harper PS. The epidemiology of Huntington's disease. *Human Genetics* 1992;89:365–376.

Harper SQ, Staber PD, He X, et al. RNA interference improves motor and neuropathological abnormalities in a Huntington's disease mouse model. *Proc Natl Acad Sci USA* 2005;102: 5820–5825.

Hayden MR, MacGregor JM, Beighton PH. The prevalence of Huntington's chorea in South Africa. *S Afr Med J* 1980;58: 193–196.

Hayden MR, Martin WR, Stoessl AJ, et al. Positron emission tomography in the early diagnosis of Huntington's disease. *Neurology* 1986;36:888–894.

Ho AK, Sahakian BJ, Brown RG, et al. for the NEST-HD Consortium. Profile of cognitive progression in early Huntington's disease. *Neurology* 2003;61:1702–1706.

Holbert S, Denghien I, Kiechle T, et al. The Gln-Ala repeat transcriptional activator CA150 interacts with huntingtin: neuropathologic and genetic evidence for a role in Huntington's disease pathogenesis. *Proc Natl Acad Sci USA* 2001;98:1811–1816.

Holmes SE, O'Hearn E, Rosenblatt A, Callahan C, et al. A repeat expansion in the gene encoding junctophilin-3 is associated with Huntington disease-like 2. *Nat Genet* 2001;29:377–378. Erratum in: *Nat Genet* 2002;30:123.

Huntington Study Group. Unified Huntington's Disease Rating Scale: reliability and consistency. *Mov Disord* 1996;11:136–142.

Huntington Study Group (2005).

Huntington's Disease Collaborative Research Group. A novel gene containing a trinucleotide repeat that is expanded and unstable on Huntington's disease chromosomes. *Cell* 1993;72: 971–983.

Ikeuchi T, Koide R, Onodera O, et al. Dentatorubral-pallidoluysian atrophy (DRPLA): Molecular basis for wide clinical features of DRPLA. *Clin Neurosci* 1995;3:23–27.

Illarioshkin SN, Igarashi S, Onodera O, et al. Trinucleotide repeat length and rate of progression of Huntington's disease. *Ann Neurol* 1994;36:630–635.

Kelly TE, Allinson P, McGlennen RC, Baker J, Bao Y. Expansion of a 27 CAG repeat allele into a symptomatic Huntington disease-producing allele. *Am J Med Genet* 1999;87:91–92.

Kieburtz K, MacDonald M, Shih C, et al. Trinucleotide repeat length and progression of illness in Huntington's disease. *J Med Genet* 1994;31:872–874.

Kirkwood SC, Siemers E, Hodes ME, Conneally PM, Christian JC, Foroud T. Subtle changes among presymptomatic carriers of the Huntington's disease gene. *J Neurol Neurosurg Psychiatry* 2000;69:773–779.

Kremer B, Clark CM, Almqvist EW, et al. Influence of lamotrigine on progression of early Huntington disease. *Neurology* 1999;53: 1000–1011.

Kremer B, Goldberg P, Andrew SE, et al. A worldwide study of the Huntington's disease mutation: the sensitivity and specificity of measuring CAG repeats. *N Engl J Med* 1994;330: 1401–1406.

Kremer 1999.

Kremer HP. Imaging Huntington's disease (HD) brains—imagine HD trials! *J Neurol Neurosurg Psychiatry* 2005;76:620.

Langbehn DR, Brinkman RR, Falush D, Paulsen JS, Hayden MR. A new model for prediction of the age of onset and penetrance for Huntington's disease based on CAG length. *Clin Genet* 2004;65: 267–77.

Le Ber I, Camuzat A, Castelnovo G, et al. Prevalence of dentatorubral-pallidoluysian atrophy in a large series of white patients with cerebellar ataxia. *Arch Neurol* 2003;60:1097–1099.

Leeflang EP, Zhang L, Tavare S, et al. Single sperm analysis of the trinucleotide repeats in the Huntington's disease gene: quantification of the mutation frequency spectrum. *Hum Mol Genet* 1995;4:1519–1526.

Leigh RJ, Newman SA, Folstein SE, Lasker AG, Jensen BA. Abnormal ocular motor control in Huntington's disease. *Neurology* 1983;33:1268–1275.

Lemiere J, Decruyenaere M, Evers-Kiebooms G, Vandenbussche E, Dom R. Cognitive changes in patients with Huntington's disease (HD) and asymptomatic carriers of the HD mutation—a longitudinal follow-up study. *J Neurol* 2004;251:935–942.

Lemiere J, Decruyenaere M, Evers-Kiebooms G, Vandenbussche E, Dom R. Longitudinal study evaluating neuropsychological changes in so-called asymptomatic carriers of the Huntington's disease mutation after 1 year. *Acta Neurol Scand* 2002;106: 131–141.

Lesca G, Goizet C, Durr A. Predictive testing in the context of pregnancy: experience in Huntington's disease and autosomal dominant cerebellar ataxia. *J Med Genet* 2002;39:522–525.

Li, Fan M, Icton CD, Chen N, et al. Role of NR2B-type NMDA receptors in selective neurodegeneration in Huntington disease. *Neurobiol Aging* 2003;24:1113–1121.

Lin B, Nasir J, Kalchman MA, et al. Structural analysis of the 5′ region of mouse and human Huntington disease genes reveals conservation of putative promoter region and di- and trinucleotide polymorphisms. *Genomics* 1995;25:707–715.

Lin B, Rommens JM, Graham RK, et al. Differential 3′ polyadenylation of the Huntington disease gene results in two mRNA species with variable tissue expression. *Hum Mol Genet* 1993;2: 1541–1545.

MacDonald ME, Vonsattel JP, Shrinidhi J, et al. Evidence for the GluR6 gene associated with younger onset age of Huntington's disease. *Neurology* 1999;12;53:1330–1332.

Marder K, Zhao H, Myers RH, et al. Rate of functional decline in Huntington's disease. *Neurology* 2000;54:452–458.

Margolis RL, Holmes SE, Rosenblatt A, et al. Huntington's disease-like 2 (HDL2) in North America and Japan. *Ann Neurol* 2004;56:670–674. Erratum in: *Ann Neurol* 2004;56:911.

Margolis RL, O'Hearn E, Rosenblatt A, et al. A disorder similar to Huntington's disease is associated with a novel CAG repeat expansion. *Ann Neurol* 2001;50:373–380.

Marshall FJ. A randomized, double-blind, placebo-controlled study of tetrabenazine in patients with Huntington's disease. *Mov Disord* 2004;19:1122.

Mayeux R, Stern Y, Herman A, Greenbaum L, Fahn S. Correlates of early disability in Huntington's disease. *Ann Neurol* 1986;20: 727–731.

McNeil SM, Novelletto A, Srinidhi J, et al. Reduced penetrance of the Huntington's disease mutation. *Hum Mol Genet* 1997;6: 775–779.

Moore RC, Xiang F, Monaghan J, et al. Huntington disease phenocopy is a familial prion disease. *Am J Hum Genet* 2001;69: 1385–1388.

Morton AJ, Wood NI, Hastings MH, Hurelbrink C, Barker RA, Maywood ES. Disintegration of the sleep-wake cycle and circadian timing in Huntington's disease. *J Neurosci* 2005;25: 157–163.

Moutou C, Gardes N, Viville S. New tools for preimplantation genetic diagnosis of Huntington's disease and their clinical applications. *Eur J Hum Genet* 2004;12:1007–1014.

Nance MA, Mathias-Hagen V, Breningstall G, Wick MJ, McGlennen RC. Analysis of a very large trinucleotide repeat in a patient with juvenile Huntington's disease. *Neurology* 1999;52: 392–394.

Nance MA, Myers RH. Juvenile onset Huntington's disease: clinical and research perspectives. *Ment Retard Dev Disabil Res Rev* 2001;7:153–157.

Naze P, Vuillaume I, Destee A, et al. Mutation analysis and association studies of the ubiquitin carboxy-terminal hydrolase L1 gene in Huntington's disease. *Neurosci Lett* 2002;2;328:1–4.

Norremolle A, Sorensen SA, Fenger K, Hasholt L. Correlation between magnitude of CAG repeat length alterations and length of the paternal repeat in paternally inherited Huntington's disease. *Clin Genet* 1995;47:113–117.

Paulsen JS, Hoth KF, Nehl C, Stierman L. Critical periods of suicide risk in Huntington's disease. *Am J Psychiatry* 2005;162: 725–731.

Paulsen JS, Ready RE, Hamilton JM, Mega MS, Cummings JL. Neuropsychiatric aspects of Huntington's disease. *J Neurol Neurosurg Psychiatry* 2001;71:310–314.

Paulsen JS, Zimbelman JL, Hinton SC, et al. fMRI biomarker of early neuronal dysfunction in presymptomatic Huntington's Disease. *AJNR Am J Neuroradiol* 2004;25:1715–1721.

Peschanski R, Bachoud-Levi A-C, Hantraye P. Integrating fetal neural transplants into a therapeutic strategy: the example of Huntington's disease. *Brain* 2004;127:1219–1228.

Piccolo I, Defanti CA, Soliveri P, et al. Cause and course in a series of patients with sporadic chorea. *J Neurol* 2003;250: 429–435.

Pillon B, Dubois B, Ploska A, Agid Y. Severity and specificity of cognitive impairment in Alzheimer's, Huntington's, and Parkinson's diseases and progressive supranuclear palsy. *Neurology* 1991;41:634–643.

Puri BK, Leavitt BR, Hayden MR, et al. Ethyl-EPA in Huntington disease: a double-blind, randomized, placebo-controlled trial. *Neurology* 2005;65:286–292.

Racette BA, Perlmutter JS. Levodopa responsive parkinsonism in an adult with Huntington's disease. *J Neurol Neurosurg Psychiatry* 1998;65:577–579.

Rampoldi L, Dobson-Stone C, Rubio JP, et al. A conserved sorting-associated protein is mutant in chorea-acanthocytosis. *Nature Genet* 2001;28:119–120.

Rasmussen A, Macias R, Yescas P, Ochoa A, Davila G, Alonso E. Huntington disease in children: genotype-phenotype correlation. *Neuropediatrics* 2000;31:190–194.

Reading SA, Dziorny AC, Peroutka LA, et al. Functional brain changes in presymptomatic Huntington's disease. *Ann Neurol* 2004;55: 879–883.

Reuter I, Hu MT, Andrews TC, et al. Late onset levodopa responsive Huntington's disease with minimal chorea masquerading as Parkinson plus syndrome. *J Neurol Neurosurg Psychiatry* 2000;68: 238–241.

Rosenblatt A, Brinkman RR, Liang KY, et al. Familial influence on age of onset among siblings with Huntington disease. *Am J Med Genet* 2001;105:399–403.

Rubinsztein DC, Leggo J, Chiano M, et al. Genotypes at the GluR6 kainate receptor locus are associated with variation in the age of onset of Huntington disease. *Proc Natl Acad Sci USA* 1997;94: 3872–3876.

Rubinsztein DC, Leggo J, Coles R, et al. Phenotypic characterization of individuals with 30–40 CAG repeats in the Huntington disease (HD) gene reveals HD cases with 36 repeats and apparently normal elderly individuals with 36-39 repeats. *Am J Hum Genet* 1996;59:16–22.

Rubio JP, Danek A, Stone C, et al. Chorea-acanthocytosis: genetic linkage to chromosome 9q21. *Am J Hum Genet* 1997;61:899–908.

Seneca S, Fagnart D, Keymolen K, et al. Early onset Huntington disease: a neuronal degeneration syndrome. *Eur J Pediatr* 2004;163:717–721.

Shoulson I. Huntington disease: functional capacities in patients treated with neuroleptic and antidepressant drugs. *Neurology* 1981;31:1333–1335.

Shoulson I, Fahn S. Huntington disease: clinical care and evaluation. *Neurology* 1979;29:1–3.

Siesling S, van Vugt JP, Zwinderman AH, et al. Unified Huntington's Disease Rating Scale: a follow up. *Mov Disord* 1998;13:915–919.

Siesling S, Vegter-van der Vlis M, Roos RA. Juvenile Huntington disease in the Netherlands. *Pediatr Neurol* 1997;17:37–43.

Simpson SA, Zoeteweij MW, Nys K, et al. Prenatal testing for Huntington's disease: a European collaborative study. *Eur J Hum Genet* 2002;10:689–693.

Snell RG, MacMillan JC, Cheadle JP, et al. Relationship between trinucleotide repeat expansion and phenotypic variation in Huntington's disease. *Nat Genet* 1993;4:393–397.

Spires TL, Grote HE, Varshney NK, et al. Environmental enrichment rescues protein deficits in a mouse model of Huntington's disease, indicating a possible disease mechanism. *J Neurosci* 2004;24:2270–2276.

Squitieri F, Andrew SE, Goldberg YP, et al. DNA haplotype analysis of Huntington disease reveals clues to the origins and mechanisms of CAG expansion and reasons for geographic variations of prevalence. *Hum Mol Genet* 1994;3:2103–2114.

Stevanin G, Camuzat A, Holmes SE, et al. CAG/CTG repeat expansions at the Huntington's disease-like 2 locus are rare in Huntington's disease patients. *Neurology* 2002;58:965–967.

Stevanin G, Fujigasaki H, Lebre AS, et al. Huntington's disease-like phenotype due to trinucleotide repeat expansions in the TBP and JPH3 genes. *Brain* 2003;126(pt 7):1599–1603.

Tabrizi SJ, Blamire AM, Manners DN, et al. Creatine therapy for Huntington's disease: clinical and MRS findings in a 1-year pilot study. *Neurology* 2003;61:141–142.

Telenius H, Almqvist E, Kremer B, et al.Somatic mosaicism in sperm is associated with intergenerational (CAG)n changes in Huntington disease. [published erratum in *Hum Mol Genet* 1995;4:974] *Hum Mol Genet* 1995;4:189–195.

Telenius H, Kremer HPH, Theilmann J, et al. Molecular analysis of juvenile Huntington disease: the major influence on (CAG)n repeat length is the sex of the affected parent. *Hum Mol Genet* 1993;2:1535–1540.

Vaddadi KS, Soosai E, Chiu E, Dingjan P. A randomised, placebo-controlled, double blind study of treatment of Huntington's disease with unsaturated fatty acids. *Neuroreport* 2002;13:29–33. Erratum in: *Neuroreport* 2002;13:inside back cover.

van Dellen A, Hannan AJ. Genetic and environmental factors in the pathogenesis of Huntington's disease. *Neurogenetics* 2004;5:9–17.

Van der Steenstraten IM, Tibben A, Roos RA, van de Kamp JJ, Niermeijer MF. Predictive testing for Huntington disease: nonparticipants compared with participants in the Dutch program. *Am J Hum Genet* 1994;55:618–625.

van Dijk JG, van der Velde EA, Roos RA, Bruyn GW. Juvenile Huntington disease. *Hum Genet* 1986;73:235–239.

Verbessem P, Lemiere J, Eijnde BO, et al. Creatine supplementation in Huntington's disease: a placebo-controlled pilot trial. *Neurology* 2003;61:925–930.

Verhagen Metman L, Morris MJ, Farmer C, et al. Huntington's disease: a randomized, controlled trial using the NMDA antagonist amantadine. Neurology 2002;59:694–699.

Vonsattel JP, Myers RH, Stevens TJ, et al. Neuropathological classification of Huntington's disease. *J Neuropathol Exp Neuro* 1985;44: 559–577.

Walker FO, Raymond LA. Targeting energy metabolism in Huntington's disease. *Lancet* 2004;364:312–313.

Watkins WS, Bamshad M, Jorde LB. Population genetics of trinucleotide repeat polymorphisms. *Hum Mol Genet* 1995;4: 1485–1491.

Wexler NS, Lorimer J, Porter J, et al. Venezuelan kindreds reveal that genetic and environmental factors modulate Huntington's disease age of onset. *Proc Natl Acad Sci USA.* 2004;101: 3498–3503.

Wiggins S, Whyte P, Huggins M, et al. The psychological consequences of predictive testing for Huntington's disease. Canadian Collaborative Study of Predictive Testing [see comments]. *N Engl J Med* 1992;327:1401–1405.

Wilson RS, Como PG, Garron DC, Klawans HL, Barr A, Klawans D. Memory failure in Huntington's disease. *J Clin Exp Neuropsychol* 1987;9:147–154.

Xia H, Mao Q, Eliason SL, Harper SQ, et al. RNAi suppresses polyglutamine-induced neurodegeneration in a model of spinocerebellar ataxia. *Nat Med* 2004;10:816–820.

Xiang F, Almqvist EW, Huq M, et al. A Huntington diseaselike neurodegenerative disorder maps to chromosome 20p. *J Hum Genet* 1998;63:1431–1438.

Chorea, Ballism, and Athetosis

Francisco Cardoso

19

This chapter aims to provide an overview of the most important conditions associated with chorea in clinical practice, with emphasis on clinical features, differential diagnosis, and management. Because some chapters in this book address Huntington's disease and related conditions, I focus the discussion on nongenetic causes of chorea. A recent publication discusses details of differential diagnosis of genetic and nongenetic causes of chorea (Cardoso et al., 2006).

DEFINITIONS AND PHENOMENOLOGY

Chorea is defined as a syndrome characterized by the continuous flow of random muscle contractions. This pattern of movement conveys a feeling of restlessness to the observer. When choreic movements are more severe, assuming a flinging, sometimes violent character, they are called *ballism*. Neurophysiologic studies confirm this overlapping of chorea and ballism, which share the same neuronal pattern, i.e., hypoactivity of the subthalamic nucleus and increased firing rate of the globus pallidum pars interna (Hamani et al., 2004). Regardless of its etiology, chorea has the same features. Thus, the differential diagnosis of its etiology relies not so much on differences in the phenomenology of the hyperkinesia but on accompanying findings.

The unpredictable nature of chorea is a feature that distinguishes it from tremor and dystonia. The former is characterized by rhythmic contractions of antagonist muscles, whereas the hallmark of dystonia is the patterned contraction resulting in abnormal postures or torsion movements. Stereotypies also are produced by repetitive contractions but, unlike tremor and dystonia, the resulting movements mimic complex motor behaviors that are part of the normal human repertoire. Tics can be readily differentiated from chorea because they also reproduce normal human movements or vocalizations, are often preceded by a local unpleasant sensation (sensory tic or prodrome), and can be voluntarily suppressed. A note of caution is necessary regarding the possibility of interpreting chorea of some body areas as tics. Such confusion is particularly common in the face, as well as in the pharynx where chorea can result in vocalizations. One isolated choreic movement also can be misinterpreted as myoclonus (a brief, lighting-like contraction with duration inferior to 200 ms), but the latter lacks the continuous flow so typical of chorea.

Athetosis describes sinuous, slow movements affecting distal limbs, particularly in the arms. There is a clear decline of the use of this term in the contemporary literature. The reason behind this tendency is the realization that athetosis is better defined as dystonia associated occasionally with some degree of chorea. As will be seen in the end of this chapter, the word *athetosis* remains employed to refer to the dyskinesia seen in patients with cerebral palsy and in those with dysfunction of proprioception.

Nongenetic Causes of Chorea

Table 19.1 contains a classification of nongenetic choreas by categories of etiology. The most common causes of sporadic chorea are drugs, pregnancy, vascular disease, thyrotoxicosis, systemic lupus erythematosus (SLE), and the primary antiphospholipid antibody syndrome (PAPS), polycythemia rubra vera, AIDS, and Sydenham's chorea (SC) (Quinn & Schrag, 1998). Although population-based epidemiologic studies are not available, a recent report provides an estimate of the relative frequency of the most important causes of nongenetic chorea. In a tertiary referral center, the authors identified the following etiologies in 42 consecutive patients

TABLE 19.1

ETIOLOGIC CLASSIFICATION OF NONGENETIC CHOREA

Vascular chorea
Autoimmune chorea
Drug-induced chorea
Metabolic chorea
Infectious chorea

with chorea: vascular-related (21 cases); drug-induced (7 cases); AIDS-related (5 cases); hyperglycemia, hyponatremia, and hypoxia (2 cases each); borreliosis, vasculitis, and SC (1 case each) (Piccolo et al., 2003). These frequencies most probably vary according to the geographic area in question. For example, at the Movement Disorders Clinic of the Federal University of Minas Gerais (MDC-UFMG), Brazil, SC accounts for two-thirds of all cases of chorea (Cardoso et al., 1997).

Vascular Chorea

Chorea is an unusual complication of acute vascular lesion, seen in less than 1% of patients with acute stroke. This hyperkinesia, often characterized as hemiballism, is usually related to ischemic or hemorrhagic lesion of the basal ganglia and adjacent white matter in the territory of the middle or the posterior cerebral artery. In contrast to common sense, the majority of patients with vascular chorea have lesions outside the subthalamus (Ghika-Schmid et al., 1997). Although vascular chorea often comes into remission spontaneously, in the acute phase patients may require treatment with such antichoreic drugs as neuroleptics or dopamine depleters. A few patients with vascular chorea may remain with persistent movement disorder. In this circumstance, they can be treated effectively with stereotactic surgery such as thalamotomy or posteroventral pallidotomy (Cardoso et al., 1995; Choi et al., 2003).

An uncommon cause of chorea is Moyamoya disease, an intracranial vasculopathy that presents with ischemic lesion or, less commonly, with hemorrhagic stroke of the basal ganglia (Gonzalez-Alegre et al., 2003). Another rare, but still reported, vascular cause of chorea is the so-called "post-pump chorea"—a complication of extracorporeal circulation. The pathogenesis of this movement disorder is believed to be related to vascular insult of the basal ganglia during the surgical procedure. The natural history of post-pump chorea is benign with spontaneous remission in most cases (Thobois et al., 2004).

Autoimmune Chorea

Sydenham's Chorea

SC, the neurological manifestation of rheumatic fever (RF), is the prototype of chorea resulting from immune mechanisms. Chorea occurs in 26% of patients with RF

(Cardoso et al., 1997). Although largely confined to areas outside North America and Western Europe, it is now drawing growing interest. This results from the possibility that a similar pathogenic mechanism may be responsible for a subset of patients with Tourette's syndrome (TS) and related conditions (Swedo et al., 1998). Despite declining incidence, SC remains the most common cause worldwide of acute chorea in children. More recently, however, outbreaks of RF with occurrence of chorea have been identified in the United States and Australia (Ayoub, 1992; Ryan et al., 2000).

The usual age at onset of SC is 8 years to 9 years, although there are reports of patients developing chorea in the third decade of life. In most series there is a female preponderance (Cardoso et al., 1997). One important clinical finding is the observation that SC is very rarely seen below age 5 years (Tani et al., 2003). Typically, patients develop this disease 4 weeks to 8 weeks after an episode of group A β-hemolytic streptococcus (GABHS) pharyngitis. It does not occur after streptococcal infection of the skin. The chorea rapidly spreads and becomes generalized, but 20% of patients remain with hemichorea (Cardoso et al., 1997; Nausieda et al., 1980). Patients display motor impersistence, particularly noticeable during tongue protrusion and ocular fixation. The muscle tone is usually decreased; in severe and rare cases (1.5% of all patients seen at the MDC-UFMG) this is so pronounced that the patient may become bedridden (chorea paralytica).

Patients with SC often display other motor findings. There are reports of common occurrence of tics in SC. However, this author finds it virtually impossible to distinguish simple tics from fragments of chorea. Even vocal tics, reported to be common in SC (Mercadante et al., 1997), are not simple to diagnose in patients with hyperkinesias. Involuntary vocalizations, simply resulting from dystonia or chorea of the pharynx or larynx, have been reported in subjects with, for instance, oromandibular dystonia or Huntington's disease (Jankovic, 2001). In a cohort of 120 SC patients followed up at the MDC-UFMG, we have identified complex tics in fewer than 4% of subjects. There is evidence that many patients with active SC have hypometric saccades, and a few of them also show oculogyric crisis.

There also has been growing interest in the behavioral abnormalities present in SC. At the MDC-UFMG, Maia et al. (2005) studied 50 healthy subjects (CG), 50 patients with RF without chorea, and 56 patients with SC. The authors found that obsessive–compulsive behavior (OCB), obsessive–compulsive disorder (OCD), and attention deficit and hyperactivity disorder (ADHD) were more frequent in SC (19%, 23.2%, 30.4%) than in CG (11%, 4%, 8%) and in RF (14%, 6%, 8%). In this study, the authors demonstrated that OCB displays little degree of interference in the performance of the activities of daily living. Comparing patients with acute and persistent SC (duration of illness greater than 2 years), ADHD was significantly more common in the latter (50% versus 16%). There was also a trend toward more OCB and OCD among subjects with more protracted forms of SC, but the difference failed to reach statistical significance. Psychosis can rarely be present in SC (Teixeira et al., 2006).

In a recent survey of 100 patients with RF, half of whom had chorea, we found that migraine is more frequent in SC (21.8%) than in normal controls (8.1%, $p = 0.02$) (Teixeira Jr et al., 2005d). This is similar to what has been described in TS (Kwack et al., 2003). In the older literature, there also are references to papilledema, central retinal artery occlusion, and seizures in a few patients with SC. A recent investigation demonstrated that the peripheral nervous system is not targeted in SC (Cardoso et al., 2004). Finally, it must be kept in mind that SC is a major manifestation of RF: Between 60% and 80% of patients display cardiac involvement, particularly mitral valve dysfunction, whereas the association with arthritis is less common, seen in 30% of subjects; however, in approximately 20% of the patients, chorea is the sole finding (Cardoso et al., 1997). The first validated scale to rate SC, the University of Minas Gerais Sydenham Chorea Rating Scale (USCRS), was published in 2005. It was designed to provide a detailed quantitative description of the performance of activities of daily living, behavioral abnormalities, and motor function of patients with SC. It comprises 27 items, and each item is scored from 0 (no symptom or sign) to 4 (severe disability or finding) (Teixeira et al., 2005b).

There is no investigation directly comparing clinical features of SC with TS. However, the studies of the latter suggest that OCD, ADHD, and other behavioral manifestations are more common and disabling in TS than in SC (Leckman, 2002). Another important clinical difference between these conditions is the observation that the vast majority of SC subjects present with carditis, whereas this complication has never been reported in TS (Cardoso et al., 1997; Leckman, 2002). Moreover, there is no indication of the existence of geographic clusters of TS in contrast with SC. It can be concluded that although there are similarities between SC and tic disorders, there remain important distinctions. This suggests that the pathogenic mechanism responsible for SC, if active in TS and related conditions, accounts for a limited number of patients with tic disorders.

The pathogenesis of SC is thought to be related to the existence of molecular mimicry between streptococcal and central nervous system antigens. It has been proposed that the GABHS infection in genetically predisposed subjects leads to the formation of crossreactive antibodies that disrupt the basal ganglia function. Several studies have demonstrated the presence of such circulating antibodies in 50% to 90% of patients with Sydenham chorea (Husby et al., 1976; Church et al., 2002). In a study of patients seen at the MDC-UFMG, we demonstrated that all patients with active SC have antibasal ganglia antibodies demonstrated by enzyme-linked immunosorbent assay (ELISA) and the Western blot test. In subjects with persistent SC, the positivity was about 60% (Church et al., 2002). It must

be emphasized that the biological value of the antibasal ganglia antibodies remains to be determined. Two recent studies suggest that they may interfere with neuronal function. In one, the authors demonstrated that immunoglobulin (IgM) of 1 patient with SC induced expression of calcium-dependent calmodulins in a culture of neuroblastoma cells. Although an interesting finding, this study (Kiroan et al., 2003) has three limitations: (1) it is an in vitro investigation, employing an artificial paradigm that does not necessarily reflect the situation observed in human patients; (2) the antibody was obtained from a single patient; and, (3) the authors studied IgM, whereas all investigations of antibasal ganglia antibodies in SC have detected immunoglobulin G (IgG). In another investigation, we demonstrated that there is a linear correlation between the increase of intracellular calcium levels in PC12 cells and antibasal ganglia antibody titer in the serum from SC patients. This result suggests that the antibodies have a pathogenic value (Teixeira et al., 2005a).

There have been recent studies that address the role of immune cellular mechanisms in SC. Investigating sera and cerebrospinal fluid (CSF) samples of SC patients of MDC-UFMG, Church and colleagues (2003) found elevation of serum interleukins 4 (IL-4) and 10 (IL-10). These are cytokines that take part in the Th2 (antibody-mediated) response. They also described IL-4 in 31% of the CSF of acute SC, whereas just IL-4 was raised in the CSF of persistent cases. The authors concluded that SC is characterized by a Th2 response. However, as they have found an elevation of IL-12 in acute SC and, more recently, we described an increased concentration of chemokines CXCL9 and CXCL10 in the serum of patients with acute SC (Teixeira et al., 2004), it can be concluded that Th1 (cell-mediated) mechanisms also may be involved in the pathogenesis of SC.

The current diagnostic criteria of SC are a modification of the Jones criteria: chorea with acute or subacute onset and lack of clinical and laboratory evidence of alternative cause are mandatory findings. The diagnosis is further supported by the presence of additional major or minor manifestations of RF (Special Writing Group, 1992; Cardoso et al., 1997; Cardoso et al., 1999). The aim of the diagnostic workup in patients suspected to have SC is threefold: (a) to identify evidence of recent streptococcal infection or acute phase reaction; (b) to search for cardiac injury associated with RF; and (c) to rule out alternative causes. Tests of acute phase reactants such as erythrocyte sedimentation rate, C-reactive protein, leukocytosis; other blood tests like rheumatoid factor, mucoproteins, protein electrophoresis; and supporting evidence of preceding streptococcal infection (increased antistreptolysin-O, antiDNAse-B, or other antistreptococcal antibodies; positive throat culture for group A *Streptococcus*; recent scarlet fever) are much less helpful in SC than in other forms of RF due to the usual long latency between the infection and onset of the movement disorder. Elevated antistreptolysin O titer may be found in populations with a high prevalence of

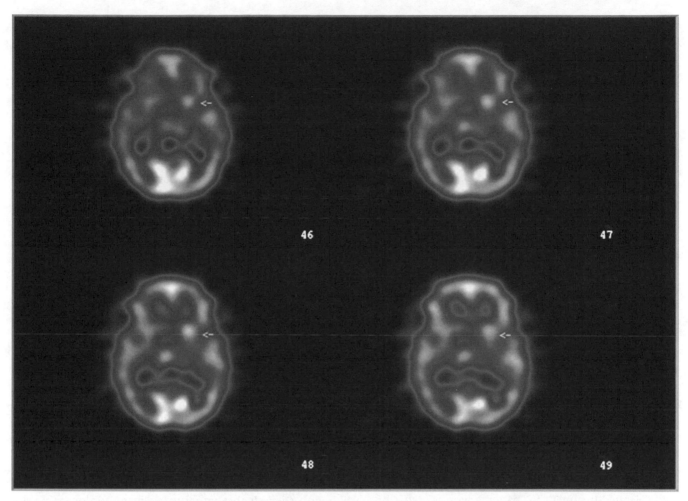

Figure 19.1 Axial sections of ^{99m}Tc-ECD of a patient with generalized chorea caused by acute Sydenham's chorea. There is hyperperfusion in the basal ganglia, particularly on the left side (*arrow*). (See color section.)

streptococcal infection. Furthermore, the antistreptolysin O titer declines if the interval between infection and RF is greater than 2 months. Anti-DNase-B titers, however, may remain elevated up to 1 year after strep pharyngitis. Heart evaluation (i.e., Doppler echocardiography) is mandatory because of the common association of SC with carditis. Serologic studies for SLE and PAPS must be ordered to rule out these conditions. EEG may show generalized slowing acutely or after clinical recovery. Spinal fluid analysis is usually normal, but it may show a slight increased lymphocyte count. In general, neuroimaging will help rule out structural causes of chorea. CT scan of the brain invariably fails to display abnormalities. Similarly, head MRI is often normal, although there are case reports of reversible hyperintensity in the basal ganglia area. In one study, the authors showed increased signal in just 2 of 24 patients, although morphometric techniques revealed mean values for the size of the striatum and pallidum larger than controls (Giedd et al., 1995). Unfortunately, these findings are of little help on an individual basis since there was an extensive overlap between controls and patients. A study reported in 2003 showed that there is a correlation between the presence of persistent lesions of the basal ganglia on MRI and tendency for a more prolonged course of the disease (Faustino et al., 2003). PET and SPECT imaging may prove to be useful tools in the evaluation, revealing transient increases in striatal metabolism (Weindl et al., 1993). In one SPECT study of 10 patients with SC, the authors showed that 6 had hyperperfusion of the basal ganglia (Barsottini et al., 2002). Figure 19.1 shows ^{99m}Tc-ECD SPECT of an SC patient with basal ganglia hyperperfusion. This contrasts with other choreic disorders (such as Huntington's disease) that are associated with hypometabolism. Of note, however, is a recent SPECT investigation that showed hyperperfusion in 2 patients with SC, whereas the remaining 5 had hypometabolism (Citak et al., 2004). It is possible that the inconsistencies in these functional imaging studies reflect heterogeneity of the population of patients. Increasing interest is now directed to autoimmune markers that may be useful for diagnosis. The test of antineuronal antibodies, however, is not commercially available, being performed only for research purposes. Preliminary evidence, moreover, suggests that these antibodies are not specific for SC. Similarly, the low sensitivity and specificity of the alloantigen D8/17, a proposed marker of susceptibility for RF and SC, render it unsuitable for the diagnosis of rheumatic chorea.

There are no controlled studies of symptomatic treatment of SC. For most authorities, however, the first choice is valproic acid, although other anticonvulsants—such as carbamazepine—also are found to be effective and well tolerated (Genel et al., 2002; Hernandez-Latorre & Roig-Quilis, 2003). Dopamine receptor blocking agents, usually pimozide, are left for patients who fail to respond to valproic acid or those rare cases with chorea paralytica. The need for caution in the use of neuroleptics in rheumatic chorea is demonstrated by a case-control study, comparing the response to these drugs in patients with SC and TS. The authors demonstrated that 5% of 100 patients with chorea developed parkinsonism, dystonia, or both, whereas these findings were not observed among patients with tics matched for age and dosage of neuroleptics (Teixeira Jr et al., 2003).

Some controversy exists as to the role of immunosuppression in the management of SC. Steroids are reserved for patients with persistent disabling chorea refractory to antichoreic agents. We reported that 25 mg/kg/day in children and 1 g/day in adults of methylprednisolone for 5 days followed by 1 mg/kg/day of prednisone is an effective and well-tolerated treatment for patients with SC refractory to conventional treatment with antichoreic drugs and penicillin (Cardoso et al., 2003). The same protocol has been shown to control chorea in patients with SC who developed side effects to neuroleptics (Teixeira Jr et al., 2005c). There are few reports describing the usefulness of plasma exchange or intravenous ImG in SC (Jordan et al., 2003). Because of the efficacy of other therapeutic agents described in the previous paragraph, potential complications, and the high cost of the latter treatment modalities, these options are usually not recommended. Finally, the most important measure in the treatment of patients with SC is secondary prophylaxis with penicillin or, if there is allergy, sulfa drugs up to age 21 years.

SC is often described as a self-limited condition that comes into remission spontaneously after a course of 8 to 9 months. However, prospective studies have shown that up to 50% of patients may remain with chorea after a follow-up of 2 years. This has been called *persistent SC* (Cardoso et al., 1999). Moreover, despite regular use of secondary prophylaxis, recurrences of SC are observed in up to 50% of subjects (Cardoso et al., 1999; Korn-Lubetzki et al., 2004). Interestingly, in many of the recurrences there is lack of association either with streptococcus infection or even anti-Basal ganglia antibodies (Harrison et al., 2004; Korn-Lubetzki et al., 2004).

Other Autoimmune Choreas

Other immunologic causes of chorea are SLE, PAPS, vasculitis, and paraneoplastic syndromes. SLE or PAPS are classically described as the prototypes of autoimmune choreas (Quinn & Schrag, 1998). However, several reports show that chorea is seen in no more than 1%–2% of large series of patients with these conditions (Asherson & Cervera, 2003; Sanna et al., 2003). In the latter study, the authors confirmed the notion that chorea and other neuropsychiatric syndromes, present in 185 of their 323 consecutive patients with SLE, are associated with antiphospholipid antibodies. Autoimmune chorea also has been reported in the context of paraneoplastic syndromes associated with anti-Hu and/or anti-CRMP5 antibodies in rare patients with small-cell lung carcinoma (Kinirons et al., 2003; Dorban et al., 2004).

Drug-Induced Chorea

Table 19.2 contains a list of drugs described in association with induction of chorea. Levodopa-induced chorea, the most common form of drug-induced chorea seen by movement disorders specialists, is discussed somewhere else in this book. There are reports of patients treated with lithium, lamotrigine, or methadone who developed chorea that remitted after discontinuation of the drugs (Das et al., 2003; Lussier & Cruciani, 2003; Stemper et al., 2003). Oral contraceptive–induced chorea has been regarded traditionally as a syndrome related to SC. It is hypothesized that hormones could potentially lead a basal ganglia previously injured during the acute phase of RF to produce chorea. A report suggests that rather than related to dopamine system dysfunction, oral contraceptive–induced chorea could be mediated by antibasal ganglia antibodies (Miranda et al., 2004). Chorea gravidarum (chorea occurring during pregnancy) also is believed to have the same pathogenesis as oral contraceptive–induced chorea (Cardoso, 2002a).

TABLE 19.2

DRUGS RELATED TO INDUCTION OF CHOREA

Alcohol
Anticholinergics
Antiepileptic agents (hydantoin, lamotrigine, valproic acid)
Antihypertensive agents (captopril, alpha-methyldopa)
Calcium channel blockers (cinnarize, flunarizine)
Cocaine
Dopamine agonists
Hormones
Levodopa
Lithium
Methadone
Neuroleptics
Stimulants (amphetamine, methyl-phenidate, pemoline)
Superselective serotonin reuptake inhibitors
    (fluoxetine, paroxetine)
Tricyclic antidepressants (imipramine)

Metabolic Chorea

Chronic acquired or non-Wilsonian hepatolenticular degeneration was the first well-characterized metabolic cause of chorea, thanks to the pioneering work of Victor and Adams. Although first described in the context of complications of alcohol abuse, it can occur in any form of acquired liver disease. The clinical picture is heterogeneous since patients may present with a variable combination of neurological and hepatic manifestations. The neurological findings include apathy, somnolence, parkinsonism, tremor, myoclonus, asterixis, and chorea. In most instances, there is a combination of different movement disorders, but a few subjects may present with isolated chorea. MRI of the brain shows not only images compatible with cavitations in the basal ganglia (hyperintense signal on T2 and hypointense on T1) but also hyperintense T1 signal in the pallidum, putamen, and upper brainstem. The latter has been interpreted as caused by deposition of manganese (Jog & Lang, 1995).

There is growing interest in the association of chorea and nonketotic hyperglycemia in type II diabetes mellitus. This condition seems particularly common among Asians since the reports in the literature almost exclusively describe patients with this ethnic background. Unlike the usual neurological manifestations of nonketotic hyperglycemia, these patients do not show change in the level of consciouness but do develop unilateral or generalized chorea–ballism. The MRI findings are characteristic with hyperintense signal of the pallidum on T1. Although their interpretation is controversial, most studies relate this image to microhemorrhages of the pallidum. Once glycemic control is achieved, there is gradual remission of chorea (Chu et al., 2002; Lin & Chang, 1994). The risk of nonketotic hyperglycemia, with or without putamenal hyperintensity on T1-weighted MRI, has been found to be increased in diabetic patients with acanthocytosis (Pisani et al., 2005).

A few patients with hyperthyroidism may develop generalized chorea or even ballism related to this endocrine dysfunction. The lack of structural changes in the brain, appearance with onset of thyrotoxicosis, and remission with endocrine control suggest that the basal ganglia dysfunction is induced by hormones (Ristic et al., 2004). Other possible metabolic causes of chorea are hypoglycemia, renal failure, and ketogenic diet (Kalita et al., 2003).

Infectious Chorea

SC could be considered as a form of infectious chorea since it is induced by GABHS. However, in this section the discussion will be limited to instances where chorea results from injury to the brain directly produced by a microorganism. HIV and its complications has constituted the most often reported infectious cause of chorea. In 1 series of 42 consecutive patients with nongenetic chorea, for instance, AIDS was found to be the cause in 12% of the subjects (Piccolo et al., 2003). In HIV-positive patients, chorea is the result of either the direct action of the virus or other mechanisms, such as opportunistic infections (toxoplasmosis, syphilis, and others) or drugs (Cardoso, 2002b). Other infections related to chorea are new variant Creutzfeldt-Jakob disease and tuberculosis (Kalita et al., 2003; McKee & Talbot, 2003).

Genetic Causes of Chorea

There are chapters of this book devoted to Huntington's disease and other genetic causes of chorea. The aim of this section is to provide the reader with clinical guidelines for differential diagnosis of hereditary conditions in which chorea is one of the key clinical features (Table 19.3).

TABLE 19.3
MOST COMMON CAUSES OF GENETIC CHOREA

Condition	Mode of Inheritance	Gene	Location
Huntington's disease	AD	IT15	4p15
Huntington's disease-like 1	AD	PRNP	20p12
Huntington's disease-like 2	AD	JPH3	16q24.3
Huntington's disease-like 3	AR	?	4915.3
Huntington's disease-like 4	AD	?	?
SCA17	AD	TBP	6q27
Neuroacanthocytosis	AR	CHAC	9q21
McLeod syndrome	X-linked recessive	XK	Xp21
Benign hereditary chorea	AD	TITF-1	14q13.1
SCA3	AD	MJD1	14q32.1
Dentato-rubral-pallido-luysian atrophy	AD	DRPLA	12p13.31
Ataxia-telangiectasia	AR	ATM	11q22-23
Wilson's disease	AR	WD	13q14.3
Ferritin-associated basal ganglia disease	AD	FTL	19p13.3

?, unknown; AD, autosomal dominant; AR, autosomal recessive; SCA17, spinocerebellar atrophy 17; SCA3, spinocerebellar atrophy 3.

Huntington' Disease and Related Conditions

Huntington' disease (HD) is the most important genetic cause of chorea. Patients with HD usually develop the first symptoms of the illness around age 40 years. The age at onset, however, may range from early childhood (Westphal variant) to the last decades of life. There is an inverse correlation between the number of CAG repeats in the HD gene (IT15 on 4p15) and age at onset. The typical clinical picture is a combination of cognitive decline, behavioral changes, and movement disorder. Patients with HD typically develop a subcortical dementia, characterized by dysexecutive syndrome, decreased verbal fluency, bradyphrenia, and relative preservation of cortical functions. The spectrum of behavioral abnormalities may include depression, apathy, aggressiveness, suicide attempts, drug addiction, inappropriate sexual behavior, and others. Chorea is just one of the possible movement disorders present in HD. It is typically observed in patients with onset in middle age, as well as in the elderly. Along the progression of the illness, chorea is usually replaced by rigidity and dystonia. A comprehensive evaluation found that the latter hyperkinesia is present in 95% of patients with HD, although it was rated as severe and constant in 16% (Louis et al., 1999). It is thought that selective degeneration of striatal neurons of the indirect pathway is associated with chorea. With progressive loss of cell bodies related to the direct pathway, there is development of dystonia (Deng et al., 2004). A clinical hallmark of HD is supranuclear ophthalmoparesis (Penney Jr et al., 1990). Longitudinal follow up of patients at risk for HD has shown that abnormalities of ocular motility often are the earliest clinical signs of this condition. Other clinical features are seizures, occasionally seen in patients with the Westphal variant, and weight loss. Some authors have interpreted the latter as evidence of energy metabolism dysfunction playing an important role in the pathogenesis of HD (Browne & Beal, 2004).

The diagnosis of HD is suspected when patients with this clinical picture have a family history consistent with autosomal dominant transmission. Neuroimaging studies show atrophy of the pallidum and the head of the caudate. SPECT and PET disclose decreased metabolism of the basal ganglia. With commercial availability of testing for the HD gene, the diagnosis of this condition became much easier. It must be emphasized, however, that to prevent potentially serious ethical problems, guidelines produced by the World Federation of Neurology should be observed before ordering the test (International Huntington Association [IHA] & World Federation of Neurology [WFN] Research Group on Huntington's Chorea, 1994). Interestingly, about 3% of patients with features typical of HD test negative for IT15. They correspond to the Huntington's-diseaselike (HD-Like) phenotype (Walker et al., 2003b). Although the genes of SCA17 (TBP) and HDL2 (JPH3) are the most commonly found mutations related to the HD-like phenotype, most patients are negative for known genes. This suggests that there is a high degree of genetic heterogeneity in the HD-like phenotype (Stevanin et al., 2003).

Although studies in experimental models of HD raise the hope of finding neuroprotective agents, to date none has been shown to change the relentlessly progressive course of HD and related conditions. There also have been attempts of cell therapy in humans. Despite the evidence of survival of transplanted fetal cells, no meaningful improvement has been noticed, and a call for a pause in the performance of these procedures was published (Albin, 2002). The treatment of patients with HD and related conditions is targeted, thus, at symptomatic control. As few, if any, controlled studies have been published, the choice of agents relies primarily on clinical experience. Chorea can be effectively treated with neuroleptics or dopamine-depleting agents such as tetrabenazine (Ondo et al., 2002). However, since they can induce parkinsonism, potentially increasing the rigidity and postural instability often seen in HD, the use of these drugs must be left for situations in which chorea is severe and disabling. Despite conflicting findings, amantadine has been shown to alleviate chorea. This effect is presumed to be mediated by amantadine's antiglutamate action (Lucetti et al., 2003). Patients with severe chorea refractory to clinical treatment may benefit from pallidotomy or deep-brain stimulation of the pallidum (Moro et al., 2004). With progression of the illness and appearance of disabling rigidity, small doses of dopamine agonists and even levodopa can be necessary. Neuroleptics in combination with antidepressants can be useful in the management of such behavioral disturbances as aggressiveness and major depression.

Neuroacanthocytosis

A clinical triad also found in HD characterizes this rare condition: movement disorder (particularly chorea), behavioral changes, and dementia. The hereditary nature and presence of atrophy of the head of the caudate on neuroimaging studies creates further confusion between the two conditions. There are, however, several features that help one to distinguish neuroacanthocytosis from HD: The condition is transmitted in an autosomal recessive manner in most patients, although there are well-documented families with autosomal dominant forms of the illness (Saiki et al., 2003); more than half of the patients have a self-mutilating oro-mandibulo-lingual dystonia with biting of the tongue; vocal tics are fairly common; parkinsonism can be the sole movement disorder; tonic–clonic generalized seizures are often present; areflexia and amyotrophy are also common; the serum level of creatine kinase is elevated; electromyography shows peripheral neuropathy; some patients have the eye-of-the-tiger sign on MRI, similar to what happens in pantothenate kinase-associated neurodegeneration; acanthocytes account for 10% or more of the peripheral red cells, although this level may vary along the timeline (Hardie et al., 1991); and the gene was found on Ch 9q21, but cases related to the HD-like 2 and other loci have been reported (Walker et al., 2003a).

McLeod Syndrome

In the past, descriptions of the clinical features of this condition mentioned the occurrence of neurological abnormalities as accidental findings. Recent studies have demonstrated, however, that progressive basal ganglia dysfunction is an integral part of the McLeod syndrome. In fact, in one report of 6 patients, 5 had chorea, tics were observed in 4, dystonia in 3, self-mutilating lip dyskinesia and seizure in 1 each (Danek et al., 2001). Atrophy of the caudate also can be seen in this condition, as exemplified by a patient followed up at the UFMG Movement Disorders Clinic (Fig. 19.2). In summary, the clinical picture of McLeod syndrome can be identical to the one observed in neuroacanthocytosis. Seizures and self-mutilating tongue dystonia are more common in the latter, whereas more patients with McLeod syndrome have myopathy and myocardiopathy. Definite distinction between the two conditions, however, can be firmly established just by the finding of the gene CHAC in neuroacanthocytosis or the low reactivity of Kell erythrocyte antigens, the hallmark of McLeod syndrome. Symptomatic management of both conditions follows the same guidelines described for HD. Because of the frequent coexistence of a seizure disorder, McLeod syndrome patients often require such antiepileptic drugs as carbamazepine or valproic acid. Injections of botulinum toxin are the only option effective to treat the self-mutilating lingual dystonia.

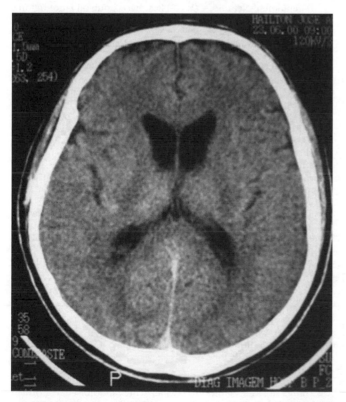

Figure 19.2 Axial section of a computerized tomography of the brain of a patient with McLeod syndrome showing bilateral atrophy of the head of the caudate.

Benign Hereditary Chorea

The clinical features of benign hereditary chorea (BHC) are onset before 5 years of age; chorea; lack of other neurological findings with exception of mild cerebellar ataxia in a few patients; course static or with spontaneous improvement after childhood; and autosomal dominant transmission. There were doubts until 2002 whether BHC existed as an independent nosologic entity (Schrag et al., 2000). The discovery of a mutation of the TITF-1 gene mutation on Ch 14q associated with this phenotype confirmed the notion of BHC (Breedveld et al., 2002a). However, many families with the clinical features previously described are negative for this gene, indicating that there is genetic heterogeneity in BHC (Breedveld et al., 2002b).

Wilson's Disease

The neurological manifestations of this rare autosomal recessive condition, caused by a mutation in the Wilson's disease (WD) gene on Ch 13q, is caused by deposition of copper in the brain, particularly in the basal ganglia and upper brainstem. Because of the existence of effective treatment with agents that chelate copper or prevent its absorption and the invariable fatal outcome in subjects with WD left untreated, it is mandatory to rule out this diagnosis in all patients with movement disorders of onset at age 40 years or less. The clinical phenotype of WD is quite variable, including parkinsonism, dystonia, tremor, chorea, and other findings. Isolated chorea, however, is seldom seen (Prashanth et al., 2004). The diagnosis is usually based on the recognition of Kayser-Fleischer ring and the typical biochemical abnormalities (low serum ceruloplasmin and elevated urine copper).

Athetosis

As mentioned at the beginning of this chapter, movement disorders experts use the term *athetosis* less and less. However, there are two situations where it is still used. The first and most common is to describe the combination of dystonia and chorea in the distal portions of limbs in patients with cerebral palsy (Morris et al., 2002). Although traditionally described as a complication of kernicterus, athetosis may happen in cerebral palsy of any cause. The phenomenology is characterized by a variable combination of dystonia, chorea, myoclonus, and spasticity. A few patients may improve with levodopa, clonazepan, baclofen, anticholinergics, or tetrabenazine. Most of them, however, are refractory to clinical treatment, and even surgical treatment has not been successful. There is one report, for example, describing the failure of deep-brain stimulation of the globus pallidus internus in alleviating chorea in four patients with cerebral palsy (Krauss et al., 2003). Finally, slow, distal, writhing movements of the fingers or toes in patients with proprioception loss are described as *pseudoathetosis*. This dyskinesia is usually described in association with peripheral neuropathy. However, central lesions resulting in impairment of proprioception (myelopathy, thalamic lesion, or others) also may cause pseudoathetosis (Sharp et al., 1994). As this movement disorder does not cause significant morbidity, no treatment is required.

ACKNOWLEDGMENTS

I thank Antonio Lúcio Teixeira Jr., M.D., Ph.D.; Débora Maia, M.D.; and Mauro César Cunningham, M.D., for their collaboration in many of the investigations of Sydenham's chorea. I also thank Cristiano Ferrari, M.D. for performing the SPECT studies of our patients with Sydenham's chorea, including the one shown in Figure 19.1.

REFERENCES

Albin RL. Fetal striatal transplantation in Huntington's disease: time for a pause. *J Neurol Neurosurg Psychiatry* 2002;73:612.

Asherson RA, Cervera R. Unusual manifestations of the antiphospholipid syndrome. *Clin Rev Allergy Immunol* 2003;25:61–78.

Ayoub EM. Resurgence of rheumatic fever in the United States: the changing picture of a preventable illness. *Postgrad Med* 1992;92:133–142.

Barsottini OG, Ferraz HB, Seviliano MM, Barbieri A. Brain SPECT imaging in Sydenham's chorea. *Braz J Med Biol Res* 2002;35:431–436.

Breedveld GJ, van Dongen JW, Danesino C, et al. Mutations in TITF-1 are associated with benign hereditary chorea. *Hum Mol Genet* 2002a;11:971–979.

Breedveld GJ, Percy AK, MacDonald ME, et al. Clinical and genetic heterogeneity in benign hereditary chorea. *Neurology* 2002b;59:579–584.

Browne SE, Beal MF. The energetics of Huntington's disease. *Neurochem Res* 2004;29:531–546.

Cardoso F. Chorea gravidarum. *Arch Neurol* 2002a;59:868–870.

Cardoso F. HIV-related movement disorders: epidemiology, pathogenesis and management. *CNS Drugs.* 2002b;16:663–668.

Cardoso F, Dornas L, Cunningham M, Oliveira JT. Nerve conduction study in Sydenham's chorea. *Mov Disord* 2004;

Cardoso F, Jankovic J, Grossman RG, Hamilton WJ. Outcome after stereotactic thalamotomy for dystonia and hemiballismus. *Neurosurgery* 1995;36:501–507.

Cardoso F, Maia D, Cunningham MC, Valença G. Treatment of Sydenham chorea with corticosteroids. *Mov Disord* 2003;18: 1374–1377.

Cardoso F, Seppi K, Mair KY, et al. Seminar on choreas. *Lancet Neurol.* 2006;5:589–602.

Cardoso F, Silva CE, Mota CC. Sydenham's chorea in 50 consecutive patients with rheumatic fever. *Mov Disord* 1997;12:701–703.

Cardoso F, Vargas AP, Oliveira LD, et al. Persistent Sydenham's chorea. *Mov Disord* 1999;14:805–807.

Choi SJ, Lee SW, Kim MC, et al. Posteroventral pallidotomy in medically intractable postapoplectic monochorea: case report. *Surg Neurol* 2003;59:486–490.

Chu K, Kang DW, Kim DE et al. Diffusion-weighted and gradient echo magnetic resonance findings of hemichorea-hemiballismus associated with diabetic hyperglycemia: a hyperviscosity syndrome? *Arch Neurol* 2002;59:448–452.

Church AJ, Cardoso F, Dale RC, et al. Anti-basal ganglia antibodies in acute and persistent Sydenham's chorea. *Neurology* 2002;59: 227–231.

Church AJ, Dale RC, Cardoso F, et al. CSF and serum immune parameters in Sydenham's chorea: evidence of an autoimmune syndrome? *J Neuroimmunol* 2003;136:149–153.

Citak EC, Gukuyener K, Karabacak NI, et al. Functional brain imaging in Sydenham's chorea and streptococcal tic disorders. *J Child Neurol* 2004;19:387–390.

Danek A, Tison F, Rubio J, et al. The chorea of McLeod syndrome. *Mov Disord* 2001;16:882–889.

Das KB, Harris C, Smyth DP, Cross JH. Unusual side effects of lamotrigine therapy. *J Child Neurol* 2003;18:479–480.

Deng YP, Albin RL, Penney JB, et al. Differential loss of striatal projection systems in Huntington's disease: a quantitative immunohistochemical study. *J Chem Neuroanat* 2004;27:143–164.

Dorban S, Gille M, Kessler R, et al. Chorea-athetosis in the anti-Hu syndrome. *Rev Neurol (Paris)* 2004;160:126–129.

Faustino PC, Terreri MT, da Rocha AJ, et al. Clinical, laboratory, psychiatric and magnetic resonance findings in patients with Sydenham chorea. *Neuroradiology* 2003;45:456–462.

Genel F, Arslanoglu S, Uran N, Saylan B. Sydenham's chorea: clinical findings and comparison of the efficacies of sodium valproate and carbamazepine regimens. *Brain Dev* 2002;24:73–76.

Ghika-Schmid F, Ghika J, Regli F, Bogousslavsky J. Hyperkinetic movement disorders during and after acute stroke: the Lausanne Stroke Registry. *J Neurol Sci* 1997;146:109–116.

Giedd JN, Rapoport JL, Kruesi MJ, et al. Sydenham's chorea: magnetic resonance imaging of the basal ganglia. *Neurology* 1995;45: 2199–2202.

Gonzalez-Alegre P, Ammache Z, Davis PH, Rodnitzky RL. Moyamoya-induced paroxysmal dyskinesia. *Mov Disord* 2003;18:1051–1056.

Hamani C, Saint-Cyr JA, Fraser J, et al. The subthalamic nucleus in the context of movement disorders. *Brain* 2004;127:4–20.

Hardie RJ, Pullon HW, Harding AE, et al. Neuroacanthocytosis: a clinical, haematological and pathological study of 19 cases. *Brain* 1991;114:13–49.

Harrison NA, Church A, Nisbet A, Rudge P, Giovannoni G. Late recurrences of Sydenham's chorea are not associated with anti-basal ganglia antibodies. *J Neurol Neurosurg Psychiatry* 2004;75:1478–1479.

Hernandez-Latorre MA, Roig-Quilis M. The efficiency of carbamazepine in a case of post-streptococcal hemichorea. *Rev Neurol (Spain)* 2003;37:322–326.

Husby G, Van De Rijn U, Zabriskie JB, et al. Antibodies reacting with cytoplasm of subthalamic and caudate nuclei neurons in chorea and acute rheumatic fever. *J Exp Med* 1976;144:1094–1110.

International Huntington Association (IHA) and the World Federation of Neurology (WFN) Research Group on Huntington's Chorea. Guidelines for the molecular genetics predictive test in Huntington's disease. *Neurology* 1994;44:1533–1536.

Jankovic J. Differential diagnosis and etiology of tics. *Adv Neurol* 2001;85:15–29.

Jog MS, Lang AE. Chronic acquired hepatocerebral degeneration: case reports and insights. *Mov Disord* 1995;10:714–722.

Jordan LC, Singer HS. Sydenham chorea in children. *Curr Treat Options Neurol* 2003;5:283–290.

Kalita J, Ranjan P, Misra UK, Das BK. Hemichorea: a rare presentation of tuberculoma. *J Neurol Sci* 2003;208:109–111.

Kinirons P, Fulton A, Keoghan M, et al. Paraneoplastic limbic encephalitis (PLE) and chorea associated with CRMP-5 neuronal antibody. *Neurology* 2003;61:1623–1624.

Kiroan CA, Suvedo SE, Heuser JS, et al. Mimicry and auto-antibody-mediated neuronal cell signaling in Sydenham Chorea. *Nat Med.* 2003;9:914–928.

Korn-Lubetzki I, Brand A, Steiner I. Recurrence of Sydenham chorea: implications for pathogenesis. *Arch Neurol* 2004;61:1261–1264.

Krauss JK, Loher TJ, Weigel R, et al. Chronic stimulation of the globus pallidus internus for treatment of non-DYT1 generalized dystonia and choreoathetosis: 2-year follow up. *J Neurosurg* 2003;98: 785–792.

Kwack C, Vuong KD, Jankovic J. Migraine headache in patients with Tourette syndrome. *Arch Neurol* 2003;60:1595–1598.

Leckman JF. Tourette's syndrome. *Lancet* 2002;360:1577–1586.

Lin JJ, Chang MK. Hemiballism-hemichorea and non-ketotic hyperglicaemia. *J Neurol Neurosurg Psychiatry* 1994;57:748–750.

Louis ED, Lee P, Quinn L, Marder K. Dystonia in Huntington's disease: prevalence and clinical characteristics. *Mov Disord* 1999;14: 95–101.

Lucetti C, Del Dotto P, Gambaccini G, et al. IV amantadine improves chorea in Huntington's disease: an acute randomised, controlled study. *Neurology* 2003;60:1995–1997.

Lussier D, Cruciani RA. Choreiform movements after a single dose of methadone. *J Pain Symptom Manage* 2003;26:688–691.

Maia DP, Teixeira AL Jr, Cunningham MCQ, Cardoso F. Obsessive compulsive behavior, hyperactivity and attention deficit disorder in Sydenham's chorea. *Neurology* 2005;64:1799–1801.

McKee D, Talbot P. Chorea as a presenting feature of variant Creutzfeldt-Jakob disease. *Mov Disord* 2003;18:837–838.

Mercadante MT, Campos MC, Marques-Dias MJ, et al. Vocal tics in Sydenham's chorea. *J Am Acad Child Adolesc Psychiatry* 1997;36:305–306.

Miranda M, Cardoso F, Giovannoni G, Church A. Oral contraceptive induced chorea: another condition associated with anti-basal ganglia antibodies. *J Neurol Neurosurg Psychiatry* 2004;75: 327–328.

Morris JG, Grattan-Smith P, Jankelowitz SK, et al. Athetosis II: the syndrome of mild athetoid cerebral palsy. *Mov Disord* 2002;17: 1281–1287.

Moro E, Lang A, Srafella AP, et al. Bilateral globus pallidus stimulation for Huntington's disease. *Ann Neurol* 2004;56:290–294.

Nausieda PA, Grossman BJ, Koller WC, et al. Sydenham's chorea: an update. *Neurology* 1980;30:331–334.

Ondo WG, Tintner R, Thomas M, Jankovic J. Tetrabenazine treatment for Huntington's disease-associated chorea. *Clin Neuropharmacol* 2002;25:300–302.

Penney Jr JB, Young AB, Shoulson I, et al. Huntington's disease in Venezuela: 7 years of follow-up on symptomatic and asymptomatic individuals. *Mov Disord* 1990;5:93–99.

Piccolo I, Defanti CA, Soliveri P, et al. Cause and course in a series of patients with sporadic chorea. *J Neurol* 2003;250:429–435.

Pisani A, Diomedi M, Rum A, Cianciulli P, Floris R, Orlacchio A, Bernardi G, Calabresi P. Acanthocytosis as a predisposing factor for non-ketotic hyperglycaemia induced chorea-ballism. *J Neurol Neurosurg Psychiatry* 2005;76:1717–1719.

Prashanth LK, Taly AB, Sinha S, Arunodaya GR, Swamy HS. Wilson's disease: diagnostic errors and clinical implications. *J Neurol Neurosurg Psychiatry* 2004;75:907–909.

Quinn N, Schrag A. Huntington's disease and other choreas. *J Neurol* 1998;245:709–716.

Ristic AJ, Svetel M, Dragasevic N, et al. Bilateral chorea-ballism associated with hyperthyroidism. *Mov Disord* 2004;19:982–983.

Ryan M, Antony JH, Grattan-Smith PJ. Sydenham chorea: a resurgence of the 1990s? *J Pediatr Child Health* 2000;36:95–96.

Saiki S, Sakai K, Kitagawa Y, et al. Mutation in the CHAC gene in a family of autosomal dominant chorea-acanthocytosis. *Neurology* 2003;61:1614–1616.

Sanna G, Bertolaccini ML, Cuadrado MJ, et al. Neuropsychiatric manifestations in systemic lupus erythematosus: prevalence and association with antiphospholipid antibodies. *J Rheumatol* 2003; 30:985–992.

Schrag A, Quinn NP, Bhatia KP, Marsden CD. Benign hereditary chorea—entity or syndrome? *Mov Disord* 2000;15:280–288.

Sharp FR, Rando TA, Greenberg SA, et al. Pseudochoreoathetosis: movements associated with loss of proprioception. *Arch Neurol* 1994;51:1103–1109.

Special Writing Group of the Committee of Rheumatic Fever, Endocarditis, and Kawasaki Disease of the Council on Cardio-Vascular Disease of the Young of the American Heart Association. Guidelines for diagnosis of rheumatic fever: Jones criteria, 1992 update. *JAMA* 1992;268:2069–2073.

Stemper B, Thurauf N, Neundorfer B, Heckmann JG. Choreoathetosis related to lithium intoxication. *Eur J Neurol* 2003;10:743–744.

Stevanin G, Fujigasaki H, Lebre AS, et al. Huntington's disease-like phenotype due to trinucleotide repeat expansions in the TBP and JPH3 genes. *Brain* 2003;126:1599–1603.

Swedo SE, Leonard HL, Garvey M, et al. Pediatric autoimmune neuropsychiatric disorders associated with streptococcal infections: clinical description of the first 50 cases. *Am J Psychiatry* 1998; 155:264–271.

Tani LY, Veasy LG, Minich LL, Shaddy RE. Rheumatic fever in children younger than 5 years: is the presentation different? *Pediatrics* 2003;112:1065–1068.

Teixeira Jr AL, Cardoso F, Maia DP, Cunningham MC. Sydenham's chorea may be a risk factor for drug induced parkinsonism. *J Neurol Neurosurg Psychiatry* 2003;74:1350–1351.

Teixeira Jr AL, Cardoso F, Souza ALS, Teixeira MM. Increased serum concentrations of monokine induced by interferon-γ/CXCL9 and interferon-γ-inducible protein 10/CXCL-10 in Sydenham's chorea patients. *J Neuroimmunol* 2004;150:157–62.

Teixeira Jr AL, Guimar„es MM, Romano-Silva MA, Cardoso F. Serum from Sydenham's chorea patients modifies intracellular calcium levels in PC12 cells by a complement independent mechanism. *Mov Disord* 2005a;20:893–895.

Teixeira Jr AL, Maia DP, Cardosa F. Psychosis following acute Sydenham's chorea. *Eur Child Adolesc Psychiatry* 2006 (E pub ahead of print).

Teixeira Jr AL, Maia DP, Cardoso F. UFMG Sydenham's chorea rating scale (USCRS): reliability and consistency. *Mov Disord* 2005b;20:585–591.

Teixeira Jr AL, Maia DP, Cardoso F. Treatment of acute Sydenham's chorea with methyl-prednisolone pulse-therapy. *Parkinsonism Relat Disord.* 2005c;11:323–330.

Teixeira Jr AL, Meira FCA, Maia DP, Cunningham MC, Cardoso F. Migraine headache in patients with Sydenham's chorea. *Cephalalgia* 2005d;25:542–544.

Thobois S, Bozio A, Ninet J, Akhavi A, Broussolle E. Chorea after cardiopulmonary bypass. *Eur Neurol* 2004;51:46–47.

Victor M, Adams RD. The effect of alcohol on the nervous system. In: Metabolic and toxic diseases of the nervous system. ARNMD 1953;32:526–536.

Walker RH, Rasmussen A, Rudnicki D, et al. Huntington's diseaselike 2 can present as chorea-acanthocytosis. *Neurology* 2003a;61: 1002–1004.

Walker RH, Jankovic J, O'Hearn E, Margolis RL. Phenotypic features of Huntington's disease-like 2. *Mov Disord* 2003b;18:1527–1530.

Weindl A, Kuwert T, Leenders KL, et al. Increased striatal glucose consumption in Sydenham's chorea. *Mov Disord* 1993;8:437–444

20

Neurodegeneration with Brain Iron Accumulation

Madhavi Thomas

INTRODUCTION

Iron is essential for normal cellular functioning in the brain. Iron-mediated cell death has been implicated in a variety of neurodegenerative disorders, including Alzheimer's disease, Parkinson's disease (PD), Friedreich's ataxia, and Huntington's disease. Hallervorden-Spatz syndrome (HSS), a childhood onset neurodegenerative movement disorder named after Julius Hallervorden and Hugo Spatz, is associated with pathologic deposition of iron in the basal ganglia (1). Hallervorden's involvement in the euthanasia program has raised serious ethical concerns regarding his research conducted during the Nazi regime in Germany and, therefore, the disorder has been renamed *neurodegeneration with brain iron accumulation* (2,3). Discovery of mutation in the pantothenate kinase II gene and the ferritin light polypeptide (FTL) chain gene in patients with inherited neurodegenerative disorders has firmly established a link between iron deposition and specific genetic and metabolic abnormality (4,5). The following discussion is an exploration of the presence of iron in the brain, both in normal and pathologic states, and clinicopathologic implications for specific movement disorders.

IRON REGULATION IN THE BRAIN

Iron, an important element for neuron survival, is an essential component of cytochrome oxidases and iron sulfur complexes of the oxidative chain; thus it plays an important role in adenosine triphosphate (ATP) production. Iron is also a cofactor for tyrosine hydroxylase and tryptophan hydroxylase, and it plays a critical role in synthesis of neurotransmitters, DNA synthesis, and energy metabolism of the cell via the tricarboxylic acid cycle (6,7).

Areas of the brain involved in motor function, such as the globus pallidus, substantia nigra, dentate nucleus, and motor cortex, contain a high concentration of iron. Iron content of white matter is greater than gray matter; oligodendrocytes and microglia have particularly high iron content (6,8). Neurons store iron in the form of ferritin, which exists as light and heavy chains. Misregulation of ferritin, such as adenine insertion in light chains, can cause inappropriate iron release and result in neurodegeneration, as seen in neuroferritinopathy. Iron has a unique property of being both an electron donor and acceptor with a potential for generating toxic-free radicals. Iron homeostasis is, therefore, critical for normal neuronal function.

There are multiple regulatory pathways for iron metabolism in the cells (see Table 20.1). The pathways of iron processing within the cell are highly complex and involve various intracellular enzymes and organelles. Several genes are involved in the regulation of iron homeostasis in the cell (6,7,8,9). The complexity of the iron regulatory system poses a challenge to our understanding of the role of iron in neurodegenerative disorders.

IRON REGULATION IN PATHOLOGIC STATES

The following discussion is separated into disorders in which there is a specific genetic mutation identified in the iron regulatory pathways and in which there is a possible

TABLE 20.1
RECEPTORS AND ENZYMES INVOLVED IN CELLULAR IRON METABOLISM

Iron Uptake

Transferrin and transferrin receptor
Melanotransferrin, hemochromatosis gene and product
Lactotransferrin and lactotransferrin receptor
Divalent cation transporter (DCT 1), metal transporter protein (MTP 1), and stimulator of iron transport (SFT)

Iron Storage

Ferritin, neuromelanin

Iron Release

Ceruloplasmin (cp)/ferroxidase, hemoxygenase-1 (HO-1)

Intracellular Iron Metabolism

Hemoxygenase-1(HO-1)
Transferrin
Ferroreductases
Possible role for Frataxin and ABC (ATP binding casette)
Possible role for Frataxin and ABC7 (ATP binding casette)

Posttranscriptional Control

Iron regulatory proteins (IRP 1, 2)
Iron responsive elements (IRE)
DCT1
Changes in redox state of the cell

---

role for iron misregulation. Specific genetic mutations in the iron regulatory pathways are seen in pantothenate kinase–associated neurodegeneration (PKAN); hypoprebetalipoproteinemia, acanthocytosis, and retinitis pigmentosa with pallidal degeneration (HARP); neuroferritinopathy; and aceruloplasminemia. The term *neurodegeneration with brain iron accumulation* (NBIA) has been proposed for these disorders (10) (Table 20.2).

DISORDERS WITH SPECIFIC GENETIC MUTATIONS IN THE IRON REGULATORY PATHWAYS

Pantothenate Kinase–Associated Neurodegeneration (PKAN)

Historical Aspects
Julius Hallervorden and Hugo Spatz first described a family containing members with childhood-onset dystonia intellectual impairment, choreoathetosis, dysarthria, and dysphagia with onset at 7–9 years and death by 16–27 years. On autopsy, the patients had rust-brown discoloration of the globus pallidus and substantia nigra pars reticulata (1). Since this original description, several cases with similar features have been described in literature.

Classification
Dooling et al. (11) in 1974 categorized these patients into three groups: familial and nonfamilial cases of HSS were included in group I (Ia and Ib, respectively), typical cases of HSS without nigral lesions were included in group II, and group III included cases that were clinically atypical but pathologically typical. A variety of clinical features in the 64 cases—including ataxia, myoclonus, tremor, retinal pigmentary changes, seizures, spasticity, dementia, hyperreflexia, and seizures—were identified, establishing for the first time the diverse clinical presentation of this disorder. Patients with familial syndrome (group 1a) had dystonia, choreoathetosis, rigidity, tremor, and hyperreflexia with relentless progression of the disease resulting in death in early adulthood. Group II included patients with clinical presentation similar to group I with pathologic changes in the globus pallidus. Group III included patients with pathological findings similar to typical cases but variable clinical presentation (11). Swaiman (12,13) proposed classification of cases described under the terminology of HSS based on age at onset into early (onset <10 years of age), late (onset between 10 and 18 years of age), and adult-onset types. Early-onset cases included those with slow and rapid progression, while late- and adult-onset cases were slowly progressive.

TABLE 20.2

NEURODEGENERATION WITH BRAIN IRON ACCUMULATION

Primary Genetic Abnormalities in Iron Metabolic Pathways

Autosomal Dominant

Neuroferritinopathy

Autosomal Recessive

1. Pantothenate kinase–associated neurodegeneration:
   i. Childhood-onset and adult-onset PKAN with PANK-2 mutation
   ii. Hypoprebetalipoproteinemia, acanthocytosis, and pallidal degeneration (HARP)
2. Disorders with clinical presentation similar to PKAN but negative for PANK-2 mutation
   i. Disorders described as Hallervorden-Spatz syndrome (HSS) in the literature
   ii. Karak syndrome
3. Aceruloplasminemia
4. Hemochromatosis

Genetic Disorders with Role in Iron Metabolism

Huntington's disease
Friedreich's ataxia
Restless legs syndrome

Involvement of Iron in Cell Death Pathways

Parkinson's disease
Alzheimer's disease

Genetics

Genetic studies in patients with HSS resulted in identification of a linkage to chromosome 20p13, and the locus was termed *neurodegeneration with brain iron accumulation type 1* (NBIA-1) (14). In 2001, Zhou et al. identified the mutation in the pantothenate kinase-2 gene (PANK-2) on chromosome 20p13 (15). Hayflick et al. suggested the term *pantothenate kinase–associated neurodegeneration* (PKAN) for those cases with mutation in the PANK-2 gene with the clinical presentation of parkinsonism or dystonia in association with pyramidal tract signs, retinitis pigmentosa, and—in some cases—intellectual impairment, with evidence of iron deposition in the basal ganglia based on imaging findings or pathology (4). PANK-2 mutation analysis included both adult- and childhood-onset cases. Mutations with predicted protein truncation were associated with a rapidly progressive early-onset form of the disease. In the adult-onset form, slowly, progressive form mutations were mainly amino acid changes. Two missense mutations—G411 R and T418 M—were the most common mutations, and G411R was a semidominant mutation (16).

Pathogenesis

Pantothenate kinase is a regulatory enzyme in coenzyme A biosynthesis. PANK-2 is important for cytosolic phosphorylation of pantothenate (vitamin B_5), N-pantothenoyl cysteine, and pantetheine. Coenzyme A, an acyl carrier, plays an important role in intermediary and fatty acid metabolism. One can hypothesize that phosphopantothenate deficiency leads to accumulation of cysteine, which undergoes rapid auto-oxidation in the presence of iron, resulting in iron-induced lipid peroxidation that leads to cell damage (15). Accumulation of cysteine due to cysteine dioxygenase deficiency has been shown in clinical studies in patients with HSS (17).

Clinical Features

Common clinical features of PKAN include parkinsonism, dystonia, tremor, cognitive abnormalities, choreoathetosis, rigidity, hyperreflexia, and retinal pigmentary changes. Atypical findings include myoclonus, tics, seizures, and ataxia. In our study of clinical heterogeneity of PKAN, we were able to identify differences in clinical presentation in patients with and without PANK-2 gene mutation. Patients with disease onset at a young age presented with dystonia while those with adult-onset disease had parkinsonism as the initial symptom (18). Some patients with clinically or pathologically diagnosed HSS may have PANK-2 mutations, but the frequency of this metabolic defect in these patients is not known. In addition to defects in the pantothenate pathway, many other metabolic or genetic abnormalities may be responsible for the clinical phenotype of HSS (18). Clinical and neuropathological features

TABLE 20.3

CLINICAL, PATHOLOGIC, AND MRI FINDINGS OF DISORDERS WITH SPECIFIC MUTATIONS IN IRON METABOLISM

Disorder	Clinical Features	Biochemical Features	Brain MRI	Pathology
PKAN	Dystonia, parkinsonism, dysarthria, gait disorder, dementia, spasticity, tics, RP, OA, chorea	Co A pathway is affected	"Eye of the tiger" sign T2 proton relaxation enhancement due to iron in GP	Iron in GP (Gpi), SN, gliosis Axonal spheroids, GCI, NFT LB's, synuclein, tau, dystrophic neurites
HARP	Dystonia, parkinsonism, choreoathetosis Retinitis Pigmentosa	Hypoprebetalipoproteinemia Acanthocytosis	"Eye of the tiger" sign	Pallidal degeneration
Neuroferritinopathy	Dystonia dysarthria, orolingual dyskinesias, lingual tremor, cerebellar signs, choreoathetosis, blepharospasm, frontal lobe dysfunction	Decreased serum ferritin Abnormal muscle biopsy	Hyperintense T2, striatum, SN, hypointense T1, GP, dentate	Iron in GP, SN Axonal spheroids, ubiquitin, tau, ferritin-positive inclusions
Aceruloplasminemia	Diabetes, ataxia, dystonia, blepharospasm, chorea, parkinsonism, tremor, retinal degeneration, dementia	Absent serum ceruloplasmin High serum ferritin Low serum copper, iron	T1,T2 hypointensities in striatum, thalamus dentate nucleus	Iron in striatum, cortex Iron in cerebellum Neuronal loss, iron in glial cells and iron in neurons

HARP, hypoprebetalipoproteinemia, acanthocytosis, retinitis pigmentosa, pallidal degeneration; PKAN, pantothenate kinase–associated neurodegeneration.

of PKAN and other disorders included under NBIA are summarized in Table 20.3.

HARP is a disorder with clinical manifestation of parkinsonism, dystonia, and choreoathetosis, in addition to the previously mentioned laboratory abnormalities. Higgins et al. (19) and Orrell et al. (20) described cases of HARP syndrome with clinical features of dystonia since childhood, in addition to the biochemical abnormalities and magnetic resonance imaging (MRI) findings of the "eye of the tiger" sign. HARP has been shown to have an arg371-to-ter (R371X) mutation in the PANK-2 gene (21). Houlden et al. (22) identified compound heterozygosity for mutations in the PANK-2 gene: a met 327-to-thr (M327T) substitution and a splice mutation. Further characterization of the mutations in other cases of HSS may help identify additional disease mechanisms.

Radiologic Findings

Brain MRI usually shows abnormalities in the globus pallidus and the substantia nigra pars reticulata. The abnormalities are better demonstrated on high-field MRI (1.5 T). Due to preferential T2 proton relaxation enhancement (i.e., very low signal intensity), MRI demonstrates iron deposition (16,23,24,25). An area of high signal intensity is sometimes seen in the central part of the pallidum and is due to the smaller amount of iron and greater amount of water content. This finding is described as the "eye of the tiger" sign (23) (Fig. 20.1).

Diagnosis

Based on clinical presentation, diagnostic criteria were proposed by Swaiman (12,13). He proposed criteria for HSS, which are similar to those for PKAN. Obligate features included progressive disease with onset within first 2 decades of life, evidence of one or more extrapyramidal features, dystonia, rigidity, and choreoathetosis, in addition to a finding of hypodense areas in the globus pallidus and substantia nigra on MRI of the brain. Corroborative features include corticospinal tract involvement, progressive intellectual impairment retinitis pigmentosa and/or optic atrophy, and family history consistent with autosomal recessive inheritance. In addition to the clinical features, abnormal cystosomes in circulating lymphocytes and/or sea-blue histiocytes on bone marrow are supportive laboratory findings. Exclusionary features for HSS include absence of extrapyramidal signs, abnormal ceruloplasmin levels, neuronal ceroid lipofuscinosis, family history of Huntington's disease, autosomal dominant movement disorder, caudate atrophy on MRI of brain, hexosaminidase A or GM1 galactosidase deficiency, and a nonprogressive course.

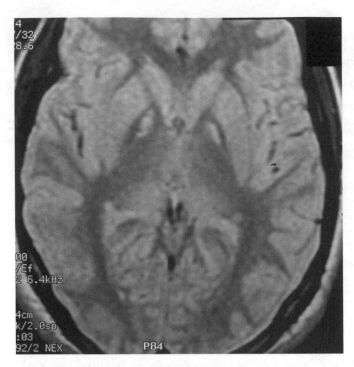

Figure 20.1 MRI brain image of patient with pantothenate kinase–associated neurodegeneration and the classic "eye of the tiger" sign.

Differential Diagnosis

Differential diagnosis of PKAN includes childhood-onset dystonias, including dopa-responsive dystonia, ceroid lipofuscinosis, and infantile neuroaxonal dystrophy.

Treatment

No specific disease-modifying treatment is available at this time. Chelating agents for removal of iron have not been successful in the past. Dystonia with parkinsonism seems to respond to dopaminergic agents, such as levodopa. Dystonia and tremor also respond to botulinum toxin injections. Seizures can be treated with anticonvulsants such as carbamazepine, and phenytoin, but newer drugs also may have a role. Rehabilitation and multidisciplinary supportive therapy are helpful in improving quality of life for patients (12,13).

Neuroferritinopathy

A recently described autosomal dominant neurodegenerative disorder, neuroferritinopathy occurs due to abnormal iron deposition in the basal ganglia associated with clinical features of dystonia and choreoathetosis, with a mutation in the gene encoding the FTL chain on chromosome 19q13.3.

Genetics and Clinical Presentation

First described in a family from Cumbria in Northern England in 2002 by Curtis et al. (5), all patients in this family had a single adenine insertion between nucleotides

460 and 461 in exon 4 of the FTL gene. Patients had low serum ferritin since the FTL chain is a major component of serum ferritin. Clinical manifestations include choreoathetosis, dystonia, spasticity, rigidity, and sometimes acute progression. One patient showed palatal tremor, oral-lingual dyskinesia, unsteadiness, and frontal lobe dysfunction (5). A French family with neuroferritinopathy was described by Chinnery et al. (26). Seven patients in this family with onset between 24–48 years had clinical manifestations of dystonia, dysarthria, chorea, parkinsonism, blepharospasm, cerebellar signs, and cognitive impairment, and some showed frontal lobe dysfunction. These patients had the same mutation as the British family. Abnormal muscle biopsy with skeletal muscle changes in mitochondrial complex I, III, IV was an additional finding in these patients. Vidal et al. (27) described cerebellar features in addition to tremor, parkinsonism, and dystonia in association with pathological findings of neuroferritinopathy. Maciel et al. (28) reported the case of a 19-year-old man with clinical features of parkinsonism, ataxia, and corticospinal signs. A mutation in the FTL gene (A96T; 134790.0013) and decreased serum ferritin were found in this patient, his mother, and his asymptomatic brother. Brain MRI showed bilateral pallidal necrosis in the patient and his mother.

Imaging Studies

MRI changes were similar in the families previously described (26). The MRI brain images show central hyperintensity on T2 weighted images in the caudate, putamen, globus pallidus, and subtantia nigra and T1 hypointensity in the globus pallidus and dentate nucleus (5,26).

Pathology

Pathological changes were similar to those of PKAN, with reddish-brown discoloration of basal ganglia. Extracellular ferritin-positive inclusions were localized to the globus pallidus, forebrain, and cerebellum. Inclusions were extracellular but colocalized with microglia, neurons, and oligodendrocytes. Pathologically, intranuclear and intracytoplasmic bodies containing FTL and ferritin heavy polypeptide (FTH1) were found in glia and subsets of neurons in the striatum and cerebellar cortex, as well as in extra neural tissue (27). Axonal spheroids were immunoreactive for neurofilaments, ubiquitin, and tau in the striatum and white matter tracts (5).

Differential Diagnosis

Autosomal dominant neurodegenerative diseases, such as Huntington's disease and dentatopallidorubroluysian atrophy, should be considered due to the presence of similar clinical features; however, in neuroferritinopathy the neurological abnormalities are associated with low serum ferritin, which would help in diagnosis.

Treatment

Mostly supportive treatment, as discussed in the section on PKAN. No curative treatments are available.

Aceruloplasminemia

Ceruloplasmin is a multicopper ferroxidase responsible for iron homeostasis in the brain. Aceruloplasminemia is an autosomal recessive disorder associated with mutations in the *ceruloplasmin* gene, resulting in iron overload in the brain and viscera. This disorder shows the effects of abnormal iron regulation due to mutations in the *ceruloplasmin* gene, linking the genetic abnormality with pathologic changes in the basal ganglia resulting from iron deposition.

Genetics

Aceruloplasminemia is caused by mutations in the *ceruloplasmin* gene itself, resulting in iron overload in the brain and other organs, and paradoxical decrease in the serum iron. Mutations were described in the exons 3, 7, 13, 15, and 18 in the *ceruloplasmin* gene on chromosome 3q23-24 (29,30,31,32,33,34,35). Iron deposition in this disorder is seen in the basal ganglia, retina, liver, and pancreas.

Clinical Features

Patients usually present with diabetes between 30–39 years of age (40% of cases), followed in the fifth decade with neurologic symptoms (71% of cases). Clinical triad of aceruloplasminemia includes retinal degeneration, diabetes mellitus, and neurological symptoms. Ataxia, blepharospasm, dystonia, tremor, parkinsonism, chorea, nystagmus, gait disorder, and rigidity are commonly seen in association with cognitive dysfunction and dementia (36,37).

Pathology

Iron deposition is seen in the striatum, cerebral cortex, and cerebellum, but the greatest iron concentration is in the liver. Measures of lipid peroxidation, such as malondialdehyde (MDA) and 4-hydroxynonenal (4-HNE), are more elevated in the putamen than in the cortex of patients. Mild atrophy of the cerebral cortex, cerebellum, midbrain tegmentum, and pons is noted on autopsy. The basal ganglia, thalamus, and dentate nucleus of the cerebellum show brownish pigmentation due to iron deposition. Microscopic examination shows iron deposition in glial cells and neurons in association with a neuronal loss in the affected areas, with the greatest cell loss in the striatum. Despite the loss of Purkinje cells in the cerebellum, the granular cell layer is unaffected. The substantia nigra and dentate nucleus have moderate neuronal loss (37,38,39).

Differential Diagnosis

One must consider Wilson's disease, Menke's disease, parkinsonism, and PKAN in the differential diagnosis due to common features of tremor, parkinsonian features, and dystonia. However, biochemical features of serum ceruloplasmin, copper, and iron would help distinguish this disorder.

Diagnosis

Absence of serum ceruloplasmin and low serum copper, low serum iron, high serum ferritin, and increased hepatic iron concentration indicate aceruloplasminemia. Characteristic T1 and T2 hypointensities on brain MRI, reflecting iron accumulation in the striatum, thalamus, and dentate nucleus, support the diagnosis of aceruloplasminemia (36,37).

Disease-Specific Treatment

Treatment options include iron chelating agents (i.e., desferrioxamine) to decrease tissue iron overload. Intravenous administration of fresh-frozen human plasma increases the serum iron content, resulting in improvement of neurologic symptoms (40).

Karak Syndrome

Mubaidin et al. (41) in 2003 reported a family from Karak with early-onset progressive cerebellar ataxia, dystonia, spasticity, and intellectual decline with cerebellar atrophy and "eye of the tiger" sign on brain MRI, in addition to findings of iron deposition in the putamen and substantia nigra. A linkage analysis showed no association with the PANK-2 gene, identifying this as yet another disorder that probably can be classified under the category of NBIA.

OTHER CLINICAL DISORDERS ASSOCIATED WITH IRON DEPOSITION IN THE BRAIN

Hemochromatosis is a hereditary disorder of iron overload in the visceral organs. Hemochromatosis can result from defects in genes encoding HFE, transferrin receptor 2, ferroportin, hepcidin, and hemojuvelin. Hepcidin, a hepatic peptide, is an iron regulatory hormone, and mutations in the gene coding for hepcidin have been shown in juvenile hemochromatosis. Ferroportin gene abnormlities also are seen in patients with hemochromatosis. Hepcidin regulates the activity of ferroportin iron transporter. When hepcidin levels are low, there is increased activity of ferroportin transporter, resulting in iron overload in cells. The known causes of hemochromatosis interrupt normal iron homeostasis. Most patients with hemochromatosis have mutations in the

HFE gene. The C282Y mutation in the HFE gene leads to iron sequestration, while the H63D mutation is less penetrant and is a susceptibility factor for hemochromatosis (42). Few case reports of parkinsonism in association with hemochromatosis have been published (43,44,45,46). A recent genetic study indicated that a higher incidence of C282Y heterozygous mutation in patients with hemochromatosis is associated with a higher incidence of parkinsonism. The numbers in this study are small, but no clear indication is given regarding correlation of clinical syndrome with MRI findings (45). Further studies are needed to investigate long-term neurologic problems in patients with hemochromatosis (43,44,45,46).

Other movement disorders, such as PD, Friedreich's ataxia, and Huntington's disease, have been associated with abnormalities in the iron pathways leading to accumulation of iron, local changes resulting in oxidative damage, and neurodegeneration. Complete discussion of these disorders is beyond the scope of this review. Searches for mutations in the FTL chain have yielded no results in PD (47). Overexpression of lactoferrin receptor and of divalent metal transporter (DMT-1) in the substantia nigra has been demonstrated in PD (48). Huntington's disease is an autosomal dominant disorder shown to have a triplet repeat expansion (CAG) in the first exon of the HD gene (coding for *huntingtin*, a protein product) localized to chromosome 4p16.3 (49). *Huntingtin* has been shown to alter proteasomal function, resulting in caspase activation via the mitochondrial cytochrome release, and it is a regulator for transferrin receptor protein (50).

Friedreich's ataxia is an autosomal recessive triplet repeat disorder characterized clinically by progressive ataxia of the limbs and trunk with onset before 25 years of age; proprioceptive loss, areflexia, and extensor plantar reflexes occur in the presence of scoliosis and cardiac abnormalities. Friedreich's ataxia is caused by mutations of the frataxin (X25) gene on chromosome 9q13 (51). Causative mutations can be homozygous unstable GAA-repeat expansion in the first intron of the frataxin gene (94%–98% of patients) or heterozygous GAA-repeat expansion in one allele of the frataxin gene and a point mutation in the other allele (52,53). Mitochondrial function depends on a continuous supply of iron to the iron-sulfur cluster (ISC) and heme biosynthetic pathways, as well as on the ability to prevent iron-catalyzed oxidative damage. Frataxin has shown specific mechanisms of sequestering and forming complexes in mitochondria that help to detoxify redox iron (54).

CONCLUSION: RESEARCH IMPLICATIONS

From the preceding discussion, we can conclude that the metabolic pathways of iron are complex processes and that even those disorders described as having primary genetic defects in proteins in iron metabolism are not well-understood. Recent articles about mitochondrial localization of PANK-2 again raise the question of whether the iron misregulation is a secondary process (55). Development of mouse models of disease with particular attention to the iron metabolic pathways has helped our understanding of certain gene defects in various disorders of iron regulatory proteins (56).

However, the critical question of whether iron misregulation is a primary or secondary event remains to be answered. Although defects in disorders such as hemochromatosis are suggestive of a systemic iron regulatory disorder, the role of iron in other primary neurodegenerative disorders, such as PD and restless legs syndrome (discussed in other chapters) (57,58), is still poorly understood. It is hoped that future genomic and proteomic studies of these disorders will add to our understanding of iron regulation in the nervous system and its role in neurodegeneration.

REFERENCES

1. Hallervorden J, Spatz H. Eigenartige Erkrankung im extrapyramidalen System mit besonderer Beteiligung des Globus pallidus und der Substantia nigra.: Ein Beitrag zu den Beziehungen zwischen diesen beiden Zentren. *Z Ges Neurol Psychiat* 1922;79:254–302.
2. Shevell M. Racial hygiene, active euthanasia, and Julius Hallervorden. *Neurology* 1992;12:2214–2219.
3. Shevell M. Hallervorden and history. *NEJM* 2003;348:3–4.
4. Zhou B, Westaway SK, Levinson B, Johnson MA, Gitschier J, Hayflick SJ. A novel pantothenate kinase gene (PANK2) is defective in Hallervorden-Spatz syndrome. *Nat Genet* 2001;28:345–349.
5. Curtis AR, Fey C, Morris CM, et al. Mutation in the gene encoding ferritin light polypeptide causes dominant adult-onset basal ganglia disease. *Nat Genet* 2001;28:350–354.
6. Connor JR, Menzies SL, Burdo JR, Boyer PJ. Iron and iron management proteins in neurobiology. *Pediatr Neurol* 2001;25:118–129.
7. Beal MF. Mitochondrial dysfunction in neurodegenerative diseases. *Biochim Bipphys Acta* 1998;1366:211–223.
8. Connor JR, Menzies SL. Relationship of iron to oligodendrocytes and myelination. *Glia* 1996;17:83–93.
9. Rouault TA. Systemic iron metabolism: a review and implications for brain iron metabolism. *Pediatr Neurol* 2001;25:130–137.
10. Hayflick SJ, Westaway SK, Levinson B, et al. Genetic, clinical and radiographic delineation of Hallervorden-Spatz syndrome. *NEJM* 2003;348:33–40.
11. Dooling EC, Schoene WC, Richardson EP Jr. Hallervorden Spatz syndrome. *Arch Neurol* 1974;30:70–83.
12. Swaiman KF. Hallervorden-Spatz syndrome and brain iron metabolism. *Arch Neurol* 1991;48:1285–1293.
13. Swaiman KF. Hallervorden-Spatz syndrome. *Pediatr Neurol* 2001;25:102–108.
14. Taylor TD, Litt M, Kramer P, et al. Homozygosity mapping of Hallervorden-Spatz syndrome to chromosome 20p12.3-p13. *Nat Genet* 1996;14:479–481.
15. Zhou B, Westaway SK, Levinson B, Johnson MA, Gitschier J, Hayflick SJ. A novel pantothenate kinase gene (PANK2) is defective in Hallervorden-Spatz syndrome. *Nat Genet* 2001;28:345–349.
16. Hayflick SJ, Westaway SK, Levinson B, et al. Genetic, clinical, and radiographic delineation of Hallervorden-Spatz syndrome. *N Engl J Med* 2003;348:33–40.
17. Perry TL, Norman MG, Yong VW, et al. Hallervorden-Spatz disease: cysteine accumulation and cysteine dioxygenase deficiency in the globus pallidus. *Ann Neurol* 1985;18:482–489.
18. Thomas M, Hayflick SJ, Jankovic J. Clinical heterogeneity of neurodegeneration with brain iron accumulation (Hallervorden Spatz syndrome) and pantothenate kinase–associated neurodegeneration. *Mov Disord* 2004;8:36–42.
19. Higgins JJ, Patterson MC, Papadopoulos NM, et al. Hypoprebetalipoproteinemia, acanthocytosis, retinitis pigmentosa, and

pallidal degeneration (HARP syndrome). *Neurology* 1992;42: 194–198

20. Orrell RW, Amrolia PJ, Heald A, et al. Acanthocytosis, retinitis pigmentosa, and pallidal degeneration: a report of three patients including the second reported case with hypoprebetalipoproteinemia (HARP syndrome). *Neurology* 1995;45:487–492

21. Ching KH, Westaway SK, Gitschier J, Higgins JJ, Hayflick SJ. HARP syndrome is allelic with pantothenate kinase-associated neurodegeneration. *Neurology* 2002;58:1673–1674.

22. Houlden H, Lincoln S, Farrer M, Cleland P, Hardy J, Orrell RW. Compound heterozygous PANK2 mutations confirm HARP and Hallervorden-Spatz syndromes are allelic. *Neurology* 2003;61: 1423–1426.

23. Savoiardo M, Halliday WC, Nardocci N, et al. Hallervorden-Spatz disease: MR and pathologic findings. *AJNR Am J Neuroradiol* 1993;14:155–162.

24. Sethi KD, Adams RJ, Loring DW, el Gammal T. Hallervorden-Spatz syndrome: clinical and magnetic resonance imaging correlations. *Ann Neurol* 1988;24:692–694.

25. Feliciani M, Curatolo P. Early clinical and imaging (high-field MRI) diagnosis of Hallervorden-Spatz disease. *Neuroradiology* 1994;36:247–248.

26. Chinnery PF, Curtis ARJ, Fey C, et al. Neuroferritinopathy in a French family with late onset dominant dystonia. *J Med Genet* 2003;40:e69.

27. Vidal R, Ghetti B, Takao M, et al. Intracellular ferritin accumulation in neural and extraneural tissue characterizes a neurodegenerative disease associated with a mutation in the ferritin light polypeptide gene. *J Neuropathol Exp Neurol* 2004;63:363–380.

28. Maciel P, Cruz VT, Constante M, et al. Neuroferritinopathy: missense mutation in FTL causing early-onset bilateral pallidal involvement. *Neurology* 2005;65:603–605.

29. Harris ZL, Takahashi Y, Miyajima H, Serizawa M, MacGillivray RT, Gitlin JD. Aceruloplasminemia: molecular characterization of this disorder of iron metabolism. *Proc Natl Acad Sci USA* 1995; 92:2539–2543.

30. Daimon M, Kato T, Kawanami T, et al. A nonsense mutation of the ceruloplasmin gene in hereditary ceruloplasmin deficiency with diabetes mellitus. *Biochem Biophys Res Commun* 1995;217: 89–95.

31. Daimon M, Susa S, Ohizumi T, et al. A novel mutation of the ceruloplasmin gene in a patient with heteroallelic ceruloplasmin gene mutation (HypoCPGM). *Tohoku J Exp Med* 2000;191: 119–125.

32. Harris ZL, Migas MC, Hughes AE, Logan JI, Gitlin JD. Familial dementia due to a frameshift mutation in the ceruloplasmin gene. *QJM* 1996;89:355–359.

33. Hatanaka Y, Okano T, Oda K, Yamamoto K, Yoshida K. Aceruloplasminemia with juvenile-onset diabetes mellitus caused by exon skipping in the ceruloplasmin gene. *Intern Med* 2003;42: 599–604.

34. Yoshida K, Furihata K, Takeda S. et al. (1995) A mutation in the ceruloplasmin gene is associated with systemic hemosiderosis in humans. *Nat Genet* 1995 9:267–272.

35. Miyajima H, Kohno S, Takahashi Y, Yonekawa O, Kanno T. Estimation of the gene frequency of aceruloplasminemia in Japan. *Neurology* 1999;53:617–619.

36. Miyajima H, Nishimura Y, Mizoguchi K, Sakamoto M, Shimizu T, Honda N. Familial apoceruloplasmin deficiency associated with blepharospasm and retinal degeneration. *Neurology* 1987;37: 761–767.

37. Miyajima H, Takahashi Y, Kono S. Aceruloplasminemia: an inherited disorder of iron metabolism. *Biometals* 2003;16:205–213.

38. Kaneko K, Yoshida K, Arima K, et al. Astrocytic deformity and globular structures are characteristic of the brains of patients with aceruloplasminemia. *J Neuropathol Exp Neurol* 2002;61: 1069–1077.

39. Kawanami T, Kato T, Daimon M, et al. Hereditary caeruloplasmin deficiency: clinicopathological study of a patient. *J Neurol Neurosurg Psychiatry* 1999;61:506–509.

40. Miyajima H, Takahashi Y, Kamata T, Shimizu H, Sakai N, Gitlin JD. Use of desferrioxamine in the treatment of aceruloplasminemia. *Ann Neurol* 1997;41:404–407.

41. Mubaidin A, Roberts E, Hampshire D, et al. Karak syndrome: a novel degenerative disorder of the basal ganglia and cerebellum. *J Med Genet* 2003;40:543–546.

42. Beutler E. Hemochromatosis: genetics and pathophysiology. *Annu Rev Med* 2006;57:331–347.

43. Buchanan DD, Silburn PA, Chalk JB, Le Couteur DG, Mellick GD. The Cys282Tyr polymorphism in the HFE gene in Australian Parkinson's disease patients. *J Neurol Neurosurg Psychiatry* 1995;59: 318–321.

44. Nielsen JE, Jensen LN, Krabbe K. Hereditary haemochromatosis: a case of iron accumulation in the basal ganglia associated with a parkinsonian syndrome. *J Neurol Neurosurg Psychiatry* 1995;59: 318–321.

45. Dekker MC, Giesbergen PC, Njajou OT, et al. Mutations in the hemochromatosis gene (HFE), Parkinson's disease and parkinsonism. *Neurosci Lett* 2002;327:91–94.

46. Costello DJ, Walsh SL, Harrington HJ, Walsh CH. Concurrent hereditary haemochromatosis and idiopathic Parkinson's disease: a case report series. *J Neurol Neurosurg Psychiatry* 2004;75:631–633.

47. Chen R, Langston JW, Chan P. Screening of ferritin light polypeptide 460-461InsA mutation in Parkinson's disease patients in North America. *Neurosci Lett* 2002;335:144–146.

48. Faucheux BA, Nillesse N, Damier P, et al. Expression of lactoferrin receptors is increased in the mesencephalon of patients with Parkinson disease. *Proc Natl Acad Sci USA.* 1995;92:9603–9607.

49. The Huntington's Disease Collaborative Research Group. A novel gene containing a trinucleotide repeat that is expanded and unstable on Huntington's disease chromosomes. *Cell* 1993;72: 971–983.

50. Hilditch-Maguire P, Trettel F, Passani LA, et al. Huntingtin: an iron-regulated protein essential for normal nuclear and perinuclear organelles. *Hum Mol Genet* 2000;9:2789–2797.

51. Campuzano V, Montermini L, Molto MD, et al. Friedreich's ataxia: autosomal recessive disease caused by an intronic GAA triplet repeat expansion [see comments]. *Science* 1996;271: 1423–1427.

52. Monros E, Molto MD, Martinez F, et al. Phenotype correlation and intergenerational dynamics of the Friedreich ataxia GAA trinucleotide repeat. *Am J Hum Genet* 1997;61:101–110.

53. Rotig A, de Lonlay P, Chretien D, et al. Aconitase and mitochondrial iron-sulphur protein deficiency in Friedreich ataxia. *Nat Genet* 1997;17:215–217.

54. O'Neill HA, Gakh O, Park S, et al. Assembly of human frataxin is a mechanism for detoxifying redox-active iron. *Biochemistry* 2005;44:537–545.

55. Johnson MA, Kuo YM, Westaway SK, et al. Mitochondrial localization of human PANK2 and hypotheses of secondary iron accumulation in pantothenate kinase-associated neurodegeneration *Ann NY Acad Sci* 2004;1012:282–298.

56. Meyron-Holtz EG, Ghosh MC, Iwai K, et al. Genetic ablations of iron regulatory proteins 1 and 2 reveal why iron regulatory protein 2 dominates iron homeostasis. *EMBO J* 2004;23:386–395.

57. Haba-Rubio J, Staner L, Petiau C, Erb G, Schunck T, Macher JP. Restless legs syndrome and low brain iron levels in patients with haemochromatosis. *J Neurol Neurosurg Psychiatry* 2005;76: 1009–1010.

58. Trenkwalder C, Paulus W, Walters AS. The restless legs syndrome. *Lancet Neurol* 2005;8:465–75.

59. Morgan NV, Westaway SK, Morton JE, et al. PLA2G6, encoding a phospholipase A(2), is mutated in neurodegenerative disorders with high brain iron. *Nat Genet* 2006;38:752–754.

60. Hayflick SJ, Hartman M, Coryell J et al. Brain MEI in neurodegeneration with brain iron accumulation with and without PANK2 mutations. *AJNR Am J Neuroradiol* 2006;27:1230–1233.

61. Bartzokis G, Tishler TA, Lu PH, et al. Brain ferritin iron may influence age- and gender-related risks of neurodegeneration. *Neurobiol Aging* 2006;22 [Epub ahead of print].

Neurologic Aspects of Wilson's Disease: Clinical Manifestations and Treatment Considerations

21

Peter LeWitt   *Ronald Pfeiffer*

Progressive hepatolenticular degeneration, or Wilson's disease (WD), though only a rare cause of movement disorders, occupies an important place in the history of neurology. Over the past century, it has evolved from a confusing, heterogeneous syndrome to a disease entity whose molecular identity is becoming rapidly ascertained. In a 1912 monograph, S. A. Kinnier Wilson, a young British neurologist at the National Hospital for Nervous Diseases, Queen Square, elucidated the key features of this previously unrecognized disease (1). His report defined this disorder from extensive analysis of 4 cases together with reexamination of 6 cases previously studied by others. Initially termed *progressive lenticular degeneration* and now synonymous with Wilson's name, WD represents one of medical science's successes in deciphering the biochemical and molecular biological basis for a systemic disease.

WD can take on a puzzling array of clinical findings that can be easy to overlook. In Wilson's day, several syndromes had been described corresponding to the same disorder he defined. These included entities termed *tetanoid chorea* by Gowers (2), *pseudosclerosis* by Westphal (3) and Strümpell

(4), and *Wohl Lues hereditaria tarde* by Homen (5). Wilson's 1912 report correctly established the relationship between liver involvement and central nervous system (CNS) disease and characterized the pathologic changes unique to this disorder. Wilson also offered insights into the basis for the distinctive types of clinical impairment. In his monograph, Wilson made no mention of the corneal opacification now recognized as nearly always present in WD with CNS involvement, nor did he have an inkling as to the role of copper, despite tissue color changes suggestive of the presence of this metal. Nonetheless, the description of *progressive lenticular degeneration* initiated a flood of clinical and laboratory research, which eventually transformed this illness from a disabling and ultimately fatal condition to a disorder with several treatment options and the potential for presymptomatic diagnosis.

Since WD is inherited as an autosomal recessive disorder, carriers of the gene develop the disease only if they are homozygous. The gene appears to be fully penetrant: All individuals homozygous for WD will develop some form of the disease (and their siblings have a 25% risk of doing so).

It is extremely unlikely for consecutive generations to be affected, although this has been described (6). Inheritance of the *WD* gene does not appear to dictate the pattern of predilection for different sites of organ involvement, age of onset, or disease severity. The gene for WD has been estimated to be carried in 1 of every 40,000 births. Based on this estimate, the number of homozygotes in the United States would be approximately 5,000 to 6,000 cases, and the carrier frequency may be as great as 1% of the population. Hence, the risk for relatives of an affected patient is 1 in 200 for offspring, 1 in 600 for nieces and nephews, and 1 in 800 for first cousins (7). Even within the same family, clinical manifestations of WD, including sites of organ involvement and age of onset, can vary greatly (8).

In the past decade, linkage analysis studies in affected families have shown that there is a single disease locus for WD, residing on chromosome 13 (9). Most aspects of clinical heterogeneity (i.e., hepatic versus neurologic presentations) probably do not seem to be determined by features of genetic heterogeneity (at least at the level of the gene locus) (7). The discovery of the human gene locus at a single marker interval, 13q14.3 (10), identified a mutation in copper- and membrane-binding ATPase, called *ATP7B*. The protein product of *ATP7B* is essential for the normal transport and intracellular distribution of copper using an ATP-dependent process (11,12). The regulation of this protein's expression by copper has recently been characterized with functional gene expression techniques in insects (13). A large variety of *ATP7B* mutation types (including frameshift, splice site, missense, and nonsense) can lead to WD (14). A further advance in studying the pathophysiology of WD has been aided by the discovery of an animal homologue, a genetic form of hepatitis in the Long Evans Cinnamon rat (15,16). With this model, which is susceptible to systemic toxicity from copper excess resembling that found in WD, various therapeutic interventions, such as hepatocyte transplantation, can be explored (17).

The pathophysiology of WD has a unitary theme in a systemic defect of copper metabolism. Copper derived from the diet is normally excreted into the bile (18). All patients with WD are unable to excrete copper to an adequate extent (19–21). The defect in copper excretion is likely a problem of protein complexing, though the exact mechanism has not been determined. WD is not necessarily due to the defect in the production of ceruloplasmin, a liver-derived copper-binding protein whose serum concentrations are generally (but not always) decreased in WD. While a useful diagnostic marker of the disease, ceruloplasmin is generated by a structural gene residing on chromosome 3. Since the gene for WD is on chromosome 13, other mechanisms must be invoked if a defect in ceruloplasmin synthesis is also involved in the pathophysiology of WD (22).

WD provided the first example of a progressive neurologic deterioration that could be explained by a neurotoxic mechanism linked to a biological defect (23). The disease appears to be solely the outcome from excessive deposition of copper, a dietary mineral whose presence in trace amounts is necessary for life. Massive amounts of copper are deposited throughout the body at sites where damage to tissues is observed, as shown by radiolabeled copper studies (24). Though WD is a systemic disorder, correction of copper excretion by means of normalizing liver function can produce full recovery, as first demonstrated by successful outcomes with autologous hepatic transplantation (25). However, removing systemic copper by any means can interrupt progression of WD and often succeeds at reversing neurologic deficits. It is unclear if any additional toxicity is conferred by the increased cerebral uptake of iron also demonstrable in WD (26).

Copper is largely bound to protein throughout the body. Brain and liver, the two organs most susceptible to copper toxicity, exert the greatest avidity for copper. Within the brain, gray matter shows high affinity for copper deposition (27). The damage copper can produce throughout the body can result in a number of clinical syndromes, as listed in Table 21.1. These manifestations of WD can begin monosymptomatically or simultaneously with other clinical features. Although its usual clinical presentations are unmistakable, WD has been observed to start in an extremely limited manner. It has been described with focal, asymmetric features, sometimes without further deficit over several years of follow-up (28,29). Missing the opportunity for diagnosis when its signs and symptoms are mild is one of the greatest challenges posed by this treatable disorder (30–32).

TABLE 21.1
SYSTEMIC MANIFESTATIONS OF WILSON'S DISEASE

Brain (atrophy, necrosis, gliosis, demyelination, central pontine myelinolysis)

Liver (cirrhosis, acute hepatitis)

Ophthalmologic (corneal Kayser-Fleischer rings; starburst cataract of lens)

Heart (cardiomyopathy)

Kidney (renal lithiasis, hematuria, hypercalcuria, nephrocalcinosis) (218, 219)

Anemia (acute hemolytic, thrombocytopenia, Heinz body anemia) (220–222)

Bone and joint disorders (rickets, osteoarthritis, recurrent arthritis, bone fragmentation, chondrocalcinosis, osteoporosis, spinal degeneration, spontaneous fractures, spontaneous rupture of Achilles tendon) (38, 52, 223–228)

Hypoparathyroidism

Hemosiderosis (229)

Pancreatic exocrine and endocrine impairment (99)

Splenic rupture (230)

Acute rhabdomyolysis (231)

MOTOR FEATURES OF NEUROLOGIC IMPAIRMENT

In addition to a thorough description of hepatolenticular degeneration as a clinical syndrome, Wilson gave a detailed analysis of its pathologic imprint on the brain. He further provided a correlation between the motor disorders and the selectivity of its damage to basal ganglia structures. These impairments include dystonic or choreic involuntary movements, tremor, dysarthria, and rigidity. Although the initial presentation of WD can be only one category of movement disorder, the typical case usually involves combinations of each of these motor features. Rarely, other types of movement disorder (such as essential tremor) can coexist in a family with WD (33).

Almost half of all WD patients with neurologic disease first experience problems in their second or third decades of life (29,30). For neurologic involvement in WD, the age of presentation tends to be older than with purely hepatic disease. However, initial neurologic presentations of WD at less than age 5 years or more than age 50 years have been described (34–39), including cases older than age 70 years (40). Most commonly, juvenile-onset WD tends to present with hepatic damage, whereas older individuals with WD are more likely to have neurologic symptomatology early in the disorder. In younger individuals WD tends to have a more rapid course than in adults (41). Considerable heterogeneity in clinical features can be found in familial involvement in WD. Another puzzling aspect of WD is the marked variety in neurologic presentations. Even with its propensity for asymmetric or focal deficits, virtually all cases of WD have some degree of bilateral pathologic change in the lenticular nuclei. The broad range of neurologic impairments in WD also can be attributed to the sometimes extensive pathologic change beyond the boundaries of the basal ganglia.

A major challenge for an early diagnosis of WD is the recognition of subtle initial clinical features. Variable signs and symptoms that are intermittent or hard to categorize can result in delayed diagnosis. It is important to recognize that in WD the excess copper load can be quite severe, even in patients with only mild neurologic impairments. Also, patients with severe liver damage may be lacking any systemic illness or evidence of CNS involvement. Even certain abrupt systemic manifestations of WD (such as hemolytic anemia or liver failure) can appear with little or no change in neurologic impairment. A sudden or gradual decline in hepatic function caused by WD can by itself generate an extrapyramidal movement disorder and encephalopathy apart from the direct damage that copper deposition can inflict on the brain. Pathologic examination can readily distinguish the two disorders. Unlike changes found in WD, hepatic encephalopathy usually is characterized by neuronal damage with a pseudoulegyric pattern but lacking the necrotic changes in the putamen or frontal gyri as found in WD (42) (see the following).

Typically, neurologic WD presents insidiously with tremor, dystonia, rigidity, dysarthria, drooling, dysphagia, unsteady gait, and mental deterioration (43). Less commonly, the neurologic syndrome can present more suddenly in association with an irregular fever, emaciation, and a seemingly toxic state. Among the most common initial signs are dysarthria—described by Wilson (44) as "a trifling indistinctness of speech"—clumsiness of the hands, and mental change ("a childishness seen in facile laughter, or irritability, or caprice"). Another series of neurologic WD (44 cases) found 12 presenting predominantly with basal ganglia–related abnormalities, 6 with cerebellar impairment, and 17 with a combination of these (45). Others have made similar observations with the types of neurologic dysfunction (46). The experience of Walshe and Yealland (30) indicated that parkinsonian signs appeared in almost half the patients. Approximately one-quarter of presentations involved a "pseudosclerotic" syndrome, resembling a common pattern of multiple sclerosis involvement by causing cerebellar outflow tremor and speech ataxia. The remainder of patients in the latter study (mostly children) presented with primarily choreic or dystonic features. The disruption of dopaminergic neurotransmission in striatal structures, as demonstrated in neuroimaging studies, is probably responsible for the development of parkinsonian features, dystonia, and dyskinesia in WD (47).

Tremor in one or both hands is probably the most common initial symptom of WD (48,49). Tremor can be unilateral or bilateral, near constant or paroxysmal, or initiated only during specific motor tasks. Most commonly, the limbs and the head are affected. The tremor in WD can affect limbs at rest, with postural maintenance, or during movement (or any combination of these). Though the action tremor can resemble that observed with cerebellar dysfunction, other signs (such as dysdiadochokinesis, nystagmus, or the Holmes rebound sign) are generally lacking. One characteristic pattern of tremor in WD involves a coarse, irregular, to-and-fro movement elicited by action. When the arms are held forward and flexed horizontally, this maneuver can bring out a proximal component of tremor activity with a "wing-beating" quality. The types of tremor found in parkinsonism and or dystonia may also occur in WD. Less commonly, tremor presents in the trunk or in the tongue (44,50). Familial (essential-type) tremor with dominant inheritance has been described as a confounding diagnostic feature in a family also affected with WD (51).

Motor dysfunction in the territory of the bulbar musculature is prominent in WD and in one series (52) was more common than tremor as an initial feature. Drooling, dysarthria, cranial dystonia, and pharyngeal dysmotility (53) all can be observed. Other types of motor impairment can involve the cranial region, especially when dystonic features develop elsewhere in the body (52). Among these are facial grimacing, blepharospasm, and tongue dyskinesia (54). A fixed, sardonic smile with retracted lips and opened jaw was illustrated in Wilson's original report (43) and is still a highly typical feature. This facial dystonia often can progress to impair closure of the mouth. Spasmodic movements of dystonia also can occur in cranial or cervical musculature. The varieties of dystonia in WD include generalized, segmental, or multifocal patterns, such as bilateral foot dystonia (55).

Virtually all untreated patients are affected by progressive disturbance of speech. Speech can be disturbed in several ways due to impaired motor control of lip, tongue, and pharyngeal muscles. In the 1955 edition of Wilson's textbook, dysarthria in this disorder "reproduces the slurring but not the staccato element of multiple sclerosis" and can progress to complete anarthria. Lesser degrees of speech impairment include indistinct articulation, loss of consonant production, a "whispering dysphonia" (56), and marked slowing in the cadence of speech (41,57). Walshe and Yealland (30) have commented on a characteristic inspiratory laugh in WD that "once heard, is never forgotten."

In early WD, there can be other types of motor impairment, some of which can be difficult to categorize. Patients tend to become clumsy and slowed at everyday tasks. Handwriting and other limb movements may reflect loss of dexterity, as evidenced by the fingers' diminished ability to tap rapidly (58). Trunk titubation, a change of posture, or a disturbance of gait are commonly observed as subtle features in mild cases. Muscle cramps with distal dysesthesias may be experienced (59). WD also can present with a typical unilateral or bilateral parkinsonian syndrome. Sometimes, clinical features initially observed do not correspond to the basal ganglia involvement, which is nearly always found in the brain. For example, ataxia has been described as the only clinical manifestation in a chronic case of WD (37). Sometimes an early manifestation of WD is an unusual task-specific difficulty, such as inability to maintain a particular head posture or to protrude the tongue (41). Sustained, abnormal postures characteristic of dystonia are especially common and, in addition to the bulbar region, can affect the trunk and limbs. The intensity of rigid dystonic posturing can be so great as to require tendon release to relieve disability.

The basis for clinical heterogeneity in presenting features is not understood (60), although it has long been recognized that some patients develop predominantly dystonic or parkinsonian features, and others are affected more with bulbar dysfunction and tremor. For this reason, WD should be highly suspect with respect to any number of categories of movement disorder. Spasticity usually does not develop, although some patients exhibit hyperreflexia and Babinski signs. An early manifestation of WD can be pseudobulbar palsy with involuntary bouts of crying or laughter (61). The latter problems, when advanced, can be highly disabling. Other types of movement disorders, such as tics and myoclonus, are generally not observed. However, in 1 case of WD that presented as a tremor disorder, there was also episodic truncal myoclonus, priapism, and seminal ejaculation that occurred several times per day (62).

Seizures

In Wilson's 1912 monograph, instances of epilepsy are described. Though seizures are not a common occurrence in WD, some reports have documented either focal or major motor seizures at any stage of the disorder (63,64). Seizures have been described in cases lacking other evidence for CNS involvement and are more common in juvenile WD patients. One large series of cases found the prevalence of seizures in a WD group to be 6.2% (65). The latter prevalence corresponds to an approximately tenfold increase over seizure occurrence in the general population. In some reports, convulsions begin to occur at initiation of decoppering treatment. Seizures sometimes can be confused with other paroxysmal movements, such as tremors or dystonia, which sometimes occur as intermittent events in WD.

BEHAVIORAL AND MENTAL STATUS FEATURES

A spectrum of changes in behavior and mental status can occur in WD. Among these are anxiety, mood alterations, impulsivity, and other psychiatric disorders. Wilson's original case reports included the description of "emotionalism," though he regarded such behavioral features to be transient. However, subsequent study of WD has shown how commonly this disorder produces an affliction of the mind. Such impairment can be evident in disturbances of school performance, personality, or behavior. Prominent abnormalities on the Minnesota Multiphasic Personality Inventory (MMPI) and other evaluations of personality traits may be found (66). Other early signs of WD include a decline in memory function or cognitive abilities (67–69). Some aspects of neuropsychological performance tend not to be impaired, such as rate of information processing (70). Patients with WD have been described as exhibiting schizophreniform or paranoid features, sometimes with hallucinations or delusional thinking (71,72). Psychiatric disorders in WD without psychotic manifestations include depression or other mood disorders, lethargy, nightmares, disinhibited behavior (such as inappropriate laughter), or loss of insight (31,69,73).

As many as 20% of patients with WD developed some form of psychiatric disturbance as an initial feature (74,75). Other studies have estimated an even greater incidence of psychiatric disturbance, such as moderate to severe depressive traits (76,77). Prior to a confirmed diagnosis of WD, another series found that 17 of 34 patients had received psychiatric treatment for various disorders, including schizophrenia, depression, and anxiety (78). Depression can be a presenting feature (79). With other types of neurologic involvement, the likelihood of a behavioral disorder is much increased. Among these are such behaviors as impulsiveness, self-injuriousness, suicidal ideation, aggressiveness, sexual preoccupations, and childishness (71). Other behavioral disturbances include irritability and a low threshold for anger. A decline in schoolwork or work performance is almost always evident (77). Antisocial or criminal behavior may occur (80). Case reports of WD appearing with anorexia nervosa (81), hypersomnia (82), or with catatonia (83) have been described. When untreated, patients with WD can experience progressive decline in cognitive abilities as a consequence of neuropathologic changes throughout the brain or as a secondary consequence of liver failure. Dementia from WD is usually irreversible. A striking finding in one study was the lack of correlation between the extent of copper toxicity and the features of neuropsychological impairments in both symptomatic and asymptomatic WD patients (78).

OPHTHALMOLOGIC FEATURES

Opaque or mottled bands of pigmentation in the peripheral cornea are characteristic of WD when it involves the CNS (84,85). Although this feature escaped recognition by Wilson, these corneal rings were discovered prior to description of hepatolenticular degeneration. Independent reports by Kayser (86) and by Fleischer (87) are the basis for the eponym now applied to these distinctive changes in the cornea, caused by deposition of copper. Eventually, clinicians came to recognize the strong connection between the corneal pigmentation and the progressive neurologic and hepatic disorder described by Wilson.

Kayser-Fleischer rings have a brownish or greenish tint and generally arise in the periphery of the cornea. Though usually they appear uniformly concentric around the cornea, these rings can be especially prominent at the upper pole (and can require lifting of the eyelid for recognition). Rarely, Kayser-Fleischer rings can be unilateral (37,88). Kayser-Fleischer rings often can be identified without magnification or special illumination, especially in individuals with blue irises. However, a definitive analysis for the presence or absence of these rings requires a careful ophthalmologic slit-lamp examination. With this magnified view of the eye, another characteristic finding in WD can be discerned, if present. The "sunflower" cataract is an opacification in the lens (89). Though a less common finding in WD than the Kayser-Fleischer ring (90), sunflower cataracts have the same significance. Using Scheimpflug photography, the clinical course of corneal and lens opacification can be followed (91).

Copper-containing granules compose the Kayser-Fleischer ring, which develops primarily in Descemet's membrane of the cornea. These rings and the sunflower cataract arise simultaneously with the onset of neurologic manifestations of WD (90). The intensity of the rings tends to decrease with institution of decoppering therapy (92) or after liver transplantation (93), occasionally disappearing

from view. The majority of cases of CNS WD demonstrate Kayser-Fleischer rings. In exceptional circumstances, they can be absent in otherwise typical cases of WD (30,36, 94–97). One report described Kayser-Fleischer rings developing only after the start of penicillamine in a subject whose clinical picture was otherwise highly typical of WD (98). Other disorders rarely give rise to corneal deposits similar in appearance to Kayser-Fleischer rings (99). These conditions include cirrhosis and other forms of biliary obstruction (100).

In WD, the eye may be affected in other ways. As an early feature of the disorder, reading may be impaired (101), possibly due to gaze distractibility or difficulty in fixation (43,102). Among the types of abnormal eye movements are a defect of supranuclear accommodation (103), a disturbance of smooth pursuit, nystagmus, episodic diplopia, and impaired convergence (29,30). Apraxia of eyelid opening (104) and slowed saccadic pursuit (105) have also been described. Presentations of neurologic WD with oculogyric crisis (106) and with progressive visual loss (107) have been described.

NEUROPATHOLOGY OF WILSON'S DISEASE

Much of Wilson's 1912 monograph on hepatolenticular degeneration was devoted to detailed pathologic analysis of the distinctive changes produced in the brain. Whereas the distribution and severity of histologic changes can differ among cases, pathologic involvement is usually most extensive in the basal ganglia, where there can be cystic or cavitary degeneration. The massive necrosis that can be found in the gross pathology of the cut brain (28,42,108) explains why neurologic impairments are often irreversible. As is evident from neuroimaging studies, the lenticular nuclei are the major targets of atrophic changes. The symmetric shrinkage of the putamen is sometimes the consequence of necrotic changes that tend to be especially prominent laterally. The entire putamen can be shrunken with cavitary necrosis and a cystic or granular appearance. Tissues in the striatum can take on a brown, red, or yellow color, though not the greenish hue sometimes seen in corneas. The pallidum also may exhibit discoloration, but these structures tend not to undergo degeneration. Flattening of the caudate nucleus may occur, though more atrophy in the putamen is usually found. Cystic or cavitary necrosis can occur beyond the lenticular nuclei in the claustrum, extreme capsule, thalamus, subthalamic nucleus, and red nucleus (28,109,110). About 10% of cases have atrophic or degenerative changes beyond the lenticular nuclei (108).

Elsewhere in the brain, WD can be associated with dilation of the lateral ventricles and generalized brain atrophy. Rarely, the major brunt of pathologic change is found in cerebral cortical gray and white matter (111–114).

Degenerative changes have been described to be most prominent in the superior and middle frontal gyri. Similar degrees of damage can extend as far back as the temporal and parietal cortex. In some cases of WD, damage to myelin has been the predominant pathologic picture. Sometimes the loss of white matter is so extensive as to suggest the presence of demyelinating disease (111,113,114). Another picture of the CNS pathology of WD involves atrophy in the brainstem and cerebellar folia (115). Atrophy can show a predilection for the superior vermis and the dentate nucleus (116). White matter lesions with the appearance of central pontine myelinolysis have been described in otherwise typical cases of WD (42,117–119), including development after liver transplantation (120).

Microscopy shows that pathologic change in WD tends to be more widespread than might be suspected from inspection of the cut brain. In particular, deeper layers of cerebral cortex and adjacent white matter are often the most affected regions. Prominent changes include capillary endothelial swelling and proliferation of glia (especially those of Alzheimer's type II) (69,108). Gliosis is most abundant in the putamen and also can be present in the globus pallidus and caudate nucleus whether or not cavitary or necrotic changes are present. Most cases of severe WD show extensive evidence of damage to myelinated fibers in association with Alzheimer's type II gliosis, extending diffusely throughout cerebral white matter. A variety of degenerative changes in glia have been described (108), including spongy changes of white matter.

Though a distinctive pathologic change, Alzheimer type II glia are not specific to WD. When observed in other forms of chronic hepatic disease in association with encephalopathy, they may not be as prominently configured in the lenticular nuclei as in WD. Another pathologic finding in most cases of WD are the Opalski cells, which appear to be derived from glia (121). Opalski cells are large, rounded cells with periodic acid–Schiff–positive staining for cytoplasmic granules and an irregularly shaped nucleus. The most common locations for Opalski cells are the cerebral cortex cells and the boundaries of lenticular nuclei cavities. When such cells are found in this configuration together with Alzheimer's type II glia, the pathologic diagnosis of WD is almost certain. Alzheimer's type I cells also can be found in WD. In one study, their presence was highly correlated to the extent of reactive astrogliosis and inversely proportional to the severity of Alzheimer's type II changes (122). Opalski cells and Alzheimer's types I and II glia may be involved in a copper detoxification process, since they express the copper binding protein metallothionein (121).

Other types of neuronal damage may be found throughout the brain, especially for larger neurons. The cerebellar pathology of WD most often consists of prominent damage to white matter surrounding the dentate nuclei and extensive (but nonspecific) loss of Purkinje cells (69). Two reports of cerebral cortex electron microscopy in WD have been published (123,124). In addition to typical degenerative changes in neurons, myelin, glia, and axons, Hirano bodies and protoplasmic astrocytes (probably Alzheimer's type II) were also found. In cortical neurons, spheroid bodies were prominent. Similar changes have appeared in the lower brainstem sensory nuclei in WD (125). Activated microglia can be found in WD, with ultrastructural changes demonstrating a number of patterns, including transitional forms between rod, ramified, and amoeboid microglia (126).

The impact of decoppering treatment was analyzed in the brains of 11 WD subjects treated chronically with penicillamine (119). For 5 of the patients, neurologic features of WD had fully resolved, and the other patients achieved marked clinical improvement. Despite continued copper chelation therapy, brain content of copper was greatly increased over control values for 8 of the 9 brains studied. Furthermore, prominent neuropathologic changes typical of WD were evident in each of the penicillamine-treated patients, despite their good neurologic outcomes. These results indicate that chelation therapy with penicillamine does not normalize brain copper content or avert either the gross or microscopic pathology associated with CNS WD. The severity of neuropathologic change and regional cerebral copper content was only weakly correlated.

NEUROPHYSIOLOGIC FINDINGS

Disruption of central conduction pathways can provide a sensitive clue to the impact of WD on the CNS. In general, this disorder does not have pathognomonic findings on any form of neurophysiologic testing, though the results of testing for evoked responses can be useful in the workup of WD (127). Usually, the electroencephalogram has not been informative, though generalized slowing and focal abnormalities may be found (128). Most cases of WD studied by electroencephalographic spectral analysis and topographic mapping have shown slowing or epileptiform activity (129). One study of evoked potentials (EPs) revealed that most WD patients with neurologic involvement had one or more findings of a prolonged EP, as did almost half of those lacking other evidence for CNS involvement (130). Delayed conduction of sensory EPs can show a variety of patterns (128). Whether or not clinical signs are present, patients with WD can have abnormal visual EPs, especially with respect to the P100 waveforms (131–133). Studies of brainstem auditory EPs have shown no abnormality (132) or else prolongation (133). A study comparing all three types of EPs found that those of brainstem auditory and somatosensory pathways were more likely to be delayed than those from the visual pathways (134). In the latter study, prolongation of an EP was determined in all severely affected patients, and in almost all of those patients moderately affected by neurologic WD. An abnormal EP also was found in more than half of those judged to be mildly affected and in 4 of 24 lacking any other clinical evidence for CNS involvement. Hence, EP can be highly sensitive to WD in the brain or spinal cord. Brainstem auditory and somatosensory EPs may also show changes in response to therapy for WD (130). Abnormalities of pattern-reversal visual evoked responses and flash electroretinograms can undergo improvement with treatment of WD (135).

Another approach that has been used for studying damage to central conduction pathways has been the study of motor EPs following magnetic stimulation of the motor cortex and the spinal roots (136). Subjects with neurologic WD, whether with demyelination or extrapyramidal features, have shown diminished or absent cortically evoked motor responses (137–139). In 1 reported case of WD, abnormal electromyographic responses evoked by transcranial magnetic brain stimulation were the only strongly abnormal neurophysiologic finding (140). These magnetically elicited motor responses became normal after a course of decoppering therapy.

DIAGNOSTIC TESTING FOR WILSON'S DISEASE

The initial hope that the deciphering of the genetic abnormality in WD would lead quickly to a simple diagnostic test has been dashed (or at best delayed) by the subsequent identification of what is now approaching 300 distinct mutations in the *ATP7B* gene (141,142). Thus, the clinician must still rely on a battery of tests to make the diagnosis, the composition of the battery varying with disease stage. Of course, clinical suspicion of this disorder is always an indispensable first step, regardless of the available laboratory tests. The protean nature of WD's clinical presentations always will make its diagnosis a challenge. Prashnath et al. address this diagnostic difficulty, noting that diagnostic errors were made by referring physicians in 192 of 307 patients with WD, and that a mean delay in diagnosis of 2 years ensued because of these errors (143). In light of the pleomorphic clinical character of WD, the diagnosis should be considered in any individual presenting with unexplained hepatic, psychiatric, or neurologic dysfunction—especially if the neurologic dysfunction involves basal ganglia or cerebellar function. Whereas this is especially true for younger individuals, the fact that WD has even been first diagnosed in individuals over age 70 (40) means that the diagnosis should be considered and excluded even in middle-aged and elderly persons with appropriate symptoms.

Liver Biopsy for Hepatic Copper Content

Liver biopsy is the most sensitive and accurate test for the diagnosis of WD. Hepatic copper content is significantly elevated in virtually all individuals with WD. Even asymptomatic, or presymptomatic, individuals will have marked elevations of hepatic copper. In WD, the major elevation of hepatic copper generally exceeds 250 mg per gram of dry tissue. However, liver biopsy is not without its diagnostic pitfalls with regard to WD. Intrahepatic copper accumulation, although present, may be undetectable by histochemical staining in more than 50% of patients in the very early stages of WD because the copper is diffusely distributed in the cytoplasm (144,145). Even when liver involvement is more advanced, copper deposition can be unevenly distributed and actually missed if the biopsy specimen is small. Thus, negative copper staining by itself does not absolutely exclude the diagnosis of WD (145).

Although elevated hepatic copper content is a sensitive diagnostic finding in WD, there also may be alternative explanations for its presence. Obstructive liver diseases—such as primary biliary cirrhosis, biliary atresia, extrahepatic biliary obstruction, primary sclerosing cholangitis, intrahepatic cholestasis of childhood, cirrhosis in native North American (Indian) children, and even chronic active hepatitis—also result in elevated hepatic copper (146–150). Copper content lower than expected—but still elevated beyond the threshold of 100 mg/g liver tissue—may be found in WD if the biopsy is obtained when copper is being released from the liver into the systemic circulation (69).

As an invasive procedure, liver biopsy is associated with a small but real morbidity. Therefore, it should be reserved for situations in which other noninvasive studies do not provide the answer. Liver biopsy is thus the diagnostic test of choice in the individual presenting solely with hepatic dysfunction, since at this stage the copper load may not have been released from the liver into the general circulation. The clinician should always keep in mind that a single determination of hepatic copper content might be misleading in WD (151).

Serum Ceruloplasmin

Ceruloplasmin originates as an inactive, non–copper-containing form, called *apoceruloplasmin*. One of the functions of *ATP7B* protein is to add 7 copper atoms to the apoceruloplasmin, producing holoceruloplasmin, which is the functionally active form of ceruloplasmin (152). Routine measurement of ceruloplasmin usually involves an immunologic assay, which measures total ceruloplasmin (apoceruloplasmin and holoceruloplasmin). Some investigators have suggested that enzymatic assay of ceruloplasmin oxidase activity, which measures only holoceruloplasmin, is a more accurate method of assessment and should be preferentially employed (152,153).

Serum ceruloplasmin determination, even when immunologically measured, is a simple and useful (though insufficient) screening test for WD. Ceruloplasmin concentrations are reduced in the majority of individuals with WD, though not in all. For 5% to 15% of WD cases, serum ceruloplasmin concentrations may be in a low normal or only slightly subnormal range (69,154). It is also helpful to remember that because ceruloplasmin is an acute-phase reactant, it is transiently elevated during pregnancy, during estrogen administration, or during infectious or inflammatory disorders (155). In such circumstances, the diagnosis of WD may be obscured by a normal serum ceruloplasmin concentration (156). Furthermore, ceruloplasmin deficiency is not unique to WD and can be found in a variety of other disorders, including Menkes disease, protein-losing enteropathy, nephrotic syndrome, sprue, and other situations in which protein and total calorie intake are insufficient (155,157). Low ceruloplasmin levels, however, are not typically found in severe hepatic cirrhosis of non-WD origin (158).

Because of these limitations, ceruloplasmin determination should not be relied on as the sole screening study for the diagnosis of WD. However, a serum ceruloplasmin level greater than 30 mg/dL (159) or 40 mg/dL (160) virtually excludes the possibility of WD.

24-Hour Urinary Copper Excretion

Urinary copper excretion serves as another useful screening study for WD. However, urinary copper concentrations may be completely normal in asymptomatic WD cases or in presentations limited to hepatic dysfunction. In the latter circumstance, copper still may be accumulating in the liver and not exiting into the circulation. In individuals with neurologic or psychiatric dysfunction, urinary copper levels consistently tend to exceed 100g/day. Obstructive liver disease, such as primary biliary cirrhosis, may also produce elevation of urinary copper (147,161).

Slit-Lamp Examination

As discussed, corneal copper deposition in the form of Kayser-Fleischer rings is an indispensable and sensitive clue to the diagnosis of WD. In fact, the lack of Kayser-Fleischer rings almost always excludes the diagnosis of neurologic or psychiatric WD (69). Only rarely is the rule transgressed. Cases in which Kayser-Fleischer rings are absent in the face of typical neurologic symptoms are known (36,95,96,98) but are exceptional (97). Although Kayser-Fleischer rings may sometimes be seen easily by direct observation, a magnified slit-lamp examination by an experienced ophthalmologist is often necessary to visualize the deposited copper. Kayser-Fleischer rings tend not to be present in individuals with purely hepatic manifestations of WD because, in this situation, the accumulating copper has not yet escaped the liver.

Serum-Free (Unbound) Copper

Serum copper concentrations, which are measurements of both bound and unbound copper, provide only limited diagnostic value for WD because total serum copper concentrations largely reflect the quantity of the copper-transporting protein ceruloplasmin. Serum copper concentrations are reduced in WD in direct correlation to ceruloplasmin reduction (69,159,162). Determination of nonceruloplasmin and, therefore, free (unbound) serum copper can be of value because this measurement represents the potentially toxic fraction of serum copper, which increases once the copper storage capabilities of the liver are exceeded (46,159). Serum-free copper can be calculated by the following formula: (Total serum copper in µg/dL) − (Ceruloplasmin in mg/dL x 3); normal concentrations are 10–15 µg/dL (32). Serum-free copper levels are useful both for diagnostic purposes and for monitoring compliance with treatment.

Radioactive Copper Studies

After an oral dose of ^{64}Cu, a normal individual will have an initial rise in the serum radioactive label as the dose enters the blood and is complexed with albumin and amino acids. The isotope concentration then drops as the ^{64}Cu is cleared from the blood by the liver. A secondary rise peaks at 48 hours from incorporation of ^{64}Cu into newly synthesized ceruloplasmin, which is then released into the bloodstream.

In WD, this secondary rise is not seen, even in individuals with normal or near-normal ceruloplasmin levels. Thus, although this study is not necessary as a screening tool for WD, it can be useful in confirming the diagnosis of WD in the few individuals for whom serum ceruloplasmin concentrations are inconclusive (163).

Neuroimaging Procedures

Abnormalities on magnetic resonance imaging (MRI) are present in virtually all individuals with WD who display neurologic dysfunction (164,165). Increased signal intensity on T2 weighted images, sometimes with a central core of decreased signal intensity, is the characteristic abnormality. Such findings most consistently involve the basal ganglia (166). Several other MRI abnormalities have been described as characteristic of WD, such as the "face of the panda" sign in the midbrain (167) and the "bright claustrum" sign (168), but these are not consistently present. Abnormal MRI findings can improve or vanish with treatment of WD (169,170). Computed tomography (CT) may also expose abnormalities in WD, but less reliably than MRI. Other aspects of neuroimaging studies, including positron emission tomography (PET) and single-photon emission computed tomography (SPECT), are reviewed (see Chapter 43).

Cerebrospinal Fluid Copper

Copper concentration in cerebrospinal fluid (CSF) is elevated in WD with neurologic dysfunction, but this test has not been used routinely nor has it been validated for the diagnosis of WD. There are indications that CSF copper offers an accurate reflection of the brain's copper load (171). During treatment for WD, CSF copper content slowly returns to normal (172). Sequential CSF copper content determinations also can provide evidence for noncompliance (173).

Genetic Testing

Testing for the *WD* gene, located on 13q14.3, can be used to augment clinical diagnosis. However, the tremendous diversity of mutations in the *ATP7B* gene in WD limits the general utility of genetic testing. The techniques involved include analysis of DNA markers amplified by polymerase chain reaction and single-strand conformational analysis (174). Cases of WD diagnosed by gene markers can lack other diagnostic features, such as Kayser-Fleischer rings (96,97). Successful recognition of WD at a presymptomatic stage is a goal for avoiding tissue damage that can precede even the earliest clinical signs and symptoms of WD. Newer techniques may eventually allow more extensive use of genetic testing for WD diagnosis (175).

Guidelines to Diagnostic Testing

Generally, Kayser-Fleischer rings will be lacking in WD subjects with symptoms or signs only of hepatic dysfunction if neurologic or psychiatric features have not developed. Furthermore, urinary copper tends not to be elevated because the liver has not started disgorging copper from the liver. Serum ceruloplasmin concentrations also cannot be relied on as a diagnostic measure. Hence, in these circumstances, liver biopsy becomes necessary for pathologic analysis and determination of hepatic copper content.

Once typical forms of neurologic or psychiatric dysfunction have appeared, liver biopsy for diagnostic purposes is generally not necessary. The diagnosis of WD can be developed by the reduced serum ceruloplasmin, the elevated urinary copper excretion, and the appearance of Kayser-Fleischer rings. Only in those unusual instances where ceruloplasmin is normal or marginally reduced might liver biopsy be required. If biopsy is not possible or if the results of biopsy are inconclusive, a radio-labeled copper incorporation study may be useful.

MANAGEMENT OF WILSON'S DISEASE

The management of WD is an arduous task that requires long-term commitment and constant vigilance on the part of both patient and physician. The lifelong compliance required for successful therapy is a major challenge for many patients. At present, all treatment for WD—with the exception of liver transplantation—is strictly empirical and must be continued without pause. In certain situations,

such as pregnancy (176) or rapid progression of neurologic disease, modification of the treatment regimen may be necessary. Four primary approaches to the management of WD are available. For each patient, the ideal treatment modality (or modalities) can vary greatly.

Dietary Therapy

Although copper can be found in small amounts in many comestibles, foods such as chocolate, nuts, shellfish, mushrooms, soy products, gelatin, and liver have an especially high content (145). Eliminating liver from the diet might seem to be a logical strategy, but a strict attempt to eliminate all copper from the diet results in an unpalatable product and offers no definite advantage beyond what can be achieved by simply forgoing high-copper-content foods (177). It is important to note that individuals with WD who have adopted strict lactovegetarian diets have achieved adequate control of copper balance without additional therapy, presumably from the reduced bioavailability of dietary copper due to the fiber and phytates abundant in the lactovegetarian diet (178). However, such a diet is poorly tolerated. Additional dietary issues are the presence of copper in drinking water (177,179), the use of water softeners that increase the copper content of the water (159), and the elemental copper present in health food vitamin/mineral supplements.

Inhibition of Intestinal Copper Absorption

In recent years, the treatment for WD has been advanced by several innovative approaches to achieving adequate copper balance by limiting absorption of copper via the gut. Prior attempts to decrease dietary copper absorption through the use of potassium iodide or potassium sulfide met with little success, but newer approaches utilizing zinc or tetrathiomolybdate are very promising (see the following).

Zinc

By itself, zinc has no direct effect on copper absorption. However, it acts indirectly on *metallothionein*, a protein with several physiologic roles. *Metallothionein* binds zinc for transport and helps to maintain its homeostasis (180). Present in many body tissues (including liver and brain), metallothionein is also found in intestinal mucosal cells (enterocytes). Metallothionein avidly binds copper (181). In the gut this protein exerts its therapeutic effect on copper balance in WD. When persistently increased amounts of zinc enter the intestine, metallothionein formation is induced in the enterocytes and excess zinc is bound by the metallothionein, thus maintaining zinc homeostasis. However, the increased amount of metallothionein in the enterocyte is also capable of binding copper since this metal is absorbed through the enterocytes. The net effect of zinc administration is a negative copper balance. The trapped copper remains in the enterocyte (along with zinc) until the cell is sloughed and excreted in the feces (179,182). Furthermore, both dietary copper and copper secreted into the gastrointestinal tract via saliva and gastric juices are trapped and ultimately eliminated (182). The induction of metallothionein by zinc is a relatively slow process (requiring 1 to 2 weeks to evolve) and results in a relatively small negative copper balance (183). Zinc administration also has been reported to inhibit lipid peroxidation by means of increasing glutathione availability (145,184).

For the treatment of WD, either zinc sulfate or zinc acetate may be employed. A dosage of 50 mg (elemental zinc) 3 times daily is generally used. However, a total daily dosage of 75 mg is probably sufficient (185,186). The marketed tablets of zinc sulfate (220 mg) contain 50 mg of elemental zinc. It is important to administer zinc on an empty stomach, separated from food intake by at least 1 hour (187).

Zinc is generally tolerated without any difficulty. However, gastric irritation may occur, especially with zinc sulfate (179,188). Sideroblastic anemia, probably resulting from impaired iron utilization, also has been described as a result of zinc therapy (189). Transient elevations of serum amylase, lipase, and alkaline phosphatase also have been attributed to zinc (186). Reductions of high-density lipoprotein cholesterol by approximately 20% in men and total cholesterol in both men and women by about 10% have been noted as well (183,190).

The virtues of zinc as a therapeutic agent in the treatment of WD have been strongly advocated by Brewer and by Hoogenraad. Despite strong evidence based on clinical experience, the role of zinc administration in the management of WD has not been established to everyone's satisfaction (191). The extremely low incidence of toxicity makes zinc an ideal therapy for the individual with WD who has not yet developed clinical symptoms (179,192). Its place in symptomatic WD is less certain. The slow onset of action of zinc probably makes it unsuitable as initial therapy for the patient with neurologic symptoms (193), but Brewer has enthusiastically promoted the use of zinc as "maintenance" therapy following initial decoppering with more potent agents (31,183,193). Other investigators, less convinced about the efficacy of zinc, suggest that zinc therapy be limited to individuals who have been unable to tolerate penicillamine or trientine (159,191).

Brewer et al. also have addressed the question of using zinc concomitantly with other agents, such as penicillamine, with different mechanisms of action. They reported that even when zinc and penicillamine are given at different times during the day, an interaction occurs: Urinary copper excretion increases and fecal copper excretion decreases, thus canceling any benefit derived from combining the two drugs (179). On the other hand, the same group of investigators has found the combination of zinc and trientine to be very effective, even in some patients who otherwise would have required liver transplantation (188).

Tetrathiomolybdate

Ammonium tetrathiomolybdate (TM) actually bridges two categories of mechanism of action in the treatment of WD. Though still experimental, TM has sufficient promise to merit discussion here. TM acts in the gut lumen, where it limits gastrointestinal absorption of copper by forming a tripartite complex with dietary copper and albumin, thus rendering the copper unavailable for absorption (195). This mechanism is especially active if TM is administered with meals. A second mode of action of TM becomes active when TM is administered without food. In this situation, TM is readily absorbed into the bloodstream, where it forms the same tripartite complex with albumin and unbound (free) copper, thus trapping and holding the copper in an inactive, nontoxic state (195).

To take advantage of this potential dual mechanism of action, TM has been administered in a regimen of 6 doses daily (3 doses with and 3 doses between meals) (195). Mealtime doses were 20 mg, whereas intermeal doses ranged from 20 mg to 60 mg. Utilized in this manner, TM produces a prompt and significant reduction in free copper in the plasma (195). In most instances, TM has been tolerated without difficulty. However, reversible bone marrow suppression has been reported (188), which may be the result of impaired erythropoiesis as a consequence of bone marrow copper depletion (Professor George Brewer, personal communication, 2002).

TM has not been utilized as a long-term agent in the management of WD, and it has been given as an 8- to 16-week course, followed by a switch to zinc maintenance therapy (193,196). It may be especially important to avoid long-term TM administration in children and adolescents, since TM has been shown to damage epiphyses in growing bone in rats (188,197). Clinical experience with TM has suggested that deterioration in neurologic function following initiation of TM therapy is much less common than with penicillamine (198).

Copper Chelation Therapy

The modern era of WD therapy began in 1951 with the introduction of British anti-Lewisite (BAL, dimercaprol) as the first effective copper-chelating agent in the management of WD (199,200). The necessity of parenteral administration and the frequent occurrence of adverse effects were serious limits to the use of BAL in the management of WD. BAL has now been replaced by orally administered copper-chelating agents, first penicillamine and then trientine.

Penicillamine

Penicillamine (dimethylcysteine), a metabolic byproduct of penicillin, was introduced into clinical usage shortly after the discovery of excess copper deposition in the pathophysiology of WD (201). Penicillamine avidly chelates copper. The complexed copper is excreted in the urine, initially producing a robust cupriuresis that diminishes with prolonged administration as the excess body load of copper is corrected. Penicillamine is the most potent agent available for the management of WD, although chronic treatment presents many possible adverse outcomes. Because alternatives to penicillamine are available, strong arguments have been made to avoid use of this drug based on the dangers of exacerbation in neurologic impairments and the high frequency of other adverse outcomes (198). Despite this, penicillamine is still widely used as a first-line treatment for initial and long-term management of WD (202).

Acute sensitivity reactions develop in 20% to 30% of individuals placed on penicillamine (203,204). These reactions tend to occur within 2 weeks of initiation of treatment and are characterized by skin rash, fever, or lymphadenopathy with associated laboratory abnormalities (eosinophilia, leukopenia, and thrombocytopenia). Fatal agranulocytosis may occur (205). In the face of an acute sensitivity reaction, penicillamine should be discontinued until the rash clears. Subsequently, it may possible to reintroduce penicillamine, beginning with very low doses and slowly escalating. One formula for reintroducing penicillamine consists of using prednisone 30 mg/day for 2 days before the start of penicillamine at a reduced dosage of 125 mg/day. Penicillamine is then increased by 125 mg at 3-day intervals to reach a daily intake of 500 mg. Over the next month, prednisone is gradually tapered and discontinued while penicillamine is progressively increased by 250 mg at 2- to 3-day intervals to reach a target dose of 1000 mg/day (206). Despite such measures, 5% to 20% of WD patients will be unable to tolerate penicillamine (31).

A formidable array of potential complications can accompany the long-term use of penicillamine. Various dermatologic problems may develop. Urticaria affects as many as one-third of treated patients (204). Penicillamine also can induce cutaneous and systemic elastic fiber damage, which may result in elastosis perforans serpiginosa, a reactive perforating dermatosis, and pseudo-pseudoxanthoma elasticum (207). Recurrent subcutaneous bleeding following incidental trauma can result in characteristic brownish skin discoloration, termed *penicillamine dermatopathy* (208). Penicillamine-induced inhibition of collagen and elastin cross-linking may be responsible for the subcutaneous bleeding (209). Impaired wound healing also may complicate chronic penicillamine therapy (210). Reduction of penicillamine dosage to 250 mg/day to 500 mg/day during perioperative periods may help to dampen this tendency (69). Other penicillamine-induced problems that have been described include nephrotic syndrome (211), Goodpasture's syndrome (212), a lupuslike syndrome (213,214), a myasthenia gravis–like syndrome (215,216), acute polyarthritis (59), thrombocytopenia (69), retinal hemorrhage (217), dysgeusia (177,218), and IgA deficiency (219). The adverse effects associated with chronic penicillamine administration may first appear after years of therapy.

Penicillamine can trigger neurologic deterioration after the start of therapy. This outcome has led to some disenchantment with using it as a primary treatment for WD (193,220). Neurologic deterioration may occur in 22% to 52% of persons receiving penicillamine (188). Moreover, when this neurologic deterioration occurs, half of patients will never regain their baseline neurologic status (221). Status dystonicus with a lethal outcome has been reported (222). Emergence of neurologic dysfunction in previously neurologically asymptomatic individuals also has been described (195,223). The mechanism for this neurologic deterioration is not clear but could be due to excessive systemic mobilization of copper that can be taken up in the brain.

There is considerable difference of opinion regarding the appropriate dosage of penicillamine. Although doses of 1000 to 2000 mg daily usually have been recommended, more modest doses have been advised, such as a starting dose of 250 mg/day (187,179). Penicillamine should be taken with meals. Supplemental pyridoxine often has been administered with penicillamine, although the need for it has not been established.

Improvement in function following initiation of treatment with penicillamine may not be discernible for 2 to 3 months. Because of this lag in clinical response, it is important to educate patients and their families so that treatment will be maintained and disillusionment in the lack of immediate effect will be avoided. Although virtually all clinical features of WD parameters may improve with penicillamine therapy, some deficits, such as dystonia and a fixed facial grimace, may be more resistant. Improvement may continue for as long as 1 to 2 years with continued therapy. Even abnormalities on neuroimaging that appear to be structural may improve with penicillamine therapy (164,165,224).

Trientine

Triethylene tetramine dihydrochloride (trientine) is an avid copper-chelating agent. It has been utilized in the management of WD since the late 1960s (225–228), although it became available in the United States more recently. Its mechanism of action is similar to penicillamine, but trientine is not quite as potent a chelating agent. This characteristic makes trientine a preferred agent over penicillamine in the opinion of some experts (193,194). However, most practitioners reserve trientine for use in individuals who have been unable to tolerate penicillamine. Trientine is generally administered 3 times a day, with total daily dose ranging from 750 mg/day to 2,000 mg/day. As with penicillamine, trientine should be administered with food.

Adverse effects appear to be less common with trientine than with penicillamine. Among the observed reactions to this drug are colitis, duodenitis (229), sideroblastic anemia (230), and lupus nephritis (227). As with penicillamine, neurologic deterioration may develop following initiation of trientine therapy (229).

Liver Transplantation

Experience with orthotopic liver transplantation in the management of WD has accumulated over the past two decades. As a potentially curative treatment, orthotopic liver transplantation has an obvious advantage over such symptomatic treatment as copper chelation. Improvement for hepatic, neurologic, psychiatric, and ophthalmologic aspects of the disorder all may be achieved from orthotopic liver transplantation. Indeed, experience has shown that copper metabolism normalizes following orthotopic liver transplantation and chelation therapy may be discontinued (231,232). Although orthotopic liver transplantation has generally been conducted with WD patients experiencing fulminant hepatic failure (for whom mortality otherwise would be 100%), this procedure also has been performed on individuals with chronic, severe hepatic insufficiency (231). Dramatic clinical improvement can be achieved from successful liver transplantation (233). One-year survival rates of 80% or greater have been documented (231,232,234,235). This success rate has led some investigators to consider orthotopic liver transplantation in individuals with stable hepatic function but deterioration in neurologic function despite trials of appropriate medications (236). Extracorporeal porcine hepatic tissue is also under investigation in WD and other disorders of hepatic failure (237).

The transplantation of liver tissue (right lobe or left lobe) from living, related, healthy donors, including mothers or fathers who would be heterozygote carriers of the WD mutation, has been successfully employed in patients with WD. The ethical dilemma in this approach, however, is the risk of complications and even death that is incurred by the healthy donor. Indeed, deaths have been reported in such individuals (238).

Potentials for Future Treatment

The search continues for additional treatment modalities that might be beneficial for individuals with WD. In a small, open-label, pilot study, captopril was reported to demonstrate modest anticopper activity, whereas sodium dimercaptosulphonate was a more potent agent (239). In a case report, cannabis afforded marked relief from dystonia in a single individual with WD (240).

Additional potentially therapeutic approaches have been investigated in animal models of WD. Bone marrow stem cell transplantation from normal littermates was effective in genotypically repopulating the liver and reducing hepatic copper levels in 24% of transplanted mice with the toxic milk mutation (241). In the Long-Evans Cinnamon (LEC) rat, producing transgenic rats by introducing the normal human *ATP7B* transgene into fertilized rat oocytes partially reversed the abnormalities of copper metabolism (242). Administration of dietary polyunsaturated fatty acids suppressed development of acute hepatitis and prolonged survival in female LEC rats (243). N-benzyl-D-glucamine dithiocarbamate, a metal chelating agent, markedly reduced tissue copper accumulation in LEC rats, while also blocking the progressive hepatocellular damage characteristic of this animal model (244). Whether any of these potential treatment approaches can be translated to humans with WD remains to be seen.

REFERENCES

1. Hoogenraad TU. S.A. Kinnier Wilson (1878–1937). *J Neurol* 2001;248:71–72.
2. Gowers WR. Tetanoid chorea. In: *A Manual of Disease of the Nervous System*. Philadelphia: P Blakiston, 1888;1059.
3. Westphal C. Über eine dem Bilde der cerebrospinalen grauen Degeneration ähnliche Erkrankung des centralen Nervensystems ohne anatomischen Befund, nebst einigen Bermerkungen über paradoxe Contraction. *Arch Psychiatr Nervenkrank* 1883; 14:87–134.
4. Strümpell A. Über die Westphal'sche Pseudosklerose und über diffuse Hirnsklerose, inbesondere bei Kindern. *Deutsch Z Nervenheilk* 1898;12:115–149.
5. Homen EA. Eine eigenthümliche bei drei Geschwistern auftretende typische Krankheit unter der Form einer progressiven Dementia, in Verbindung mit ausgedehnten Gefässveränderungen (Wohl Lues hereditaria tarda). *Arch Psychiatr Nervenkrank* 1892; 24:191–228.
6. Firneisz G, Szonyi L, Ferenci P, et al. Wilson disease in two consecutive generations: an exceptional family. *Am J Gastroenterology* 2001;96:2269–2271.
7. LeWitt PA, Brewer GJ. Wilson's disease (progressive hepaticolenticular degeneration). In: Calne DB, ed. *Neurodegenerative Disorders*. Philadelphia: WB Saunders, 1994:667–683.
8. Takeshita Y, Shimizu N, Yamaguchi Y, et al. Two families with Wilson disease in which siblings showed different phenotypes. *J Hum Genet* 2002;47:543–547.
9. Houwen RH, Roberts EA, Thomas GR, et al. DNA markers for the diagnosis of Wilson disease. *J Hepatol* 1993;17:269–276.
10. Tanzi RE, Petrukhin K, Chernov I, et al. The Wilson disease gene is a copper transporting ATPase with homology to the Menkes disease gene. *Nat Genet* 1993;5:344–350.
11. Tsivkovskii R, Efremov RG, Lutsenko S. The role of the invariant His-1069 in folding and function of the Wilson's disease protein, the human copper-transporting ATPase ATP7B. *J Biol Chem* 2003; 278:13,302–13,308.
12. Fatemi N, Sarkar B. Molecular mechanism of copper transport in Wilson disease. *Environ Health Perspect* 2002;110(suppl 5):695–698.
13. Lutsenko S, Efremov RG, Tsivkovskii R, Walker JM. Human copper-transporting ATPase ATP7B (the Wilson's disease protein): biochemical properties and regulation. *J Bioenerg Biomembr* 2002;34:-351–362.
14. Loudianos G, Lovicu M, Solinas P, et al. Delineation of the spectrum of Wilson disease mutations in the Greek population and the identification of six novel mutations. *Genet Test* 2000;4: 399–402.
15. Sasaki N, Hayashizaki Y, Muramatsu M, et al. The gene responsible for LEC hepatitis, located on rat chromosome 16, is the homolog to the human Wilson disease gene. *Biochem Biophys Res Commun* 1994;202:512–518.
16. Yamaguchi Y, Heiny ME, Shimizu N, et al. Expression of the Wilson disease gene is deficient in the Long-Evans Cinnamon rat. *Biochem J* 1994;301(pt 1):1–4.
17. Malhi H, Irani AN, Rajvanshi P, et al. KAPT channels regulate mitogenically induced proliferation in primary rat hepatocytes and human liver cell lines: implications for liver growth control and potential therapeutic targeting. *J Biol Chem* 2000;275: 26,050–26,057.
18. Cartwright GE, Wintrobe MM. Copper metabolism in normal subjects. *Am J Clin Nutr* 1964;14:224–232.

19. O'Reilly S, Weber PM, Oswald M, et al. Abnormalities of the physiology of copper in Wilson's disease. III. The excretion of copper. *Arch Neurol* 1971;25:28–32.

20. Frommer DJ. Defective biliary excretion of copper in Wilson's disease. *Gut* 1974;15:125–129.

21. Gibbs K, Walshe JM. Biliary excretion of copper in Wilson's disease. *Lancet* 1980;2:538–539.

22. Iyengar V, Brewer GJ, Dick Rd, et al. Studies of cholecystokinin-stimulated biliary secretions reveal a high molecular weight copper-binding substance in normal subjects that is absent in patients with Wilson's disease. *J Lab Clin Med* 1988;111:267–274.

23. Cumings JN. The copper and iron content of brain and liver in the normal and in hepatolenticular degeneration. *Brain* 1948;71:410–415.

24. Walshe JM, Potter G. The pattern of whole body distribution of radioactive copper (^{67}Cu, ^{64}Cu) in Wilson's disease and various control groups. *Q J Med* 1977;46:445–462.

25. Groth CG, Dubois RS, Corman J, et al. Hepatic transplantation in Wilson's disease. *Birth Defects* 1973;9:106–108.

26. Bruehlmeier M, Leenders KL, Vontobel P, et al. Increased cerebral iron uptake in Wilson's disease: a 52Fe-citrate PET study. *J Nucl Med* 2000;41:781–787.

27. Warren PJ, Earl CJ, Thompson RHS. The distribution of copper in human brain. *Brain* 1960;83:709–717.

28. Dastur DK, Manghani DK. Wilson's disease: inherited cuprogenic disorder of liver, brain, kidney. In: Goldensohn E, Appel SH, eds. *Scientific Foundations of Neurology*. Philadelphia: Lea & Febiger, 1977;1033–1051.

29. Sternlieb I, Giblin DR, Scheinberg IH. Wilson's disease. In: Marsden CD, Fahn S, eds. *Movement Disorders 2*. New York: Butterworth, 1985;288–302.

30. Walshe JM, Yealland M. Wilson's disease: the problem of delayed diagnosis. *J Neurol Neurosurg Psychiatr* 1992;55:692–696.

31. Brewer GJ, Yuzbasiyan-Gurkan V. Wilson disease. *Medicine* 1992;71:139–164.

32. Brewer GJ. *Wilson's Disease: A Clinician's Guide to Recognition, diagnosis, and Management*. Boston: Kluwer Academic Publishers, 2001.

33. Quinn NP, Marsden CD. Coincidence of Wilson's disease with other movement disorders in the same family. *J Neurol Neurosurg Psychiatry* 1986;49:221–222.

34. Fitzgerald M, Gross JB, Goldstein NP, et al. Wilson's disease of late adult onset. *Mayo Clin Proc* 1975;50:438–442.

35. Czlonkowska A, Rodo M. Late onset Wilson's disease. *Arch Neurol* 1981;38:729–730.

36. Ross ME, Jacobson IM, Dienstag JL, et al. Late onset Wilson's disease with neurologic involvement in the absence of Kayser-Fleischer rings. *Ann Neurol* 1985;17:411–413.

37. Madden JW, Ironside JW, Triger DR, et al. An unusual case of Wilson's disease. *Q J Med* 1985;55:63–73.

38. Pilloni L, Lecca S, Coni P, et al. Wilson's disease with late onset. *Dig Liver Dis* 2000;32:180.

39. Kumagi T, Horiike N, Michitaka K, et al. Recent clinical features of Wilson's disease with hepatic presentation. *J Gastroenterol* 2004;39:1165–1169.

40. Ala A, Borjigin J, Rochwarger A, Schilsky M. Wilson disease in septuagenarian siblings: raising the bar for diagnosis. *Hepatology* 2005;41:668–670.

41. Purdon Martin J. Wilson's disease. In: Vinken PJ, Bruyn GW, Klawans HL, eds. *Handbook of Clinical Neurology*. New York: American Elsevier, 1968:267–278.

42. Shiraki H. Comparative neuropathologic study of Wilson's disease and other types of hepatocerebral disease. In: Bergsma D, Scheinberg IH, Sternlieb I, eds. *Wilson's Disease* (Birth Defects Original Article Series, vol 4.). New York: The National Foundation–March of Dimes, 1968;64–73.

43. Wilson SAK. Progressive lenticular degeneration: a familial nervous disease associated with cirrhosis of the liver. *Brain* 1912;34:295–509.

44. Wilson SAK. Progressive lenticular degeneration (hepatolenticular degeneration, Wilson's disease). In: Bruce AN, ed. *Neurology*, 2nd ed. Baltimore: Williams & Wilkins, 1955;941–967.

45. Dobyns WB, Goldstein NP, Gordon H. Clinical spectrum of Wilson's disease (hepatolenticular degeneration). *Mayo Clin Proc* 1979;54:35–42.

46. Stremmel W, Meyerrose K-W, Niederau K, et al. Wilson disease: clinical presentation, treatment, and survival. *Ann Intern Med* 1991;115:720–726.

47. Barthel H, Sorger D, Kuhn HJ, et al. Differential alteration of the nigrostriatal dopaminergic system in Wilson's disease investigated with [123I]ss-CIT and high-resolution SPET. *Eur J Nucl Med* 2001;28:1656–1663.

48. Walshe JM. Wilson's disease (hepatolenticular degeneration). In: Vinken PJ, Bruyn GW, Klawans HL, eds. *Handbook of Clinical Neurology*, vol 27. New York: American Elsevier, 1976;379–414.

49. Walshe JM. Wilson's disease. In: Vinken PJ, Bruyn GW, Klawans HL, eds. *Handbook of Clinical Neurology*. New York: American Elsevier, 1986;223–238.

50. Topaloglu H, Gucuyener K, Orkun C, et al. Tremor of tongue and dysarthria as the sole manifestation of Wilson's disease. *Clin Neurol Neurosurg* 1990;92:295–296.

51. Nicholl DJ, Ferenci P, Polli C, et al. Wilson's disease presenting in a family with an apparent dominant history of tremor. *J Neurol Neurosurg Psychiatry* 2001;70:514–516.

52. Starista-Rubinstein S, Young AB, Kluin K, et al. Clinical assessment of 31 patients with Wilson's disease: correlations with structural changes on magnetic resonance imaging. *Arch Neurol* 1987;44:365–370.

53. Gulyas AE, Salazar-Grueso EF. Pharyngeal dysmotility in a patient with Wilson's disease. *Dysphagia* 1988;2:230–234.

54. Liao KK, Wang SJ, Kwan SY, et al. Tongue dyskinesia as an early manifestation of Wilson disease. *Brain Devel* 1991;13:451–453.

55. Svetel M, Kozic D, Stefanova E, et al. Dystonia in Wilson's disease. *Mov Disord* 2001;16:719–723.

56. Parker N. Hereditary whispering dysphonia. *J Neurol Neurosurg Psychiatry* 1985;48:218–224.

57. Berry WR, Darley FL, Aronson AE, et al. Dysarthria in Wilson's disease. *J Speech Hearing Res* 1974;17:169–183.

58. Davis LJ, Goldstein NP. Psychologic investigation of Wilson's disease. *Mayo Clin Proc* 1974;49:409–499.

59. Golding DN, Walshe JM. Arthropathy of Wilson's disease: study of clinical and radiological features in 32 patients. *Ann Rheum Dis* 1977;36:99–111.

60. Denny-Brown D. Hepato-lenticular degeneration (Wilson's disease). *N Engl J Med* 1964;270:1149–1156.

61. Mingazzini G. Über das Zwangsweinen und lachen. *Klin Wochenschr (Wien)* 1928;41:998–1002.

62. Nair KR, Pillai PG. Trunkal myoclonus with spontaneous priapism and seminal ejaculation in Wilson's disease. *J Neurol Neurosurg Psychiatry* 1990;53:174.

63. Smith CK, Mattson RH. Seizures in Wilson's disease. *Neurology* 1967;17:1121–1123.

64. Chu N-S. Clinical, CT, and evoked potential manifestations in Wilson's disease with cerebral white matter involvement. *Clin Neurol Neurosurg* 1989;91:45–51.

65. Dening TR, Berrios GE, Walshe JM. Wilson's disease and epilepsy. *Brain* 1988;111:1139–1155.

66. Portala K, Westermark K, Ekselius L, et al. Personality traits in treated Wilson's disease determined by means of the Karolinska Scales of Personality (KSP). *Eur Psychiatry* 2001;16:362–371.

67. Knehr CA, Bearn AG. Psychological impairment in Wilson's disease. *J Nerv Ment Dis* 1956;124:251–255.

68. Goldstein NP, Ewert JC, Randall RV, et al. Psychiatric aspects of Wilson's disease (hepatolenticular degeneration): results of psychometric tests during long-term therapy. *Am J Psychiatry* 1968;124:1555–1561.

69. Scheinberg IH, Sternlieb I. *Wilson's disease: major problems in internal medicine*, vol 23. Philadelphia: WB Saunders, 1984.

70. Littman E, Medalia A, Senior G, et al. Rate of information processing in patients with Wilson's disease. *J Neuropsychiatr Clin Neurosci* 1995;7:68–71.

71. Dening TR. Psychiatric aspects of Wilson's disease. *Br J Psychiatry* 1985;147:677–682.

72. Scheinberg IH, Sternlieb I, Richman J. Psychiatric manifestations of Wilson's disease. *Birth Defects Orig Art Ser* 1968;4:85–86.

73. Hawkes ND, Mutimer D, Thomas GA. Generalised oedema, lethargy, personality disturbance, and recurring nightmares in a young girl. *Postgrad Med J* 2001;77:529,537–539.

74. Medalia A, Scheinberg IH. Psychopathology in patients with Wilson's disease. *Am J Psychiatry* 1989;146:662–664.

75. Jackson GH, Meyer A, Lippmann S. Wilson's disease: psychiatric manifestations may be the clinical presentation. *Postgrad Med* 1994;95:135–138.

76. Portala K, Westermark K, von Knorring L, et al. Psychopathology in treated Wilson's disease determined by means of CPRS expert and self-ratings. *Acta Psychiatr Scand* 2000;101:85–86,104–109.

77. Akil M, Brewer GJ. Psychiatric and behavioral abnormalities in Wilson's disease. *Adv Neurol* 1995;65:171–178.

78. Rathbun JK. Neuropsychological aspects of Wilson's disease. *Int J Neurosci* 1996;85:221–229.

79. Keller R, Torta R, Lagget M, et al. Psychiatric symptoms as late onset of Wilson's disease: neuroradiological findings, clinical features and treatment. *Ital J Neurol Sci* 1999;20:49–54.

80. Kaul A, McMahon D. Wilson's disease and offending behaviour—a case report. *Med Sci Law* 1993;33:353–358.

81. Gwirtsman HE, Prager J, Henkin R. Case report of anorexia nervosa associated with Wilson's disease. *Int J Eating Disord* 1993;13:241–244.

82. Firneisz G, Szalay F, Halasz P, et al. Hypersomnia in Wilson's disease: an unusual symptom in an unusual case. *Acta Neurol Scand* 2001;101:286–288.

83. Davis EJ, Borde M. Wilson's disease and catatonia. *Brit J Psychiatry* 1993;162:256–259.

84. Heckmann JG, Lang CJ, Neundorfer B, et al. Neuro/Images: Kayser-Fleischer corneal ring. *Neurology* 2000;54:1839.

85. Patel AD, Bozdech M. Wilson disease. *Arch Ophthalmol* 2001;119:1556–1557.

86. Kayser B. Über einen Fall von angeborener grünlicher Verfärbung der Cornea. *Klin Monatsb Augenheilk* 1902;40:22–25.

87. Fleischer B. Über eine der "Pseudosklerose" nahestehende bisher unbekannte Krankheit (gekenn zeichnet durch Tremor, psychische Störungen, braunliche Pigmententierung, bestimmter Gewebe, insobesondere suh der Hornhautperipherie, Lebercirrhose). *Deutsch Z Nervenheilkr* 1912;44:179–201.

88. Innes JR, Strachan IM, Triger DR. Unilateral Kayser-Fleischer ring. *Br J Ophthalmol* 1979;70:469–470.

89. Goyal V, Tripathi M. Sunflower cataract in Wilson's disease. *J Neurol Neurosurg Psychiatry* 2000;69:133.

90. Wiebers DO, Hollenhorst RW, Goldstein NP. The ophthalmologic manifestations of Wilson's disease. *Mayo Clin Proc* 1977;52:409–416.

91. Obara H, Ikoma N, Sasaki K, et al. Usefulness of Scheimpflug photography to follow up Wilson's disease. *Ophthalmic Res* 1995;27(suppl 1):100–103.

92. Sussman W, Sternlieb IH. Disappearance of Kayser-Fleischer rings. *Arch Ophthalmol* 1969;82:738–741.

93. Song HS, Ku WC, Chen CL. Disappearance of Kayser-Fleischer rings following liver transplantation. *Transplant Proc* 1992;24:1483–1485.

94. Heckmann J, Saffer D. Abnormal copper metabolism: another "non-Wilson's" case. *Neurology* 1988;38:1493–1594.

95. Oder W, Grimm G, Kollegger H, et al. Neurological and neuropsychiatric spectrum of Wilson's disease: a prospective study of 45 cases. *J Neurol* 1991;238:281–287.

96. Vidaud D, Assouline B, Lecoz P, et al. Misdiagnosis revealed by genetic linkage analysis in a family with Wilson disease. *Neurology* 1996;46:1485–1486.

97. Demirkiran M, Jankovic J, Lewis RA, et al. Neurologic presentation of Wilson disease without Kayser-Fleischer rings. *Neurology* 1996;46:1040–1043.

98. Weilleit J, Kiechl SG. Wilson's disease with neurological impairment but no Kayser-Fleischer rings. *Lancet* 1991;337:1426.

99. Frommer D, Morris J, Sherlock S, et al. Kayser-Fleischer-like rings in patients without Wilson's disease. *Gastroenterology* 1977;72:1331–1335.

100. Fleming CR, Dickson ER, Wahner HW, et al. Pigmented corneal rings in non-Wilsonian liver disease. *Ann Intern Med* 1977;86:285–288.

101. Hyman NM, Phuapradit P. Reading difficulty as a presenting symptom in Wilson's disease. *J Neurol Neurosurg Psychiatry* 1979;42:478–480.

102. Lennox G, Jones R. Gaze distractibility in Wilson's disease. *Ann Neurol* 1989;25:415–417.

103. Klinqele TG, Newman SA, Burde RM. Accommodation defect in Wilson's disease. *Am J Ophthalmol* 1980;90:22–24.

104. Keane JR. Lid-opening apraxia in Wilson's disease. *J Clin Neuro-Ophthalmol* 1988;8:31–33.

105. Kirkham TH, Kamin DF. Slow saccadic eye movements in Wilson's disease. *J Neurol Neurosurg Psychiatry* 1974;37:191–194.

106. Lee MS, Kim YD, Lyoo CH. Oculogyric crisis as an initial manifestation of Wilson's disease. *Neurology* 1999;52:1714–1715.

107. Gow PJ, Peacock SE, Chapman RW. Wilson's disease presenting with rapidly progressive visual loss: another neurologic manifestation of Wilson's disease? *J Gastroenterol Hepatol* 2001;16:699–701.

108. Schulman S. Wilson's disease. In: Minkler J, ed. *Pathology of the Nervous System*. New York: McGraw-Hill, 1968;1139–1151.

109. Owen CA Jr. *Wilson's Disease: The Etiology, Clinical Aspects, and Treatment of Inherited Toxicosis*. Park Ridge, NJ: Noyes Publications, 1981;1–215.

110. Duchen LW, Jacobs JM. Nutritional deficiencies and metabolic disorders. In: Adams JH, Corsellis JAN, Duchen LW, eds. *Greenfield's Neuropathology*, 4th ed. New York: John Wiley & Sons, 1984;595–599.

111. Schulman S, Barbeau A. Wilson's disease: a case with almost total loss of cerebral white matter. *J Neuropathol Exp Neurol* 1963;22:105–119.

112. Richter RB. Pallidal component in hepatolenticular degeneration. *J Neuropathol Exp Neurol* 1948;7:1–18.

113. Ishino H, Takashi M, Hayashi Y, et al. A case of Wilson's disease with enormous cavity formation of cerebral white matter. *Neurology* 1972;22:905–909.

114. Miyakawa T, Murayama E. An autopsy case of the "demyelinating type" of Wilson's disease. *Acta Neuropathol* 1976;35:235–241.

115. Miskolczy D. Wilson'she Krankheit und Kleinhirn. *Arch Psych Nervenkr* 1932;97:27–63.

116. Bielschowsky M, Hallervorden J. Symmetrische Einschmelzungsherde in Stirnhim beim Wilson Pseudosklerose Komplex. *J Psych Neurol* 1931;42:177–189.

117. Popoff N, Budzilovich G, Goodgold A, et al. Hepatocerebral degeneration: its occurrence in the presence and in the absence of abnormal copper metabolism. *Neurology* 1965;15:919–930.

118. Seitelberger F. Zentrale pontin Myelinolyse. *Schweiz Arch Neurol Neurochir Psych* 1973;112:285–297.

119. Horoupian DS, Sternlieb I, Scheinberg IH. Neuropathological findings in penicillamine-treated patients with Wilson's disease. *Clin Neuropathol* 1988;7:62–67.

120. Lui CC, Chen CL, Chang YF, et al. Subclinical central pontine myelinolysis after liver transplantation. *Transplant Proc* 2000;32:2215–2516.

121. Bertrand E, Lewandowska E, Szpak GM, et al. Neuropathological analysis of pathological forms of astroglia in Wilson's disease. *Folia Neuropathol* 2001;39:73–79.

122. Ma KC, Ye ZR, Fang J, et al. Glial fibrillary acidic protein immunohistochemical study of Alzheimer I and II astrogliosis in Wilson's disease. *Acta Neurol Scand* 1988;78:290–296.

123. Foncin JF. Pathologie ultrastructurale de la glie chez l'homme. In: *Proceedings of the 6th International Congress of Neuropathology*. Paris: Masson et Cie, 1970;377–390.

124. Anzil AP, Herrlinger H, Blinzinger K, et al. Ultrastructure of brain and nerve biopsy tissue in Wilson disease. *Arch Neurol* 1974;31:94–100.

125. Jellinger K. Neuroaxonal dystrophy: its natural history and related disorders. In: Zimmerman HM, ed. *Progress in Neuropathology*, vol 2. New York: Grune & Stratton, 1973;129–180.

126. Lewandowska E, Wierzba-Bobrowicz T, Kosno-Kruszewska E, et al. Ultrastructural evaluation of activated forms of microglia in human brain in selected neurological diseases (SSPE, Wilson's disease and Alzheimer's disease). *Folia Neuropathol* 2004;42:81–91.

127. Chu N-S. Sensory evoked potentials in Wilson's disease. *Brain* 1986;109:491–506.

128. Giagheddu M, Tamburini G, Piga M, et al. Comparison of MRI, EEG, Eps, and ECD-SPECT in Wilson's disease. *Acta Neurol Scand* 2001;103:71–81.

129. Chu N-S, Chu CC, Tu SC, et al. EEG spectral analysis and topographic mapping in Wilson's disease. *J Neurol Sci* 1991;106:1–9.

130. Grimm G, Oder W, Prayer L, et al. Evoked potentials in assessment and follow-up of patients with Wilson's disease. *Lancet* 1990;336:963–964.

131. Aiello I, Sau GF, Cacciotto R, et al. Evoked potentials in patients with non-neurological Wilson's disease. *J Neurol* 1992;239:65–68.

132. Butinar D, Trontelj JV, Khuraibet AJ, et al. Brainstem auditory evoked potentials in Wilson's disease. *J Neurol Sci* 1990;95:163–169.

133. Satishchandra P, Swamy HS. Visual and brain stem auditory evoked responses in Wilson's disease. *Acta Neurol Scand* 1989;79:108–113.

134. Grimm G, Madl C, Katzenschlager R, et al. Detailed evaluation of evoked potentials in Wilson's disease. *EEG Clin Neurophysiol* 1992;82:119–124.

135. Satishchandra P, Ravishankar Naik K. Visual pathway abnormalities Wilson's disease: an electrophysiological study using electroretinography and visual evoked potentials. *J Neurol Sci* 2000;176:13–20.

136. Perretti A, Pellecchia MT, Lanzillo B, et al. Excitatory and inhibitory mechanisms in Wilson's disease: investigation with magnetic motor cortex stimulation. *J Neurol Sci* 2001;192:35–40.

137. Chu N-S. Motor evoked potentials in Wilson's disease: early and late motor responses. *J Neurol Sci* 1990;99:259–269.

138. Meyer BU, Britton TC, Benecke R. Wilson's disease: normalization of cortically evoked motor responses with treatment. *J Neurol* 1991;238:327–330.

139. Berardelli A, Inghilleri M, Priori A, et al. Involvement of corticospinal tract in Wilson's disease: a study of three cases with transcranial stimulation. *Mov Disord* 1990;5:334–337.

140. Meyer BU, Britton TC, Bischoff C, et al. Abnormal conduction in corticospinal pathways in Wilson's disease: investigation of nine cases with magnetic brain stimulation. *Mov Disord* 1991;6:320–323.

141. Velez-Pardo C, Del Rio MJ, Moreno S, Ramirez-Gomez L, Correa G, Lopera F. New mutation (T123P) of the ATP7B gene associated with neurologic and neuropsychiatric dominance onset of Wilson's disease in three unrelated Colombian kindred. *Neuroscience Letters* 2004;367:360–364.

142. Kenney D, Cox D. Wilson Mutation Data Base. Available at http://www.uofa-medical-genetics.org/wilson/index.php. Accessed April 2005.

143. Prashanth LK, Taly AB, Sinha S, Arunodaya GR, Swamy HS. Wilson's disease: diagnostic errors and clinical implications. *J Neurol Neurosurg Psychiatry* 2004;75:907–909.

144. Pilloni L, Lecca S, Van Eyken P, et al. Value of histochemical stains for copper in the diagnosis of Wilson's disease. *Histopathology* 1998;33:28–33.

145. Langner C , Denk H. Wilson disease. *Virchows Arch* 2004;445:111–118.

146. Smallwood RA, Williams HA, Rosenauer VM. Liver copper levels in liver disease: studies using neutron activation analysis. *Lancet* 1968;2:1310–1313.

147. LaRusso NF, Summerskill WH, McCall JT. Abnormalities of chemical tests for copper metabolism in chronic active liver disease: differentiation from Wilson's disease. *Gastroenterology* 1976;70:653–655.

148. Benson GD. Hepatic copper accumulation in primary biliary cirrhosis. *Yale J Biol Med* 1979;52:83–88.

149. Evans J, Newman S, Sherlock S. Liver copper levels in intrahepatic cholestasis of childhood. *Gastroenterology* 1978;75:875–878.

150. Tanner MS, Portmann B, Mowat AP, et al. Increased hepatic copper concentration in Indian childhood cirrhosis. *Lancet* 1979;1:1203–1205.

151. Song YM, Chen MD. A single determination of liver copper concentration may misdiagnose Wilson's disease. *Clin Biochem* 2000;33:589–590.

152. MacIntyre G, Gutfreund KS, Martin WRW, Camicioli R, Cox DW. Value of an enzymatic assay for the determination of serum ceruloplasmin. *J Lab Clin Med* 2004;144:294–301.

153. Walshe JM, Clinical Investigations Standing Committee of the Association of Clinical Biochemists. Wilson's disease: the importance of measuring serum caeruloplasmin non-immunologically. *Ann Clin Biochem* 2003;40(pt 2):115–121.

154. Yuce A, Kocak N, Ozen H, et al. Wilson's disease patients with normal ceruloplasmin levels. *Turk J Pediatr* 1999;41:99–102.

155. Gibbs K, Walshe JM. A study of the ceruloplasmin concentrations found in 75 patients with Wilson's disease, their kinships and various control groups. *Q J Med* 1979;48:447–463.

156. Sternlieb I, Scheinberg IH. Chronic hepatitis as a first manifestation of Wilson's disease. *Ann Intern Med* 1972;76:59–64.

157. Weiner WJ, Lang AE. *Movement Disorders: A Comprehensive Survey.* Mt. Kisco, NY: Futura, 1989;257–291.

158. Lan C, Ropert M, Laine F, et al. Serum ceruloplasmin and ferroxidase activity are not decreased in hepatic failure related to alcoholic cirrhosis: clinical and pathophysiological implications. *Alcohol Clin Exp Res* 2004;28:775–779.

159. Yarze JC, Martin P, Munoz SJ, et al. Wilson's disease: current status. *Am J Med* 1992;92:643–654.

160. Snow B. Laboratory diagnosis and monitoring of Wilson's disease. *Neurological aspects of Wilson's disease.* Taken from American Academy of Neurology Course Number 411, 1995;25–30.

161. Frommer DJ. Urinary copper excretion and hepatic copper concentrations in liver disease. *Digestion* 1981;21:169–178.

162. Cumings JN. Trace metals in the brain and in Wilson's disease. *J Clin Pathol* 1968;21:1–7.

163. Sternlieb I, Scheinberg IH. The role of radiocopper in the diagnosis of Wilson's disease. *Gastroenterology* 1979;77:138–142.

164. Thuomas KA, Aquilonius SM, Bergstrom K, et al. Magnetic resonance imaging of the brain in Wilson's disease. *Neuroradiology* 1993;35:134–141.

165. Roh JK, Lee TG, Wie BA, et al. Initial and follow-up brain MRI findings and correlation with the clinical course in Wilson's disease. *Neurology* 1994;44:1064–1068.

166. Magalhaes ACA, Caramelli P, Menezes JR, et al. Wilson's disease: MRI with clinical correlation. *Neuroradiology* 1994;36:97–100.

167. Hitoshi S, Iwata M, Yoshikawa K. Midbrain pathology of Wilson's disease: MRI analysis of three cases. *J Neurol Neurosurg Psychiatry* 1991;54:624–626.

168. Sener RN. The claustrum on MRI: normal anatomy, and the bright claustrum as a new sign in Wilson's disease. *Pediatr Radiol* 1993;23:594–596.

169. Alanen A, Komu M, Penttinen M, et al. Magnetic resonance imaging and proton MR spectroscopy in Wilson's disease. *Br J Radiol* 1999;72:749–756.

170. Stefano Zagami A, Boers PM. Disappearing "face of the giant panda." *Neurology* 2001;56:665.

171. Hartard C, Weisner B, Dieu C, et al. Wilson's disease with cerebral manifestations: monitoring therapy by CSF copper concentration. *J Neurol* 1993;241:101–107.

172. Stuerenburg HJ. CSF copper concentrations, blood–brain barrier function, and ceruloplasmin synthesis during the treatment of Wilson's disease. *J Neural Transm* 2000;107:321–329.

173. Stuerenburg HJ, Eggers C. Early detection of non-compliance in Wilson's disease by consecutive copper determination in cerebrospinal fluid. *J Neurol Neurosurg Psychiatry* 2000;69:701–702.

174. Butler P, McIntyre N, Mistry PK. Molecular diagnosis of Wilson disease. *Mol Genet Metab* 2001;72:223–230.

175. Huster D, Weizenegger M, Kress S, Mossner J, Caca K. Rapid detection of mutations in Wilson disease gene ATP7B by DNA strip technology. *Clin Chem Lab Med* 2004;42:507–510.

176. Furman B, Bashiri A, Wiznitzer A, et al. Wilson's disease in pregnancy: five successful consecutive pregnancies of the same woman. *Eur J Obstet Gynecol Reprod Biol* 2001;96:232–234.

177. Shoulson I, Goldblatt D, Plassche W, et al. Some therapeutic observations in Wilson's disease. *Adv Neurol* 1983;37:239–246.

178. Brewer GJ, Yuzbasiyan-Gurkan V, Dick R, et al. Does a vegetarian diet control Wilson's disease? *J Am Coll Nutr* 1993;12:527–530.

179. Brewer GJ, Yuzbasiyan-Gurkan V. Wilson's disease. In: Klawans HL, Goetz CG, Tanner CM, eds. *Textbook of Clinical Neuropharmacology and Therapeutics.* New York: Raven Press, 1992;191–205.

180. Ebadi M. Metallothionein and other zinc-binding proteins in brain. *Meth Enzymol* 1991;205:363–387.

181. Day FA, Panemangalore M, Brady FO. In vivo and ex vivo effects of copper on rat liver metallothionein. *Proc Soc Exp Biol Med* 1981;168:306–310.

182. Brewer GJ, Hill GM, Prasad AS, et al. Oral zinc therapy for Wilson's disease. *Ann Intern Med* 1983;99:314–320.

183. Brewer GJ, Yuzbasiyan-Gurkan V, Lee DY. Molecular genetics and zinc-copper interactions in human Wilson's disease and canine copper toxicosis. In: Prasad AS, ed. *Essential and Toxic Trace Elements in Human Health and Disease: An Update.* New York: Wiley-Liss, 1993;129–145.

184. Farinati F, Cardin R, D'Inca R, Naccarato R, Sturniolo GC. Zinc treatment prevents lipid peroxidation and increases glutathione availability in Wilson's disease. *J Lab Clin Med* 2003;141:372–377.

185. Brewer GJ, Yuzbasiyan-Gurkan V, Johnson V, et al. Treatment of Wilson's disease with zinc. XI. Interaction with other anticopper agents. *J Am Coll Nutr* 1993;12:26–30.

186. Brewer GJ, Yuzbasiyan-Gurkan V, Johnson V, et al. Treatment of Wilson's disease with zinc. XII. Dose regimen requirements. *Am J Med Sci* 1993;305:199–202.

187. Brewer GJ, Yuzbasiyan-Gurkan V, Dick R. Zinc therapy of Wilson's disease. 8. Dose response studies. *J Trace Elem Exp Med* 1990;3:227–234.

188. Walshe JM, Yealland M. Chelation treatment of neurological Wilson's disease. *Q J Med* 1993;86:197–204.

189. Simon SR, Branda RF, Tindle BH, et al. Copper deficiency and sideroblastic anaemia associated with zinc ingestion. *Am J Hematol* 1988;28:181–183.

190. Hooper PL, Visconti L, Garry PJ, et al. Zinc lowers high-density lipoprotein-cholesterol levels. *JAMA* 1980;244:1960–1961.

191. Lipsky MA, Gollan JL. Treatment of Wilson's disease: in D-penicillamine we trust—what about zinc? *Hepatology* 1987;7:593–595.

192. Brewer GJ, Yuzbasiyan-Gurkan V, Lee DY, et al. Treatment of Wilson's disease with zinc. 6. Initial treatment studies. *J Lab Clin Med* 1989;114:633–638.

193. Brewer GJ. Practical recommendations and new therapies for Wilson's disease. *Drugs* 1995;50:240–249.

194. Askari FK, Greenson J, Dick RD, Johnson VD, Brewer GJ. Treatment of Wilson's disease with zinc. XVIII. Initial treatment of the hepatic decompensation presentation with trientine and zinc. *J Lab Clin Med* 2003;142:385–390.

195. Brewer GJ, Dick RD, Johnson V, et al. Treatment of Wilson's disease with ammonium tetrathiomolybdate. I. Initial therapy in 17 neurologically affected patients. *Arch Neurol* 1994;51:545–554.

196. Brewer GJ. Neurologically presenting Wilson's disease: epidemiology, pathophysiology and treatment. *CNS Drugs* 2005;19:185–192.

197. Spence JA, Suttle NF, Wenham G, et al. A sequential study of the skeletal abnormalities which develop in rats given a small dietary supplement of ammonium tetrathiomolybdate. *J Comp Pathol* 1980;90:139–153.

198. Brewer GJ. Penicillamine should not be used as initial therapy in Wilson's disease. *Mov Disord* 1999;14:551–554.

199. Denny-Brown D, Porter H. The effect of BAL (2,3 dimercaptopropanol) on hepatolenticular degeneration (Wilson's disease). *N Engl J Med* 1951;245:917–925.

200. Cumings JN. The effects of BAL in hepatolenticular degeneration. *Brain* 1951;74:10–22.

201. Walshe JM. Penicillamine: a new oral therapy for Wilson's disease. *Am J Med* 1956;21:487–495.

202. Walshe JM. Penicillamine: the treatment of first choice for patients with Wilson's disease. *Mov Disord* 1999;14:545–550.

203. Sternlieb I, Scheinberg IH. Penicillamine therapy in hepatolenticular degeneration. *JAMA* 1964;189:748–754.

204. Haggstrom GC, Hirschowitz BI, Flint A. Long-term penicillamine therapy for Wilson's disease. *South Med J* 1980;73:530–531.

205. Corcos JM, Soler-Bechera J, Mayer K, et al. Neutrophilic agranulocytosis during administration of penicillamine. *JAMA* 1964;189:265–268.

206. Chan C-Y, Baker AL. Penicillamine hypersensitivity: successful desensitization of a patient with severe hepatic Wilson's disease. *Am J Gastroenterol* 1994;89:442–443.

207. Becuwe C, Dalle S, Ronger-Savle S, et al. Elastosis perforans serpiginosa associated with pseudo-pseudoxanthoma elasticum during treatment of Wilson's disease with penicillamine. *Dermatology* 2005;210:60–63.

208. Sternlieb I, Fisher M, Scheinberg IH. Penicillamine-induced skin lesions. *J Rheumatol* 1981;8(suppl 7):149–154.

209. Nimni ME. Mechanism of inhibition of collagen cross-linking by penicillamine. *Proc R Soc Med* 1977;70(suppl 3):65–72.

210. Morris JJ, Seifter E, Rettura G, et al. Effect of penicillamine upon wound healing. *J Surg Res* 1969;9:143–149.

211. Hirschman SZ, Isselbacher KJ. The nephrotic syndrome as a complication of penicillamine therapy of hepatolenticular degeneration (Wilson's disease). *Ann Intern Med* 1965;62: 1297–1300.

212. Sternlieb I, Bennett B, Scheinberg IH. D-Penicillamine induced Goodpasture's syndrome in Wilson's disease. *Ann Intern Med* 1975;82:673–675.

213. Walshe JM. Penicillamine and the SLE syndrome. *J Rheumatol* 1981;8(suppl 7):155–160.

214. Lin HC, Hwang KC, Lee HJ, et al. Penicillamine induced lupus-like syndrome: a case report. *J Microbiol Immunol Infect* 2000;33: 202–204.

215. Czlonkowska A. Myasthenia syndrome during penicillamine treatment. *Br Med J* 1975;2:726–727.

216. Narayanan CS, Behari M. Generalized myasthenia gravis following use of D-pencillamine in Wilson's disease. *J Assoc Physicians (India)* 1999;47:648.

217. Bigger JF. Retinal hemorrhages during penicillamine therapy of cystinuria. *Am J Ophthalmol* 1968;66:954–955.

218. Henkin RI, Keiser HR, Jaffe IA, et al. Decreased taste sensitivity after D-penicillamine reversed by copper administration. *Lancet* 1967;2:1268–1271.

219. Proesman W, Jaeken J, Eckels R. D-penicillamine-induced IgA deficiency in Wilson's disease. *Lancet* 1976;2:804–805.

220. Brewer GJ, Turkay A, Yuzbasiyan-Gurkan V. Development of neurologic symptoms in a patient with asymptomatic Wilson's disease treated with penicillamine. *Arch Neurol* 1994;51:304–305.

221. Brewer GH, Terry CA, Aisen AM, et al. Worsening of neurological syndrome in patients with Wilson's disease with initial penicillamine therapy. *Arch Neurol* 1987;44:490–494.

222. Svetel M, Sternic N, Pejovic S, et al. Penicillamine-induced lethal status dystonicus in a patient with Wilson's disease. *Mov Disord* 2001;16:568–569.

223. Glass JD, Reich SG, DeLong MR. Wilson's disease: development of neurological disease after beginning penicillamine therapy. *Arch Neurol* 1990;47:595–596.

224. Williams FJB, Walshe JM. Wilson's disease: an analysis of the cranial computerized tomographic appearances found in patients and the changes in response to treatment with chelating agents. *Brain* 1981;104:735–752.

225. Walshe JM. The management of penicillamine nephropathy in Wilson's disease: a new chelating agent. *Lancet* 1969;2:1401–1402.

226. Walshe JM. Copper chelation in patients with Wilson's disease: a comparison of penicillamine and triethylene tetramine hydrochloride. *Q J Med* 1973;42:441–452.

227. Walshe JM. Treatment of Wilson's disease with trientine (triethylene tetramine) dihydrochloride. *Lancet* 1982;1:643–647.

228. Walshe JM. Assessment of the treatment of Wilson's disease with triethylene tetramine 2HCL (Trien 2HCl). In: Sarkar B, ed. *Biological Aspects of Metal Related Diseases.* New York: Raven Press, 1983;243–261.

229. Dahlman T, Hartvig P, Lofholm M, et al. Long-term treatment of Wilson's disease with triethylene tetramine dihydrochloride (trientine). *Q J Med* 1995;88:609–616.

230. Condamine L, Hermine O, Alvin P, et al. Acquired sideroblastic anaemia during treatment of Wilson's disease with triethylene tetramine dihydrochloride. *Br J Hematol* 1993;83:166–168.

231. Schilsky ML, Scheinberg IH, Sternlieb I. Liver transplantation for Wilson's disease: indications and outcome. *Hepatology* 1994;19: 583–587.

232. Rela M, Heaton ND, Vougas V, et al. Orthotopic liver transplantation for hepatic complications of Wilson's disease. *Br J Surg* 1993;80:909–911.

233. Bax RT, Hassler A, Luck W, et al. Cerebral manifestation of Wilson's disease successfully treated with liver transplantation. *Neurology* 1998;51:863–865.

234. Chen CL, Kuo YC. Metabolic effects of liver transplantation in Wilson's disease. *Transplant Proc* 1993;25:2944–2947.

235. Emre S, Atillasoy EO, Ozdemir S, et al. Orthotopic liver transplantation for Wilson's disease: a single-center experience. *Transplantation* 2001;72:1232–1236.

236. Mason AL, Marsh W, Alpers DH. Intractable neurological Wilson's disease treated with orthotopic liver transplantation. *Dig Dis Sci* 1993;38:1746–1750.

237. Mazariegos GV, Kramer DJ, Lopez RC, et al. Safety observations in phase I clinical evaluation of the Excorp Medical Bioartificial Liver Support System after the first four patients. *ASAIO J* 2001;47:471–475.

238. Wang X-H, Zhang F, Li X-C, et al. Eighteen living related liver transplants for Wilson's disease: a single-center. *Transplant Proc* 2004;36:2243–2245.

239. Wang XP, Yang RM, Ren MS, Sun BM. Anticopper efficacy of captopril and sodium dimercaptosulphonate in patients with Wilson's disease. *Funct Neurol* 2003;18:149–153.

240. Uribe Roca MC, Micheli F, Viotti R. Cannabis sativa and dystonia secondary to Wilson's disease. *Mov Disord* 2005;20:113–115.

241. Allen KJ, Cheah DM, Lee XL, et al. The potential of bone marrow stem cells to correct liver dysfunction in a mouse model of Wilson's disease. *Cell Transplant* 2004;13:765–773.

242. Meng Y, Miyoshi I, Hirabayashi M, et al. Restoration of copper metabolism and rescue of hepatic abnormalities in LEC rats, an animal model of Wilson disease, by expression of human ATP7B gene. *Biochem Biophys Acta* 2004;1690:208–219.

243. Du C, Fujii Y, Ito M, et al. Dietary polyunsaturated fatty acids suppress acute hepatitis, alter gene expression and prolong survival of female Long-Evans Cinnamon rats, a model of Wilson disease. *J Nutr Biochem* 2004;15:273–280.

244. Shimada H, Takahashi M, Shimada A, et al. Protection from spontaneous hepatocellular damage by N-benzyl-D-glucamine dithiocarbamate in Long-Evans Cinnamon rats, an animal model of Wilson's disease. *Toxicol Appl Pharmacol* 2005;202:59–67.

Neuropathology of Parkinsonian Disorders

22

Dennis W. Dickson

The most common parkinsonian disorders can be assigned to one of two categories based on biochemical abnormalities in tau protein or synuclein. As a group, these disorders have been termed tauopathies and synucleinopathies (1). Tau protein, which is the major component of neurofibrillary tangles (NFTs) in Alzheimer's disease (AD), was initially considered a neuronal protein, but tau-positive glial lesions are increasingly recognized in parkinsonian disorders (2). The discovery of mutations in the tau gene *(MAPT)*, located on chromosome 17, and their relationship to frontotemporal dementia with parkinsonism (FTDP-17) (3) has lead to renewed interest in tau and development of animal models of tau pathology (4) that offer promise for improved diagnosis and management of these disorders. Synuclein was discovered as a nonamyloid component of senile plaques in AD (5). Subsequently, α-synuclein was discovered to be a member of a family of related proteins, including β-synuclein and γ-synuclein, which are either not expressed in the brain or not considered to be directly involved in neurodegeneration. Consequently, in this discussion, synuclein refers to α-synuclein. Interest in synuclein was fueled by the discovery that its gene, which is located on chromosome 4, was mutated in rare familial forms of Parkinson's disease (PD) (6). Subsequently, synuclein was shown to be present in Lewy bodies (LBs) (7) and glial inclusions were shown to be present in multiple system atrophy (MSA) (8).

Although tau and synuclein are neuronal proteins, they also are expressed in pathologic astrocytes and oligodendroglia. They are heat-stable proteins with potential for protein–protein interactions (9). In addition to their physiologic binding partners (e.g., binding of tau to tubulin), they also have a tendency to self-associate to form pathologic fibrils, and known mutations in each molecule favor fibril formation. The best characterized posttranslational modification of tau and synuclein is phosphorylation. Many protein kinases have been shown to phosphorylate tau, but only a

limited set of kinases phosphorylate synuclein (10). It is of interest that one of the most common genetic causes of PD, LRRK2, also has putative protein kinase properties (11). Phosphorylation of tau modifies its binding to tubulin, but little is known about the effects of phosphorylation of synuclein. Tau and synuclein in pathologic lesions are ubiquitinated (12). Although ubiquitination may be merely an adaptive cellular response, it also may have a role in the normal life cycle of these molecules and may contribute directly to pathogenesis of the inclusions. Given evidence that parkin, another molecule involved in familial juvenile-onset parkinsonism, is a ubiquitin ligase and involved in proteasome-mediated proteolysis (13), additional studies are required to understand the role of ubiquitin in normal cellular physiology of tau and synuclein and in parkinsonian disorders.

Synuclein and tau inclusions in neurons and glia are the neuropathologic hallmarks of the major parkinsonian disorders. Tau is present in NFTs, as well as in other neuronal inclusions in the tauopathies. Similarly, synuclein is present not only in LBs and Lewy neurites but also in Lewy-like neuronal inclusions in MSA. Tau-positive glial inclusions include oligodendroglial coiled bodies, tufted astrocytes, and astrocytic plaques (2). Synuclein-positive oligodendroglial cytoplasmic inclusions are the histopathologic hallmark of MSA (14).

SYNUCLEINOPATHIES

Lewy Body Disorders: Parkinson's Disease and Dementia with Lewy Bodies

In this discussion, PD and dementia with Lewy bodies (DLB) are used as clinical terms, whereas Lewy body disease (LBD) is used as a pathologic term. The clinical features of PD are bradykinesia, rigidity, tremor, postural instability, autonomic dysfunction, and bradyphrenia.

The most common pathologic finding in PD is LBD, but occasionally progressive supranuclear palsy (PSP), MSA, or other disorders present clinically with a syndrome indistinguishable from PD. The clinical features of DLB include dementia, extrapyramidal signs, visual hallucinations, and a fluctuating course (15). The pathologic findings in DLB include LBs and varying degrees of Alzheimer's-type pathology. Overlap between these two clinical syndromes is vexing in that dementia can occur late in the course of PD. Whether DLB and dementia in PD are distinct clinico-pathologic entities is an area of current study.

Lewy Bodies and Lewy Neurites

LBs are concentric hyaline cytoplasmic inclusions in specific vulnerable populations of neurons (Fig. 22.1). Although most LBs are single and spherical, some neurons have multiple or pleomorphic LBs. In some regions of the brain, such as the dorsal motor nucleus of the vagus, similar inclusions within neuronal processes are referred to as *intraneuritic LBs*. Intraneuritic LBs can be detected in routine histopathologic preparations and should be distinguished from Lewy neurites, which are not visible with routine histopathology. Lewy neurites were first described in the hippocampus (16) but also are found in other regions of the brain, including the amygdala, cingulate gyrus, and temporal cortex.

Ultrastructural studies of LBs demonstrate non–membrane-bound, granulofilamentous structures. The central region of the LB is usually amorphous, dense material that lacks discernible detail, whereas the periphery has radially arranged 10-nm-diameter filaments (17). At the electron microscopic level, Lewy neurites also have 10 nm filaments, but they lack a dense core and the filaments are more haphazardly arranged (16).

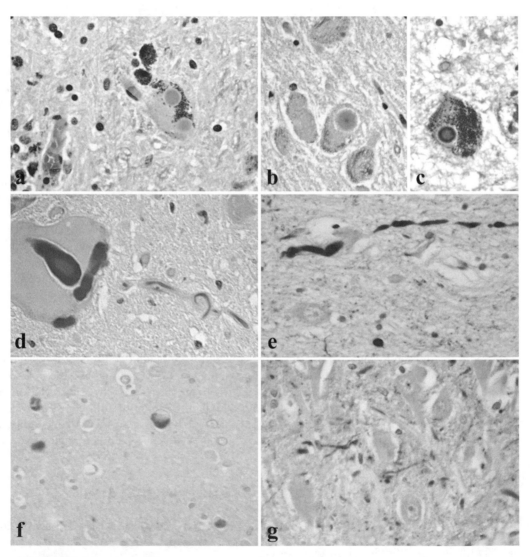

Figure 22.1   Lewy bodies (LBs) are concentric hyaline inclusions in pigmented neurons of the substantia nigra **(A)** and other brainstem nuclei, such as the dorsal raphe **(B)**. They are immunostained with ubiquitin **(C)**. LBs are also found within neuritic processes, such as in the dorsal motor nucleus of the vagus **(D)** and in the basal forebrain **(E)**. Synuclein immunostaining reveals intraneuritic LBs **(E)**, cortical LBs **(F)**, and Lewy neurites in the hippocampus **(G)**.

Neurons that are most vulnerable to LBs include the monoaminergic neurons of the substantia nigra, locus ceruleus, and dorsal motor nucleus of the vagus, as well as cholinergic neurons in the basal forebrain. LBs are rarely detected in the basal ganglia or thalamus but are common in the hypothalamus, especially the posterior and lateral hypothalamus, and the brainstem reticular formation. The oculomotor nuclear complex is also vulnerable. In the pons, the dorsal raphe and subpeduncular nuclei are often affected, but neurons of the pontine base are not. LBs have not been described in the cerebellar cortex. In the spinal cord, the neurons of the intermediolateral cell column are most vulnerable. LBs can be found in the autonomic ganglia, including the submucosal ganglia of the lower esophagus. Neurons in the anterior olfactory nucleus in the olfactory bulb also are vulnerable.

The spread of synuclein pathology in PD has recently been proposed by Braak and coworkers (18), with initial stages of the disease process affecting neurons in the medulla and olfactory bulb, with later spread to the locus ceruleus, substantia nigra, basal forebrain, and limbic structures. The final stage is characterized by LBs in multimodal cortical association areas. The validity of this staging scheme has been confirmed in recent studies (18a, 18b). The progression suggests that clinically overt PD should be preceded by nonmotor manifestations, such as olfactory, autonomic, or gastrointestinal disturbances.

In contrast to typical or classical LBs, cortical LBs are more difficult to detect with routine histology. They tend to be found in small nonpyramidal neurons in lower cortical layers. Similar lesions in the substantia nigra are referred to as "pale bodies." Ultrastructural studies of cortical LBs demonstrate poorly organized granulofilamentous structures rather than the radial arrangement of filaments in classical LBs. Not all cortical regions are equally vulnerable to cortical LBs. The frontal and temporal multimodal association and limbic cortices are most vulnerable, with the amygdala being the most vulnerable of all. LBs are only

rarely detected in primary cortices. Regions with the densest accumulation of cortical LBs are the insular cortex and the parahippocampal and cingulate gyri.

Both classical and cortical LBs share immunocytochemical characteristics. Antibodies to neurofilament were first to be shown to label LBs (19), but most neurofilament antibodies label only a subset of LBs. Ubiquitin is present in most classical and cortical LBs (20), but the most specific method of detecting LBs and Lewy neurites is synuclein immunocytochemistry (21).

Only a few biochemical studies on LBs have been reported due to the paucity of LBs in a given volume of brain tissue and their solubility properties. Lewy bodies are structurally unstable and disrupted upon attempted biochemical purification (22). Initial biochemical studies suggested that a major protein constituent of LBs was a 68-kd protein that had cross-reactivity with neurofilament protein (23). More recent studies suggest that the major structural component of LBs is α-synuclein (24), and in vitro studies have demonstrated that α-synuclein aggregates to form filaments similar to those seen in LBs (25). Other notable proteins localized to LBs are chaperone proteins and proteins involved in ubiquitin-proteasomal degradation (26).

Pathology of Parkinson's Disease

The brain is usually grossly unremarkable until the brainstem is sectioned; then loss of neuromelanin pigmentation in the substantia nigra and locus ceruleus becomes apparent (Fig. 22.2). The histologic correlate of pigment loss is neuronal loss in the substantia nigra pars compacta. In typical PD, as in most other disorders associated with parkinsonism, the neuronal loss is usually most marked in the ventrolateral tier of neurons, which is known to project to the striatum. Striatal pathology is not apparent with routine histologic methods. Neuronal loss in the substantia nigra is accompanied by astrocytosis and microglial activation. Neuromelanin pigment is often found in the cytoplasm of macrophages, and occasionally neurons can be detected undergoing neu-

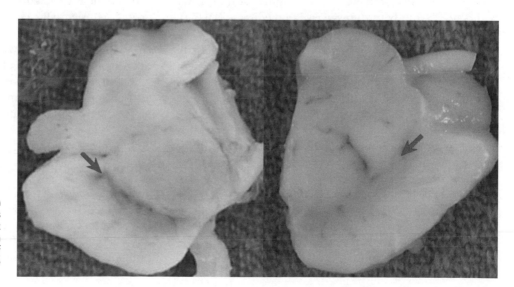

Figure 22.2 The midbrain of a control case (*left*) and a Parkinson's disease case (*right*). Note the black pigment in the substantia nigra in the control case and the loss of pigment in the Parkinson case (*arrows*).

ronophagia, or phagocytosis by macrophages. LBs and pale bodies are found in residual neurons. Similar pathology is also played out in the locus ceruleus and the dorsal motor nucleus of the vagus. The basal forebrain is also vulnerable to neuronal loss and LBs. The neocortex usually does not have LBs, but limbic areas, particularly the amygdala, may have some. Depending on the age of the individual, varying degrees of Alzheimer's-type pathology may be detected; however, if the person is not demented, such pathology usually falls within the range expected for his or her age. Some individuals may have abundant senile plaques but few or no NFTs and a low NFT stage (see the following).

Diffuse Lewy Bodies Disease and the Neuropathology of Dementia in Parkinson's Disease

In the London Parkinson's brain bank series, pathologic findings considered to account for dementia in PD included subcortical pathology (39%), coexistent AD (29%), and diffuse LBD (26%) (27). The basal forebrain cholinergic system is the subcortical region most often implicated in dementia, and neurons in this region are damaged in both AD and LBD. Neuronal loss in the basal nucleus is consistently found in PD, especially PD with dementia (28). As previously mentioned, the basal nucleus is also vulnerable to LBs. Not surprisingly, cholinergic deficits are found in LBD (29). Cholinergic deficits may contribute to dementia in PD in those patients who do not have concurrent AD or cortical LBs. Although recent studies have shown that virtually all PD brains have a few cortical LBs (30), they are usually not widespread and are not numerous in nondemented PD cases (30,31,32). When found in PD, cortical LBs are usually detected in the limbic cortices (e.g., cingulate gyrus) and not detected in association cortices of the frontal, temporal, and parietal lobes. In contrast, several studies have shown that cortical LBs can be numerous and widespread in PD with dementia (30,31,32). Furthermore, the density of cortical LBs has been shown to correlate with the severity of dementia in some studies (33). Patients with widespread cortical Lewy bodies are said to have diffuse Lewy body disease (DLBD). Kosaka and coworkers were the first to use the term *DLBD*, and Kosaka subsequently subdivided DLBD into pure and common forms. The latter is associated with coexistent Alzheimer's-type pathology (34). Some investigators use the term DLBD for cases in which cortical LBs are found in the absence of any Alzheimer's-type pathology, referring to cases with LBs and Alzheimer's-type pathology as the Lewy body variant of AD (35). Brains with cortical LBs confined to the limbic lobe are classified as *transitional LBD*, whereas those with LBs confined to brainstem and diencephalon are said to have *brainstem LBD*. Nondemented PD subjects have brainstem or, occasionally, transitional LBD, whereas PD patients with dementia often have DLBD or transitional LBD.

The entorhinal cortex is unusually susceptible to degeneration in parkinsonian disorders, as well as in aging and AD. In the AD staging scheme of Braak and Braak (36), the entorhinal cortex is among the first areas of the brain to show NFTs. In this staging scheme, six stages are described, with the initial stages being clinically silent. In most cases of DLBD, the Braak stage is lower (stage IV or less) than in comparably demented subjects with AD (stage IV or greater) but usually more than in nondemented controls (stage III or less) (37).

Senile plaques are complicated lesions composed of extracellular deposits of amyloid and localized glial and neuronal changes (38). Given the fact that development of senile plaques is nearly inevitable with aging, it is not surprising that many patients with DLBD, especially those age 60 years or older, have variable numbers of senile plaques. Since clinicopathologic studies have shown that some clinically normal elderly people may have many senile plaques but no NFTs (38), a diagnosis of AD requires the presence of both senile plaques and NFTs (39). Furthermore, there are striking morphologic differences between senile plaques in aging compared and those in AD. In AD, senile plaques differ not only in the nature of the amyloid peptides and reactive glial changes but also in the presence of neuritic elements (i.e., neuritic plaques). In aging and most cases of DLBD, the most prevalent type of plaques are so-called *diffuse plaques*, whereas *neuritic plaques* are the hallmark of AD. The importance of neuritic plaques and NFTs has been adopted by the National Institute of Aging/Reagan Institute criteria in pathologic diagnosis of AD (39). This makes a diagnosis of AD in the setting of LBD more stringent. It is no longer possible to diagnose AD in someone with dementia and LBs who has plaques but no NFTs; thus, the concept of *Lewy body variant of AD* must be revisited.

Lewy Bodies in Aging and Alzheimer's Disease

Postmortem studies of asymptomatic elderly humans demonstrate LBs, most often limited to pigmented brainstem nuclei, in up to 10% of the elderly population (40). A certain degree of parkinsonism is practically synonymous with motor aging, and it is possible that the structural correlate of age-related extrapyramidal signs may be incidental brainstem LBs. However, this remains hypothetical. The pathologic substrate of extrapyramidal signs occurring late in the course of otherwise typical AD has been the focus of only a limited number of pathologic studies. Although it is commonly assumed that LBs account for extrapyramidal features and gait problems in AD, NFT in the substantia nigra were the best correlate in two studies (41,41a).

Multiple System Atrophy

The term *multiple system atrophy* is used for a nonheritable neurodegenerative disease characterized by parkinsonism, cerebellar ataxia, and idiopathic orthostatic hypotension. The concept of MSA unifies three separate entities: olivopontocerebellar atrophy, Shy-Drager syndrome, and striatonigral degeneration. MSA has an average age of onset between age 30 and 50 years and a disease duration that runs in the decades (42). In contrast to other spinocerebellar degenerations, there is no known genetic risk factor or genetic locus in MSA.

Neuropathology of Multiple System Atrophy

The MSA brain shows varying degrees of atrophy of the cerebellum, cerebellar peduncles, pons, and medulla, as well as atrophy and discoloration of the posterolateral putamen and loss of pigment in the ventrolateral substantia nigra (Fig. 22.3). The histopathologic findings include neuronal loss, gliosis, and microvacuolation, involving the putamen, substantia nigra, cerebellum, olivary nucleus, pontine base, and intermediolateral cell column of the spinal cord. White matter inevitably shows demyelination, with the brunt of the changes affecting white matter tracts in affected areas. Recent immunohistochemical studies suggest that white matter pathology may be more widespread than previously suspected (43).

Lantos and coworkers first described oligodendroglial inclusions in MSA and named them glial cytoplasmic inclusions (GCIs) (14). GCIs can be detected with silver stains, such as the Gallyas stain, but are best seen with antibodies to synuclein, where they appear as flame- or sickle-shaped inclusions in oligodendrocytes (Fig. 22.4). In addition to synuclein immunoreactivity, GCIs are consistently immunoreactive for ubiquitin and variably immunoreactive for tubulin, α-β crystallin, and tau (14). At the ultrastructural level, GCIs are non–membrane-bound cytoplasmic inclusions composed of filaments (7–10 nm) and granular material that often coats the filaments (44). GCIs are distinctly different from the oligodendroglial inclusions, so-called coiled bodies (45) that are found in the tauopathies (see discussion below). Most tau antibodies readily stain coiled bodies, but GCIs are usually negative. GCIs are specific for MSA and have not been found in other neurodegenerative diseases. Glial inclusions somewhat similar to GCIs are sometimes detected in LBD, but they are never widespread or numerous (46). In addition to GCIs, synuclein-immunoreactive lesions are also detected in some neurons in MSA. The distribution of neuronal inclusions in MSA is decidedly different from LBD in that the most vulnerable neuronal populations are neurons in the inferior olivary nucleus, pontine base, and putamen, which are neurons rarely affected in LBD. Biochemical studies of synuclein in MSA have shown changes in its solubility (47) similar to solubility changes in LBD and tau in the tauopathies.

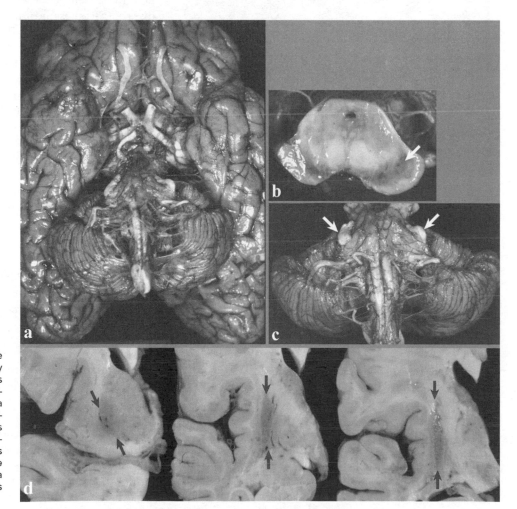

Figure 22.3 The base of the brain in multiple system atrophy shows marked atrophy of the pons (**a**) with loss of pigment in the lateral part of the substantia nigra (**b**, *arrow*). Note the relative prominence of the trigeminal nerves (*arrows* in **c**) due to pontine atrophy. On coronal sections, there is atrophy and discoloration in the lateral putamen (*arrows*) with a gradient of severity that increases caudally (**d**, *left to right*).

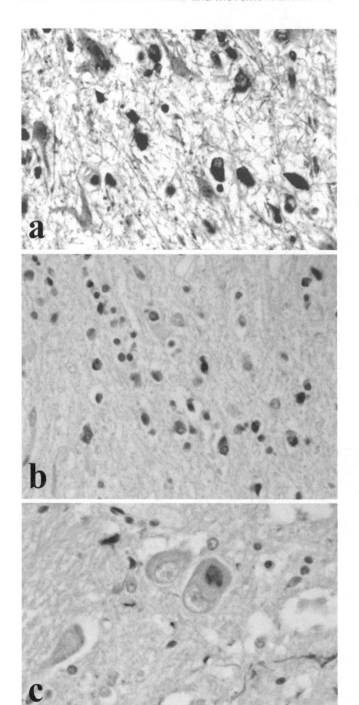

Figure 22.4   Gallyas silver stain reveals dense, round to crescent-shaped glial cytoplasmic inclusions (GCIs) in multiple system atrophy **(a)** and numerous GCIs in affected areas with synuclein immuno-stains **(b)**. Synuclein also occasionally reveals Lewy-like neuronal inclusions **(c)** and neuritic processes (*lower right*) in the pontine base.

TAUOPATHIES

Introduction

Tau abnormalities are increasingly considered to play a crucial role in a group of neurodegenerative diseases known as the *tauopathies*. PSP and CBD are the most common sporadic tauopathies. Other tauopathies include Pick's disease, fron-

totemporal dementia and parkinsonism linked to chromosome 17 (FTDP-17), postencephalitic parkinsonism (PEP), Guam parkinsonism–dementia complex (Guam PDC), and dementia pugilistica. All tauopathies involve neurodegeneration of specific neuronal populations with filamentous tau protein aggregates in neurons and glia. Many are associated with clinical features of parkinsonism. Some are sporadic (Pick's disease, PSP, CBD, PEP, Guam PDC, dementia pugilistica), whereas others are hereditary (FTDP-17).

PSP and CBD were first reported in the 1960s (48,49), and the term *corticobasal degeneration* was coined in the 1980s (50). Molecular and genetic studies have identified similar changes in PSP and CBD. Furthermore, PSP and CBD share clinical and pathologic features, but notable differences warrant their current separation as clinicopathologic entities. Although individuals with CBD and PSP have bradykinesia, rigidity, and gait abnormalities, neither group has demonstrated a sustained clinical response to levodopa. Rest tremor, one of the cardinal clinical features of PD, is uncommon in PSP and CBD. Motor abnormalities in PSP are usually symmetric, while asymmetry is the hallmark of CBD. Focal cortical signs, such as apraxia and aphasia, are common in CBD but rare in PSP. Dementia is common in CBD and may be one of the most common presentations, but it is not prominent in PSP. Supranuclear gaze palsy occurs early in most cases of PSP but is uncommon and a late feature in CBD.

Pathologically, both PSP and CBD include neuronal and glial lesions composed of tau protein. Although the anatomic distribution of lesions shows overlap, the overall pattern differs (51). Cortical and cerebral white matter are more affected in CBD, whereas the diencephalon and brainstem are more affected in PSP. The morphology of the typical neuronal and glial lesions is distinctive in PSP and CBD (52).

Yet biochemical studies of tau protein show indistinguishable alterations in PSP and CBD (53). In both disorders, there is evidence of enrichment of abnormal insoluble tau isoforms (4R tau) derived from specific tau mRNA splice forms (forms that include the alternatively spliced exon 10, which encodes one of four conserved repeats in the microtubule binding domain). There is also evidence of similar predisposition with respect to genetic variants in the tau gene, *MAPT* (54,55,55a).

Neuropathology of Progressive Supranuclear Palsy

Gross examination of the brain often shows frontal and midbrain atrophy. The third ventricle and aqueduct of Sylvius may be dilated. The substantia nigra shows loss of pigment, while the locus ceruleus is better preserved. The subthalamic nucleus is smaller than expected (Fig. 22.5). The superior cerebellar peduncle and the hilus of the cerebellar dentate nucleus may be atrophic and gray due to myelinated fiber loss (Fig. 22.6).

Microscopic findings include neuronal loss and fibrillary gliosis affecting multiple brain regions. The nuclei with the most marked and consistent pathology are the

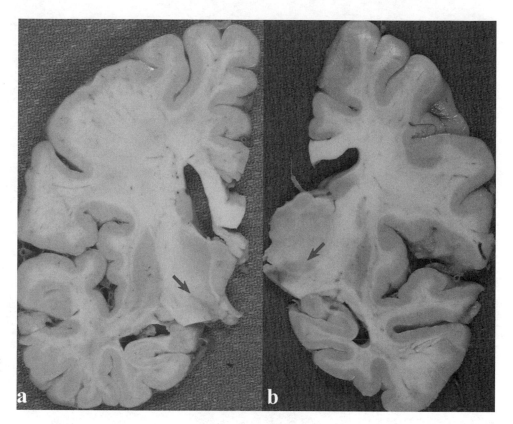

Figure 22.5 The subthalamic nucleus (*arrows*) is markedly atrophic in progressive supranuclear palsy **(a)** in comparison with normal **(b)**.

globus pallidus, subthalamic nucleus, and substantia nigra. Other parts of the basal ganglia, diencephalon, and brainstem are affected to a variable degree.

In addition to the changes visible with routine histologic methods, silver stains (e.g., Gallyas stain) or immunostaining for tau reveal NFTs and glial lesions (Fig. 22.7). NFTs in PSP often have a rounded or globose appearance, but flame-shaped NFTs are also detected. Special stains demonstrate a variety of inclusions in both neurons and glia, including pretangles, neuropil threads, and tufts of abnormal fibers. Pretangles are neurons with nonfilamentous granular cytoplasmic tau immunoreactivity that may be precursors to NFTs. Tufts of abnormal fibers, also known as *tufted astrocytes*, are most common in the motor cortex and striatum. They are fibrillary lesions within astrocytes based on double immunolabeling of tau and glial fibrillary acidic protein. Tufted astrocytes account for much of the cortical pathology observed in PSP. Tau immunohistochemistry also reveals tau-positive fibers, so-called *neuropil threads*, and small round glial cells in the white matter, which are oligodendroglial inclusions based on double immunolabeling with tau and oligodendroglial markers. Threadlike processes in white matter are not as numerous in PSP as in CBD, but have been shown with immunoelectron microscopy in both disorders to be in axons, as well as glial processes (56). In gray matter, neuropil threads are less common in PSP than in AD and CBD.

The NFTs in PSP may be distinguished from NFTs in AD by the paucity of ubiquitin immunoreactivity. The same is true for CBD. They also have far less fluorescence with thioflavin-S stains. In fact, NFT may be completely missed if thioflavin-S is the only means used to evaluate neuropathology in PSP and CBD. Since NFTs in AD and CBD are composed of tau (57), the observed differences must reflect differences in packing, conformation, or posttranslational modification.

Whereas NFTs in AD are composed mostly of 22-nm-diameter paired helical filaments (PHFs) and a minor

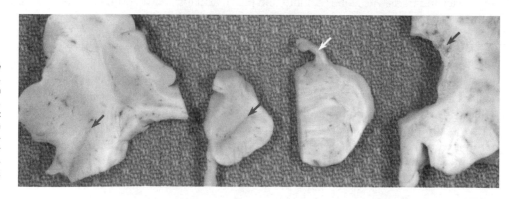

Figure 22.6 Sections of the diencephalon, midbrain, pons, medulla, and cerebellar dentate in progressive supranuclear palsy. Note the small subthalamic nucleus (*arrow*), loss of pigment in the substantia nigra (*arrow*), atrophy of the superior cerebellar peduncle (*white arrow*), and atrophy and discoloration of the hilus of the dentate nucleus (*arrow*).

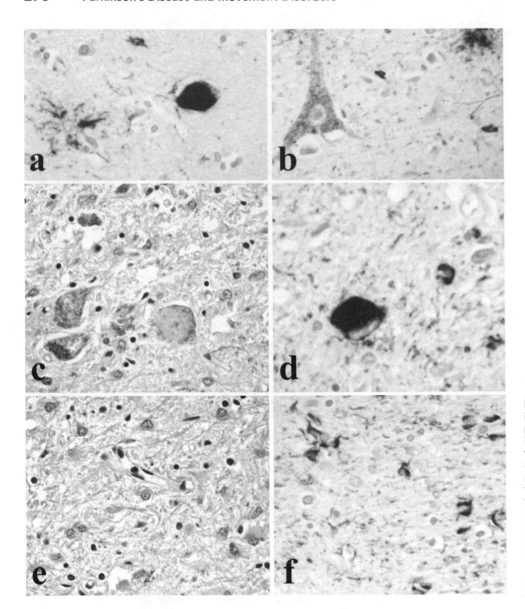

Figure 22.7 Tau immunostaining reveals a range of lesions in progressive supranuclear palsy, including a globose neurofibrillary tangle (NFT) (**a**, *right*) and tufted astrocytes (**a**, *left*) in the caudate; pretangles (**b**, *left*), NFTs, and tufted astrocytes (**b**, *top right*) in the motor cortex. The substantia nigra has neuronal loss with extraneuronal neuromelanin pigment (**c**) and NFTs (**d**). The subthalamic nucleus has neuronal loss and dense fibrillary gliosis (**e**). Tau immunostaining shows many coiled bodies in white matter tracts (**f**).

component of 15- to 18-nm-diameter straight filaments, NFTs in PSP are composed of 15- to 18-nm-diameter straight filaments. The abnormal filaments in glial cells in PSP also contain straight filaments.

The distribution of pathology is highly characteristic of PSP. Pathologic diagnosis is contingent on pathology in specific nuclei and tracts. The globus pallidus and pars reticularis of the substantia nigra may show—in addition to neuronal loss, gliosis, and NFTs—extensive iron pigment deposition and granular neuroaxonal spheroids. The striatum and thalamus, especially the ventral anterior and lateral nuclei, may show gliosis. The basal nucleus of Meynert usually show mild cell loss and many pretangles. The brainstem regions that are affected include the superior colliculus, periaqueductal gray matter, oculomotor nuclei, locus ceruleus, pontine nuclei, pontine tegmentum, vestibular nuclei, medullary tegmentum, and inferior olives. The cerebellar dentate nucleus is frequently affected and may show grumose degeneration, a type of neuronal degeneration associated with clusters of degenerating presynaptic terminals around dentate neurons. The dentatorubrothalamic pathway consistently shows fiber loss. The cerebellar cortex is preserved, but there may be mild Purkinje cell loss with scattered axonal torpedoes. Coiled bodies are common in the cerebellar white matter. The spinal cord, where neuronal inclusions can be found in anterior horn and intermediolateral cells, is often affected.

Cortical gray matter is less affected than deep gray matter, but lesions are increasingly recognized in the cortex, especially the perirolandic region (58). Neocortical NFTs and tufted astrocytes are concentrated in the motor cortex. Recent studies suggest that cortical pathology may be more widespread in cases of PSP with atypical features, such as dementia (59). The white matter beneath the motor cortex often has coiled bodies. More widespread cerebral white matter pathology is uncommon in PSP. This contrasts with CBD, where white matter lesions are numerous and widespread.

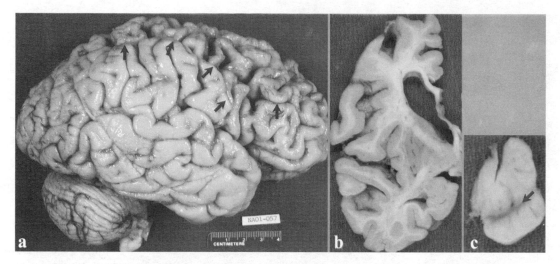

Figure 22.8   The cortical atrophy in corticobasal degeneration is often most marked in the superior frontal gyrus and superior parietal lobule (**a**, *arrows*). On coronal sections, the frontal horn is dilated, while the temporal horn of the lateral ventricle is normal (**b**). The lateral part of the substantia nigra (*arrow*) may show pigment loss (**c**).

The limbic lobe is preserved in PSP. The neurofibrillary pathology in the hippocampus is variable and not inherent to PSP, but rather more consistent with concurrent age-related pathology. An exception is the frequent involvement of the dentate gyrus granule neurons in PSP (58).

Neuropathology of Corticobasal Degeneration

Gross examination of the brain characteristically reveals subtle asymmetric atrophy of cortical gyri, most marked in pre- and post-central regions (Fig. 22.8). The atrophy is not as sharply circumscribed or as severe as in Pick's disease. Dorsal frontoparietal atrophy merges with less severe atrophy in ventral frontal and posterior parietal regions, whereas the temporal and occipital cortical regions are usually preserved. The brainstem does not have the consistent atrophy found in PSP, but pigment loss is common in the substantia nigra. In contrast to PSP, the superior cerebellar peduncle and the subthalamic nucleus are also normal on gross examination.

The cerebral white matter in affected areas is often attenuated and may have a gray discoloration. The corpus callosum is sometimes thinned, and the frontal horn of the lateral ventricle is frequently dilated. The anterior limb of the internal capsule may show attenuation as well, but other white matter tracts, such as the optic tract, anterior commissure, and fornix, are preserved.

Microscopic examination of atrophic regions of the frontoparietal cortex shows moderately severe nerve cell loss with superficial spongiosis, gliosis, and subcortical myelin pallor. Thioflavin-S fluorescence and silver staining fail to reveal senile plaques or NFTs. These findings are not dissimilar to those of nonspecific focal cortical degenerations; however, several histologic features readily distinguish CBD from nonspecific focal cortical degenerations, most notably the presence of many achromatic or ballooned neurons. Ballooned neurons are swollen and vacuolated neurons found in middle and lower cortical layers. They lack apparent Nissl substance, which was the basis for the term *achromasia*. Ballooned neurons in anterior cingulate, amygdala, and claustrum have less diagnostic significance because they can be found in several disorders, most notably argyrophilic grain disease disorder named in honor of Braak, who discovered it. (60).

Ballooned neurons are strongly immunoreactive for phosphorylated neurofilaments and α-β crystallin (Fig. 22.9). They show variable immunoreactivity for tau and ubiquitin. Ultrastructurally, the cytoplasm of the ballooned neurons contains haphazardly arranged 9- to 16-nm-diameter filaments, interspersed with other cytoplasmic elements.

Neurons in atrophic cortical areas also have pleomorphic tau-immunoreactive lesions. In some neurons, tau is densely packed into a small inclusion body somewhat reminiscent of a Pick body or a small NFT (Fig. 22.9). In other neurons, the filamentous inclusions are more dispersed and disorderly. In contrast to NFTs of AD where lesions are readily detected with a host of diagnostic silver stains and even with thioflavin fluorescent microscopy, the neuronal lesions in CBD are negative with thioflavin-S. Neurofibrillary lesions in brainstem monoaminergic nuclei, such as the locus ceruleus and substantia nigra, sometimes resemble globose NFTs but may also be ill-defined amorphous inclusions.

In addition to fibrillary lesions in the perikarya of neurons, the neuropil of CBD invariably contains an assortment of threadlike tau-immunoreactive cell processes (61). A small fraction of threadlike structures are double labeled with neurofilament antibodies, which indicates that many threadlike lesions in CBD are in glial processes. They are usually profuse in affected areas of gray and white matter. The predominance of tau immunoreactivity in cell processes is an important attribute of CBD and a useful feature in

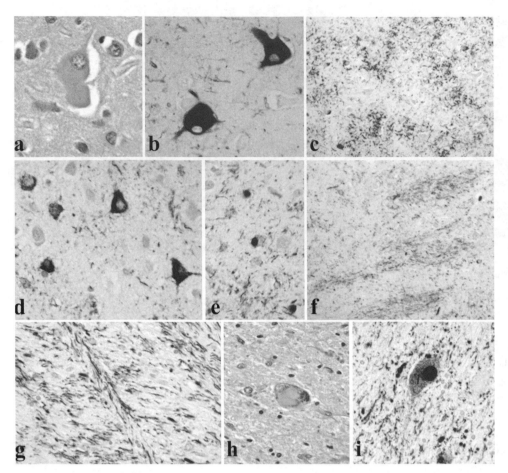

Figure 22.9 Ballooned neurons have swelling of perikarya and proximal processes **(a)** and immunoreactivity with α-β crystallin **(b)**. Tau immunostaining of the cortex shows annual clusters of cell processes, which are astrocytic plaques **(c)**. Neuronal inclusions are diverse **(d)** and some resemble Pick bodies **(e)**. White matter tracts, such as pencil fibers in the striatum **(f)** and the internal capsule near the thalamic fasciculus **(g)**, have many tau-positive threadlike processes. Neurons in the substantia nigra contain eosinophilic corticobasal bodies **(h)** that are tau positive **(i)**.

differentiating it from other disorders (62). In other disorders with which CBD can be confused, tau-related pathology is more often located in cell bodies (e.g., NFTs and Pick bodies) and the proximal cell processes of neurons and glia.

The most characteristic tau-immunoreactive astrocytic lesion in CBD is an annular cluster of short stubby processes with fuzzy outlines that may be highly suggestive of a neuritic plaque (61) (Fig. 22.9). These lesions, in contrast to Alzheimer's plaques, do not contain amyloid. In further contradistinction, the tau filaments are found not in neuronal but rather in glial processes. These lesions are termed *astrocytic plaques*. Astrocytic plaques differ from the tufted astrocytes seen in PSP, and the two lesions do not coexist in the same brain (52). The astrocytic plaque may be the most specific histopathologic lesion of CBD.

In addition to cortical pathology, deep gray matter is consistently affected in CBD. The globus pallidus and putamen show mild neuronal loss with gliosis. The nucleus basalis of Meynert has minimal neuronal loss and pretangles. Thalamic nuclei may also be affected, particularly the ventrolateral nucleus. In the basal ganglia, threadlike processes are often extensive in the pencil fibers of the striatum. There also may be astrocytic plaques in the striatum. Pretangles are common in the striatum and globus pallidus. The internal capsule often has many threadlike processes, especially in the vicinity of the thalamic fasciculus. The

subthalamic nucleus usually has a normal neuronal population, but a few neurons may have tau inclusions, and there may be a number of threadlike lesions in the nucleus. Fibrillary gliosis typical of PSP is uncommon in the subthalamic nucleus in CBD.

The substantia nigra usually shows moderate to severe nerve cell loss with extraneuronal neuromelanin and gliosis. Many of the remaining neurons contain NFTs, which have also been termed *corticobasal bodies*. The locus ceruleus and raphe nuclei have similar inclusions. In contrast to PSP, where neurons in the pontine base almost always have at least a few NFTs, the pontine base is largely free of NFTs in CBD. In comparison, tau inclusions in glia and in cell processes are common in the pontine base in CBD. NFTs are also detected in the tegmental gray matter. The cerebellum has mild Purkinje cell loss and axonal torpedoes. There is also mild neuronal loss in the dentate nucleus, but grumose degeneration is much less common than in PSP.

In CBD, the filaments have a paired helical appearance at the electron microscopic level, but the diameter is wider and the periodicity is longer than the paired helical filaments of AD (63). These structures have been referred to as *twisted ribbons*. Similar filaments are found in some cases of FTDP-17, particularly those associated with overexpression of specific isoforms of tau containing an extra repeat in the microtubule binding domain (4R tau) (64). Similar to

PSP, tau in CBD is enriched in tau isoforms containing the domain encoded by exon 10 of the tau gene, *MAPT*.

Neuropathology of Other Parkinsonian Disorders with Neurofibrillary Tangles

Several other disorders with parkinsonism are associated with NFTs and can be considered among the tauopathies. These are uncommon disorders that in some cases have nearly disappeared, but they are discussed here from a historical perspective.

Postencephalitic Parkinsonism

Parkinsonism following encephalitis lethargica during the influenza pandemic between 1916 and 1926 is known as *postencephalitic parkinsonism* (PEP) (65). The acute stage of this illness was characterized by a somnolent state, for which the disorder is named, that, in some cases, progressed to coma. Other clinical features included oculomotor palsy, myoclonus, and masked facies. During the recovery phase, parkinsonian rigidity developed, with the most characteristic clinical features being oculogyric crises (65). The pathology in the acute stage was characterized by inflammation and hyperemia that was widespread, but marked in basal ganglia and brainstem. Neuronal loss was present in the locus ceruleus, substantia nigra, oculomotor nuclei, and lentiform nucleus. Dystrophic calcification was also described in affected areas (65). Evaluation of brains of subjects long after the disease occurred has revealed NFTs in the cortex, basal ganglia, thalamus, hypothalamus, substantia nigra, brainstem tegmentum, and cerebellar dentate nucleus (66,67). The distribution of the pathology overlaps with PSP, and in recent studies, it has not been possible to distinguish the two disorders by histopathologic analysis alone (66,67). Biochemical studies of tau that accumulates in PEP has not been reported, but the NFTs resemble those seen in AD, so it is reasonable to assume that abnormal tau in PEP is composed of a mixture of 3R and 4R tau. Tau-immunopositive glial lesions have not been reported in PEP.

Parkinsonism Dementia Complex in Guam

An unusually high incidence of Parkinsonism dementia complex (PDC) has been reported since the 1950s in the native Chamorro population of Guam (68). Some individuals also have amyotrophic lateral sclerosis (ALS), and the natives refer to the complex of PDC with ALS as "lytico-bodig." The incidence of the disorder has declined in recent years for unknown reasons, and the etiology remains unknown despite intensive epidemiologic and genetic research. The disorder has a geographic distribution on Guam, but the basis for this is not known. Some studies suggest that ALS on Guam is no different from ALS in other populations (69). On the other hand, PDC and the pathologic substrate of PDC—namely, widespread cortical and brainstem NFTs—is distinctly different from PD with dementia.

The gross findings in PDC are notable for cortical atrophy affecting the frontal and temporal lobes, as well as atrophy of the hippocampus and the tegmentum of the rostral brainstem (70). These areas typically have neuronal loss and gliosis with many NFTs in residual neurons. Extracellular NFTs are also numerous. In the cortex, NFTs show a laminar distribution different from that of AD, with more NFTs in superficial cortical layers in Guam PDC and in lower cortical layers in AD (71). The hippocampus has severe pathology with numerous NFTs. Interestingly, NFTs are also found in nondemented Chamorros at a higher frequency than in Western populations (72). The substantia nigra and locus ceruleus have neuronal loss and NFTs (Fig. 22.10). The basal nucleus and large neurons in the striatum are also vulnerable to NFTs. Lewy bodies are not detected, but some neurons in the amygdala may have synuclein-immunoreactive lesions (73). Biochemically and morphologically, NFTs in Guam PDC are indistinguishable from those in AD (74). Immunohistochemically, they are similar with all antibodies that have been tested to tau and other NFT-associated molecules; at the electron microscopic level, the filaments in the NFTs are 22-nm-diameter paired helical filaments; and biochemically, they contain insoluble tau composed of a mixture of 3R tau and

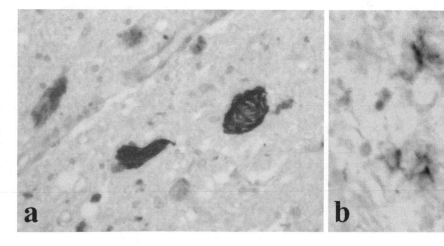

Figure 22.10 In Guam parkinsonism-dementia complex, there is marked neuronal loss in the substantia nigra, and Gallyas silver stain reveals neurofibrillary tangles in the few residual neurons **(a)**. The silver stain also reveals granular hazy astrocytes in parkinsonism-dementia complex **(b)**. (Slides courtesy of Asao Hirano, Montefiore Hospital, The Bronx, New York.)

4R tau. Recently, an unusual type of tau-immunoreactive astrocyte, so-called granular *hazy inclusions*, has been noted in Guam PDC (75).

Dementia Pugilistica

An akinetic rigid syndrome with dysarthria and dementia is sometimes the long-term outcome of repeated closed-head trauma, as is seen in professional boxers. The pathology on gross examination, other than lesions that can be attributed to trauma (e.g., subdural membrane and cortical contusions), is characterized by fenestration or cavum of the septum pellucidum (76). The substantia nigra may also show pigment loss. Microscopically, there are NFTs that are similar to those found in AD. They are found in brainstem monoaminergic nuclei but also in the cortex and hippocampus. In the cortex, they may be clustered around blood vessels (77). At the electron microscopic level, they are composed of paired helical filaments; biochemically, the abnormal insoluble tau extracted from affected brain regions is composed of a mixture of 3R tau and 4R tau (78).

REFERENCES

1. Hardy J, Gwinn-Hardy K. Genetic classification of primary neurodegenerative disease. *Science* 1998;282:1075–1078.
2. Chin SSM, Goldman JE. Glial inclusions in CNS degenerative diseases. *J Neuropathol Exp Neurol* 1996;55:499–508.
3. Hutton M, Lendon CL, Rizzu P, et al. Association of missense and 5'-splice-site mutations in tau with the inherited dementia (FTDP-17). *Nature* 1998;393:702–705.
4. Lewis J, McGowan E, Rockwood J, et al. Neurofibrillary tangles, amyotrophy and progressive motor disturbance in tau mutant (P301L) transgenic mice. *Nat Genet* 2000;25:402–405.
5. Iwai A, Masliah E, Yoshimoto M, et al. The precursor protein of non-Aβ component of Alzheimer's disease amyloid is a presynaptic protein of the central nervous system. *Neuron* 1995;14:467–475.
6. Polymeropoulos MHC, Leroy E, Ide SE, et al. Mutation in the alpha-synuclein gene identified in families with Parkinson's disease. *Science* 1997;276:2045–2047.
7. Spillantini MG, Schmidt ML, Lee VM, et al. Alpha-synuclein in Lewy bodies. *Nature* 1997;388:839–840.
8. Arima K, Ueda K, Sunohara N, et al. NACP/α-synuclein immunoreactivity in fibrillary components of neuronal and oligodendroglial cytoplasmic inclusions in the pontine nuclei in multiple system atrophy. *Acta Neuropathol* 1998;96:439–444.
9. Dickson DW. Tau and synuclein and their role in neuropathology. *Brain Pathol* 1999;9:657–661.
10. Dickson DW. α-Synuclein and the Lewy body disorders. *Curr Opin Neurol* 2001;14:423–432.
11. Zimprich A, Biskup S, Leitner P, et al. Mutations in LRRK2 cause autosomal-dominant parkinsonism with pleomorphic pathology. *Neuron* 2004;44:601–607.
12. Dickson DW, Yen S-H. Ubiquitin, the cytoskeleton and neurodegenerative diseases. In: Mayer RJ, Brown IR, eds. Heat Shock or Stress Proteins and the Nervous System. London: Academic Press, 1994;235–262.
13. Kitada T, Asakawa S, Hattori N, et al. Mutations in the parkin gene cause autosomal recessive juvenile parkinsonism. *Nature* 1998;392:605–608.
14. Lantos PL. The definition of multiple system atrophy: a review of recent developments. *J Neuropathol Exp Neurol* 1998;57:1099–1111.
15. McKeith IG, Dickson DW, Lowe J, et al. Diagnosis and management of dementia with Lewy bodies. Third report of the DLB consortium. *Neurology* 2005;65:1863–1872.
16. Dickson DW, Ruan D, Crystal H, et al. Hippocampal degeneration differentiates diffuse Lewy body disease (DLBD) from Alzheimer's disease: light and electron microscopic immunocytochemistry of CA2-3 neurites specific to DLBD. *Neurology* 1991;41:1402–1409.
17. Galloway PG, Mulvihill P, Perry G. Filaments of Lewy bodies contain insoluble cytoskeletal elements. *Am J Pathol* 1992;140:809–815.
18. Braak H, Ghebremedhin E, Rub U, et al. Stages in the development of Parkinson's disease-related pathology. *Cell Tissue Res* 2004;318:121–134.
18a. Muller CM, de Vos RA, Maurage CA, et al. Staging of sporatic Parkinson disrelated alpha-synuclein pathology: inter- and intrarater reliability. *J Neuropathol Exp Neurol* 2005;64:623–628.
18b. Klos KJ, Ahlskog JE, Josephs KA, et al. Alpha-synuclein pathology in the spinal cords of neurological asymptomatic aged individuals. *Neurology* 2006;66:1100–1102.
19. Goldman JE, Yen S-H, Chiu F-C, et al. Lewy bodies of Parkinson's disease contain neurofilament antigens. *Science* 1983;221:1082–1084.
20. Kuzuhara S, Mori H, Izumiyama N, et al. Lewy bodies are ubiquitinated: a light and electron microscopic immunocytochemical study. *Acta Neuropathol* 1988;75:345–353.
21. Irizarry MC, Growdon W, Gomez-Isla T, et al. Nigral and cortical Lewy bodies and dystrophic nigral neurites in Parkinson's disease and cortical Lewy body disease contain α-synuclein immunoreactivity. *J Neuropathol Exp Neurol* 1998;57:334–337.
22. Iwatsubo T, Yamaguchi H, Fujimuro M, et al. Purification and characterization of Lewy bodies from the brains of patients with diffuse Lewy body disease. *Am J Pathol* 1996;148:1517–1529.
23. Pollanen MS, Bergeron C, Weyer L. Detergent-insoluble Lewy body fibrils share epitopes with neurofilament and tau. *J Neurochem* 1992;58:1953–1956.
24. Baba M, Nakajo S, Tu PH, et al. Aggregation of alpha-synuclein in Lewy bodies of sporadic Parkinson's disease and dementia with Lewy bodies. *Am J Pathol* 1998;152:879–884.
25. Conway KA, Harper JD, Lansbury PT. Accelerated in vitro fibril formation by a mutant alpha-synuclein linked to early-onset parkinson's disease. *Nat Med* 1998;4:1318–1320.
26. Pollanen MS, Dickson DW, Bergeron C: Pathology and biology of the Lewy body. *J Neuropathol Exp Neurol* 1993;52:183–191.
27. Hughes AJ, Daniel SE, Blankson S, et al. A clinicopathologic study of 100 cases of Parkinson's disease. *Arch Neurol* 1993;50:140–148.
28. Whitehouse PJ, Hedreen JC, White CL III, et al. Basal forebrain neurons in dementia of parkinson's disease. *Ann Neurol* 1983;13:243–248.
29. Dickson DW, Davies P, Mayeux R, et al. Diffuse Lewy body disease: neuropathological and biochemical studies of six patients. *Acta Neuropathol* 1987;75:8–15.
30. Mattila PM, Roytta M, Torikka H, et al. Cortical Lewy bodies and Alzheimer-type changes in patients with Parkinson's disease. *Acta Neuropathol* 1998;95:576–582.
31. Hurtig HI, Trojanowski JQ, Galvin J, et al. Alpha-synuclein cortical Lewy bodies correlate with dementia in Parkinson's disease. *Neurology* 2000;54:1916–1921.
32. Apaydin H, Ahlskog JE, Parisi JE, et al. Parkinson's disease neuropathology: later-developing dementia and loss of the levodopa response. *Arch Neurol* 2002;59:102–112.
33. Lennox G, Lowe JS, Landon M, et al. Diffuse Lewy body disease: correlative neuropathology using anti-ubiquitin immunocytochemistry. *J Neurol Neurosurg Psychiatry* 1989;52:1236–1247.
34. Kosaka K. Diffuse Lewy body disease in Japan. *J Neurol* 1990;237:197–204.
35. Hansen L, Salmon D, Galasko D, et al. Lewy body variant of Alzheimer's disease: a clinical and pathological entity. *Neurology* 1990;40:1–8.
36. Braak H, Braak E. Neuropathological staging of Alzheimer-related changes. *Acta Neuropathol* 1991;82:239–259.
37. Jellinger KA, Bancher C. Dementia with Lewy bodies: relationships to Parkinson's and Alzheimer's diseases. In: Perry RH, McKeith IG, Perry EK, eds. Dementia with Lewy Bodies. Cambridge: Cambridge University Press, 1996;268.

38. Dickson DW. Pathogenesis of senile plaques. *J Neuropathol Exp Neurol* 1997;56:321–354.

39. Hyman BT, Trojanowski JQ. Consensus recommendations for the postmortem diagnosis of Alzheimer disease from the National Institute on Aging and the Reagan Institute Working Group on diagnostic criteria for the neuropathological assessment of Alzheimer disease. *J Neuropathol Exp Neurol* 1997; 56:1095–1097.

40. Forno LS. Concentric hyaline intraneuronal inclusions of Lewy body type in the brains of elderly persons (50 incidental cases): relationship to parkinsonism. *J Am Geriatr Soc* 1969; 17:557–575.

41. Liu Y, Stern Y, Chun MR, et al. Pathological correlates of extrapyramidal signs in Alzheimer's disease. *Ann Neurol* 1997;41: 368–374.

41a.Schneider JA, Li JL, Li Y, et al. Substantia nigra tangles are related to gait impairment in older persons. *Ann Neurol* 2006;59:166–173.

42. Wenning GK, Tison F, Ben Shlomo Y, et al. Multiple system atrophy: a review of 203 pathologically proven cases. *Mov Disord* 1997;12:133–147.

43. Matsuo A, Akiguchi I, Lee GC, et al. Myelin degeneration in multiple system atrophy detected by unique antibodies. *Am J Pathol* 1998;153:735–744.

44. Kato S, Nakamura H. Cytoplasmic argyrophilic inclusions in neurons of pontine nuclei in patients with olivopontocerebellar atrophy: immunohistochemical and ultrastructural studies. *Acta Neuropathol* 1990;79:584–594.

45. Braak H, Braak E. Cortical and subcortical argyrophilic grains characterize a disease associated with adult onset dementia. *Neuropathol Appl Neurobiol* 1989;15:13–26.

46. Wakabayashi K, Hayashi S, Yoshimoto M, et al. NACP/alpha-synuclein-positive filamentous inclusions in astrocytes and oligodendrocytes of Parkinson's disease brains. *Acta Neuropathol* 2000;99:14–20.

47. Dickson DW, Liu W-K, Hardy J, et al. Widespread alterations of alpha-synuclein in multiple system atrophy. *Am J Pathol* 1999;155: 1241–1251.

48. Steele JC, Richardson JC, Olszewski J. Progressive supranuclear palsy: a heterogenous degeneration involving the brainstem, basal ganglia and cerebellum with vertical gaze and pseudobulbar palsy, nuchal dystonia, and dementia. *Arch Neurol* 1964;10: 333–339.

49. Rebeiz JJ, Kolodny EH, Richardson EP Jr. Corticodentatonigral degeneration with neuronal achromasia. *Arch Neurol* 1968;18: 20–33.

50. Gibb WRG, Luthert PJ, Marsden CD. Corticobasal degeneration. *Brain* 1989;112:1171–1192.

51. Feany MB, Mattiace LA, Dickson DW. Neuropathologic overlap of progressive supranuclear palsy, Pick's disease and corticobasal degeneration. *J Neuropathol Exp Neurol* 1996;55:53–67.

52. Komori T. Tau-positive glial inclusions in progressive supranuclear palsy, corticobasal degeneration, and Pick's disease. *Brain Pathol* 1999;9:663–679.

53. Buee L, Delacourte A. Comparative biochemistry of tau in progressive supranuclear palsy, corticobasal degeneration, FTDP-17 and Pick's disease. *Brain Pathol* 1999;9:681–693.

54. Baker M, Litvan I, Houlden H, et al. Association of an extended haplotype in the tau gene with progressive supranuclear palsy. *Hum Mol Genet* 1999;8:711–715.

55. Di Maria E, Tabaton M, Vigo T, et al. Corticobasal degeneration shares a common genetic background with progressive supranuclear palsy. *Ann Neurol* 2000;47:374–377.

55a.Rademakers R, Melquist S, Cruts M, et al. High density SNP haplotyping suggests altered regulation of tau gene expression in progressive supranuclear palsy. *Hum Mol Genet* 2005;14: 3281–3292.

56. Arima K, Nakamura M, Sunohara N, et al. Ultrastructural characterization of the tau-immunoreactive tubules in the oligodendroglial perikarya and their inner loop processes in progressive supranuclear palsy. *Acta Neuropathol* 1997;93:558–566.

57. Schmidt ML, Huang R, Martin JA, et al. Neurofibrillary tangles in progressive supranuclear palsy contain the same tau epitopes identified in Alzheimer's disease PHF-tau. *J Neuropathol Exp Neurol* 1996;55:534–539.

58. Hof PR, Delacourte A, Bouras C. Distribution of cortical neurofibrillary tangles in progressive supranuclear palsy: a quantitative analysis of six cases. *Acta Neuropathol* 1992;84:45–51.

59. Bigio EH, Brown DF, White CL III. Progressive supranuclear palsy with dementia: cortical pathology. *J Neuropathol Exp Neurol* 1999;58:359–364.

60. Tolnay M, Probst A. Ballooned neurons expressing alpha B-crystallin as a constant feature of the amygdala in argyrophilic grain disease. *Neurosci Lett* 1998;246:165–168.

61. Feany MB, Dickson DW. Widespread cytoskeletal pathology characterizes corticobasal degeneration. *Am J Pathol* 1995;146: 1388–1396.

62. Dickson DW, Bergeron C, Chin SS, et al. Office of Rare Diseases neuropathologic criteria for corticobasal degeneration. *J Neuropathol Exp Neurol* 2002;61: 935–946.

63. Dickson DW, Liu W-K, Ksiezak-Reding H, et al. Neuropathologic and molecular considerations. In: Litvan I, Goetz CG, Lang AE, eds. Corticobasal Degeneration and Related Disorders (Advances in Neurology, vol 82.). New York: Lippincott Williams & Wilkins, 2000;9–27.

64. Spillantini MG, Bird TD, Ghetti B. Frontotemporal dementia and parkinsonism linked to chromosome 17: a new group of tauopathies. *Brain Pathol* 1998;8:387–402

65. Oppenheimer DR. Disease of the basal ganglia, cerebellum, and motor neurons. In: Blackwood W, Corsellis JAN, eds. Greenfield's Neuropathology, 3rd ed. London: Edward Arnold, 1976;609–622.

66. Geddes JF, Hughes AJ, Lees AJ, et al. Pathological overlap in cases of parkinsonism associated with neurofibrillary tangles: a study of recent cases of postencephalitic parkinsonism and comparison with progressive supranuclear palsy and Guamanian parkinsonism-dementia complex. *Brain* 1993;116:281–302.

67. Litvan I, Hauw JJ, Bartko JJ, et al. Validity and reliability of the preliminary NINDS neuropathologic criteria for progressive supranuclear palsy and related disorders. *J Neuropathol Exp Neurol* 1996;55:97–105.

68. Hof PR, Nimchinsky EA, Buee-Scherrer V, et al. Amyotrophic lateral sclerosis/parkinsonism-dementia complex of Guam: quantitative neuropathology, immunohistochemical analysis of neuronal vulnerability, and comparison with related neurodegenerative disorders. *Acta Neuropathol* 1994;88:397–404.

69. Oyanagi K, Makifuchi T, Ohtoh T, et al. Amyotrophic lateral sclerosis of Guam: the nature of the neuropathological findings. *Acta Neuropathol* 1994;88:405–412.

70. Oyanagi K, Makifuchi T, Ohtoh T, et al. Topographic investigation of brain atrophy in parkinsonism-dementia complex of Guam: a comparison with Alzheimer's disease and progressive supranuclear palsy. *Neurodegeneration* 1994;3:301–304.

71. Hof PR, Perl DP, Loerzel AJ, et al. Neurofibrillary tangle distribution in the cerebral cortex of parkinsonism-dementia cases from Guam: differences with Alzheimer's disease. *Brain Res* 1991;564:306–313.

72. Anderson FH, Richardson EP Jr, Okazaki H, et al. Neurofibrillary degeneration on Guam: frequency in Chamorros and non Chamorros with no known neurological disease. *Brain* 1979;102: 65–77.

73. Yamazaki M, Arai Y, Baba M, et al. Alpha-synuclein inclusions in amygdala in the brains of patients with the parkinsonism-dementia complex of Guam. *J Neuropathol Exp Neurol* 2000;59: 585–591.

74. Buee-Scherrer V, Buee L, Hof PR, et al. Neurofibrillary degeneration in amyotrophic lateral sclerosis/parkinsonism-dementia complex of Guam. Immunochemical characterization of tau proteins. *Am J Pathol* 1995;146:924–932.

75. Oyanagi K, Makifuchi T, Ohtoh T, et al. Distinct pathological features of the Gallyas- and tau-positive glia in the parkinsonism-dementia complex and amyotrophic lateral sclerosis of Guam. *J Neuropathol Exp Neurol* 1997;56:308–316.

76. Graham DI, Gennarelli TA. Trauma. In: Graham DI, Lantos PL, eds. Greenfield's Neuropathology, 6th ed. London: Arnold, 1997;197–263.

77. Geddes JF, Vowles GH, Nicoll JA, et al. Neuronal cytoskeletal changes are an early consequence of repetitive head injury. *Acta Neuropathol* 1999;98:171–178.

78. Schmidt ML, Zhukareva V, Newell KL, et al. Tau isoform profile and phosphorylation state in dementia pugilistica recapitulate Alzheimer's disease. *Acta Neuropathol* 2001;101:518–524.

Mitochondria in Movement Disorders

23

Anthony H.V. Schapira

INTRODUCTION

Mitochondria are intracellular organelles ubiquitous among eukaryotic cells. Their functions are diverse, but their main responsibility is the production of energy for cellular metabolism. They contain their own DNA, which is inherited along maternal lines, and mutations are a recognized cause of human disease. The involvement of mitochondria in movement disorders is extensive and includes diseases due to mutations of mitochondrial DNA (mtDNA), mutations of nuclear-encoded proteins that are transported to mitochondria, and the effects of mitochondrial toxins, both endogenous and exogenous.

MITOCHONDRIAL STRUCTURE

Mitochondria are double-membraned organelles with an intermembranous space and a matrix that lies within the folded inner membrane. The matrix contains up to several thousand mtDNA molecules. MtDNA is a small, circular, double-stranded molecule 16,493 bases long encoding two ribosomal RNAs, 22 transfer RNAs, and 13 proteins (Fig. 23.1). These proteins are all part of the oxidative phosphorylation (OXPHOS) system (see Table 23.1). MtDNA remains dependent on the nucleus for the production of proteins involved in its transcription, translation, replication, and repair. Thus, although mitochondria have some element of independence in having their own DNA, they remain dependent upon the nucleus for the function of mtDNA and also for the production of all mitochondrial proteins other than the 13 produced by mtDNA.

MtDNA-encoded proteins are translated on mitochondrial ribosomes and incorporated directly into complexes I, III, IV, and V on the inner membrane. Nuclear-encoded proteins are translated on cytosolic ribosomes and are imported into the mitochondrion through a complex receptor and transport system. For many proteins, this involves an N-terminal amino targeting sequence that interacts with membrane receptors and signals the carrier protein's import into the mitochondrion. The signaling sequence is then cleaved and the protein trafficked to the appropriate mitochondrial compartment. Some proteins are incorporated into the outer mitochondrial membrane and others directly into the intermembranous space.

Four respiratory chain complexes (I–IV) and ATPase (complex V) constitute the OXPHOS system. These proteins are embedded in the inner mitochondrial membrane and comprise a total of approximately 85 subunits, 72 being encoded by nuclear DNA and 13 by mtDNA. The OXPHOS system is not only responsible for ATP production but is also an important source of superoxide radicals. Defects of the OXPHOS system have the potential not only to cause a failure of energy metabolism but also to increase free radical mediated damage.

MtDNA continuously replicates, and this function is therefore independent of cell cycle phases. MtDNA replication involves mtDNA polymerase gamma (POLG), thymidine kinase 2, and deoxyguanosine kinase. MtDNA transcription is necessary for the initiation of replication.

MtDNA is highly polymorphic with numerous differences in sequence between individuals of the same ethnic group, but more so between members of different ethnic groups. MtDNA haplotypes are based upon specific patterns of polymorphisms and appear to have some influence upon the prevalence of certain diseases and the expression of certain mitochondrial mutations, e.g., Parkinson's disease (PD) (see below), senescence,

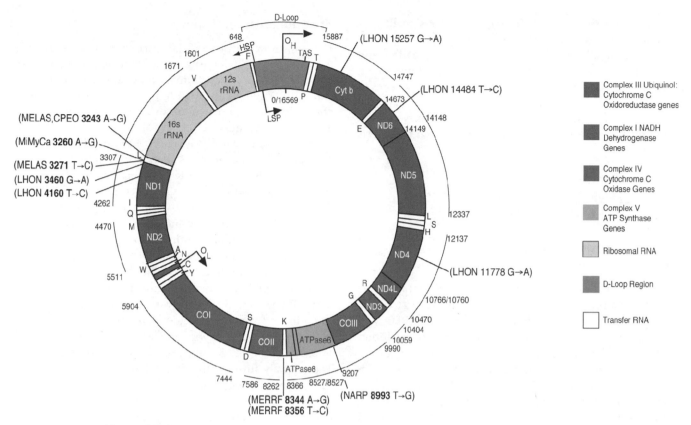

Figure 23.1 Schematic representation of human mitochondrial DNA and the respiratory chain. Included are the genes for respiratory chain proteins and for ribosomal and transfer RNAs. The O_H and O_L are the origins of heavy and light strand replication, respectively. Location of the more common mitochondrial DNA mutations are indicated. (See color section).

and the expression of Leber hereditary optic neuropathy (LHON) mutations.

MtDNA is inherited through the female line, although there has been one report of paternal inheritance of a mtDNA microdeletion in a complex I gene (1). MtDNA mutations are often present in heteroplasmic form, i.e., coexisting with normal wild-type mtDNA. The proportion of mutant to wild type may vary among individuals and among tissues of the same individual. There is a relationship between the mutant load and the degree of biochemical defect, although this is both tissue dependent and recessive; i.e., from studies undertaken so far, 5%–20% of wild-type mtDNA can compensate at the biochemical level.

Mitochondria are randomly segregated at cell division, including oogenesis, and during this process, a random segregation or partitioning of wild-type and mutant mtDNA takes place, which results in a varying proportion of wild-type and mutant molecules in daughter cells. When this process occurs through oogenesis, it does so through a narrow passage, whereby only a small proportion of the mtDNA population is transmitted. A high proportion of mutant load in the oocyte population would result in a high proportion of offspring at risk of developing disease.

The primary function of mitochondria is to support aerobic respiration and to provide energy substrates adenosine triphosphate (ATP) for intracellular metabolic pathways. More recently, mitochondria have been shown to play an

TABLE 23.1

THE RESPIRATORY CHAIN AND OXIDATIVE PHOSPHORYLATION SYSTEM

Complex	Enzyme Activity	Number of Subunits	MtDNA Encoded Subunits
Complex I	NADH ubiquinone reductase	43	7
Complex II	Succinate ubiquinone reductase	4	—
Complex III	Ubiquinol cytochrome c reductase	11	1
Complex IV	Cytochrome c oxidase	13	3
Complex V	ATP synthase	14	2

important role in cell signaling, particularly in signaling for apoptotic cell death. Mitochondria host a number of metabolic pathways, including the Krebs cycle, β-oxidation, and lipid and cholesterol synthesis. In the context of movement disorders, it is noteworthy that the basal ganglia are sites of high OXPHOS demand, a feature that renders them particularly susceptible to factors that interfere with oxygen delivery directly, e.g., hypoxia, or indirectly through the effects of toxins.

MITOCHONDRIAL DNA MUTATIONS AND MOVEMENT DISORDERS

Chronic Progressive External Ophthalmoplegia

Generally, chronic progressive external ophthalmoplegia (CPEO) is a predominantly myopathic disorder. However, encephalopathic features may also occur with CPEO, and there have been reports of dementia, seizures, myoclonus, and stroke-like episodes (2,3). In a study of 66 patients, 55% had CPEO with muscle weakness but no major central nervous system (CNS) disease. Of these, 61% had additional minor features including salt and pepper retinopathy, with preserved acuity in 45%, mild limb or gait ataxia in 41%, extensor plantars in 23%, sensorineural deafness in 23%, and infrequent seizures in 5%.

In Kearns-Sayre syndrome (KSS), CPEO is accompanied by pigmentary retinopathy and one or more of the following: complete heart block, a cerebrospinal fluid (CSF) protein level above 1 g/l, and ataxia (4). Other cardiac conduction defects described in KSS include left anterior hemiblock, right bundle branch block, and type II atrioventricular block (5). The diagnostic criteria state an age of onset below 20 years, but improved identification of cases has revealed later onset in some cases. In pure CPEO, ophthalmoplegia and ptosis may be the only manifestations of this mitochondrial myopathy; however it is more commonly associated with symptoms such as limb weakness, fatigue, or retinopathy. These cases are often referred to as *CPEO plus*, and the term *Kearns-Sayre syndrome* is reserved for cases in which the preceding diagnostic criteria are met. In a study of 52 patients, the majority had both ptosis and ophthalmoplegia, with the former occurring in isolation.

MtDNA from CPEO/KSS patients shows large single deletions detectable in DNA extracted from muscle samples, but blood mtDNA analysis usually is normal. These deletions are found in 80% of those with KSS, and 70% of those with CPEO (6,7,8). MtDNA duplications are also occasionally found in less abundance (8). Histological examination of muscle reveals ragged red fibers (RRFs) and a mosaic pattern of COX negative fibers. It is essential that a portion of the muscle obtained at biopsy is sent for mtDNA analysis. Patients with mtDNA deletions present as sporadic cases (9).

Encephalomyopathies

The common mitochondrial encephalopathies include myopathy, encephalopathy, lactic acidosis, and stroke-like episodes (MELAS) and myoclonic epilepsy and RRFs (MERRF). MELAS can include psychomotor retardation, ataxia, cognitive impairment, deafness, diabetes mellitus, and limb weakness. Optic atrophy, dystonia, chorea, peripheral neuropathy, myoclonus, pigmentary retinopathy, spasticity, and progressive external ophthalmoplegia (PEO) have also been reported in MELAS patients since the original description. Of all cases meeting the clinical criteria for MELAS, 80% are positive for an A to G transition at base pair 3243 within the transfer RNA (tRNA) LeuUUR gene (10,11,12). A large number of different mutations have also been found to result in the MELAS phenotype. A G13513A mutation in the ND5 gene was also associated with recurrent focal cortical brain hematomas in a child with MELAS (13). Conversely, of all cases with the 3243 mutation from an unselected population of 17 patients with mitochondrial myopathy, 50% were found to fulfill the criteria for MELAS at the time of clinical assessment (10). Theoretically, further cases could develop these clinical features with the passage of time.

The core clinical features of MERRF are myoclonus, ataxia, and seizures. Myoclonus is often the presenting symptom and may be induced by action, noise, or photic stimulation. Seizure types are variable but include drop attacks, focal seizures, and photo-sensitive tonic–clonic seizures (14,15). Myopathy is usually either mild, subclinical, or absent. RRFs are seen on muscle biopsy in the majority of patients but not all. Additional associated features have been reported in varying numbers of patients. These include ophthalmoplegia, ptosis, deafness, peripheral neuropathy, headache, foot deformity, optic atrophy, and cervical lipomas. An insidiously progressive dementia may occur later in the disease course. Furthermore, the vast majority of the clinical features seen in the other mitochondrial encephalomyopathies have been reported in patients with MERRF. These include short stature, involuntary movements, episodic hemicranial headache, cardiomyopathy, spastic paraparesis, and psychomotor retardation (2,15,16,17).

The most commonly detected mutation, found in approximately 80% of cases fulfilling the clinical criteria for MERRF, is at position 8344 within the tRNA Lys and was first reported by Shoffner in 1990 (10,18,19). It was detected in three independent MERRF pedigrees, was absent in 75 controls, alters a highly conserved nucleotide, and is heteroplasmic, thus fulfilling the criteria for a pathogenic mutation as opposed to a silent polymorphism. In vitro studies using cybrids have confirmed its pathogenic role (20). Other mutations within the same tRNA gene [T8356C(17) and G8363C(21)] are also described in association with MERRF. Insertion of a C nucleotide at position 7472 in the tRNA Serine UCN gene results in a syndrome of hearing loss, ataxia, and myoclonus that is very similar to MERRF (22). MERRF also has been reported in patients harboring multiple mtDNA deletions (23), and overlap syndromes with features of both MERRF and MELAS have been reported for the T7572C and T8356C tRNA Serine UCN mutations. Retinopathy has been found only in MERRF cases with mtDNA mutations other than the most common A8344G mutation (2,10,24).

Neurogenic Weakness Ataxia and Retinal Pigmentation

The key features of neurogenic weakness ataxia and retinal pigmentation (NARP), a mitochondrial encephalomyopathy, are peripheral neuropathy, ataxia, retinitis pigmentosa, seizures, and dementia (25). A spectrum of neurological findings has been described in NARP, including migraine and mental retardation (25,26,27,28,29,30,31). Clinical features are variable, as is the age of onset, which in one series varied between 1 and 32 years (32,33). Inheritance is maternal.

The most common mutation is a T to G transversion at nucleotide position 8993. This causes a change from the highly conserved leucine to arginine within subunit 6 of the mitochondrial F_0F_1 ATP synthase. Patients with NARP usually have mutant mtDNA levels above 80%. With mutant mtDNA levels below 75%, patients usually suffer from pigmentary retinopathy alone, or suffer migraines, or are asymptomatic (25,30). This illustrates the good correlation between mutant load and disease severity that is not present in the majority of the other mitochondrial encephalomyopathies.

RRFs and other morphological mitochondrial hallmarks are lacking in muscle biopsies from patients with NARP (25). There is, therefore, an overlap between NARP and some nonmitochondrial neurodegenerative disorders, such as Refsum's disease and Usher's syndrome, which share the clinical features of hearing loss, ataxia, and visual impairment due to retinitis pigmentosa. Lactic acidosis may also be absent in NARP. Muscle weakness is often mild and may be masked by the presence of ataxia. Reduced complex V activity has been found in cultured cells from affected patients (26,34), but no in vivo evidence of ATPase deficiency has been reported in patients carrying the NARP mutation. Biochemical analysis of muscle samples may fail to reveal a respiratory chain or OXPHOS defect, however, since complex V (ATP synthase) activity is rarely measured routinely.

Leigh Syndrome

Leigh syndrome (LS) is a subacute, necrotizing encephalomyelopathy characterized by bilateral symmetrical focal necrotic lesions within the thalamus, extending into the pons, inferior olives, and spinal cord. The clinical features of LS are psychomotor retardation, hypotonia, failure to thrive, respiratory abnormalities, oculomotor disturbances, optic atrophy, seizures, and lactic acidosis. Biochemical abnormalities include defects of OXPHOS (35), particularly complex I (36) or complex IV (37,38), and deficiency of the pyruvate

dehydrogenase complex (39) and biotinidase deficiency (40). The majority of LS cases are believed to result from nuclear gene defects (34,41). This has been confirmed for cases of LS with PDH complex deficiency (41), complex I (42), and complex II (43). Complex IV deficient LS results from mutations of the Surf or other assembly genes (44,45,46). Nuclear gene defects are also presumed to be causal for cases of LS with biotinidase deficiency. Up to 20% of LS patients have the T to G, or T to C, mtDNA mutation at position 8993 within the ATPase 6 gene of complex V (47,48,49,50,51). Mutant loads are above 90%, and lower levels of this mutation are associated with the NARP syndrome. High levels of the A3243G MELAS mutation and the A8344G MERRF mutation have also been reported in LS (52,53,54). Other mtDNA mutations described include G1644T within the tRNA Val gene (55) and deletions (53,56,57) and depletion of mtDNA levels (58). The ATPase 6 mutations T8851C and T9176C are also associated with bilateral striatal necrosis and with maternally inherited LS (14,59,60).

Leber Hereditary Optic Neuropathy

LHON is characterized clinically by bilateral sequential acute or subacute visual failure due to degeneration of the retinal ganglion cells and their axons. Three mtDNA mutations—G11778A, G3460A, and T14484C located in the *MTND4*, *MTND1*, and *nMTND6* genes, respectively—account for approximately 95% of cases. The G11778A mutation is the most common, being present in 56% of cases; the G3460A is in 31%, and the T14484C is in 6.3% (61). The disease occurs predominantly in young men, usually with little or no visual recovery, although the T14484C mutation is generally associated with better prognosis. A range of "secondary" or "intermediate" polymorphisms may modify expression (62). More recently, additional mutations in *MTND1* and *MTND6* have been described (63,64), with the C4171A mutation in *MTND1* being associated with significant visual recovery. All these LHON mutations are all usually present in homoplasmic or high heteroplasmic proportions. Additional features include dystonia and striatal degeneration as reported in some families, especially with point mutations G14459A, A11696G, and T14596A in the mitochondrial complex I subunit genes (65,66).

NUCLEAR GENE MUTATIONS AND MITOCHONDRIAL MOVEMENT DISORDERS

Mitochondrial DNA Polymerase Gamma Mutations

MtDNA polymerase gamma (POLG) is a heterodimer comprising a 140kDa alpha subunit and a 41kDa beta subunit. It is located within the inner mitochondrial membrane and is essential for mtDNA replication. The alpha subunit is catalytic and contains both polymerase and exonuclease activities; the beta subunit facilitates DNA binding and promotes DNA synthesis (67). Mutations of POLG have been associated with a range of clinical phenotypes, including PD. Autosomal dominant or recessive inheritance of CPEO with age of onset ranging from 10–54 years was followed some years later (range 6–40 years) by the development of an asymmetric, L-dopa–responsive bradykinetic rigid syndrome together with resting tremor in some patients. Additional features included variable limb, pharyngeal, or facial weakness; cataracts; ataxia; peripheral neuropathy; and premature ovarian failure (68). Muscle biopsy demonstrated ragged red, cytochrome oxidase negative fibers in all patients with multiple mtDNA deletions on Southern blotting. Symmetrically reduced striatal 18F-β-CFT was seen in two patients. Brain histology was available on a further two patients, and both showed severe loss of substantia nigral dopaminergic neurons but without the development of Lewy bodies or other synuclein aggregates. Four families had the same A2864G mutation inherited in autosomal fashion in three, with a founder effect in the fourth. Mutations in the exonuclease or polymerase portions of the gene were identified in the autosomal recessive families. A further patient with autosomal dominant PEO-parkinsonism and an A2492G mutation has been reported (69).

Friedreich's Ataxia

Friedreich's ataxia (FRDA) is an autosomal recessive disease characterized clinically by a progressive gait and limb ataxia, absence of deep tendon reflexes, and loss of position and vibration sense in the lower limbs. Skeletal abnormalities, cardiac hypertrophy, and, to a lesser degree, diabetes and optic atrophy are also present in FRDA patients.

FRDA is inherited in an autosomal recessive pattern with over 95% of patients having a homozygous expansion of a GAA triplet repeat (6–34 GAA repeats expanded to between 67–1700 in patients) in intron 1 of the FRDA gene on chromosome 9 (70). Most of the remaining patients are compound heterozygotes with the GAA expansion in one allele and point mutations in the other (71).

The size of the GAA repeat appears to influence the clinical phenotype with a significant inverse relationship between the size of the smaller GAA repeat and the age of onset (72,73). Homozygous GAA repeat expansions resulted in decreased frataxin mRNA levels in patients' lymphoblasts and fibroblasts (74,75). This correlated with lower levels of frataxin protein in skeletal muscle, cerebellum, and cerebral cortex from patients with FRDA. In addition, frataxin protein levels have been shown to be inversely decreased in proportion to the GAA repeat size in FRDA lymphoblasts (76).

While the normal function of frataxin is not known, the analysis of the protein sequence identified a predicted N-terminal mitochondrial targeting sequence (76) and a stretch of highly conserved amino acids in the C terminal half of the protein (77). Evidence from the knockout of the frataxin homologue in yeast cells, mice models, and patient samples suggests that frataxin deficiency results in impaired mitochondrial respiratory chain function, mitochondrial iron accumulation, decreased MtDNA levels, and increased oxidative stress.

Dysfunction of the mitochondrial respiratory chain was observed in yeast YFH1 mutants (78,79), conditional frataxin knockout transgenic mice (80), and postmortem heart and skeletal muscle from FRDA patients (81,82). The pattern of respiratory chain dysfunction (complexes I, II, and III) is reminiscent of that caused by oxidative stress caused by knockout of the manganese superoxide dismutase (83) or secondary to excitotoxicity in Huntington's disease (84). However, all the activities decreased in FRDA contain iron–sulphur (Fe–S) clusters, which led to the proposal that an abnormality of Fe–S cluster synthesis may be responsible for these defects. As the decrease in mitochondrial respiratory chain (MRC) activities preceded the iron accumulation in the conditional frataxin knockout transgenic mouse model of FRDA (80), the likely mechanism involves decreased Fe–S synthesis, which may then be exacerbated in the longer term by secondary oxidative damage. The concurrent loss of mtDNA (81,85) may also contribute to the MRC defects, which may be secondary to increased oxidative damage.

An in vivo technique that can measure high-energy phosphorous compounds (phosphocreatine and ATP) in heart and skeletal muscle is 31 phosphorous magnetic resonance spectroscopy (31P MRS). In skeletal muscle, phosphocreatine (PCr) levels fall during exercise, and the analysis of the rate at which PCr levels recover following exercise (Vmax) is a measure of the efficiency of OXPHOS (86). The PCr/ATP ratio is used as a good measure of energy availability in the heart (87). Analysis with 31P MRS of FRDA patients revealed markedly decreased OXPHOS in the heart (88) and skeletal muscle, with the latter correlating with the size of the smallest GAA repeat (89). These data underscore the role of mitochondrial dysfunction in FRDA and suggest it is playing a primary role in disease pathogenesis.

A conditional knockout mouse model of muscle frataxin lead to death at 10–12 weeks (80,90). Abnormalities began at week 4 with a 50% reduction in complex II activity; cardiac function remained normal at that time. By week 5, however, there was an increase in left ventricular mass, left ventricular systolic and diastolic diameter, and a 24% reduction in the shortening fraction. At week 6, cardiac output was down 15%, and there was evidence of abnormal mitochondrial morphology. Week 7 showed a 67% decrease in shortening fraction and a surprising reduction in oxidized protein. By week 8, cardiac output was 67% of control, and complex II activity was down 80%, but there was no evidence of mitochondrial iron accumulation. At week 9, mitochondrial iron was elevated but lipid peroxidation was decreased. Idebenone treatment (90 mg/kg/day) delayed the onset of cardiac abnormalities by only 1 week and prolonged lifespan by 10%. The therapy had no protective effect on complex II activity.

The potential protective effect of antioxidant treatment in this murine model was assessed by overexpression of copper–zinc (Cu-Zn) superoxide dismutase (SOD) and an manganese (Mn) SOD mimetic. However, there was no evidence of a protective effect on the development or severity of the cardiomyopathy, and no benefit on survival (91). Mn SOD protein expression fell by approximately 50% compared to controls in the heart at 10 weeks. There was no increase in oxidized protein levels in either the heart or cerebellum. These results indicate that frataxin deficiency does not lead to oxidative stress and alternative mechanisms may be involved in mediating the neurodegeneration associated with deficiencies of Fe–S proteins.

Vitamin E is a naturally occurring lipid-soluble antioxidant distributed throughout cellular membranes, and it is particularly abundant in mitochondrial membranes. Vitamin E treatment has been shown to increase vitamin E levels in a variety of tissues, including brain, muscle, and heart (92). It has been used to treat cardiovascular disease, PD, cancers, and ataxia with vitamin E deficiency (AVED) with varying degrees of success (93,94,95,96). The treatment of FRDA patients with vitamin E has been reported only in conjunction with coenzyme Q10 (CoQ10). CoQ10 is naturally found in cells, and up to 5 mg/day may be consumed in an average diet (CoQ is very rich in soybean oil, meat, and fish). CoQ10 is readily taken up into the blood (97), the brain (98), and the liver (92), although other reports suggest dietary CoQ10 levels do not influence tissue CoQ10 levels in the rat (99). CoQ10 may reduce vitamin E; therefore, when combined in a therapy, it may act synergistically (100). We have assessed the efficacy of long-term treatment of 10 patients with FRDA with high doses of vitamin E (2100 IU/day) and CoQ10 (400mg/day). After 6 months, 31P MRS data indicated that heart and skeletal muscle energetics were significantly improved (101). Data from a 4-year follow-up to this study showed the enhanced energy levels were maintained, clinical parameters were stabilized or improved in 7 out of 10 patients, and heart fraction shortening had improved (102).

Idebenone is a short-chain analogue of CoQ10, is well tolerated by humans, crosses the blood–brain barrier (103), has been reported to be a relatively good antioxidant (104), and has been used in a variety of diseases with some benefits (105,106). The effect of idebenone upon cardiac hypertrophy in FRDA patients was assessed using echocardiography, but other clinical improvements were not reported. After 6 months of treatment, cardiac hypertrophy was decreased in up to half the patients tested, although this was not always associated with improved fraction shortening (107). Another assessment of idebenone failed to identify improvements in skeletal muscle 31P MRS or echocardiographic parameters (108), although this may reflect the short time scale used.

COENZYME Q10 DEFICIENCY

CoQ10 is a lipophilic component of the respiratory chain that transfers electrons from complexes I and II, and from fatty acids and branched-chain amino acids via flavin-linked dehydrogenases, to complex III (Fig. 23.2). The first report of human disease associated with CoQ10 deficiency was in a patient with encephalomyopathy and recurrent myoglobinuria with RRFs and changes of lipid storage on muscle biopsy (109). Relatively severe CoQ10 deficiency was then described in six patients with early-onset (age range birth to 16 years) myopathy and ataxia (110). Seizures, weakness, and mental retardation were described in some, and cerebellar atrophy was found in all. Genetic testing for Friedreich's ataxia and spinocerebellar ataxia was negative, and inheritance was consistent with an autosomal recessive pattern. Muscle biopsy in these patients showed nonspecific abnormalities only and, in particular, no evidence of mitochondrial pathology. Residual muscle CoQ10 levels were 26%–35% of normal. Administration of CoQ10 (300–3000 mg/day) resulted in significant improvement in the ataxia.

Subsequent assay of muscle CoQ10 levels in 135 patients with genetically undefined childhood-onset ataxia identified significantly reduced levels in 10% (111). All patients had cerebellar atrophy, and some had seizures, developmental delay, and pyramidal features. Lactic acidosis in the ataxic patients is rare, and in contrast to the myopathic form, the muscle biopsy may appear normal. The same group subsequently described muscle CoQ10 deficiency in two brothers with adult-onset (ages 29 and 39 years) progressive cerebellar ataxia with cerebellar atrophy and hypergonadotrophic hypogonadism. Muscle morphology showed neurogenic changes only. CoQ10 dosage of 750–1200mg/day resulted in improved ataxia, neurophysiology, and normal testosterone levels within 2 months in these patients.

PARKINSON'S DISEASE

The first direct association between mitochondrial dysfunction and idiopathic PD was made with the discovery in 1989 of a complex I defect in substantia nigra from patients with PD (112,113). This study has been expanded since then, and results to date show that there is a specific circa 35% complex I deficiency in the substantia nigra in PD. This defect in complex I activity does not appear to

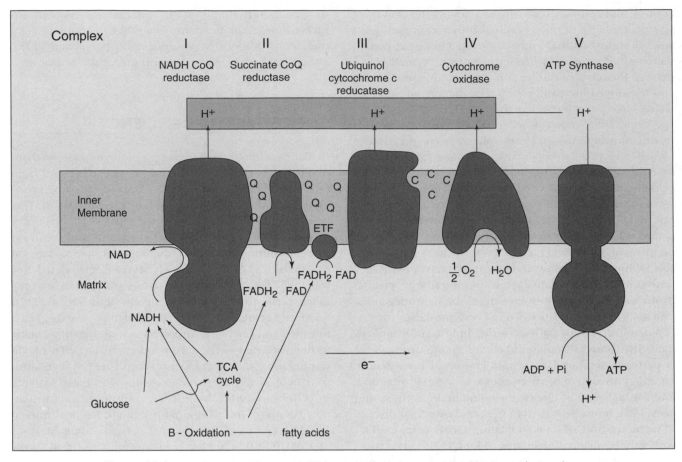

Figure 23.2 The functional features of the mitochondrial respiratory chain in oxidative phosphorylation system. ADP, adenosine diphosphate; ATP, adenosine triphosphate; CoQ, ubiquinone; e-, electron; ETF, electron transfer flavoprotein; FAD, flavin adenine dinucleotide; FADH$_2$, the reduced form of flavin adenine dinucleotide; NAD, nicotinamide adenine dinucleotide; NADH, the reduced form of nicotinamide-adenine dinucleotide; Pi, inorganic phosphate; TCA, tricarboxylic acid cycle.

affect any other part of the respiratory chain. In addition, no defect in mitochondrial activity has been identifiable in any other part of the brain in PD, including the caudate putamen, globus pallidus, tegmentum, cortex, cerebellum, or substantia innominata (114).

This observation provided a direct biochemical link between idiopathic PD and the 1-methyl-4-phenyl-1,2,3,6-tetrahydropyridine (MPTP) model of this disorder. The toxic metabolite of MPTP—1-methyl-4-phenylpyridinium (MPP$^+$)—inhibits complex I in a concentration-dependent but reversible manner. Prolonged exposure of submitochondrial particles to MPP$^+$, however, results in more severe and irreversible inhibition of complex I when electron flow through the chain is prevented by inhibition of cytochrome oxidase (complex IV). This severe and irreversible inhibition can be prevented with free radical scavengers (115). Free radicals can damage the respiratory chain. In vitro studies suggest that both complexes I and III are particularly affected, while in vivo studies suggest that complex IV and, less so, complex I are inhibited (116,117,118,119).

Following the report of complex I deficiency in PD substantia nigra, respiratory chain abnormalities were described in skeletal muscle mitochondria from PD patients. This particular area has proved very contentious, with several groups describing either similar defects or no abnormality whatsoever (120). Two magnetic resonance spectroscopy studies on skeletal muscle mitochondrial function in PD have shown conflicting results (121,122).

Finally, mitochondrial complex I deficiency was also identified in platelet mitochondria of PD patients (123). In contrast to the conclusions regarding skeletal muscle, there is a consensus among several laboratories that complex I deficiency does exist in PD platelet mitochondria. The majority of studies, however, suggest that this deficiency, as least based on a group-to-group analysis, is modest (circa 20%–25%) (120).

The cause of the complex I defect in PD remains unknown. As virtually all the brains taken from PD patients had been exposed to L-dopa, an important question related to whether L-dopa caused the complex I deficiency. There was no relationship between the level of complex I defect and prior L-dopa exposure. Furthermore, there is no deficiency of complex I activity in PD striatum, an area high in dopamine (124). L-dopa does not appear to cause any deficiency of complex I activity in platelet mitochondria, which again might be expected given the relatively high circulating levels of L-dopa in the periphery. Most importantly, it has been shown that patients with multiple system atrophy (MSA) who have taken L-dopa in quantities and for duration comparable to patients with PD have no defect of mitochondrial activity in their substantia nigra (125). Also, cell loss in the substantia nigra is at least as severe in MSA as it is in PD; thus, one would expect that, if the mitochondrial defect in PD were simply a reflection of this degeneration, the same abnormality should be present in MSA. Its absence in MSA, therefore, suggests that its presence in PD is the result of a more specific cause than simple cell loss.

Alternatives for the cause of the complex I deficiency in PD include an mtDNA mutation or nuclear gene mutations of mitochondrial proteins. Following the identification of the complex I defect in PD, several studies investigated the structure of mtDNA in tissues from PD patients. An early study suggested increased levels of the common deletion in the PD brain (126). However, this study did not use age-matched controls, and the increase in the common deletion was, in fact, no greater than would be expected from the aging process. Other studies using properly matched controls found no increase in this mitochondrial mutation in PD substantia nigra (127,128). Several studies have sequenced mtDNA in PD, but all these have involved small numbers of unselected patients (129,130,131,132,133,134,135,136). Although some reports have suggested an increased frequency of certain mtDNA polymorphisms in PD, this has not been replicated in other studies (137,138).

The relationship between mitochondrial dysfunction, mtDNA, and PD has been highlighted further by the recent description of mtDNA abnormalities in PD patients. Occasional mtDNA point mutations have been identified in PD, but these have not been present in the general PD population. Thus, their association with PD may represent merely part of the wide clinical spectrum of mtDNA mutations and may not necessarily imply a more common role in sporadic PD. POLG mutations have been described in patients with CPEO and PD with RRFs and multiple mtDNA deletions, but mutations of this gene have not been found in sporadic PD (139). A mutation in the mtDNA 12S RNA was found in a patient with maternally inherited early-onset PD, deafness, and neuropathy (140). Several studies have sequenced mtDNA in PD patients, and no consistent mutation has been described (141). However, none of the studies to date have focused on PD patients with complex I deficiency. Two studies have demonstrated a relationship between mtDNA haplotypes and the risk for developing PD. The first showed a reduced risk for PD in individuals with haplotypes J and K (142),

and the second showed a 22% decrease in PD in those with the UKJT haplotype cluster (143). In contrast, a smaller study reported an increased risk for PD with haplotypes J and T (144).

Two studies have used genetic transplantation with cells lacking mtDNA (rho zero cells) to investigate the potential for PD mtDNA to determine the complex I defect. In one study, unselected PD patients' cells were fused and grown in mixed culture (145). In the other, PD patients were selected on the basis of demonstrating a peripheral complex I deficiency. These patients' cells were then fused with rho zero cells and grown both in mixed and clonal cultures (146). In both, mtDNA transferred from the PD patients induced a complex I defect in the recipient cybrid cells. These results indicate that the mtDNA in these patients caused the complex I deficiency through either inherited or somatic mutations. Further experiments suggested that the recipient cells also developed abnormal calcium handling and a lower mitochondrial membrane potential.

Genetic causes of familial PD affect mitochondrial function. For instance, α-synuclein overexpression inhibits mitochondrial activity (147,148), *parkin*-knockout mice have a striatal respiratory chain defect (149), *parkin*-knockout flies have skeletal muscle mitochondrial abnormalities (150), and *parkin*-positive PD patients have complex I deficiency (151). Overexpression models of *parkin* have shown localization of the protein to mitochondria (152). DJ1 is a mitochondrial protein and thought to play a role in antioxidant defenses (153). Most recently, mutations in the PINK1 gene, which causes autosomal dominant PD, have been described, and the protein product localizes to the mitochondrion (154,155). The function of PINK1 is not known, but it is a protein kinase whose mutations enhance sensitivity to UPS inhibitors and lower the threshold to apoptotic cell death. Thus, the current pathogenetic model of PD reflects a complex network of interacting biochemical abnormalities that are, in turn, a consequence of genetic and environmental factors.

Thus, there is substantial evidence that mitochondria play an important role in both the etiology and pathogenesis of PD. This relationship between mitochondrial dysfunction and PD has been exploited in an attempt to develop treatment that might favorably influence the progression of the disease. CoQ10 both enhances respiratory chain function and scavenges free radicals and, therefore, might be predicted to have a beneficial effect upon PD pathogenesis. A pilot study using three doses of CoQ10 in early, untreated PD patients showed that the highest dose (1200mg/day) produced a statistically significant improvement in clinical scores compared to placebo at 16 months (156). As noted by the authors, this result must be regarded as provisional, and CoQ10 will be the subject of further study alone or in combination with other putative disease-modifying therapies.

DYSTONIA

Movement disorders—dystonia, in particular—are known to occur more frequently than expected in patients with primary mitochondrial diseases (2). Several families with maternally inherited LHON with dystonia and mutations in mtDNA genes encoding complex I subunits have been described (157,158,159). A specific and reproducible deficiency of complex I activity in patients with sporadic focal dystonia (160,161) has been identified but not in patients with generalized dystonia linked or not to the dystonia-1 gene (162).

A nuclear-encoded mitochondrial protein defect has now been identified in one particular type of dystonia. Deafness dystonia (Mohr-Tranebjaerg) syndrome is an X-linked disorder characterized by progressive sensorineural deafness, cortical blindness, dystonia, dysphagia, and paranoia (163). Deafness dystonia syndrome is due to deletion or truncation of a gene (DFN-1) encoding an 11kDa protein: DDPI. This protein has been identified recently, through homology studies, as a component of the mitochondrial import system (164). It is not yet known which proteins are affected by this import defect, nor whether OXPHOS is compromised, although the clinical phenotype is reminiscent of other mitochondrial encephalopathies.

HUNTINGTON'S DISEASE

Huntington's disease (HD) is an autosomal dominant neurodegenerative disorder characterized clinically by chorea, ataxia, and dementia and pathologically by the loss of gamma aminobutyric acid- and enkephalin-containing neurons of the striatum. HD usually presents in early to middle adult life, although both juvenile and late-onset forms are recognized. The mutation responsible is an abnormally expanded (>36) cytosine-adenine-guanine (CAG) repeat in the huntingtin gene on chromosome 4. Knockout of the huntingtin gene results in early fetal death in mice, implying a critical role in embryogenesis (165). The gene product, *huntingtin*, is a widely expressed 349kDa protein of unknown function (166). Cultured cells expressing mutant *huntingtin* molecules have intranuclear inclusions (167), which also are seen in the brains of patients with HD (168) and in Huntington transgenic mice (169).

Excitotoxicity has been suggested to play an important role in neuronal cell death in HD (170). This is dependent upon glutamate excitation of N-methyl-D-aspartate receptors, inward flow of calcium, activation of nitric oxide synthase, and nitric oxide generation. Nitric oxides—particularly peroxynitrite, the product of the reaction of nitric oxide with superoxide O_2—are free radicals that can damage tissues. An important factor in this sequence is the release of the energy-dependent magnesium blockade of N-methyl-D-aspartate (NMDA) receptors, thus rendering ambient levels of glutamate excitotoxic. Evidence for a defect of mitochondrial function in HD arises from a variety of sources, including reduced striatal and cerebral-cortical glucose utilization as detected by positron emission tomography (PET) and increased lactic acid concentrations as detected by magnetic resonance spectroscopy (171,172), although the latter is not a universal finding (173). Biochemical analyses by several groups have demonstrated a severe respiratory chain defect: deficiency of complexes II and III and IV (174,175), in addition to a 90% decrease in aconitase activity (176). R6/2 HD transgenic mice also have evidence of striatal deficiencies of complex IV and aconitase (177).

The development of such severe defects of mitochondrial respiratory chain and aconitase function must be secondary to the primary huntingtin gene defect. The question arises whether this is a causal relationship or the consequence of alternative biochemical and pharmacological events. *Huntingtin* is expressed in muscle and, at a low level, in fibroblasts and lymphoblasts. Mitochondrial respiratory chain and aconitase activities were normal in fibroblasts and platelets from patients with HD (174). Magnetic resonance spectroscopy in muscle of patients with HD has been reported to be abnormal (172). This finding has recently been confirmed and also decreased rates of ATP synthesis (which correlated with the length of the CAG repeat, i.e., the longer the repeat, the worse the defect) were found in the muscle of both symptomatic and presymptomatic patients with HD (178).

The presence of mitochondrial defects in HD brain and skeletal muscle, in particular the correlation of the latter with the length of the CAG repeats, suggests that mutant *huntingtin* may have a direct role in inducing mitochondrial abnormalities. These observations are supported by the protective effects of creatine in the R6/2 transgenic mouse (179) and have been the basis for a trial in the United States of ubiquinone therapy in HD.

WILSON'S DISEASE

Wilson's disease (WD) is an autosomal recessive disorder that results in liver disease in 40% of affected patients, neurological dysfunction (dystonia, rigidity, and parkinsonism) in 40%, and psychiatric disease in 20% of patients. The WD gene on 13q14.3 codes for a protein that functions as a P-type ATPase localized in both the Golgi network (180) and possibly in mitochondria (181). We have recently identified severe defects of respiratory chain function, particularly complexes I, II, and III, and aconitase deficiency in liver samples from patients with WD (182). This pattern of enzyme defect, identical to that seen in FRDA and to that found in the superoxide dismutase 2 knockout mouse (183), suggests that free radical formation and oxidative damage may contribute to the pathogenesis of cirrhosis in WD. This might be expected as copper, which accumulates in the liver in WD, may substitute for iron in free-radical–generating reactions. The results suggest that effective antioxidant therapy may be helpful in WD patients.

CONCLUSION

Mitochondria play a critical role in cellular metabolism, and it is clear that defects in biochemical pathways hosted by mitochondria result in a wide spectrum of human disease. Movement disorders are particularly well-represented among these, and this may reflect the vulnerability of the basal ganglia to abnormal energy metabolism. Treatment remains a challenge. For some of the diseases discussed in this chapter, mitochondrial involvement is secondary, while in others, the cause is a mutation in a mitochondrial protein, whether encoded by mtDNA or nuclear DNA. Targeting effective drugs, e.g., antioxidants, to the mitochondrion is an evolving science that offers promise for improving cell function in diseases such as PD, FRDA, and some of the mitochondrial myopathies.

REFERENCES

1. Leonard JV, Schapira AH. Mitochondrial respiratory chain disorders II: neurodegenerative disorders and nuclear gene defects. *Lancet* 2000;355:389–394.
2. Truong DD, Harding AE, Scaravilli F, Smith SJ, Morgan-Hughes JA, Marsden CD. Movement disorders in mitochondrial myopathies: a study of nine cases with two autopsy studies. *Mov Disord* 1990;5:109–117.
3. Quade A, Zierz S, Klingmuller D. Endocrine abnormalities in mitochondrial myopathy with external ophthalmoplegia. *Clin Investig* 1992;70(5):396–402.
4. Berenberg RA, Pellock JM, DiMauro S, et al. Lumping or splitting? "Ophthalmoplegia-plus" or Kearns-Sayre syndrome? *Ann Neurol* 1977;1:37–54.
5. Roberts NK, Perloff JK, Kark RA. Cardiac conduction in the Kearns-Sayre syndrome (a neuromuscular disorder associated with progressive external ophthalmoplegia and pigmentary retinopathy): report of 2 cases and review of 17 published cases. *Am J Cardiol* 1979;44:1396–1400.
6. Holt IJ, Harding AE, Morgan-Hughes JA. Deletions of muscle mitochondrial DNA in patients with mitochondrial myopathies. *Nature* 1988;331:717–719.
7. Holt IJ, Harding AE, Cooper JM, et al. Mitochondrial myopathies: clinical and biochemical features of 30 patients with major deletions of muscle mitochondrial DNA. *Ann Neurol* 1989;26:699–708.
8. Moraes CT, DiMauro S, Zeviani M, et al. Mitochondrial DNA deletions in progressive external ophthalmoplegia and Kearns-Sayre syndrome. *N Engl J Med* 1989;320:1293–1299.
9. Zeviani M, Moraes CT, DiMauro S, et al. Deletions of mitochondrial DNA in Kearns-Sayre syndrome. *Neurology* 1998;51:1525.
10. Hammans SR, Sweeney MG, Brockington M, Morgan-Hughes JA, Harding AE. Mitochondrial encephalopathies: molecular genetic diagnosis from blood samples. *Lancet* 1991;337:1311–1313.
11. De Volder A, Ghilain S, de Barsy T, Goffinet AM. Brain metabolism in mitochondrial encephalomyopathy: a PET study. *J Comput Assist Tomogr* 1988;12:854–857.
12. Kobayashi Y, Momoi MY, Tominaga K, et al. A point mutation in the mitochondrial tRNA(Leu)(UUR) gene in MELAS (mitochondrial myopathy, encephalopathy, lactic acidosis and stroke-like episodes). *Biochem Biophys Res Commun* 1990;173:816–822.
13. Penisson-Besnier I, Reynier P, Asfar P, et al. Recurrent brain hematomas in MELAS associated with an ND5 gene mitochondrial mutation. *Neurology* 2000;55:317–318.
14. Hammans SR, Sweeney MG, Brockington M, et al. The mitochondrial DNA transfer RNA(Lys)A→G(8344) mutation and the syndrome of myoclonic epilepsy with ragged red fibres (MERRF): relationship of clinical phenotype to proportion of mutant mitochondrial DNA. *Brain* 1993;116(pt 3):617–632.
15. Berkovic SF, Carpenter S, Evans A, et al. Myoclonus epilepsy and ragged-red fibres (MERRF). 1. A clinical, pathological, biochemical, magnetic resonance spectrographic and positron emission tomographic study. *Brain* 1989;112(pt 5):1231–1260.
16. Fukuhara N, Tokiguchi S, Shirakawa K, Tsubaki T. Myoclonus epilepsy associated with ragged-red fibres (mitochondrial abnormalities): disease entity or a syndrome? Light- and electron-microscopic studies of two cases and review of literature. *J Neurol Sci* 1980;47:117–133.
17. Tulinius MH, Holme E, Kristiansson B, Larsson NG, Oldfors A. Mitochondrial encephalomyopathies in childhood. II. Clinical manifestations and syndromes. *J Pediatr* 1991;119:251–259.
18. Shoffner JM, Lott MT, Lezza AM, Seibel P, Ballinger SW, Wallace DC. Myoclonic epilepsy and ragged-red fiber disease (MERRF) is associated with a mitochondrial DNA tRNA(Lys) mutation. *Cell* 1990;61:931–937.
19. Zeviani M, Amati P, Bresolin N, et al. Rapid detection of the A→G(8344) mutation of mtDNA in Italian families with myoclonus epilepsy and ragged-red fibers (MERRF). *Am J Hum Genet* 1991;48:203–211.
20. Enriquez JA, Chomyn A, Attardi G. MtDNA mutation in MERRF syndrome causes defective aminoacylation of tRNA(Lys) and premature translation termination. *Nat Genet* 1995;10:47–55.
21. So N, Berkovic S, Andermann F, Kuzniecky R, Gendron D, Quesney LF. Myoclonus epilepsy and ragged-red fibres (MERRF). 2. Electrophysiological studies and comparison with other progressive myoclonus epilepsies. *Brain* 1989;112(pt 5):1261–1276.
22. Tiranti V, Chariot P, Carella F, et al. Maternally inherited hearing loss, ataxia and myoclonus associated with a novel point mutation in mitochondrial tRNASer(UCN) gene. *Hum Mol Genet* 1995;4:1421–1427.
23. Blumenthal DT, Shanske S, Schochet SS, et al. Myoclonus epilepsy with ragged red fibers and multiple mtDNA deletions. *Neurology* 1998;50:524–525.
24. Morgan-Hughes JA, Hayes DJ, Clark JB, et al. Mitochondrial encephalomyopathies: biochemical studies in two cases revealing defects in the respiratory chain. *Brain* 1982;105(pt 3):553–582.
25. Holt IJ, Harding AE, Petty RK, Morgan-Hughes JA. A new mitochondrial disease associated with mitochondrial DNA heteroplasmy. *Am J Hum Genet* 1990;46:428–433.
26. Tsairis P, Engel W, Kark P. Familial myoclonic epilepsy syndrome associated with skeletal muscle mitochondrial abnormalities. (Abstract). *Neurology* 1973;23:408.
27. Takeda S, Wakabayashi K, Ohama E, Ikuta F. Neuropathology of myoclonus epilepsy associated with ragged-red fibers (Fukuhara's disease). *Acta Neuropathol (Berl)* 1988;75:433–440.
28. Ortiz RG, Newman NJ, Shoffner JM, Kaufman AE, Koontz DA, Wallace DC. Variable retinal and neurologic manifestations in patients harboring the mitochondrial DNA 8993 mutation. *Arch Ophthalmol* 1993;111:1525–1530.
29. Fryer A, Appleton R, Sweeney M, et al. Mitochondrial DNA 8993 (NARP) mutation presenting with a heterogeneous phenotype including "cerebral palsy." *Arch Dis Child* 1994;71:419–422.
30. Makela-Bengs P, Suomalainen A, Majander A, et al. Correlation between the clinical symptoms and the proportion of mitochondrial DNA carrying the 8993 point mutation in the NARP syndrome. *Pediatr Res* 1995;37:634–639.
31. Puddu P, Barboni P, Mantovani V, et al. Retinitis pigmentosa, ataxia, and mental retardation associated with mitochondrial DNA mutation in an Italian family. *Br J Ophthalmol* 1993;77:84–88.
32. Uziel G, Moroni I, Lamantea E, et al. Mitochondrial disease associated with the T8993G mutation of the mitochondrial ATPase 6 gene: a clinical, biochemical, and molecular study in six families. *J Neurol Neurosurg Psychiatry* 1997;63:16–22.

33. Chowers I, Lerman-Sagie T, Elpeleg ON, Shaag A, Merin S. Cone and rod dysfunction in the NARP syndrome. *Br J Ophthalmol* 1999;83:190–193.

34. Vazquez-Memije ME, Shanske S, Santorelli FM, et al. Comparative biochemical studies in fibroblasts from patients with different forms of Leigh syndrome. *J Inherit Metab Dis*1996;19:43–50.

35. DiMauro S, De Vivo DC. Genetic heterogeneity in Leigh syndrome. *Ann Neurol* 1996;40:5–7.

36. van Erven PM, Gabreels FJ, Ruitenbeek W, Renier WO, Fischer JC. Mitochondrial encephalomyopathy: association with an NADH dehydrogenase deficiency. *Arch Neurol* 1987;44:775–778.

37. Willems JL, Monnens LA, Trijbels JM, et al. Leigh's encephalomyelopathy in a patient with cytochrome c oxidase deficiency in muscle tissue. *Pediatrics* 1977;60:850–857.

38. Van Coster R, Lombres A, De Vivo DC, et al. Cytochrome c oxidase-associated Leigh syndrome: phenotypic features and pathogenetic speculations. *J Neurol Sci* 1991;104:97–111.

39. Kretzschmar HA, DeArmond SJ, Koch TK, et al. Pyruvate dehydrogenase complex deficiency as a cause of subacute necrotizing encephalopathy (Leigh disease). *Pediatrics* 1987;79:370–373.

40. Baumgartner ER, Suormala TM, Wick H, et al. Biotinidase deficiency: a cause of subacute necrotizing encephalomyelopathy (Leigh syndrome): report of a case with lethal outcome. *Pediatr Res* 1989;26:260–266.

41. Matthews PM, Marchington DR, Squier M, Land J, Brown RM, Brown GK. Molecular genetic characterization of an X-linked form of Leigh's syndrome. *Ann Neurol* 1993;33:652–655.

42. Loeffen J, Smeitink J, Triepels R, et al. The first nuclear-encoded complex I mutation in a patient with Leigh syndrome. *Am J Hum Genet* 1998;63:1598–1608.

43. Bourgeron T, Rustin P, Chretien D, et al. Mutation of a nuclear succinate dehydrogenase gene results in mitochondrial respiratory chain deficiency. *Nat Genet* 1995;11:144–149.

44. Tiranti V, Hoertnagel K, Carrozzo R, et al. Mutations of SURF-1 in Leigh disease associated with cytochrome c oxidase deficiency. *Am J Hum Genet* 1998;63:1609–1621.

45. Zhu Z, Yao J, Johns T, et al. SURF1, encoding a factor involved in the biogenesis of cytochrome c oxidase, is mutated in Leigh syndrome. *Nat Genet* 1998;20:337–343.

46. Sue CM, Karadimas C, Checcarelli N, et al. Differential features of patients with mutations in two COX assembly genes, SURF-1 and SCO2. *Ann Neurol* 2000;47:589–595.

47. Ciafaloni E, Santorelli FM, Shanske S, et al. Maternally inherited Leigh syndrome. *J Pediatr* 1993;122:419–422.

48. Santorelli FM, Shanske S, Macaya A, DeVivo DC, DiMauro S. The mutation at nt 8993 of mitochondrial DNA is a common cause of Leigh's syndrome. *Ann Neurol* 1993;34:827–834.

49. De Vries DD, van Engelen BG, Gabreels FJ, Ruitenbeek W, van Oost BA. A second missense mutation in the mitochondrial ATPase 6 gene in Leigh's syndrome. *Ann Neurol* 1993;34:410–412.

50. Santorelli FM, Shanske S, Jain KD, Tick D, Schon EA, DiMauro S. A T→C mutation at nt 8993 of mitochondrial DNA in a child with Leigh syndrome. *Neurology* 1994;44:972–974.

51. Cox GB, Fimmel AL, Gibson F, Hatch L. The mechanism of ATP synthase: a reassessment of the functions of the b and a subunits. *Biochim Biophys Acta* 1986;849:62–69.

52. Petty RK, Harding AE, Morgan-Hughes JA. The clinical features of mitochondrial myopathy. *Brain* 1986;109 (pt 5):915–938.

53. Rahman S, Blok RB, Dahl HH, et al. Leigh syndrome: clinical features and biochemical and DNA abnormalities. *Ann Neurol* 1996;39:343–351.

54. Koga Y, Yoshino M, Kato H. MELAS exhibits dominant negative effects on mitochondrial RNA processing. *Ann Neurol* 1998;43:835.

55. Chalmers RM, Lamont PJ, Nelson I, et al. A mitochondrial DNA tRNA(Val) point mutation associated with adult-onset Leigh syndrome. *Neurology* 1997;49:589–592.

56. Yamamoto M, Clemens PR, Engel AG. Mitochondrial DNA deletions in mitochondrial cytopathies: observations in 19 patients. *Neurology* 1991;41:1822–1828.

57. Yamadori I, Kurose A, Kobayashi S, Ohmori M, Imai T. Brain lesions of the Leigh-type distribution associated with a mitochondriopathy of Pearson's syndrome: light and electron microscopic study. *Acta Neuropathol (Berl)* 1992;84:337–341.

58. Morris AA, Taanman JW, Blake J, et al. Liver failure associated with mitochondrial DNA depletion. *J Hepatol* 1998;28:556–563.

59. De Meirleir L, Seneca S, Lissens W, Schoentjes E, Desprechins B. Bilateral striatal necrosis with a novel point mutation in the mitochondrial ATPase 6 gene. *Pediatr Neurol* 1995;13:242–246.

60. Thyagarajan D, Shanske S, Vazquez-Memije M, De Vivo D, DiMauro S. A novel mitochondrial ATPase 6 point mutation in familial bilateral striatal necrosis. *Ann Neurol* 1995;38:468–472.

61. Man PY, Griffiths PG, Brown DT, Howell N, Turnbull DM, Chinnery PF. The epidemiology of Leber hereditary optic neuropathy in the North East of England. *Am J Hum Genet* 2003;72:333–339.

62. Wallace DC, Brown MD, Lott MT. Mitochondrial DNA variation in human evolution and disease. *Gene* 1999;238:211–230.

63. Valentino ML, Barboni P, Ghelli A, et al. The ND1 gene of complex I is a mutational hot spot for Leber hereditary optic neuropathy. *Ann Neurol* 2004;56:631–641.

64. Valentino ML, Avoni P, Barboni P, et al. Mitochondrial DNA nucleotide changes C14482G and C14482A in the ND6 gene are pathogenic for Leber's hereditary optic neuropathy. *Ann Neurol* 2002;51:774–778.

65. Jun AS, Brown MD, Wallace DC. A mitochondrial DNA mutation at nucleotide pair 14459 of the NADH dehydrogenase subunit 6 gene associated with maternally inherited Leber hereditary optic neuropathy and dystonia. *Proc Natl Acad Sci USA* 1994;91: 6206–6210.

66. De Vries DD, Went LN, Bruyn GW, et al. Genetic and biochemical impairment of mitochondrial complex I activity in a family with Leber hereditary optic neuropathy and hereditary spastic dystonia. *Am J Hum Genet* 1996;58:703–711.

67. Filosto M, Mancuso M, Nishigaki Y, et al. Clinical and genetic heterogeneity in progressive external ophthalmoplegia due to mutations in polymerase gamma. *Arch Neurol* 2003;60:1279–1284.

68. Luoma P, Melberg A, Rinne JO, et al. Parkinsonism, premature menopause, and mitochondrial DNA polymerase gamma mutations: clinical and molecular genetic study. *Lancet* 2004;364: 875–882.

69. Mancuso M, Filosto M, Oh SJ, DiMauro S. A novel polymerase gamma mutation in a family with ophthalmoplegia, neuropathy, and Parkinsonism. *Arch Neurol* 2004;61:1777–1779.

70. Campuzano V, Montermini L, Molto MD, et al. Friedreich's ataxia: autosomal recessive disease caused by an intronic GAA triplet repeat expansion. *Science* 1996;271:1423–1427.

71. Pook MA, Al Mahdawi SA, Thomas NH, et al. Identification of three novel frameshift mutations in patients with Friedreich's ataxia. *J Med Genet* 2000;37):E38.

72. Durr A, Cossee M, Agid Y, et al. Clinical and genetic abnormalities in patients with Friedreich's ataxia. *N Engl J Med* 1996;335:1169–1175.

73. Filla A, De Michele G, Cavalcanti F, et al. The relationship between trinucleotide (GAA) repeat length and clinical features in Friedreich ataxia. *Am J Hum Genet* 1996;59:554–560.

74. Bidichandani SI, Ashizawa T, Patel PI. The GAA triplet-repeat expansion in Friedreich ataxia interferes with transcription and may be associated with an unusual DNA structure. *Am J Hum Genet* 1998;62:111–121.

75. Wong A, Yang J, Cavadini P, et al. The Friedreich's ataxia mutation confers cellular sensitivity to oxidant stress which is rescued by chelators of iron and calcium and inhibitors of apoptosis. *Hum Mol Genet* 1999;8:425–430.

76. Campuzano V, Montermini L, Lutz Y, et al. Frataxin is reduced in Friedreich ataxia patients and is associated with mitochondrial membranes. *Hum Mol Genet* 1997;6:1771–1780.

77. Dhe-Paganon S, Shigeta R, Chi YI, Ristow M, Shoelson SE. Crystal structure of human frataxin. *J Biol Chem* 2000;275:30,753–30,756.

78. Foury F, Cazzalini O. Deletion of the yeast homologue of the human gene associated with Friedreich's ataxia elicits iron accumulation in mitochondria. *FEBS Lett* 1997;411:373–377.

79. Koutnikova H, Campuzano V, Foury F, Dolle P, Cazzalini O, Koenig M. Studies of human, mouse and yeast homologues indicate a mitochondrial function for frataxin. *Nat Genet* 1997;16: 345–351.

80. Puccio H, Simon D, Cossee M, et al. Mouse models for Friedreich ataxia exhibit cardiomyopathy, sensory nerve defect and Fe-S enzyme deficiency followed by intramitochondrial iron deposits. *Nat Genet* 2001;27:181–186.

81. Bradley JL, Blake JC, Chamberlain S, Thomas PK, Cooper JM, Schapira AH. Clinical, biochemical and molecular genetic correlations in Friedreich's ataxia. *Hum Mol Genet* 2000;9:275–282.
82. Rotig A, de Lonlay P, Chretien D, et al. Aconitase and mitochondrial iron-sulphur protein deficiency in Friedreich ataxia. *Nat Genet* 1997;17:215–217.
83. Melov S, Coskun P, Patel M, et al. Mitochondrial disease in superoxide dismutase 2 mutant mice. *Proc Natl Acad Sci USA* 1999;96:846–851.
84. Tabrizi SJ, Workman J, Hart PE, et al. Mitochondrial dysfunction and free radical damage in the Huntington R6/2 transgenic mouse. *Ann Neurol* 2000;47:80–86.
85. Babcock M, de Silva D, Oaks R, et al. Regulation of mitochondrial iron accumulation by Yfh1p, a putative homolog of frataxin. *Science* 1997;276:1709–1712.
86. Kemp GJ, Taylor DJ, Thompson CH, et al. Quantitative analysis by 31P magnetic resonance spectroscopy of abnormal mitochondrial oxidation in skeletal muscle during recovery from exercise. *NMR Biomed* 1993;6:302–310.
87. Ingwall JS, Kramer MF, Fifer MA, et al. The creatine kinase system in normal and diseased human myocardium. *N Engl J Med* 1985;313:1050–1054.
88. Lodi R, Rajagopalan B, Blamire AM, et al. Cardiac energetics are abnormal in Friedreich ataxia patients in the absence of cardiac dysfunction and hypertrophy: an in vivo 31P magnetic resonance spectroscopy study. *Cardiovasc Res* 2001;52:111–119.
89. Lodi R, Cooper JM, Bradley JL, et al. Deficit of in vivo mitochondrial ATP production in patients with Friedreich ataxia. *Proc Natl Acad Sci USA* 1999;96:11,492–11,495.
90. Seznec H, Simon D, Monassier L, et al. Idebenone delays the onset of cardiac functional alteration without correction of Fe-S enzymes deficit in a mouse model for Friedreich ataxia. *Hum Mol Genet* 2004;13:1017–1024.
91. Seznec H, Simon D, Bouton C, et al. Friedreich ataxia: the oxidative stress paradox. *Hum Mol Genet* 2005;14:463–474.
92. Zhang Y, Aberg F, Appelkvist EL, Dallner G, Ernster L. Uptake of dietary coenzyme Q supplement is limited in rats. *J Nutr* 1995;125:446–453.
93. Stephens NG, Parsons A, Schofield PM, Kelly F, Cheeseman K, Mitchinson MJ. Randomised controlled trial of vitamin E in patients with coronary disease: Cambridge Heart Antioxidant Study (CHAOS). *Lancet* 1996;347:781–786.
94. Shoulson I. DATATOP: a decade of neuroprotective inquiry. Parkinson Study Group. Deprenyl and tocopherol antioxidative therapy of parkinsonism. *Ann Neurol* 1998;44(suppl1):S160–S166.
95. Bostick RM, Potter JD, McKenzie DR, et al. Reduced risk of colon cancer with high intake of vitamin E: the Iowa Women's Health Study. *Cancer Res* 1993;53:4230–4237.
96. Gabsi S, Gouider-Khouja N, Belal S, et al. Effect of vitamin E supplementation in patients with ataxia with vitamin E deficiency. *Eur J Neurol* 2001;8:477–481.
97. Folkers K, Moesgaard S, Morita M. A one year bioavailability study of coenzyme Q10 with 3 months withdrawal period. *Mol Aspects Med* 1994;15(suppl):S281–S285.
98. Matthews RT, Yang L, Browne S, Baik M, Beal MF. Coenzyme Q10 administration increases brain mitochondrial concentrations and exerts neuroprotective effects. *Proc Natl Acad Sci USA* 1998;95:8892–8897.
99. Reahal S, Wrigglesworth J. Tissue concentrations of coenzyme Q10 in the rat following its oral and intraperitoneal administration. *Drug Metab Dispos* 1992;20:423–427.
100. Ernster L, Dallner G. Biochemical, physiological and medical aspects of ubiquinone function. *Biochim Biophys Acta* 1995;1271:195–204.
101. Lodi R, Hart PE, Rajagopalan B, et al. Antioxidant treatment improves in vivo cardiac and skeletal muscle bioenergetics in patients with Friedreich's ataxia. *Ann Neurol* 2001;49:590–596.
102. Hart PE, Lodi R, Rajagopalan B, et al. Antioxidant treatment of patients with Friedreich ataxia: four-year follow-up. *Arch Neurol* 2005;62:621–626.
103. Nagai Y, Yoshida K, Narumi S, Tanayama S, Nagaoka A. Brain distribution of idebenone and its effect on local cerebral glucose utilization in rats. *Arch Gerontol Geriatr* 1989;8:257–272.

104. Mordente A, Martorana GE, Minotti G, Giardina B. Antioxidant properties of 2,3-dimethoxy-5-methyl-6-(10-hydroxydecyl)-1,4-benzoquinone (idebenone). *Chem Res Toxicol* 1998;11:54–63.
105. Gutzmann H, Hadler D. Sustained efficacy and safety of idebenone in the treatment of Alzheimer's disease: update on a 2-year double-blind multicentre study. *J Neural Transm Suppl* 1998;54:301–310.
106. Ranen NG, Peyser CE, Coyle JT, et al. A controlled trial of idebenone in Huntington's disease. *Mov Disord* 1996;11:549–554.
107. Hausse AO, Aggoun Y, Bonnet D, et al. Idebenone and reduced cardiac hypertrophy in Friedreich's ataxia. *Heart* 2002;87:346–349.
108. Schulz JB, Dehmer T, Schols L, et al. Oxidative stress in patients with Friedreich ataxia. *Neurology* 2000;55:1719–1721.
109. Ogasahara S, Engel AG, Frens D, Mack D. Muscle coenzyme Q deficiency in familial mitochondrial encephalomyopathy. *Proc Natl Acad Sci USA* 1989;86:2379–2382.
110. Musumeci O, Naini A, Slonim AE, et al. Familial cerebellar ataxia with muscle coenzyme Q10 deficiency. *Neurology* 2001;56:849–855.
111. Lamperti C, Naini A, Hirano M, et al. Cerebellar ataxia and coenzyme Q10 deficiency. *Neurology* 2003;60:1206–1208.
112. Schapira A, Cooper J, Dexter D. Mitochondrial complex 1 deficiency in Parkinson's disease. *Ann Neurol* 1989;26:122–123.
113. Schapira AH, Cooper JM, Dexter D, Jenner P, Clark JB, Marsden CD. Mitochondrial complex I deficiency in Parkinson's disease. *Lancet* 1989;1:1269.
114. Schapira AH, Mann VM, Cooper JM, et al. Anatomic and disease specificity of NADH CoQ1 reductase (complex I) deficiency in Parkinson's disease. *J Neurochem* 1990;55:2142–2145.
115. Cleeter MW, Cooper JM, Darley-Usmar VM, Moncada S, Schapira AH. Reversible inhibition of cytochrome c oxidase, the terminal enzyme of the mitochondrial respiratory chain, by nitric oxide: implications for neurodegenerative diseases. *FEBS Lett* 1994;345:50–54.
116. Hillered L, Ernster L. Respiratory activity of isolated rat brain mitochondria following in vitro exposure to oxygen radicals. *J Cereb Blood Flow Metab* 1983;3:207–214.
117. Zhang Y, Marcillat O, Giulivi C, Ernster L, Davies KJ. The oxidative inactivation of mitochondrial electron transport chain components and ATPase. *J Biol Chem* 1990;265:16,330–16,336.
118. Benzi G, Curti D, Pastoris O, Marzatico F, Villa RF, Dagani F. Sequential damage in mitochondrial complexes by peroxidative stress. *Neurochem Res* 1991;16:1295–1302.
119. Thomas PK, Cooper JM, King RH, et al. Myopathy in vitamin E deficient rats: muscle fibre necrosis associated with disturbances of mitochondrial function. *J Anat* 1993;183(pt3):451–461.
120. Schapira AH. Evidence for mitochondrial dysfunction in Parkinson's disease: a critical appraisal. *Mov Disord* 1994;9:125–138.
121. Taylor DJ, Krige D, Barnes PR, et al. A 31P magnetic resonance spectroscopy study of mitochondrial function in skeletal muscle of patients with Parkinson's disease. *J Neurol Sci* 1994;125:77–81.
122. Penn AM, Roberts T, Hodder J, Allen PS, Zhu G, Martin WR. Generalized mitochondrial dysfunction in Parkinson's disease detected by magnetic resonance spectroscopy of muscle. *Neurology* 1995;45:2097–2099.
123. Parker WD Jr, Boyson SJ, Parks JK. Abnormalities of the electron transport chain in idiopathic Parkinson's disease. *Ann Neurol* 1989;26:719–723.
124. Cooper JM, Daniel SE, Marsden CD, Schapira AH. L-dihydroxyphenylalanine and complex I deficiency in Parkinson's disease brain. *Mov Disord* 1995;10:295–297.
125. Gu M, Gash MT, Cooper JM, et al. Mitochondrial respiratory chain function in multiple system atrophy. *Mov Disord* 1997;12:418–422.
126. Ikebe S, Tanaka M, Ohno K, et al. Increase of deleted mitochondrial DNA in the striatum in Parkinson's disease and senescence. *Biochem Biophys Res Commun* 1990;170:1044–1048.
127. Schapira AH, Holt IJ, Sweeney M, Harding AE, Jenner P, Marsden CD. Mitochondrial DNA analysis in Parkinson's disease. *Mov Disord* 1990;5:294–297.
128. Lestienne P, Nelson I, Riederer P, Reichmann H, Jellinger K. Mitochondrial DNA in postmortem brain from patients with Parkinson's disease. *J Neurochem* 1991;56:1819.

129. Kosel S, Grasbon-Frodl EM, Hagenah JM, Graeber MB, Vieregge P. Parkinson disease: analysis of mitochondrial DNA in monozygotic twins. *Neurogenetics* 2000;2:227–230.

130. Ozawa T, Tanaka M, Ino H, et al. Distinct clustering of point mutations in mitochondrial DNA among patients with mitochondrial encephalomyopathies and with Parkinson's disease. *Biochem Biophys Res Commun* 1991;176:938–946.

131. Ikebe S, Tanaka M, Ozawa T. Point mutations of mitochondrial genome in Parkinson's disease. *Brain Res Mol Brain Res* 1995;28:281–295.

132. Richter G, Sonnenschein A, Grunewald T, Reichmann H, Janetzky B. Novel mitochondrial DNA mutations in Parkinson's disease. *J Neural Transm* 2002;109:721–729.

133. Simon DK, Pulst SM, Sutton JP, Browne SE, Beal MF, Johns DR. Familial multisystem degeneration with parkinsonism associated with the 11778 mitochondrial DNA mutation. *Neurology* 1999;53:1787–1793.

134. Brown MD, Shoffner JM, Kim YL, et al. Mitochondrial DNA sequence analysis of four Alzheimer's and Parkinson's disease patients. *Am J Med Genet* 1996;61:283–289.

135. Kapsa RM, Jean-Francois MJ, Lertrit P, et al. Mitochondrial DNA polymorphism in substantia nigra. *J Neurol Sci* 1996;144:204–211.

136. Vives-Bauza C, Andreu AL, Manfredi G, et al. Sequence analysis of the entire mitochondrial genome in Parkinson's disease. *Biochem Biophys Res Commun* 2002;290:1593–1601.

137. Shoffner JM, Brown MD, Torroni A, et al. Mitochondrial DNA variants observed in Alzheimer disease and Parkinson disease patients. *Genomics* 1993;17:171–184.

138. Lucking CB, Kosel S, Mehraein P, Graeber MB. Absence of the mitochondrial A7237T mutation in Parkinson's disease. *Biochem Biophys Res Commun* 1995;211:700–704.

139. Taanman JW, Schapira AH. Analysis of the trinucleotide CAG repeat from the DNA polymerase gamma gene (POLG) in patients with Parkinson's disease. *Neurosci Lett* 2005;376:56–59.

140. Thyagarajan D, Bressman S, Bruno C, et al. A novel mitochondrial 12SrRNA point mutation in parkinsonism, deafness, and neuropathy. *Ann Neurol* 2000;48:730–736.

141. Tan EK, Khajavi M, Thornby JI, Nagamitsu S, Jankovic J, Ashizawa T. Variability and validity of polymorphism association studies in Parkinson's disease. *Neurology* 2000;55:533–538.

142. Van der Walt JM, Nicodemus KK, Martin ER, et al. Mitochondrial polymorphisms significantly reduce the risk of Parkinson disease. *Am J Hum Genet* 2003;72:804–811.

143. Pyle A, Foltynie T, Tiangyou W, et al. Mitochondrial DNA haplogroup cluster UKJT reduces the risk of PD. *Ann Neurol* 2005;57:564–567.

144. Ross OA, McCormack R, Maxwell LD, et al. Mt4216C variant in linkage with the mtDNA TJ cluster may confer a susceptibility to mitochondrial dysfunction resulting in an increased risk of Parkinson's disease in the Irish. *Exp Gerontol* 2003;38:397–405.

145. Swerdlow RH, Parks JK, Miller SW, et al. Origin and functional consequences of the complex I defect in Parkinson's disease. *Ann Neurol* 1996;40:663–671.

146. Gu M, Cooper JM, Taanman JW, Schapira AH. Mitochondrial DNA transmission of the mitochondrial defect in Parkinson's disease. *Ann Neurol* 1998;44:177–186.

147. Hsu LJ, Sagara Y, Arroyo A, et al. Alpha-synuclein promotes mitochondrial deficit and oxidative stress. *Am J Pathol* 2000;157:401–410.

148. Lee SJ. Alpha-synuclein aggregation: a link between mitochondrial defects and Parkinson's disease? *Antioxid Redox Signal* 2003;5:337–348.

149. Palacino JJ, Sagi D, Goldberg MS, et al. Mitochondrial dysfunction and oxidative damage in parkin-deficient mice. *J Biol Chem* 2004;279:18,614–18,622.

150. Greene JC, Whitworth AJ, Kuo I, Andrews LA, Feany MB, Pallanck LJ. Mitochondrial pathology and apoptotic muscle degeneration in Drosophila parkin mutants. *Proc Natl Acad Sci USA* 2003;100:4078–4083.

151. Muftuoglu M, Elibol B, Dalmizrak O, et al. Mitochondrial complex I and IV activities in leukocytes from patients with parkin mutations. *Mov Disord* 2004;19:544–548.

152. Darios F, Corti O, Lucking CB, et al. Parkin prevents mitochondrial swelling and cytochrome c release in mitochondria-dependent cell death. *Hum Mol Genet* 2003;12:517–526.

153. Canet-Aviles RM, Wilson MA, Miller DW, et al. The Parkinson's disease protein DJ-1 is neuroprotective due to cysteine-sulfinic acid-driven mitochondrial localization. *Proc Natl Acad Sci USA* 2004;101:9103–9108.

154. Valente EM, Abou-Sleiman PM, Caputo V, et al. Hereditary early-onset Parkinson's disease caused by mutations in PINK1. *Science* 2004;304:1158–1160.

155. Beilina A, Van Der BM, Ahmad R, et al. Mutations in PTEN-induced putative kinase 1 associated with recessive parkinsonism have differential effects on protein stability. *Proc Natl Acad Sci USA* 2005;102:5703–5708.

156. Shults CW, Oakes D, Kieburtz K, et al. Effects of coenzyme Q10 in early Parkinson disease: evidence of slowing of the functional decline. *Arch Neurol* 2002;59:1541–1550.

157. Howell N, Kubacka I, Xu M, McCullough DA. Leber hereditary optic neuropathy: involvement of the mitochondrial ND1 gene and evidence for an intragenic suppressor mutation. *Am J Hum Genet* 1991;48:935–942.

158. De Vries DD, Went LN, Bruyn GW, et al. Genetic and biochemical impairment of mitochondrial complex I activity in a family with Leber hereditary optic neuropathy and hereditary spastic dystonia. *Am J Hum Genet* 1996;58:703–711.

159. Benecke R, Strumper P, Weiss H. Electron transfer complex I defect in idiopathic dystonia. *Ann Neurol* 1992;32:683–686.

160. Schapira AH, Warner T, Gash MT, Cleeter MW, Marinho CF, Cooper JM. Complex I function in familial and sporadic dystonia. *Ann Neurol* 1997;41:556–559.

161. Benecke R, Strümper P, Weiss H. Electron transfer complex I defect in idiopathic dystonia. *Ann Neurol* 1992;32:683–686.

162. Tabrizi SJ, Cooper JM, Schapira AH. Mitochondrial DNA in focal dystonia: a cybrid analysis. *Ann Neurol* 1998;44:258–261.

163. Tranebjaerg L, Schwartz C, Eriksen H, et al. A new X linked recessive deafness syndrome with blindness, dystonia, fractures, and mental deficiency is linked to Xq22. *J Med Genet* 1995;32:257–263.

164. Koehler CM, Leuenberger D, Merchant S, Renold A, Junne T, Schatz G. Human deafness dystonia syndrome is a mitochondrial disease. *Proc Natl Acad Sci USA* 1999;96:2141–2146.

165. Zeitlin S, Liu JP, Chapman DL, Papaioannou VE, Efstratiadis A. Increased apoptosis and early embryonic lethality in mice nullizygous for the Huntington's disease gene homologue. *Nat Genet* 1995;11:155–163.

166. Trottier Y, Lutz Y, Stevanin G, et al. Polyglutamine expansion as a pathological epitope in Huntington's disease and four dominant cerebellar ataxias. *Nature* 1995;378:403–406.

167. Martindale D, Hackam A, Wieczorek A, et al. Length of huntingtin and its polyglutamine tract influences localization and frequency of intracellular aggregates. *Nat Genet* 1998;18:150–154.

168. Roos RA, Bots GT. Nuclear membrane indentations in Huntington's chorea. *J Neurol Sci* 1983;61:37–47.

169. Davies SW, Turmaine M, Cozens BA, et al. Formation of neuronal intranuclear inclusions underlies the neurological dysfunction in mice transgenic for the HD mutation. *Cell* 1997;90:537–548.

170. Beal MF. Does impairment of energy metabolism result in excitotoxic neuronal death in neurodegenerative illnesses? *Ann Neurol* 1992;31:119–130.

171. Kuwert T, Lange HW, Langen KJ, Herzog H, Aulich A, Feinendegen LE. Cortical and subcortical glucose consumption measured by PET in patients with Huntington's disease. *Brain* 1990;113(pt5):1405–1423.

172. Koroshetz WJ, Jenkins BG, Rosen BR, Beal MF. Energy metabolism defects in Huntington's disease and effects of coenzyme Q10. *Ann Neurol* 1997;41:160–165.

173. Hoang TQ, Bluml S, Dubowitz DJ, et al. Quantitative proton decoupled 31P MRS and 1H MRS in the evaluation of Huntington's and Parkinson's diseases. *Neurology* 1998;50:1033–1040.

174. Gu M, Gash MT, Mann VM, Javoy-Agid F, Cooper JM, Schapira AH. Mitochondrial defect in Huntington's disease caudate nucleus. *Ann Neurol* 1996;39:385–389.

175. Browne SE, Bowling AC, MacGarvey U, et al. Oxidative damage and metabolic dysfunction in Huntington's disease: selective vulnerability of the basal ganglia. *Ann Neurol* 1997;41:646–653.

176. Tabrizi SJ, Cleeter MW, Xuereb J, Taanman JW, Cooper JM, Schapira AH. Biochemical abnormalities and excitotoxicity in Huntington's disease brain. *Ann Neurol* 1999;45:25–32.

177. Tabrizi SJ, Workman J, Hart PE, et al. Mitochondrial dysfunction and free radical damage in the Huntington R6/2 transgenic mouse. *Ann Neurol* 2000;47:80–86.

178. Lodi R, Schapira AH, Manners D, et al. Abnormal in vivo skeletal muscle energy metabolism in Huntington's disease and dentatorubropallidoluysian atrophy. *Ann Neurol* 2000;48:72–76.

179. Ferrante RJ, Andreassen OA, Jenkins BG, et al. Neuroprotective effects of creatine in a transgenic mouse model of Huntington's disease. *J Neurosci* 2000;20:4389–4397.

180. Schaefer M, Hopkins RG, Failla ML, Gitlin JD. Hepatocyte-specific localization and copper-dependent trafficking of the Wilson's disease protein in the liver. *Am J Physiol* 1999;276:3 (pt1): G639–G646.

181. Lutsenko S, Cooper MJ. Localization of the Wilson's disease protein product to mitochondria. *Proc Natl Acad Sci USA* 1998;95: 6004–6009.

182. Gu M, Cooper JM, Butler P, et al. Oxidative-phosphorylation defects in liver of patients with Wilson's disease. *Lancet* 2000;356:469–474.

183. Melov S, Coskun P, Patel M, et al. Mitochondrial disease in superoxide dismutase 2 mutant mice. *Proc Natl Acad Sci USA* 1999;96:846–851.

Tremors: Differential Diagnosis, Pathophysiology, and Therapy

24

Günther Deuschl　　*Jens Volkmann*　　*Jan Raethjen*

Tremor is a rhythmic oscillation of at least one functional body region. Although neurologists are mainly confronted with pathologic tremors, one should keep in mind that any movement is accompanied by normal physiologic tremor. This mostly invisible oscillation is assumed to be necessary for fast movements, as the onset of voluntary movements coincides usually with the peak of the tremor burst in normal tremor. The limits between normal and pathologic tremors can be difficult to define. A pragmatic clinical approach is to define abnormal tremor whenever it is visible to the naked eye or if any frequencies occur that are lower than normal tremor.

PHENOMENOLOGY AND TERMINOLOGY OF TREMOR

Clinical analysis and classification of tremor depend critically on a definition of the activation conditions during which tremor occurs, because, for example, resting tremor will otherwise be used by clinicians with a different meaning. The following definitions and related criteria are based on the consensus statement of the Movement Disorder Society on tremor (1).

Resting tremor occurs in a body part that is not voluntarily activated and is completely supported against gravity. The amplitude of tremor must increase during (mental and sometimes motor) activation (counting backward, Stroop test, gait, movements of the contralateral hand); the tremor amplitude must diminish or disappear during the onset of voluntary activation (1); and the tremor can reoccur after a certain time period (2). Mental activation increases the amplitude of many tremors, but only resting tremor is triggered in the relaxed limbs. Resting tremor often but not always responds to dopaminergic treatment. Resting tremor is a separate tremor entity generated by central mechanisms unique to this symptom.

Action tremor is any tremor occurring on voluntary contraction of muscle. This includes postural, isometric, and kinetic tremor.

Postural tremor is present while voluntarily maintaining a position against gravity. A rare variant of postural tremor is *position-specific postural or position-sensitive* tremor. *Isometric tremor* occurs as a result of muscle contraction against a rigid stationary object (e.g., a heavy table). This form of force tremor can occur in isolation or together with other tremor symptoms and may be the cause of separate complaints.

Kinetic tremor occurs during any voluntary movement. Kinetic tremor may occur in non-goal-directed and goal-directed movements.

Simple kinetic tremor occurs during voluntary movements that are not goal directed and is contrasted to tremor during goal-directed movements (intention tremor).

Intention tremor is present when the amplitude increases during visually guided movements toward a target and if typical fluctuations of the amplitude (velocity) of the tremor occur.

Whenever a tremor increases substantially during the pursuit of a target or goal, it can be assumed that a disturbance of the cerebellum or its afferent or efferent pathways is present (3). Typically, tremor amplitude fluctuates significantly as the target is approached. It can be difficult to distinguish between intention tremor and ataxia in some patients.

Task-specific kinetic tremor may appear or become exacerbated during specific activities. Occupational tremors and primary writing tremor are examples of this kind of tremor.

CLINICAL ASSESSMENT OF TREMOR PATIENTS

The description of a particular tremor should include the following aspects (1): The topography of tremor (head, chin, jaw, vocal cords, upper/lower extremity, body, etc.), the activation condition of tremor (rest, posture, non-goal-directed movements, goal-directed movements, specific tasks) and the frequency of tremor (low: <4 Hz, medium: 4–7 Hz, high: >7 Hz). The general neurological examination has a great impact on the differential diagnosis of tremor. For obvious reasons, it should be documented if akinesia, rigidity (including Froment's sign for the upper and lower extremity and coactivation sign of psychogenic tremor), postural abnormalities, dystonia, spasticity, ataxia, and signs of neuropathy are present. Specific data from the medical history should include information on the onset of tremor, family history, alcohol sensitivity, associated diseases, medications, and drug use/abuse.

Several rating scales have been proposed. Generally, it is necessary to distinguish between resting and action tremors, which are associated with different complaints. Moreover, specific problems arise from the variability of tremor. For resting tremor, the Unified Parkinson's Disease Rating Scale (UPDRS) has been proposed. For postural and intention tremor, two partially overlapping scales have been proposed (4,5), including a motor score and a disability scale. A related disability test has been validated (6). Portable instruments for field studies to assess tremor have been validated (7), and quantitative measures with accelerometry, EMG (8,9), and graphic tablets (10,11) have been developed and partly validated.

SYNDROME CLASSIFICATION AND MANAGEMENT OF TREMOR PATIENTS

From a clinical standpoint, a classification of tremor that would allow us to identify the etiology by means of the clinical features of a tremor is desirable. However, different etiologies can have similar clinical presentations, making such an approach unsuccessful. On the other hand, distinct tremor etiologies (such as parkinsonian tremor or essential tremor) can have variable clinical expressions. Thus, we can separate distinct tremor syndromes that are frequent or that can be separated as phenomenological entities. The Movement Disorder Society has proposed a classification that, in some cases, implies a clear-cut etiology, but in others, it describes a syndrome, leaving the etiology open. The different syndromes in this classification are defined on the basis of clinical observations without additional laboratory tests. The clinical classifications, their frequency ranges, and the activating conditions are summarized in Figure 24.1. Some of the etiologies of tremor are listed in Table 24.1.

Normal Tremor

Physiologic tremor is present in every normal subject during posture and action. Its frequency for hand tremor is between 6 and 12 Hz. Normal finger tremor can sometimes be seen with the naked eye. Mechanical and, sometimes, central oscillations cause this tremor (9,12,13).

Enhanced physiologic tremor (EPT) is a visible, predominantly postural, and high-frequency tremor of short duration (<2 years). Evidence for a neurological disease related to tremor must be excluded.

This definition covers many tremor etiologies, typically those elicited by endogenous or exogenous intoxication producing postural tremor (Table 24.1). These etiologies are mostly reversible, provided that the cause of the tremor is identified and corrected. Some standard laboratory tests that may be considered for etiologic diagnosis in these patients are summarized in Table 24.2. This form of tremor overlaps with the category of drug-induced and toxic tremors (see the following).

Pathophysiology: The mechanism underlying essential palatal tremor (EPT) is mainly mechanical tremor aggravated by reflex activation or central oscillations (9,14). Hyperthyroidism is an example for a reflex activation as the hormone sensitizes muscle spindles and subsequently aggravates muscle reflexes causing tremor (15). Amitriptyline, an antidepressant, activates the central oscillator of physiologic tremor, thereby eliciting EPT (16).

Treatment: Whenever causal treatment is not available or does not suppress tremor sufficiently, propranolol or other beta blockers are recommended.

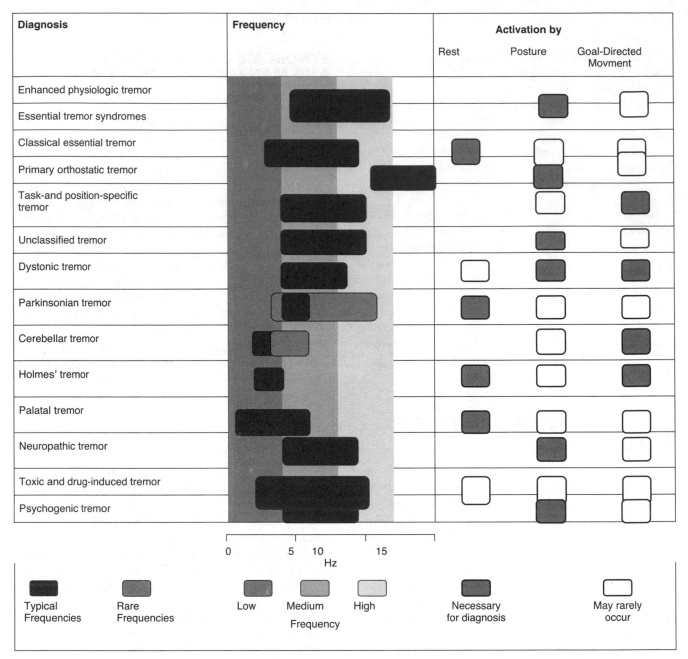

Figure 24.1 The clinical forms of tremors. Deuschl G, Bain P, Brin M, Ad Hoc Scientific Committee. Consensus statement of the Movement Disorder Society on Tremor. *Mov Disord* 1998;13:2–23.

TABLE 24.1

ETIOLOGIC CLASSIFICATION OF TREMOR

1. Hereditary, Degenerative and Idiopathic Diseases

Parkinson's disease	R, P
Pallido-nigral degeneration	P
Multiple system atrophy	
Olivo-ponto-cerebellar atrophy	R, P, I
Striato-nigral degeneration	R, P, I
Wilson's disease	R, P, I
Progressive pallidum atrophy	R
Huntington's disease	R, P, I
Benign hereditary chorea	P, I
Fahr's syndrome	R, I
Paroxysmal dystonic choreoathetosis	I
Familial intention tremor and lipofuscinosis	I
Ramsay Hunt syndrome	P, I
Ataxia teleangiectasia	P

(Continued)

TABLE 24.1
CONTINUED

Fragile X syndrome; Fragile X permutation	P, I	Lead	P (R, I)
Dystonia musculorum deformans	P	CO	P (R, I)
Segawa dystonia	P	Manganese	P (R, I)
Spasmodic torticollis	P	Arsenic	P (R, I)
Meige syndrome	P	Cyanide	P
Essential myoclonus und tremor	P, I	Naphthalene	P, I
Essential tremor	P, I	Alcohol	P, I
Hereditary chin tremor	P, I	Phosphor	P (R, I)
Task-specific tremors:		Toluene	P
Writer's tremor		DDT	P (R, I)
Voice tremor		Lindan	P, I
"Golfers"-tremor ("yips")		Kepone	P, I
Laughing tremor		Dioxins	P
Klinefelter's syndrome	P, I		

2. Cerebral Diseases of Various Etiologies

6. Drugs

Infectious diseases and other inflammations		Centrally acting substances	
Multiple sclerosis	R, P, I	Neuroleptics	R, P
Neurolues	R, P, I	Reserpine	R, P
Neuroborreliosis	R, P, I	Tetrabenazine	R, P
HIV infection	P	Metoclopramide	R, P
FSME	P, I	Antidepressants (especially tricyclics)	P
Tick-borne encephalitis		Lithium	R, P, I
Smallpox, measles	P	Cocaine	P
Typhus	P	Alcohol	P, I
Space-occupying lesions		Sympathomimetics	
Tumors	R, P, I	Adrenaline	P, I
Cysts	R, P, I	Bronchodilators (β-agonists, e.g., Formoterol)	P, I
Hematoma	R, P, I	Theophylline	P
AV-malformations	R, P, I	Caffeine	P
Cerebrovascular insults	R, P, I	Teeine	P
Trauma	R, P, I	Dopamine	P
		Steroids	
		Progesterone (medroxyprogesterone acetate)	R, P

3. Metabolic Diseases

		Antiestrogens (tamoxifen)	P
Hyperthyroidism	P	Adrenocorticosteroids	P
Hyperparathyroidism	R, P	Miscellaneous	
Magnesium deficiency	R, P	Valproate	P
Hypocalcemia	R, I	Perhexiline	R, P
Hyposodiumemia	P	Antiarrhythmics (amiodarone)	P
Hypoglycemia	P	Mexiletine, procainamide	P
Disturbed liver function		Calcitonine	P
Chronic hepatocerebral degeneration	P, I	Thyroid hormones	P
Hepatic encephalopathy	P, I	Cytostatics (vincristin, adriablastin,	P, I
Kidney disturbances	P, I	cytosinarabinoside, ifosfanide)	
Vitamin B12 deficiency	R, P, I	Immunodepressants (cyclosporine A)	P
Eosinophilia-myalgia syndrome	P, I		

7. Others

4. Peripheral Neuropathies and Similar Disorders

		Emotions (anxiety, stress)	P
Charcot-Marie-Tooth disease	P, I	Fatigue	P
Roussy-Levy syndrome	P	Cooling	P
Chronic demyelinating neuropathies	P	Trauma of the periphery/reflex sympathetic dystrophy	
Guillain-Barré syndrome	P	Reflex dystrophy	P, I
Gammopathia (IgM, IgG)	P	High-pressure neurological syndrome	P
Malabsorption neuropathy	P	Withdrawal of drugs	P
Polyneuropathy of various origins	P	Withdrawal of alcohol	P, I
(diabetes, uremia, porphyria)		Withdrawal of cocaine	R
HIV-associated neuropathy	P	Psychogenic tremor	R, P, I
Spinal muscle atrophy	P		

5. Toxins

Nicotine	P
Mercury	P (R, I)

Adapted from Elble RJ, Brilliant M, Leffler K, Higgins C. Quantification of essential tremor in writing and drawing. *Mov Disord* 1996; 11:70–78. I, Intention tremor; R, Rest tremor; P, Postural tremor.

TABLE 24.2
LABORATORY CHECK OF SYMPTOMATIC TREMORS

T3, T4, TRH
Na+, K+, Ca++, Cl-
gamma-GT, GOT, GPT, cholinesterase
creatinine, urea, glucose
cortisol,[a] parathormon[a]
24h copper excretion + ceruloplasmin[a]
toxicologic tests*

[a] These tests are to be performed only when clinically suggested.

Therapy studies are available for only a few specific tremors that are classified as enhanced physiologic tremors: Valproate tremors seem to respond to propranolol but not to amantadine, cyproheptadine, diphenhydramine, and benztropine (17,18). The general treatment of hyperthyroidism has been addressed in various studies (19), but none of them has specifically studied the treatment of tremor. The following drugs and dosages have been applied in these patients: propranolol (160 mg/day), atenolol (200 mg/day), metoprolol (200 mg/day), acebutolol (400 mg/day), oxprenolol (160 mg/day), nadolol (80 mg/day), timolol (20 mg/day). Lithium tremor also has been shown to respond to beta blockers (20). Tremor in drug-induced parkinsonism does not respond to propranolol (21). Some patients with postural tremors in the setting of peripheral neuropathies respond to propranolol.

Essential Tremor

Essential tremor (ET) has evolved into two different meanings during the past years. On one hand, the term describes a tremor syndrome classically defined by an often hereditary monosymptomatic tremor (1), and this is the most common movement disorder. On the other hand, there are tremors of unknown origin (*idiopathic* or *essential*) but with distinct clinical characteristics that usually can be separated on clinical grounds from classical ET but also have been labeled as *essential* tremors. To cover these two groups in a single classification, the Movement Disorder Society proposes to separate these tremors into *classical essential tremor* and the other well-defined but nevertheless idiopathic tremor syndromes. In addition, the patients who cannot yet be classified unequivocally are classified as *indeterminate postural tremor syndromes*.

Classical Essential Tremor

Classical ET is a monosymptomatic, predominant postural and action tremor that is usually slowly progressive over time. The diagnostic criteria and the differential diagnoses are listed in Table 24.3. It is the most frequent movement disorder. Prevalence rates vary between 0.4% and 5.6% (22, 23). In 60% of the patients, the condition is autosomal dominant. Twin studies suggest a strong heritability above 90% and an almost complete penetrance above 60 years of age (24,25). Genes causing ET have not yet been identified, but linkage has been found in different families on chromosome 2 (26), chromosome 3 (27), and chromosome 4 (28). Recently, a missense mutation of the HS1-BP3 gene on chromosome 2 locus has been suggested to be pathogenetically related with ET (29), but subsequent studies have cast doubt on this observation as the mutation has been found with similar frequency in Parkinson's disease (PD) and normal controls (30). This protein seems to regulate the activation of tyrosine and tryptophan hydroxylase. On chromosome 3, a gain of function-mutation of the DRD3 gene is considered to be responsible (31). Not only genetic influences have been suggested to cause ET; possible environmental factors or toxins have been searched for, and increased blood levels of lead (32) and higher beta-carboline alkaloids were found, compared with controls (32,33). These substances

TABLE 24.3
GUIDELINES FOR THE DIAGNOSIS OF ESSENTIAL TREMOR

Core Criteria	Secondary Criteria	Red Flags
1. Bilateral action tremor of the hands and forearms (but not rest tremor) 2. Absence of other neurological signs, with the exception of the cogwheel phenomenon 3. May have isolated head tremor with no abnormal posture	1. Long duration (>3 years) 2. Family history 3. Beneficial response to ethanol	1. Unilateral tremor, focal tremor, leg tremor, gait disturbance, rigidity, bradykinesia, rest tremor 2. Sudden or rapid onset 3. Current drug treatment that might cause or exacerbate tremor 4. Isolated head tremor with abnormal posture (head tilt or turning)

This table is based on the following sources: (1) Spieker S, Loschmann P, Jentgens C, Boose A, Klockgether T, Dichgans J. Tremorlytic activity of budipine: a quantitative study with long-term tremor recordings. *Clin Neuropharmacol* 1995;18:266–272. (2) Deuschl G, Koester B. Diagnose und Behandlung des Tremors. In: Conrad B, Ceballos-Baumann AO, eds. Bewegungsstörungen in der Neurologie, Stuttgart/New York: Thieme Verlag, 1996;222–253.

are normal body constituents but may be tremorogenic. The significance of these findings is still unknown.

About 50%–90% of the patients improve with ingestion of alcohol. The condition may begin at a very early age, and the incidence is increasing above age 40 years, with a mean onset of 35–45 years in different studies and an almost complete penetrance at the age of 60 (33,34). The topographic distribution shows hand tremor in 94%, head tremor in 33%, voice tremor in 16%, jaw tremor in 8%, facial tremor in 3%, leg tremor in 12%, and tremor of the trunk in 3% of the patients (33,34,35). In some of the topographic regions (e.g., head, vocal cords, and chin), tremor may occur in isolation (36) (Table 24.3).

Usually, ET is mainly a postural tremor, but rarely even resting tremors do occur (37,38) that are not related to an abnormality of dopaminergic function (39) or a specific dopaminergic degeneration (40). In almost half of the patients, intention tremor (41) occurs together with other signs of cerebellar dysfunction, such as ataxia and movement overshoot. These patients often also have a disturbance of tandem gait that is even clinically visible (42,43). Oculomotor abnormalities do not belong to the spectrum of abnormalities. The severity of tremor increases slowly over years. All the patients are disabled to some extent, and most are socially handicapped due to the tremor. Up to 25% of the patients seeking medical attention must change jobs or have to retire from work (43,44,45).

Additional subtle abnormalities of different functions have been found: a slight abnormality of olfaction (45,46) unrelated to resting tremor, hearing abnormalities (46,47), and a subclinical vestibulocerebellar affection of oculomotor functions (47,48). Moreover, several studies found subtle neuropsychological deficits in attention and select executive functions (49,50,51), which have been interpreted to reflect a frontal or cerebello-thalamo-cortical dysfunction (51). There are also hints at a consistent abnormality of personality (52). However, signs of a progressive dementia have not been substantiated in any study.

Pathophysiology: Classical ET is most likely due to central oscillations (53,54) arising in the Guillain-Mollaret triangle. Experimental evidence in animal tremor models suggests the inferior olive to function abnormally in this condition. Recent studies in patients have pointed to a functional abnormality of the cerebellum based on cerebellar disturbances of hand movements (41), gait (42), and eye movements (47). This is further strengthened by MRI-spectroscopic abnormalities of the cerebellar cortex compatible with neuronal damage (55,56). These findings indicate a hitherto undetermined pathologic process of cerebellar function that is most likely related to the disease. However, morphologic abnormalities have not been found in pathoanatomic studies so far (40), except for preliminary data in a few patients showing signs of Purkinje-cell degeneration (57). Thus, either a functional disturbance (e.g., abnormal receptor function or,

less likely, a neurodegenerative process) is responsible for this abnormality. An example of such a receptor abnormality has been shown in a knockout mouse model of the alpha 1 subunit of the GABA receptor (58) exhibiting trembling that can be improved with various tremor drugs. The cerebellar Purkinje cells exhibited a loss of all responses to synaptic or exogenous GABA, but no differences in abundance, gross morphology, or spontaneous synaptic activity were observed (59).

TREATMENT OF TREMOR

(Also see Table 24.4: The Treatment of Essential Tremor.)

Tremor of the hands: Propranolol and primidone are clearly the drugs of first choice for this indication, and both have been carefully studied (60). Propranolol was introduced in 1971 (61) for the treatment of ET. Drugs with predominant β-1 effects have been shown to be less effective than those acting on the β-2 receptor, and none has proved superior to propranolol. Only 25% of the patients maintain their initial good response for 2 years. Contraindications are cardiac insufficiency or arrhythmia and diabetes. As propranolol acts on the peripheral (reflex) component of tremors, it is helpful for many other tremors, such as Parkinson's or cerebellar tremor (62,63). Primidone is efficient for essential tremor (64), but tachyphylaxis may occur. The major problems are early adverse effects with nausea, dizziness, sedation, and headache. The combination of propranolol and prinmidone is recommended whenever one of the drugs is insufficient. Arotinolol has been tested in a crossover study with an effects similar to propranolol (65). Gabapentine also appears effective, following two double-blind studies (66,67), but another double-blind study showed no convincing effect (68). Topiramate has been shown to be effective in a small, double-blind study (69). Levetiracetam is just now being explored for the treatment of ET, and open single-dose studies are promising (70,71). Acetazolamide (and methazolamide) are not significantly better than placebo (72). Alprazolam is helpful in ET (73). Clonazepam is recommended for patients with predominant action and intention tremor in ET (74) but ineffective in uncomplicated essential tremor (75). Botulinum toxin at a dosage of 50 units or 100 units Botox has a significant but clinically limited effect and carries a high risk of a clinically meaningful but completely reversible paresis (76). (For drug dosages, also see Table 24.5.)

Meanwhile, surgery is the accepted treatment for patients with severe disability being resistant to medical treatment. Two multicenter studies have shown that thalamic deep-brain stimulation is effective (77,78,79), and one study has shown that deep-brain stimulation of the ventral intermediate nucleus (VIM) has a better effect than VIM-thermocoagulation and even fewer side effects (80). The selection of patients for surgery is a crucial point for a good therapeutic effect.

TABLE 24.4

THE TREATMENT OF ESSENTIAL TREMOR

	Drug	Dosage	Remarks
1st choice	Propranolol	(30–320 mg, 3 doses) (standard or long-acting)	Contraindications: cardiac, pulmonary, diabetes, etc. Hand and head tremor
1st choice	Primidone	(62.5–500 mg, single dose in the evening)	Hand and head tremor Preferentially for patients with age >60 years
1st choice	Combination: propranolol/ primidone	Maximum dosage for each	Always try before using 2nd- and 3rd-choice drugs
2nd choice	Arotinilol	(10–30 mg)	Crossover study with propranolol
2nd choice	Gabapentine	1800–2400 mg/day	Conflicting results of 3 double-blind studies: 1 without, 2 with benefit
2nd choice	Topiramate	<400 mg	So far small double-blind study only
2nd choice	Clonazepam	0.75–6 mg	For predominant kinetic tremor
3rd choice	Botulinum toxin		Double-blind study with a significant result, but weakness as a significant side effect
3rd choice	Clozapine	Test: 12.5 mg, 30–50 mg daily	Less well-documented effect than for Parkinson's disease, often ineffective
Last choice	Surgery		VIM stimulation or thalamotomy

TABLE 24.5

DOSAGES OF VARIOUS SUBSTANCES APPLIED FOR THE TREATMENT OF TREMOR

	Initial Dose	Increase in Steps	Maximum Dose
L-dopa			
L-dopa + benserazid	62.5 mg	62.5 mg/d	750 mg
L-dopa + carbidopa	50 mg	50 mg/d	600 mg
Dopaminagonists			
Bromocriptine	5 mg	5 mg/w	20 mg
Lisuride	0.1 mg	0.1 mg/w	1.2 mg
α-dihydroergocryptine	10 mg	10 mg/w	90 mg
Pergolide	0.15 mg	0.10 mg/d	3.0 mg
Pramipexol	1.5 mg	0.5 mg/w	4.5 mg
Ropinirole	3 mg	1.5 mg/d	15 mg
Cabaserile	2 mg	1 mg/w	6 mg
Anticholinergics			
Bornaprine	3 mg	3 mg/w	12 mg
Biperiden	1 mg	2 mg/w	12 mg
Metixen	7.5 mg	7.5 mg/w	60 mg
Trihexyphenidyl	1 mg	2 mg/w	10 mg
Beta Blockers			
Propranolol	30 mg	30 mg/w	240 mg
Nadolol	10 mg	30 mg/w	120 mg
Miscellaneous			
Amantadine	100 mg	100 mg/d	300 mg
Primidone	62.5 mg	125 mg/d	500 mg
Clonazepam	0.5 mg	0.5 mg/d	6 mg
Alprazolam	0.75 mg	0.75 mg/d	4 mg
Clozapine	12.5 mg	12.5 mg/d	75 mg

For some substances (e.g., anticholinergics), a slow titration is strictly recommended. d, day; w, week.

Head and voice: Pharmacological treatment of essential head and voice tremor is less efficient than treatment for hand tremor. Propranolol and primidone, each alone or both combined, have been recommended (81,82) for essential head tremor. Clonazepam is often recommended for this indication, but careful studies are not available. One of the promising therapies for head tremor is the local injection of botulinum toxin (83). Deep-brain stimulation is also effective for head and voice tremor. As bilateral thalamotomies carry a high risk of dysarthria, mostly bilateral VIM stimulation is applied (78,84,85,86). (Also see Table 24.4.)

VARIANTS OF ESSENTIAL TREMOR

The following clinical entities can be separated on clinical grounds, although much of the pathophysiological background of these tremors remains unknown and reclassifications may be necessary in the future.

Primary Writing Tremor and Other Task- or Position-Specific Tremors

Tremor during writing without other manifestations of tremor or other neurological disease is called *primary writing tremor.* After initial observation (87), two forms of writing tremor have been described (88). *Task-specific tremor* is characterized by tremor appearing only during writing (type A). Position-specific tremor occurs when the hand position used in writing is adopted (type B).

Several other conditions are often summarized under the topic of task- or position-specific tremors. The patients suffering from these tremors, such as musicians and sportsmen, mostly perform motor activities at the highest level. They develop tremor in their professional activity (e.g., piano playing), but other skilled movements (eating, handling delicate objects, etc.) remain unaffected. Common examples are the tremors in golfers (89,90) and the tremors occurring in pianists (91,92).

Pathophysiology: The pathophysiological interpretation of these syndromes is controversial. The relation between dystonic tremor and writing tremor is not yet clearly defined, and some interpret it as a form of focal dystonia (93). Others did not find evidence for dystonia and consider it to be an idiopathic condition separate from dystonia, a specific overuse syndrome or a focal form of essential tremor (94).

Treatment: The treatment of task-specific tremors is difficult. Propranolol and local injections of botulinum toxin have been proposed. Physical therapy, abstinence from the tremor-producing tasks, and a later retraining are often the most valuable help for these patients. Successful treatment of one patient with drug-resistant primary writing tremor with thalamotomy (95) and, more recently, thalamic deep-brain stimulation (96), respectively, have been described.

Isolated Voice Tremor

The clinical diagnosis of isolated vocal tremor can be put forward if the tremor is limited to the voice. Such isolated voice tremor (97) occurs in two variants. The first resembles spasmodic dysphonia with a dysphonic and trembling voice and is often considered to be a form of focal dystonia of the vocal cord (98,99). The second presents with a pure voice tremor and is considered a form of essential tremor (33,34,35,100). Dystonic tremulous voice tremor is more likely to occur if the tremor is not present during emotional speech production or singing. In our experience this feature is not present in voice tremor in the setting of ET. Voice tremor also occurs in cerebellar disease or classical ET, together with further tremor manifestations, and thus it does not fit with the definition of isolated voice tremor. The pathophysiology of voice tremor is unknown.

Treatment: This is another condition that is difficult to treat. Essential voice tremor can sometimes be improved with propranolol and primidone. Dystonic voice tremor can often be very successfully treated with local injections into the vocal cord of botulinum toxin (101,102); this also has been shown to be effective for essential voice tremor (103). Thalamic deep-brain stimulation also often reduces voice tremor (104), but isolated voice tremor is rarely an indication for surgery.

Isolated Chin Tremor

Isolated chin tremor is a rare, autosomal dominant hereditary tremor syndrome characterized by attacks of high-frequency tremor of the mentalis muscles or of the chin, typically starting in early childhood (105). A genetic linkage has been found (106). Isolated chin tremor may be reclassified in the future among the myoclonia or channelopathies, rather than among the tremors. Slow-frequency chin tremors often occur in PD and sometimes in ET.

Treatment: Reports on the treatment of chin trembling are rare. Mostly, specific treatment is not necessary. One case has been treated with botulinum toxin (107).

Primary Orthostatic Tremor

Primary orthostatic tremor (OT) is a unique tremor syndrome (108,109) that has been observed until now only in patients over 40 years of age. It is characterized by a subjective feeling of unsteadiness during stance but only in severe cases during gait. Some patients show sudden falls. None of the patients has problems when sitting and lying. The clinical findings are sparse, often limited to a visible and sometimes only palpable fine-amplitude rippling of the leg (quadriceps) muscles. The diagnosis can be confirmed by electromyographic recordings (e.g., from the quadriceps femoris muscle) with a typical 13–18 Hz pattern. All the leg, trunk, and arm muscles show this pattern, which in many cases is absent during tonic innervation when sitting and lying (110,111,112). OT occurs more often in PD, and secondary forms have been described (113).

The diagnosis of OT is critically dependent on the electromyographic demonstration of this electromyography (EMG) pattern, as other tremors during stance (e.g., essential, parkinsonian, or cerebellar tremors of the legs) can present with similar complaints.

Pathophysiology: There is strong evidence that OT is a central tremor because the high-frequency EMG pattern is highly coherent in all the trembling muscles. Recent studies have shown that OT also may be present during maneuvers that do not involve stance (114), and the time relation of the muscle jerks shows a task-specific plasticity (115). All the muscles on both sides of the body are involved and are coherent, and this is the strongest evidence for a central tremor. The oscillator of this tremor is unknown. Due to the unique coherence of all the muscles of both sides and the brainstem and that resetting of the tremor was only possible with electrical stimulation over the posterior fossa but not over the cortex, this tremor has been considered a brainstem tremor. This view has recently been questioned (116).

Treatment: OT has been documented to be responsive to clonazepam and primidone. Valproate and propranolol were applied in single cases with variable success. Abnormalities of dopaminergic innervation of the striatum have been described (117), although L-dopa has not shown efficiency consistently (117,118). According to small double-blind studies (119,120) and our own experience, gabapentine seems to have an excellent and most consistent beneficial effect (121). Meanwhile, we use it as the drug of first choice for orthostatic tremor (1800–2400 mg/day). Another efficient drug is clonazepam.

Dystonic Tremor

Dystonic tremor is still an entity that is being debated, and different definitions have been proposed by clinicians (122,123,124). Tremor in dystonia has been proposed as a forme fruste of essential tremor (125); however, it is not yet clear if they share common genes (the *DYT1* locus is already excluded) (124) or, at least, pathophysiologic mechanisms.

There are clinical features that separate these tremors. Dystonic tremor is defined (126) as a postural/kinetic tremor usually not seen during complete rest and occurring in an extremity or body part that is affected by dystonia. These are usually focal tremors with irregular amplitudes and variable frequencies (mostly below 7 Hz).

Some patients exhibit focal tremors even without overt signs of dystonia. These focal tremors have been included among dystonic tremors (127) because some of them later evolve into dystonia. In many patients with dystonic tremors, antagonistic gestures lead to a reduction of the tremor amplitude. This is well-known for dystonic head tremor in the setting of spasmodic torticollis showing tremor reduction when the patient touches the head or only lifts the arm, whereas essential head tremor does not show this sign (124).

Dystonic tremor and *tremor associated with dystonia* can be different because unspecific postural tremors occur in extremities not involved in dystonia. Hand tremor in patients with otherwise uncomplicated idiopathic spasmodic torticollis is a typical example for this (128).

Pathophysiology: The pathophysiology of tremors in dystonia is unknown. It may be related to the same basal ganglia abnormality as dystonia itself (126).

Treatment: A positive effect of propranolol has been described previously in studies of dystonic head tremor. The effectivity of botulinum toxin for dystonic head (129) and hand (76) tremor, as well as in tremulous spasmodic dysphonia, is well-documented. Severe cases in the setting of a generalized dystonia have been treated successfully with deep-brain stimulation of the pallidum or ventrolateral thalamus (130). Tremor associated with dystonia often responds to the medication for classical ET. (For drug dosages, see Table 24.5)

TREMORS IN PARKINSON'S DISEASE

Most patients with PD present with any kind of tremor. Resting tremor with pill rolling is typical. In addition to resting tremor, up to 40% of patients have different forms of postural and action tremor (131,132,133), which can occur in isolation or together with resting tremor. Thus, tremor in PD cannot be generally defined by the tremor characteristics itself. Tremor in PD is assumed, if the patient has PD according to the brain bank criteria, including bradykinesia, and if the patient has any form of pathological tremor.

A wide range of clinical presentations of tremors can be found in PD. For clinical simplicity, they have been subdivided strictly according to their clinical symptoms (1). Unilateral tremors or leg tremors are more likely to be due to PD (134).

Type I: Classical Parkinsonian Tremor

Type I classical parkinsonian tremor occurs with the same frequency either as resting tremor or as resting and postural/action tremor. Pure resting tremor does occur in a significant portion of patients. The frequency of pure resting tremor is mostly 4–6 Hz, but in the early stage of the disease, much higher resting tremor frequencies can be found (135,136). In other patients, the resting tremor is combined with a kinetic tremor of the same frequency, and amplitude increases with mental stress, with contralateral movements, or during gait. When a voluntary movement is initiated, the tremor is temporarily suppressed and reoccurs after a few seconds with the hands outstretched (1,2). The clinical observations fit with the hypothesis that this postural/kinetic tremor (with similar frequencies for rest and postural/kinetic tremors) is a continuation of the resting tremor under postural and or action conditions. The frequencies for resting and postural/action tremor can be considered to be equal if they do not differ by more than 1.5 Hz. With some experience, this difference in frequency can be seen clinically.

Type II: Resting and Postural/Action Tremors of Different Frequencies

In some patients, the postural/action tremor has a frequency higher and nonharmonically related to the resting tremor.

A mild form of action tremor is present in almost every parkinsonian patient. This can be seen during slow flexion/extension movements. This postural/action tremor can be extremely disabling. Some patients have a predominant postural tremor in addition to their resting tremor. The postural/action tremor has a higher frequency nonharmonically related to the resting tremor. This form is rare (<15% of patients with PD) and has often been described as a combination of an ET with PD (135,136). Some of these patients had their postural tremor long before the onset of other symptoms of PD.

Type III: Pure Postural/Action Tremor

Isolated postural and action tremors are rare but do occur in PD. They have been assigned as ET variants or have been found to be indistinguishable from enhanced physiologic tremor. A relation of this form of tremor with rigidity seems possible (132).

Only the resting tremor component is by itself a positive diagnostic criterion for PD according to the brain bank criteria, but other tremors are often seen in PD. The differential diagnosis between PD and classical essential tremor can be difficult to make, especially in the early stage of the condition. It has been estimated that 20% of the patients with ET are misdiagnosed for PD and vice versa. (Some

of the differential diagnostic criteria are summarized in Table 24.6.)

Type IV: Monosymptomatic Tremor at Rest

Some patients exhibit a resting and postural tremor without overt signs of bradykinesia or rigidity. Thus, the clinical findings are not sufficient to diagnose PD, although there is positron emission tomograpy (PET) evidence that these patients have a dopaminergic deficit (137) and—as in full-blown PD—the distance between the substantia nigra and the red nucleus was reduced (138). These patients are often difficult to treat. Monosymptomatic tremor at rest is thus defined (1) by the following:

(i)   Pure or predominant resting tremor
(ii) No signs of bradykinesia, rigidity, or problems with stance; stability sufficient to diagnose PD
(iii) Duration of the tremor of at least 2 years

Pathophysiology: Dopamine depletion in the striatum is the hallmark of PD, but the pathophysiology of parkinsonian tremor is still being debated. The most extreme hypotheses argue about peripheral versus central nervous system origin, intrinsic cellular oscillator versus network oscillators, and basal-ganglia–based pathophysiology versus cerebello-thalamic–based pathophysiology. Recent studies support the view that parkinsonian symptoms are most likely due to abnormal synchronous oscillating neuronal activity within the basal ganglia. Peripheral factors play only a minor role in the generation, maintenance, and modulation of PD tremor and other signs. The most likely candidates producing these oscillations are the weakly coupled neural networks of the basal ganglia–thalamocortical loops. However, present evidence supports the view that the basal ganglia loops are influenced by other neuronal structures and systems, and that the tuning of these loops by cerebello-thalamic mechanisms and by other modulator neurotransmitter systems entrain the abnormal

TABLE 24.6

CLINICAL CRITERIA TO SEPARATE ESSENTIAL AND PARKINSONIAN TREMOR

	Essential Tremor	Parkinson's Disease
Hereditary tremor	+++	-
Head tremor	+++	-
Voice tremor	+++	-
Sensitivity to alcohol	+++	-
Classical resting tremor	+	++
Predominant unilateral tremor	+	+++
Leg tremor	+	+++
Rigididy (not only Fromment's sign)	+	++
Sensitivity to L-dopa	-	+++

-, usually not present; + to +++, degree commonly observed.

TABLE 24.7
SUGGESTIONS FOR THE TREATMENT OF TREMORS IN PARKINSON'S DISEASE

Tremor Type	1. Step	2. Step	3. Step
Classical parkinsonian tremor or monosymptomatic rest tremor	L-dopa Dopaminagonists Anticholinergics	Amantadine Propranolol Clozapine	Subthalamic nucleus stimulation
Rest and postural tremor with different frequencies	Propranolol Primidon	Dopamine Dopaminagonists Anticholinergics Clozapine	Subthalamic nucleus stimulation
Isolated action tremor	Propranolol Anticholinergics	Amantadine	

synchronized oscillations. Resting tremor in PD is most likely due to abnormal central oscillators within the basal ganglia (139). The pathophysiology of action tremors in PD is unknown.

Treatment: Due to the different forms of tremor in PD, the clinical characteristics of the tremor have to be taken into account. Our personal approach to the treatment of patients is included in Table 24.7. (For drug dosages, see Table 24.5.)

L-dopa is the most effective treatment for the majority of symptoms in PD. Among the tremors in PD, mainly the resting tremor is improved but other forms may also respond. Generally, the effect on tremor is highly variable in patients with PD, and the tremor may worsen, especially for the action tremor with frequencies different from the resting tremor frequency. All the available double-blind studies of different dopamine agonists failed to demonstrate a superior effect of one or the other agonist on tremor, although all of them obviously have a significant effect. For pramipexol a double-blind study has shown a favorable effect on tremor (140). Although the treatment of tremors with anticholinergics is often recommended, there have been only a few double-blind studies. The anticholinergic bornaprine has been found to be effective in 2 double blind-studies (141,142). Trihexyphenidyl has been tested alone and compared with amantadine and L-dopa (133). Possible side effects are dry mouth, visual disturbances, constipation, glaucoma, disturbance of micturation, and memory deficits. Especially in elderly subjects confusional states that are reversible after cessation of the drug can occur. Discontinuation may induce a severe rebound effect. One study has provided ample evidence that patients treated with anticholinergics have a higher incidence of Alzheimer's pathology (143).

The favorable effect of clozapine on rest tremor has been confirmed in several studies (144,145) that have shown a good effect on resting tremor, even when other drugs failed (146). No tolerance has been observed over 6 months. The dosage was 18–75 mg. Major side effects are sedation and leukopenia as a serious, even lethal complication in some patients.

Functional neurosurgery is a useful treatment for some patients who cannot be treated otherwise. Thalamic thermocoagulation or deep brain stimulation (DBS) of the VIM improves tremor but not akinesia. Lesional surgery cannot be applied bilaterally due to speech disturbances (but DBS can) and is therefore no longer the surgical treatment of first choice (80). Pallidotomy and stimulation of the pallidum also improve tremor. Subthalamic nucleus (STN) stimulation does successfully improve tremor (147,148) but also akinesia and rigidity and is, therefore, presently the preferred surgery by far. Further controlled studies are necessary (Table 24.5).

CEREBELLAR TREMOR SYNDROMES

Cerebellar tremor is often used synonymously with *intention tremor*, although various clinical forms of tremor have been described in cerebellar disorders (149,150). There is general agreement that the most common form of cerebellar tremor is intention tremor.

The following conditions have to be fulfilled for the diagnosis of cerebellar tremor:

(i) Pure or dominant intention tremor, often unilateral
(ii) Tremor frequency below 5 Hz (mostly below 4 Hz)
(iii) Postural tremor may be present, but no resting tremor

Another tremor that is most likely due to pathology of the cerebellum or its afferent/efferent pathways is known as *titubation*. It is a slow-frequency oscillation of the whole body and/or head depending on postural innervation. During movement, the amplitude usually increases and its victims are severely incapacitated (149). The most common causes for intention tremor and titubation are multiple sclerosis, brain trauma with infratentorial damage, and (hereditary) ataxias. Both intention tremor and titubation are symptomatic tremors. The most extensive study of tremor in multiple sclerosis (MS) (151) has confirmed that rest tremor never occurs in MS and that about 50% of MS patients suffer from cerebellar tremor, with 27%

exhibiting significant disability and 10% exhibiting incapacitating tremors.

All other forms of tremor (postural tremor, stance tremors, etc.) are only accepted as being of cerebellar origin if other signs of cerebellar dysfunction are seen in the patient. Cerebellar tremor can be considered as a symptomatic tremor. The major differential diagnoses are atypical forms of essential tremor and some symptomatic tremor etiologies, such as Wilson's disease. The pathophysiological basis of cerebellar tremor is believed to be abnormal feedforward or feedback mechanisms (long-loop reflexes).

Treatment: Cerebellar tremors are difficult to treat and good results are rare. Double-blind studies are rare. Studies with cholinergic substances (physostigmine; lecitine, a precurser of choline) have shown improvement in some patients but have failed in the majority. Isoniazid failed to show significant results (152). In some patients, 5-HTP has been found to be effective (153). Another recent proposal has been to administer amantadine. Open studies or single-case observations have shown favorable results with propranolol, clonazepam, carbamazepine, and trihexyphenidyl. Limited improvements have been observed after loading of the shaking extremity, but most clinicians do not do that because the patients adapt rapidly to the new weight. Probably the best symptomatic improvement can be obtained with thalamotomy and also with stereotactic high-frequency stimulation in selected patients (155–157). Functional outcome after stereotaxy, however, greatly varies and depends on the presence of other motor symptoms of the disease. In a recent study (158). patients with MS tremor with a frequency above 3 Hz and significant tremor-related disabilities were found to respond favorably. Accelerometric recordings in this study may have helped to distinguish patients with predominant MS tremor from those with tremor and ataxia. The long-term follow-up in a larger cohort has not yet been assessed.

Holmes Tremor

Rubral tremor, midbrain tremor, myorhythmia, and Benedikt's syndrome are tremors that are all due to a lesion of the central nervous system (CNS), mainly in the midbrain. To avoid definitions that include topographic relations, the Consensus Statement of the Movement Disorder Society has proposed to label this well-defined tremor as *Holmes tremor,* because G. Holmes was among the first to describe it (159). The following criteria define this tremor (1):

(i) The presence of both resting and intention tremor. In many patients, postural tremor is also present. The tremor rhythm is often not as regular as for other tremors, giving the impression of jerky movements.
(ii) Slow frequency, mostly below 4.5 Hz.
(iii) If the date of the lesion is known (e.g., a cerebrovascular accident), a variable delay between the lesion and the first occurrence of the tremor is typical (mostly 2 weeks until 2 years).

Holmes tremor is among the most disabling forms of tremor because it disturbs rest and much voluntary and involuntary movement. It mainly affects the hands and the proximal arm and is mostly a unilateral tremor.

Pathophysiology: It is generally accepted that Holmes tremor is a symptomatic tremor due to lesions that seem to be centered in the brainstem/cerebellum and the thalamus. However, lesions of the involved fiber tracts in other regions may cause a similar clinical phenomenology.

The pathophysiological basis of Holmes tremor is a combined lesion of the cerebello-thalamic and nigrostriatal systems. Autopsy data (160), PET data (161), and clinical observations (162,163) suggest that it develops following a combined lesion of these two pathways. Central oscillators cause this tremor. It seems likely that the rhythm of resting tremor is usually blocked during voluntary movements by the cerebellum. If this cerebellar compensation is absent, the rhythm of rest tremor spills into movements (163), thereby producing the low-frequency intention tremor.

Involuntary movements after thalamic stroke: A specific tremor syndrome associated with thalamic lesions has been presented often in the past but was recently further analyzed with modern imaging techniques (164–166). The label *thalamic tremor* (164) has been used for this novel entity. A more detailed study has shown that this tremor is part of a specific dystonia–athetosis–chorea–action tremor following lateral–posterior thalamic strokes (165,166). The combination of tremor, dystonia, and a severe sensory loss seems to be the important clue for the diagnosis of this stroke. The tremor itself is a mixture of action tremor with an intentional component and dystonia in the setting of a well-recovered severe hemiparesis. Proximal segments are often involved. This tremor syndrome also develops with a certain delay after the initial insult.

Treatment: No generally accepted therapy is available. Nevertheless, treatment is successful in a higher percentage than for patients with cerebellar tremor. Some patients respond to levodopa, anticholinergics, or clonazepam. (For drug dosages, see also Table 24.5.) The effect of functional neurosurgery for this tremor syndrome is poorly documented. Such patients have been operated on, but they are diagnosed as posttraumatic tremors or poststroke tremors, and the clinical features are not described in detail. Several patients received thalamic DBS (167).

PALATAL TREMOR SYNDROMES

Palatal tremor was classified earlier among the myoclonias (palatal myoclonus) (168), but as it is rhythmic it has been reclassified among the tremors. Palatal tremor can be separated into two forms (169,170).

Symptomatic palatal tremor (SPT) is characterized by the following features (1):

(i) Preceding brainstem/cerebellar lesion with subsequent olivary pseudohypertrophy (which can be demonstrated by MRI).

(ii) Rhythmic movements of the soft palate (levator veli palatini) and often other brainstem-innervated or extremity muscles. This is clinically visible as a rhythmic movement of the edge of the palate.

A specific subgroup characterized by a slowly progressive condition with progressive ataxia and palatal tremor (PAPT) has been more clearly delineated recently (171).

Essential palatal tremor (EPT) is characterized by the following:

(i) Absent CNS lesion and absent olivary pseudohypertrophy.

(ii) Rhythmic movements of the soft palate (tensor veli palatini), usually with an ear click. The tensor contraction is visible as a movement of the roof of the palate. Extremity or eye muscles are not involved.

The pathophysiologic basis is believed to be autonomous oscillations of the inferior olive in SPT (172) and is unknown for EPT.

Besides these two classical forms, further rhythmic movement disorders of the palate and neighboring structures may occur that have not yet been classified.

Treatment: The disability of patients with SPT is due mostly to other clinical symptoms of the underlying cerebellar lesion. The rhythmic palatal movement in SPT does not cause discomfort or disability for the patient except when the eyes are involved or when there is an extremity tremor.

Oscillopsia is only rarely to be treated sufficiently. Single cases have been described with a favorable response to clonazepam. Other oral drugs that have been proposed are trihexyphenidyl and valproate. Botulinum toxin has been used for the treatment of oscillopsia. The toxin can be injected either into the retrobulbar fat tissue or into specific muscles that can be targeted selectively (173,174). So far no controlled studies are available. In our hands, this treatment is helpful for some patients but is not always accepted for long-term use.

For the treatment of extremity tremors, only single case reports have been described to respond to clonazepam (175) or trihexiphenidyl (176).

The only complaint of patients with EPT is the ear click. A number of medications have been reported to be successful: valproate (177), trihexyphenidyl (176), and flunarizine (178). Sumatriptane also has been found to be effective in a few patients (179–181) but was ineffective in another (182). The antagonism of 5-HTP-receptors may thus play a role, at least for some patients. As a long-term therapy, this drug is not suited for various reasons. Presently, the most established therapy is the treatment of the click by injection of botulinum toxin into the tensor veli palatini (183). Low dosages

of botulinum toxin (e.g., 4–10 units Botox) are injected under electromyographic guidance either transpalatally or transnasally. The critical point is to ascertain, with endoscopy and electromyography through an EMG injection needle isolated until the tip, that the needle is definitely placed within the tensor muscle. Spread of botulinum toxin in the soft palate or overly large dosages can otherwise cause severe side effects. Although we have never seen any such complications in our patients, it must be mentioned that the injection of botulinum toxin into the palatal muscles in rabbits has been introduced as an animal model for middle ear infections. (For drug dosages, see Table 24.5.)

DRUG-INDUCED AND TOXIC TREMOR SYNDROMES

Drug-induced tremors can present with the whole range of clinical features of tremors, depending on the drug and, probably, on the individual disposition of the patients. The most common form is enhanced physiologic tremor following, for example, sympathomimetics or antidepressants (see Table 24.1). Another frequent form is parkinsonian tremor following neuroleptic or, more generally, antidopaminergic drugs (dopamine-receptor blockers, dopamine-depleting drugs such as reserpine, flunarizine, etc). Intention tremor may occur following e.g., lithium intoxication. The withdrawal tremor from alcohol or other drugs has been characterized as enhanced physiologic tremor with tremor frequencies mostly above 6 Hz. However, this has to be separated from the intention tremor of chronic alcoholism, which is most likely related to cerebellar damage following alcohol ingestion (184). This often comes with a 3-Hz stance tremor that has been assigned to anterior lobe damage due to chronic alcoholism (185). (The etiologies of toxic tremors are summarized in Table 24.1.)

A specific variant is *tardive tremor,* which is associated with long-term neuroleptic treatment (186,187). The risk factors for developing this tremor are not well-known, but many clinicians believe that female patients with essential tremor and older age have a higher risk of developing it. This tremor's frequency range is 3–5 Hz, and it is most prominently a postural tremor, but it is also present at rest and during goal-directed movements.

Treatment: The treatment for drug-induced and toxic tremors is usually to stop the medication or toxin ingestion. Treatment attempts for tardive tremor have been made with trihexyphenidyl or clozapine with some success.

TREMOR SYNDROMES IN PERIPHERAL NEUROPATHY

Several peripheral neuropathies tend to develop tremors more often than others. Dysgammaglobulinemic neuropathies and chronic Guillain-Barré syndrome are the most frequent causes, but many other neuropathies have been found to be associated with tremor (188,189) (see Table 24.1). The tremors are mostly postural and action tremors. The frequency in hand muscles can be lower than in proximal arm muscles. It it is important to note that abnormal position sense is not a necessary condition for the diagnosis. The pathophysiology of this tremor is believed to be due to the abnormal interaction of peripheral and central factors (190).

Treatment: No convincing therapies are reported for this type of tremor. Successful treatment of the neuropathy only rarely improves the tremor. In our experience, propranolol and primidone have been helpful for some patients at dosages similar to those for essential tremor. One patients was successfully implanted with DBS electrodes (191).

PSYCHOGENIC TREMOR

Psychogenic tremors have different clinical presentations. The following criteria suggest psychogenic tremor (192–197):

(i) Sudden onset of the condition and/or remissions.
(ii) Unusual clinical combinations of resting and postural/intention tremors.
(iii) Decrease of tremor amplitude during distraction.
(iv) Variation of tremor frequency during distraction or during voluntary movements of the contralateral hand with an externally paced frequency different from the tremor frequency (entrainment).
(v) Coactivation sign of psychogenic tremor. This is tested at the wrist. Variable, voluntarylike force can be felt in both directions of movement.
(vi) Somatization in the past history.

The most consistent signs for the diagnosis of psychogenic tremor are the coactivation sign, a positive entrainment maneuver, or both. These are the signs present in the vast majority of patients because only a limited number of normal motor control mechanisms exist to perform rhythmic movements. Voluntary-like movements can be detected with the entrainment test. Rhythmic clonuslike movements based on cocontraction of antagonist muscles can be detected by the coactivation sign. This may easily explain the motor control mechanisms underlying these tremors (197), but it does not allow conclusions on the underlying psychological mechanisms.

Treatment: No studies are available on treatment effects in psychogenic tremor (192). Psychotherapy is helpful only in the minority of patients. During World War I, many patients were treated successfully with hypnosis (198). Today such treatment is of only limited value. We recommend physiotherapy, aiming at a decontraction of the muscles during voluntary movements. We also administer propranolol at medium or high dosages to desensitize the muscle spindles, which is necessary to maintain the clonus mechanism in these patients.

DIFFERENTIAL DIAGNOSIS

Rhythmic Myoclonus and Cortical Tremor/Myoclonus

Rhythmic myoclonus is a syndrome that has been proposed by several authors (199) as intermittent brief muscle jerks, irregular or rhythmic, arising in the central nervous system with a low frequency (usually below 5 Hz) and topographically limited to segmental levels.

This type of hyperkinesia is not yet well defined, and the present definition is preliminary. Rhythmic myoclonus cannot be clearly distinguished from tremor (especially from myorhythmia/rubral tremor and thalamic tremor). Sometimes the driving muscle contractions are very brisk, so that there are longer pauses between individual jerks. This has been put forward as a feature for the differential diagnosis (199). The present definition does also not separate epilepsia partialis continua from rhythmic myoclonus.

Cortical tremor is considered a specific form of rhythmic myoclonus (200,201). It presents with high-frequency, irregular, tremorlike postural and action myoclonus. On electrophysiological analysis, cortical tremor shows the typical features of cortical myoclonus with a related electroencephalogram (EEG) spike preceding the EMG jerks, and often with enhanced long-loop reflexes and/or giant somatosensory evoked potentials (SEPs). This form is mostly hereditary but also has been described in corticobasal degeneration (202,203) and after focal lesions (204) or celiac disease (205).

Clonus

Clonus is a rhythmic movement, mostly around one joint (but sometimes of a whole extremity), that is elicited through the stretch reflex loop. Clonus increases in strength (or amplitude) in response to maneuvers affecting the stretch reflex (206). Clonus is only rarely misinterpreted as tremor. On clinical examination, passive stretching of the muscles increases the force of clonus but not of tremor. This is the best criterion for separating the conditions. In terms of pathophysiology, it is still debated if clonus also depends on a central oscillator or if it is only based on segmental reflex circuits.

Asterixis (Negative Myoclonus)

Asterixis is a negative myoclonus with sudden lapses of innervation. When the EMG pauses are long (>200 ms), typical flapping tremor during tonic contraction will result.

When the pauses are shorter, the clinical phenomenology can resemble a somewhat irregular high-frequency enhanced physiologic tremor.

Asterixis can occur either as a focal or a generalized condition and is usually a symptomatic movement disorder. Unilateral asterixis is often due to focal lesions of the contralateral hemisphere, and bilateral asterixis is commonly due to endocrine dysfunction, intoxication and various focal lesions (207). The diagnosis should be confirmed with polymyographic recordings from different muscles of one extremity showing synchronous pauses of innervation.

Epilepsia Partialis Continua

Epilepsia partialis continua (EPC) is a focal epilepsy that can produce (mostly low-frequency) rhythmic jerks of an extremity. Thus, it can be misinterpreted as tremor. Resting and, rarely, postural/intention tremors (e.g., Holmes tremor) can be mimicked by EPC. Lack of a history for tremor, a medical history for epilepsy and presence of EEG spikes, short EMG bursts, and jerk-locked averaging are helpful to identify this movement disorder.

PATHOPHYSIOLOGY OF TREMORS

The clinical spectrum of tremors is broad. Nevertheless, the pathophysiologic principles underlying these different entities are limited. A full description of our present knowledge of the origin of tremor is beyond the scope of this chapter (for reviews, see 54,208), but the following summarizes the basic principles.

Four different mechanisms have been proposed to produce tremor:

1. Mechanical oscillations of the extremity
2. Reflexes eliciting and maintaining oscillations
3. Central oscillators to guarantee various normal physiologic functions (Central oscillators functioning abnormally are believed to produce tremor.)
4. Tremulous central motor command because central feed-forward or feedback loops are altered

There is much evidence that one of these mechanisms is mainly responsible for a particular form of tremor. However, several of these mechanisms may play a role in the same patient at the same time (209).

The *first mechanism* is based on simple mechanical properties of any mass–spring system: A mass (extremity) coupled with a spring of a certain stiffness (joint and muscles) will oscillate after mechanical perturbation. Thus, the hand or arm held against gravity will oscillate with a resonance frequency that can be demonstrated with lightweight accelerometers. The resonance frequency differs for different joints, mainly due to the different mass of the oscillating mechanical parts: fingers, approximately 20 Hz; hand, 7–9 Hz; forearm, 3–4 Hz; shoulder, 1–2.5 Hz (53). Several factors have been identified as mediating the initial pertubations of this passive system. These include cardioballistic oscillations of the extremities, unsteadiness of any postural innervation, and unfused contractions of single motor units that cause a rhythmic modulation of the muscle force. These unfused contractions of the motor units cause, by themselves, a rhythmic activation of the muscle–tendon system that is subsequently synchronized to the resonance frequency. In technical terms, the extremity is behaving like a damped oscillator. The resonance frequency can be determined when the frequency of postural tremor is measured with a sensitive accelerometer. This becomes more evident if the resonance frequency is reduced by loading the extremity.

The *second mechanism* is reflex activation of tremor. The basic idea is that the oscillation of a limb will activate muscle receptors that elicit several afferent volleys. These volleys will evoke stretch reflexes that activate the muscles through homonymous and heteronymous pathways. If this reflex burst is appropriately timed, it can represent the next burst of muscle activity of a tremor rhythm. This will subsequently elicit the next afferent volley and thereby produce ongoing tremor. Such a reflex mechanism can be enhanced by two mechanisms: (a) by synchronizing or increasing the afferent volley, thus producing a stronger reflex response or (b) by increasing the reflex gain. In fact, such mechanisms are likely to occur in humans. For example, adrenaline or thyroid hormones sensitize the muscle spindles leading to a more synchronized and stronger afferent volley, thereby increasing tremor amplitude.

The *third mechanism* producing tremor involves a central oscillator. Specific cell populations within the central nervous system have the capacity to fire repetitively due to special properties of their membrane potential (210). For example, cell groups in the thalamus can fire in the "relay mode," i.e., they show normal spatial and temporal summation of the membrane potential, including spikes, as long as they get inputs from other sources. Under certain circumstances, however, they can fire in an "oscillating mode," which is characterized by specific changes of the membrane conductance for calcium. Cells of the inferior olive show continuous spontaneous activity based on this mechanism. Oscillations of single cells within the CNS are not sufficient to produce a visible tremor in the periphery, but if several cells are synchronized, a strong synchronized volley can reach the motoneuronal pool and produce muscle tremor. One mechanism synchronizing the activity of a cell group is electrotonic coupling through gap junctions between different cells, which has been demonstrated for the inferior olive. If this coupling is strong, rhythmic activation of one cell will activate other cells, but there are a number of other ways in which oscillations can build up in the CNS (211). In the pathological state, different mechanisms may act together to lock large cell groups in the tremor rhythm. From magnetoencephalography (MEG)/ EEG and deep-brain recordings in humans, it has become clear that central tremor rhythms are represented in deep-brain nuclei, as well as in the cortex (212–217). Thus pathological tremors likely emerge from different reverberating and pathologically synchronized (218) subcortical loops, for which the motor cortex is the primary output station. The importance of cortical involvement for tremor transmission to the periphery is currently under debate, and subcortical outputs seem to play a role, at least intermittently (219,220).

Whether the tremor of a particular patient is due to a central or a mechanical reflex mechanisms can be assessed when comparing the frequency of the EMG synchronization when the extremity is loaded or unloaded.

As a *fourth mechanism*, it has been proposed that abnormal functioning of the cerebellum might produce tremor (221,222). This need not be due to the activation of a cerebellar oscillator, but it is more likely due to altered characteristics of feed-forward or feedback loops. Cooling or lesioning experiments have shown that deep cerebellar nuclei have to be affected to produce this type of abnormality. Meanwhile, it is well-established in animals (222,223) and humans that one of the striking abnormalities in cerebellar dysfunction is a delay of the second and third phase of the triphasic pattern of ballistic movements (223,224) or a delay of the reflexes regulating stance control (225). During goal-directed movements, this will cause the breaking movement to occur late and will, thereby, produce an overshoot and, thereby, will produce a quasirhythmic movement that is compatible with intention tremor. However, this does not exclude the existence of a separate central oscillator related to cerebellar tremor.

ELECTROPHYSIOLOGICAL TOOLS FOR DIAGNOSIS AND MONITORING OF TREMORS

Electromyography of Tremors

The diagnosis of tremors can be confirmed with electromyographic examinations. Surface electromyography is sufficient, and needle recordings are rarely necessary. Electromyography is the best method to identify those muscles and limb segments that are involved in tremor (52). The electromyographic assessment of tremors is the most reliable method in cases with primary orthostatic tremor to confirm or exclude asterixis in cases of high-frequency irregular "tremors."

Electromyography can be helpful for the diagnosis of dystonic tremor and to assess the tremor frequency for various tremors. The value of EMG exams is limited for the differential diagnosis of essential and parkinsonian tremor.

Quantitative Tremor Analysis

The analysis of the accelerogram and EMG of hand tremor with spectral analysis can be used to assess the frequency and amplitude of tremor during standardized maneuvers.

This helps to quantify both the amplitude and the frequency of tremor for documentation or objective control of treatment. It also may be used for diagnostic purposes. This procedure is well established (53). The mathematical and technical requirements are not trivial and bear some pitfalls (226). It can be assessed if the tremor of a particular patient is due to a central or a reflex mechanism by comparing the frequency of the EMG synchronization (227) when the extremity is loaded with 1000 g or unloaded (see Fig. 24.2). A special computer program has been developed for this analysis (8). The results of these tests can be interpreted in the following way:

1. *No synchronization of the EMG, despite rhythmic oscillation of the limb, is recorded with accelerometry.* The frequency of oscillation decreases when an inertial load is applied to the limb because the resonance frequency of the hand-mass system is lowered. The EMG spectrum is flat because there is no significant contribution from the stretch reflex or central oscillation at the time of tremor recording. This is characteristic of normal mechanical tremor (Fig. 24.2A).

2. *Synchronization is found in the EMG, and the frequencies of the accelerometry and the EMG both decrease and are equal.* Hence, the oscillating musculoskeletal system dictates the frequency of motor-unit entrainment through somatosensory feedback (reflexes). This is the outcome in some patients with enhanced physiologic tremor (Fig. 24.2B).

3. *In the unloaded condition, limb oscillation and EMG have the same or slightly different frequencies, but in the loaded condition the frequency of the accelerometric peak decreases away from the frequency of the EMG. The latter oscillation is interpreted as a central oscillation.* This is the most common outcome in patients with mild essential tremor, but identical results are obtained from some normal people with prominent 8–12-Hz tremor (Fig. 24.2C). In this situation, EMG frequencies below 8 Hz clearly are in favor of beginning essential tremor (228).

4. *The mechanical oscillation and EMG entrainment have the same frequency in the loaded and unloaded conditions.* This is a sign of definite pathologic central oscillations, and it occurs in almost all central tremors. Higher harmonics may occur, but they are of no diagnostic value (Figs. 24.2 and 24.3).

Graphic Tablet Analysis

Graphic tablets have been introduced for the analysis of writing tremor and to measure the severity of action and intention tremor (10,229). They can be used for diagnostic purposes and especially for treatment monitoring.

Long-Term Recordings of Tremor

Long-term recordings of tremor EMG have been made for one or several days. This is of special interest for the study of drug effects (230).

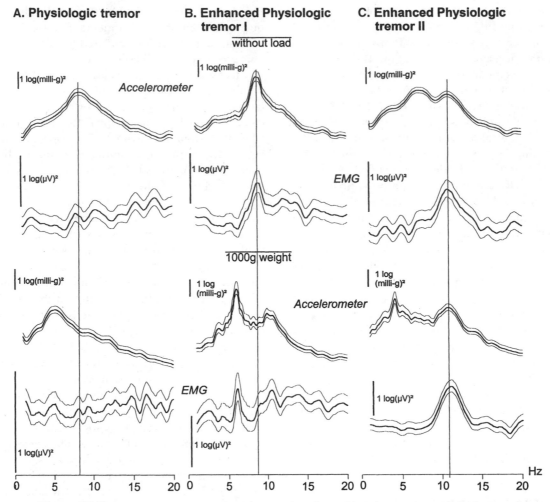

Figure 24.2 Representative examples of spectral analysis of hand tremor recordings in normal subjects. The first and third traces in each row show the spectrum of accelerometry and the second and fourth traces show the spectrum of the extensor electromyogram (EMG). The records without and with a weight of 1000 g attached to the dorsum of the hand are shown. A majority of normal subjects had no peak in the EMG, and the accelerometer peak (corresponding to the resonance frequency) has a lower frequency after loading **(A)**. For some patients the frequency of the EMG peak is decreasing with the accelerometer-peak **(B)** indicating that this portion of the tremor is due to reflex activation. In this particular paper there is an additional central component at 11 Hz. Finally, a significant portion of normal subjects has a central tremor component **(C)**. This is assumed because an EMG synchronization appears at a frequency of 11.5 Hz with corresponding peaks in the spectrum of the accelerogram. The weight-dependent resonance component shows a lower frequency after loading.

CONCLUSIONS

During the previous decade, significant advances have been achieved in tremor research and most of the tremor syndromes have been defined clinically. Still, many clinical studies today are hampered by the fact that inhomogeneous patient populations are included. Advances in the treatment of tremors also have been significant. New medications and, especially, surgical techniques, including deep-brain stimulation, allow treatment of patients who cannot be treated otherwise. The pathophysiology of tremor is still unclear for many of the conditions, and we are confident that progress in this field will improve the therapy of tremor in the near future.

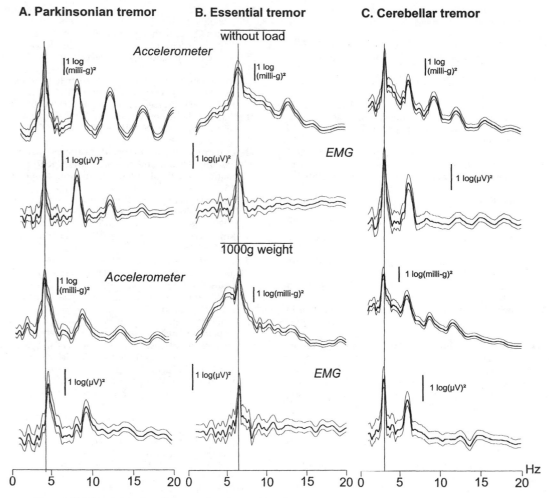

Figure 24.3 Examples of spectral analysis of hand tremor in patients. Typical parkinsonian tremor **(A)** shows a dominant frequency with several upper harmonics. Loading does not change the frequency. Similar findings can be obtained in patients with essential tremor **(B)**. Cerebellar tremor also shows mostly constant frequencies after loading. Load-independent constant frequencies in the electromyogram spectrum are interpreted to reflect a central tremor generator.

REFERENCES

1. Deuschl G, Bain P, Brin M, Adhoc-Scientific-Committee. Consensus statement of the Movement Disorder Society on Tremor. *Mov Disord* 1998;13:2–23.
2. Jankovic J, Schwartz KS, Ondo W. Re-emergent tremor of Parkinson's disease. *J Neurol Neurosurg Psychiatry* 1999;67:646–650.
3. Hallett M. Overview of human tremor physiology. *Mov Disord* 1998;13:43–48.
4. Fahn S, Tolosa E, Marin C. Clinical rating scale for tremor. In: Jankovic J, Tolosa E eds. Parkinson's Disease and Movement Disorders. Baltimore: Williams and Wilkins, 1993; 271–280.
5. Bain PG, Findley LJ, Atchison P, et al. Assessing tremor severity. *J Neurol Neurosurg Psychiatry* 1993;56:868–873.
6. Louis ED, Barnes LF, Wendt KJ, et al. Validity and test-retest reliability of a disability questionnaire for essential tremor. *Mov Disord* 2000;15:516–523.
7. Louis ED, Yousefzadeh E, Barnes LF, Yu Q, Pullman SL, Wendt KJ. Validation of a portable instrument for assessing tremor severity in epidemiologic field studies. *Mov Disord* 2000;15:95–102.
8. Lauk M, Timmer J, Lucking CH, Honerkamp J, Deuschl G. A software for recording and analysis of human tremor. *Comput Methods Programs Biomed* 1999;60:65–77.
9. Elble R, Deuschl G. Tremor. In: Brown WF, Bolton CF, Aminoff MJ, eds. *Neuromuscular Function and Disease, II.* Philadelphia: W.B. Saunders Comp., 2002;1759–1780.
10. Elble RJ, Sinha R, Higgins C. Quantification of tremor with a digitizing tablet. *J Neurosci Methods* 1990;32:193–198.
11. Pullman SL. Spiral analysis: a new technique for measuring tremor with a digitizing tablet. *Mov Disord* 1998;13:85–89.

12. Marsden CD. Origins of normal and pathologic tremor. In: Findley LJ, Capildeo R, eds. *Movement Disorders: Tremor.* London: Macmillan Press, 1984;37–84.

13. Schnitzler A, Gross J, Timmermann L. Synchronised oscillations of the human sensorimotor cortex. *Acta Neurobiol Exp* 2000;60: 271–287.

14. Deuschl G, Bergman H. Pathophysiology of nonparkinsonian tremors. *Mov Disord* 2002;17:S41–48.

15. Marsden CD, Gimlette TM, McAllister RG, Owen DA, Miller TN. Effect of beta-adrenergic blockade on finger tremor and Achilles reflex time in anxious and thyrotoxic patients. *Acta Endocrinol (Copenh)* 1968;57:353–362.

16. Raethjen J, Lemke MR, Lindemann M, Wenzelburger R, Krack P, Deuschl G. Amitriptyline enhances the central component of physiological tremor. *J Neurol Neurosurg Psychiatry* 2001;70: 78–82.

17. Karas BJ, Wilder BJ, Hammond EJ, Bauman AW. Treatment of valproate tremors. *Neurology* 1983;33:1380–1382.

18. Perucca E. Pharmacological and therapeutic properties of valproate: a summary after 35 years of clinical experience. *CNS Drugs* 2002;16:695–714.

19. Feely J, Peden N. Use of beta-adrenoceptor blocking drugs in hyperthyroidism. *Drugs* 1984;27:425–446.

20. Gelenberg AJ, Jefferson JW. Lithium tremor. *J Clin Psychiatry* 1995;56:283–287.

21. Metzer WS, Paige SR, Newton JE. Inefficacy of propranolol in attenuation of drug-induced parkinsonian tremor. *Mov Disord* 1993;8:43–46.

22. Louis ED, Ottman R. How familial is familial tremor? The genetic epidemiology of essential tremor. *Neurology* 1996;46:1200–1205.

23. Louis ED, Marder K, Cote L, et al. Differences in the prevalence of essential tremor among elderly African Americans, whites, and Hispanics in northern Manhattan, NY. *Arch Neurol* 1995;52: 1201–1205.

24. Tanner CM, Goldman SM, Lyons KE, et al. Essential tremor in twins: an assessment of genetic vs. environmental determinants of etiology. *Neurology* 2001;57:1389–1391.

25. Lorenz D, Frederiksen H, Moises H, Kopper F, Deuschl G, Christensen K. High concordance for essential tremor in monozygotic twins of old age. *Neurology* 2004;62:208–211.

26. Higgins JJ, Pho LT, Nee LE. A gene (ETM) for essential tremor maps to chromosome 2p22-p25. *Mov Disord* 1997;12: 859–864.

27. Gulcher JR, Jonsson P, Kong A, et al. Mapping of a familial essential tremor gene, FET1, to chromosome 3q13. *Nat Genet* 1997;17: 84–87.

28. Farrer M, Gwinn-Hardy K, Muenter M, et al. A chromosome 4p haplotype segregating with Parkinson's disease and postural tremor. *Hum Mol Genet* 1999;8:81–85.

29. Higgins JJ, Lombardi RQ, Pucilowska J, Jankovic J, Tan EK, Rooney JP. A variant in the HS1-BP3 gene is associated with familial essential tremor. *Neurology* 2005;64:417–421.

30. Deng H, Le WD, Guo Y, Huang MS, Xie WJ, Jankovic J. Extended study of A265G variant of HS1BP3 in essential tremor and Parkinson's disease. *Neurology* 2005;65:651–652.

31. Jeanneteau F, Funalot B, Jankovic J, et al. A functional variant of the D3 dopamine receptor is associated with risk and age-at-onset of essential tremor. *PNAS* 2006;103: 10753–10758.

32. Louis ED, Jurewicz EC, Applegate L, et al. Association between essential tremor and blood lead concentration. *Environ Health Perspect* 2003;111:1707–1711.

33. Louis ED, Zheng W, Jurewicz EC, et al. Elevation of blood beta-carboline alkaloids in essential tremor. *Neurology* 2002;59: 1940–1944.

34. Lou JS, Jankovic J. Essential tremor: clinical correlates in 350 patients. *Neurology* 1991;41:234–238.

35. Bain PG, Findley LJ, Thompson PD, et al. A study of hereditary essential tremor. *Brain* 1994;117:805–824.

36. Koller WC, Busenbark K, Miner K. The relationship of essential tremor to other movement disorders: report on 678 patients. Essential Tremor Study Group. *Ann Neurol* 1994;35:717–23.

37. Jankovic J. Essential tremor: clinical characteristics. *Neurology* 2000;54:S21–S25.

38. Koller WC. Diagnosis and treatment of tremors. *Neurol Clin* 1984;2:499–514.

39. Cohen O, Pullman S, Jurewicz E, Watner D, Louis ED. Rest tremor in patients with essential tremor: prevalence, clinical correlates, and electrophysiologic characteristics. *Arch Neurol* 2003;60: 405–410.

40. Asenbaum S, Pirker W, Angelberger P, Bencsits G, Pruckmayer M, Brucke T. [123I]beta-CIT and SPECT in essential tremor and Parkinson's disease. *J Neural Transm* 1998;105:1213–1228.

41. Rajput A, Robinson CA, Rajput AH. Essential tremor course and disability: a clinicopathologic study of 20 cases. *Neurology* 2004;62:932–936.

42. Deuschl G, Wenzelburger R, Loffler K, Raethjen J, Stolze H. Essential tremor and cerebellar dysfunction clinical and kinematic analysis of intention tremor. *Brain* 2000;123(pt 8): 1568–1580.

43. Stolze H, Petersen G, Raethjen J, Wenzelburger R, Deuschl G. The gait disorder of advanced essential tremor. *Brain* 2001;124: 2278–2286.

44. Koller W, Cone S, Herbster G. Caffeine and tremor. *Neurology* 1987;37:169–172.

45. Louis ED, Barnes L, Albert SM, et al. Correlates of functional disability in essential tremor. *Mov Disord* 2001;16:914–920.

46. Louis ED, Jurewicz EC. Olfaction in essential tremor patients with and without isolated rest tremor. *Mov Disord* 2003;18:1387–1389.

47. Ondo WG, Sutton L, Dat Vuong K, Lai D, Jankovic J. Hearing impairment in essential tremor. *Neurology* 2003;61:1093–1097.

48. Helmchen C, Hagenow A, Miesner J, et al. Eye movement abnormalities in essential tremor may indicate cerebellar dysfunction. *Brain* 2003;126:1319–1332.

49. Lombardi WJ, Woolston DJ, Roberts JW, Gross RE. Cognitive deficits in patients with essential tremor. *Neurology* 2001;57: 785–790.

50. Lacritz LH, Dewey R, Jr., Giller C, Cullum CM. Cognitive functioning in individuals with "benign" essential tremor. *J Int Neuropsychol Soc* 2002;8:125–129.

51. Troster AI, Woods SP, Fields JA, et al. Neuropsychological deficits in essential tremor: an expression of cerebello-thalamo-cortical pathophysiology? *Eur J Neurol* 2002;9:143–151.

52. Chatterjee A, Jurewicz EC, Applegate LM, Louis ED. Personality in essential tremor: further evidence of non-motor manifestations of the disease. *J Neurol Neurosurg Psychiatry* 2004;75: 958–961.

53. Elble RJ, Koller WC. *Tremor.* Baltimore, London: The Johns Hopkins University Press, 1990.

54. Deuschl G, Raethjen J, Lindemann M, Krack P. The pathophysiology of tremor. *Muscle Nerve* 2001;24:716–735.

55. Pagan FL, Butman JA, Dambrosia JM, Hallett M. Evaluation of essential tremor with multi-voxel magnetic resonance spectroscopy. *Neurology* 2003;60:1344–1347.

56. Louis ED, Shungu DC, Chan S, Mao X, Jurewicz EC, Watner D. Metabolic abnormality in the cerebellum in patients with essential tremor: a proton magnetic resonance spectroscopic imaging study. *Neurosci Lett* 2002;333:17–20.

57. Benabid AL, Wallace B, Mitrofanis J, et al. Therapeutic electrical stimulation of the central nervous system. *C R Biol* 2005;328: 177–186.

58. Kralic JE, Criswell HE, Osterman JL, et al. Genetic essential tremor in gamma-aminobutyric acidA receptor alpha1 subunit knockout mice. *J Clin Invest* 2005;115:774–779.

59. Jankovic J, Noebels JL. Genetic mouse models of essential tremor: are they essential? *J Clin Invest* 2005;115:584–586.

60. Findley LJ. Essential tremor. *Br J Hosp Med* 1986;35:388, 390–392.

61. Winkler GF, Young RR. The control of essential tremor by propranolol. *Transac Am Neurol Ass* 1971;96:66–68.

62. Koller WC. Long-acting propranolol in essential tremor. *Neurology* 1985;35:108–110.

63. Meert TF. Pharmacological evaluation of alcohol withdrawal-induced inhibition of exploratory behaviour and supersensitivity to harmine-induced tremor. *Alcohol Alcohol* 1994;29: 91–102.

64. Findley LJ, Cleeves L, Calzetti S. Primidone in essential tremor of the hands and head: a double blind controlled clinical study. *J Neurol Neurosurg Psychiatry* 1985;48:911–915.

65. Lee KS, Kim JS, Kim JW, Lee WY, Jeon BS, Kim D. A multicenter randomized crossover multiple-dose comparison study of arotinolol and propranolol in essential tremor. *Parkinsonism Relat Disord* 2003;9:341–347.

66. Gironell A, Kulisevsky J, Barbanoj M, Lopez-Villegas D, Hernandez G, Pascual-Sedano B. A randomized placebo-controlled comparative trial of gabapentin and propranolol in essential tremor. *Arch Neurol* 1999;56:475–480.

67. Alusi SH, Worthington J, Glickman S, Findley LJ, Bain PG. Evaluation of three different ways of assessing tremor in multiple sclerosis. *J Neurol Neurosurg Psychiatry* 2000;68:756–760.

68. Pahwa R, Lyons K, Hubble JP, et al. Double-blind controlled trial of gabapentin in essential tremor. *Mov Disord* 1998;13:465–467.

69. Connor GS. A double-blind placebo-controlled trial of topiramate treatment for essential tremor. *Neurology* 2002;59:132–134.

70. Bushara KO, Malik T, Exconde RE. The effect of levetiracetam on essential tremor. *Neurology* 2005;64:1078–1080.

71. Sullivan KL, Hauser RA, Zesiewicz TA. Levetiracetam for the treatment of essential tremor. *Mov Disord* 2005;20:640.

72. Busenbark K, Pahwa R, Hubble J, Hopfensperger K, Koller W, Pogrebra K. Double-blind controlled study of methazolamide in the treatment of essential tremor (published erratum in *Neurology* 1993;43:1910). *Neurology* 1993;43:1045–1047.

73. Huber SJ, Paulson GW. Efficacy of alprazolam for essential tremor. *Neurology* 1988;38:241–243.

74. Biary N, Koller W. Kinetic predominant essential tremor: successful treatment with clonazepam. *Neurology* 1987;37:471–474.

75. Thompson C, Lang A, Parkes JD, Marsden CD. A double-blind trial of clonazepam in benign essential tremor. *Clin Neuropharmacol* 1984;7:83–88.

76. Brin MF, Lyons KE, Doucette J, et al. A randomized, double masked, controlled trial of botulinum toxin type A in essential hand tremor. *Neurology* 2001;56:1523–1528.

77. Koller W, Pahwa R, Busenbark K, et al. High-frequency unilateral thalamic stimulation in the treatment of essential and parkinsonian tremor. *Ann Neurol* 1997;42:292–299.

78. Limousin P, Speelman JD, Gielen F, Janssens M. Multicentre European study of thalamic stimulation in parkinsonian and essential tremor. *J Neurol Neurosurg Psychiatry* 1999;66:289–296.

79. Pahwa R, Lyons KL, Wilkinson SB, et al. Bilateral thalamic stimulation for the treatment of essential tremor. *Neurology* 1999;53:1447–1450.

80. Schuurman PR, Bosch DA, Bossuyt PM, et al. A comparison of continuous thalamic stimulation and thalamotomy for suppression of severe tremor (see comments). *N Engl J Med* 2000;342:461–468.

81. Massey EW, Paulson GW. Essential vocal tremor: clinical characteristics and response to therapy. *South Med J* 1985;78:316–317.

82. Calzetti S, Sasso E, Negrotti A, Baratti M, Fava R. Effect of propranolol in head tremor: quantitative study following single-dose and sustained drug administration. *Clin Neuropharmacol* 1992;15:470–476.

83. Pahwa R, Busenbark K, Swanson HE, et al. Botulinum toxin treatment of essential head tremor. *Neurology* 1995;45:822–824.

84. Pollak P, Benabid AL, Krack P, Limousin P, Benazzouz A. Deep brain stimulation. In: Jankovic J, Tolosa E, eds. Parkinson's disease and movement disorders, Baltimore: Williams & Wilkins, 1998:1085–1102.

85. Koller WC, Lyons KE, Wilkinson SB, Pahwa R. Efficacy of unilateral deep brain stimulation of the VIM nucleus of the thalamus for essential head tremor. *Mov Disord* 1999;14:847–850.

86. Ondo W, Almaguer M, Jankovic J, Simpson RK. Thalamic deep brain stimulation: comparison between unilateral and bilateral placement. *Arch Neurol* 2001;58:218–222.

87. Rothwell JC, Traub MM, Marsden CD. Primary writing tremor. *J Neurol Neurosurg Psychiatry* 1979;42:1106–1114.

88. Bain PG, Findley LJ, Britton TC, et al. Primary writing tremor. *Brain* 1995;116:203–209.

89. McDaniel KD, Cummings JL, Shain S. The "yips": a focal dystonia of golfers. *Neurology* 1989;39:192–195.

90. Sachdev P. Golfers' cramp: clinical characteristics and evidence against it being an anxiety disorder. *Mov Disord* 1992;7:326–332.

91. Turjanski N, Pirtosek Z, Quirk J, et al. Botulinum toxin in the treatment of writer's cramp. *Clin Neuropharmacol* 1996;19:314–320.

92. Ross MH, Charness ME, Sudarsky L, Logigian EL. Treatment of occupational cramp with botulinum toxin: diffusion of toxin to adjacent noninjected muscles. *Muscle Nerve* 1997;20:593–598.

93. Elble RJ, Moody C, Higgins C. Primary writing tremor: a form of focal dystonia? *Mov Disord* 1990;5:118–126.

94. Kachi T, Rothwell JC, Cowan JM, Marsden CD. Writing tremor: its relationship to benign essential tremor. *J Neurol Neurosurg Psychiatry* 1985;48:545–550.

95. Ohye C, Miyazaki M, Hirai T, Shibazaki T, Nakajima H, Nagaseki Y. Primary writing tremor treated by stereotactic selective thalamotomy. *J Neurol Neurosurg Psychiatry* 1982;45:988–997.

96. Racette BA, Dowling J, Randle J, Mink JW. Thalamic stimulation for primary writing tremor. *J Neurol* 2001;248:380–382.

97. Hachinski VC, Thomsen IV, Buch NH. The nature of primary vocal tremor. *Can J Neurol Sci* 1975;2:195–197.

98. Aminoff MJ, Dedo HH, Izdebski K. Clinical aspects of spasmodic dysphonia. *J Neurol Neurosurg Psychiatry* 1978;41:361–365.

99. Barkmeier JM, Case JL, Ludlow CL. Identification of symptoms for spasmodic dysphonia and vocal tremor: a comparison of expert and nonexpert judges. *J Commun Disord* 2001;34:21–37.

100. Koller WC, Glatt S, Biary N, Rubino FA. Essential tremor variants: effect of treatment. *Clin Neuropharmacol* 1987;10:342–350.

101. Blitzer A, Brin MF, Stewart C, Aviv JE, Fahn S. Abductor laryngeal dystonia: a series treated with botulinum toxin. *Laryngoscope* 1992;102:163–167.

102. Ludlow CL. Treatment of speech and voice disorders with botulinum toxin. *JAMA* 1990;264:2671–2675.

103. Warrick P, Dromey C, Irish JC, Durkin L, Pakiam A, Lang A. Botulinum toxin for essential tremor of the voice with multiple anatomical sites of tremor: a crossover design study of unilateral versus bilateral injection. *Laryngoscope* 2000;110:1366–1374.

104. Taha JM, Janszen MA, Favre J. Thalamic deep brain stimulation for the treatment of head, voice, and bilateral limb tremor. *J Neurosurg* 1999;91:68–72.

105. Danek A. Geniospasm: hereditary chin trembling. *Mov Disord* 1993;8:335–338.

106. Jarman PR, Wood NW, Davis MT, et al. Hereditary geniospasm: linkage to chromosome 9q13-q21 and evidence for genetic heterogenicity. *Am J Hum Genet* 1997;61:928–933.

107. Gordon K, Cadera W, Hinton G. Successful treatment of hereditary trembling chin with botulinum toxin. *J Child Neurol* 1993;8:154–156.

108. Pazzaglia P, Sabattini L, Lugaresi E. Su di un singolare disturbo della stazione eretta (osservazione di tre casi). *Riv Freniatria* 1970;96:450–457.

109. Heilman KM. Orthostatic tremor. *Arch Neurol* 1984;41:880–881.

110. Thompson PD, Rothwell JC, Day BL, et al. The physiology of orthostatic tremor. *Arch Neurol* 1986;43:584–587.

111. Deuschl G, Lücking CH, Quintern J. Orthostatischer Tremor: Klinik, Pathophysiologie und Therapie. *Z EEG EMG* 1987;18:13–19.

112. McManis PG, Sharbrough FW. Orthostatic tremor: clinical and electrophysiologic characteristics. *Muscle Nerve* 1993;16:1254–1260.

113. Gerschlager W, Munchau A, Katzenschlager R, et al. Natural history and syndromic associations of orthostatic tremor: a review of 41 patients. *Mov Disord* 2004;19:788–795.

114. Boroojerdi B, Ferbert A, Foltys H, Kosinski CM, Noth J, Schwarz M. Evidence for a non-orthostatic origin of orthostatic tremor. *J Neurol Neurosurg Psychiatry* 1999;66:284–288.

115. McAuley JH, Britton TC, Rothwell JC, Findley LJ, Marsden CD. The timing of primary orthostatic tremor bursts has a task-specific plasticity. *Brain* 2000;123:254–266.

116. Norton JA, Wood DE, Day BL. Is the spinal cord the generator of 16-Hz orthostatic tremor? *Neurology* 2004;62:632–634.

117. Katzenschlager R, Costa D, Gerschlager W, et al. [123I]-FP-CIT-SPECT demonstrates dopaminergic deficit in orthostatic tremor. *Ann Neurol* 2003;53:489–496.

118. Wills AJ, Brusa L, Wang HC, Brown P, Marsden CD. Levodopa may improve orthostatic tremor: case report and trial of treatment. *J Neurol Neurosurg Psychiatry* 1999;66:681–684.

119. Onofrj M, Thomas A, Paci C, D'Andreamatteo G. Gabapentin in orthostatic tremor: results of a double-blind crossover with placebo in four patients. *Neurology* 1998;51:880–882.

120. Evidente VG, Adler CH, Caviness JN, Gwinn KA. Effective treatment of orthostatic tremor with gabapentin. *Mov Disord* 1998;13:829–831.

121. Rodrigues JP, Edwards DJ, Walters SE, et al. Gabapentin can improve postural stability and quality of life in primary orthostatic tremor. *Mov Disord* 2005;20:865–870.

122. Jedynak CP, Bonnet AM, Agid Y. Tremor and idiopathic dystonia. *Mov Disord* 1991;6:230–236.

123. Vidailhet M, Jedynak CP, Pollak P, Agid Y. Pathology of symptomatic tremors. *Mov Disord* 1998;13:49–54.

124. Masuhr F, Wissel J, Muller J, Scholz U, Poewe W. Quantification of sensory trick impact on tremor amplitude and frequency in 60 patients with head tremor. *Mov Disord* 2000;15:960–964.

125. Marsden CD. Dystonia: the spectrum of the disease. *Res Publ Assoc Res Nerv Ment Dis* 1976;55:351–367.

126. Deuschl G. Dystonic tremor. *Rev Neurol (Paris)* 2003;159:900–905.

127. Rivest J, Marsden CD. Trunk and head tremor as isolated manifestations of dystonia. *Mov Disord* 1990;5:60–65.

128. Deuschl G. Tremor-Syndrome. In: H. C. Hopf H. Schliack eds. *Neurologie in Klinik und Praxis, II.* Stuttgart/New York: Thieme Verlag, 1992;4.53–4.73.

129. Jankovic J, Schwartz K. Botulinum toxin treatment of tremors. *Neurology* 1991;41:1185–1188.

130. Coubes P, Roubertie A, Vayssiere N, Hemm S, Echenne B. Treatment of DYT1-generalised dystonia by stimulation of the internal globus pallidus. *Lancet* 2000;355:2220–2221.

131. De Jong H. Action tremor in Parkinson's disease. *J Nerv Ment Dis* 1926;64:1,ff.

132. Findley LJ, Gresty MA, Halmagyi GM. Tremor, the cogwheel phenomenon and clonus in Parkinson's disease. *J Neurol Neurosurg Psychiatry* 1981;44:534–546.

133. Koller WC. Pharmacologic treatment of parkinsonian tremor. *Arch Neurol* 1986;43:126–127.

134. Chaudhuri KR, Buxton-Thomas M, Dhawan V, Peng R, Meilak C, Brooks DJ. Long duration asymmetrical postural tremor is likely to predict development of Parkinson's disease and not essential tremor: clinical follow up study of 13 cases. *J Neurol Neurosurg Psychiatry* 2005;76:115–117.

135. Deuschl G, Lücking CH. Tremor and electrically elicited long-latency reflexes in early stages of Parkinson's disease. In: Riederer P, ed. *Early diagnosis and preventive therapy of Parkinson's disease.* Wien, New York: Springer Verlag, 1989;103–110.

136. Koller WC, Vetere OB, Barter R. Tremors in early Parkinson's disease. *Clin Neuropharmacol* 1989;12:293–297.

137. Brooks DJ, Playford ED, Ibanez V, et al. Isolated tremor and disruption of the nigrostriatal dopaminergic system: an 18F-dopa PET study (see comments). *Neurology* 1992;42:1554–1560.

138. Chang MH, Chang TW, Lai PH, Sy CG. Resting tremor only: a variant of Parkinson's disease or of essential tremor. *J Neurol Sci* 1995;130:215–219.

139. Bergman H, Deuschl G. Pathophysiology of Parkinson's disease: from clinical neurology to basic neuroscience and back. *Mov Disord* 2002;17:S28–S40.

140. Pogarell O, Gasser T, van Hilten JJ, et al. Pramipexole in patients with Parkinson's disease and marked drug resistant tremor: a randomised, double blind, placebo controlled multicentre study. *J Neurol Neurosurg Psychiatry* 2002;72:713–720.

141. Cantello R, Riccio A, Gilli M, et al. Bornaprine vs placebo in Parkinson disease: double-blind controlled cross-over trial in 30 patients. *Ital J Neurol Sci* 1986;7:139–143.

142. Piccirilli M, D'Alessandro P, Testa A, Piccinin GL, Agostini L. Bornaprine in the treatment of parkinsonian tremor. *Riv Neurol* 1985;55:38–45.

143. Perry EK, Kilford L, Lees AJ, Burn DJ, Perry RH. Increased Alzheimer pathology in Parkinson's disease related to antimuscarinic drugs. *Ann Neurol* 2003;54:235–238.

144. Pakkenberg H, Pakkenberg B. Clozapine in the treatment of tremor. *Acta Neurol Scand* 1986;73:295–297.

145. Fischer PA, Baas H, Hefner R. Treatment of parkinsonian tremor with clozapine. *J Neural Transm* 1990;2:233–238.

146. Jansen EN. Clozapine in the treatment of tremor in Parkinson's disease. *Acta Neurol Scand* 1994;89:262–265.

147. Sturman MM, Vaillancourt DE, Metman LV, Bakay RA, Corcos DM. Effects of subthalamic nucleus stimulation and medication on resting and postural tremor in Parkinson's disease. *Brain* 2004;127(pt 9):2131–2143.

148. Krack P, Batir A, Van Blercom N, et al. Five-year follow-up of bilateral stimulation of the subthalamic nucleus in advanced Parkinson's disease. *N Engl J Med* 2003;349:1925–1934.

149. Fahn S. Cerebellar tremor: clinical aspects. In: Findley LJ, Capildeo R, eds. *Movement disorders: tremor.* London: Macmillan, 1984;355–364.

150. Hallett M, Massaquoi SG. Physiologic studies of dysmetria in patients with cerebellar deficits. *Can J Neurol Sci* 1993; 20(suppl 3):S83–S92.

151. Alusi SH, Worthington J, Glickman S, Bain PG. A study of tremor in multiple sclerosis. *Brain* 2001;124:720–730.

152. Hallett M, Ravits J, Dubinsky RM, Gillespie MM, Moinfar A. A double-blind trial of isoniazid for essential tremor and other action tremors. *Mov Disord* 1991;6:253–256.

153. Rascol A, Clanet M, Montastruc JL, Delage W, Guiraud-Chaumeil B. L-5-H-tryptophan in the cerebellar syndrome treatment. *Biomed* 1981;35:112–113.

154. Fox P, Bain PG, Glickman S, Carroll C, Zajicek J. The effect of cannabis on tremor in patients with multiple sclerosis. *Neurology* 2004;62:1105–1109.

155. Van Manen J. Stereotaxic operations in cases of hereditary and intention tremor. *Acta Neurochir (Wien)* 1974;21:49–55.

156. Wishart HA, Roberts DW, Roth RM, et al. Chronic deep brain stimulation for the treatment of tremor in multiple sclerosis: review and case reports. *J Neurol Neurosurg Psychiatry* 2003;74:1392–1397.

157. Lozano AM. VIM thalamic stimulation for tremor. *Arch Med Res* 2000;31:266–269.

158. Alusi SH, Aziz TZ, Glickman S, Jahanshahi M, Stein JF, Bain PG. Stereotactic lesional surgery for the treatment of tremor in multiple sclerosis: a prospective case-controlled study. *Brain* 2001;124:1576–1589.

159. Holmes G. On certain tremors in organic cerebral lesions. *Brain* 1904;27:327–375.

160. Masucci EF, Kurtzke JF, Saini N. Myorhythmia: a widespread movement disorder: clinicopathological correlations. *Brain* 1984;107:53–79.

161. Remy P, de Recondo A, Defer G, et al. Peduncular "rubral" tremor and dopaminergic denervation: a PET study (see comments). *Neurology* 1995;45:472–477.

162. Krack P, Deuschl G, Kaps M, Warnke P, Schneider S, Traupe H. Delayed onset of "rubral tremor" 23 years after brainstem trauma. *Mov Disord* 1994;9:240–242.

163. Deuschl G, Wilms H, Krack P, Wurker M, Heiss WD. Function of the cerebellum in Parkinsonian rest tremor and Holmes' tremor. *Ann Neurol* 1999;46:126–128.

164. Miwa H, Hatori K, Kondo T, Imai H, Mizuno Y. Thalamic tremor: case reports and implications of the tremor-generating mechanism. *Neurology* 1996;46:75–79.

165. Lehericy S, Grand S, Pollak P, et al. Clinical characteristics and topography of lesions in movement disorders due to thalamic lesions. *Neurology* 2001;57:1055–1066.

166. Kim JS. Delayed onset mixed involuntary movements after thalamic stroke: clinical, radiological and pathophysiological findings. *Brain* 2001;124:299–309.

167. Nikkhah G, Prokop T, Hellwig B, Lucking CH, Ostertag CB. Deep brain stimulation of the nucleus ventralis intermedius for Holmes (rubral) tremor and associated dystonia caused by upper brainstem lesions: report of two cases. *J Neurosurg* 2004;100:1079–1083.

168. Lapresle J. Rhythmic palatal myoclonus and the dentato-olivary pathway. *J Neurol* 1979;220:223–230.

169. Deuschl G, Mischke G, Schenck E, Schulte-Mönting J, Lücking CH. Symptomatic and essential rhythmic palatal myoclonus. *Brain* 1990;113:1645–1672.

170. Deuschl G, Toro C, Valls SJ, Zeffiro T, Zee DS, Hallett M. Symptomatic and essential palatal tremor. 1. Clinical, physiological and MRI analysis. *Brain* 1994;117:775–788.

171. Samuel M, Torun N, Tuite PJ, Sharpe JA, Lang AE. Progressive ataxia and palatal tremor (PAPT): clinical and MRI assessment with review of palatal tremors. *Brain* 2004;127:1252–1268.
172. Lapresle J. Palatal myoclonus. Adv Neurol 1986;43:265–273.
173. Repka MX, Savino PJ, Reinecke RD. Treatment of acquired nystagmus with botulinum neurotoxin A. *Arch Ophthalmol* 1994;112:1320–1324.
174. Leigh RJ, Averbuch HL, Tomsak RL, Remler BF, Yaniglos SS, Dell'Osso LF. Treatment of abnormal eye movements that impair vision: strategies based on current concepts of physiology and pharmacology. *Ann Neurol* 1994;36:129–141.
175. Bakheit AM, Behan PO. Palatal myoclonus successfully treated with clonazepam (letter) (see comments). *J Neurol Neurosurg Psychiatry* 1990;53:806.
176. Jabbari B, Scherokman B, Gunderson CH, Rosenberg ML, Miller J. Treatment of movement disorders with trihexyphenidyl. *Mov Disord* 1989;4:202–212.
177. Borggreve F, Hageman G. A case of idiopathic palatal myoclonus: treatment with sodium valproate. *Eur Neurol* 1991;31:403–404.
178. Cakmur R, Idiman E, Idiman F, Baklan B, Ozkiziltan S. Essential palatal tremor successfully treated with flunarizine. *Eur Neurol* 1997;38:133–134.
179. Scott BL, Evans RW, Jankovic J. Treatment of palatal myoclonus with sumatriptan. *Mov Disord* 1996;11:748–751.
180. Jankovic J, Scott BL, Evans RW. Treatment of palatal myoclonus with sumatriptan. *Mov Disord* 1997;12:818.
181. Gambardella A, Quattrone A. Treatment of palatal myoclonus with sumatriptan (letter). *Mov Disord* 1998;13:195.
182. Pakiam AS, Lang AE. Essential palatal tremor: evidence of heterogeneity based on clinical features and response to sumatriptan. *Mov Disord* 1999;14:179–180.
183. Deuschl G, Lohle E, Heinen F, Lücking C. Ear click in palatal tremor: its origin and treatment with botulinum toxin. *Neurology* 1991;41:1677–1679.
184. Lefebre-D'Amour M, Shahani BT, Young RR. Tremor in alcoholic patients. *Prog Clin Neurophisiol* 1978;5:160–164.
185. Diener HC, Dichgans J. Pathophysiology of cerebellar ataxia. *Mov Disord* 1992;7:95–109.
186. Stacy M, Jankovic J. Tardive tremor. *Mov Disord* 1992;7:53–57.
187. Ebersbach G, Tracik F, Wissel J, Poewe W. Tardive jaw tremor. *Mov Disord* 1997;12:460–462.
188. Smith IS. The natural history of chronic demyelinating neuropathy associated with benign IgM paraproteinaemia. A clinical and neurophysiological study. *Brain* 1994;117:949–957.
189. Ghosh A, Young AC. Early tremor seen in IgG-paraproteinaemic neuropathy. *J Neurol* 2001;248:225–226.
190. Bain PG, Britton TC, Jenkins IH, et al. Tremor associated with benign IgM paraproteinaemic neuropathy. *Brain* 1996;119:789–799.
191. Ruzicka E, Jech R, Zarubova K, Roth J, Urgosik D. VIM thalamic stimulation for tremor in a patient with IgM paraproteinaemic demyelinating neuropathy. *Mov Disord* 2003;18:1192–1195.
192. Koller W, Lang A, Vetere OB, et al. Psychogenic tremors. *Neurology* 1989;39:1094–1099.
193. Deuschl G, Koster B, Lucking CH, Scheidt C. Diagnostic and pathophysiological aspects of psychogenic tremors. *Mov Disord* 1998;13:294–302.
194. Kim YJ, Pakiam AS, Lang AE. Historical and clinical features of psychogenic tremor: a review of 70 cases. *Can J Neurol Sci* 1999;26:190–195.
195. McAuley J, Rothwell J. Identification of psychogenic, dystonic, and other organic tremors by a coherence entrainment test. *Mov Disord* 2004;19:253–267.
196. Zeuner KE, Shoge RO, Goldstein SR, Dambrosia JM, Hallett M. Accelerometry to distinguish psychogenic from essential or parkinsonian tremor. *Neurology* 2003;61:548–550.
197. Raethjen J, Kopper F, Govindan RB, Volkmann J, Deuschl G. Two different pathogenetic mechanisms in psychogenic tremor. *Neurology* 2004;63:812–815.
198. Kretschmer E. Die Gesetze der willkürlichen Reflexverstärkung in ihrer Bedeutung für das Hysterie- und Simulationsproblem. *Zsch ges Neurol und Psychiat* 1918;41:354–385.
199. Silfverskiöld BP. Rhythmic myoclonias including spinal myoclonus. In: Fahn S, Marsden CD, VanWoert M, eds. *Advances in neurology, 43.* New York: Raven Press, 1986:275–285.
200. Ikeda A, Kakigi R, Funai N, Neshige R, Kuroda Y, Shibasaki H. Cortical tremor: a variant of cortical reflex myoclonus. *Neurology* 1990;40:1561–1565.
201. Toro C, Pascual LA, Deuschl G, Tate E, Pranzatelli MR, Hallett M. Cortical tremor: a common manifestation of cortical myoclonus. *Neurology* 1993;43:2346–2353.
202. Chen R, Ashby P, Lang AE. Stimulus-sensitive myoclonus in akinetic-rigid syndromes. *Brain* 1992;115:1875–1888.
203. Thompson PD, Day BL, Rothwell JC, Brown P, Britton TC, Marsden CD. The myoclonus in corticobasal degeneration: evidence for two forms of cortical reflex myoclonus. *Brain* 1994;44:578–591.
204. Wang HC, Hsu WC, Brown P. Cortical tremor secondary to a frontal cortical lesion. *Mov Disord* 1999;14:370–374.
205. Fung VS, Duggins A, Morris JG, Lorentz IT. Progressive myoclonic ataxia associated with celiac disease presenting as unilateral cortical tremor and dystonia. *Mov Disord* 2000;15:732–734.
206. Jung R. Physiologische Untersuchungen über den Parkinson tremor und andere Zitterformen beim Menschen. *Zsch ges Neurol und Psychiat* 1941;173:263–332.
207. Kim JS. Involuntary movements after anterior cerebral artery territory infarction. *Stroke* 2001;32:258–261.
208. Deuschl G, Raethjen J, Baron R, Lindemann M, Wilms H, Krack P. The pathophysiology of parkinsonian tremor: a review. *J Neurol* 2000;247(suppl 5):V33–V48.
209. Young RR, Hagbarth KE. Physiological tremor enhanced by manoeuvres affecting the segmental stretch reflex. *J Neurol Neurosurg Psychiatry* 1980;43:248–256.
210. Llinas R. Rebound excitation as the physiological basis for tremor: a biophysical study of the oscillatory properties of mammalian central neurons in vitro. In: Findley LJ, Capildeo R, eds. *Movement disorders: tremor.* London: Macmillan, 1984:339–351.
211. Schnitzler A, Gross J. Normal and pathological oscillatory communication in the brain. *Nat Rev Neurosci* 2005;6:285–296.
212. Volkmann J, Joliot M, Mogilner A, et al. Central motor loop oscillations in parkinsonian resting tremor revealed by magnetoencephalography. *Neurology* 1996;46:1359–1370.
213. Hua SE, Lenz FA, Zirh TA, Reich SG, Dougherty PM. Thalamic neuronal activity correlated with essential tremor. *J Neurol Neurosurg Psychiatry.* 1998;64:273–276.
214. Hurtado JM, Gray CM, Tamas LB, Sigvardt KA. Dynamics of tremor-related oscillations in the human globus pallidus: a single case study. *Proc Natl Acad Sci USA* 1999;16:1674–1679.
215. Hellwig B, Haussler S, Lauk M, et al. Tremor-correlated cortical activity detected by electroencephalography. *Clin Neurophysiol* 2000;111:806–809.
216. Raethjen J, Lindemann M, Dumpelmann M, et al. Corticomuscular coherence in the 6–15 Hz band: is the cortex involved in the generation of physiologic tremor? *Exp Brain Res* 2002;142:32–40.
217. Timmermann L, Gross J, Dirks M, Volkmann J, Freund HJ, Schnitzler A. The cerebral oscillatory network of parkinsonian resting tremor. *Brain* 2003;126:199–212.
218. Bergman H, Feingold A, Nini A, et al. Physiological aspects of information processing in the basal ganglia of normal and parkinsonian primates. *Trends Neurosci* 1998;21:32–38.
219. Halliday DM, Conway BA, Farmer SF, Shahani U, Russell AJ, Rosenberg JR. Coherence between low-frequency activation of the motor cortex and tremor in patients with essential tremor. *Lancet* 2000;355:1149–1153.
220. Hellwig B, Haussler S, Schelter B, et al. Tremor-correlated cortical activity in essential tremor. *Lancet* 2001;357:519–523.
221. Elble RJ, Randall JE. Motor-unit activity responsible for 8- to 12-Hz component of human physiological finger tremor. *J Neurophysiol* 1976;39:370–383.
222. Flament D, Hore J. Comparison of cerebellar intention tremor under isotonic and isometric conditions. *Brain Res* 1988;439:179–186.
223. Hore J, Wild B, Diener HC. Cerebellar dysmetria at the elbow, wrist, and fingers. *J Neurophysiol* 1991;65:563–571.
224. Hallett M, Shahani BT, Young RR. EMG analysis of patients with cerebellar deficits. *J Neurol Neurosurg Psychiatry* 1975;38:1163–1169.
225. Mauritz KH, Schmitt C, Dichgans J. Delayed and enhanced long latency reflexes as the possible cause of postural tremor in late cerebellar atrophy. *Brain* 1981;104:97–116.

226. Timmer J, Lauk M, Pfleger W, Deuschl G. Cross-spectral analysis of physiological tremor and muscle activity. I. Theory and application to unsynchronized electromyogram. *Biol Cybern* 1998;78: 349–357.

227. Raethjen J, Pawlas F, Lindemann M, Wenzelburger R, Deuschl G. Determinants of physiologic tremor in a large normal population. *Clin Neurophysiol* 2000;111:1825–1837.

228. Elble RJ, Higgins C, Elble S. Electrophysiologic transition from physiologic tremor to essential tremor. *Mov Disord* 2005;25.

229. Elble RJ, Brilliant M, Leffler K, Higgins C. Quantification of essential tremor in writing and drawing. *Mov Disord* 1996;11: 70–78.

230. Spieker S, Loschmann P, Jentgens C, Boose A, Klockgether T, Dichgans J. Tremorlytic activity of budipine: a quantitative study with long-term tremor recordings. *Clin Neuropharmacol* 1995;18: 266–272.

231. Deuschl G, Koester B. Diagnose und Behandlung des Tremors. In: Conrad B, Ceballos-Baumann AO, eds. Bewegungsstörungen in der Neurologie, Stuttgart/New York: Thieme Verlag, 1996; 222–253.

232. Bain P, Brin M, Deuschl G, et al. Criteria for the diagnosis of essential tremor. *Neurology* 2000;54:S7.

233. Elble RJ. Diagnostic criteria for essential tremor and differential diagnosis. *Neurology* 2000;54:S2–S6.

Dystonic Disorders

25

Joseph Jankovic

HISTORICAL PERSPECTIVE

The primary objective of this chapter is to provide an updated review on the diagnosis, classification, etiology, and pathophysiology of dystonia. Therapeutic approaches are covered separately (see Chapter 26). One of the earliest descriptions of dystonia was provided by Gowers in 1888, who coined the term *tetanoid chorea* to describe the movement disorder in two siblings later found to have Wilson's disease (1,2) (Table 25.1). The term *dystonia musculorum deformans,* coined by Oppenheim in 1911, was criticized because fluctuating muscle tone was not necessarily characteristic of the disorder, the term *musculorum* incorrectly implied that the involuntary movement was due to a muscle disorder, and not all patients became deformed. Until recently, the term *torsion dystonia* has been used in the literature, but since *torsion* is part of the definition of dystonia, the term *torsion dystonia* seems redundant and, hence, the simple term *dystonia* is preferred.

PHENOMENOLOGY AND DIFFERENTIAL DIAGNOSIS OF DYSTONIA

Dystonia is currently defined as a neurological syndrome characterized by involuntary, sustained, patterned, and often repetitive muscle contractions of opposing muscles, causing twisting movements or abnormal postures. Traditional descriptions of dystonia emphasize that the muscle contractions are sustained and that rapid dystonic movements are often not recognized. These rapid movements resemble myoclonus, and the term *myoclonic dystonia* is sometimes applied when the movements are fast and repetitive. Myoclonic dystonia, a rapid dystonic movement,

should be differentiated from the syndrome of myoclonus-dystonia, an autosomal dominant, alcohol-responsive disorder manifested by coexisting dystonia and myoclonus, where the myoclonus occurs in body parts not necessarily affected by dystonia (3,4).

A characteristic feature of dystonia that helps to distinguish it from the other hyperkinetic movement disorders is the fact that dystonic movements, whether slow or rapid, are repetitive and patterned. The term *patterned* refers to the repeated involvement of the same group of muscles. Thus, a patient with cervical dystonia manifested by torticollis to the left tends to always have the same abnormal pattern and direction of movement (i.e., turning of the head to the left) during the course of the disease. Although additional muscles may subsequently be involved, the pattern usually remains the same. This is in contrast to chorea, which consists of brief movements that occur continuously and flow randomly from one body part to another.

Tics are brief and intermittent movements (motor tics) or sounds (vocal tics) (5). In contrast to dystonia, tics can be more easily suppressed, are usually abrupt rather than continual, and are often preceded by a subjective, compulsive urge or sensation (premonitory sensation) that is temporarily relieved after the tic has been executed. The phenomenology of tics ranges from brief, lightninglike jerks (clonic tics) to more sustained contractions (tonic or dystonic tics). Although these latter tics resemble dystonic movements, they can be differentiated easily from dystonic movements, particularly when clonic tics or other features of Tourette's syndrome are present.

The diagnosis of dystonia is often complicated by the coexistence of tremor. Two basic types of tremor can occur in patients with dystonia: postural (essential-like) and dystonic. Postural tremor in the hands, phenomenologically

TABLE 25.1

MILESTONES IN THE HISTORY OF DYSTONIA

Year	Author	Description
1887	Wood	Facial and oromandibular dystonia
1888	Gowers	Tetanoid chorea—2 siblings, later found to have Wilson's disease
1901	Destarac	Torticollis spasmodique—a 17-year-old girl with torticollis, tortipelvis, writer's cramp, foot cramps, improved by sensory tricks, exacerbated by motor activity
1903	Leszynsky	Hysterical spasms and gait
1908	Hunt	Myoclonia of the trunk, tic spasms, hystericia
1908	Schwalbe	Hereditary tonic, crampus syndrome, maladie des tics—rapid movements; recognized the familial nature of dystonia in Jewish siblings (Lewin family); used scopolamine
1911	Ziehen	Torsion neurosis—did not believe it to be hysterical; observed that "convulsive movements increased during voluntary movement" and during emotional excitement
1911	Oppenheim	Dystonia musculorum deformans and dysbasia lordotica progressive, "monkey" or "dromedary" gait, "mobile spasms," sustained posturing, spasms, fluctuating muscle tone, rapid movement resembling tremor, chorea, and athetosis
1911	Flatau and Sterling	Progressive torsion spasm—noted hereditary, repetitive pattern, jerky; Jewish patients of high intelligence; objected to the term *deformans* because not all patients become disfigured and objected to the term *musculorum* because it implied a muscle condition
1912	Fraenkel	Rapid, twisting, sustained movement, tortipelvis
1912	Wilson	Hepatolenticular degeneration—clonic or tic-like spasms, choreiform and athetoid movements
1916	Hunt	Slow, twisting or clonic, rhythmic movements
1919	Mendel	Torison dystonia—review of literature; 33 patients; "a morbid disease entity"
1920	Taylor	Dystonia lenticularis, postural (myostatic) and kinetic forms of dystonia
1926	Davidenkow	Myoclonic dystonia—rapid tic-like movements
1929	Wimmer	"Not a disease but only a syndrome"—seen in Wilson's disease, postencephalitic, perinatal brain damage
1944	Herz	Idiopathic dystonia as a disease entity—15 personal cases and 105 from the literature; "slow, long-sustained, turning movements"; alternating "myorhythmia" or "very rapid, tic-like twitchings"
1958	Cooper	Thalamotomy
1959	Zeman	Autosomal dominant
1960	Zeman et al.	Formes frustes of dystonia
1962	Denny-Brown	Fixed or relatively fixed attitude
1967	Zeman and Dyken	No specific neuropathology in dystonia brains
1976	Marsden	Blepharospasm is a form of focal dystonia
1983	Fahn	High-dose anticholinergic therapy
1983	Jankovic and Patel	Blepharospasm-oromandibular dystonia secondary to rostral brainstem-diencephalic lesion
1985	Scott et al.	Botulinum toxin for blepharospasm
1989	Ozeliue et al.	Gene for autosomal dominant dystonia linked to chromosome 9q32–34 (*DYT1*)
1989		Botulinum toxin type A approved by the U.S. Food and Drug Administration
1994	Ichinose et al.	Mutations in the GTP-cyclohydrolase 1 gene on chromosome 14q22.1–22.2 in autosomal dominant dopa-responsive dystonia
1995		Mutation in the *TH* gene on chromosome 11p15.5 causes autosomal recessive form of dopa-responsive dystonia
1996		Third International Dystonia Symposium
1997	Ozelius et al.	Dystonia gene (*DYT1*) encodes an ATP-binding protein
1999	Nygaard et al.	A gene for myoclonus-dystonia mapped to chromosome 7q21–q23
1999		Botulinum toxin type A and botulinum toxin type B approved for the management of cervical dystonia by the U.S. Food and Drug Administration
2001	Zimrich et al.	Myoclonic dystonia localized to 7q21 gene coding for ε-sarcoglycan
2005		Prospective, controlled study of GPi DBS in dystonia

identical to essential tremor (ET), is present in one-quarter of patients with cervical dystonia (6). Whether the hand tremor seen in 10%–85% of patients with cervical dystonia represents an enhanced physiologic tremor, ET, dystonic tremor, or some other form of postural tremor is unknown. Although patients referred to a movement dis-

orders clinic have disorders more severe and atypical than the general population of patients with ET-like tremor, the true prevalence of dystonia in patients with ET tremor is clearly higher than in the general population. Furthermore, a number of large families have been described in which some members have only ET while others have only dystonia and still others have the combination of dystonia and ET (7). Münchau et al. (8) studied 11 patients with classic ET and compared them to 19 patients with cervical dystonia and arm tremor. They found that the latency of second agonist burst during ballistic wrist flexion movements occurred later in ET patients than in those with arm tremor–associated cervical dystonia. Furthermore, the latter group had a greater variability in reciprocal inhibition than the ET group. Patients with normal presynaptic inhibition had onset of their arm tremor simultaneously with their cervical dystonia (mean age 40 years), whereas patients with reduced or absent presynaptic inhibition had onset at an earlier age (mean 14 years) and the interval between the onset of the tremor and of cervical dystonia was longer (mean 21 years). These findings suggest that the mechanisms of arm tremor in patients with ET and cervical dystonia are different. In some patients, head and trunk tremor (usually of slow, 2- to 5-Hz frequency) may precede the onset of dystonia and may be the initial manifestation of focal dystonia (dystonic tremor) (9). Certain task-specific (e.g., writing) tremors may actually represent forms of focal dystonia (10). Rarely, cerebellar and parkinsonian tremors can be associated with dystonia, and dystonia may be the presenting finding of Parkinson's disease (PD) or such other parkinsonian disorders as progressive supranuclear palsy (PSP) and corticobasal degeneration (11,12).

Dystonia is either a symptom of an underlying disorder or a specific disease entity (Table 25.2). When no etiologic factor can be identified, the dystonia is referred to as primary dystonia. Primary dystonia can be either sporadic or inherited and is not associated with any cognitive, pyramidal, cerebellar, or sensory abnormalities. When there is an associated neurological abnormality, such as parkinsonism, dementia, corticospinal tract signs, and other disturbances besides dystonia, the term *dystonia-plus* may be appropriate (Table 25.2).

Classification of Dystonia

Dystonia can be classified according to (a) severity, (b) clinical characteristics, (c) distribution, (d) age at onset, and (e) etiology (13) (Fig. 25.1).

Classification by Severity

Dystonic movements can occur at rest but are usually exacerbated by voluntary motor activity (action dystonia). One form of action dystonia is the task-specific focal dystonia present only during specific activity. This type of dystonia is exemplified best by writer's cramp (graphospasm) (14). Other specific activities known to induce dystonic movements or postures include holding a cup or utensils in certain positions, cutting food, typing, and other skilled actions required in certain occupations or sports, including playing musical instruments, such as piano and violin, and use of the lips, tongue, and teeth in embouchure (15,16), auctioneering (17), golfing (18), and other specific activities (19). The severity of dystonia varies from a task- or position-specific dystonia to status dystonicus and dystonic storm, causing a breakdown of the contracting muscles and a life-threatening myoglobinuria (20).

The intensity of dystonic movements can be influenced by various conditions. For example, voluntary motor activity, such as walking, running, writing, talking, and performing specific motor tasks, can intensify dystonia. Furthermore, dystonia often increases with stress and fatigue. On the other hand, dystonic movements sometimes can be relieved by rest, self-hypnosis, and various sensory tricks (geste antagonistique) or counterpressure, such as touching the chin or the occiput to help overcome torticollis (21). Using electromyography (EMG) to study muscle contractions in patients with cervical dystonia, Schramm et al. (22) proposed a two-phase model in which abnormal head posture is first normalized by counterpressure or volitional antagonisitic muscle activity and then the position is stabilized by sensory tricks. Patients with generalized dystonia, particularly involving the trunk and legs, note marked improvement when they walk backward. Rarely, dystonia improves during activity. With this so-called paradoxical dystonia, the patient actively moves the affected body part in an attempt to relive the dystonia. This voluntary movement can be mistaken for restlessness or akathisia, particularly when the dystonia affects the trunk. The type of dystonia that is most typically relieved by voluntary movement, such as speaking, is blepharospasm. Dystonic movements usually cease during sleep but may be recorded during lighter stages of sleep; however, dystonic postures may persist during all stages of sleep.

Classification by Clinical Characteristics

Although dystonic movements are usually continual, the timing and intensity of the movements can be influenced by various factors, including emotion, fatigue, relaxation, and motor activity. In some patients, dystonia fluctuates so much that it may be almost absent in the morning and become pronounced and disabling in the afternoons and evenings. This diurnal dystonia may be associated with parkinsonian features and characteristically improves dramatically with levodopa therapy—hence the term *dopa-responsive dystonia* (DRD) (23). The genetics and classification of DRD are discussed later in this chapter.

Another type of fluctuating dystonia is paroxysmal dystonia, characterized by sudden onset or an exacerbation of dystonic movements lasting seconds to hours (24; also see Chapter 34) (Table 25.3). We favor a classification for this group of disorders that is based chiefly on precipitating events, which categorizes the attacks as either nonkinesigenic or kinesigenic paroxysmal dyskinesia. In contrast to paroxysmal nonkinesigenic dystonia (PND), which occurs unpredictably without any particular precipitant, paroxysmal kinesigenic dystonia (PKD) is induced by a sudden movement. In addition, paroxysmal exertional dystonia (PED) follows prolonged physical exertion, and paroxysmal

TABLE 25.2
ETIOLOGIC CLASSIFICATION OF DYSTONIA

I. *Primary dystonia*
   A. Sporadic
   B. Inherited (all autosomal dominant)
      Classic (Oppenheim's) dystonia (common in Ashkenazi Jews, DYT1—9q34)
      Childhood- and adult-onset cranial-cervical-limb dystonia (DYT6—8p21–22)
      Adult-onset cervical and other focal dystonia (DYT—18p)

II. *Secondary dystonia (dystonia-plus syndromes)*
   A. Sporadic
      Parkinson's disease
      Progressive supranuclear palsy
      Multiple system atrophy
      Corticobasai degeneration
   B. Inherited
      1. Autosomal dominant
         Dopa-responsive dystonia (DRD) (DYT5—GTP cyclohydrolase I 14q22.1)
         Dystonia-myoclonus (11q23)
         Alternating hemiplegia of childhood
         Dystonia-ataxia (SCA types 3 and 6)
      2. Autosomal recessive
         Dopa-responsive dystonia (11p11.5)
         Tyrosine hydroxylase deficiency (chromosome –21)
         Biopterin deficiency diseases
         Aromatic amino acid decarboxylase deficiency (dopamine agonist-responsive dystonia)

III. *Heredogenerative diseases* (typically not pure dystonia)
   A. X-linked recessive
      Lubag (X-linked dystonia parkinsonism, DYT3—Xq12–Xq21)
      Pelizaeus-Merzbacher disease
      Lesch-Nyhan syndrome
      Dystonia-deafness (Xq22)
      Deafness, dystonia, retardation, blindness
   B. Autosomal dominant
      Rapid-onset dystonia-parkinsonism
      Juvenile parkinsonism-dystonia
      Huntington's disease (*IT15*–4p 16.3)
      Spinocerebellar degenerations (SCA1–SCA8)
      Dentatorubropallidoluysian atrophy
      Hereditary spastic paraplegia with dystonia
      Thalamo-olivary degeneration with Wernicke's encephalopathy
   C. Autosomal recessive
      Wilson's disease (CU-ATPase–13q14.3)
      Neurodegeneration with brain iron accumulation type 1 or pantothenate kinase–associated neurodegeneration (formerly Hallervorden-Spatz disease–20p12.3–p13)
      Hypoprebetalipoproteinemia, acanthocytosis, retinitis pigmentosa, and pallidal degeneration (HARP syndrome)
      Ataxia telangiectasia
      Associated with metabolic disorders
      1. Amino acid disorders
         Glutaric acidemia
         Methylmalonic acidemia
         Homocystinuria
         Hartnup disease
         Tyrosinosis
      2. Lipid disorders
         Metachromatic leukodystrophy

Ceroid lipofuscinosis
         Niemann-Pick type C (dystonic lipidosis, "sea blue" histiocytosis)
         Gangliosidoses G_{M1}, G_{M2} variants
         Hexosaminidase A and B deficiency
      3. Other metabolic disorders
         Biopterin deficiency diseases
         Triose phosphate isomerase deficiency
         Aromatic amino acid decarboxylase deficiency (dopamine agonist-responsive dystonia)
         Biotin-responsive basal ganglia disease
   D. Mitochondrial
      Leigh's disease
      Leber's disease
   E. Unknown inheritance
      Neuroacanthocytosis
      Rett's syndrome
      Intraneuronal inclusion disease
      Infantile bilateral striatal necrosis
      Familial basal ganglia calcifications
      Hereditary spastic paraplegia with dystonia
      Deletion of 18q

Due to a known specific cause
   Perinatal cerebral injury and kernicterus: athetoid cerebral palsy, delayed-onset dystonia
   Infection: viral encephalitis, encephalitis lethargica, Reye's syndrome; subacute sclerosing panencephalitis; Creutzfeldt-Jakob disease; HIV infection
   Other: tuberculosis, syphilis, acute infectious torticollis
   Drugs: levodopa and dopamine agonists, dopamine receptor—blocking drugs, fenfluramine, anticonvulsants, flecainide, ergots, some calcium channel blockers
   Toxins: MN, CO, CS_2, cyanide, methanol, disulfiram, 3-nitropropionic acid, wasp sting toxin
   Metabolic: hypoparathyroidism
   Paraneoplastic brainstem encephalitis
   Vitamin E deficiency
   Primary antiphospholipid syndrome
   Cerebrovascular or ischemic injury, Sjögren's syndrome
   Multiple sclerosis
   Central pontine myelinolysis
   Brainstem lesions
   Spinal cord lesions
   Syringomyelia
   Brain tumor
   Arteriovenous malformation
   Head trauma and brain surgery (thalamotomy)
   Lumbar stenosis
   Peripheral trauma (with causalgia)
   Electrical injury

IV. *Other hyperkinetic syndromes associated with dystonia*
   A. *Tic disorders with dystonic tics*
   B. *Paroxysmal dyskinesias*
      1. Paroxysmal kinesigenic dyskinesia (16p11.2–q12.1)
      2. Paroxysmal nonkinesigenic dyskinesia (2q33–35)
      3. Paroxysmal exertional dyskinesia (16p12–q12)
      4. Paroxysmal hypnogenic dyskinesia (20q13.2–13.3)

V. *Psychogenic*

VI. *Pseudodystonia*

(Continued)

TABLE 25.2
CONTINUED

Atlantoaxial subluxation	Congenital Klippel-Feil syndrome
Syringomyelia	Isaacs' syndrome
Arnold-Chiari malformation	Sandifier's syndrome
Trochlear nerve palsy	Satoyoshi's syndrome
Vestibular torticollis	Stiff-man syndrome
Posterior fossa mass	Dupuytren's contractures
Soft-tissue neck mass	Trigger digits
Congenital postural torticollis	Ventral hernia

SCA, spinocerebellar ataxia; DRD, dopa-responsive dystonia.

hypnogenic dystonia (PHD) occurs only during sleep. These paroxysmal episodes usually last only a few seconds to minutes and may be exacerbated by stress, extreme temperatures, menses, and other factors. Some paroxysmal dystonias are also associated with seizures and ataxia. The relationship between paroxysmal dystonia and epilepsy is further supported by the observation that dystonic movements can occur during certain seizures (ictal dystonia) (25) and that PKD responds well to anticonvulsant drugs (24).

In addition to the idiopathic fluctuating dystonias there are many other causes of paroxysmal or fluctuating dystonias, including seizures, multiple sclerosis, thyrotoxicosis, migraines, transient ischemic attacks, aminoacidurias, and other metabolic disorders (Table 25.2). Inherited errors of metabolism, such as aromatic amino acid decarboxylase deficiency, should be considered in patients with fluctuating (diurnal) dystonia, particularly if it starts in infancy and if accompanied by axial hypotonia, athetosis, ocular convergence spasm, oculogyric crises, and limb rigidity (26). Patients with aromatic amino acid decarboxylase deficiency fail to respond to levodopa but may obtain substantial benefit from dopamine agonists. The disorder is inherited in an autosomal recessive pattern and the gene maps to 7p12.1–p12.3 (27). Levodopa therapy, acute dystonic reactions to neuroleptics, and gastroesophageal reflux are other examples of intermittent fluctuating dystonia. Another example of intermittent paroxysmal dystonia is oculogyric crisis, characterized by a

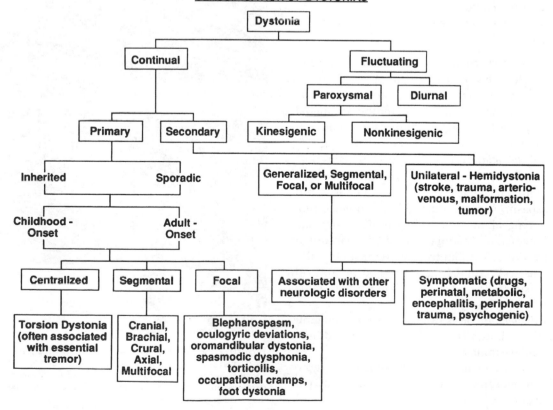

Figure 25.1 Algorithm for the classification of dystonias.

TABLE 25.3			
PAROXYSMAL DYSKINESIAS			
	PKD	**PND**	**PED**
Male/female ratio	4:1	3:2	1:2(?)
Age at onset (yr)	5–15(1–35)	<5 (0–25)	2–20
Inheritance	AD, sporadic	AD, sporadic	AD
Duration of attacks	<5 min	Minutes–hours	5–30 min
Frequency of attacks	100/d–1/mo	3/d–2/yr	1/d–1/mo
Associated features	Dystonia, chorea, epilepsy	Chorea, dystonia, ataxia	Dystonia, chorea
Asymmetry	++	+	
Ability to suppress attacks	+++	+++	
Inducing or precipitating factors	Sudden movement; startle; hyperventilation; fatigue; stress	Alcohol; caffeine; exercise; excitement	Prolonged exercise, stress, caffeine, fatigue
Medical therapy	Phenytoin; carbamazepine; barbiturates; acetazolamide	Clonazepam; oxazepam	

AD, autosomal dominant; d, day; min, minutes; mo, month; PKD, paroxysmal kinesigenic dyskinesia (dystonia); PND, paroxysmal nonkinesigenic dyskinesia (dystonia); PED, paroxysmal exertional dyskinesia dystonia).

sudden, transient, conjugate eye deviation, often seen as part of the postencephalitic parkinsonism syndrome, Tourette's syndrome, drug-induced dystonia, or tardive dyskinesia (28). There are many other causes of paroxysmal dystonias, and these should be pursued particularly in patients with atypical features (29).

Classification by Distribution

Dystonia may be classified according to distribution into one of five categories:

1. *Focal dystonia* affects a single body part and is exemplified by cervical dystonia (torticollis); occupational cramp (e.g., writer's cramp); foot dystonia; oculogyric deviations; blepharospasm; oromandibular, lingual, pharyngeal, and laryngeal dystonia (spasmodic dysphonia); and some forms of bruxism and trismus.
2. *Segmental dystonia* affects one or more contiguous body parts. Examples of segmental dystonia include craniocervical dystonia, characterized by the combination of blepharospasm, facial–oromandibular, lingual, pharyngeal, laryngeal, and cervical dystonia. Other categories of segmental dystonia include brachial (one or both arms with or without the involvement of axial or cranial muscles), crural (one leg plus trunk or both legs), and axial (neck and trunk with or without cranial muscles).
3. *Multifocal dystonia* involves two or more noncontiguous body parts (such as a combination of oromandibular dystonia and dystonia of a leg).
4. *Generalized dystonia* consists of segmental crural dystonia and dystonia in at least one additional body part (Figs. 25.2 and 25.3).

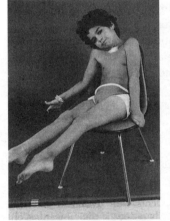
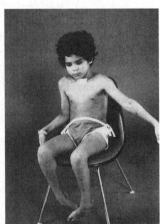
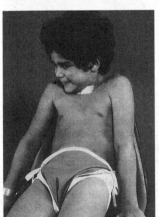
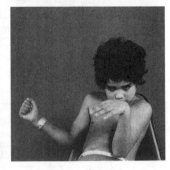

Figure 25.2 An 8-year-old boy with severe inherited generalized dystonia causing myoglobinuria. Tracheostomy was performed because he required prolonged paralysis with curare to prevent further rhabdomyolysis. (Photo courtesy of Joseph Jankovic and Penn, 1982.)

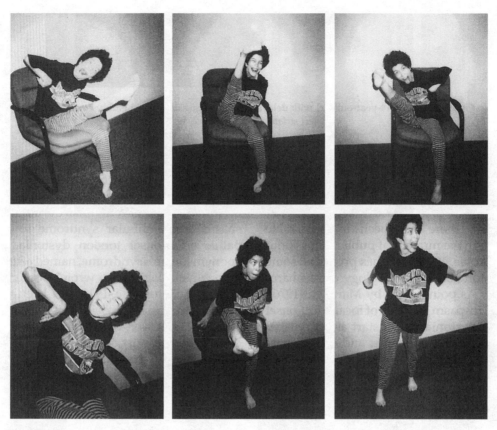

Figure 25.3 A 33-year-old woman with severe, generalized primary dystonia, progressive since age 4.

5. *Hemidystonia* (unilateral dystonia) involves only half of the body and is usually associated with a structural lesion in the contralateral basal ganglia, particularly the putamen (Figs. 25.4 and 25.5).

Based on a combined series of about 8,000 patients with dystonia evaluated at the Movement Disorders Clinic at Baylor College of Medicine (Houston) and New York-Presbyterian Medical Center (New York) about two-thirds of patients have focal dystonia, one-fourth have segmental dystonia, and one-fourth have either generalized hemidystonia or multifocal dystonia. Cervical dystonia represents about one-half of all patients, cranial dystonia (blepharospasm and oromandibular dystonia) one-fourth, and laryngeal or limb dystonia one-fourth. However, this distribution may not be typical for the general population of dystonic individuals because, by virtue of referral to a specialty clinic, this population is biased toward more severe and atypical cases. It is likely, for example, that dystonic writer's cramp is much more common in the general population than is indicated by these figures. Several rating scales, including the Toronto Western Spasmodic Torticollis Scale (TWSTRS) (30,31), Barry-Albright Dystonia (BAD) Scale (32), Burke-Fahn-Marsden Scale (33), Unified Dystonia Rating Scale (UDRS),

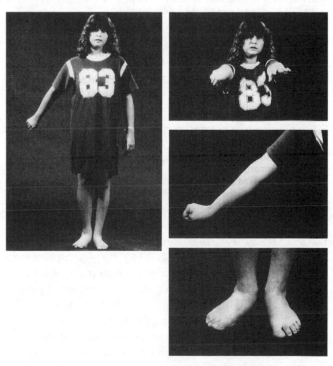

Figure 25.4 A 14-year-old girl with delayed-onset progressive right hemidystonia due to left striatal injury at age 2.

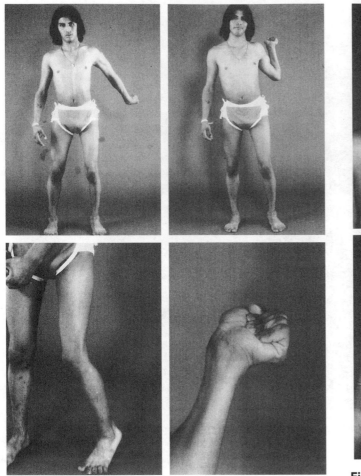

Figure 25.5 Dystonic abduction and extension of the left arm and flexion of the left hand associated with left hemidystonia due to right putamenal postencephalitic lesion.

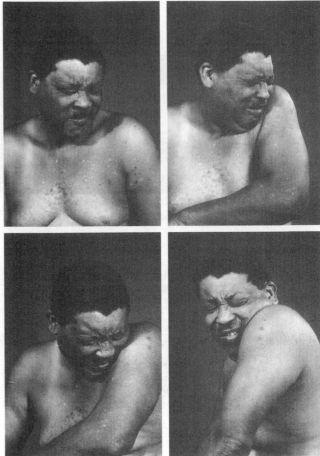

Figure 25.6 Patient with craniocervical dystonia showing blepharospasm, oromandibular dystonia, torticollis, and left shoulder shrug.

Jankovic Blepharospasm Rating Scale (34), Blepharospasm Disability Scale (35), Cranial Dystonia Questionnaire (36) are currently used to assess the severity of dystonia.

Cranial Dystonia

Since craniocervical structures are most frequently affected by dystonia, the characteristic clinical features of craniocervical dystonia will be emphasized. Blepharospasm, an involuntary bilateral eye closure produced by spasmodic contractions of the entire (pretarsal, preseptal, and periorbital) orbicularis oculi muscles, is often accompanied by dystonic movements of the eyebrows and of the paranasal, facial, masticatory, labial, lingual, oral, pharyngeal, laryngeal, and cervical muscles (Fig. 25.6). Blepharospasm usually affects women (3:1 in comparison to men) older than 50 years (37). Blepharospasm is often exacerbated by exposure to bright light, wind, and air pollution, as well as by movement and stress. Although some patients with blepharospasm may seem somewhat anxious and talkative, there is no evidence that blepharospasm is associated with any overt psychopathology (38). When it occurs only in response to certain stimuli, such as sudden visual threat or

auditory or tactile stimuli, the term *reflex blepharospasm* is used. Reflex blepharospasm is also seen in premature infants and patients with various parkinsonian syndromes, nondominant temporoparietal lobe lesions (Fisher's sign), and a variety of ocular disorders, including blepharitis, conjunctivitis, iritis, and dry-eye syndrome. Eventually patients have difficulty reading, watching television, driving, and performing other daily activities that depend on normal vision. Various "tricks," such as pulling on an upper eyelid, pinching the neck, talking, humming, or singing, can transiently relieve the involuntary eye closure in some patients. Because of the fluctuating symptoms, exacerbation by emotional stimuli, and frequent association with logorrhea, anxiety, and depression, there is a tendency to label blepharospasm as a psychogenic problem.

A form of focal adult-onset torsion dystonia, blepharospasm can start as an isolated movement of the eyelids. If blepharospasm occurs alone, without the involvement of other craniocervical structures, then the term *essential blepharospasm* might be appropriate. However, in the vast majority of blepharospasm patients, the other facial, pharyngeal, or cervical muscles are also involved, and the term *craniocervical dystonia* best describes the condition. The eponym Meige syndrome, named after the French neurologist who wrote about craniocervical dystonia in 1910, has been used in the literature to describe this movement disorder. However, Horatio Wood, a Philadelphia neurologist, described facial and oromandibular dystonias in 1887, 23 years before Meige. Therefore, the generic term *craniocervical dystonia* is more appropriate for this disorder.

In addition to dystonia, other conditions can lead to closure of the eyelids, such as ptosis due to weakness or paralysis of the levator palpebrae muscle or the smooth muscle of Müller. Some patients are unable to open their eyes because they cannot "activate" the levator palpebrae muscles. This is analogous to the motor blocks or the freezing phenomenon experienced by some, and the terms *apraxia of eyelid opening* and *eyelid freezing* have been used to describe this disorder. Apraxia of eyelid opening may occur in isolation without any other motor deficits, or it may be combined with blepharospasm or associated with parkinsonian disorders. The inability to open one's eyes has been attributed to absence of contraction or even inhibition of the levator palpebrae (despite compensatory frontalis contraction), but others have argued that this sign was caused by isolated contraction of the pretarsal orbicularis oculi. In some cases electromyographic (EMG) recording from the levator palpebrae and orbicularis oculi muscles is required to differentiate this persistent pretarsal orbicularis oculi contraction from the levator inhibition.

Oromandibular dystonia may cause jaw closure with trismus and bruxism, or involuntary jaw opening or deviation, interfering with speaking and chewing and often causing severe pain or discomfort due to secondary temporomandibular joint syndrome (39–41) (Fig. 25.7). Many patients have noted that various maneuvers (sensory tricks) and dental prosthetic devices relieve their jaw spasms,

particularly jaw closure dystonia (42). Oromandibular dystonia may follow jaw injury or surgery and may be complicated by secondary dental wear and temporomandibular joint syndrome (43). Besides primary or peripherally induced dystonia, oromandibular dystonia may be associated with or secondary to a variety of neurodegenerative disorders, such as neuroacanthocytosis (44), Huntington's disease (44), and brainstem lesions (45). Oromandibular dystonia should be differentiated from hemifacial or hemimasticatory spasm, tetany, tetanus, trismus, and mechanical disorder of the jaw or the temporomandibular joint (40,46).

Blepharospasm is usually idiopathic, but many cases are associated with lesions in the rostral brainstem or the basal ganglia (47). A variety of lesions in this area, including stroke, multiple sclerosis, encephalitis, thalamotomy, hydrocephalus, and autoimmune and other disorders can produce craniocervical dystonia. An abnormal excitatory drive from the basal ganglia to the facial and other motor brainstem nuclei has been proposed as a mechanism of the blepharospasm seen after lesions in the midbrain–diencephalic area (48). Some support for this hypothesis is provided by neurophysiologic studies demonstrating increased amplitude and duration of the R1 and R2 blink response and increased duration of the corneal reflex in blepharospasm patients. In addition, acoustic reflex abnormalities have been found in 87% of patients with craniocervical dystonia (49).

As in other forms of dystonia, genetic factors might also be important in craniocervical dystonia. Besides idiopathic or familial forms, some patients with craniocervical dystonia have secondary dystonias (50). These include drug-induced dystonia, such as that seen after withdrawal from dopamine-blocking agents (tardive dystonia) (51,52) or caused by levodopa and other drugs known to produce abnormal involuntary movements. Furthermore, an injury

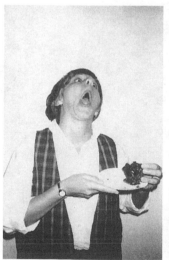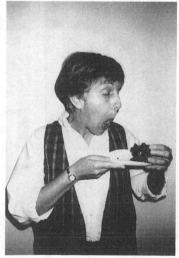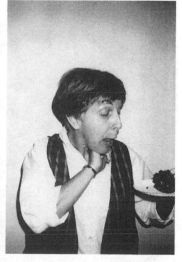

Figure 25.7 Patient with oromandibular jaw-opening dystonia that interferes with her ability to eat.

to or surgery on the eye, jaw, teeth, and other facial structures can trigger blepharospasm or oromandibular dystonia (43). A corneal lesion has been found to enhance the gain of blink reflex and as such has been proposed as an animal model for dystonic blepharospasm (53). Postmortem studies of brains of patients with craniocervical dystonia usually show no specific pathology. Some postmortem studies of brains of patients with primary adult-onset dystonia have demonstrated a significant increase in copper levels and a reduction of copper-transporting Menkes protein in the lentiform nuclei (as well as reduced Menkes mRNA copies and lower copper levels in leukocytes) compared with controls (54).

Cervical Dystonia

Cervical dystonia is the most common form of focal dystonia encountered in a movement disorders clinic (55). In addition to turning (torticollis), flexing (anterocollis), or extending (retrocollis) of the neck, the head might be shifted forward or off the midline to either side or tilted toward one shoulder (Fig. 25.8). Frequently, the shoulder is elevated and displaced anteriorly on the side toward which the chin is pointing. In 300 patients with cervical dystonia studied at Baylor College of Medicine (Houston), 61% of whom were women, the mean age was 49.7 years and the mean duration of dystonia was 7.8 years (56). Torticollis was present in 82%, laterocollis in 42%, retrocollis in 29%, and anterocollis in 25%. A majority (66%) of the patients had a combination of these abnormal postures; in addition, scoliosis was present in 39%. In addition to cervical involvement, 16% of patients had oral

dystonia, 12% mandibular dystonia, 10% hand/arm dystonia, and 10% blepharospasm.

While in some patients the head deviation produced by cervical dystonia is constant, the majority display "spasmodic" contractions of the neck muscles that cause rhythmic, jerky movements of the head in the direction of the most active muscles. These muscles can be identified readily by palpation, which reveals not only the active contractions but also hypertrophy (Fig. 25.9). However, if not performed properly, such an examination can be misleading and may fail to differentiate between the agonist and compensating antagonist muscles, both of which typically contract simultaneously in dystonia. To identify the most involved muscles, we find it helpful to instruct the patient to close his or her eyes and to allow the head to "draw" or deviate into the most comfortable position without any active volitional resistance. EMG recordings of the cervical muscles can be helpful in such an evaluation (57). Blocking the active contraction of the agonist by local injection of an anesthetic or by botulinum toxin (BTX) causes a reduction in the activity in the antagonist muscle. On the other hand, paralyzing the antagonist muscles should not alter the contraction of the agonist.

Patients with cervical dystonia have been found to have an increased risk of secondary degenerative changes of the upper cervical spine, particularly on the side ipsilateral to the head tilt (58). This cervical arthritis can contribute to the pain, limitation of head movement, and poor response to BTX and surgical therapy. Evidence of secondary cervical radiculopathy was noted in 32% of the patients at Baylor (56). One patient developed left arm paralysis due to a

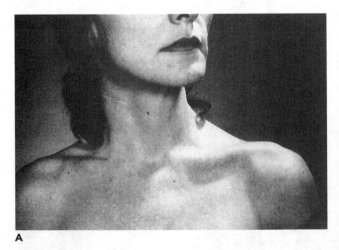

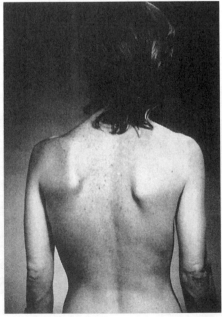

Figure 25.8 A: Patient with torticollis that persists even after right sternocleidomastoid myectomy. **B:** Same patient with torticollis showing the segmental involvement of the upper trunk and left scapula.

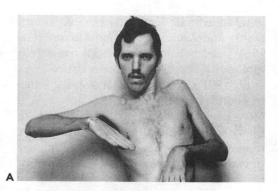
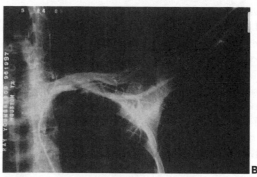

Figure 25.9 **A:** A 23-year-old schizophrenic man with tardive torticollis and a hypertrophy of the left sternocleidomastoid muscle causing marked left arm weakness and atrophy due to thoracic outlet syndrome. **B:** An arteriogram showing occlusion of the left subclavian artery, compressed by enlarged left neck muscles.

thoracic outlet syndrome produced by a hypertrophied left sternocleidomastoid muscle (Fig. 25.9). The arm weakness improved after a myotomy of the muscle. Torticollis accompanied by pain seems to have a less favorable prognosis and response to therapy than painless torticollis. Some investigators also have postulated central mechanisms for the pain associated with cervical dystonia (59). In addition to pain, some patients with cervical dystonia also have dysphagia due to delayed swallow initiation (60).

Cervical dystonia is often exacerbated during periods of stress or fatigue and is usually relieved by relaxation and various sensory maneuvers. Although some series have reported that up to 23% of patients with spasmodic torticollis achieve spontaneous and lasting remission, a remission rate of 10% is probably more accurate. Remission, if it occurs, is most frequently noted during the first 3 years after the onset of symptoms and is more likely in patients with spasmodic or "jerky" dystonia than in patients with constant neck deviation. However, in the vast majority of patients cervical dystonia is a lifelong disorder, and in about 20% of patients it progresses to segmental or generalized dystonia. Similar to other forms of dystonia, the abnormal muscle contractions that produce head deviation can be temporarily controlled by a variety of sensory tricks, such as touching the chin, face, or back of the head. In a study of 50 patients with cervical dystonia known to have at least 1 sensory trick, 54% of them had 2 to 5 tricks and 82% had a reduction of head deviation at least 30% (61). Although this observation suggests that cervical dystonia can be influenced by altering the proprioceptive input, the exact mechanism of the counterpressure, sensory trick, or geste antagoniste phenomenon is not known (21,22). In one study of patients with cervical dystonia, using H215O positron emission tomography (PET), Naumann et al. (62) found that keeping the head in primary position by application of a sensory trick decreased motor cortical activation (including the anterior part of the supplementary motor cortex) contralateral to the side to which the head tends to turn. In addition, the sensory trick

is associated with increased activation of the parietal cortex ipsilateral to the direction of dystonic head rotation.

The pathophysiologic mechanisms underlying cervical dystonia have not been elucidated. While some studies have suggested primary disturbance in the vestibular system, other studies concluded that the vestibular hyperactivity noted in some patients with cervical dystonia was secondary (63). Some investigators found that patients with torticollis seemed to relate straight ahead to the orientation of their trunks rather than their heads, thus implying faulty processing of the afferent signals from the vestibular apparatus and from proprioceptors in the neck (64). It is possible when torticollis patients utilize a sensory trick that they provide needed additional proprioceptive input to restore their head position. The repetitive head movement seen particularly in phasic cervical dystonia may result in disruption of normal vestibular input and a perception of impaired dynamic equilibrium (65). An involvement of the midbrain in the pathogenesis of cervical dystonia has been suggested by reports of torticollis secondary to midbrain lesions and posterior fossa and spinal cord tumors (66).

Similar to other forms of idiopathic dystonia, genetic mechanisms seem to have an important role in the pathogenesis of cervical dystonia. A family history of some movement disorder was present in 44% (dystonia in 20% and tremor in 32%) of the patients studied at Baylor (56), and a family history of dystonia was present in 12% of the Columbia-Presbyterian patients (67). Tardive dystonia was the cause in 6%, and 11% had onset of their dystonia after a neck trauma. Central and peripheral trauma has been implicated not only in the etiology of some cases of cervical dystonia but also in other forms of focal dystonia (68,69). In contrast to the mobile dystonic posture, seen typically in patients with primary dystonia, the posttraumatic, peripherally induced dystonia is often characterized by a fixed posture, absence of sensory tricks and activation maneuvers, focal muscle hypertrophy, and severe causalgia, sometimes referred to as *complex regional pain syndrome* (CRPS) (68).

Laryngeal Dystonia

The career of a teacher, a trial attorney, or a professional singer can be prematurely terminated with the development of laryngeal dystonia (spasmodic dysphonia). Despite growing evidence in support of neurological origin, the symptoms are attributed still too often to psychogenic causes. Dystonia of the larynx may cause excessive and uncontrolled closing of the vocal folds (adductor spasmodic dysphonia), producing effortful and strained voice interrupted by frequent breaks in phonation (voiceless pauses). The abductor form of spasmodic dysphonia is much less common, consisting of prolonged vocal fold openings producing breathy and whispering voice and phonatory pauses extending into vowels. Adductor spasmodic dysphonia is caused by hyperadduction of the thyroarytenoid vocalis complex, and the abductor form of spasmodic dysphonia is due to contractions of the posterior cricoarytenoid muscle. Whereas nearly all cases of adductor spasmodic dysphonia are thought to represent a form of focal dystonia, many cases of abductor dysphonia are thought to be of psychogenic origin. Spasmodic dysphonia often begins as a task-specific focal (laryngeal) dystonia affecting either the speaking voice or the singing voice, but the symptoms usually progress to involve both of them. Many patients with spasmodic dysphonia also have voice tremor, and in some cases isolated voice tremor precedes by several years the onset of spasmodic dysphonia. Patients with spasmodic dysphonia also may complain of difficulties breathing, and respiratory muscles may be affected in dystonia even without laryngeal involvement (70). Respiratory involvement in dystonia may be manifested by deep inspiratory gasps, loud breathing, respiratory arrests, and respiratory dysregulation.

Limb Dystonia

Idiopathic limb dystonia usually starts as an action dystonia, whereas secondary dystonia may begin as dystonia at rest. The task-specific, focal dystonia seen in many occupational cramps is the most common example of idiopathic arm dystonia. This type of focal dystonia often occurs in association with writing, typing, and feeding; during certain sports-related activities; and during the playing of musical instruments (14,15). Like cervical dystonia, the distal, focal, task-specific dystonias are often associated with either dystonic or essential-type tremor. Such dystonic tremor occurs only during a specific action, and the tremor may not be evident when arms are outstretched in front of the body or when placed in any other position.

In children, the legs are often involved as the initial site of primary generalized dystonia; however, they are affected only rarely in adult dystonic patients. When dystonia affects the foot of an adult, one should consider the possibility of PD or a parkinsonian syndrome as the cause (11). The striatal foot deformity, with unilateral equinovarus dystonic posture of the foot and extension of the big toe (sometimes confused with Babinski's sign), may be seen in as many as

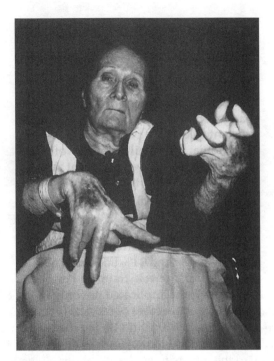

Figure 25.10 "Striatal" dystonic deformity in a woman with Parkinson's disease.

half of patients with PD. In addition to the striatal foot, some PD have a striatal hand deformity, often confused with rheumatoid arthritis (Fig. 25.10). We also have observed patients in whom foot or leg dystonia was the initial manifestation of the stiff-man syndrome, associated with positive antibodies against glutamic acid dehydrogenase (71).

Trunk Dystonia

Trunk dystonia can result in scoliosis, lordosis, kyphosis, tortipelvis, and opisthotonic posturing (Fig. 25.11). At onset, the truncal movements may be seen during walking or running, but in the advanced stages of disease the trunk deformities become fixed and present even when the patient is sitting or lying. As a result of trunk dystonia many patients have a bizarre gait, phenomenologically linked to gaits of various animals; hence the terms *dromedary-like*, *monkey-like*, and *duck-like* gait. Various sensory tricks, such as placing hands in pockets, behind the neck or back, or on the hip, might enable the patient to walk relatively normally. Also, running or walking backward or dancing might improve the truncal dystonia and dystonic gait. A study of 18 patients with adult-onset, severe, predominantly axial primary dystonia showed that, similar to the other adult-onset dystonias, this form of dystonia tends to remain focal (72).

Hemidystonia

In contrast to other types of dystonias, which are usually idiopathic, about 75% of patients with hemidystonia have computed tomography (CT) or magnetic resonance

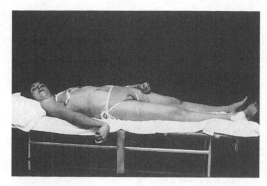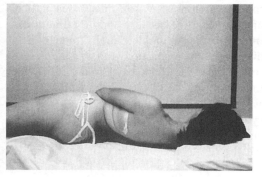

Figure 25.11 Young woman with severe generalized, predominantly trunk, tardive dystonia.

imaging (MRI) evidence of contralateral basal ganglia lesion, a history of hemiparesis, or both. Infarction or hemorrhage involving the basal ganglia, particularly the putamen, preceded onset of hemidystonia in one-third of patients; other causes included perinatal trauma, head trauma, infarction, thalamotomy, encephalitis, AIDS, neurodegenerative disorders, arteriovenous malformation, and porencephalic cyst (Fig. 25.5) (73–76). In 190 cases of hemidystonia reviewed by Chuang et al. (76), stroke, trauma, and perinatal injury were responsible for most cases. Although a relatively long delay of several years is somewhat typical for dystonia related to perinatal injury (77,78), the latency between the acute lesion and subsequent onset of dystonia is often less than 6 months in adult patients. It has been postulated that contralateral dystonia results from striatal lesions, particularly in the putamen or the striatopallidothalamic pathway (78). Because the corticospinal tract is spared for the most part, the abnormal input into the premotor cortex is expressed as dystonic movements. Rarely, hemidystonia may be associated with hemiparkinsonism and hemiatrophy (11,76,79).

Classification by Age at Onset

Whereas childhood-onset dystonias often become generalized, adult-onset dystonias tend to remain focal or segmental. In the majority of patients with childhood-onset dystonia, the disorder progresses into generalized dystonia, whereas patients with adult-onset movements only rarely manifest generalized dystonia.

Classification by Etiology

When dystonia occurs as an isolated neurologic disorder without any evidence of cognitive abnormalities, seizures, weakness, sensory or cerebellar deficit, or other movement disorders, it is classified as primary dystonia (previously referred to as idiopathic torsion dystonia). Primary dystonia can be either sporadic or inherited. The genetic forms of dystonia are discussed in another section.

Secondary dystonias, caused by a specific structural or metabolic etiologic factor, are usually associated with additional neurologic findings; therefore, the secondary dystonias are often classified as *dystonia-plus syndromes* (11,50). Whereas primary dystonia usually begins gradually as an action dystonia, secondary dystonias often begin suddenly and occur at rest from the onset (Table 25.4). Secondary dystonia may occur after a specific event such as head trauma, encephalitis, stroke, brain surgery, or exposure to certain drugs or toxins and in association with a variety of systemic and neurodegenerative disorders (50,80). Virtually all metabolic or structural lesions of the brain, particularly if they involve the putamen, other basal ganglia, the rostral brainstem, and upper cervical lesions, have been associated with dystonia (Table 25.1). In a multivariate analysis of 202 patients with adult-onset primary dystonia, the Italian Movement Disorders Study Group identified the following for the development of dystonia: head or facial trauma with loss of consciousness, family history of dystonia, family history of tremor, and local body injury and dystonia of the same body part (81). Although genetic predisposition has been suggested to play a role in some cases of secondary dystonia, the presence of the *DYT1* haplotype does not seem to contribute to secondary dystonia (82).

TABLE 25.4
SECONDARY (SYMPTOMATIC) DYSTONIA

1. Etiologic history: perinatal problems, encephalitis, head/neck trauma, peripheral injury, toxin/drug exposure
2. Sudden onset and rapid progression
3. Onset in infancy
4. Cranial onset in childhood
5. Onset in legs in adulthood
6. Abnormal neurologic findings: dementia, apraxia, seizures, ocular/visual disturbance, ataxia, weakness, amyotrophy, spasticity, areflexia, sensory deficit, parkinsonism, dysautonomia, systemic and skeletal abnormalities
7. Hemidystonia
8. Fixed posture
9. Early speech involvement
10. Evidence for psychogenic etiology
11. Abnormal brain imaging
12. Abnormal laboratory studies

Of the secondary dystonias, Wilson's disease is particularly important to recognize because early treatment can result in a complete or nearly complete abolishment of neurologic and liver problems associated with this autosomal recessive disease (83; also see Chapter 17). In one study, dystonia was found in 10 of 27 (37%) patients with Wilson's disease and was the presenting sign in 4 (15%) (83). All children and young adults with dystonia should have their serum ceruloplasmin tested and should have a slit-lamp examination. If the results are abnormal or questionable, then 24-hour urine copper excretion and a liver biopsy for morphology and copper content should be carried out.

One of the most important causes of secondary dystonia is drug-induced dystonia. The dopamine receptor–blocking drugs or neuroleptics (e.g., the major tranquilizers, metoclopramide) can cause not only an acute transient dystonic reaction but a persistent dystonic disorder (tardive dystonia) (51,84). Brain injury is another important cause of dystonia (69). In some cases, there may be a latency of several months or years from the time of the brain injury to the onset of dystonia (77,78). Among the metabolic causes of dystonia, homocystinuria has been attracting more attention, particularly because homocystinuria has been associated with dystonia and patients with primary dystonia have been found to have abnormally high levels of plasma homocystine in comparison with age- and sex-matched controls (85).

Besides central etiologic factors, which presumably account for the vast majority of dystonias, peripherally induced dystonia caused by an injury to a nerve or a nerve root, often associated with reflex sympathetic dystrophy, is being increasingly recognized as an important cause of focal and segmental dystonia (68,86), although this is still a topic of debate (87).

About 40% of all patients with dystonia have been previously misdiagnosed as having a psychogenic illness, but less than 5% have a psychogenic cause (88). The differentiation between psychogenic and neurologic dystonia represents one of the most formidable challenges facing the clinical neurologist. Because primary dystonia is not associated with any laboratory abnormalities, diagnosis of psychogenic dystonia must be based on positive criteria; it is not sufficient merely to exclude other causes. Certain clues usually provide evidence of a psychogenic etiology (Table 25.5). These include false weakness, false sensory symptoms, multiple somatizations, self-inflicted injuries, bizarre movements or pseudoseizures, obvious psychiatric illness, and other features that are incongruous with typical dystonia (89; also see Chapter 36). Relief of dystonia with psychotherapy, powerful suggestion, placebo, or physiotherapy virtually excludes a neurological cause because complete and permanent remissions are rare in organic forms of dystonia. Improvement under hypnosis or with amobarbital is not particularly helpful because both can ameliorate even neurological dystonia. On the other hand, acute exacerbation and relief of the dystonia by a powerful suggestion coupled with intravenous or oral

TABLE 25.5
PSYCHOGENIC DYSTONIA

1. Incongruous (nonpatterned) movements and postures
2. Markedly fluctuating or intermittent dystonia
3. Inconsistent weakness
4. Inconsistent sensory deficit
5. Multiple somatizations (pain)
6. Self-inflicted injuries
7. Psychiatric disturbance
8. Response to placebo and suggestions
9. Marked distractibility
10. Other abnormal movements, including bizarre gait

placebo provides important support for the diagnosis of psychogenic dystonia (90). Some patients with psychogenic dystonia undergo a variety of invasive and surgical procedures and may develop Munchausen syndrome. Using PET functional imaging, Halligan et al. (91) found that hypnotic paralysis and conversion hysteria activated the contralateral anterior cingulate and orbitofrontal cortex, which, they suggested, represented neural activity responsible for inhibiting the subject's voluntary attempt to move the limb. This may provide clues as to the psychophysiologic mechanisms of conversion or psychogenic disorders, including psychogenic dystonia. Other physiological markers, including cortical inhibition and cutaneous silent period, although abnormal when compared to healthy controls, were not different when patients with psychogenic and organic dystonia were compared, suggesting that these abnormal findings represent a consequence of rather than a cause of dystonia or that they are endophenotypic abnormalities that predispose to both types of dystonia (91a).

Genetics

Despite the variable presentation and phenotypic heterogeneity of dystonia, many families with genetic forms of dystonia have been characterized genetically, and a genetic classification of dystonia is evolving rapidly (Table 25.6). Most cases of childhood-onset dystonia are inherited, usually in an autosomal dominant pattern. The most important advance in the understanding of autosomal dystonia has been identification of a DNA marker (TOR1A, DYT1) in the q32-34 region of chromosome 9 in a large non-Jewish kindred (92). Subsequently, a 3-bp (GAG) deletion was identified in the fifth exon of the TOR1A gene in the 9q34 locus coding for a novel 332-amino-acid, ATP-binding protein (torsinA), resulting in a loss of a pair of glutamic acid residues (93). This important discovery not only enabled DNA testing for the abnormal TOR1A (DYT1) gene but launched fruitful research into the cellular mechanisms of this form of dystonia. In addition to the 3-bp GAG deletion, an 18-bp deletion that would remove 6-amino-acid residues close to the carboxy terminus of torsinA was discovered in one patient with dystonia, myoclonus, and tics (94).

TABLE 25.6
GENETIC CLASSIFICATION OF DYSTONIAS

Disease	Dystonia Type	Pattern of Inheritance	Chromosome Region	Gene Locus	Protein
Oppenheim's torsion dystonia	PTD, onset <40 yrs, 30% penetrance	AD	9q34	DYT1	TorsinA
Early-onset (unconfirmed)	PTD, Spanish gypsies	AR	Not mapped	DYT2	Not identified
Lubag's disease (X-linked dystonia-parkinsonism)	Heredo-degenerative dystonia; onset <55 yrs, Filipinos (Lubag), cranial (stridor), limb, mosaic striatal gliosis	X-linked recessive	Xq13.1	DYT3	Multiple transcript system
Whispering dystonia	PTD, Australian family	AD	Not mapped	DYT4	Not identified
Dopa-responsive dystonia	Dystonia-plus, onset <16 yrs, gait disorder, parkinsonism, spasticity, diurnal variation	AD	14q22.1	DYT5	GTP cyclohydrolase I
Cranio-cervical dystonia	PTD, onset childhood–adulthood, Mennonite/Amish, cranial (dysarthria, dysphonia), cervical, limb	AD	8p21–q22	DYT6	Not identified
Familial torticollis	PTD, cranial, cervical, spasmodic dysphonia, hand tremor	AD	18p	DYT7	Not identified
Paroxysmal dystonic choreoathetosis (nonkinesigenic) (Mount-Rebak)	Paroxysmal dystonia, choreoathetosis, onset: childhood	AD	2q33–q35	DYT8	Myofibrillogenesis regulator 1
Paroxysmal dyskinesias with spasticity	Paroxysmal dystonia, ataxia, spasticity	AD	1p21	DYT9	Not identified
Paroxysmal kinesigenic dyskinesia	Paroxysmal dystonia, choreoathetosis	AD	16p11.2–q12.1	DYT10	Not identified
Myoclonus-dystonia	Dystonia-plus, alcohol-responsive, OCD, drug addiction	AD	7q21–q23	DYT11	Epsilon-sarcoglycan
Rapid-onset dystonia-parkinsonism	Dystonia-plus, onset: adulthood, childhood	AD	19q13	DYT12	Na+/K+-ATPase alpha3
Cervical-cranial-brachial	PTD, cranial-cervical, upper limb, jerky, onset: adulthood, childhood	AD	1p36	DYT13	Not identified
Dopa-responsive dystonia	Dystonia-plus, parkinsonism, Swiss family	AD	14q13	DYT14	Not identified
Myoclonus-dystonia	Dystonia-plus, alcohol-responsive	AD	18p11	DYT15	Not identified
Wilson's disease	Dystonia, tremor, other movement disorders, liver disease	AR	13q14.3		Copper-transporting P-type ATPase (ATP7B)
Neurodegeneration with brain iron accumulation (Hallervorden-Spatz disease)	Dystonia, dementia, seizures	AR	20p12.3–p13		Pantothenate kinase (PANK2)
AA decarboxylase deficiency	Dystonia, hyppotonia, aculogyric crises, infancy	AR	7p12.1–p12.3		

AA, Amino Acid; AD, Autosomal Dominant; AR, Autosomal Recessive.

TOR1A, which encodes torsinA, is a member of a large gene family including TOR1B, TOR2A, and TOR2B. TorsinA is expressed widely in the brain, particularly in the hippocampus, substantia nigra pars compacta, and cerebellum (95,96). Although the function of torsinA is still not fully understood and its role in the pathogenesis of primary dystonia remains unknown, the protein is a 332-amino-acid member of the AAA+ (ATPases associated with a variety of cellular activities) superfamily of chaperone proteins with ATPase activity predominantly expressed in dopaminergic neurons (97). AAA+ ATPases share Mg2+-ATP binding domain, a AAA-specific region of homology, and a typical 6-membered oligomeric ring structure (98). This doughnutlike ring is situated in the lumen of the endoplasmic reticulum (ER), with each monomer tethered to the ER membrane via the N terminus. The loss of glutamic acid residue in the C terminus apparently prevents closure of the ring or prevents interaction with some partner protein. The wild-type torsinA protein is found throughout the cytoplasm and neurites with a high degree of colocalization with the ER. In contrast, the mutant protein forms multiple, large inclusions composed of ER-derived membrane whorls in cultured cells (99,100) but not in the brains of patients with *DYT1* dystonia (101). However, no alterations in torsinA immunohistochemistry, such as cytoplasmic aggregations or colocalization of torsinA with ER, have been found in brains of patients with *DYT1* dystonia (101). Furthermore, mutant torsinA has been found to colocalize with vesicular monomaine transporter 2 (VMAT2) and, therefore, may interfere with normal dopaminergic transmission (102). More recent studies suggest that torsinA accumulates in the nuclear envelope, a structure contiguous with cytoplasmic ER (103). In another study of 4 genetically confirmed *DYT1* dystonias, perinuclear inclusion bodies in the midbrain reticular formation and periaqueductal gray of the pedunculopontine nucleus, cuneiform nucleus, and griseum centrale mesencephali have been found (104). These inclusions stained positive for ubiquitin, torsinA, and the nuclear envelope protein lamin A/C. In addition, tau/ubiquitin-immunoreactive aggregates were found in the substantia nigra pars compacta and locus coeruleus. These findings support the notion that *DYT1* dystonia is associated with impaired protein handling, particularly in the brainstem nuclei, such as the pedunculopontine nucleus (105). Transgenic *TOR1A* mice have been developed with a variable phenotype including hyperkinetic circling behavior (106,107). Neurons, but not nonneuronal cell types, from both torsinA null and homozygous disease mutant "knock-in" mice contain severely abnormal nuclear membranes (108).

TorsinA has been found in Lewy bodies, the cytoplasmic inclusions typically found in patients with PD (109). It is also of interest that TorsinA has 25%–30% homology to the 100/Clp proteases family of heat-shock proteins (HSPs), which are normally responsible for protecting the cells from a variety of stresses (e.g., heat, trauma, toxins). It is, therefore,

interesting to speculate whether central or peripheral trauma somehow alters the brain's HSP and eventually leads to the expression of dystonia in an individual who otherwise would be asymptomatic (nonpenetrant) (68,110). TorsinA also shares features with ATPases that are involved in vesicle fusion, mitochondrial function, and protein translocation. Thus, current evidence suggests that the mutant torsinA interferes with the integrity of the ER, membrane trafficking, downstream regulation of vesicular release, and metabolic-energy processes of the cells (98,99). Some preliminary results in PC12 cell lines suggest that torsinA may have a neuroprotective role in making the cells more resistant to the effects of the proteasome inhibitor MG132 (217). *TOR1A* "knock-in" and "knock-down" mice have demonstrated some subtle behavioral changes manifested by increased reactivity in the open field and deficient response habituation but no dystonia; the "knock-out" mice do not survive (218).

The single GAG deletion mutation in the *TOR1A (DYT1)* gene is apparently responsible for the vast majority of typical early-onset dystonia, and it accounts for approximately 90% of such cases in the Ashkenazi Jewish population (111). The mutation was probably introduced in the Ashkenazi Jewish population about 350 years ago in Lithuania or Byelorussia (112). This population has a five- to tenfold increase in incidence of early-onset dystonia compared with a control population, and the estimated frequency of the disease in this population is 1:3,000 to 1:9,000. The *DYT1* GAG mutation may be detected even in patients with primary dystonia without family history (113). About one-third of those carrying the *DYT1* gene express it clinically (30%–40% penetrance). However, using 18F-fluorodeoxyglucose PET, Eidelberg et al. (110) found an abnormal metabolic pattern in asymptomatic carriers of the *DYT1* gene that was similar to that of symptomatic individuals, indicating that the penetrance of the *DYT1* gene is considerably greater than previously assumed.

Typically *DYT1* dystonia presents as a childhood-onset dystonia usually starting in the foot or hand and gradually progressing to generalized dystonia. However, there are many exceptions to this typical presentation; the phenotype may range from simple focal dystonia, such as writer's cramp, to cervical dystonia, to severe, life-threatening dystonia (dystonic storm) (20,114). An analysis of clinical features and genetic status of 267 patients with primary dystonia indicated that the clinical feature most highly correlated with *DYT1* GAG deletion carrier status in patients with onset of dystonia before age 26 (115). Using this age-at-onset limit, the specificity of the *DYT1* test is 63% in Ashkenazi Jews and 43% in non-Jews. In addition to testing for *DYT1* mutation in patients with primary dystonia whose age of onset is earlier than 26 years, Bressman et al. (115) recommend the use of this test in patients with onset after age 26 if there are affected relatives who exhibit dystonia at an early age.

In addition to the *DYT1* dystonia, several other genetic forms of primary torsion dystonia have been identified and designated as *DYT6*, *DYT7*, and *DYT13*. A gene locus in the 8p21–q22 region has been identified in a large German-American Mennonite family with craniocervical and limb dystonia (116). This dystonia, designated as *DYT6*, 8p21–q22, is clinically similar to *DYT1* although the involvement is more generalized and it includes the head and neck. A *DYT7* designation was assigned to the locus on chromosome 18p in a German family with adult-onset, autosomal dominant inheritance predominantly manifested by cervical dystonia and spasmodic dysphonia (117). However, subsequent studies by the same group caused some doubts about this association (118). Three patients monosomic for large parts of chromosome 18p displayed a syndrome of mental retardation, mildly dysmorphic appearance, short stature, and dystonia. Two patients showed blepharospasm, oromandibular dystonia, and cervical dystonia, whereas the third exhibited cervical dystonia, axial dystonia, arm rigidity, and dystonic posturing of the right upper extremity. Genetic analysis revealed that the common deleted area spanned a 49.6-centimorgan distance and included the *DYT7* locus. The authors note that "dystonia in these patients may be caused by haploinsufficiency of the *DYT7* gene, a new dystonia gene on 18p, or may result from developmental brain anomalies" (119). Another genetic primary torsion dystonia, designated *DYT13* and mapped to chromosome 1p36.13–36.22 in an Italian family, is manifested as craniocervical or upper limb dystonia (120). In addition to these gene abnormalities, several studies have demonstrated various polymorphisms, including the dopamine receptor D5 gene (121).

In one family with myoclonic dystonia (also referred to as myoclonus-dystonia), the gene locus was mapped to 7q21–q31 (122). The average age at onset was 6 to 8 years with action-induced myoclonus or dystonia. The myoclonus was usually not startle sensitive, but in all patients it was alcohol responsive. Symptoms tend to stabilize in adulthood, although some have developed associated psychiatric symptoms such as depression, anxiety, and obsessive–compulsive disorder. Another family with alcohol-responsive myoclonus-dystonia (122a) syndrome has been recently reported to have a Val154Ile missense mutation in the D2 dopamine receptor *(DRD2)* gene on chromosome 11q23 and has been designated *DYT11*, but this mutation was not found in 5 other families with myoclonus-dystonia syndrome (3). In contrast, positive lod scores were found in all 3 families with myoclonus-dystonia and 1 with essential myoclonus, indicating that chromosome 7q21–q31 is a major locus for myoclonus-dystonia syndrome (123). Using a positional cloning approach, Zimprich et al. (124) identified 5 different heterozygous loss-of-function mutations in the 7q21 gene for epsilon-sarcoglycan (SGCE), expressed in all brain regions examined. SGCE is 1 of 5 members of the sarcoglycan family encoding transmembrane components of trophin-glycoprotein complex, which links that cytoskeleton to the extracellular matrix. It is possible that the loss of SGCE alters the normal neuronal architecture, leading to changes in "wiring" of the normal neuronal circuitry. The 7q and 11q23 loci have been excluded in a large Canadian family with autosomal dominant dystonia-myoclonus, but a linkage to a novel 5-Mb region on chromosome 18p11 has been identified (125).

DRD, designated as *DYT5* and inherited in an autosomal dominant pattern, typically presents during early childhood (onset 1 to 12 years) with foot dystonia during walking or running; later, patients may show signs of parkinsonism. The gene for the most common form of DRD was mapped to a locus on chromosome 14 by Nygaard et al. (126) in 1993, and the following year Ichinose et al. (127) discovered 4 independent mutations in the GTP-cyclohydrolase 1 (GCH1) gene (128). GCH1 is the enzyme that catalyzes the first step in the synthesis of tetrahydrobiopterin (BH4), the natural cofactor for tyrosine hydroxylase (TH), tryptophan hydroxylase, and phenylalanine hydroxylase (128). This gene defect results in impaired synthesis of dopamine by nigral neurons without degeneration (hypomelanization without neuronal cell loss) (129). GCH1 mutation seems to have a higher penetrance in women than men, thus accounting for the female preponderance in this disorder (130). In about 40% of families, members affected with DRD do not appear to have the GCH1 mutation (131), or the mutation may lie outside the coding region (132). Furukawa et al. (133) found a large heterozygous deletion in the GCH1 gene that cannot be detected by the usual genomic DNA sequence analysis and might account for some "mutation-negative" patients with dominantly inherited DRD. Well over 100 independent mutations in the GCH1 gene producing different phenotypes have been described (128,134–136). It has been postulated that the decreased GCH1 activity in the autosomal dominant form of DRD may be due to a dominant negative effect of the mutant GCH1, thus inhibiting the expression of the wild-type protein and reducing the normal enzyme activity, which also may account for the phenotypic heterogeneity of DRD (23). As a result of this dominant-negative mechanism, a single mutation may decrease GCH1 activity to less than 50% of normal (137). Another possibility is that the decreased levels of GCH1 mRNA and protein cause inactivation of one allele of the GCH1 gene (128).

Because of the large number of GCH1 mutations, a simple DNA test as a diagnostic tool is not going to be readily available and, therefore, alternate diagnostic methods are being sought. Endogenous neopterin levels are low in unstimulated lymphoblasts, but this may not be a reliable test for all cases of DRD since GCH1 mutation may not necessarily affect GCH1 enzyme activity (138). Cerebrospinal fluid (CSF) biopterin and neopterin levels are reduced by 20% to 30% in patients with DRD due to GCH1 deficiency. A phenylalanine loading protocol has been proposed to determine if there is a defect in BH4, which is an essential cofactor not only for TH but also for phenylalanine hydroxylase (139). Patients with DRD have a significantly higher phenylalanine-to-tyrosine ratio, whereas biopterin levels are decreased at baseline and after a load of 100 mg/kg of oral phenylalanine. It is not yet clear how sensitive and specific this test is as a diagnostic tool for this form of dystonia. Furthermore, it is important to recognize that not all patients with DRD have a defect in the GCH1 gene (140).

PET studies have a limited usefulness in confirming the diagnosis of DRD, but they may be helpful in differentiating DRD from juvenile PD in that the latter shows evidence of reduced fluorodopa uptake, whereas fluorodopa uptake is usually normal in patients with DRD. Results of [^{123}I]-CIT single-photon emission computed tomography (SPECT) are also normal, indicating normal striatal dopamine transporter (DAT) (141). Interestingly, striatal D2 receptor binding is increased in symptomatic and asymptomatic carriers of the DRD gene mutation, possibly as a homeostatic response to the dopaminergic deficit.

Although diurnal variation, characterized by worsening of symptoms as the day progresses and relief after sleep, is a typical feature of DRD, such marked fluctuation is present only in one-half of patients with DRD. Because DRD patients often present with developmental motor delay, stiff gait, and marked postural instability, they often are misdiagnosed initially as having cerebral palsy or parkinsonism. Some patients with DRD, however, do have motor delay, and such patients may represent compound heterozygotes. The motor and psychiatric phenotype of DRD keeps expanding. For example, a late-onset (>30 years of age), adult form of DRD has been reported with mild dystonia, with the additional presence of depression, obsessive–compulsive behavior, sleep disorder, and other psychiatric problems (142).

Patients with DRD usually continue to respond well to relatively low doses of carbidopa/levodopa (usual dose is 1 to 3 tablets of 25/100 mg per day) without developing motor fluctuations, although some patients report a wearing-off effect, with recurrence of dystonia and parkinsonism 6 to 8 hours after the last levodopa dose (143). In 1 study of 20 patients with DRD, 20% of the patients exhibited mild levodopa-induced dyskinesia (144). In contrast to PD, the short-duration response to levodopa dosing seems to develop more slowly and persists for a longer time (145). Most patients with DRD also improve with anticholinergic drugs (146).

GCH1 mutation is occasionally present in patients who do not exhibit the typical symptoms of DRD. The clinical phenotype and spectrum of manifestations of GCH1 mutation now have been extended to include focal dystonia, intermittent dystonia, and dystonia with onset during the first week of life (140,147). However, the clinical spectrum of the DRD phenotype may include parkinsonism with levodopa-induced dyskinesia, spastic paraplegia, scoliosis (148), and absence of dystonia (135). The diagnosis is further complicated by the identification of mutations in

the *parkin* gene on chromosome 6 in some patients with otherwise typical DRD (135). In addition to the motor signs, some patients with DRD exhibit a variety of psychiatric symptoms, such as depression and anxiety, and some families also exhibit deafness (149).

Although the presentation and course of DRD are highly variable, at least 3 types of GCH1 deficiency have been proposed: (a) heterozygote manifested chiefly by limb dystonia responding to levodopa; (b) compound heterozygote manifested by limb dystonia with developmental motor delay responding to the combination of levodopa and BH4; and (c) homozygote manifested by mental retardation, developmental motor delay, limb dystonia and truncal hypotonia, elevated plasma phenylalanine, low plasma and CSF biopterin; the clinical features respond to the combination of levodopa, BH4, and 5-hydroxytryptophan (150) (Table 25.7). Studies have shown that BH4 and neopterin are markedly decreased in the brains of patients with DRD (151).

About 40% of all patients with otherwise typical DRD with diurnal variation do not have a mutation in the coding region of the GCH1 gene, and some of these patients may have an autosomal recessive form of DRD due to mutations in the TH gene on chromosome 11p15.5 (128,134,152). While in the autosomal dominant DRD the TH enzyme activity is decreased to 2% to 20% of normal, in the autosomal recessive form the activity is reduced to 30% to 40% of normal and the heterozygotes are normal. A point mutation in this gene, inherited in an autosomal recessive pattern, has resulted in 85% to 98% reduction in the activity of TH and parkinsonism/dystonia phenotype (128). Some members of the family with autosomal recessive DRD have severe dysarthria, rigidity, and progressive contractures, only partially relieved by levodopa. The autosomal recessive TH-deficient form of DRD may start in infancy or early childhood and responds completely to low doses of levodopa. In addition to dystonia, patients with autosomal recessive TH deficiency suffer from mental retardation, developmental delay, limb rigidity, truncal hypotonia, parkinsonism, and overt hyperphenylalaninemia. Furukawa et al. (153) described a 10-year-old boy, a compound heterozygote for a novel mutation in the TH gene, who had levodopa-responsive spastic paraplegia and whose father had exercise-induced stiffness.

Other dystonias resulting from inborn errors of metabolism affecting the dopamine biosynthetic pathway include dihydropteridine reductase deficiency and aromatic amino acid decarboxylase deficiency. A disorder with subacute encephalopathy, dysarthria, dysphagia, possible ophthalmoparesis, dystonia, parkinsonism, and quadriparesis responsive to biotin has been described (154). About one-half of patients with DRD have no family history, and some of these sporadic cases may represent incomplete penetrance of GCH1 mutation or independent de novo mutation (150). The penetrance of GCH1 mutation is much higher in females (87% to 100%) than in males (38% to 55%) and in young versus older individuals.

TABLE 25.7
DIFFERENTIAL DIAGNOSIS OF CHILDHOOD DYSTONIA

	Primary Dystonia	DRD	Juvenile PD
Onset	>6	<12	<20
Gender	M = F	F > M	M > F
Foot dystonia	40%–60%	100%	>50%
Arm dystonia	45%–65%	5%–75%	<10%
Axial dystonia	15%–65%	5%–50%	<5%
Bradykinesia	0	+++	++++
Rest tremor	0	+	+++
Diurnal	0	++	0
L-dopa response	0	++++	+++
Dyskinesias	0	+	+++
Pet F-dopa	NL	NL	
Beta CIT SPECT	NL	NL	
CSF biopterin	NL		
Phenylalanine test	NL	ABNL	NL
Progression	+++	0	++++

DRD, dopa-responsive dystonia; PET, positron emission tomography; SPECT, single photon emission computed tomography; PD, Parkinson's disease.

Besides DRD, dystonia may be associated with parkinsonism in the syndrome *rapid-onset dystonia-parkinsonism* (RDP) (155,156). This autosomal dominant disorder is characterized by rapid development of focal, segmental, or unilateral dystonia, often over a period of hours or days, involving primarily the cranial structures and upper limbs. It is often associated with bulbar symptoms (particularly dysarthria and dysphagia), bradykinesia, postural instability, other parkinsonian features, and depression. The progression is relatively slow, and patients respond poorly to dopaminergic therapy. PET studies suggest that there is no degeneration of dopamine nerve terminals and no loss of dopamine reuptake sites. Some members of the RDP family may involve only mild writer's cramp or subtle parkinsonism. Neuroimaging studies are usually normal, and CSF homovanillic acid levels have been reported as low. Mutations in the Na+/K+-ATPase alpha3 gene ATP1A3 were later associated with RDP (156,157).

X-linked recessive dystonia, called *Lubag's disease* and classified as DYT3, has been reported only in natives of Panay Island in the Philippines. The gene causing this form of inherited dystonia has been mapped to the pericentromeric region of the X chromosome, Xq12–Xq21 (158). Some brains of patients with this dystonia-parkinsonism syndrome have been found to have a mosaic pattern of striatal gliosis (159).

Leber's disease is another X-linked recessive disorder that has been seen in association with dystonia (160,161); a mitochondrial abnormality has been considered to be the underlying pathogenic mechanism in this disorder. Putaminal necrosis with "striatal slits" on MRI has been reported in some members of a large kindred with Leber's hereditary optic atrophy and spastic dystonia (162). Features of Leber's disease, including progressive dystonia and striatal necrosis, also have been observed in Leigh's syndrome, another mitochondrial striatopallidal disease with yet undetermined genetic defect (163). Another X-linked dystonia, linked to Xq22 locus, is associated with early-onset deafness, cognitive impairment, and corticospinal tract involvement (164,165). Similar to Lubag's disease, this X-linked dystonia–deafness syndrome is associated with a mosaic pattern of neuronal loss and gliosis in the striatum. Another form of dystonia associated with deafness, as well as blindness and mental retardation, is Mohr-Tranebjaerg syndrome (DFN1/MTS), which has been found to be due to a mutation in the gene on X chromosome that codes for the deafness–dystonia peptide (DDP1). DDP1 is a mitochondrial intermembrane space protein similar to Tim8p, 1 of 5 proteins that function as chaperones guiding hydrophobic proteins across the aqueous inner mitochondrial membrane (166,167).

In addition to finding gene markers on chromosomes 8 and 9 for idiopathic dystonia, gene markers or mutations have been identified in a number of secondary dystonias. The Wilson's disease gene has been localized to the long arm of chromosome 13; it encodes copper-transporting P-type ATPase and has been termed *ATP7B* (168). Numerous mutations already have been identified, and most patients carry at least 2 mutations (169). The Wilson's disease gene has a frequency of about 0.005 and a carrier frequency of about 0.01 (see Chapter 17). Linkage analyses initially localized Hallervorden-Spatz disease to the gene on 20p12.3–p13; subsequently, 7-bp deletion and various missense mutations were identified in the coding sequence of gene PANK2 with homology to pantothenate kinase (170). Because of the recent discovery of Hallervorden's terrible past and his shameless involvement in active euthanasia, the disorder has been renamed *neurodegeneration with brain iron accumulation type 1* (NBIA-1) or pantothenate kinase–associated neurodegeneration (PKAN) (171). Finally, many of the spinocerebellar atrophies, particularly type 3 and type 6, have been associated with dystonia (172).

Epidemiology

In a large series of patients with primary dystonia studied in Europe, female predominance was found in all anatomic categories, except for writer's cramp (173). Based on an epidemiologic study in the population living in Rochester, Minnesota, the incidence of dystonia has been estimated to be 2 per million persons per year for generalized dystonia and 24 per million persons per year for focal dystonia (174). The prevalence of dystonia has been estimated to be 3.4 per 100,000 for generalized dystonia and 30 per 100,000 for focal dystonia. The prevalence of generalized dystonia among Jews of Eastern European ancestry (Ashkenazi) living in Israel was 6.8/100,000, double that of the U.S. population (175). In northern England the prevalence has been estimated to be 1.42 per 100,000 for generalized dystonia and 12.9 per 100,000 for focal dystonia (176).

Pathophysiology

The pathophysiology of dystonia is not well understood, but progress has been made as a result of novel neurophysiologic and imaging techniques (177–179). Excessive co-contraction of antagonist muscles is one of the physiologic hallmarks of dystonia. The co-contraction in dystonia is apparently produced by abnormal synchronization of presynaptic inputs to antagonist motor neuron pools (180). In addition to co-contraction, there is an "overflow" of contractions to adjacent or remote muscles, which is particularly noticeable during a volitional movement of the affected limb. The third characteristic of dystonia is the paradoxical contraction of passively shortened muscles (the Westphal's phenomenon). However, this phenomenon is not specific for dystonia and is also seen in spasticity and in parkinsonian disorders. Using the H-reflex technique, reciprocal inhibition, normally a triphasic event lasting up to 1 second, was reduced in patients in several studies of patients with dystonia (179). Although the exact mechanism of this abnormality is not understood, a disturbed presynaptic inhibition of 1A afferents from the flexor muscles has been proposed as a possible explanation. The neurophysiologic findings, including increased duration of both the long latency stretch reflex and the first burst of agonist EMG activity in ballistic movements, suggest that lack of inhibition or excess excitation in both reflex and voluntary movement is the underlying mechanism of dystonia. Abnormalities in early and late long-latency reflex responses have been found in focal dystonia, and these can be influenced by BTX injections, suggesting involvement of peripheral mechanisms (181). Several investigators have demonstrated increased amplitude and duration of the R1 and R2 blink responses not only in patients with blepharospasm but also in those with cervical and other dystonias. These findings have been interpreted as being indicative of enhanced excitatory drive to the rostral brainstem or reduced spinal and brainstem inhibition.

Abnormal processing of muscle spindle input has been suggested as an important element in the pathophysiology of dystonia. Dystonia may be precipitated or exacerbated by vibration that activates sensory fibers, particularly Ia spindle afferents (182). This can be blocked by lidocaine, which blocks the gamma motor neurons. In some studies, however, vibration improves cervical dystonia. Vibration induces presynaptic inhibition and the tonic vibration reflex (TVR), a polysynaptic spinal cord reflex. The observation that dystonic patients have abnormal perception of motion, but not position, in response to a 50-Hz vibratory stimulus was interpreted as evidence for abnormal muscle spindle afferent processing in dystonia (183).

Several studies have suggested that cortical excitability is increased in dystonia (177,184,185). Using transcranial magnetic stimulation (TMS) and recording from the flexor carpi radialis muscles bilaterally, Ikoma et al. (184) found that the area of the motor-evoked potentials (MEPs) to the M wave was increased in patients with dystonia, providing evidence of increased cortical motor excitability in dystonia. Using similar techniques, but recording from orbicularis oculi and perioral muscles, Currà et al. (185) found shortened silent period in patients with blepharospasm and other types of cranial dystonia reflecting hyperexcitability of cortical inhibitory neurons in cranial dystonia. This can be modified by BTX injections into dystonic muscles (186). Patients with writer's cramp have been shown to have a deficiency in the negative slope that follows the Bereitschaftspotential, suggesting failure to achieve normal motor cortex activation in dystonia. The deficient activation of the premotor cortex in patients with writer's cramp has been thought to be due to a dysfunction of the premotor cortical network coupled with a loss of inhibition during generation of motor commands (187). Using the Bereitschaftspotential, Yazawa et al. (188) found that patients with focal hand dystonia had abnormal cortical preparatory process for voluntary muscle relaxation or motor inhibition. Studying scalp electroencephalographic (EEG) oscillations in response to self-paced simple index finger abduction movements, Toro et al. (189) found that patients with writer's cramp had less reduction in 20- to 30-Hz EEG (beta rhythm) power compared with controls. Since this EEG activity in the sensorimotor region is related to ongoing muscle activity, the observed abnormality in movement-related EEG desynchronization provides additional evidence for motor-cortical involvement in focal dystonia.

More and more studies seem to indicate that the excessive activation of antagonists, overflow into synergists, and prolongation of muscle activation are due to a deficiency of inhibition (190). This has been demonstrated at the level of the motor cortex, brainstem, and spinal cord. TMS studies, using the paired-pulse technique, found evidence of defective intracortical inhibition in patients with dystonia. In addition to a disorder of movement execution, there is growing evidence that dystonia is a sensory disorder as well as a disorder of movement preparation (190). The evidence for the latter includes (a) loss of EEG negativity of the movement-related cortical potential; (b) movement-related EEG desynchronization; (c) deficient contingent negative variation (CNV), which is the EEG period between a warning signal (S1) and a go signal (S2) (189); and (d) inappropriate modulation of the N30 between S1 and S2 in that instead of the normal reduction (gating) of N30 during the premovement period there is no such gating in patients with dystonia (although normal gating does occur during movement) (191). Assessment of spatial discrimination thresholds also has been used to detect asymptomatic individuals at risk for dystonia, and the demonstrated sensory abnormalities have been thought to represent endophenotype (192). The role of cortical reorganization in response to altered or repetitive peripheral input in the pathophysiology of dystonia is gaining increased recognition among neurophysiologists, neuroanatomists, and neurobiologists (68,193). Byl et al. (194) provided evidence for involvement of the somatosensory cortex in dystonia. They trained monkeys to perform repetitive hand-grip opening and closing and found, by electrophysiologic mapping of primary somatosensory cortical area 3b, marked dedifferentiation and enlargement of the normal cortical representation of the hand, breakdown of the normal sharply segregated areas of representation, and a change in the cortical topography. Since this cortical area has connections not only with other cortical areas but also with the putamen, the alterations described in the preceding paradigm may have implications for development of peripherally induced movement disorders, such as dystonia, associated with repetitive strain injuries (overusage syndromes). Although evidence that anatomic reorganization within the somatosensory cortex leads to a change in function is still lacking (195), it is possible that deafferentation as a result of peripheral injury not only may cause topographic reorganization but also may lead to abnormal function manifested by dystonia. Indeed, Lenz and Byl (196) found that the receptive fields in the ventral caudal (sensory) thalamus were 3 times larger in patients with dystonia than in those with ET. The notion that abnormal central nervous system plasticity is involved in the development of dystonia is also supported by the alteration in the somatosensory homunculus in patients with focal hand dystonia, as demonstrated by topographic mapping using the N20 peak of somatosensory-evoked potentials (197). As a result of these and other studies, there is growing support for the concept of cortical reorganization as a pathogenetic mechanism for some forms of dystonia.

According to this notion, environmental experience, such as repetitive motion (e.g., continuous practicing by musicians), prolonged restriction of focal movement, or limb amputation, changes the brain's representation of the periphery. Studies by Sanger et al. (198), as well as by others, have led some investigators to conclude that "fusion of representational zones is at the core of dystonia" (199).

The involvement of basal ganglia and their cortical projections in dystonia is also supported by the finding of reduced glucose metabolism, as demonstrated by PET scans, in the basal ganglia, in the frontal projection field of the mediodorsal thalamic nucleus, and in the frontal cortex of patients with primary dystonia. Blood-flow PET and activation studies suggest that the chief alteration in primary dystonia is overactivity of the planning (rostral) portion of the supplemental motor area (SMA), prefrontal area, and caudate nucleus, whereas the motor executive (caudal) portions of the SMA and the motor cortex are underactive. These findings have been interpreted as evidence of thalamofrontal disinhibition and abnormal central sensorimotor processing in dystonia (179). It is of interest that an ablative lesion or high-frequency stimulation of the globus pallidus can produce as well as improve dystonia, suggesting that it is the pattern of discharge in the basal ganglia rather than the location or frequency of discharge that is pathophysiologically relevant to dystonia. Using the 18F-fluorodeoxyglucose PET scan, Eidelberg et al. (200) found lentiform-thalamic metabolic dissociation, supporting the notion that dystonic movements may arise from excessive activity of the direct putamenopallidal inhibitory pathway. In a subsequent study, Eidelberg et al. (110) demonstrated 2 patterns of metabolic abnormality in patients with dystonia: (a) increased activity in the lentiform nuclei, cerebellum, and SMA, found in dystonic patients without evident dystonia during sleep (movement free, or MF) and (b) increased metabolic activity in the midbrain, cerebellum, and thalamus, found only in patients who exhibited dystonia at rest while awake (movement related, or MR). Various neurophysiologic and imaging studies provide additional support for the observation that in dystonia there is reduced pallidal inhibition of the thalamus that may explain the overactivity of medial and prefrontal cortical areas and underactivity of the primary motor cortex (177). In comparison with normal or parkinsonian primates, the globus pallidus pars interna (GPi) discharges in patients with dystonia seem to be lower in frequency and more irregular, with more bursting and pauses, and the receptive fields to passive and active movements seem to be widened (201). Although the physiologic studies, based on lower mean discharge rates in globus pallidus pars externa (GPe) and GPi suggest an overactivity of both direct (striatum–GPi) and indirect (striatum–GPe–GPi) pathway (202), dopamine-receptor ligand studies suggest increased activity in the direct and decreased activity in the indirect pathway. In either case, pallidotomy (202,203) and GPi deep-brain stimulation

(204) appear to be effective procedures for patients with dystonia, perhaps because they disrupt the abnormal GPi pattern and thus reduce cortical overactivation, characteristic of dystonia.

Pathoanatomy and Biochemistry

Although in most patients with dystonia no specific abnormality can be identified by neuroimaging or autopsy studies, there is convincing evidence supporting central origin (basal ganglia, brainstem, or both) for this movement disorder. Lesions, particularly in the putamen and GPi, have been associated with dystonia (74). In one anatomic-clinical study using three-dimensional MRI, dystonic spasms were associated with a lesion in the striatopallidal complex, whereas myoclonic dystonia was associated with lesions in the thalamus, particularly ventral intermediate and ventral caudal nuclei (205). In another study, using three-dimensional T1-weighted MRI, striatopallidal dystonia was attributed to lesions within the sensorimotor part of the striatopallidal complex and thalamic dystonia was associated with lesions in the centromedial or the ventral intermediate nuclei (78). Imaging studies usually do not show any specific abnormalities, but a 10% enlargement of the putamen was found in patients with focal dystonia (206). Although this finding probably reflects a response to the dystonia, it could also indicate early gliosis in the lentiform nucleus.

Despite high *DYT1* mRNA expression in the substantia nigra pars compacta of normal brains, the *DYT1* mutation is not associated with significant change in the nigrostriatal DA system, which may explain the lack of response to levodopa (133). Only a mild reduction in striatal 18F-dopa uptake was demonstrated in some patients with familial primary dystonia and in DRD. Perlmutter et al. (207) found about a 30% reduction in D2 receptor density as estimated by PET scans of patients with hand dystonia using 18F-spiperone. In patients with secondary dystonia due to midbrain damage, Vidailhet et al. (48) demonstrated evidence of dopaminergic dysfunction using 18F-dopa and three-dimensional MRI. Using two-dimensional J-resolved magnetic resonance spectroscopy to study brain gamma-aminobutyric acid (GABA) levels in 7 patients with focal dystonia, Levy and Hallett (208) showed a significant decrease in GABA levels in the contralateral sensorimotor cortex and lentiform nucleus.

Biochemical analysis of brains of 2 patients with generalized childhood-onset dystonia showed a 30% to 80% reduction in norepinephrine concentration in the posterior and lateral hypothalamus and a fourfold increase in the red nucleus (209). Similar biochemical changes were noted in the brain of a 68-year-old woman with a 7-year history of blepharospasm, oromandibular dystonia, spasmodic dysphonia, and anterocollis (210). Neuronal loss in the lateral tegmentum and the compensatory increase in norepinephrine levels (via the locus coeruleus) in the projection areas were hypothesized as an explanation for these changes in norepinephrine. The other neurotransmitters were less affected. Additional postmortem examinations must be performed before it can be concluded that these changes in norepinephrine are pathophysiologically related to dystonia. Although the morphology is normal, copper and manganese content are increased in the lentiform nucleus of brains of 3 patients with primary adult-onset dystonia (211).

Pathology

Although autopsy studies of brains of patients with primary dystonia have found no specific pathology, some brains of patients with atypical dystonia have shown a mosaic pattern of striatal gliosis. Similar changes were reported in a 34-year-old Filipino man with X-linked dystonia-parkinsonism (Lubag's disease) (159). Studies of patients with secondary dystonia have identified lesions involving the basal ganglia, particularly the putamen, and the rostral brainstem (50).

Animal Models of Dystonia

Various animal models of dystonia have implicated a dysfunction in the basal ganglia, thalamus, cerebellum, and brainstem (106–108,212). The red nucleus, other rostral brainstem structures, and the cerebellum have been implicated in the pathogenesis not only of human dystonia but also of mouse and rat mutant dystonia. Pharmacologically induced dystonia has been studied in monkeys rendered parkinsonian by unilateral infusion of 1-methyl-4-phenyl-1,2,3,6-tetrahydropyridine (MPTP) into the right common carotid artery (213). Using this model, these investigators demonstrated a marked increase in 2-deoxyglucose uptake in the basal ganglia, including the subthalamic nucleus, but decreased uptake in the subcortical structures that receive output from the basal ganglia, such as the anterior/ventral lateral thalamic complex and lateral habenula. The authors concluded that dystonia was characterized by increased activity in the basal ganglia outflow pathways. Other studies in MPTP-treated monkeys have provided evidence that D2 receptor stimulation is not only important for antiparkinsonian activity but also may result in dystonia; activation of the D1 receptors appears to be important in the genesis of chorea (214). Delayed-onset progressive dystonia has been reported following subacute 3-nitroproprionic acid treatment in monkeys (215).

Pseudodystonia

Besides dystonia due to central nervous system dysfunction and peripherally induced dystonia, there are many other causes of abnormal postures that resemble dystonia. These syndromes should be differentiated from true dystonia and are classified here as pseudodystonias (Table 25.2).

Examples include disorders associated with muscle stiffness and continuous muscle contractions (see Chapter 33), such as stiff-man syndrome (216), Isaacs' syndrome, Satoyoshi's syndrome, and others. Another example of pseudodystonia is flexor tendon entrapment of the digits, also referred to as trigger finger and trigger thumb (195). Characterized by sudden, painful or painless, snapping or locking of the thumb or fingers, this disorder is usually due to thickening of the digits A1 (proximal) annular pulley or other tendon abnormalities at the different finger joints.

REFERENCES

1. Goetz CG, Chmura TA, Lanska DJ. History of dystonia: part 4 of the MDS-sponsored history of movement disorders exhibit, Barcelona, June 2000. *Mov Disord* 2001;16:339–345.
2. Grundmann K. Primary torsion dystonia. *Arch Neurol* 2005;62:682–685.
3. Klein C, Gurvich N, Sena-Esteves M, et al. Evaluation of the role of the D2 dopamine receptor in myoclonus dystonia. *Ann Neurol* 2000;47:369–373.
4. Grimes DA, Bulman D, George-Hyslop PS, et al. Inherited myoclonus-dystonia: evidence supporting genetic heterogeneity. *Mov Disord* 2001;16:106–110.
5. Jankovic J. Tourette's syndrome. *N Engl J Med* 2001;345:1184–1192.
6. Jankovic J. Essential tremor: a heterogeneous disorder. *Mov Disord* 2002;17:638–644.
7. Jankovic J, Beach J, Pandolfo M, et al. Familial essential tremor in four kindreds: prospects for genetic mapping. *Arch Neurol* 1997;54:289–294.
8. Münchau A, Schrag A, Chuang C, et al. Arm tremor in cervical dystonia differs from essential tremor and can be classified by onset age and spread of symptoms. *Brain* 2001;124:1765–1776.
9. Jedynak CP, Bonnet AM, Agid Y. Tremor and idiopathic dystonia. *Mov Disord* 1991;6:230–236.
10. Soland VL, Bhatia KP, Volonte MA, et al. Focal task-specific tremors. *Mov Disord* 1996;11:665–670.
11. Ashour R, Tintner R, Jankovic J. "Striatal" hand and foot deformities in Parkinson's disease. *Lancet Neurol* 2005;4:423–431.
12. Ashour R, Jankovic J. Joint and skeletal deformities in Parkinson's disease, multiple system atrophy, and progressive supranuclear palsy. *Mov Disord* 2006 (in press).
13. Fahn S, Bressman S, Marsden CD. Classification of dystonia. *Adv Neurol* 1998;78:1–10.
14. Jedynak PC, Tranchant C, Zegers de Beyl. Prospective clinical study of writer's cramp. *Mov Disord* 2001;16:494–499.
15. Frucht SJ, Fahn S, Greene PE, et al. The natural history of embouchure dystonia. *Mov Disord* 2001;16:899–906.
16. Jabusch HC, Zschucke D, Schmidt A, Schuele S, Altenmuller E. Focal dystonia in musicians: treatment strategies and long-term outcome in 144 patients. *Mov Disord* 2005;20:1623–1626.
17. Scolding NJ, Smith SM, Sturman S, et al. Auctioneer's jaw: a case of occupational oromandibular hemidystonia. *Mov Disord* 1995;10:508–509.
18. Adler CH, Crews D, Hentz JG, Smith AM, Caviness JN. Abnormal co-contraction in yips-affected but not unaffected golfers: evidence for focal dystonia. *Neurology* 2005;64:1813–1814.
19. Rosenbaum F, Jankovic J. Task-specific focal dystonia and tremor. *Neurology* 1988;38:522–527.
20. Opal P, Tintner R, Jankovic J, et al. Intrafamilial phenotypic variability of the DYT1 dystonia: from asymptomatic *TOR1A* gene carrier status to dystonic storm. *Mov Disord* 2002;17:339–345.
21. Jahanshahi M. Factors that ameliorate or aggrevate spasmodic torticollis. *J Neurol Neurosurg Psychiatry* 2000;68:227–229.
22. Schramm A, Reiners K, Naumann M. Complex mechanisms of sensory tricks in cervical dystonia. *Mov Disord* 2004;19:452–458.
23. Segawa M. Hereditary progressive dystonia with marked diurnal fluctuation. *Brain Dev* 2000;22(suppl):S65–S80.
24. Jankovic J, Demirkiran M. Classification of paroxysmal dyskinesias and ataxias. In: Fahn S, Frucht SJ, Truong DD, Hallett M, eds. *Myoclonus and paroxysmal dyskinesias. Adv Neurol*, vol 89, Philadelphia: Lippincott Williams & Wilkins, 2002:387–400.
25. Dupont S, Semah F, Boon P, et al. Association of ipsilateral motor automatisms and contralateral dystonic posturing. *Arch Neurol* 1999;56:927–932.
26. Swoboda KJ, Hyland K, Goldstein DS, et al. Clinical and therapeutic observations in aromatic L-amino acid decarboxylase deficiency. *Neurology* 1999;53:1205–1211.
27. Chang YT, Sharma R, Marsh JL, et al. Levodopa-responsive aromatic L-amino acid decarboxylase deficiency. *Ann Neurol* 2004;55:435–438.
28. FitzGerald P, Jankovic J. Tardive oculogyric crises. *Neurology* 1989;39:1434–1437.
29. Blakeley J, Jankovic J. Secondary causes of paroxysmal dyskinesias. In: Fahn S, Frucht SJ, Truong DD, Hallett M, eds. Myoclonus and Paroxysmal Dyskinesias, *Adv Neurol*, vol 89, Philadelphia: Lippincott Williams & Wilkins, 2002:401–420.
30. Comella CL, Stebbins GT, Goetz CG, et al. Teaching tape for the motor section of the Toronto Western Spasmodic Torticollis Scale. *Mov Disord* 1997;12:570–575.
31. Consky ES, Lang AE. Clinical assessments of patients with cervical dystonia. In: Jankovic J, Hallett M, eds. *Therapy with botulinum toxin*. New York: Marcel Dekker, 1994;211–237.
32. Barry MJ, VanSwearingen JM, Albright AL. Reliability and responsiveness of the Barry-Albright Dystonia Scale. *Dev Med Child Neurol* 1999;41,404–41,411.
33. Comella CL, Leurgans S, Wuu J, Stebbins GT, Chmura T. Rating scales for dystonia: a multicenter assessment. *Mov Disord* 2003;18:303–312.
34. Jankovic J, Orman J. Botulinum A toxin for cranial-cervical dystonia: a double-blind, placebo-controlled study. *Neurology* 1987;37:616–623.
35. Lindeboom R, de Haan R, Aramideh M, et al. The blepharospasm disability scale: an instrument for the assessment of functional health in blepharospasm. *Mov Disord* 1995;10:444–449.
36. Muller J, Wissel J, Kemmler G, et al. Craniocervical dystonia questionnaire (CDQ-24): development and validation of a disease-specific quality of life instrument. *J Neurol Neurosurg Psychiatry* 2004;75:749–753.
37. Jankovic J. Blepharospasm. In: Gilman S, ed. *Medlink.com*. La Jolla, Calif: Arbor Publishing, 2005.
38. Scheidt CE, Schuller B, Rayki O, et al. Relative absence of psychopathology in benign essential blepharospasm and hemifacial spasm. *Neurology* 1996;47:43–45.
39. Wooten-Watts M, Tan E-K, Jankovic J. Bruxism and cranial-cervical dystonia: is there a relationship? *Cranio* 1999;17:1–6.
40. Tan EK, Jankovic J. Bilateral hemifacial spasm: a report of 5 cases and a literature review. *Mov Disord* 1999;14:345–349.
41. Jankovic J. Oromandibular dystonia. In: Gilman S, ed. *Medlink.com*. La Jolla, Calif: Arbor Publishing, 1999, 2000, 2001, 2002c.
42. Frucht S, Fahn S, Ford B, et al. A geste antagoniste device to treat jaw-closing dystonia. *Mov Disord* 1999;14:883–886.
43. Sankhla C, Lai E, Jankovic J. Peripherally induced oromandibular dystonia. *J Neurol Neurosurg Psychiatry* 1998;65:722–728.
44. Tan E-K, Jankovic J, Ondo W. Bruxism in Huntington's disease. *Mov Disord* 2000;15:171–173.
45. Dietrichs E, Heier MA, Nakstad PH. Jaw-opening dystonia presumably caused by a pontine lesion. *Mov Disord* 2000;15:1026–1028.
46. Wang A, Jankovic J. Hemifacial spasm: clinical correlates and treatments. *Muscle Nerve* 1998;21:1740–1747.
47. Hallett M, Daroff RB. Blepharospasm: report of a workshop. *Neurology* 1996;46:1213–1218.
48. Vidailhet M, Dupel C, Lehericy S, et al. Dopaminergic dysfunction in midbrain dystonia: anatomoclinical study using three-dimensional magnetic resonance imaging and fluorodopa F18 positron emission tomography. *Arch Neurol* 1999;56:982–989.
49. Lew H, Jordan C, Jerger J, et al. Acoustic reflex abnormalities in cranial-cervical dystonia. *Neurology* 1992;42:594–597.
50. Hartmann A, Pogarell O, Oertel WH. Secondary dystonia. *J Neurol* 1998;245:511–518.
51. Adityanjee, Aderibigbe YA, Jampala VC, Mathews T, et al. The current status of tardive dystonia. *Biol Psychiatry* 1999;45:715–730.

52. Van Harten NP, Kahn RS. Tardive dystonia. *Schizophrenia Bull* 1999;25:741–748.

53. Schicatano EJ, Basso MA, Evinger C. Animal model explains the origins of the cranial dystonia benign essential blepharospasm. *J Neurophysiol* 1997;77:2842–2846.

54. Kruse N, Berg D, Francis MJ, et al. Reduction of Menkes mRNA and copper leukocytes of patients with primary adult-onset dystonia. *Ann Neurol* 2001;49:405–408.

55. Dauer WT, Burke RE, Greene P, et al. Current concepts on the clinical features, aetiology, and management of idiopathic cervical dystonia. *Brain* 1998;121:547–560.

56. Jankovic J, Leder S, Warner D, et al. Cervical dystonia: clinical findings and associated movement disorders. *Neurology* 1991;41: 1088–1091.

57. Deuschl G, Heinen F, Kleedorfer B, et al. Clinical and polymyographic investigation of spasmodic torticollis. *J Neurol* 1992; 239:9–15.

58. Chawda SJ, Münchau A, Johnson D, et al. Pattern of premature degenerative changes of the cervical spine in patients with spasmodic torticollis and the impact on the outcome of selective peripheral denervation. *J Neurol Neurosurg Psychiatry* 2000;68: 465–471.

59. Kutvonen O, Dastidar P, Nurmikko T. Pain in spasmodic torticollis. *Pain* 1997;69:279–286.

60. Münchau A, Good CD, McGowan S, et al. Prospective study of swallowing function in patients with cervical dystonia undergoing selective peripheral denervation. *J Neurol Neurosurg Psychiatry* 2001;71:67–72.

61. Muller J, Wissel T, Masuhr F, et al. Clinical characteristics of the geste antagoniste in cervical dystonia. *J Neurol* 2001;248: 478–482.

62. Naumann M, Magyar-Lehmann S, Reiners K, et al. Sensory tricks in cervical dystonia: perceptual dysbalance of parietal cortex modulates frontal motor programming. *Ann Neurol* 2000;47: 322–328.

63. Münchau A, Bronstein AM. Role of the vestibular system in the pathophysiology of spasmodic torticollis. *J Neurol Neurosurg Psychiatry* 2001;71:285–288.

64. Anastasopoulos D, Bhatia K, Bronstein AM, et al. What is straight ahead to a patient with torticollis? *Brain* 1998;121:91–101.

65. Müller J, Ebersbach G, Wissel J, et al. Disturbance of dynamic balance in phasic cervical dystonia. *J Neurol Neurosurg Psychiatry* 1999;67:807–810.

66. Krauss JK, Toops EG, Jankovic J, et al. Symptomatic and functional outcome of surgical treatment of cervical dystonia. *J Neurol Neurosurg Psychiatry* 1997;63:642–648b.

67. Chan J, Brin MF, Fahn S. Idiopathic cervical dystonia: clinical characteristics. *Mov Disord* 1991;6:119–126.

68. Jankovic J. Can peripheral trauma induce dystonia and other movement disorders? Yes! *Mov Disord* 2001;16:7–12.

69. Krauss JK, Jankovic J. Head injury and posttraumatic movement disorders. *Neurosurgery* 2002;50:927–940.

70. Lagueny A, Burband P, Le Masson G, et al. Involvement of respiratory muscles in adult-onset dystonia: a clinical and electrophysiologic study. *Mov Disord* 1995;10:708–713.

71. Blum P, Jankovic J. Stiff-person syndrome: an autoimmune disease. *Mov Disord* 1991;6:12–20.

72. Bhatia KP, Quinn NP, Marsden CD. Clinical features and natural history of axial predominant adult onset primary dystonia. *J Neurol Neurosurg Psychiatry* 1997;63:788–791.

73. Krauss JK, Kiriyanthan GD, Borremans JJ. Cerebral arteriovenous malformations and movement disorders. *Clin Neurol Neurosurg* 1999;101:92–99.

74. Münchau A, Mathen D, Cox T, et al. Unilateral lesions of the globus pallidus: report of four patients presenting with focal or segmental dystonia. *J Neurol Neurosurg Psychiatry* 2000;69: 494–498.

75. Lehéricy S, Grand S, Pollak P, et al. Clinical characteristics and topography of lesions in movement disorders due to thalamic lesions. *Neurology* 2001;57:1055–1066.

76. Chuang C, Fahn S, Fruch SJ. The natural history and treatment of acquire hemidystonia: report of 33 cases and review of literature. *J Neurol Surg Psychiatry* 2002;72:59–67.

77. Scott B, Jankovic J. Delayed-onset progressive movement disorders. *Neurology* 1996;46:68–74.

78. Kim JS. Delayed onset mixed involuntary movements after thalamic stroke: clinical, radiological, and pathophysiological findings. *Brain* 2001;124:299–309.

79. Greene PE, Bressman SB, Ford B, et al. Parkinsonism, dystonia, and hemiatrophy. *Mov Disord* 2000;15:537–541.

80. Janavs J, Aminoff MJ. Dystonia and chorea in acquired systemic disorders. *J Neurol Neurosurg Psychiatry* 1998;65:436–445.

81. Defazio G, Berardelli A, Abbruzzese G, et al. Possible risk factors for primary adult onset dystonia: a case-control investigation by the Italian Movement Disorders Study Group. *J Neurol Neurosurg Psychiatry* 1998;64:25–32.

82. Bressman SB, de Leon D, Raymond D, et al. Secondary dystonia and the *DYT1* gene. *Neurology* 1997;48:1571–1577.

83. Svetel M, Kozic D, Stefanoval E, et al. Dystonia in Wilson's disease. *Mov Disord* 2001;16:719–723.

84. Jankovic J. Tardive syndromes and other drug-induced movement disorders. *Clin Neuropharmacol* 1995;18:197–214.

85. Müller T, Woitalla D, Hunsdiek A, et al. Elevated plasma levels of homocystein in dystonia. *Acta Neurol Scand* 2000;101: 388–390.

86. Topp KS, Byl NN. Movement dysfunction following repetitive hand opening and closing: anatomical analysis in owl monkeys. *Mov Disord* 1999;14:295–306.

87. Weiner WJ. Can peripheral trauma induce dystonia? No! *Mov Disord* 2001;16:13–22.

88. Owens DG. Dystonia: a potential psychiatric pitfall. *Br J Psychiatry* 1990;156:620–634.

89. Brown P, Thompson PD. Electrophysiologic aids to the diagnosis of psychogenic jerks, spasms, and tremor. *Mov Disord* 2001;16:595–599.

90. Monday K, Jankovic J. Psychogenic myoclonus. *Neurology* 1993;43:349–352.

91. Halligan PW, Athwal BS, Oakley DA, et al. Imaging hypnotic paralysis: implications for conversion hysteria. *Lancet* 2000;355: 986–987.

91a. Espay AJ, Morgante F, Purzner J, et al. Cortical and spinal abnormalities in psychogenic dystonia. *Ann Neurol* 2006;59:825–834.

92. Kramer PL, Ozelius L, de Leon D, et al. Dystonia gene in Ashkenazi Jewish population located on chromosome 9q32-34. *Ann Neurol* 1990;27:114–120.

93. Ozelius LJ, Hewett JW, Page CE, et al. The early onset torsion dystonia gene [*DYT1*] encodes an ATP-binding protein. *Nat Genet* 1997;17:40–48.

94. Leung JC, Klein C, Friedman J, et al. Novel mutation and polymorphisms in the TOR1A (*DYT1*) gene in atypical, early onset dystonia and polymorphisms in dystonia and early onset parkinsonism. *Neurogenetics* 2001;3:133–143.

95. Konakova M, Huynh DP, Yong W, et al. Cellular distribution of torsinA and torsinB in normal human brain. *Arch Neurol* 2001;58:921–927.

96. Walker RH, Brin MF, Sandu D, et al. Distribution and immunohistochemical characterization of torsinA immunoreactivity in rat brain. *Brain Res* 2001;900:348–354.

97. Ozelius LJ, Page CE, Klein C, et al. The TOR1A (*DYT1*) gene family and its role in early onset torsion dystonia. *Genomics* 1999;62:377–384.

98. Breakfield XO, Kamm C, Hanson PI. TorsinA: movement at many levels. *Neuron* 2001;31:9–12.

99. Hewett J, Gonzalez-Agosti C, Slater D, et al. Mutant torsinA, responsible for early-onset torsion dystonia, forms membrane inclusions in cultured neural cells. *Hum Mol Genet* 2000;9: 1404–1414.

100. Kustedjo K, Bracey MH, Cravatt BF. TorsinA and its torsin dystonia–associated mutant forms are lumenal glycoproteins that exhibit distinct subcellular localizations. *J Biol Chem* 2000;275: 27,933–27,939.

101. Walker RH, Brin MF, Sandu D, et al. TorsinA immunoreactivity in brains of patients with *DYT1* and non-*DYT1* dystonia. *Neurology* 2002;58:120–124.

102. Placzek MR, Misbahuddin A, Taanman J-W, Cooper JM, Warner TT. Mutant torsinA, which causes early onset childhood dystonia, associated with vesicular monoamine transporter in cultured human neuroblastoma cells. *European J Neurol* 2003;10(suppl 1):80–81.

103. Gonzalez-Alegre P, Bode N, Davidson BL, Paulson HL. Silencing primary dystonia: lentiviral-mediated RNA interference therapy for *DYT1* dystonia. *J Neurosci* 2005;25:10,502–10,509.

104. McNaught KS, Kapustin A, Jackson T, et al. Brainstem pathology in *DYT1* primary torsion dystonia. *Ann Neurol* 2004;56:540–547.

105. Mena-Segovia J, Bolam JP, Magill PJ. Pedunculopontine nucleus and basal ganglia: distant relatives or part of the same family? *Trends Neurosci* 2004;27:585–588.

106. Shashidharan P, Sandu D, Potla U, et al. Transgenic mouse model of early-onset *DYT1* dystonia. *Hum Mol Genet* 2005;14:125–133.

107. Jinnah HA, Hess EJ, Ledoux MS, Sharma N, Baxter MG, Delong MR. Rodent models for dystonia research: characteristics, evaluation, and utility. *Mov Disord* 2005;20:283–292.

108. Goodchild RE, Kim CE, Dauer WT. Loss of the dystonia-associated protein torsinA selectively disrupts the neuronal nuclear envelope. *Neuron* 2005;48:923–932.

109. Sharma N, Hewett J, Ozelius LJ, et al. A close association of torsinA and alpha-synuclein in Lewy bodies: a fluorescence resonance energy transfer study. *Am J Pathol* 2001;159:339–344.

110. Eidelberg D, Moeller JR, Antonini A, et al. Functional brain networks in *DYT1* dystonia. *Ann Neurol* 1998;44:303–312.

111. Valente EM, Warner TT, Jarman PR, et al. The role of *DYT1* in primary torsion dystonia in Europe. *Brain* 1998;121:2335–2339.

112. Risch N, DeLeon D, Ozelius L, et al. Genetic analysis of idiopathic torsion dystonia in Ashkenazi Jews and their recent descent from small founder population. *Nat Genet* 1995;9:152–159.

113. Brassat D, Camuzat A, Vidailhet M, et al. Frequency of the *DYT1* mutation in primary torsion dystonia without family history. *Arch Neurol* 2000;57:333–335.

114. Kamm C, Naumann M, Mueller J, et al. The *DYT1* GAG deletion is infrequent in sporadic and familial writer's cramp. *Mov Disord* 2000;15:1238–1241.

115. Bressman SB, Sabatti C, Raymond D, et al. The *DYT1* phenotype and guidelines for diagnostic testing. *Neurology* 2000;54:1746–1752.

116. Almasy L, Bressman SB, Raymond D, et al. Idiopathic torsion dystonia linked to chromosome 8 in two Mennonite families. *Ann Neurol* 1997;42:670–673.

117. Leube B, Hendgen T, Kessler KR, et al. Sporadic focal dystonia in northwest Germany: molecular basis on chromosome 18p. *Ann Neurol* 1997;42:111–114.

118. Leube B, Auburger G. Questionable role of adult-onset focal dystonia among sporadic dystonia patients. *Ann Neurol* 1998;44:984–986.

119. Klein C, Page CE, LeWitt P, et al. Genetic analysis of three patients with an 18p- syndrome and dystonia. *Neurology* 1999;52:649–651a.

120. Valente EM, Bentivoglio AR, Cassetta E, et al. *DYT13*, a novel primary torsion dystonia locus, maps to chromosome 1p36.13-36.32 in an Italian family with cranial-cervical or upper limb onset. *Ann Neurol* 2001;49:362–366.

121. Placzek MR, Misbahuddin A, Chadhuri KR, et al. Cervical dystonia is associated with a polymorphism in the dopamine (D5) receptor gene. *J Neurol Neurosurg Psychiatry* 2001;71:262–264.

122. Nygaard TG, Raymond D, Chen C, et al. Localization of a gene for myoclonus-dystonia to chromosome 7q21-q23. *Ann Neurol* 1999;46:794–798.

122a. Gerrits MC, Foncke EM, de Haan R, et al. Phenotype-genotype correlation in Dutch patients with myoclonus-dystonia. *Neurology* 2006;66:759–761.

123. Vidailhet M, Tassin J, Durif F, et al. A major locus for several phenotypes of myoclonus-dystonia on chromosome 7q. *Neurology* 2001;56:1213–1216.

124. Zimprich A, Grabowski M, Asmus F, et al. Mutations in the gene encoding varepsilon-sarcoglycan cause myoclonus-dystonia syndrome. *Nat Genet* 2001;29:66–69.

125. Grimes DA, Han F, Lang AE, et al. A novel locus for inherited myoclonus-dystonia on 18p11. *Neurology* 2002;59:1183–1186.

126. Nygaard TG, Wilhelmsen KC, Risch NJ, et al. Linkage mapping of dopa-responsive dystonia (DRD) to chromosome 14q. *Nat Genet* 1993;5:386–391.

127. Ichinose H, Ohye T, Takahi E, et al. Hereditary progressive dystonia with marked diurnal fluctuation caused by mutations in the GTP cyclohydrolase I gene. *Nat Genet* 1994;8:236–242.

128. Ichinose H, Suzuki T, Inagaki H, et al. Molecular genetics of dopa-responsive dystonia. *Biol Chem* 1999;380:1355–1364.

129. Rajput AH, Gibb WRG, Zhong XH, et al. DOPA-responsive dystonia: pathological and biochemical observations in a case. *Ann Neurol* 1994;35:396–402.

130. Furukawa Y, Lang AE, Trugman JM, et al. Gender-related penetrance and de novo GTP-cyclohydrolase I gene mutations in dopa-responsive dystonia. *Neurology* 1998;50:1015–1020b.

131. Nygaard TG, Wooten GF. Dopa-responsive dystonia: some pieces of the puzzle are still missing. *Neurology* 1998;50:853–855.

132. Tamaru Y, Hirano M, Ito H, et al. Clinical similarities of hereditary progressive/dopa responsive dystonia caused by different types of mutations in the GTP cyclohydrolase I gene. *J Neurol Neurosurg Psychiatry* 1998;64:469–473.

133. Furukawa Y, Guttman M, Sparagana SP, et al. Dopa-responsive dystonia due to a large deletion in the GTP cyclohydrolase I gene. *Ann Neurol* 2000;47:517–520.

134. Furukawa Y, Kish SJ. Dopa-responsive dystonia: recent advances and remaining issues to be addressed. *Mov Disord* 1999;14:709–715.

135. Tassin J, Dürr A, Bonnet A-M, et al. Levodopa-responsive dystonia: GTP cyclohydrolase I or parkin mutations? *Brain* 2000;123:1112–1121.

136. Steinberger D, Korinthenber R, Topka H, et al. Dopa-responsive dystonia: mutation analysis of GCH1 and analysis of therapeutic doses of L-dopa. *Neurology* 2000;55:1735–1737.

137. Hwu W-L, Chiou Y-W, Lai S-Y, et al. Dopa-responsive dystonia is induced by a dominant-negative mechanism. *Ann Neurol* 2000;48:609–613.

138. Bezin L, Nygaard TG, Neville JD, et al. Reduced lymphoblast neopterin detects GTP cyclohydrolase dysfunction in dopa-responsive dystonia. *Neurology* 1998;50:1021–1027.

139. Hyland K, Fryburg JS, Wilson WG, et al. Oral phenylalanine loading in dopa-responsive dystonia: a possible diagnostic test. *Neurology* 1997;48:1290–1297.

140. Bandman O, Valente EM, Holmans P, et al. Dopa-responsive dystonia: a clinical and molecular genetic study. *Ann Neurol* 1998;44:649–656.

141. Jeon BS, Jeong J-M, Park S-S, et al. Dopamine transporter density measured by ^{123}I-CIT single-photon emission tomography is normal in dopa-responsive dystonia. *Ann Neurol* 1998;43:792–800.

142. Van Hove JL, Steyaert J, Matthijs G, et al. Expanded motor and psychiatric phenotype in autosomal dominant Segawa syndrome due to GTP cyclohydrolase deficiency. *J Neurol Neurosurg Psychiatry* 2006;77:18–23.

143. Dewey RB, Muenter MD, Kishore A, et al. Long-term follow-up of levodopa responsiveness in generalized dystonia. *Arch Neurol* 1998;55:1320–1323.

144. Hwang WJ, Calne DB, Tsui JK, et al. The long-term response to levodopa in dopa-responsive dystonia. *Parkinsonism Relat Disord* 2001;8:1–5.

145. Nutt JG, Nygaard TG. Response to levodopa treatment in dopa-responsive dystonia. *Arch Neurol* 2001;58:905–910.

146. Jarman PR, Bandmann O, Marsden CD, et al. GTP cyclohydrolase I mutations in patients with dystonia responsive to anticholinergic drugs. *J Neurol Neurosurg Psychiatry* 1997;63:304–308.

147. Steinberger D, Topla H, Fischer D, et al. GCH1 mutation in a patient with adult-onset oromandibular dystonia. *Neurology* 1999;52:877–879.

148. Furukawa Y, Kish SJ, Lang AE. Scoliosis in a dopa-responsive dystonia family with a mutation of the GTP cyclohydrolase I gene. *Neurology* 2000;54:2187.

149. Hahn H, Trant MR, Brownstein MJ, et al. Neurologic and psychiatric manifestations in a family with a mutation in exon 2 of the guanosine triphosphate-cyclohydrolase gene. *Arch Neurol* 2001;58:749–755.

150. Furukawa Y, Kish SJ, Bebin EM, et al. Dystonia with motor delay in compound heterozygotes for GTP-cyclohydrolase I gene mutations. *Ann Neurol* 1998;44:10–16a.

151. Furukawa Y, Nygaard TG, Gutlich M, et al. Striatal biopterin and tyrosine hydroxylase protein production in dopa-responsive dystonia. *Neurology* 1999;53:1032–1041.

152. De Rijk-van Andel JF, Gabreëls FJM, Geurtz B, et al. L-dopa-responsive infantile hypokinetic rigid parkinsonism due to tyrosine hydroxylase deficiency. *Neurology* 2000;55:1926–1928.

153. Furukawa Y, Graf WD, Wong H, et al. Dopa-responsive dystonia simulating spastic paraplegia due to tyrosine hydroxylase (TH) gene mutations. *Neurology* 2001;56:260–263.

154. Ozand PT, Gascon GG, Essa MA, et al. Biotin-responsive basal ganglia disease: a novel entity. *Brain* 1998;121:1267–1279.

155. Brashear A, DeLeon D, Bressman SB, et al. Rapid-onset dystonia-parkinsonism in a second family. *Neurology* 1997;48:1086.

156. Pittock SJ, Joyce C, O'Keane V, et al. Rapid-onset dystonia-parkinsonism: a clinical and genetic analysis of a new kindred. *Neurology* 2000;55:991–995.

157. De Carvalho Aguiar P, Sweadner KJ, et al. Mutations in the Na+/K+-ATPase alpha3 gene ATP1A3 are associated with rapid-onset dystonia parkinsonism. *Neuron* 2004;43:169–175.

158. Wilhelmsen KC, Weeks DE, Nygaard TG, et al. Genetic mapping of "Lubag" (X-linked dystonia-parkinsonism) in a Filipino kindred to the pericentromeric region of the X chromosome. *Ann Neurol* 1991;2:124–131.

159. Waters CH, Faust PL, Powers J, et al. Neuropathology of Lubag (X-linked dystonia parkinsonism). *Mov Disord* 1993;8:387–390.

160. Marsden CD, Lang AE, Quinn NP, et al. Familial dystonia and visual failure with striatal CT lucencies. *J Neurol Neurosurg Psychiatry* 1986;49:500–509.

161. Novotny EJ, Gurparkash S, Wallace DC, et al. Leber's disease and dystonia: a mitochondrial disease. *Neurology* 1986;36:1053–1060.

162. Bruyn GW, Vielvoye GJ, Went LN. Hereditary spastic dystonia: a new mitochondrial encephalopathy? *J Neurol Sci* 1991;103:195–202.

163. Caparros-Lefebvre D, Destee A, Petit H. Late onset familial dystonia: could mitochondrial deficits induce a diffuse lesioning process of the whole basal ganglia system? *J Neurol Neurosurg Psychiatry* 1997;63:196–203.

164. Hayes MW, Ouvrier RA, Evans W, et al. X-linked dystonia-deafness syndrome. *Mov Disord* 1998;13:303–308.

165. Ujike H, Tanabe Y, Takehisa Y, et al. A family with X-linked dystonia-deafness syndrome with a novel mutation of the DDP gene. *Arch Neurol* 2001;58:1004–1007.

166. Koehler CM, Leuenberger D, Merchant S, et al. Human deafness dystonia syndrome is a mitochondrial disease. *Proc Natl Acad Sci USA* 1999;96:2141–2146.

167. Swerdlow RH, Wooten GF. A novel deafness/dystonia peptide gene mutation that causes dystonia in female carriers of Mohr-Tranebjaerg syndrome. *Ann Neurol* 2001;50:537–540.

168. Bull P, Thomas GR, Forbes J, et al. The Wilson disease gene is a putative copper transporting P-type ATPase similar to the Menkes disease gene. *Nat Genet* 1993;5:327–337.

169. Xu P, Liang X, Jankovic J, et al. Identification of a high frequency of mutation at exon 8 of ATP7B gene in Chinese population with Wilson's disease by fluorescent PCR. *Arch Neurol* 2001;58:1879–1882.

170. Valentino P, Annesi G, Ciro Candiano IC, et al. Genetic heterogeneity in patients with pantothenate kinase-associated neurodegeneration and classic magnetic resonance imaging eye-to-the-tiger pattern. *Mov Disord* 2006;21:252–254.

171. Thomas M, Hayflick SJ, Jankovic J. Clinical heterogeneity of neurodegeneration with iron accumulation–1 (Hallervorden-Spatz syndrome) and pantothenate kinase associated neurodegeneration (PKAN). *Mov Disord* 2004;19:36–42.

172. Sethi KD, Jankovic J. Dystonia in spinocerebellar ataxia type 6. *Mov Disord* 2002;17:150–153.

173. Epidemiologic Study of Dystonia in Europe (ESDE) Collaborative Group. Sex-related influences on the frequency and age of onset of primary dystonia. *Neurology* 1999;53:1871–1873.

174. Nutt JG, Muenter MD, Melton J, et al. Epidemiology of dystonia in Rochester, Minnesota. In: Fahn S, Marsden CD, Calne DB, eds. *Dystonia: advances in neurology*, vol. 50. New York: Raven Press, 1988:361–365.

175. Zilber N, Korczyn AD, Kahana E, et al. Inheritance of idiopathic torsion dystonia among Jews. *J Med Genet* 1984;21:13–20.

176. Duffey P, Butler AG, Hawthorne MR, et al. The epidemiology of primary dystonia in the North of England. In: Fahn S, Marsden CD, DeLong DR, eds. *Dystonia 3: advances in neurology*, vol 78. Philadelphia: Lippincott–Raven Publishers, 1998:121–125.

177. Berardelli A, Rothwell JC, Hallett M, et al. The pathophysiology of primary dystonia. *Brain* 1998;121:1195.

178. Crossman AR, Brotchie JM. Pathophysiology of dystonia. In: Fahn S, Marsden CD, DeLong DR, eds. *Dystonia 3: advances in neurology*, vol 78. Philadelphia: Lippincott–Raven Publishers, 1998:19–25.

179. Hallett M. Physiology of dystonia. *Adv Neurol* 1998;78:11–18.

180. Farmer SF, Sheean GL, Mayston MJ, et al. Abnormal motor unit synchronization of antagonist muscles underlies pathological co-contraction in upper limb dystonia. *Brain* 1998;121:801–814.

181. Naumann M, Reiners K. Long-latency reflexes of hand muscles in idiopathic focal dystonia and their modification by botulinum toxin. *Brain* 1997;120:409–416.

182. Kaji R, Rothwell JC, Katayama M, et al. Tonic vibration reflex and muscle afferent block in writer's cramp. *Ann Neurol* 1995;38:155–162.

183. Grünewald RA, Yoneda Y, Shipman JM, et al. Idiopathic focal dystonia: a disorder of muscle spindle afferent processing? *Brain* 1997;120:2179–2185.

184. Ikoma K, Sami A, Mercuri B, et al. Abnormal cortical motor excitability in dystonia. *Neurology* 1996;46:1371–1376.

185. Currà A, Romaniello A, Berardelli A, et al. Shortened cortical silent period in facial muscles of patients with cranial dystonia. *Neurology* 2000;54:130–135.

186. Gilio F, Curra A, Lorenzano C, et al. Effects of botulinum toxin type A on intracortical inhibition in patients with dystonia. *Ann Neurol* 2000;48:20–26.

187. Ibáñez V, Sadato N, Karp B, et al. Deficient activation of the motor cortical network in patients with writer's cramp. *Neurology* 1999;53:96–105.

188. Yazawa S, Ikeda A, Kaji R, et al. Abnormal cortical processing of voluntary muscle relaxation in patients with focal hand dystonia studied by movement-related potentials. *Brain* 1999;122:1357–1366.

189. Toro C, Deuschl G, Hallett M. Movement-related electroencephalographic desynchronization in patients with hand cramps: evidence for motor cortical involvement in focal dystonia. *Ann Neurol* 2000;47:456–461.

190. Hallett M. Disorder of movement preparation in dystonia. *Brain* 2000;123:1765–1766.

191. Murase N, Kaji R, Shimazu H, et al. Abnormal premovement gating of somatosensory input in writer's cramp. *Brain* 2000;123:1813–1829.

192. O'Dwyer JP, O'Riordan S, Saunders-Pullman R, et al. Sensory abnormalities in unaffected relatives in familial adult-onset dystonia. *Neurology* 2005;65:938–40.

193. Meunier S, Garnero L, Ducorps A, et al. Human brain mapping in dystonia reveals both endophenotypic traits and adaptive reorganization. *Ann Neurol* 2001;50:521–527.

194. Byl NN, Merzenich MM, Jenkins WM. A primate genesis model of focal dystonia and repetitive strain injury. I: Learning-induced dedifferentiation of the representation of the hand in the primary somatosensory cortex in adult monkeys. *Neurology* 1996;47:508–520.

195. Moore CEG, Schady W. Investigation of the functional correlates of reorganization within the human somatosensory cortex. *Brain* 2000;123:1883–1895.

196. Lenz FA, Byl NN. Reorganization in the cutaneous core of the human thalamic principal somatic sensory nucleus (ventral caudal) in patients with dystonia. *J Neurophysiol* 1999;82:3204–3212.

197. Bara-Jimenez W, Catalan MJ, Hallett M, et al. Abnormal somatosensory homunculus in dystonia of the hand. *Ann Neurol* 1998;44:828–831.

198. Sanger TD, Merzenich MM. Computational model of the role of sensory disorganization in focal task-specific dystonia. *J Neurophysiol* 2000;84:2458–2464.

199. Elbert T, Heim S. A light and a dark side. *Nature* 2001;411:139.

200. Eidelberg D, Moeller JR, Ishikawa T, et al. The metabolic topography of idiopathic torsion dystonia. *Brain* 1995;118: 1473–1484.
201. Hashimoto T, Tada T, Nakazato F, et al. Abnormal activity in the globus pallidus in off-period dystonia. *Ann Neurol* 2001;49: 242–245.
202. Vitek JL, Chockkan V, Zhang J-Y, et al. Neuronal activity in the basal ganglia in patients with generalized dystonia and hemiballism. *Ann Neurol* 1999;46:22–35.
203. Ondo WG, Desaloms M, Jankovic J, et al. Surgical pallidotomy for the treatment of generalized dystonia. *Mov Disord* 1998;13: 693–698.
204. Krauss JK, Loher TJ, Pohle T, et al. Pallidal deep brain stimulation in patients with cervical dystonia and sever cervical dyskinesias with cervical myelopathy. *J Neurol Neurosurg Psychiatry* 2002;72:249–256.
205. Lehéricy S, Vidailhet M, Dormont D, et al. Striatopallidal and thalamic dystonia: a magnetic resonance imaging anatomoclinical study. *Arch Neurol* 1996;53:241–250.
206. Black KJ, Öngür D, Perlmutter JS. Putamen volume in idiopathic focal dystonia. *Neurology* 1998;51:819–824.
207. Perlmutter JS, Stambuk MK, Markham J, et al. Decreased [18F]spiperone binding in putamen in idiopathic focal dystonia. *Neuroscience* 1997;17:843–850.
208. Levy LM, Hallett M. Impaired brain GABA in focal dystonia. *Ann Neurol* 2002;51:93–101.
209. Hornykiewicz O, Kish SJ, Becker LE, et al. Brain neurotransmitters in dystonia musculorum deformans. *N Engl J Med* 1986;315: 347–353.
210. Jankovic J, Svendsen CN, Bird ED. Brain neurotransmitters in dystonia. *N Engl J Med* 1987;316:278–279.
211. Becker G, Berg D, Rausch W-D, et al. Increased tissue copper and manganese content in the lentiform nucleus in primary adult-onset dystonia. *Ann Neurol* 1999;46:260–263.
212. Richter A, Löscher W. Pathophysiology of idiopathic dystonia: findings from genetic animal models. *Progr Neurobiol* 1998;54: 633–677.
213. Mitchell IJ, Luquin R, Boyce S, et al. Neural mechanisms of dystonia: evidence from a 2-deoxyglucose uptake study in a primate model of dopamine agonist-induced dystonia. *Mov Disord* 1990;5:49–54.
214. Boyce S, Rupniak NMJ, Steventon MJ, et al. Differential effects of D1 and D2 agonists in MPTP-treated primates: functional implications for Parkinson's disease. *Neurology* 1990;40: 927–933.
215. Palfi S, Leventhal L, Goetz CG, et al. Delayed onset of progressive dystonia following subacute 3-nitroprionic acid treatment in Cebus apella monkeys. *Mov Disord* 2000;15: 524–530.
216. Murinson BB. Stiff-man syndrome: GABA, GAD, and mechanisms of disease. *Neuroscientist* 2000;6:147–150.
217. Shashidharan P, Paris N, Sandu D, et al. Overexpression of torsinA in PC12 cells protects against toxicity. *J Neurochem* 2004;88:1019–1025.
218. Goodchild RE, Kim CE, Dauer WT. Loss of the dystonia-associated protein torsinA selectively disrupts the neuronal nuclear envelope. *Neuron* 2005;48:923–932.

Treatment of Dystonia

26

Stacy Horn   Cynthia L. Comella

Dystonia is a central nervous system (CNS) disorder that causes excessive, sustained muscular contractions of both agonist and antagonist muscles. The sustained contractions cause repetitive twisting movements that may be fast or slow. Dystonia is often aggravated by activity, and the sustained muscular contractions may cause pain. Treatment for dystonia is required when functional or social impairment occurs. The treatment strategies for dystonia include pharmacological and nonpharmacological means and are directed to the type of dystonia present. The pathophysiology of dystonia is incompletely understood and has made the creation of therapeutic options difficult.

TREATMENT

Treatment strategies are varied and include oral medication, chemodenervation, surgical approaches, limb immobilization and orthosis, and physical therapy. The most effective treatment for secondary dystonia is to focus on the underlying etiologic factor, but standard symptomatic treatment regimens may be effective when necessary. Management of dystonia can be difficult. Medical therapy may be effective for generalized, hemisegmental, focal, or tardive dystonias. Patients do not consistently respond to one type of therapy, and multiple strategies may be necessary before an effective therapy can be found. The most common medical therapies for dystonia are listed with their typical dosages in Table 26.1. Each of these therapies is detailed in the following sections. An algorithm of treatment options is provided in Figure 26.1.

ORAL MEDICATIONS

Anticholinergic medications constitute the only class of drugs assessed in controlled clinical trials of dystonia and have been found to be effective for the treatment of dystonia (1). The first beneficial reports of anticholinergic medications in dystonia were reported 30 years ago (2). Since that time, anticholinergic medications have often been used. Anticholinergic medications are often the first choice of medical therapy used in adults and the second medication trial in most children and adolescents, after levodopa. When high doses of anticholinergic agents were used, beneficial responses were observed. Although children tolerated these high doses without significant side effect, adults treated with higher doses frequently experienced intolerable side effects (2).

Anticholinergic medications were shown to be effective in one double-blind prospective crossover trial. In this study, 31 patients with mostly generalized primary or secondary dystonia and a mean age of 19 years were studied using trihexyphenidyl in dosages up to 30 mg/day. Twenty-two patients had clinical improvement in their dystonia using the Fahn-Marsden scale (3). The adverse effects in this younger patient group were mostly mild and transient, limiting upward escalation of dosing in only 4 patients. It was the older patients in this study who experienced dose-limiting memory loss. The side effects of the anticholinergic medications are problematic and are best managed by initiating treatment with a low dose with a gradual upward titration until benefit or intolerable adverse effects occur. In children, it is frequently possible to reach the high dose of anticholinergic medications in those patients in whom benefit is most likely to occur. Fahn has noted that the majority of patients need a minimum of 40 mg/day of trihexyphenidyl for clinical

TABLE 26.1

FREQUENTLY USED ORAL MEDICATIONS IN THE MANAGEMENT OF DYSTONIA

Medication	Typical Starting Dosage (mg/day)	Typical Therapeutic Dosage (mg/day)
Trihexyphenidyl	1–2	Up to 120
Benztropine	0.5–1	Up to 8
Baclofen	5–10	Up to 120
Clonazepam	0.5–1	Up to 5
Levodopa	100	Up to 800
Tetrabenazine	25	Up to 75

response (4), although children may require dosages of trihexyphenidyl up to 120 mg/day. Open-label trials of anticholinergic medications in adults and children confirmed this clinical suspicion (4). Anticholinergic medications are effective in approximately 50% of children and 40% of adults (4). A retrospective study of 358 dystonia patients treated with anticholinergic medications found that 43% had a good response and that younger patients fared better. Furthermore, these investigators observed that patients treated within 5 years of the onset of their illness were more likely to have a clinical response than were patients treated after 5 years of illness (5). Patients with mild dystonia were found to have a better response to anticholinergic medications than patients

with severe disease, such as those who are wheelchair bound (6). No differences in response could be found in terms of gender. Cross-sectional observations have shown that the therapeutic response to anticholinergic medications did not differ in patients with primary dystonia or with secondary dystonia. Therapeutic response to anticholinergic therapy is thought to wane over time. A retrospective study showing a good initial therapeutic response waned after 15 months, although therapeutic response lasted a median of 38 months in childhood onset dystonia (5). Side effects of anticholinergic medications include memory loss, dry mouth, confusion, hallucinations, exacerbation of acute angle glaucoma, and sedation.

The muscle relaxant *baclofen* may be useful for generalized, hemisegmental, segmental, focal, or tardive dystonia. Baclofen, an agonist of GABA, is thought to work through binding of the l isomer to the $GABA_B$ presynaptic receptor, inhibiting calcium influx and reducing the release of the excitatory transmitters glutamate and aspartate (7). In a retrospective chart review of 358 patients treated for dystonia, 108 patients were treated with baclofen, and 20% had a good therapeutic response. The daily dose of baclofen ranged from 25 mg to 120 mg, with an average daily dose of 82 mg. There was no difference in therapeutic response between familial and nonfamilial cases of dystonia. Patients with blepharospasm had the best response to baclofen when all regional body distributions of dystonia

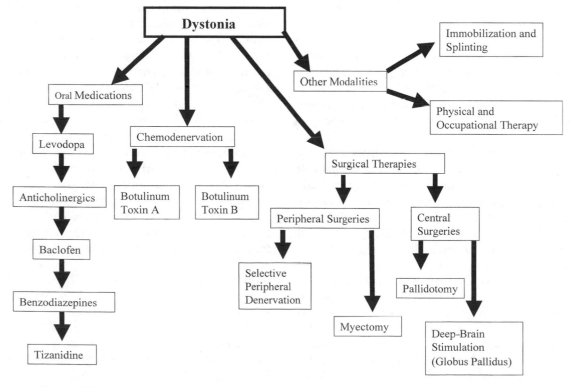

Figure 26.1 Algorithm of options for treatment of dystonia.

were taken into account. In contrast to the anticholinergic agents, duration of illness prior to institution of therapy did not affect outcome of treatment with baclofen; neither did gender or ethnic background. Patients with an onset of dystonia in adulthood displayed a better response to baclofen than patients with an onset of dystonia in childhood (5). In general, baclofen is less effective than anticholinergic medications for managing dystonia (1). In other retrospective studies, 13% of patients with generalized dystonia were found to have a good therapeutic response to baclofen (8). As with the anticholinergic drugs, baclofen is best tolerated when started at low doses and optimized to therapeutic response or untoward side effects. The combination of baclofen and anticholinergics may be more effective for controlling the symptoms of dystonia than either drug alone (9). The side-effect profile of baclofen includes sedation, weakness, and memory loss. If baclofen is to be stopped, it must be slowly withdrawn as serious withdrawal effects, including seizures and encephalopathy, may occur with abrupt discontinuation.

Benzodiazepines may be useful for generalized, hemisegmental, segmental, focal, or tardive dystonia. These medications are thought to work through the enhancement of GABA in the CNS. There are many choices of medications in this class, but the most commonly used is clonazepam because of its long half-life. Benzodiazepines may effectively treat dystonias, but they are generally found to be less effective than anticholinergics or baclofen. It has been suggested that benzodiazepines are most efficacious for management of secondary dystonias (5). The typical effective dosage for clonazepam is 2.5–12 mg/day. No differences were found in treatment responses among ethnic groups or genders. Age of onset of dystonia did not affect treatment outcomes (8). The major side effects of benzodiazepines include sedation and memory loss. When used in combination, the effects and side effects of these medications may be additive. If administered chronically, these medications should be discontinued slowly to prevent withdrawal. Sudden withdrawal of benzodiazepines can potentially cause seizures.

Levodopa is an effective agent for the treatment of dopa-responsive dystonia in which small doses may provide almost complete relief of symptoms for prolonged periods. Dopa-responsive dystonia is a childhood- or adolescent-onset dystonia associated with parkinsonism and diurnal fluctuations. These patients have a deficiency of tyrosine hydroxylase and have a dramatic and sustained response to levodopa therapy, with an average dosage of 500–1,000 mg/day. Levodopa is frequently used as a first-line therapy in cases of childhood- and adolescent-onset dystonia because a small percentage of these patients will have dopa-responsive dystonia. Full benefit from levodopa has been reported to occur within days of initiation of treatment. Minor abnormalities of gait may persist after levodopa administration, but most patients will achieve a marked improvement in symptoms (10). Levodopa is

generally well tolerated, with nausea being the most frequent but often transient side effect.

Dopamine agonists also have been used in the management of dystonia. Dopamine agonists have been studied in a double-blind crossover trial in 8 patients with cervical dystonia. The results of this study did not show statistically significant improvement in the treatment group as compared with placebo. Three patients had improvement while taking a dopamine agonist, but only 2 patients had sustained improvement for more than a year. No consistent patient demographics could identify responders to this therapy. The major side effects of the dopamine agonists include nausea, orthostasis, confusion, delusions, hallucinations, drowsiness, and memory impairment (11).

Dopamine receptor antagonists have been found to be of benefit in approximately 35% of patients assessed retrospectively, but the possibility of causing tardive dyskinesia with long-term use of these agents strongly deters physicians from prescribing them. Tetrabenazine is a monoamine-depleting and dopamine receptor–blocking medication that has been used effectively to treat a variety of movement disorders. This medication has not been approved by the U.S. Food and Drug Administration but is available in Canada and Europe. Tetrabenazine has been used in patients with focal, segmental, generalized, and tardive dystonia, and it has been shown in one small double-blind crossover study to be useful for dystonia. In that study, 12 patients with dystonia were treated with tetrabenazine or placebo. Each patient was treated for 3 or more weeks at a maximal dosage of 200 mg/day. Nine patients had clinical improvement in their dystonia (12). A subsequent study assessed the longitudinal effects of tetrabenazine on dystonia and showed that of 201 patients with idiopathic and tardive dystonia treated for 2 to 3 years, 45.4% of primary dystonia patients and 73% of tardive dystonia patients had benefit, albeit mild, during long-term therapy. The therapeutic dose range was 25–75 mg/day. The major side effects seen with tetrabenazine included depression, sedation, parkinsonism, orthostatic hypotension, insomnia, and akathisia (13).

Clozapine has been studied in open-label fashion in small numbers of patients with focal, generalized, and tardive dystonia. Clozapine is an atypical, centrally acting dopaminergic blocking medication associated with minimal occurrence of drug-induced parkinsonism and no reports of tardive dyskinesia. Clozapine has affinity for multiple receptors, including H1, muscarinic, 5-HT$_2$, 5-HT$_3$, α_1-adrenergic, α_2-adrenergic, D1, D2, and D5. The probable mechanism of efficacy of clozapine is the blockade of D1 receptors. The blockade of D1 receptors may reduce the relative overactivity of the direct pathway that occurs in dystonia (14). One study of 5 patients found a 30% improvement in their clinical symptoms using the Fahn-Marsden scale. Patients began to experience clinical improvement after 3 weeks of therapy. Patients experienced clinical benefit after taking 75–400 mg/day (15).

In contrast, an open-label trial of 10 patients with dystonia failed to show clinically statistical benefit with 100 mg/day of clozapine (16). The discrepancy between studies may be due to dosage differences. A controlled study is needed to evaluate the usefulness of this drug. The side effects of clozapine include life-threatening neutropenia requiring weekly complete blood counts, orthostatic hypotension, sedation, and seizures.

Other oral medications include tizanidine, which has not been extensively studied in dystonia but may be helpful in some patients. Tizanidine is a centrally acting potent noradrenergic α_2-receptor agonist. This chemical causes direct impairment of excitatory amino acid release from spinal interneurons and a concomitant inhibition of the facilitatory ceruleo-spinal pathways (17). Ten patients with cranial dystonia were studied in an open-label single-blind study using dosages of 28–36 mg/day. Five patients did not complete the trial due to untoward side effects. Of the 5 patients who completed the trial, 2 patients had unsustained benefit and 3 patients had no benefit. Tizanidine was found to be ineffective for managing cranial dystonia in this small trial. Side effects were common in this study and included sedation, orthostasis, dry mouth, weakness, nausea, and skin rash. A large-scale double-blind trial is needed to help ascertain the effectiveness of tizanidine in dystonia. Other oral medications that have been suggested in anecdotal case series to improve dystonia include gabapentin, cyclobenzaprine, and carbamazepine (18). Overall, there is insufficient evidence and a lack of controlled trials for most oral treatments for dystonia.

CHEMICAL DENERVATION

The localized paralytic effects of botulinum toxin have been useful in controlling the clinical symptoms of dystonia. Botulinum toxin is the product of *Clostridium botulinum*, an anaerobic bacteria, that is purified and injected into affected muscles. There are 7 serotypes of botulinum toxin: A through G. Only 2 strains are commercially available for clinical use: types A and B. The first clinical use of botulinum toxin was for strabismus in 1980. Botulinum toxin therapy is useful for treating focal and segmental dystonia. It also can be useful in generalized dystonia if focal areas are resistant to medications or if there are localized painful muscle spasms. Botulinum toxin therapy does not alter the underlying CNS dysfunction but weakens overactive muscles that cause the involuntary movements, disability, pain, and dystonia. Botulinum toxin binds to receptor sites on the presynaptic cholinergic terminals and is internalized into the nerve ending. Once internalized, the toxin inhibits the exocytosis of acetylcholine (19). The mechanism of action of botulinum toxin is the presynaptic enzymatic cleavage of intracellular proteins responsible for membrane fusion. By interrupting the cascade of protein interactions, the vesicle membranes cannot fuse with the presynaptic membrane to release the vesicle-sequestered acetylcholine. The lack of acetylcholine in the neuromuscular junction results in a chemical denervation of the muscle (20). Botulinum toxin serotype A as BOTOX or Dysport was the only commercially available toxin until 2000, when botulinum toxin type B, Myobloc, was approved for clinical use. Most clinical experience has, therefore, been with serotype A. Clinical effect is typically seen within one week after injection, peaking at 2 to 4 weeks after injection and lasting approximately 3 to 4 months (19). Botulinum toxin is a foreign protein and may serve as an antigen. In some patients, this may lead to the development of neutralizing antibodies and resistance to the effects of the toxin.

Botulinum toxin type A has been assessed in randomized, double-blind, placebo-controlled trials for cervical dystonia and blepharospasm. One of the early controlled studies was completed with 55 cervical dystonia patients and showed that botulinum toxin was superior to placebo with 61% of treated patients having clinical improvement (21). Several subsequent trials have demonstrated similar improvement following botulinum toxin in various forms of dystonia (22–25). Currently, botulinum toxin is considered the treatment of choice for many focal dystonias, including blepharospasm, oromandibular dystonia, spasmodic dysphonia, and cervical dystonia (19). Although effective for the treatment of limb and occupational dystonias, these disorders do not respond as well, likely because of the weakness of muscles involved in fine motor movements. Botulinum toxin type A has been compared to trihexyphenidyl in a double-blind trial for cervical dystonia. This study showed the superiority of botulinum toxin injections over the most efficacious oral medication for cervical dystonia (26). Botulinum toxin injections when administered with the correct dosage in the appropriate muscles are generally well tolerated without any significant systemic effects. The most frequent side effects of botulinum toxin therapy include pain and bruising at the injection site, weakness, dysphagia, and a flu-like syndrome following injection. The expense of this therapy and the need to administer toxin at 3- to 4-month intervals, as well as the availability of skilled practitioners, are drawbacks of this treatment.

Botulinum toxin type B is a serotype that has been used in the management of cervical dystonia. The first study of botulinum toxin type B included 109 patients with botulinum type A responsiveness in a randomized, double-blind, placebo-controlled trial. This trial showed statistically significant clinical improvement in patients treated with botulinum toxin type B over placebo (27). Botulinum toxin type B therapy was also studied in cervical dystonia patients with type A resistance. This study included 77 patients and again showed statistically significant improvement in clinical dystonia over placebo. The clinical effect of botulinum toxin type B was 12 to 16 weeks. The main side effects of botulinum toxin type B include dry mouth, weakness, dysphagia, and pain at the injection site (28).

Both types of botulinum toxin have been proven effective for controlling cervical dystonia. A randomized, double-blind trial of botulinum toxin types A and B in 139 subjects with cervical dystonia using Toronto Western Spasmodic Torticollis Scale (TWSTRS) as a primary measure showed that both strains were equally effective at 4 weeks (29). The rate of side effects was increased in the botulinum toxin type B group, especially dry mouth and dysphagia. Botulinum toxin type A lasted longer than botulinum toxin type B: 14 weeks versus 12 weeks. In the future, other strains of botulinum toxin may be studied to help control the symptoms of dystonia.

SURGICAL THERAPY

Surgical therapies for dystonia are available when medical therapies are inadequate. Surgical therapies include peripheral procedures and CNS procedures. These procedures are listed in Table 26.2.

Peripheral surgeries have been useful primarily in blepharospasm and cervical dystonia. Patients with cervical dystonia who have developed botulinum toxin resistance or whose symptoms cannot be controlled with medication may benefit from peripheral surgical procedures. Peripheral surgical procedures include rhizotomy, ramisectomy, and myotomy. Rhizotomies and ramisectomies address cervical dystonia by selectively denervating and weakening the overactive musculature. Myotomies attempt to control symptoms of dystonia by partial sectioning of selected muscles. These therapies were employed more frequently prior to the clinical use of botulinum toxin therapy. A retrospective chart review of 58 patients with rhizotomies for cervical dystonia showed that 85% had marked improvement in their clinical condition (30,31). A long-term follow-up study of 46 patients with staged, selected peripheral surgical procedures, including rhizotomy, ramisectomy, and myotomy were studied. These patients were followed for an average of 6.5 years postoperatively and

TABLE 26.2
SURGICAL THERAPIES IN DYSTONIA

Peripheral Surgical Procedures
Rhizotomy
Ramisectomy
Myotomy
Intrathecal baclofen

CNS Ablative Procedures
Pallidotomy
Thalamotomy

Deep-Brain Stimulation Procedures
Globus pallidus pars interna stimulation
Ventrolateral thalamic stimulation

assessed using TWSTRS. Forty-eight percent of patients achieved an excellent long-term outcome, and 42% of patients had a moderate to mild long-term response to peripheral surgical therapies for cervical dystonia (32). The risks of these procedures include paralysis of arm elevation, neck weakness, and dysphagia.

Peripheral surgical procedures for blepharospasm have included selective nerve avulsions (33) and myectomy (34). These have been variably successful, often giving rise to a cosmetically unappealing result. Recently, muscle graft augmentation after protractor myectomy has shown good results in an open-label report (35). Doxorubicin is also under investigation as a treatment for blepharospasm, but the safety of this procedure requires further evaluation (36).

Another surgical procedure used for the management of intractable generalized dystonia is intrathecal baclofen. In this procedure, a reservoir with a pump is implanted in the subcutaneous tissue and baclofen is pumped into the intrathecal space via a catheter. Although intrathecal baclofen is effective for lower-limb spasticity, its effects on primary dystonia have been discouraging. There are additional anecdotal reports of success in small numbers of patients (30,31,37). A recent large case series showed benefit in 77 generalized dystonia patients that persisted for more than 2 years, but 38% had surgical complications and 26% had adverse effects (38). In contrast, a retrospective study of 25 patients with severe segmental or generalized dystonia failed to show statistically significant clinical improvement using blinded evaluators of videotapes before and after implantation of an intrathecal baclofen pump (39). This was also seen in another retrospective trial with blinded evaluators of 14 patients with primary and secondary dystonia receiving intrathecal baclofen (40). The risks of this procedure include overdosage, respiratory depression, pump malfunction, programming errors, infection, and catheter breakage. Other drawbacks include the lack of general availability and expense.

Central nervous system surgeries have been utilized in dystonia for many years. These therapies are typically reserved for patients who fail medical therapy. CNS surgical procedures for dystonia were found incidentally in the late 1950s when it was noticed that ablative surgery improved dystonia in Parkinson's disease (PD) patients (41). Ablative procedures involve making lesions in specific areas of the brain. Thalamotomy was the first CNS procedure to show favorable results. Targeted nuclei within the thalamus have included the ventral intermedius, the posterior ventromedial, and the posterior ventrolateral. Initial reports indicated a moderate to marked clinical improvement in 70% of patients. Subsequent studies have failed to reproduce these findings. One study of 16 generalized dystonia patients showed benefit in only 4 (42) and residual dysarthria or hemiparesis in a significant percentage of those who underwent thalamotomy. A prospective study that included 56 dystonia patients showed that only

34% of patients had 50% improvement in their clinical symptoms (43). This improvement was most prominent in distal limbs and did not change midline symptoms. The complications of bilateral thalamotomy include dysarthria, hemiparesis, pseudobulbar palsy, ataxia, paresthesias, and personality changes. Improvement of dystonic symptoms in patients with PD following pallidotomy prompted clinical trials in dystonia. A small open-label study in 8 generalized dystonia patients showed marked clinical benefit in 6 and mild to moderate improvement in 2 (44). These patients had improvement immediately following surgery and continued to improve over the next 3 months with a 62% change in dystonia scores. Adverse events were mild and included transient weakness. A comparison of thalamotomy and pallidotomy in patients with dystonia suggested that the globus pallidus was a better target, with improved outcome over thalamotomy (45).

More recently, deep-brain stimulator implantation into the globus pallidus has been investigated for dystonia. The technique involves the bilateral implantation of microelectrode stimulating wires into the globus pallidus. The wires from the electrodes are burrowed under the skin and connected to pacemakers placed in the subcutaneous tissues of the upper chest or abdomen. The pacemaker is programmed until symptom control is achieved. Multiple case series were reported to show benefit in patients with generalized dystonia and cervical dystonia (46). Benefit appeared to be sustained for at least 2 years (47–50). This procedure was shown to be most effective in patients with primary dystonia and of minimal benefit to those with secondary dystonia (51). Recently, a double-blinded controlled study of bilateral pallidal stimulation was reported in 22 patients with generalized dystonia. This study confirmed that bilateral deep-brain stimulation was an effective treatment with an acceptable safety profile for dystonia (52). There has been controversy over which operation should be performed in dystonia: ablation or deep-brain stimulation. Each procedure has its advantages and disadvantages. The advantages of ablative procedures include a less intensive follow-up period and a reduced cost. The drawbacks of ablative procedures include destruction of brain tissue and a high incidence of side effects with bilateral procedures, including dysarthria, dysphagia, and pseudobulbar palsy. The advantages of deep-brain stimulation include preservation of brain tissue and the opportunity to perform bilateral procedures. The drawbacks of this procedure include the need for an experienced surgeon and programmer, the cost of the procedure and the equipment, the need for battery changes almost annually, and the frequent adjustments to the programming, in addition to the possibility of equipment malfunction, lead breakage, and infection. Both ablative and microelectrode stimulation procedures may cause intracranial hemorrhage, hemiparesis, and cognitive changes.

IMMOBILIZATION AND ORTHOTIC THERAPIES

Prolonged limb immobilization in the management of focal upper-extremity dystonia has been investigated. Eight patients with medically resistant idiopathic focal dystonia were studied in an open-label fashion with focal splinting of the affected limb for 4 to 5 weeks. Each patient underwent 6 assessments for severity of dystonia and objective motor performance using the Arm Dystonia Disability Scale, the Tubiana and Chamagne Score, and subjective improvement using the Self-Rating Score. Each patient was studied at baseline, during the immobilization, and following the immobilization. The longest follow-up was 12 months. This study found that at 24 weeks 3 patients had a moderate objective improvement and 4 patients had marked objective improvement (53). The proposed mechanism for efficacy involves the pathophysiologic changes that occur in focal upper-extremity dystonia. These changes include enlargement and smearing of the cortical areas representing the affected muscles (54–57). Immobilization may promote inactivity-dependent plastic changes in the overrepresented cortical areas and thus help to restore normal cortical representation (58). These initial results are promising, but additional large-scale studies are needed to confirm these results. The major side effect experienced with limb immobilization is muscular weakness following removal of the splint that gradually improves with activity.

A second series of case reports describes the usefulness of orthotic devices in the treatment of idiopathic writer's cramp. In each of 5 patients, a thermoplastic hand orthosis designed to substitute the use of distal musculature for more proximal musculature was constructed for each patient. Reportedly, adaptation to the device was easily achieved and improved the handwriting in each of the 5 patients. It was also reported that patients had immediate reoccurrence of their symptoms when writing without the orthosis (59). Further investigations are necessary to confirm the efficacy of hand orthosis for writer's cramp.

ADJUNCT THERAPIES

Physical and occupational therapy can be helpful adjuncts to treatment. A recent hypothesis is that occupational dystonia may arise secondary to aberrant learning and performance of motor tasks. Specific therapy to retrain motor activities has been beneficial in descriptive series (60) and is being investigated in ongoing clinical trials.

Physical therapy also can be beneficial to help with gait, transfers, strengthening, and stretching to prevent contractures. Physical therapy can help patients to understand their limitations and to set goals. Physical therapy also teaches patients how to live safely with their disabilities.

Occupational therapy can be helpful in identifying devices to assist patients with dystonia. These devices allow patients to regain some of their independence and to perform tasks that otherwise would have been impossible.

FUTURE PERSPECTIVES

The development of imaging techniques that allow direct assessments of brain interactions and networks and the development of animal models for dystonia will enhance the understanding of the pathophysiologic mechanisms of dystonia. Genetic identification of different forms of dystonia also has enhanced our understanding of specific disease processes. As more of these genetic forms with their abnormal gene products are elucidated, our understanding of the pathophysiology of this disease will increase. A greater understanding of the underlying pathophysiology of dystonia will facilitate the creation of new medications and therapeutic modalities. New surgical techniques have allowed treatment of refractory generalized dystonia without destruction of brain tissue. On the horizon are such treatment strategies as gene therapy and stem cell research. The treatment of dystonia is likely to undergo important advances as these scientific advances are applied in this area.

REFERENCES

1. Bressman SB. Dystonia update. *Clin Neuropharmacol* 2000;23: 239–251.
2. Fahn S. High-dosage anticholinergic therapy in dystonia. *Adv Neurol* 1983;37:177–188.
3. Burke RE, Fahn S, Marsden CD. Torsion dystonia: a double-blind, prospective trial of high-dosage trihexyphenidyl. *Neurology* 1986;36:160–164.
4. Fahn S. Generalized dystonia: concept and treatment. *Clin Neuropharmacol* 1986;9(suppl 2):S37–S48.
5. Greene P, Shale H, Fahn S. Experience with high dosages of anticholinergic and other drugs in the treatment of torsion dystonia. *Adv Neurol* 1988;50:547–556.
6. Burke RE, Fahn S. Double-blind evaluation of trihexyphenidyl in dystonia. *Adv Neurol* 1983;37:189–192.
7. Davidoff RA. Antispasticity drugs: mechanisms of action. *Ann Neurol* 1985;17:107–116.
8. Greene P, Shale H, Fahn S. Analysis of open-label trials in torsion dystonia using high dosages of anticholinergics and other drugs. *Mov Disord* 1988;3:46–60.
9. Greene P. Baclofen in the treatment of dystonia. *Clin Neuropharmacol* 1992;15:276–288.
10. Nygaard TG, Trugman JM, de Yebenes JG, Fahn S. Dopa-responsive dystonia: the spectrum of clinical manifestations in a large North American family. *Neurology* 1990;40:66–69.
11. Teravainen H, Calne S, Burton K, Beckman J, Calne DB. Efficacy of dopamine agonists in dystonia. *Adv Neurol* 1988;50:571–578.
12. Jankovic J. Treatment of hyperkinetic movement disorders with tetrabenazine: a double-blind crossover study. *Ann Neurol* 1982;11:41–7.
13. Jankovic J, Beach J. Long-term effects of tetrabenazine in hyperkinetic movement disorders. *Neurology* 1997;48: 358–362.
14. Trugman JM, Leadbetter R, Zalis ME, Burgdorf RO, Wooten GF. Treatment of severe axial tardive dystonia with clozapine: case report and hypothesis. *Mov Disord* 1994;9:441–446.
15. Karp BI, Goldstein SR, Chen R, Samii A, Bara-Jimenez W, Hallett M. An open trial of clozapine for dystonia. *Mov Disord* 1999;14: 652–657.
16. Burbaud P, Guehl D, Lagueny A, Petiteau F, Bioulac B. A pilot trial of clozapine in the treatment of cervical dystonia. *J Neurol* 1998;245:329–331.
17. Coward DM. Tizanidine: neuropharmacology and mechanism of action. *Neurology* 1994;44(suppl 9):S6–S10; discussion S10–S11.
18. Jankovic J. Dystonia: medical therapy and botulinum toxin. *Adv Neurol* 2004;94:275–286.
19. Jankovic J. Botulinum toxin in clinical practice. *J Neurol Neurosurg Psychiatry* 2004;75:951–957.
20. Comella CL, Pullman SL. Botulinum toxins in neurological disease. *Muscle Nerve* 2004;29:628–644.
21. Greene P, Kang U, Fahn S, Brin M, Moskowitz C, Flaster E. Double-blind, placebo-controlled trial of botulinum toxin injections for the treatment of spasmodic torticollis. *Neurology* 1990;40:1213–1218.
22. Lu CS, Chen RS, Tsai CH. Double-blind, placebo-controlled study of botulinum toxin injections in the treatment of cervical dystonia. *J Formos Med Assoc* 1995;94:189–192.
23. Moore AP, Blumhardt LD. A double blind trial of botulinum toxin "A" in torticollis, with one year follow up. *J Neurol Neurosurg Psychiatry* 1991;54:813–816.
24. Gelb DJ, Lowenstein DH, Aminoff MJ. Controlled trial of botulinum toxin injections in the treatment of spasmodic torticollis. *Neurology* 1989;39:80–84.
25. Cole R, Hallett M, Cohen LG. Double-blind trial of botulinum toxin for treatment of focal hand dystonia. *Mov Disord* 1995;10:466–471.
26. Brans JW, Lindeboom R, Snoek JW, et al. Botulinum toxin versus trihexyphenidyl in cervical dystonia: a prospective, randomized, double-blind controlled trial. *Neurology* 1996;46: 1066–1072.
27. Brashear A, Lew MF, Dykstra DD, et al. Safety and efficacy of NeuroBloc (botulinum toxin type B) in type A-responsive cervical dystonia. *Neurology* 1999;53:1439–1446.
28. Brin MF, Lew MF, Adler CH, et al. Safety and efficacy of NeuroBloc (botulinum toxin type B) in type A-resistant cervical dystonia. *Neurology* 1999;53:1431–1438.
29. The Dystonia Study Group. A randomized, double-blind study comparing botulinum toxin serotypes A and B for the treatment of cervical dystonia. *Neurology* 2005;65:1423–1429.
30. Friedman AH, Nashold BS, Jr., Sharp R, Caputi F, Arruda J. Treatment of spasmodic torticollis with intradural selective rhizotomies. *J Neurosurg* 1993;78:46–53.
31. Krauss JK, Koller R, Burgunder JM. Partial myotomy/myectomy of the trapezius muscle with an asleep-awake-asleep anesthetic technique for treatment of cervical dystonia. Technical note. *J Neurosurg* 1999;91:889–891.
32. Krauss JK, Toups EG, Jankovic J, Grossman RG. Symptomatic and functional outcome of surgical treatment of cervical dystonia. *J Neurol Neurosurg Psychiatry* 1997;63: 642–648.
33. Fante RG, Frueh BR. Differential section of the seventh nerve as a tertiary procedure for the treatment of benign essential blepharospasm. *Ophthal Plast Reconstr Surg* 2001;17:276–280.
34. Bettez M, Lavertu P. Periorbital myectomy for essential blepharospasm. *J Otolaryngol* 1986;15:306–309.
35. Yen MT, Anderson RL, Small RG. Orbicularis oculi muscle graft augmentation after protractor myectomy in blepharospasm. *Ophthal Plast Reconstr Surg* 2003;19:287–296.
36. Wirtschafter JD, McLoon LK. Long-term efficacy of local doxorubicin chemomyectomy in patients with blepharospasm and hemifacial spasm. *Ophthalmology* 1998;105: 342–346.
37. Diederich NJ, Comella CL, Matge G, Becker G, Schiltz F, Metz H. Sustained effect of high-dose intrathecal baclofen in primary generalized dystonia: a 2-year follow-up study. *Mov Disord* 1997;12:1100–1102.
38. Albright AL, Barry MJ, Shafton DH, Ferson SS. Intrathecal baclofen for generalized dystonia. *Dev Med Child Neurol* 2001;43:652–657.

39. Ford B, Greene P, Louis ED, et al. Use of intrathecal baclofen in the treatment of patients with dystonia. *Arch Neurol* 1996;53: 1241–1246.

40. Walker RH, Danisi FO, Swope DM, Goodman RR, Germano IM, Brin MF. Intrathecal baclofen for dystonia: benefits and complications during six years of experience. *Mov Disord* 2000;15:1242–1247.

41. Cooper IS. 20-year followup study of the neurosurgical treatment of dystonia musculorum deformans. *Adv Neurol* 1976;14:423–452.

42. Andrew J, Fowler CJ, Harrison MJ. Stereotaxic thalamotomy in 55 cases of dystonia. *Brain* 1983;106(pt 4):981–1000.

43. Yamashiro K, Tasker RR. Stereotactic thalamotomy for dystonic patients. *Stereotact Funct Neurosurg* 1993;60:81–85.

44. Ondo WG, Desaloms JM, Jankovic J, Grossman RG. Pallidotomy for generalized dystonia. *Mov Disord* 1998;13:693–698.

45. Yoshor D, Hamilton WJ, Ondo W, Jankovic J, Grossman RG. Comparison of thalamotomy and pallidotomy for the treatment of dystonia. *Neurosurgery* 2001;48:818–824; discussion 824–826.

46. Katayama Y, Fukaya C, Kobayashi K, Oshima H, Yamamoto T. Chronic stimulation of the globus pallidus internus for control of primary generalized dystonia. *Acta Neurochir Suppl* 2003;87: 125–128.

47. Coubes P, Cif L, El Fertit H, et al. Electrical stimulation of the globus pallidus internus in patients with primary generalized dystonia: long-term results. *J Neurosurg* 2004;101: 189–194.

48. Krauss JK, Loher TJ, Weigel R, Capelle HH, Weber S, Burgunder JM. Chronic stimulation of the globus pallidus internus for treatment of non-dYT1 generalized dystonia and choreoathetosis: 2-year follow up. *J Neurosurg* 2003;98:785–792.

49. Vitek JL, Zhang J, Evatt M, et al. GPi pallidotomy for dystonia: clinical outcome and neuronal activity. *Adv Neurol* 1998;78:211–219.

50. Bittar RG, Yianni J, Wang S, et al. Deep brain stimulation for generalised dystonia and spasmodic torticollis. *J Clin Neurosci* 2005;12:12–16.

51. Eltahawy HA, Saint-Cyr J, Giladi N, Lang AE, Lozano AM. Primary dystonia is more responsive than secondary dystonia to pallidal interventions: outcome after pallidotomy or pallidal deep brain stimulation. *Neurosurgery* 2004;54:613–619; discussion 619–621.

52. Vidailhet M, Vercueil L, Houeto JL, et al. Bilateral deep-brain stimulation of the globus pallidus in primary generalized dystonia. *N Engl J Med* 2005;352:459–467.

53. Priori A, Pesenti A, Cappellari A, Scarlato G, Barbieri S. Limb immobilization for the treatment of focal occupational dystonia. *Neurology* 2001;57:405–409.

54. Thickbroom GW, Byrnes ML, Stell R, Mastaglia FL. Reversible reorganisation of the motor cortical representation of the hand in cervical dystonia. *Mov Disord* 2003;18:395–402.

55. Byrnes ML, Mastaglia FL, Walters SE, Archer SA, Thickbroom GW. Primary writing tremor: motor cortex reorganisation and disinhibition. *J Clin Neurosci* 2005;12:102–104.

56. Pujol J, Roset-Llobet J, Rosines-Cubells D, et al. Brain cortical activation during guitar-induced hand dystonia studied by functional MRI. *Neuroimage* 2000;12:257–267.

57. Elbert T, Rockstroh B. Reorganization of human cerebral cortex: the range of changes following use and injury. *Neuroscientist* 2004;10:129–141.

58. Liepert J, Tegenthoff M, Malin JP. Changes of cortical motor area size during immobilization. *Electroencephalogr Clin Neurophysiol* 1995;97:382–386.

59. Tas N, Karatas GK, Sepici V. Hand orthosis as a writing aid in writer's cramp. *Mov Disord* 2001;16:1185–1189.

60. Byl NN, McKenzie A. Treatment effectiveness for patients with a history of repetitive hand use and focal hand dystonia: a planned, prospective follow-up study. *J Hand Ther* 2000;13: 289–301.

Tics and Tourette's Syndrome

27

Joseph Jankovic

Tourette's syndrome (TS) is a neurological disorder manifested by motor, vocal, or phonic tics that, in most cases, start in childhood and are often accompanied by obsessive–compulsive disorder (OCD), attention deficit-hyperactivity disorder (ADHD), poor impulse control, and other comorbid behavioral problems (1,2). Once considered a rare psychiatric curiosity, TS is now recognized as a relatively common and complex neurobehavioral disorder. Many notable historical figures, including Dr. Samuel Johnson and possibly Wolfgang Amadeus Mozart, are thought to have been afflicted with TS.

The clinical expression of this genetic disorder varies from one individual to another, fluctuations in symptoms are seen within the same individual, and different manifestations occur in various family members (3). This variable expression from one individual to another, even within members of the same family, contributes to diagnostic confusion. Without a specific biologic marker, the diagnosis depends on a careful evaluation of the patient's symptoms and signs by an experienced clinician. However, many patients remain undiagnosed, or their symptoms are wrongly attributed to habit, allergies, asthma, dermatitis, hyperactivity, nervousness, and many other conditions (4,5).

PHENOMENOLOGY OF TICS

Tics, the clinical hallmark of TS, are relatively brief and intermittent movements (motor tics) or sounds (vocal or phonic tics). The term *phonic tic* is preferable because not all sounds produced by TS patients involve the vocal cords. Although both types of tics must be present for the diagnosis of TS, this division into motor and phonic tics is arbitrary because phonic tics are actually motor tics involving respiratory, laryngeal, pharyngeal, oral, and nasal musculature. Motor tics typically consist of sudden, often repetitive, movements, gestures, and utterances that mimic fragments of normal behavior (1). To understand better the categorization of tics and how they fit in the general schema of movement disorders, it may be helpful to provide a simple classification of movements. All movements can be categorized into one of four classes:

1. *Voluntary:* (a) intentional (planned, self-initiated, internally generated); (b) externally triggered (in response to some external stimulus, e.g., turning head toward a loud noise or withdrawing hand from a hot plate).
2. *Semivoluntary* (unvoluntary): (a) induced by inner sensory stimulus (e.g., need to "stretch" a body part); (b) induced by unwanted feeling or compulsion (e.g., compulsive touching or smelling).
3. *Involuntary:* (a) nonsuppressible (e.g., reflexes. seizures, myoclonus); (b) suppressible (tics, tremor, dystonia, chorea, stereotypy).
4. *Automatic:* learned motor behaviors performed without conscious effort (e.g., walking or speaking); automatic, learned behaviors appear to be encoded in the sensorimotor portion of the striatum (6), which also may have a role in the generation of tics as learned voluntary motor skills may be incorporated into a tic repertoire.

Tics may be simple or complex. Simple motor tics involve only one group of muscles and cause brief jerklike movements. They are usually abrupt in onset and rapid (clonic tics), but they may be slower and cause a briefly sustained abnormal posture (dystonic tics) or an isometric contraction (tonic tics) (7). Examples of simple clonic motor tics include blinking, nose twitching, and head jerking. Simple dystonic tics include blepharospasm, oculogyric movements, bruxism, sustained mouth opening, torticollis, and shoulder rotation; the tensing of abdominal or limb muscles is an example of tonic tic. Dystonic (and tonic) muscle contraction may be responsible for blocking tics, which are due to prolonged tonic or dystonic tics that interrupt ongoing motor activity, such as speech, or to a sudden inhibition of motor activity. We and others have drawn attention to the presence of tics and dystonia in the same family, providing evidence for a possible etiologic relationship between TS and primary dystonia (8).

Motor (particularly dystonic) and phonic tics are preceded by premonitory sensations in more than 80% of patients (9). This premonitory phenomenon consist of localizable sensations or discomforts, such as a "burning feeling" in the eye before a blink, "tension or crick in the neck" relieved by stretching of the neck or jerking of the head, "feeling of tightness or constriction" relieved by arm or leg extension, "nasal stuffiness" before a sniff, "dry or sore throat" before throat clearing or grunting, and "itching" before a rotatory movement of the scapula. The observed movement or sound sometimes occurs in response to these premonitory phenomena, and this "intentional" or "unvoluntary" component of the movement may be a useful feature differentiating tics from other hyperkinetic movement disorders, such as myoclonus and chorea. Chee and Sachdev (10) suggest that "sensory tics," which we and others refer to as "premonitory sensations," "represent the subjectively experienced component of neural dysfunction below the threshold for motor and phonic tic production." Besides the local or regional premonitory sensations, this premonitory phenomenon may be nonlocalizable, less specific, and a poorly described feeling, such as an urge, anxiety, anger, and other psychic sensations. Many patients report that they have to repeat a particular movement to relieve the uncomfortable urge until "it feels good." The "just right" feeling has been associated with compulsive behavior, and as such the "unvoluntary" movement may be regarded as a "compulsive tic."

Complex motor tics consist of coordinated, sequenced movements resembling normal motor acts or gestures that are inappropriately intense and timed. They may be seemingly nonpurposeful, such as head shaking or trunk bending, or they may seem purposeful, such as touching, throwing, hitting, jumping, and kicking. Additional examples of complex motor tics include gesturing "the finger" and grabbing or exposing one's genitalia (copropraxia) or imitating gestures (echopraxia). Burping, vomiting, and retching have been described as part of the clinical picture of TS, but it is not clear whether this phenomenon represents a complex tic or some other behavioral manifestation of TS (11). Complex motor tics may be difficult to differentiate from compulsions, which frequently accompany tics, particularly in TS. A complex, repetitive movement may be considered a compulsion when it is preceded by, or associated with, a feeling of anxiety or panic, as well as an irresistible urge to produce the movement or sound

because of fear that if it is not promptly or properly executed "something bad" will happen. However, this distinction is not always possible, particularly when the patient is unable to verbalize such feelings. Some coordinated movements resemble complex motor tics but may actually represent "pseudovoluntary" movements (parakinesias) designed to camouflage the tics by incorporating them into seemingly purposeful acts, such as adjusting one's hair during a head jerk.

Simple phonic tics typically consist of sniffing, throat clearing, grunting, squeaking, screaming, coughing, blowing, and sucking sounds. Complex phonic tics include linguistically meaningful utterances and verbalizations, such as shouting of obscenities or profanities (coprolalia), repetition of someone else's words or phrases (echolalia), and repetition of one's own utterances, particularly the last syllable, word, or phrase in a sentence (palilalia). Some TS patients also manifest sudden and transient cessation of all motor activity (blocking tics) without alteration of consciousness.

In contrast to other hyperkinetic movement disorders, tics are usually intermittent and may be repetitive and stereotypic (Table 27.1). Tics may occur as short-term bouts or bursting or as long-term waxing and waning (12). They vary in frequency and intensity, often changing distribution. Typically, tics can be suppressed volitionally, although this may require intense mental effort. Suppressibility, while typical of tics, has been well documented in other hyperkinetic movement disorders but to a lesser degree. Using functional magnetic resonance imaging (MRI), Peterson et al. (13) showed decreased neuronal activity during periods of suppression in the ventral globus pallidus, putamen, and thalamus. There was increased activity in the right caudate nucleus, right frontal cortex, and other cortical areas normally involved in the inhibition of unwanted impulses (prefrontal, parietal, temporal, and cingulate cortices). Besides temporary suppressibility, tics are also characterized by suggestibility and exacerbation with stress, excitement, boredom, fatigue, and exposure to heat. Tics also may increase during relaxation following a period of stress.

In contrast to other hyperkinetic movement disorders that are usually completely suppressed during sleep, motor and phonic tics may persist during all stages of sleep (14,15). When they are concentrating on mental or physical tasks (such as when playing a video game or during orgasm), many patients note a reduction in their tics. Others have increased frequency and intensity of their tics when distracted, especially when they no longer have the need to suppress the tics. Tics are also typically exacerbated by dopaminergic drugs and by CNS stimulants, including methylphenidate and cocaine (16). Finally, it should be noted that there is a broad spectrum of movements that may be present in patients with TS and that may be confused with tics, such as akathisia, chorea, dystonia, compulsive movements, and fidgeting as part of hyperactivity associated with ADHD (7,17,18).

TABLE 27.1
DIFFERENTIAL DIAGNOSIS OF TICS

Classification	Differential Diagnosis
A. *Simple motor tics*	
1. Clonic	Myoclonus
	Chorea
	Seizures
2. Dystonic	Dystonic
	Athetosis
3. Tonic	Muscle spasms and cramps
B. *Complex motor tics*	Mannerisms
Stereotypies	
Restless legs	
Seizures	

Phenomenology

Abrupt	Myoclonus
Chorea	
Hyperreflexia	
Paroxysmal dyskinesia	
Seizures	
Sensory phenomenon	Akathisia stereotypy
(urge → relief)	Restless legs syndrome
	Dystonia
Perceived as voluntary	Akathisia
Suppressibility	All hyperkinesias but less
	than tics
Decrease with distraction	Akathisia
	Psychogenic movements
Increase with stress	Most hyperkinesias
Increase with relaxation	Parkinsonian tremor
(after period of stress)	
Multifocal, migrate	Chorea
	Myoclonus
Fluctuate spontaneously	Paroxysmal dyskinesias
	Seizures
Present during sleep	Myoclonus (segmental)
	Periodic movements
	Painful legs/moving toes
	Other hyperkinesias
	Seizures

Clinical Features of Tourette's Syndrome

Motor Symptoms

TS, the most common cause of tics, is manifested by a broad spectrum of motor and behavioral disturbances. This clinical heterogeneity often causes diagnostic difficulties and presents a major challenge in genetic linkage studies. To aid in the diagnosis of TS, the Tourette's Syndrome Classification Study Group (TSCSG) (19) formulated the following criteria for definite TS:

a. Both multiple motor and one or more phonic tics must be present at some time during the illness, although not necessarily concurrently.
b. Tics must occur many times a day, nearly every day, or intermittently throughout a period of more than a year.
c. The anatomic location, number, frequency, type, complexity, or severity of tics must change over time.
d. Onset must be before age 21.
e. Involuntary movements and noises cannot be explained by other medical conditions.
f. Motor and/or phonic tics must be directly witnessed by a reliable examiner at some point during the illness or be recorded by videotape or cinematography.

Probable TS type 1 meets all the criteria except b and d. Probable TS type 2 meets all the criteria except a, and it includes either single motor tic with phonic tics or multiple motor tics with possible phonic tics. In contrast to the criteria outlined by the fourth edition of the Diagnostic and Statistical Manual of Mental Disorders (DSM-IV) (20), the TSCSG criteria do not include a statement about "impairment." There is considerable controversy about the DSM-IV criterion requiring that "marked distress or significant impairment in social, occupational, or other important areas of functioning" be present. Therefore, patients with mild tics that do not produce impairment would not satisfy the diagnostic criteria for TS according to DSM-IV. That particular criterion will be deleted from the DSM-V edition.

Kurlan (21) suggested another set of diagnostic criteria for genetic studies and introduced the term *Tourette disorder* for patients who have "functional impairment." However, this does not take into account the marked fluctuations in symptoms and severity; some patients may be relatively asymptomatic at one time and clearly functionally impaired at another time. The Tourette Syndrome Association's International Genetic Collaboration developed the Diagnostic Confidence Index (DCI), which consists of 26 "confidence factors" with weights given to each and a maximal total score of 100. The most heavily weighted diagnostic confidence factors include history of coprolalia, complex motor or vocal tics, a waxing and waning course, echo phenomenon, premonitory sensations, an orchestrated sequence, and age at onset. The DCI was found to be a useful instrument in assessing the lifetime likelihood of developing TS (22). Several instruments, some based on ratings of videotapes, have been developed to measure and quantitate tics, but they all have some limitations (23,24).

The clinical criteria are designed to assist in accurate diagnosis, in genetic linkage studies, and in differentiating TS from other tic disorders (Table 27.2) (17). A body of evidence supports the notion that many patients, if not all, with other forms of idiopathic tic disorders represent one end of the spectrum in a continuum of TS. The most common and mildest of the idiopathic tic disorders is the *transient tic disorder* (TTD) of childhood. This disorder is essentially identical to TS except that the symptoms last for less than a year and, therefore, the diagnosis can be made only in retrospect. *Chronic multiple tic disorder* (CMTD) is also similar to TS, but these patients have only motor or, less commonly, only phonic tics lasting at least a year.

TABLE 27.2
CAUSES OF TICS

I. Primary

A. *Sporadic*
   1. Transient motor *or* phonic tics (<1 yr)
   2. Chronic motor *or* phonic tics (>1 yr)
   3. Adult-onset (recurrent) tics
   4. Tourette's syndrome
   5. Primary dystonia

B. *Inherited*
   1. Tourette's syndrome
   2. Huntington disease
   3. Primary dystonia
   4. Neuroacanthocytosis
   5. Hallervorden-Spatz syndrome
   6. Tuberous sclerosis
   7. Wilson's disease
   8. Duchenne's muscular dystrophy

II. Secondary

A. Infections; encephalitis, Creutzfeldt-Jakob disease, neurosyphilis, Sydenham's chorea
B. Drugs: amphetamines, methylphenidate, pemoline, levodopa, cocaine, carbamazepine, phenytoin, phenobarbital, lamotrigine, antipsychotics and other dopamine receptor–blocking drugs (tardive tics, tardive tourettism)
C. Toxins: carbon monoxide
D. Developmental: static encephalopathy, mental retardation syndromes, chromosomal abnormalities, autistic spectrum disorders (Asperger's syndrome)
E. Chromosomal disorders: Down syndrome, Kleinfelter's syndrome, XYY karyotype, fragile X, triple X, 9p mosaicism, partial trisomy 16, 9p monosomy, citrullinemia, Beckwith-Wiedemann syndrome
F. Other: head trauma, stroke, neurocutaneous syndromes, schizophrenia, neurodegenerative diseases

III. Related Manifestations and Disorders

1. Stereotypies/habits/mannerisms
2. Self-injurious behaviors
3. Motor restlessness
4. Akathisia
5. Compulsions
6. Excessive Startle
7. Jumping Frenchman

Chronic single tic disorder (CSTD) is the same as CMTD, but these patients have only a single motor or phonic tic. This separation into TTD, CMTD, and CSTD seems artificial because all can occur in the same family and probably represent a variable expression of the same genetic defect.

Although the TSCSG diagnostic criteria require that onset occur before the age of 21, nearly all patients with TS have symptoms before age 12. In 36% to 48% of patients, the initial symptom is eye blinking, followed by tics involving the face and head. Blink rate in persons with TS is about double that in normal, age-matched controls (25). During the course of the disorder, nearly all patients exhibit tics involving the face or head; two-thirds have tics in the

arms; and one-half have tics involving the trunk or legs. According to one study, the average age at onset of tics is 5.6 years, and the tics usually become most severe at age 10; by 18 years of age one-half of the patients are tic free (26). In a study of 58 adults diagnosed with TS during childhood, Goetz et al. (27) found that tics persisted in all patients but were moderate or severe in only 24%, although 60% had moderate or severe tics during the course of the disorder. Tic severity during childhood had no predictive value for the future course, but patients with mild tics during the preadult period had mild tics during adulthood. Although the vast majority of tics in adults represent recurrences of childhood-onset tics, rare patients may have their first tic occurrence during adulthood (28). In these adults with new-onset tics, it is important to search for secondary causes, such as infection, trauma, cocaine use, and neuroleptic exposure (17,28). Poor motor control, which can lead to poor penmanship and, at times, almost illegible handwriting, may contribute to the academic difficulties faced by many patients with TS. Tics, though rarely disabling, can be quite troublesome for TS patients because they cause embarrassment, interfere with social interactions, and at times can be quite painful or uncomfortable. Rarely, they can cause secondary neurologic deficits, such as cervical compressive myelopathy in patients with violent head and neck tics (29).

Vocalizations have been reported as the initial symptom in about one-third of all patients, with throat clearing being the most common initial phonic tic (30). Phonic tics can be troublesome for patients and those around them, particularly when they consist of loud, shrieking sounds. In addition to involuntary noises, some patients have speech dysfluencies that resemble developmental stuttering, and up to one-half of all patients with developmental stuttering have been thought to have undiagnosed TS (31). Coprolalia, perhaps the most recognizable and certainly one of the most distressing symptom of TS, is actually present in only one-half of patients. When describing the distress caused by his severe coprolalia, one of our patients remarked that immediately after shouting an obscenity he reaches out with his hand in an attempt to "catch the word and bring it back before others can hear it." This symptom appears to be markedly influenced by cultural background. Although in one retrospective analysis of 112 children with TS, only 8% exhibited coprolalia (33), the true prevalence of coprolalia in TS children and adults is only about 50% in the U.S. population, even when mental coprolalia (without actual utterance) is included. Coprolalia has been reported to occur in only 26% of Danish and 4% of Japanese patients (30). Copropraxia has been found in about 20% of patients, echolalia in 30%, echopraxia in 25%, and palilalia in 15%.

Except for the presence of tics, the neurologic examination in patients with TS is usually normal. In one casecontrol study, TS patients were found to have a shorter duration of saccades, but the saccades were performed with a greater mean velocity than normal controls and were associated with fewer correct antisaccade responses, suggesting a mild oculomotor disturbance in TS (32). Although the ability to inhibit reflexive saccades is normal, TS patients make more timing errors, indicating an inability to appropriately inhibit or delay planned motor programs (34).

Behavioral Symptoms

In addition to motor and phonic tics, patients with TS often exhibit a variety of behavioral symptoms, particularly ADHD and OCD (Fig. 27.1). Diagnosis of ADHD and OCD is based on clinical history; there are no laboratory or other tests that reliably diagnose these neurobehavioral disorders (35,36) (Table 27.3). These comorbid behavioral conditions often interfere with learning and with academic and work performance. In contrast to tics, ADHD and obsessional symptom severity are significantly associated with impaired social and emotional adjustment (37). The clinician should be skilled not only in the recognition and management of ADHD but also in documenting the ADHD-related deficits (38). Such documentation is essential for parents and educators to provide the optimal educational setting for the affected individual.

Since nearly all studies on the frequency of associated features have been based on a population of TS patients referred to physicians (usually specialists), there is a selection bias; therefore, accurate figures on the prevalence of these behavioral disorders in TS patients are not available. It has been estimated that 3% to 6% of the school-age population suffers from ADHD (36), and probably most patients with TS have had symptoms of ADHD, OCD, or both sometime during the course of their illnesses (39).

The symptoms of ADHD may be the initial manifestations of TS and may precede the onset of motor and phonic tics by about 3 years. Despite growing publicity about ADHD, there is little evidence of widespread overdiagnosis or overtreatment of this disorder (36). Based on an interview of 1,596 children, ages 9 to 17, in Rochester and Monroe County (New York) schools, tics were identified in 339 (21%) after 60 to 150 minutes of observation (40). The investigators found the following behavioral problems more frequently ($p < 0.05$) in children with tics than in those without tics: OCD, ADHD, separation anxiety, overanxious disorder, simple phobia, social phobia, agoraphobia, mania, major depression, and oppositional defiant behavior. Also, children with tics were younger (mean age: 12.5 vs. 13.3 years) and were more likely to require special education services (27 vs. 19.8%).

There are three types of ADHD: predominantly inattentive, predominantly hyperactive–impulsive, and combined (Table 27.3) (41). Although attention deficit is certainly one of the most common and disabling symptoms of TS, in many patients the inability to pay attention is due not only to a coexistent ADHD but also to uncontrollable intrusions of thoughts. Some patients are unable to pay attention because of a compulsive fixation of gaze. For example, while sitting in a classroom or a theater or during a conversation, the gaze becomes fixed on a particular object and, despite concentrated effort, patients are unable to break the fixation. As a result, they miss the teacher's lesson or a particular action in a play. Another reason for impaired attention in some TS patients is mental concentration exerted in an effort to suppress tics. Yet another cause for inattention is the sedative effect of anti-TS medications. It is, therefore, important to determine which

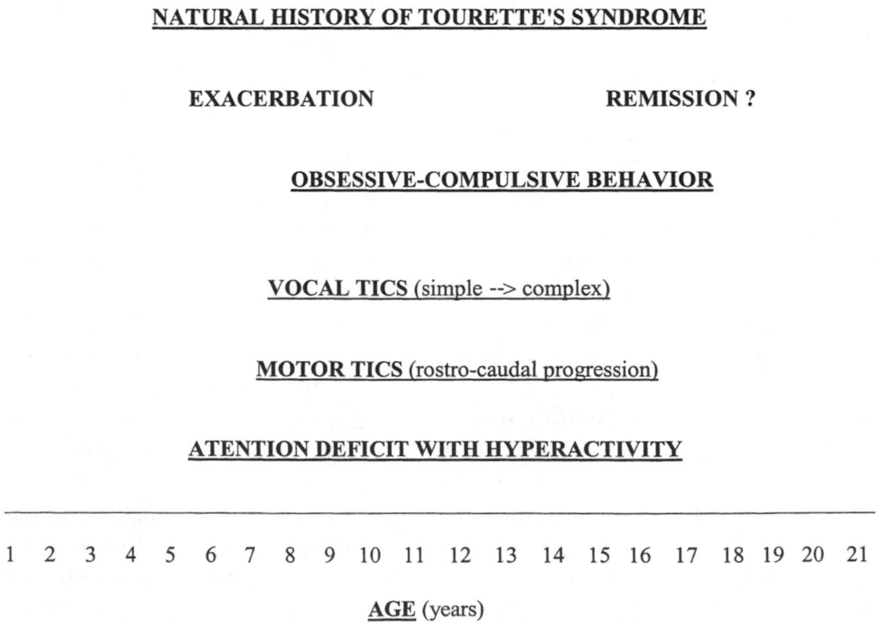

NATURAL HISTORY OF TOURETTE'S SYNDROME

EXACERBATION   REMISSION ?

OBSESSIVE-COMPULSIVE BEHAVIOR

VOCAL TICS (simple --> complex)

MOTOR TICS (rostro-caudal progression)

ATENTION DEFICIT WITH HYPERACTIVITY

1   2   3   4   5   6   7   8   9   10   11   12   13   14   15   16   17   18   19   20   21

AGE (years)

Figure 27.1 Progression of symptoms during the course of Tourette's syndrome.

TABLE 27.3

ATTENTION-DEFICIT HYPERACTIVITY DISORDER/HYPERKINETIC DISORDER (ICD-10 AND DSM-IV)

Inattention (IN)	Hyperactivity (H)	Impulsivity (IMP)
Fails to attend to details	Fidgets with hands or feet	Talks excessively
Difficulty sustaining attention	Leaves seat in classroom	Blurts out answers
Does not seem to listen	Rins about or climbs	Difficulty waiting turn
Fails to finish	Difficulty playing quietly	Interrupts or intrudes on others
Difficulty organising tasks	Motor excess ("on the go")	
Avoids sustained effort	Talks excessively	
Loses things		
Distracted by external stimuli		
Forgetful		

ADHD Diagnostic Subtypes (DSM-IV)

Combined: 6 or more from the IN domain and 6 or more from the H/IMP domain
Inattentive: 6 or more from the IN domain and fewer than 6 from the H/IMP domain
Hyperactive/impulsive: 6 or more from H/IMP domain and fewer than 6 from the IN domain

HKD (ICD-10)

6 or more from the IN domain, 3 or more from the H domain, 1 or more from the IMP domain

ADHD, attention-deficit hyperactivity disorder; HKD, hyperkinetic disorder; ICD-10, *International Classification of Diseases*, 10th ed.; DSM-IV, *Diagnostic and Statistical Manual of Mental Disorders*, 4th ed.

mechanism or mechanisms are most likely responsible for the patient's attention deficit. Although genetics clearly plays a key role in the mechanism of attention deficit disorder (ADD) and ADHD, the gene(s) or other causes have not been fully elucidated. In a genome scan of 106 families, including 128 affected sibling pairs with estimated heritability of 60% to 80%, multipoint Maximum Likelihood Score (MLS) values higher than 1 suggested the possibility of a gene locus on chromosomes 4, 9, 10, 11, 12, 16, and 17 (42). One study showed that children and adolescents with ADHD, compared to those without ADHD, are more likely to have major injuries and asthma, and their 9-year medical costs are double (43).

Although OCD frequently occurs alone without other features of TS (44), it is now well accepted that OCD is part of the spectrum of neurobehavioral manifestations in TS (44,45). With an estimated lifetime prevalence of 2% to 3% (46) and an incidence of 0.55 per 1,000 person-years (47), OCD is one of the most common causes of disability. The instrument used most frequently to measure the severity of OCD is the Yale-Brown Obsessive-Compulsive Scale (48). A distinction should be made between obsessive–compulsive symptoms or traits, obsessive–compulsive personality disorder, and OCD. Obsessions are characterized by intense, intrusive thoughts, such as concerns about bodily wastes and secretions; unfounded fears; a need for exactness, symmetry, evenness, and/or neatness; excessive religious concerns; perverse sexual thoughts; and intrusions of words, phrases, or music. Compulsions consist of a subjective urge to perform meaningless and irrational rituals, such as checking, counting, cleaning, washing, touching, smelling,

hoarding, and rearranging. Leckman et al. (49) have drawn attention to the frequent occurrence of the "just right" perception in patients with OCD and TS. Whereas obsessional slowness accounts for some of the school problems experienced by TS patients, cognitive slowing (bradyphrenia) is also a contributing factor (50). In contrast to primary OCD in which the symptoms relate chiefly to hygiene and cleanliness, the obsessive symptoms associated with TS usually involve concerns with symmetry, violent aggressive thoughts, forced touching, fear of harming self or others, and a need to say or do things "just right" (51). A principal-components factor analysis of 13 categories used to group types of obsessions and compulsions in the Yale-Brown Obsessive-Compulsive Scale symptom checklist identified the obsessions and checking and the symmetry and ordering factors as particularly common in patients with tic disorders (52). In addition to an idiopathic sporadic or familial disorder and TS, OCD has been reported to occur as a result of a variety of lesions in the frontal-limbic-subcortical circuits (53,54). Although both ADHD and OCD are regarded as integral findings of the syndrome, only OCD has been shown to be genetically linked to TS (55). A pathogenic link between TS and OCD also is suggested by the finding in one study that 59% of 54 patients with OCD had a lifetime history of tics and 14% fulfilled the criteria for TS during the 2- to 7-year follow-up (56).

One of the most troublesome symptoms of TS is poor impulse control manifested sometimes by inability to control anger, as a result of which many patients may exhibit frequent, and sometimes violent, temper outbursts and rages. Indeed, many behavioral symptoms of TS, including some complex tics, coprolalia, copropraxia, and many behavioral problems, can be explained by loss of normal inhibitory mechanisms (disinhibition) manifested by poor impulse control. Rarely, TS patients exhibit inappropriate sexual aggressiveness, as well as antisocial, oppositional, and even violent, unlawful, or criminal behavior. Indeed, TS serves as a model medical disorder that may predispose one to engage in uncontrollable and offensive behaviors that are misunderstood by the law-abiding community and legal justice system. The social and legal aspects of TS have yet to be investigated, but there is growing concern regarding media misrepresentation that attributes violent criminal behavior in certain individuals to TS. Although TS should not be used as an "excuse" to justify unlawful or criminal behaviors, studies are needed to determine whether TS-related symptoms and neurobehavioral comorbidities predispose individuals with TS to engage in such behaviors. Often the avolitional nature of behaviors in response to involuntary internal thought and emotional patterns is supported by the subsequent remorse and lack of secondary gain. This suggests that the preponderance of unlawful acts committed by TS patients are not premeditated but may result from a variety of TS-related mechanisms, such as poor impulse control, OCD associated with addictive behavior (e.g., drugs, alcohol, gambling), and ADD and distractibility (e.g., motor vehicle accidents). In one study, TS accounted for 2% of all cases referred for forensic psychiatric investigation in Stockholm, Sweden, between 1990 and 1995; 15% of offenders had ADHD, 15% had Pervasive Developmental Disorder (PDD), and 3% had Asperger's syndrome (57).

Focal frontal lobe dysfunction, demonstrated in TS by various functional and imaging studies, has been associated with an impulsive subtype of aggressive behavior (58). It has been postulated that impulse disorders stem from exaggerated reward-, pleasure-, or arousal-seeking brain centers, resulting in failure of inhibition. Animal studies of rats with lesions of the nucleus accumbens core, the brain region noted for reward and reinforcement, showed that the lesioned rats preferred small immediate rewards to larger delayed rewards (59). In addition to the ventromedial prefrontal cortices, lesions in the amygdala also have been known to cause alterations in decision-making processes and disregard for consequences (60).

One of the most distressing symptoms of TS is a self-injurious behavior, reported in up to 53% of all patients (30,61). A common form of self-injurious behavior is damage of skin by compulsive biting, scratching, cutting, engraving, or hitting (particularly in the eye and throat), often accompanied by an irresistible urge (obsession) (4). Thus, self-injurious behavior appears to be related to OCD, which has treatment implications.

The TS gene(s) may, in addition to tics, ADHD, and OCD, be expressed in a variety of behavioral manifestations, including learning and conduct disorders, schizoid and affective disorders, antisocial behaviors, oppositional defiant disorder, anxiety, depression, conduct disorder,

severe temper outbursts, rage attacks, impulse control problems, inappropriate sexual behavior, and other psychiatric problems (62). Personality disorder and depression have been reported in 64% of patients with TS (63). Besides comorbid behavioral conditions, TS has been reported to be frequently associated with migraine headaches, which may be related to the coexistent OCD (64). The Tourette International Consortium Database, which at the time of its publication in 2000 included information on 3,500 patients with TS collected from 64 centers from around the world, showed that only 12% of patients with TS had no other disorders; ADHD was seen in 60%, symptoms of OCD in 59%, anger control problems in 37%, sleep disorder in 25%, learning disability in 23%, mood disorder in 20%, anxiety disorder in 18%, and self-injurious behavior in 14% (65).

Pathogenesis

Neurophysiology

Although the pathogenic mechanisms of TS are unknown, the weight of evidence supports organic rather than psychogenic origin (66,67). Despite the observation that some tics may be, at least in part, voluntary, physiologic studies suggest that tics are not mediated through normal motor pathways utilized for willed movements. About 20% of patients with TS have exaggerated startle responses, which may fail to habituate with repetition (68). Using back-averaging techniques, Karp et al. (69) documented premotor negativity in 2 of 5 patients with simple motor tics. Although the investigators could not correlate the presence of Bereitschaftspotential with the premonitory sensation, the physiology of the premovement phenomenon requires further study.

Functional MRI studies in patients with TS have shown decreased neuronal activity during periods of suppression in the ventral globus pallidus, putamen, and thalamus and increased activity in the right caudate nucleus, right frontal cortex, and other cortical areas normally involved in the inhibition of unwanted impulses (prefrontal, parietal, temporal, and cingulate cortices) (70). In another study utilizing functional MRI, Serrien et al. showed marked reduction or absence of activity in secondary motor areas while the patients attempted to maintain a stable grip-load force control (71). The authors interpreted the findings as ongoing activation of the secondary motor areas reflecting patients' involuntary urges to move. In a study of children with ADHD, functional MRI showed increased frontal activation and reduced striatal activation on various tasks, and an enhancement of striatal function after treatment with methylphenidate (72). Transcranial magnetic stimulation (TMS) studies have demonstrated shortened cortical silent period and defective intracortical inhibition (determined in a conditioning test paired-stimulus paradigm) in patients with TS (73) and OCD (74), thus providing possible explanation for intrusive phenomena. Subsequent studies using the same technique have demonstrated that patients with tic-related OCD have more abnormal motor cortex excitability than OCD patients without tics (75). TMS studies also have demonstrated that TS children have a shorter cortical silent period but that their intracortical inhibition is not different from that of controls, although intracortical inhibition is reduced in children with ADHD (76). There is evidence of additive inhibitory deficits, as demonstrated by reduced intracortical inhibition and shortened cortical silent period in children with TS and comorbid ADHD. Both short-interval intracortical inhibition and short-interval afferent inhibition were reduced in 8 patients with TS (ages 24–38 years) as compared to 10 matched healthy controls (77).

Sleep studies have provided additional evidence that some tics are truly involuntary (14,15). Polysomnographic studies in TS patients recorded motor and phonic tics in various stages of sleep and have found that some patients with TS have alterations of arousal; decreased percentage of stage 3/4 (slow-wave) sleep; decreased percentage of rapid eye movement (REM) sleep; paroxysmal events in stage 4 sleep with sudden intense arousal, disorientation, and agitation; restless legs syndrome; periodic leg movement during sleep; and other sleep-related disorders, including sleep apnea, enuresis, sleep walking and sleep talking, nightmares, myoclonus, bruxism, and other disturbances (78–81).

Neuroimaging

Although standard anatomic neuroimaging studies in TS are unremarkable, using special volumetric, metabolic, blood flow, ligand, and functional imaging techniques, several interesting findings have been reported that have strong implications for the pathophysiology of TS (70). Careful volumetric MRI studies have suggested that the normal asymmetry of the basal ganglia is lost in TS. Frederickson et al. (81) found evidence of smaller gray matter volumes in left frontal lobes of patients with TS, further supporting the findings of loss of normal left–right asymmetry. Quantitative MRI studies have found subtle but possibly important reduction in the volume of caudate nuclei in patients with TS. In 10 pairs of monozygotic twins, the right caudate was smaller in the more severely affected individuals, providing evidence for the role of environmental events in the pathogenesis of TS (82). In contrast, the corpus callosum has been found to be larger in children with TS than in normal controls (83). Subsequent study has showed that this finding was gender related and was present only in boys with TS (84). In another study, caudate volumes have been reported to correlate significantly and inversally with the severity of tics and OCD in early adulthood (85).

Positron emission tomography (PET) scanning has shown variable rates of glucose utilization in basal ganglia, compared with controls. In one study, 18F-fluorodeoxyglucose (FDG) PET has shown evidence of increased metabolic activity in the lateral premotor and supplementary motor association cortices and in the midbrain (pattern 1), and decreased metabolic activity in the caudate and thalamic areas (limbic basal ganglia–thalamocortical projection system) (pattern 2) (86). Pattern 1 is reportedly associated with tics, and pattern 2 correlates with the overall severity of TS. In contrast to dystonia, characterized by lentiform nucleus–thalamic metabolic dissociation, attributed to overactivity of the direct striatopallidal inhibitory pathway, the pattern of TS is characterized by concomitant metabolic reduction in striatal and thalamic function. The authors suggested that this pattern could be explained by a reduction in the indirect pathway resulting in reduction in subthalamic nucleus activity. Using event-related [^{15}O]H$_2$O PET combined with time-synchronized audio- and videotaping in 6 patients with TS, Stern et al. (87 found increased activity in the sensorimotor, language, executive, paralimbic, and frontal-subcortical areas that were temporarily related to the motor and phonic tics and the irresistible urge that precedes these behaviors. Rauch et al. (88) showed bilateral medial temporal (hippocampal/parahippocampal) activation on PET in patients with OCD, compared with normal controls, and absence of activation of inferior striatum, seen in normal controls. Various neuroimaging studies also have demonstrated moderate reduction in the size of the corpus callosum, basal ganglia (particularly the caudate and globus pallidus), and frontal lobes (89) and striatal hypoperfusion (72) in patients with ADHD.

Neurochemistry

Neurochemical studies of TS have been hampered by the unavailability of postmortem brain tissue. Biochemical abnormalities in the few postmortem brains that have been studied include low serotonin, low glutamate in the internal globus pallidus, and low cyclic adenosine monophosphate (cAMP) in the cortex (90). An alteration in the central neurotransmitters in TS also has been suggested, chiefly because of relatively consistent responses to modulation of the dopaminergic system. Dopamine antagonists and depletors generally have an ameliorating effect on tics, whereas drugs that enhance central dopaminergic activity exacerbate tics. Low levels of homovanillic acid in cerebrospinal fluid, coupled with a favorable response to dopamine receptor–blocking drugs, have been interpreted as evidence in support of the notion that tics and TS are due to supersensitive dopamine receptors; however, postmortem binding studies of dopamine receptors have failed to provide support for this hypothesis (90). Using [^{11}C]raclopride PET and amphetamine stimulation, Singer et al. (91) found evidence for increased dopamine release in the putamen of patients with TS. They postulate that in TS there is increased activity of the dopamine transporter leading to increased dopamine concentration in the dopamine terminals and to a stimulus-dependent increase in dopaminergic transmission. Support for this hypothesis has been provided by the PET imaging studies using [^{11}C]dihydrotetrabenazine (DTBZ)—a type 2 vesicular monoamine transporter (VMAT-2)—as a ligand to quantify striatal monoaminergic innervation in patients with TS ($n = 19$) and control subjects ($n = 27$) (92). With voxel by voxel analysis, the investigators found increased DTBZ binding in the ventral striatum (right > left) in patients with TS compared to age-matched controls. A postmortem examination of 2 brains of patients with typical childhood onset TD and 1 with adult-onset tics, showed that the prefrontal cortex rather than the striatum showed most abnormalities, including increased D2 receptor protein, as well as increases in dopamine transporter (DAT), VAMP-2, and α-2A (93).

Functional neuroimaging studies have been used to aid in the understanding of neurotransmitter and receptor alterations in TS. Using [^{123}I]β-carboxymethoxy-3-β-(4-iodophenyl)tropane (CIT) single-photon emission computed tomography (SPECT), Malison et al. (94) demonstrated a mean increase of 37% in binding of this dopamine transporter ligand in the striatum in 5 adult patients with TS, compared with age-matched controls. In contrast, Heinz et al. (95) found no difference in [^{123}I] β-CIT binding in the midbrain, thalamus, or basal ganglia between 10 TS patients and normal control subjects. There was, however, a significant negative correlation between the severity of phonic tics and β-CIT binding in the midbrain and thalamus. In another study involving 12 adult TS patients, β-CIT scans showed evidence of increased dopamine transporter binding (96). Combining SPECT and MRI, Wolf et al. (97) found 17% greater binding of IBZM, a D2 receptor ligand, in the caudate (but not putamen) nucleus in 5 of the more affected monozygotic twins discordant for TS. It is important to note that 2 of the 5 subjects were taking neuroleptics for up to 6 weeks prior to the SPECT studies. Nevertheless, these findings, if confirmed by other studies of neuroleptic-naive patients, support the notion that the presynaptic dopamine function is enhanced in TS. This may, in turn, lead to reduced inhibitory pallidal output to the mediodorsal thalamus. However, the observation that in patients with Parkinson's disease (PD) the severity of childhood-onset tics was not influenced by the development of parkinsonism or by its treatment with levodopa argues against the role of dopamine in the pathogenesis of TS symptoms (98). This is supported by the results of PET ligand studies showing normal D2 receptor density (99). Furthermore, Meyer et al. (100) used PET imaging of (+)-α-[^{11}C]dihydrotetrabenazine to determine the density of VMAT2, a cytoplasm-to-vesicle transporter linearly related to monoaminergic nerve terminal density unaffected by medications, in 8 TS patients and 22 controls. This study showed no significant difference in terminal density between patients and controls, thus failing to provide support for the concept of increased striatal innervation. However, these studies do not exclude the possibility of abnormal regulation of dopamine release and uptake. In a small sample of TS patients, PET studies have demonstrated a 25% increase in accumulations of fluorodopa in the left caudate ($p = 0.03$) and a 53% increase in accumulations in the right midbrain ($p = 0.08$) (101). These findings indicate possible dopaminergic dysfunction in the cells of origin and in the dopaminergic terminals, suggesting increased activity of dopa decarboxylase.

Despite some limitations and inconsistencies, the imaging, ligand, and biochemical studies provide support for the hypothesis that the corticostriatothalamocortical circuit has an important role in the pathogenesis of TS and related disorders (1,70). The dorsolateral prefrontal circuit, which links Brodmann's areas 9 and 10 to the dorsolateral head of the caudate, appears to be involved with executive functions (manipulation of previously learned knowledge, abstract reasoning, organization, verbal fluency, and problem solving; closely related to intelligence, education, and social exposure) and motor planning. An abnormality in this circuit has been implicated in ADHD. The lateral orbitofrontal circuit originates in the inferior lateral prefrontal cortex (area 10) and projects to the ventral medial caudate. An abnormality in this circuit is associated with personality changes, mania, disinhibition, and irritability. Lastly, the anterior cingulate circuit arises in the cingulate gyrus (area 24) and projects to the ventral striatum, which also receives input from the amygdala, hippocampus, medial orbitofrontal cortex, and the entorhinal and perirhinal cortices. A variety of behavioral problems, including OCD, may be linked to an abnormality in this circuit.

Reduced metabolism or blood flow to the basal ganglia, particularly in the ventral striatum, most often in the left hemisphere, has been demonstrated in a majority of studies involving TS subjects. These limbic areas are thought to be involved in impulse control, reward contingencies, and executive functions, and these behavioral functions appear to be abnormal in most patients with TS. Future imaging and ligand studies should include children, a population that has been largely excluded because of ethical considerations. The studies should also rigorously characterize comorbid disorders and take into consideration potential confounding variables, such as the secondary effects of chronic illness, medications, and so forth.

Immunology

The potential role of immunologic mechanisms and, specifically, antineuronal antibodies is currently being explored in a variety of neurologic disorders, including TS (102,103). Several studies have suggested that exacerbations of TS symptoms correlated with an antecedent group A β-hemolytic streptococcus (GABHS) infection (demonstrated by elevated antistreptococcal titers) and the presence of serum antineuronal antibodies. Epitopes of streptococcal M proteins have been found to cross-react with human brain, particularly the basal ganglia, and may be pathogenetically important in various neurologic disorders, such as Sydenham's chorea, TS-like syndrome, dystonia, and parkinsonism (104). Development of dyskinesias (paw and floor licking, head and paw shaking) and phonic utterances has been reported in rodents after the microinfusion of dilute immunoglobulin G (IgG) from TS subjects into their striatum, and intrastriatal microinfusion of TS sera or IgG in rats produced stereotypies and episodic utterances, analogous to involuntary movements seen in TS (103). In 10 patients with poststreptococcal acute disseminated encephalomyelitis (PSADEM) following exposure to GABHS, Dale et al. (104) showed antibasal ganglia antibodies in all with 3 dominant bands—60, 67, and 80 kd. Furthermore, MRI showed hyperintense basal ganglia in 80% of the patients. The B lymphocyte antigen D8/17 is considered to be a marker for rheumatic fever but is also frequently overexpressed in patients with tics, OCD, and autism (105). In one study, children and adults with TS had significantly higher serum levels of antineuronal antibodies against putamen but not caudate or globus pallidus, in comparison with controls (106). However, the potential relevance of this finding has been questioned because there is no relationship between the presence of antineuronal antibodies and age at onset, severity of tics, or presence of comorbid disorders. Trifiletti and Packard (107) have confirmed the presence of a specific brain protein with a molecular weight of 83 kd that is recognized by antibodies in the serum of 80% to 90% of patients with TS or OCD (107). They concluded that there might be a subset of patients with TS and OCD, perhaps up to 10% of all cases, in whom a streptococcal infection triggers the onset of symptoms. In a large case-control study of 150 patients with tics and 150 controls, Cardona and Orefici (108) found a correlation between the occurrence of tics and prior exposure to streptococcal antigens and also found that the severity of tic disorder correlates with the magnitude of the serologic response to streptococcal antigens measured by ASO titers (38% of children with tics compared with 2% of control subjects had ASO titers >500 IU ($p < 0.001$). In another study involving 25 adult patients with TS and 25 healthy controls, increased antibody titers against streptococcal M12 and M19 proteins were found in the TS group, compared with healthy controls (109). At this time there is no evidence that serum autoantibodies differentiate pediatric autoimmune neuropsychiatric disorders associated with streptococcal infections (PANDAS) and TS from controls (110).

Variably referred to as PANDAS or as pediatric infection-triggered autoimmune neuropsychiatric disorders (PITANDS), this area is one of the most controversial topics in the pediatric neurologic and psychiatric literature (107,111). Nevertheless, the concept of *postinfectious* OCD is gradually seeping into the literature, even though definite proof is still lacking (112). Untreated GABHS infection is often complicated by rheumatic fever, within 10 to 14 weeks, and by Sydenham's chorea, within several months. Several studies have provided evidence for an overlap between TS and Sydenham's chorea with tics and OCD being manifested in both disorders. It is, therefore, not

clear whether TS and OCD are independent sequelae of GABHS or whether the observed symptoms of TS and OCD are manifestations of Sydenham's chorea. Although this intriguing hypothesis requires further study, plasmapheresis (PEX), intravenous IgG, and immunosuppressant therapies are currently being investigated in the management of TS. In a study of 30 children in whom OCD or tics were presumably triggered or exacerbated by GABHS, there were striking improvements in various measures of OCD after administration of intravenous immunoglobulin (IVIG) and in tics after plasma exchange (113). Twenty-nine children with PANDAS were randomized in a partially double-blind fashion (no sham PEX) to an IVIG, IVIG placebo (saline), or PEX group. One month after treatment, the severity of obsessive–compulsive symptoms were improved by 58% and 45% in the PEX and IVIG groups, respectively, compared with only 3% in the IVIG control. In contrast, tic scores were improved only after PEX treatment; reductions of 49% (PEX), 19% (IVIG), and 12% (IVIG placebo) were noted. Improvements in both tics and obsessive–compulsive symptoms were sustained for 1 year. However, there was no control PEX group, and the control comparisons were limited to the 1-month visit. Furthermore, there was no relationship between rate of antibody removal and therapeutic response. Until the results of this study are confirmed, these treatment modalities are not justified in patients with TS. Furthermore, because of uncertainties about the possible cause-and-effect relationship between GABHS and tics and OCD, an antibiotic treatment for acute exacerbations of these symptoms is currently considered unwarranted (111).

Genetics

Finding a genetic marker, and ultimately the responsible gene, has been the highest priority in TS research during the past decade. Unfortunately, despite a concentrated effort by many investigators, the TS gene has thus far eluded this intensive search. A systematic genome scan using 76 affected sib-pair families with a total of 110 sib-pairs showed two regions, 4q and 8p, with lod scores of 2.38 and 2.09, respectively; 4 additional regions, on chromosomes 1, 10, 13, and 19, had lod scores greater than 1.0 (114). McMahon et al. (115) examined 175 members of a large, 4-generation TS family, plus 16 spouses who married into this family. Interestingly, they found evidence of TS in 36% of the family members and in 31% of the married-in spouses (some form of tic was found in 67% and 44%, respectively). Multivariate analysis showed that tics were more severe in the offspring of both parents with tics. This study raises the possibility of assortative mating in TS (in this case, like marry like), in contrast to random, nonassortative mating presumed in the general population. Thus bilineal transmission may lead to frequent homozygosity and high density of TS in some families. Using rigorous diagnostic criteria, we found that 25% of our TS patients had both parents with some features of TS: tics, 8%; OCD,

4%; and ADD, 12% (116). We compared our TS patients with a control population of 1,142 students, observed in second-, fifth-, and eighth-grade classrooms. In contrast to 5% frequency of ADD in 1 parent of controls, the occurrence of tics in at least 1 parent of TS cases was 31%, ADD 45%, and OCD 41%. Among all parents of TS cases, tics were present in 24%, OCD in 25%, and ADD in 34%, whereas only 3% of parents of controls exhibited ADD. Bilineal transmission violates the standard principle of 1 trait/1 locus and may explain why a gene marker has not yet been identified in TS despite intense collaborative research. Our results are similar to those of Lichter et al. (117) who found bilineal transmission in 6% of patients; tics or OCD represented bilineally in 22%. In a large family study and segregation analysis, Walkup et al. (118) provided evidence for a mixed model of inheritance rather than a simple autosomal model of inheritance. This complex model of inheritance suggests that the majority of TS patients have 2 copies of the gene, 1 from each parent. This is consistent with the observation that both parents of many TS patients are affected.

Twin studies, showing 89% concordance for TS and 100% concordance for either TS or CMTD, provide strong support for the genetic etiology of TS (90). How much influence environmental factors have on the phenotypic expression of this disorder is not known. Leckman et al. (119) in a search for nongenetic factors in the pathogenesis of TS found that maternal life stress, nausea, and vomiting during the first trimester of pregnancy were some of the perinatal factors that influenced the expression of the TS gene. In a study of 16 pairs of monozygotic twins, 94% of whom were concordant for tics, low birth weight was a strong predictor of tic severity, supporting a relationship between birth weight and phenotypic expression of TS (120). A major advance in the search for the elusive TS gene or genes has been made by the discovery of a frameshift mutation in the Slit and Trk-like 1 (SLITRK1) gene on chromosome 13q31.1 (121). These variants were absent in 172 other TS and in 3600 control chromosomes. The SLITRK1 gene has been found to be expressed in brain regions previously implicated in TS, such as the cortex; the hippocampus; thalamic, subthalamic, and globus pallidus nuclei; striatum; and cerebellum. It also appears to play a role in dendritic growth. Although we did not find a mutation in the SLITRK1 gene in any of our TS patients, suggesting that this gene abnormality is a rare cause of TS (121a) the gene discovery represents an important step forward in search of cellular mechanisms of TS.

Epidemiology

Discovery of a disease-specific marker will be helpful not only in improving our understanding of this complex neurobehavioral disorder but also in clarifying the epidemiology of TS (122). The prevalence rates have varied markedly and have been estimated to be as high as 4.2% when all types of tic disorders are included (123). There are many reasons for this wide variation, the most important of which are different ascertainment methods, different study populations, and different clinical criteria. Since about one-third of patients with tics do not recognize their presence, it is difficult to derive more accurate prevalence figures for TS without a well-designed door-to-door survey. Our own observational study involved 1,142 children in second, fifth, and eighth grades of general school population, among whom 8 (0.7%) had some evidence of TS (116). In another school-based study involving 167 randomly selected 13- and 14-year-olds in United Kingdom high schools, the prevalence of TS based on DSMIII-R was estimated at 3%, but 18% screened positive for tics (124). Kurlan et al. (125) found that 27% of 341 special-education students had tics, compared with 19.7% of 1,255 students in regular classroom programs; the incidence of TS was 7% and 3.8%, respectively. In another study, based on an interview of 1,596 children, Kurlan et al. (40) found that 339 (21%) had tics. Children with tics were younger, more likely to be male and attend special education classes, and more likely to have a lower mean IQ.

Hypothesis

A unifying hypothesis for the pathogenesis of TS suggests that TS represents a developmental disorder resulting in dopaminergic hyperinnervation of the ventral striatum and the associated limbic system. Although highly speculative, it is possible that the genetic defect in TS somehow interferes with normal apoptosis during development, resulting in the increased innervation of the ventral striatum and other limbic areas (126). This implies that the genetic defect interferes somehow with the programmed cell suicide needed to control cell proliferation in normal development and growth. The link between the basal ganglia and the limbic system may explain the frequent association of tics and complex behavioral problems, and a dysfunction in the Cortico-Striatal-Thalamic-Cortical (CSTC) circuitry seems to provide the best explanation for the most fundamental behavioral disturbance in TS, namely, loss of impulse control and a state of apparent disinhibition. There are currently no animal models of TS, except for some families of horses with equine self-mutilation syndrome with features resembling human TS (127). However, future genetic studies should provide insights into the pathogenesis of this complex neurobehavioral disorder and lead to animal models on which this and other hypotheses can be tested.

TREATMENT

The first step in the management of patients with TS is proper education of the patients, relatives, teachers, and other individuals who frequently interact with the patient regarding the nature of the disorder. School principals, teachers, and students can be helpful in implementing the therapeutic strategies. In addition, parents and the physician should work as partners in advocating the best possible school environment for the child. This may include extra break periods and a refuge area to "allow" release of tics, waiving time limitations on tests or adjusting timing of tests to the morning, and other measures designed to relieve stress. National and local support groups, particularly the Tourette Syndrome Association, can provide additional information and can serve as a valuable resource for the patient and his or her family (see For Further Information). Counseling and behavioral modification may be sufficient for those with mild symptoms. However, medications may be considered when symptoms begin to interfere with peer relationships, social interactions, academic or job performance, or activities of daily living. Because of the broad range of neurologic and behavioral manifestations and the varying severity of TS, treatment must be individualized and tailored specifically to the needs of the patient (Table 27.4) (128–130).

Before discussing pharmacologic therapy of TS symptoms, it is appropriate to make a few remarks about behavioral therapy (131). Different forms of behavioral modification have been recommended since the disorder was first described, but until recently few studies of behavioral treatments had been subjected to rigorous scientific scrutiny. Most of the reported studies suffer from poor or unreliable assessments, small sample size, short follow-up, lack of controls, no validation of compliance, and other methodologic flaws. Given these limitations, the following behavioral techniques have been reported to provide at least some benefit (131):

a. *Massed (negative) practice:* Voluntary and effortful repetition of the tic leads to a buildup of a state termed *reactive inhibition*, at which point the subject is forced to rest and not perform the tic due to an accumulation of "negative habit."

b. *Operant techniques/contingency management:* Tic-free intervals are positively reinforced, and tic behaviors are punished.

c. *Anxiety management techniques:* Relaxation training.

d. *Exposure-based treatment:* Desensitization to address tic triggering phenomena, such as premonitory sensory urges.

e. *Awareness training:* Direct visual feedback, self-monitoring, and awareness enhancement techniques, such as saying the letter "T" after each tic.

f. *Habit reversal training:* Consisting of reenactment of tic movements while looking in a mirror, training to detect and increase awareness of one's tics, identification of high-risk situations, training to isometrically contract the tic-opposing muscles, and recognition of and resistance to tic urges.

Wilhelm et al. (132) studied 32 patients with TS who were randomly assigned to 14 sessions of either habit reversal (awareness training, self-monitoring, relaxation training,

TABLE 27.4

PHARMACOLOGY OF TOURETTE'S SYNDROME

Drugs	Initial Dosage (mg/d)	Clinical Effect
Dopamine receptor blockers		Tics
1. Fluphenazine	1	+++
2. Pimozide	2	+++
3. Haloperidol	0.5	+++
4. Risperidone	0.5	++
5. Ziprasidone	20	++
6. Thiothixene	1	++
7. Trifluoperazine	1	++
8. Molindone	5	++
Dopamine depleters		Tics
1. Tetrabenazine	25	++
CNS Stimulants		ADHD
1. Methylphenidate	5	+++
2. Concerta	18	+++
3. Metadate CD	20	+++
4. Metadate ER	20	+++
5. Ritalin SR	20	+++
6. Adderall	10	+++
7. Pemoline	18.75	++
8. Dextroamphetamine	5	++
9. Dexedrine spansules	20	++
		Impulse control
Noradrenergic drugs		ADHD
1. Clonidine	0.1	++
2. Guanfacine	1.0	++
Serotonergic drugs		OCD
1. Fluoxetine	20	+++
2. Clomipramine	25	+++
3. Sertraline	50	+++
4. Paroxetine	20	+++
5. Fluvoxamine	50	+++
6. Venlafaxine	25	+++

+, minimal improvement; ++, moderate; +++, marked improvement, ADHD, attention-deficit hyperactivity disorder; OCD, obsessive–complusive disorder.

competing response training, and contingency management) or supportive psychotherapy. The 16 patients assigned to the habit reversal group "improved significantly" and "remained significantly improved over pretreatment at 10-month follow-up." This approach has been also found useful in the management of phonic tics (133). It is not clear whether patients without premonitory urges would benefit from this form of therapy. There is also some concern whether the mental effort required to fully comply with habit reversal training could actually interfere with the patient's attention and learning. Given the demands on patient, therapist, and parents for time and effort, it is not surprising that even if effective the benefits of habit reversal training are usually only temporary. However, the previously described therapies may be useful ancillary techniques in patients whose response to other therapies, including pharmacotherapy, is not entirely satisfactory.

Management of Tics

The goal of treatment should not be to completely eliminate all tics but to achieve a tolerable suppression. Because of the variability of tics in terms of severity, frequency, and distribution, the assessment of efficacy of a therapeutic intervention on tics is often problematic. A number of tic rating scales have been utilized, but none of them is ideal. Although at-home videotapes can be used to capture tics that are not appreciated by patients or when patients are examined in the clinic, video-based tic rating scales have many shortcomings (23).

Despite these limitations, controlled and open trials have shown that of the pharmacologic agents used for tic suppression, the dopamine receptor–blocking drugs (neuroleptics) are clearly most effective (62,130,134) (Table 27.4). Haloperidol (Haldol) and pimozide (Orap) are the only neuroleptics actually approved by the U.S. Food and Drug Administration for the management of TS. In one randomized, double-blind, controlled study, pimozide was found to be superior to haloperidol with respect to efficacy and side effects (135). We prefer fluphenazine (Prolixin) as the first-line anti-tic pharmacotherapy because it appears to have a lower incidence of sedation and other side effects (136). If fluphenazine fails to adequately control tics, we substitute risperidone (Risperdal) or pimozide. We usually start with fluphenazine, risperidone, and pimozide at 1 mg at bedtime and increase by 1 mg every 5 to 7 days. If these drugs fail to adequately control tics, then we try haloperidol, thioridazine (Mellaril), trifluoperazine (Stelazine), molindone (Moban), or thiothixene (Navane). Risperidone, a neuroleptic with both dopamine and serotonin blocking properties, has been shown to be effective in reducing tic frequency and intensity in most (137) but not all studies (138). It is not clear whether the atypical neuroleptics, such as clozapine (Clozaril), olanzapine (Zyprexa), or quetiapine (Seroquel), will be effective in the management of tics and other manifestations of TS. Quetiapine, a dibenzothiazepine that blocks not only D1 and D2 receptors but also $5\text{-}HT_{1A}$ and $5\text{-}HT_2$ receptors, has been reported to provide beneficial effects in some patients with TS, but the clinical improvement may not be sustained. Ziprasidone (Geodon), the most recently studied atypical neuroleptic, a potent blocker of both D2 and D3, as well as $5\text{-}HT_{2A}$, $5\text{-}HT_{2C}$, $5\text{-}HT_{1A}$, $5\text{-}HT_{1D}$, and α_1 receptors, was found to decrease tic severity by 35%, compared with a 7% change in the placebo group (139). Similar to pimozide, ziprasidone may prolong the QT interval but has an advantage over other atypical neuroleptics in that it is less likely to cause weight gain. The clinical significance of prolonged QT interval is controversial, but it may be associated with torsades de pointes, which potentially can degenerate into

ventricular fibrillation and sudden death. Besides pimozide and ziprasidone, other drugs that can prolong the QT interval include haloperidol, risperidone, thioridazine, and desipramine. Tetrabenazine, a monoamine-depleting and dopamine receptor–blocking drug, is a powerful anti-tic drug, but regrettably it is not readily available in the United States (140). This drug has been effective in the management of TS and has an advantage over conventional neuroleptics in that it does not cause tardive dyskinesias. Drugs used in the management of tics include sulpiride, tiapride, metoclopramide, piquindone, and others (130,134).

The side effects associated with neuroleptics, such as sedation, depression, weight gain, and school phobia, seem to be somewhat less common with fluphenazine than with haloperidol and the other neuroleptics (137). The most feared side effects of chronic neuroleptic therapy include tardive dyskinesia and hepatotoxicity. In addition, pimozide may prolong the QT interval, and, therefore, patients treated with the drug must undergo an electrocardiographic examination before starting therapy. We repeat the electrocardiographic examination about 3 months later and annually thereafter. It is important to note that certain antibiotics, such as clarithromycin, can raise the blood levels of pimozide and indirectly contribute to the drug's cardiotoxicity. Tardive dyskinesia, usually manifested by stereotypic involuntary movements, is only rarely persistent in children. However, tardive dystonia, a variant of tardive dyskinesias most frequently encountered in young adults, may persist and occasionally progresses to a generalized and disabling dystonic disorder. Other movement disorders associated with neuroleptics include bradykinesia, akathisia, and acute dystonic reactions (141). Therefore, careful monitoring of patients is absolutely essential and, whenever possible, the dosage should be reduced or even discontinued during periods of remission or during vacations.

Several nonneuroleptic treatments have been reported to be effective in the treatment of tics. In one study, 24 patients with TS (ages 7 to 17 years), who were medication free for 4 weeks prior to treatment, were randomized to receive either placebo or pergolide for 6 weeks, followed by a 2-week washout, and then crossed over to the other treatment arm (142). Although the authors conclude that "pergolide appears to be a safe and efficacious treatment for TS in children," this result may seem paradoxical in view of the well-known beneficial effects of dopamine receptor blockers. In a follow-up, randomized, placebo-controlled trial, they concluded that "pergolide appeared to be an efficacious and safe medication for tic reduction in children, and may also improve attention deficit hyperactivity disorder symptoms" (143). Ropinirole, another dopamine agonist, also has been found to be effective in the treatment of TS (144). These findings seem paradoxical in view of the well-known beneficial effects of dopamine receptor blockers. It is possible, however, that the observed effects of dopamine agonists could be mediated by their action on dopamine D2 autoreceptors, thus reducing endogenous dopamine turnover.

Clonazepam is another drug that is sometimes useful in patients with TS, particularly in the management of clonic tics. Since some of the premonitory sensations resemble obsessions and the tics may be viewed as "compulsive" movements, anti-OCD medications also may be helpful. Management of the premonitory sensations may lead to improvement of these tics. Since sex steroids affect the expression of TS gene and modulate multiple neurotransmitter systems, antiandrogens have been tried in the treatment of patients with TS. Flutamide, an acetanilide nonsteroidal androgen antagonist, has been found in one double-blind, placebo-controlled study to modestly and transiently reduce motor, but not phonic, tics with a mild improvement in associated symptoms of OCD (145). Because of potentially serious side effects, such as diarrhea and fulminant hepatic necrosis, this drug should be reserved for those patients in whom tics remain a disabling problem despite optimal anti-tic therapy. Ondansetron, a selective 5-HT$_3$ antagonist at 8 to 16 mg/day for 3 weeks, has been associated with a decrease in severity of tics (146). Baclofen, a GABA$_B$ autoreceptor agonist, has been found to markedly decrease the severity of motor and phonic tics in 95% of 264 patients with TS (147); however, a double-blind, placebo-controlled, crossover trial of 9 patients with TS showed that the beneficial response to baclofen was due to improvement in overall impairment score rather than a reduction of tic activity (148). Donepezil, a noncompetitive inhibitor of acetylcholinesterase, has been reported anecdotally to suppress tics (149).

Ever since the discovery that cannabinoids markedly potentiate neuroleptic-induced hypokinesis in rats and that their effects on the extrapyramidal motor system may be mediated through nicotinic cholinergic receptors, interest has been growing in nicotine as a treatment for various movement disorders, including TS (150,151). Mecamylamine (Inversine), an antihypertensive agent with central antinicotinic properties, was initially shown to improve tics and behavioral problems in 11 of 13 patients with TS at doses up to 5 mg/day (150,151). However, a subsequent double-blind, placebo-controlled study failed to demonstrate a significant benefit on the symptoms associated with TS (152). Finally, there have been several anecdotal reports of marijuana helping various symptoms of TS. This is consistent with the finding that cannabinoid receptors are densely located in the output nuclei of the basal ganglia and that activation of these receptors increases GABAergic transmission and inhibition of glutamate release (153). Some patients clearly benefit when taking the cannabinoid analog dronabinol (Marinol) at a dosage of 2.5 to 10 mg twice a day.

Motor tics may be successfully managed with botulinum toxin (BTX) injections in the affected muscles. Such focal chemodenervation ameliorates not only the involuntary movements but also the premonitory sensory component. I initially treated 10 TS patients with BTX injections into the involved muscles, and all experienced moderate to marked improvement in the intensity and frequency of their tics (154). Subsequent experience with a large number of patients has confirmed the beneficial effects of BTX injections in the management of motor and phonic tics, including severe coprolalia (155,156). Furthermore, those patients in whom premonitory sensations preceded the onset of tics noted lessening of these sensory symptoms. The benefits last on the average 3 to 4 months, and there are usually no serious complications. In a study of 35 patients treated for troublesome or disabling tics in 115 sessions, the mean peak effect response was 2.8 (range 0 to 4) (156). The mean duration of benefit was 14.4 weeks (up to 45). Latency to onset of benefit was 3.8 days (up to 10). Mean duration of tics prior to initial injections was 15.3 years (range 1 to 62), and mean duration of follow-up was 21.2 months (range 1.5 to 84). Of 25 patients with notable premonitory sensory symptoms, 20 (84%) derived marked relief of these symptoms from BTX (mean benefit: 70.6%). Patients reported an overall global response of 62.7%. We concluded that BTX is effective and well tolerated in the management of tics. An additional and consistent finding was the relief of disturbing premonitory sensations. In a placebo-controlled study of 18 patients with simple motor tics, Marras et al. (157) found a 39% reduction in the number of tics per minute within 2 weeks after injection with BTX, as compared with a 6% increase in the placebo group. In addition, there was a significant reduction in urge scores with BTX compared with an increase in the placebo group. However, this preliminary study lacked the power to show significant differences in other measured variables, such as severity score, tic suppression, pain, and patient global impression. Furthermore, the full effect of BTX may not have been appreciated at only 2 weeks; a single treatment protocol does not reflect the clinical practice of evaluating patients after several adjustments in dose and site of injection; and the patients' complaints were relatively mild since they "did not rate themselves as significantly compromised by their treated tics" at baseline (158). A larger sample and longer follow-up will be needed to further evaluate the efficacy of BTX in the management of tics and to demonstrate that this treatment offers clinically meaningful benefit.

Surgical treatment of TS is controversial, and the overall experience of stereotactic surgery in the management of tics has been somewhat disappointing. Experience with 17 TS patients, median age 23 years (range 11 to 40), treated with ablative procedures between 1970 and 1998 was reviewed by Babel et al. (159). Unilateral zona incerta and ventrolateral/lamella medialis (VL/LM) lesioning was used, and occasionally second surgery on the contralateral side was performed. The authors concluded that the procedures "sufficiently" reduced both motor and phonic tics. Transient complications were reported in 68% of patients, and only 1 patient suffered permanent complications. Although stereotactic surgery has not been found to be generally useful in the management of tics (see discussion of surgical treatment of OCD), a preliminary report of a 42-year-old man with severe motor and phonic tics controlled by high-frequency deep-brain stimulation of the thalamus and other targets, such as globus pallidus internus, in subsequent patient is quite encouraging (160–163). An increasing number of reports have provided evidence that deep brain stimulation (DBS) involving the thalamus, globus pallidus, and other targets may be a very effective strategy to treat uncontrollable tics (143–145).

Management of Behavioral Symptoms

Attention-Deficit Hyperactivity Disorder

Behavioral modification, school and classroom adjustments, and other approaches described previously may be useful in selected patients for the management of behavioral problems associated with TS. However, pharmacologic therapy is required when the symptoms of ADHD impair interpersonal relationships and interfere with academic or occupational performance (164). The NIMH Collaborative Multimodal Treatment Study of Children with ADHD found medication superior to behavioral treatment (165).

Central nervous system (CNS) stimulants—such as methylphenidate (Ritalin), controlled-release methylphenidate (Concerta), controlled-delivery methylphenidate (Metadate CD), dexmethylphenidate (Focalin), d-amphetamine (Dexedrine), a mixture of amphetamine salts with a 75:25 ratio of d- and l-amphetamine (Adderall), and pemoline (Cylert)—are clearly the most effective agents in the management of ADHD. The initial dose for methylphenidate is 5 mg in the morning, and the dose can be gradually advanced up to 20–60 mg/day (0.3–0.7 mg/kg per dose). Methylphenidate has been found to be useful not only in the management of attention deficit but also as a short-term therapy for conduct disorders (166). Doses of d-amphetamine are usually one-half of those of methylphenidate. Pemoline should be given as a single morning dose that is approximately 6 times the daily dose of methylphenidate. These drugs usually have a rapid onset of action but also have a relatively short half-life. The long-acting preparations, such as Ritalin SR (20 mg), are less reliable and less effective than 2 doses of standard preparation. Dexedrine Spansule has the advantage of a greater range of available doses (5 mg, 10 mg, 15 mg). Some studies (167,168) suggest that l-amphetamine is better tolerated, produces less anorexia and sedation, and may be longer lasting than methyl-phenidate and can be administered as a one-time (morning) dose. Only future studies will determine the utility of the new formulation of methylphenidate using a novel controlled-release delivery system designed for once-daily oral dosing (Concerta: 18–36 mg methylphenidate; Metadate CD: 20 mg methylphenidate). Metadate CD is formulated to release 6 mg of methylphenidate from immediate-release (IR) and 14 mg from extended-release (ER) beads. Tolerance, while rare, is more likely to occur with the long-acting formulations, but this has not been demonstrated in patients with ADHD. In addition to the possible development of tolerance, potential side effects of these stimulant drugs include nervousness, irritability, insomnia, anorexia, abdominal pain, and headaches. In one study, d-amphetamine was found to cause more insomnia and negative emotional symptoms than methylphenidate (169). Pemoline can rarely produce chemical hepatitis and even fulminant liver failure. Liver enzymes should be assessed before administration, but because the onset of hepatitis is unpredictable, routine laboratory studies are not useful. Parents should be instructed to notify the physician if nausea, vomiting, lethargy, malaise, or jaundice appears. Although growth retardation has been suggested by some studies, this effect, if present at all, is minimal and probably clinically insignificant.

CNS stimulants may exacerbate or precipitate tics in up to 25% of patients. However, if the symptoms of ADHD are troublesome and interfere with a patient's functioning, it is reasonable to use these CNS stimulants and to titrate the dosage to the lowest effective level (Table 27.4). More recent studies suggest that while CNS stimulants may exacerbate tics when they are introduced into the anti-TS treatment regimen, with continued use these drugs can be well tolerated without tic exacerbation (170–173). The dopamine receptor–blocking drugs can be combined with the CNS stimulants if the latter produce unacceptable exacerbation of tics. If one stimulant is ineffective or poorly tolerated, another stimulant should be tried.

Although initially thought to work by raising brain levels of dopamine, more recent studies have suggested that methylphenidate's beneficial effects on ADHD are mediated via the serotonin system (174). A strain of mice with inactivated gene for dopamine transporter (DAT) has been described to exhibit behavioral symptoms similar to those in children with ADHD. Mice hyperactivity was markedly ameliorated by methylphenidate, and this improvement correlated with an increase in brain serotonin. Other investigators have provided evidence that ADHD is a "noradrenergic disorder" (175). Although it has been suggested that long-term use of CNS stimulants may lead to substance abuse, some studies have demonstrated that untreated ADHD is a significant risk factor for substance abuse and that management of ADHD with CNS stimulants significantly reduces the risk for substance abuse disorder (176).

The α_2 agonists and tricyclic antidepressants are also useful in the management of ADHD, particularly if CNS stimulants are not well tolerated or are contraindicated. Clonidine (Catapres), a presynaptic α_2-adrenergic agonist used as an antihypertensive because it decreases plasma norepinephrine, improves symptoms of ADHD and impulse control. Although a multicenter controlled clinical trial showed that clonidine is an effective anti-tic drug (173), our experience has suggested that the perceived benefit may be due not to a specific anti-tic efficacy but rather to a nonspecific anxiolytic effect or its beneficial effect on comorbid disorders (see the following). The usual starting dose is 0.1 mg at bedtime, and the dosage is gradually increased up to 0.5 mg/day in 3 divided doses. The drug is also available as a transdermal patch (Catapres TTS-1, TTS-2, TTS-3, corresponding to 0.1, 0.2, and 0.3 mg) that should be changed once a week, using a different skin location. Side effects include sedation, light-headedness, headache, dry mouth, and insomnia. Because of its sedative effects, some clinicians use clonidine as a nighttime soporific agent. Although the patch can cause local irritation, it seems to cause fewer side effects than oral clonidine.

Another drug increasingly used in the management of ADHD and impulse control problems is guanfacine (Tenex), available as 1-mg or 2-mg tablets. The initial dose is 0.5 mg at bedtime with gradual increases, as needed, to final doses up to 4–6 mg/day. Pharmacologically similar to clonidine, guanfacine may be effective in patients in whom clonidine failed to control the behavioral symptoms. Guanfacine may have some advantages over clonidine in that it has a longer half-life, appears to be less sedating, and produces less hypotension. It also seems to be more selective for the α_2-noradrenergic receptor and binds more selectively to the postsynaptic α_{2A}-adrenergic receptors located in the prefrontal cortex. Although both clonidine and guanfacine appear to be effective in the management of attention deficit with and without hyperactivity, they appear to be particularly useful in the management of oppositional, argumentative, impulsive, and aggressive behavior. The most frequently encountered side effects include sedation, dry mouth, itchy eyes, dizziness, headaches, fatigability, and postural hypotension. We have also found deprenyl or selegiline (Eldepryl), a monoamine oxidase B inhibitor, to be effective in controlling the symptoms of ADHD without exacerbating tics (177). It is not clear how deprenyl improves symptoms of ADHD, but the drug is known to metabolize into amphetamines. Other drugs frequently used in relatively mild cases of ADHD include imipramine (Tofranil), nortriptyline (Pamelor), and desipramine (Norpramin). Because of potential cardiotoxicity, electrocardiographic or cardiologic evaluation may be needed before initiation of desipramine therapy, and follow-up electrocardiography should be performed every 3 to 6 months. It is not yet known whether nonstimulant drugs, such as modafinil or atomoxetine (inhibitor of presynaptic norepinephrine transporter) (178), will be useful in the management of ADHD associated with TS. In a study of 148 children and adolescents with ADHD and comorbid tic disorders, atomoxetine improved measures of ADHD and reduced tics compared to placebo (179).

Obsessive–Compulsive Disorder

The role of cognitive–behavioral psychotherapy in the management of OCD has not been well defined, but this approach is gaining more acceptance particularly when used in combination with pharmacotherapy (44,180). Although imipramine and desipramine have been reported to be useful in the management of OCD, the most effective drugs are the selective serotonin reuptake inhibitors (SSRIs) (181). These include fluoxetine (Prozac), fluvoxamine (Luvox), clomipramine (Anafranil), paroxetine (Paxil), sertraline (Zoloft), venlafaxine (Effexor), and citalopram (Celexa). The initial dosage of clomipramine is 25 mg at bedtime, and the dosage can be gradually increased up to 250 mg/day, using 25-, 50-, or 75-mg capsules after meals or at bedtime. Fluoxetine, paroxetine, and citalopram should be started at 20 mg after breakfast, and the dosage can be increased up to 80 mg/day. In contrast to clomipramine and fluvoxamine, the other SSRIs should be started as a morning (after breakfast) dose. Although comparative trials have been lacking, meta-analyses have provided some useful information. In one such analysis, venlafaxine was found to be particularly effective in the management of depression and inducing remission, compared with the other SSRIs, possibly because of its dual effect of inhibiting both serotonin and noradrenaline (182). In addition to its antidepressant and anti-OCD effects, fluvoxamine has been found to be an effective treatment for children and adolescents with social phobia and anxiety, a relatively common comorbidity in patients with TS (183). Sudden explosive attacks of rage, which occur in a considerable proportion of patients with TS, have been found to respond to SSRIs, such as paroxetine (184). Certain drugs, such as lithium and buspirone, have been reported to augment the SSRIs, but there is little information about the potential synergistic effects of different SSRIs. When a combination of drugs, or polypharmacy, is used, it is prudent to discuss with the patients potential adverse reactions, including the serotonin syndrome (confusion, hypomania, agitation, myoclonus, hyperreflexia, sweating, tremor, diarrhea, and fever), withdrawal phenomenon, and possible extrapyramidal side effects.

In patients with extremely severe and disabling OCD in whom optimal pharmacologic therapy has failed, psychosurgery, limbic leucotomy or cingulotomy, or anterior capsulotomy may be considered as a last resort (185). Although some pilot studies suggest that stereotactic infrathalamic lesions or deep-brain stimulation can improve OCD (160), long-term results are lacking.

FOR FURTHER INFORMATION

Tourette Syndrome Association (TSA)
42-40 Bell Boulevard
Bayside, NY 11361
Tel: 718-224-2999
http://neuro-www2.mgh.harvard.edu/tsa/tsamain.nclk

RELATED WEB SITES

http://www.ed.gov

http://www.nih.gov

http://www.wemove.org

Obsessive Compulsive Foundation: http://www.ocfoundation.org

Children and Adults with Attention Deficit Disorder: http://www.chadd.org

ADDITIONAL WEB SITES

http://www.cw.bc.ca

http://www.medscape.com

REFERENCES

1. Jankovic J. Tourette's syndrome. *N Engl J Med* 2001;345: 1184–1192.
2. Singer HS. Tourette's syndrome: from behaviour to biology. *Lancet Neurol* 2005;4:149–159.
3. Kurlan R. Hypothesis II: Tourette's syndrome is part of a clinical spectrum that includes normal brain development. *Arch Neurol* 1994;51:1145–1150.
4. Jankovic J, Sekula SL, Milas D. Dermatological manifestations of Tourette's syndrome and obsessive-compulsive disorder. *Arch Dermatol* 1998;134:113–114.
5. Hogan MB, Wilson NW. Tourette's syndrome mimicking asthma. *J Asthma* 1999;36:253–256.
6. Jog MS, Kubota Y, Connolly CI, et al. Building neural representations of habits. *Science* 1999;286:1745–1749.
7. Jankovic J. Phenomenology and classification of tics. *Neurol Clin North Am* 1997;15:267–275.
8. Németh AH, Mills KR, Elston JS, et al. Do the same genes predispose to Gilles de la Tourette syndrome and dystonia? Report of a new family and review of the literature. *Mov Disord* 1999;14:826–831.
9. Kwak C, Dat Vuong K, Jankovic J. Premonitory sensory phenomenon in Tourette's syndrome. *Mov Disord* 2003;18:1530–1533.
10. Chee K-Y, Sachdev P. A controlled study of sensory tics in Gilles de la Tourette syndrome and obsessive-compulsive disorder using a structured interview. *J Neurol Neurosurg Psychiatry* 1997;62:188–192.
11. Rickards H, Robertson MM. Vomiting and retching in Gilles de la Tourette syndrome: a report of ten cases and a review of the literature. *Mov Disord* 1997;12:531–535.
12. Peterson BS, Leckman JF. The temporal dynamics of tics in Gilles de la Tourette syndrome. *Biol Psychiatry* 1998;44:1337–1348.
13. Peterson BS, Skudlarski P, Anderson AW, et al. A functional magnetic resonance imaging study of tic suppression in Tourette syndrome. *Arch Gen Psychiatry* 1998;54:326–333.
14. Rothenberger A, Kostanecka T, Kinkelbur J, et al. Sleep and Tourette syndrome. In: Cohen D, Jankovic J, Goetz C, eds. *Tourette syndrome: advances in neurology*, vol. 85. Philadelphia: Lippincott Williams & Wilkins, 2001:245–260.
15. Hanna PA, Jankovic J. Sleep and tic disorders. In: Chokroverty S, Hening Walters A, eds. *Sleep and movement disorders*. Woburn, MA: Butterworth-Heinemann, 2003:464–471.
16. Cardoso FEC, Jankovic J. Cocaine related movement disorders. *Mov Disord* 1993;8:175–178.
17. Jankovic J, Mejia NI. Tics associated with other disorders. In: Walkup J, Mink J, Hollenbeck P, eds. *Tourette syndrome. Adv Neurol.* Lippincott Williams & Wilkins, 2006:61–68.
18. Kompoliti K, Goetz CG. Hyperkinetic movement disorders misdiagnosed as tics in Gilles de la Tourette syndrome. *Mov Disord* 1998;13:477–480.
19. The Tourette Syndrome Classification Study Group. Definitions and classification of tic disorders. *Arch Neurol* 1993;50: 1013–1016.
20. American Psychiatric Association. *Diagnostic and statistical manual of mental disorders*, 4th ed. Washington, DC, 1994:100–105.
21. Kurlan R. Diagnostic criteria for genetic studies of Tourette syndrome. *Arch Neurol* 1997;54:517–518.
22. Robertson MM, Banerjee S, Kurlan R, et al. The Tourette Syndrome Diagnostic Confidence Index: development and clinical associations. *Neurology* 1999;53:2108–2112.
23. Goetz CG, Leurgans S, Chumara TA. Home alone: methods to maximize tic expression for objective videotape assessments in Gilles de la Tourette syndrome. *Mov Disord* 2001;16:693–697.
24. Goetz CG, Kampoliti K. Rating scales and quantitative assessment of tics. In: Cohen DJ, Jankovic J, Goetz CG, eds. *Tourette syndrome: advances in neurology*, vol. 85. Philadelphia: Lippincott Williams & Wilkins, 2001:31–42.
25. Tulen JHM, Azzolini M, De Vries JA, et al. Quantitative study of spontaneous eye blinks and eye tics in Gilles de la Tourette's syndrome. *J Neurol Neurosurg Psychiatry* 1999;67:800–802.
26. Leckman JF, Zhang H, Vitale A, et al. Course of tic severity in Tourette syndrome: the first two decades. *Pediatrics* 1998;102: 14–19.
27. Goetz CG, Tanner CM, Stebbins GT, et al. Adult tics in Gilles de la Tourette's syndrome: description and risk factors. *Neurology* 1992;42:784–788.
28. Chouinard S, Ford B. Adult onset tic disorders. *J Neurol Neurosurg Psychiatry* 2000;68:738–743.
29. Krauss JK, Jankovic J. Severe motor tics causing cervical myelopathy in Tourette's syndrome. *Mov Disord* 1996;11:563–566.
30. Robertson MM. The Gilles de la Tourette syndrome: the current status. *Br J Psychiatry* 1989;154:147–169.
31. Abwender DA, Trinidad K, Jones KR, et al. Features resembling Tourette's syndrome in developmental stutterers. *Brain Language* 1998;62:455–464.
32. Farber RH, Swerdlow NR, Clementz BA. Saccadic performance characteristics and the behavioural neurology of Tourette's syndrome. *J Neurol Neuorsurg Psychiatry* 1999;66:305–312.
33. Goldenberg JN, Brown SB, Weiner WJ. Coprolalia in younger patients with Gilles de la Tourette syndrome. *Mov Disord* 1994;9:622–625.
34. LeVasseur AL, Flanagan JR, Riopelle RJ, et al. Control of volitional and reflexive saccades in Tourette's syndrome. *Brain* 2001;124: 2045–2058.
35. Swanson JM, Sergeant JA, Taylor E, et al. Attention-deficit hyperactivity disorder and hyperactivity disorder. *Lancet* 1998;351: 429–433.
36. Goldman LS, Genel M, Bezman RJ, et al. Diagnosis and treatment of attention-deficit/hyperactivity disorder in children and adolescents. *JAMA* 1998;279:1100–1107.
37. Carter AS, O'Donnell DA, Schultz RT, et al. Social and emotional adjustment in children affected with Gilles de la Tourette's syndrome associations with ADHD and family functioning. *J Child Psychol Psychiatry* 2000;41:215–223.
38. Richard MM, Finkel MF, Cohen MD. Preparing reports documenting attention deficit/hyperactivity disorder for students in post-secondary education: what neurologists need to know. *Neurologist* 1998;4:277–283.
39. Coffey BJ, Park KS. Behavioral and emotional aspects of Tourette syndrome. *Neurol Clin North Am* 1997;15:277–290.
40. Kurlan R, Como PG, Miller B, et al. The behavioral spectrum of tic disorders: a community-based study. *Neurology* 2002;59:414–420.
41. Dulcan M, AACAP Works Group on Quality Issues. Practice parameters for the assessment and treatment of children, adolescents, and adults with attention-deficit/hyperactivity disorder. *J Am Acad Child Adolesc Psychiatry* 1997;36:10(suppl):85S–121S.
42. Smalley SL, Fisher SE, Francks C, et al. Genome-wide scan in attention deficit hyperactivity disorders (AHD). *Am J Hum Genet* 2001;69:535 (abstract).
43. Leibson CL, Katusic SK, Barbaresi WJ, et al. Use and costs of medical care for children and adolescents with and without attention-deficit/hyperactivity disorder. *JAMA* 2001;285:60–66.
44. Micallef J, Blin O. Neurobiology and clinical pharmacology of obsessive-compulsive disorder. *Clin Neuropharmacol* 2001;24: 191–207.
45. Stein D. The neurobiology of obsessive-compulsive disorder. *Neuroscientist* 1996;2:300–305.

46. Snider LA, Swedo SE. Pediatric obsessive-compulsive disorder. *JAMA* 2000;284:3104–3106.
47. Nestadt G, Bienvenu OJ, Cai G, et al. Incidence of obsessive-compulsive disorder in adults. *J Nerv Ment Dis* 1998;186:401–406.
48. Scahill L, Riddle MA, McSwiggin-Hardin M, et al. Children's Yale-Brown Obsessive Compulsive Scale: reliability and validity. *J Am Acad Child Adolesc Psychiatry* 1997;36:844–852.
49. Leckman JF, Walker DE, Goodman WK, et al. "Just right" perceptions associated with compulsive behavior in Tourette's syndrome. *Am J Psychiatry* 1994;151:675–680.
50. Singer HS, Schuerholz LJ, Denckla MB. Learning difficulties in children with Tourette's syndrome. *J Child Neurol* 1995;10:558–561.
51. Eapen V, Robertson MM, Alsobrook JP, et al. Obsessive-compulsive symptoms in Gilles de la Tourette syndrome and obsessive compulsive disorder: differences by diagnosis and family history. *Am J Med Genet* 1997;74:432–438.
52. Leckman JF, Grice DE, Boardman J, et al. Symptoms of obsessive-compulsive disorder. *Am J Psychiatry* 1997;154:911–917b.
53. Berthier ML, Kulisevsky J, Gironell A, et al. Obsessive-compulsive disorder associated with brain lesions: clinical phenomenology, cognitive function, and anatomic correlates. *Neurology* 1996;47: 353–361.
54. Kwak C, Vuong KD, Jankovic J: Premonitory sensory phenomenon in Tourette's syndrome. *Mov Disord* 2003;18:1530–1533.
55. Alsobrook JP, Pauls DL. The genetics of Tourette syndrome. *Neurol Clin N Am* 1997;15:381–394.
56. Leonard H. Tourette syndrome and obsessive compulsive disorder. In: Chase T, Friedhoff A, Cohen DJ, eds. *Tourette's syndrome: advances in neurology.* New York: Raven Press, 1992:83–94.
57. Siponmaa L, Kristiansson M, Jonson C, et al. Juvenile and young adult mentally disordered offenders: the role of child neuropsychiatric disorders. *J Am Acad Psychiatry Law* 2001;29:420–426.
58. Brower M, Price B. Neuropsychiatry of frontal lobe dysfunction in violent and criminal behavior: a critical review. *J Neurol Neurosurg Psychiatry* 2001;71:720–726.
59. Cardinal R, Pennicott D, Sugathapala C, et al. Impulsive choice induced in rats by lesions of the nucleus accumbens core. *Science* 2001;292:2499–2501.
60. Bechara A, Tranel D, Damasio H. Characterization of the decision-making deficit of patients with ventromedial prefrontal cortex lesions. *Brain* 2000;123:2189–2202.
61. Robertson M, Doran M, Trimble M, et al. The treatment of Gilles de la Tourette syndrome by limbic leucotomy. *J Neurol Neurosurg* 1990;53:691–694.
62. Robertson MM. Tourette syndrome, associated conditions, and the complexities of treatment. *Brain* 2000;123:425–462.
63. Robertson MM, Banerjee S, Fox Hiley PJ, et al. Personality disorder and psychopathology in Tourette's syndrome: a controlled study. *Br J Psychiatry* 1997;171:283–286.
64. Kwak C, Jankovic J. Migraine headache in Tourette syndrome. *Ann Neurol* 2001;50(suppl 1):S21–S22.
65. Freeman RD, Fast DK, Burd L, et al. Tourette Syndrome International Database Consortium. An international perspective on Tourette syndrome: selected findings from 3,500 individuals in 22 countries. *Dev Med Child Neurol* 2000;42:436–447.
66. Leckman JF, Peterson BS, Anderson GM, et al. Pathogenesis of Tourette's syndrome. *J Child Psychol Psychiatry* 1997;38:119–142a.
67. Palumbo D, Maughan A, Kurlan R. Hypothesis III: Tourette syndrome is only one of several causes of a developmental basal ganglia syndrome. *Arch Neurol* 1997;54:475–483.
68. Stell R, Thickbroom GW, Mastaglia FL. The audiogenic startle response in Tourette's syndrome. *Mov Disord* 1995;10:723–730.
69. Karp BI, Porter S, Toro C, et al. Simple motor tics may be preceded by a premotor potential. *J Neurol Neurosurg Psychiatry* 1996;61: 103–106.
70. Peterson BS. Neuroimaging studies of Tourette syndrome: a decade of progress. In: Cohen DJ, Jankovic J, Goetz CG, eds. *Tourette syndrome: advances in neurology,* vol. 85. Philadelphia: Lippincott Williams & Wilkins, 2001:179–196.
71. Serrien DJ, Nirkko AC, Loher TJ, et al. Movement control of manipulative tasks in patients with Gilles de la Tourette syndrome. *Brain* 2002;125:290–300.
72. Vaidya C, Austin G, Kirkorian G, et al. Selective effects of methylphenidate in attention deficit hyperactivity disorder: a functional magnetic resonance study. *Proc Natl Acad Sci USA* 1998;95:14,494–14,499.
73. Ziemann U, Paulus W, Rothenbgerger A. Decreased motor inhibition in Tourette's disorder: evidence from transcranial magnetic stimulation. *Am J Psychiatry* 1997;154:1277–1284.
74. Greenberg BD, Ziemann U, Harmon A, et al. Decreased neuronal inhibition in cerebral cortex in obsessive-compulsive disorder on transcranial magnetic stimulation. *Lancet* 1998;352:881–882.
75. Greenberg BD, Ziemann U, Cora-Locatelli G, et al. Altered cortical excitability in obsessive-compulsive disorder. *Neurology* 2000;54:142–147.
76. Moll GH, Heinrich H, Troo GE, et al. Children with comorbid attention-deficit-hyperactivity disorder and tic disorder: evidence for additive inhibitory deficits with the motor systems. *Ann Neurol* 2001;49:393–396.
77. Orth M, Amann B, Robertson MM, Rothwell JC. Excitability of motor cortex inhibitory circuits in Tourette syndrome before and after single dose nicotine. *Brain* 2005;128:1292–1300.
78. Voderholzer U, Müller N, Haag C, et al. Periodic limb movements during sleep are a frequent finding in patients with Gilles de la Tourette's syndrome. *J Neurol* 1997;244:521–520.
79. Picchietti DL, Underwood DJ, Farris WA, et al. Further studies on periodic limb movement disorder and restless legs syndrome in children with attention-deficit hyperactivity disorder. *Mov Disord* 1999;14:1000–1007.
80. Chokroverty S, Jankovic J. Restless legs syndrome: a disease in search of identity. *Neurology* 1999;52:907–910.
81. Frederickson KA, Cutting LE, Kates WR, et al. Disproportionate increases of white matter in right frontal lobe in Tourette syndrome. *Neurology* 2002;58:85–89.
82. Hyde TM, Stacey ME, Copoola R, et al. Cerebral morphometric abnormalities in Tourette's syndrome: a quantitative MRI study of monozygotic twins. *Neurology* 1995;45:1176–1182.
83. Baumgardner TL, Singer HS, Denckla MB, et al. Corpus callosum morphology in children with Tourette syndrome and attention. *Neurology* 1996;47:477–482.
84. Mostofsky SH, Wendlandt J, Cutting L, et al. Corpus callosum measurement in girls with Tourette syndrome. *Neurology* 1999;53: 1345–1347.
85. Bloch MH, Leckman JF, Zhu H, Peterson BS. Caudate volumes in childhood predict symptom severity in adults with Tourette syndrome. *Neurology* 2005;65:1253–1258.
86. Eidelberg D, Moeller JR, Antonini A, et al. The metabolic anatomy of Tourette's syndrome. *Neurology* 1997;48:927–934.
87. Stern E, Silbersweig DA, Chee K-Y, et al. A functional neuroanatomy of tics in Tourette syndrome. *Arch Gen Psychiatry* 2000;57:741–748.
88. Rauch SL, Savage CR, Alpert NM, et al. Probing striatal function in obsessive-compulsive disorder: a PET study of implicit sequence learning. *J Neuropsychiatry Clin Neurosci* 1997;9:568–573.
89. Filipek P, Semrud-Clikeman M, Steinggard RJ, et al. Volumetric MRI analysis comparing subjects having attention deficit-hyperactivity disorder with normal controls. *Neurology* 1997;48:589–601.
90. Singer HS. Current issues in Tourette syndrome. *Mov Disord* 2000;15:1051–1063.
91. Singer HS, Szymanski S, Giuliano J, et al. Elevated intrasynaptic dopamine release in Tourette's syndrome measured by PET. *Am J Psychiatry* 2002;159:1329–1336.
92. Albin RL, Koeppe RA, Bohnen NI, et al. Increased ventral striatal monoaminergic innervation in Tourette syndrome. *Neurology* 2003;61:310–315.
93. Minzer K, Lee O, Hong JJ, Singer HS. Increased prefrontal D2 protein in Tourette syndrome: a postmortem analysis of frontal cortex and striatum. *J Neurol Sci* 2004;219:55–61.
94. Malison RT, McDougl CJ, van Dyck CH, et al. [^{123}I]β-CIT SPECT imaging of striatal dopamine transporter binding in Tourette's disorder. *Am J Psychiatry* 1995;152:1359–1361.
95. Heinz A, Knable MB, Wolf SS, et al. Tourette's syndrome. [^{123}I]β-CIT SPECT correlates of vocal tic severity. *Neurology* 1998;51: 1069–1074.
96. Müller-Vahl KR, Berding G, Brücke T, et al. Dopamine transporter binding in Gilles de la Tourette syndrome. *J Neurol* 2000;247: 514–520.

97. Wolf S, Jones DW, Knable MB, et al. Tourette syndrome: prediction of phenotypic variation in monozygotic twins by caudate nucleus D2 receptor binding. *Science* 1996;273:1225–1227.

98. Kumar R, Lang AE. Coexistence of tics and parkinsonism: evidence for non-dopaminergic mechanisms in tic pathogenesis. *Neurology* 1997;49:1699–1701.

99. Turjanski N, Sawle GV, Playford ED, et al. PET studies of the presynaptic and postsynaptic dopaminergic system in Tourette's syndrome. *J Neurol Neurosurg Psychiatry* 1994;57:688–692.

100. Meyer P, Bohnen NI, Minshima S, et al. Striatal presynaptic monoaminergic vesicles are not increased in Tourette's syndrome. *Neurology* 1999;53:371–374.

101. Ernst M, Zametkin AJ, Jons PH, et al. High presynaptic dopaminergic activity in children with Tourette's disorder. *J Am Acad Child Adolesc Psychiatry* 1999;38:86–94.

102. Hallett JJ, Kiesling LS. Neuroimmunology of tics and other childhood hyperkinesias. *Neurol Clin North Am* 1997;15:333–344.

103. Hallett JJ, Harling-Berg CJ, Knopf PM, et al. Anti-striatal antibodies in Tourette syndrome cause neuronal dysfunction. *J Neuroimmunol* 2000;111:195–202.

104. Dale R, Church AJ, Cardoso F, et al. Poststreptococcal acute disseminated encephalomyelitis with basal ganglia involvement and auto-reactive antibasal ganglia antibodies. *Ann Neurol* 2001;50:588–595.

105. Hoekstra PJ, Bijzet J, Limburg PC, et al. Elevated D8/17 expression on B lymphocytes, a marker of rheumatic fever, measured with flow cytometry in tic disorder patients. *Am J Psychiatry* 2001;158:605–610.

106. Singer HS, Giuliano JD, Hansen BH, et al. Antibodies against human putamen in children with Tourette syndrome. *Neurology* 1998;50:1618–1624.

107. Trifiletti RR, Packard AM. Immune mechanisms in pediatric neuropsychiatric disorders: Tourette's syndrome, OCD, and PANDAS. *Child Adolesc Psychiatr Clin North Am* 1999;8:767–775.

108. Cardona F, Orefici G. Group A streptococcal infections and tic disorders in an Italian pediatric population. *J Pediatr* 2001;138:71–75.

109. Müller N, Kroll B, Schwartz MJ, et al. Increased titers of antibodies against streptococcal M12 and M19 proteins in patients with Tourette's syndrome. *Psychiatry Res* 2001;101:187–193.

110. Singer HS, Hong JJ, Yoon DY, Williams PN. Serum autoantibodies do not differentiate PANDAS and Tourette syndrome from controls. *Neurology* 2005;65:1701–1707.

111. Kurlan R. Tourette's syndrome and "PANDAS": Will the relation bear out? *Neurology* 1998;50:1530–1534.

112. Leonard H, Swedo SE, Garvey M, et al. Postinfectious and other forms of obsessive-compulsive disorder. *Child Adolesc Psychiatr Clin North Am* 1999;8:497–511.

113. Perlmutter SJ, Leitman SF, Garvey MA, et al. Therapeutic plasma exchange and intravenous immunoglobulin for obsessive-compulsive disorder and tic disorders in childhood. *Lancet* 1999;354:1153–1158.

114. The Tourette Syndrome Association International Consortium on Genetics. A complete genome screen in sib-pairs affected by Gilles de la Tourette syndrome. *Am J Hum Genet* 1999;65:1428–1436.

115. McMahon WM, van der Wetering BJ, Filoux F, et al. Bilineal transmission and phenotypic variations of Tourette's disorder in a large pedigree. *J Am Acad Child Adolesc Psychiatry* 1996;35:672–680.

116. Hanna PA, Janjua FN, Contant CF, et al. Bilineal transmission in Tourette syndrome. *Neurology* 1999;53:813–818.

117. Lichter DG, Dmochowski J, Jackson LA, et al. Influence of family history on clinical expression of Tourette's syndrome. *Neurology* 1999;52:308–316.

118. Walkup JT, LaBuda MC, Singer HS, et al. Family study and segregation analysis of Tourette syndrome: evidence for a mixed model of inheritance. *Am J Hum Genet* 1996;59:684–693.

119. Leckman JF, Dolnansky ES, Hardin MT, et al. Perinatal factors in the expression of Tourette's syndrome: an exploratory study. *J Am Acad Child Adolesc Psychiatry* 1990;29:220–226.

120. Hyde TM, Aaronson BA, Randolph C, et al. Relationship of birth weight to the phenotypic expression of Gilles de la Tourette's syndrome in monozygotic twins. *Neurology* 1992;42:652–658.

121. Abelson JF, Kwan KY, O'Roak BJ. Sequence variants in SLITRK1 are associated with Tourette's syndrome. *Science* 2005;310:317–320.

122. Scahill L, Tanner C, Dure L. The epidemiology of tics and Tourette syndrome in children and adolescents. In: Cohen DJ, Jankovic J, Goetz CG, eds. *Tourette syndrome: advances in neurology*, vol. 85. Philadelphia: Lippincott Williams & Wilkins, 2001:261–272.

123. Costello EJ, Angold A, Burns BJ, et al. The Great Smokey Mountains Study of Youth: goals, design, methods, and the prevalence of DSM-III-R disorders. *Arch Gen Psychiatry* 1996;53:1129–1136.

124. Mason A, Banerjee S, Zeitlin H, et al. The prevalence of Tourette syndrome in a mainstream school population. *Dev Med Child Neurol* 1998;40:292–296.

125. Kurlan R, McDermott MP, Deeley C, et al. Prevalence of tics in schoolchildren and association with placement in special education. *Neurology* 2001;57:1383–1388.

126. Itoh K, Suzuki K, Bise K, et al. Apoptosis in the basal ganglia of the developing human nervous system. *Acta Neuropathol* 2001;101:92–100.

127. Dodman NH, Normile JA, Shuster L, et al. Equine self-mutilation syndrome (57 cases). *JAVM* 1994;204:1219–1223.

128. Jankovic J. Gilles de la Tourette syndrome. In: Rakel RE, ed. Conn's current therapy. Philadelphia: WB Saunders, 1999:915–919.

129. Lang AE. Update on the treatment of tics. In: Cohen DJ, Jankovic J, Goetz CG, eds. *Tourette syndrome: advances in neurology*, vol. 85. Philadelphia: Lippincott Williams & Wilkins, 2001:355–362.

130. Jimenez-Jimenez FJ, Garcia-Ruiz PJ. Pharmacological options for the treatment of Tourette's disorder. *Drugs* 2001;61: 2207–2220.

131. Piacentini J, Chang S. Behavioral treatment for Tourette syndrome and tic disorders. In: Cohen DJ, Jankovic J, Goetz CG, eds. *Tourette syndrome: advances in neurology*, vol. 85. Philadelphia: Lippincott Williams & Wilkins, 2001:319–332.

132. Wilhelm S, Deckersbach T, Coffey BJ, Bohne A, Peterson AL, Baer L. Habit reversal versus supportive psychotherapy for Tourette's disorder: a randomized controlled trial. *Am J Psychiatry* 2003;160: 1175–1177.

133. Woods DW, Twohig MP, Flessner CA, Roloff TJ. Treatment of vocal tics in children with Tourette syndrome: investigating the efficacy of habit reversal. *J Appl Behav Anal* 2003;36:109–112.

134. Silay Y, Jankovic J. Emerging drugs in Tourette syndrome. *Expert Opini Emerging Drugs* 2005;10:365–380.

135. Sallee FR, Nesbit L, Jackson C, et al. Relative efficacy of haloperidol and pimozide in children and adolescents. *Am J Psychiatry* 1997;154:1057–1062.

136. Silay YS, Vuong KD, Jankovic J. The efficacy and safety of fluphenazine in patients with Tourette syndrome. *Neurology* 2004;62(suppl 5):A506.

137. Bruun RD, Budman CL. Risperidone as a treatment for Tourette's syndrome. *J Clin Psychiatry* 1996;57:29–31.

138. Robertson MM, Scull DA, Eapen V, et al. Risperidone in the treatment of Tourette syndrome: a retrospective case note study. *J Psychopharmacol* 1996;10:317–320.

139. Sallee FR, Kurlan R, Goetz CG, et al. Ziprasidone treatment of children and adolescents with Tourette's syndrome: a pilot study. *J Am Acad Child Adolesc Psychiatry* 2000;39:292–299.

140. Kenney C, Jankovic J. Tetrabenazine in the treatment of hyperkinetic movement disorders. *Expert Rev Neurotherapeutics* 2006;6:7–17.

141. Jankovic J. Tardive syndromes and other drug-induced movement disorders. *Clin Neuropharmacol* 1995;18:197–214.

142. Gilbert DL, Sethuraman G, Sine L, et al. Tourette's syndrome improvement with pergolide in a randomized, double-blind crossover trial. *Neurology* 2000;54:1310–1315.

143. Gilbert DL, Dure L, Sethuraman G, Raab D, Lane J, Sallee FR. Tic reduction with pergolide in a randomized controlled trial in children. *Neurology* 2003;60:606–611.

144. Anca MH, Giladi N, Korczyn AD. Ropinirole in Gilles de la Tourette syndrome. *Neurology* 2004;62:1626–1627.

145. Peterson BS, Zhang H, Anderson GM, et al. A double-blind, placebo-controlled, crossover trial of an antiandrogen in the treatment of Tourette's syndrome. *J Clin Psychopharmacol* 1998;18:324–331.

146. Toren P, Laor N, Cohen DJ, et al. Ondansetron treatment in patients with Tourette's syndrome. *Int Clin Psychopharmacol* 1999;14:373–376.

147. Awaad Y. Tics in Tourette syndrome: new treatment options. *J Child Neurol* 1999;14:316–319.
148. Singer HS, Wendlandt J, Krieger M, et al. Baclofen treatment in Tourette syndrome: a double-blind, placebo-controlled, crossover trial. *Neurology* 2001;56:599–604.
149. Hoopes SP. Donezepil for Tourette's disorder and ADHD. *J Clin Psychopharmacol* 1999;19:381–382.
150. Sanberg PR, Shytle RD, Silver AA. Treatment of Tourette's syndrome with mecamylamine. *Lancet* 1998;352:705–706.
151. Silver AA, Shytle RD, Sanberg PR. Mecamylamine in Tourette's syndrome: a two-year retrospective case study. *J Child Adolesc Psychopharmacol* 2000;10:59–68.
152. Silver AA, Shytle RD, Sheehan D, et al. A multi-center, double-blind placebo controlled safety and efficacy study of mecamylamine (inversine) monotherapy for Tourette syndrome. *J Am Acad Child Adolesc Psychiatry* 2001;40:1103–1110.
153. Müller-Vahl KR, Kolbe H, Schneider U, et al. Cannabis in movement disorders. *Forsch Komplementarmed* 1999;6(suppl 3):23–27.
154. Jankovic J. Botulinum toxin in the treatment of dystonic tics. *Mov Disord* 1994;9:347–349.
155. Scott BL, Jankovic J, Donovan DT. Botulinum toxin into vocal cord in the treatment of malignant coprolalia associated with Tourette's syndrome. *Mov Disord* 1996;11:431–433.
156. Kwak CH, Hanna PA, Jankovic J. Botulinum toxin in the treatment of tics. *Arch Neurol* 2000;57:1190–1193.
157. Marras C, Andrews D, Sime EA, et al. Botulinum toxin for simple motor tics: a randomized, double-blind, controlled clinical trial. *Neurology* 2001;56:605–610.
158. Kurlan R. New treatments for tics? *Neurology* 2001;56:580–581.
159. Babel TB, Warnke PC, Ostertag CB. Immediate and long term outcome after infrathalamic and thalamic lesioning for intractable Tourette's syndrome. *J Neurol Neurosurg Psychiatry* 2001;70:666–671.
160. Vandewalle V, Van Der Linden C, Groenegen HJ, et al. Stereotactic treatment of Gilles de la Tourette syndrome by high frequency stimulation of thalamus. *Lancet* 1999;353:724.
161. Temel Y, Visser-Vandewalle V. Surgery in Tourette syndrome. *Mov Disord* 2004;19:3–14.
162. Houeto JL, Karachi C, Mallet L, et al. Tourette's syndrome and deep brain stimulation. *J Neurol Neurosurg Psychiatry* 2005;76:992–995.
163. Shahed J, Poysky J, Kenney C, et al. Bilateral GPi deep brain stimulation for Tourette syndrome: *Neurology* 2006;66:A366.
164. Riddle MA, Carlson J. Clinical psychopharmacology for Tourette syndrome and associated disorders. In: Cohen DJ, Jankovic J, Goetz CG, eds. *Tourette syndrome: advances in neurology*, vol. 85. Philadelphia: Lippincott Williams & Wilkins, 2001: 343–354.
165. The MTA Cooperative Group. A 14-month randomized clinical trial of treatment strategies for attention-deficit/hyperactivity disorder: The MTA Cooperative Group. Multimodal Treatment Study of Children with ADHD. *Arch Gen Psychiatry* 1999;56:1073–1086.
166. Klein RG, Abikoff H, Klass E, et al. Clinical efficacy of methylphenidate in conduct disorder with and without attention deficit hyperactivity disorder. *Arch Gen Psychiatry* 1997;54:1073–1080.
167. Manos MJ, Short EJ, Findling RL. Differential effectiveness of methylphenidate and Adderall in school-age youths with attention-deficit/hyperactivity disorder. *J Am Acad Child Adolesc Psychiatry* 1999;38:813–819.
168. Pliszka SR, Browne RG, Olvera RL, et al. A double-blind, placebo-controlled study of Adderall and methylphenidate in the treatment of attention-deficit/hyperactivity disorder. *J Am Acad Child Adolesc Psychiatry* 2000;39:619–626.
169. Efron D, Jarman F, Barker M, et al. Side effects of methylphenidate and dextroamphetamine in children with attention deficit hyperactivity disorder: a double-blind, crossover trial. *Pediatrics* 1997;100:662–666.
170. Gadow KD, Sverd J, Sprafkin J, et al. Long-term methylphenidate therapy in children with comorbid attention-deficit hyperactivity and chronic multiple tic disorder. *Arch Gen Psychiatry* 1999;56:330–336.
171. Law SF, Schachtar RT. Do typical clinical doses of methylphenidate cause tics in children treated for attention-deficit hyperactivity disorder? *J Amer Acad Child Adolesc Psychiatry* 1999;38:944–951.
172. Kurlan R. Methylphenidate to treat ADHD is not contraindicated in children with tics. *Mov Disord* 2002;17:5–6.
173. The Tourette's Syndrome Study Group. Treatment of ADHD in children with tics: a randomized controlled trial. *Neurology* 2002;58:527–536.
174. Gainetdinov RR, Wetsel WC, Jones SR, et al. Role of serotonin in the paradoxical calming effect of psychostimulants in hyperactivity. *Science* 1999;283:397–401.
175. Biederman J, Spencer T. Attention-deficit/hyperactivity disorder (ADHD) as a noradrenergic disorder. *Biol Psychiatry* 1999;46:1234–1242.
176. Biederman J, Wilens T, Mick E, et al. Pharmacotherapy of attention-deficit/hyperactivity disorder reduces risk of substance abuse disorder. *Pediatrics* 1999;104:e20b.
177. Feigin A, Kurlan R, McDermott MP, et al. A controlled trial of deprenyl in children with Tourette's syndrome and attention deficit hyperactivity disorder. *Neurology* 1996;46:965–968.
178. Michelson D, Faries D, Wernicke J, et al. Atomoxetine in the treatment of children and adolescents with attention-deficit/hyperactivity disorder: a randomized, placebo-controlled, dose-response study. *Pediatrics* 2001;108:1–9.
179. Allen AJ, Kurlan RM, Gilbert DL, et al. Atomoxetine treatment in children and adolescents with ADHD and comorbid tic disorders. *Neurology* 2005;65:1941–1949.
180. March JS, Franklin M, Nelson A, et al. Cognitive-behavioral psychotherapy for pediatric obsessive-compulsive disorder. *J Child Psychology* 2001;30:8–18.
181. Grados MA, Riddle MA. Pharmacologic treatment of childhood obsessive-compulsive disorder: from theory to practice. *J Child Psychology* 2001;30:67–79.
182. Thase ME, Entsua AR, Rudolph RL. Remission rates during treatment with venlafaxine or selective serotonin reuptake inhibitors. *Br J Psychiatry* 2001;178:234–241.
183. The Research Unit on Pediatric Psychopharmacology Anxiety Study Group. Fluvoxamine for the treatment of anxiety disorders in children and adolescents. *N Engl J Med* 2001;344:1279–1285.
184. Bruun RD, Budman CL. Paroxetine treatment of episodic rages associated with Tourette's disorder. *J Clin Psychiatry* 1998;59:581–584.
185. Rauch SL, Baer L, Cosgrove GR, et al. Neurosurgical treatment of Tourette's syndrome: a critical review. *Compr Psychiatry* 1995;36:141–156.

Myoclonus and Startle Syndromes

28

Hiroshi Shibasaki

Myoclonus is defined as sudden, brief, jerky, shocklike, involuntary movements arising from the central nervous system and involving the extremities, face, and trunk. Most myoclonic jerks are caused by abrupt muscle contraction (positive myoclonus), but abrupt movements are also caused by sudden cessation of muscle contraction associated with the silent period of the electromyographic (EMG) discharges (negative myoclonus) (1).

Myoclonus can be classified from various aspects, but it is commonly classified with respect to the underlying physiologic mechanism or causative factor (2,3). According to its possible origin in the central nervous system, myoclonus is classified in three main categories: cortical, subcortical, and spinal (Table 28.1) (3). Of these three categories, cortical myoclonus is most commonly encountered, and it is most important because patients with this form of myoclonus also tend to suffer from generalized convulsions. This is mainly related to the fact that cortical myoclonus in most cases is based on the pathologic hyperexcitability of the sensory cortex, the motor cortex, or both. Moreover, cortical myoclonus is more often disabling to patients and intractable to treatment than other forms of myoclonus. Cortical myoclonus is seen in a variety of diseases and syndromes (Table 28.2). Progressive myoclonus epilepsies (PMEs) have various diseases as their underlying causes, and they are mostly hereditary. There are significant differences in the relative frequency of those diseases among different regions of the world. There has been significant advance in the genetic studies of hereditary diseases causing PME (Table 28.3) (4).

As for the term Ramsay Hunt syndrome, which used to be applied to PMEs of undetermined causation, in 1990 the Marseille Consensus Group (5) recommended that this category be discarded. The last two categories of PMEs listed in Table 28.2 now replace Ramsay Hunt syndrome; these

disorders are referred to as *PMEs of unknown cause* when seizures are frequent and severe and as *progressive myoclonic ataxias* when seizures are infrequent and mild. Celiac disease has been added as a cause of progressive myoclonic ataxia (6). The neuropathological findings reported in an autopsied case of celiac disease consisted of atrophy of the cerebellar hemispheres but no abnormality in the cerebrum (6). Guerrini et al. (7) reported Angelman syndrome as a cause of PME. Furthermore, they demonstrated cortical reflex myoclonus in 9 of 10 patients with Rett's syndrome (8).

As will be described in detail later in this chapter, the pathophysiology of cortical myoclonus can be studied by using various electrophysiological techniques (3). In contrast, the diagnosis of subcortical myoclonus depends largely on exclusion of cortical myoclonus. As listed in Table 28.1, the subcortical myoclonus contains various subgroups, and some of them share common features with other kinds of involuntary movements, such as tremor and dystonia. Quinn (9) in 1996 reviewed the literature related to essential myoclonus and hypothesized that hereditary essential myoclonus and dominantly inherited myoclonic dystonia, both of which dramatically respond to alcohol, might be the same disease, although the proof must come from genetic studies. Zimprich et al. (10) in 2001 discovered that mutations in the gene encoding the epsilon-sarcoglycan gene cause myoclonus–dystonia syndrome. However, these mutations explain only a part of the dominantly inherited dystonia–myoclonus syndrome (11). Pathophysiology of myoclonus in dystonia–myoclonus syndrome has not been well elucidated. Occasional association of this condition with epilepsy in families with epsilon-sarcoglycan gene mutation might suggest that myoclonus in this condition might be of cortical origin (12).

Startle syndrome was categorized into subcortical myoclonus because it was demonstrated to be based on the

TABLE 28.1
PATHOPHYSIOLOGIC CLASSIFICATION OF MYOCLONUS

Cortical
   Spontaneous cortical myoclonus
   Cortical reflex myoclonus
   Epilepsia partialis continua

Subcortical
   Essential myoclonus
   Periodic myoclonus
   Dystonic myoclonus
   Palatal myoclonus
   Reticular reflex myoclonus
   Startle syndrome
   Drug-induced myoclonus

Spinal
   Segmental
   Propriospinal

TABLE 28.3
MAJOR FORMS OF PROGRESSIVE MYOCLONUS EPILEPSY AND THEIR GENE ABNORMALITY

Disorder	Locus/ Chromosome	Gene Product
Unverricht-Lundborg	EPM1/21q22.3	Cystatin B
Lafora's disease	EPM2A/6q24	Laforin (dual-specificity phosphatase)
	EPM2B/6p22.3	Malin
MERRF	MTTK/mtDNA	tRNA^{Lys}
Sialidosis	NEU1/6p21	Neuraminidase 1
DRPLA	DRPLA/12p13	Atrophin 1
Neuronal ceroid lipofuscinosis		
Infantile	CLN1/1p32	Palmitoyl-protein thioesterase 1
Late infantile	CLN2/11p15	Tripeptidyl peptidase 1
Juvenile	CLN3/16p12	CLN3 (membrane protein of unknown function)

MERFF, myoclonic epilepsy associated with ragged red fibers; DRPLA, dentatorubral-pallidoluysian atrophy. Modified from Lehesjoki A-E. Molecular background of progressive myoclonus epilepsy. *EMBO J* 2003;22:3473–3478, with the help of Dr. Lehesjoki.

stimulus-sensitive hyperexcitability of lower brainstem centers (13,14). However, in this chapter it will be dealt with as an independent category, with special emphasis placed on the recent advance in its genetic studies.

Various drugs have been reported to cause myoclonic jerks (2,15,16). These include anticonvulsants such as vigabatrin and valproate, chronically abused alcohol, methyl ethyl ketone, the anesthetic agent propofol, the antipsychotic drug clozapine, the antidiarrheic bismuth subsalicylate, and serotomimetic agents such as trazodone, isocarboxazide, and methylphenidate hydrochloride. Most

TABLE 28.2
DISEASES UNDERLYING CORTICAL MYOCLONUS

Progressive myoclonus epilepsy
  Unverricht-Lundborg epilepsy
  Lafora's disease
  Neuronal ceroid lipofuscinosis
  Myoclonus epilepsy associated with ragged red fibers (MERRF)
  Lipidosis
  Dentatorubral-pallidoluysian atrophy (DRPLA)
  Familial adult myoclonic epilepsy
  Angelman syndrome
  Celiac disease
  Progressive myoclonus epilepsies of unknown cause
  Progressive myoclonic ataxias
Juvenile myoclonic epilepsy
Postanoxic myoclonus (Lance-Adams syndrome)
Alzheimer's disease
Creutzfeldt-Jakob disease (advanced stage)
Metabolic encephalopathy
Corticobasal ganglionic degeneration
Olivopontocerebellar atrophy
Rett's syndrome

drug-induced myoclonus is dose dependent. Although detailed electrophysiological findings have not been reported, most of them seem to be of subcortical origin because the electroencephalogram (EEG) does not show any myoclonus-related spike.

In spinal myoclonus, two representative forms are known: segmental spinal myoclonus and propriospinal myoclonus. Segmental spinal myoclonus is often rhythmic or periodic and can be stimulus sensitive. One form of segmental spinal myoclonus is diaphragmatic flutter or respiratory myoclonus, first described by Antony van Leeuwenhoek, the inventor of the microscope (17). However, segmental spinal myoclonus will not be covered here due to lack of recent progress in the field. Since Chapter 29 of this volume is entirely devoted to the pharmacology and management of myoclonus, this aspect of myoclonus will not be discussed here.

CORTICAL MYOCLONUS

Myoclonus of cortical origin is characterized clinically by brief jerks of extremity and facial muscles that are enhanced by posturing and actions (movements) and are commonly sensitive to stimulus. Electrophysiologically, it is characterized by (a) an associated EMG discharge of short duration (usually less than 50 ms), (b) an EEG spike preceding the myoclonus by a short interval (20 ms in case of hand myoclonus) and localized to the area of the contralateral central region corresponding to the involved muscle (around C3 or C4 of the International 10–20 System for hand myoclonus and around Cz for foot myoclonus), and (c) significant enhancement of early cortical components of the somatosensory-evoked responses, often accompanied by enhanced long-latency, long-loop EMG response (C-reflex) (3,18–21).

Most electrophysiological studies suggest abnormal hyperexcitability of the sensory or motor cortex, or both, underlying the cortical myoclonus. Among various sensory modalities, most patients are predominantly sensitive to the somesthetic stimuli, although some patients also show increased sensitivity to photic stimuli (22,23).

Hyperexcitability of the Somatosensory Cortex

Giant somatosensory-evoked potentials (SEPs) are attributable to the pathological enhancement of physiological

components of SEPs seen in normal subjects but not to the development of abnormal SEP components (20,21,24,25). By analyzing the scalp distribution and the time relationship of the subcomponents of giant SEPs following electrical stimulation of the peripheral nerves in patients with cortical reflex myoclonus, Ikeda et al. (25) in 1995 demonstrated that not only the components P30 and N30, which are derived from the tangentially oriented dipole source within area 3b in the posterior bank of the central sulcus, but also the components P25 and N35, which are localized to the central region probably arising from the radially oriented dipole source(s) in the crown of the postcentral gyrus (area 1 or 2), are enhanced to different degrees, depending on the individual patient (Fig. 28.1). By using a specially devised instrument for selectively activating the muscle afferents, Mima et al. (26) demonstrated that in some patients with cortical reflex myoclonus the proprioception-induced SEPs are also enhanced. In view of the previously reported experimental data suggesting that the impulses arising from muscle afferents arrive mainly at area 3a and that those from tactile

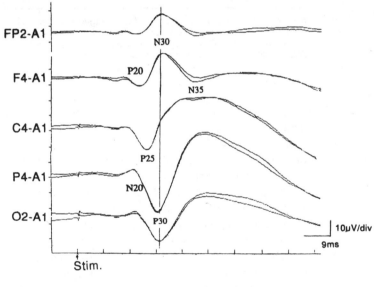

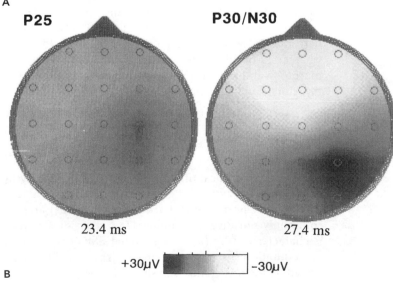

Figure 28.1 Somatosensory-evoked potentials (SEPs) in a patient with cortical reflex myoclonus. **A:** Left median nerve stimulation. **B:** Scalp topography of each component of giant SEPs. P25 and N35 are seen as a single positive and negative peak, respectively, at the right peri-rolandic area. N30-P30 is seen as a pair of two fields of opposite polarities across the right central sulcus. (From Ikeda A, Shibasaki H, Nagamine T, et al. Peri-rolandic and fronto-parietal components of scalp-recorded giant SEPs in cortical myoclonus. *Electroenceph Clin Neurophysiol* 1995;96:300–309. With permission.) (See color section.)

inputs arrive mainly at areas 3b, 1 and 2, the preceding finding is in agreement with the conclusion drawn by Ikeda et al. (25) based on the scalp distribution of giant SEPs following electrical stimulation of the peripheral nerve trunk. In contrast, nociceptive stimuli presented by applying a CO_2 laser beam to skin did not enhance the pain SEP even in those patients who showed giant SEP in response to electrical stimulation of the peripheral nerves (27). However, previous studies using pain SEP were focused on the N2 and P2 components because of the technical difficulty of recording an earlier component, N1, which was shown to be generated in the primary somatosensory cortex. As the N2 and P2 components are believed to be generated in the second somatosensory cortex (SII) (28), the preceding finding suggests that the SII is not hyperreactive in cortical myoclonus.

Hyperexcitability of the Primary Motor Cortex

The temporal and spatial relation between cortical myoclonus and its EEG correlates can be studied by the use of the jerk-locked back-averaging technique (29). This technique may disclose the myoclonus-related cortical activity that is not detectable on the conventional EEG–EMG polygraphic record. Certain similarities between the EEG spike preceding the spontaneous cortical myoclonus and the giant SEP following electrical stimulation of the peripheral nerve have been pointed out in terms of waveform, time relation to the EMG discharge (spike to spontaneous myoclonus versus giant SEP to C-reflex), and topography over the scalp (18,20,30). This observation led to the postulation that the giant SEP seen in cortical reflex myoclonus might contain the motor or efferent component in it (18,20,30). This concept was substantiated by the studies of giant SEPs using magnetoencephalography (MEG). Although the main component of the giant somatosensory-evoked magnetic fields was generated in area 3b, a certain component (P25m) was shown to arise from the precentral gyrus, thus supporting the preceding hypothesis (Fig. 28.2) (31).

As for the MEG correlates of the premyoclonus spike, Uesaka et al. (32) in 1996 studied by MEG 6 patients with cortical reflex myoclonus and 1 with epilepsia partialis continua. The spike was estimated as a single-current dipole in the postcentral gyrus in 5 of the 6 patients with cortical reflex myoclonus, and in the remaining patient 2 dipoles were detected, one each in the precentral and postcentral gyri. These facts suggested the possible origin of cortical myoclonus also in the postcentral gyrus. In the patient with epilepsia partialis continua, a single dipole was estimated in the precentral gyrus (32). Mima et al. (33) in 1998 studied 6 patients with cortical myoclonus due to various causes by jerk-locked back-averaging of MEG and identified the generator source of the pre-myoclonus activity in the contralateral precentral gyrus in all the cases, although the

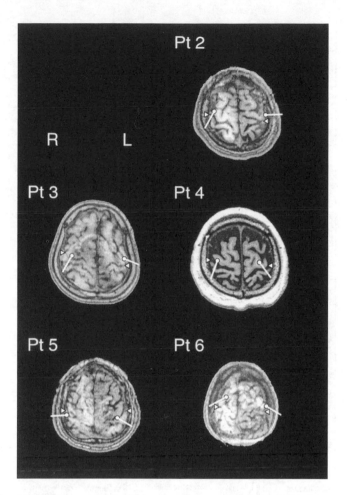

Figure 28.2 Equivalent current dipoles (ECDs) of the P25m component calculated from the averaged magnetoencephalographic responses to electric stimulation of the median nerves at wrist in 5 patients with cortical reflex myoclonus. The sources are located in the precentral gyrus in all cases. The ECDs of the initial cortical component N20m were localized in the postcentral gyrus in all cases (data not shown). White spots and bars indicate the location of the ECD and their direction. Triangles show the central sulcus. (From Mima T, Nagamine T, Nishitani N, et al. Cortical myoclonus: sensorimotor hyperexcitability. *Neurology* 1998;50:933–942. With permission.)

direction of the current flow was different among cases (Figs. 28.3 and 28.4). This finding confirmed the important role of the precentral cortex in generating spontaneous myoclonus although the activation pattern may not be consistent among patients. It is especially noteworthy that, in some patients, jerk-locked back-averaging of MEG disclosed myoclonus-related cortical activity that was not detectable on the jerk-locked averaged EEG (33).

Silen et al. (34) in 2000, by using MEG, analyzed the reactivity of the approximately 20-Hz cortical rhythm to electrical stimulation of the peripheral nerves as an index for the functional state of the primary motor cortex in patients with Unverricht-Lundborg epilepsy. In the patient group they found a loss of significant rebounds of the cortical rhythm, which occur following a transient decrease of the rhythm in

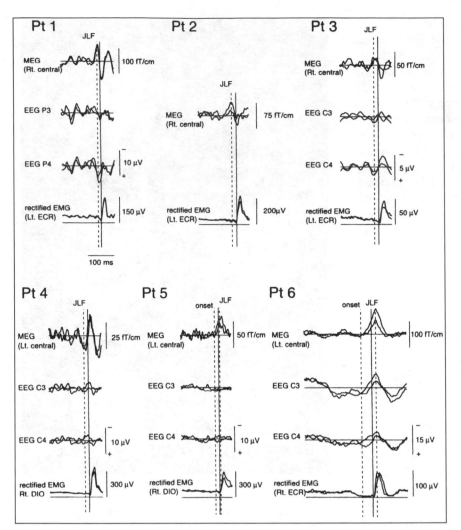

Figure 28.3 Waveforms of magnetoencephalograms and electroencephalograms simultaneously recorded and back-averaged with respect to the onset of hand myoclonus in 6 patients with cortical myoclonus. In Patient 4 (Pt 4) and Patient 5 (Pt 5), the back-averaged electroencephalograms show no myoclonus-related activity, whereas the corresponding magnetoencephalograms show a cortical activity time locked to myoclonus. (From Mima T, Nagamine T, Ikeda A, et al. Pathogenesis of cortical myoclonus studied by magnetoencephalography. *Ann Neurol* 1998;43:598–607. With permission.)

response to the stimulation in normal subjects (Fig. 28.5) (34). Since the 20-Hz rebounds are believed to reflect increased cortical inhibition, their loss in this condition was interpreted as indicating decreased GABAergic inhibition in the motor cortex in those patients (34). By contrast, Mochizuki et al. (35) reported the enhancement of the late component of the somatosensory-evoked high-frequency oscillations (500–700 Hz) in patients with cortical myoclonus.

Brown et al. (36) in 1991, by analyzing the time relation among myoclonic jerks of various muscles and the time relation between those myoclonic jerks and the EEG correlates in patients with cortical myoclonus, suggested the spread of myoclonus-related cortical activities through the motor strip within one hemisphere and across the two hemispheres through the corpus callosum. In 1996, Brown et al. extended their study to clarify the excitability of the motor cortex by using transcranial magnetic stimulation (TMS) in two groups of patients with cortical myoclonus; one group consisted of spreaders (patients with multifocal and bilateral or generalized cortical myoclonus) and the

other of nonspreaders (patients with just multifocal cortical myoclonus) (37). They found lower motor thresholds to single magnetic shocks at rest in spreaders than in nonspreaders or healthy subjects. Furthermore, by using paired magnetic stimulation at interstimulus intervals of 1 to 6 ms, they found less ipsilateral inhibition and less transcallosal inhibition in the spreaders than in the nonspreaders or healthy subjects. These findings were interpreted to suggest that abnormalities in ipsilateral and transcallosal inhibition may facilitate the spread of the cortical myoclonic activity responsible for bilateral and generalized jerks (37).

As regards the interhemispheric interaction, Hanajima et al. (38) in 2001 studied effects of the conditioning stimulus over the ipsilateral motor cortex on responses in the hand muscle to the test stimulus over the contralateral motor area, and they found facilitation at interstimulus intervals of 4–6 ms (early facilitation) in patients with myoclonus epilepsy, which was not seen in normal subjects. In addition, they found inhibition at interstimulus intervals of 8–20 ms (late inhibition) in normal subjects, but it was absent in the patients (Fig. 28.6).

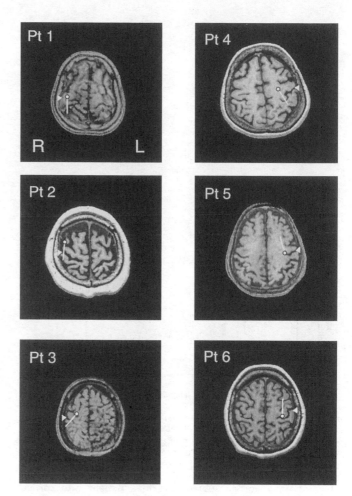

Figure 28.4 Equivalent current dipoles (ECDs) of cortical activity preceding myoclonus of hand in 6 patients with cortical myoclonus, calculated from the magnetic fields obtained by jerk-locked back averaging (the same data as shown in Fig. 28.3). The sources are located in the precentral cortex in all cases, although the direction of the current dipole is different (posterior in the first 4 cases and anterior in the last 2 cases). Triangles indicate the central sulcus. (From Mima T, Nagamine T, Ikeda A, et al. Pathogenesis of cortical myoclonus studied by magnetoencephalography. *Ann Neurol* 1998;43:598–607. With permission.)

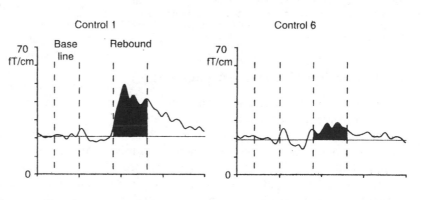

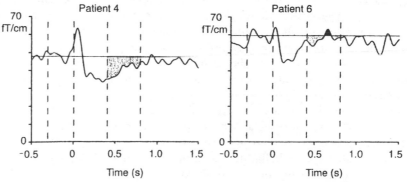

Figure 28.5 Changes in the approximately 20-Hz magnetoencephalographic activity following electric stimulation of median nerves in normal subjects (*top panel*) and 2 patients with Unverricht-Lundborg progressive myoclonus epilepsy (*Patients 4 and 6*). Activity of this frequency band shows rebounds (*dark grey shadow*) 400 to 800 ms after stimulus (time 0) in normal subjects, whereas it is suppressed (*light gray shadow*) in patients. (From Silen T, Forss N, Jensen O, et al. Abnormal reactivity of the ~20-Hz motor cortex rhythm in Unverricht-Lundborg type progressive myoclonus epilepsy. *Neuroimage* 2000;12:707–712. With permission.)

A.

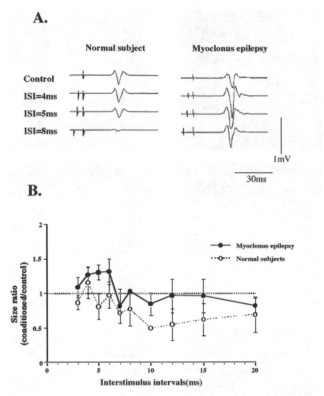

B.

Figure 28.6 Lack of interhemispheric inhibition in the motor cortex in patients with cortical myoclonus, as demonstrated by abnormal effects of the conditioning transcranial magnetic stimulation (TMS) over the ipsilateral motor cortex. **A:** Motor-evoked potentials following TMS of the contralateral motor cortex preceded by that of the ipsilateral motor cortex by short intervals (4–8 ms) in a normal subject and in a patient with cortical myoclonus. **B:** Time course of interhemispheric inhibition in patients with cortical myoclonus (*closed circle*) and in normal subjects (*open circle*). Note the early facilitation and loss of the late inhibition in the patients. (From Hanajima R, Ugawa Y, Okabe S, et al. Interhemispheric interaction between the hand motor areas in patients with cortical myoclonus. *Clin Neurophysiol* 2001;112: 623–626. With permission.)

Rhythm Formation of Cortical Myoclonus

Cortical myoclonus usually occurs irregularly. However, in some cases it involves the same muscles repetitively, and even rhythmically, thus clinically resembling tremor. Recently, several conditions have attracted attention in this regard. Familial adult myoclonic epilepsy (FAME) has been reported mainly in Japan under various names, such as benign epilepsy with essential myoclonus, benign familial myoclonic epilepsy, cortical tremor, and familial cortical myoclonic tremor (39). It is characterized by autosomal dominant inheritance, relatively late onset, relatively benign postural-action myoclonus involving small muscles of hands resembling essential tremor, and infrequent occurrence of generalized convulsions, but it fulfills all the electrophysiological criteria of cortical reflex myoclonus (39). In 2004 van Rootselaar et al. (40) reported neuropathological findings in an autopsied case of this condition, which showed cerebellar degeneration with somal sprouting and loss of dendritic trees in Purkinje cells, and

those findings were strikingly similar to those seen in spinocerebellar ataxia type 6. The genetic locus of this disease in a Japanese family was defined on chromosome 8q23.3-q24.1 (41–43). More recently, families presenting with similar clinical picture have been reported from Europe with chromosome location at 2p11.1-q12.2, suggesting genetic heterogeneity of this unique condition (44,45).

Myoclonic jerks seen in patients with corticobasal ganglionic degeneration are often rhythmic. This condition is characterized by rigid akinetic syndrome associated with apraxia, myoclonic jerks, and cortical sensory loss, all of which start asymmetrically. Electrophysiological abnormalities are also quite asymmetric. One of the unique features of electrophysiological findings in this condition is a slightly shorter latency of the C-reflex or evoked myoclonus by peripheral stimulation as compared with the ordinary form of cortical reflex myoclonus (46). Another feature is reduction of the SEP amplitudes except for the initial cortical component (N20 in the case of median nerve stimulation at wrist) (46,47). The latter finding is compatible with the cortical sensory loss that is clinically demonstrated in the majority of these cases. Furthermore, both the spontaneous and reflex myoclonic jerks in this condition tend to repeat themselves at an approximate rate of once every 70 to 90 ms, or they may occur as trains of jerks. Because this interval is too long for the reverberating circuit between the cortex and the periphery, it is believed to be due to the repetitive excitation of the sensorimotor cortex (39,46,47). Lu et al. (47) in 1998 studied 2 patients with this disease by TMS of the motor cortex and found shortening of the induced EMG silent period predominantly on the affected side, suggesting impairment of the inhibitory system in the motor cortex.

Guerrini et al. (7) in 1996 reported 11 patients, aged 3 to 28 years, with Angelman syndrome, which is due to lack of genetic contribution from maternal chromosome 15q11-13. It manifests severe mental retardation, ataxic gait, tremors, and jerky movements. It is noteworthy that this chromosomal region encompasses three $GABA_A$ receptor subunit genes. All patients exhibited quasi-continuous rhythmic myoclonus involving mainly hands and face, accompanied by rhythmic 5- to 10-Hz EEG activity. Burst-locked EEG averaging disclosed a pre-myoclonus transient preceding the burst by 19 ± 5 ms. Although no giant SEP or C-reflex was observed, it was thought to arise in the cortex. Recently, rhythmic cortical myoclonus was described in a patient with HIV-related encephalopathy (48).

The mechanism underlying the rhythm formation in cortical myoclonus has not been clarified yet. Thompson et al. (46) gave TMS over the motor cortex in 13 patients with corticobasal degeneration. In 8 of them, they found 2 successive motor-evoked potentials about 70 ms apart in response to a single magnetic stimulation and only 1 motor-evoked potential with normal short latency in 5 patients. Electrical stimulation did not elicit these double EMG responses, supporting the concept of rhythm generation at the cortical level. Valzania et al. (49) in 1999 applied paired pulse TMS at 110% of the resting motor threshold for both stimuli to patients with PME and found facilitation at 50 ms, which was in strong contrast with normal subjects. Manganotti et al. (50) in 2001 used electrical stimulation of digital nerve delivered at 3 times the sensory threshold, followed by TMS in patients with PME, and found facilitation at interstimulus intervals of 25 to 40 ms whereas a significant MEP inhibition was seen from 25 to 50 ms in normal subjects.

Brown et al. (51) in 1999 studied 8 patients with cortical myoclonus by analyzing the coherence between EEG and EMG activities. They found significant coherence between the EMG and the contralateral and vertex EEG in the frequency ranges (15–30 Hz and 30–60 Hz) during weak muscle contraction in normal subjects, as well as in 6 patients, and in 3 of the latter group they also found significant coherence at higher frequencies (up to 175 Hz). Based on the coherence data, they estimated the conduction time from the cortex to the muscles of the forearm, hand, and foot to be 14, 25, and 35 ms, respectively. Thus, the cortical drive seems to synchronize muscle discharges over a broader range of frequencies in some patients with cortical myoclonus as compared with normal subjects. In corticobasal degeneration, however, Grosse et al. (52) studied EEG-EMG coherence, as well as EMG-EMG coherence in 5 patients with clinical diagnosis of this condition, and found negligible corticomuscular coherence despite a dramatically exaggerated EMG-EMG coherence. They concluded that the myoclonic jerks in this condition may not be due to an exaggerated cortical drive.

Negative Myoclonus

Negative myoclonus, or asterixis, occurs when a muscle contraction is suddenly interrupted. It can be either cortical or subcortical in origin (1). It is often seen in association with metabolic or toxic encephalopathy, but unilateral asterixis is seen most commonly in association with ischemic or hemorrhagic disorders, especially those involving the thalamus. Within the thalamus, ventral lateral or lateral posterior thalamus seems to be responsible for the unilateral pure asterixis (53). Lance and Adams (54) in 1963 clearly documented in their patients with posthypoxic myoclonus the association of positive myoclonus with the EEG spike and that of the EMG silent period (negative myoclonus) with the EEG slow wave, suggesting its cortical origin. In 1994, Shibasaki et al. (55) reported 4 cases of negative myoclonus elicited by peripheral stimulation, with or without associated positive myoclonus. In those cases, presentation of a single electric shock to the median nerve at the wrist while the wrist was maintained in extended position evoked the giant SEP on the EEG and a clear silent period on the EMG, resulting in sudden wrist drop. It was clearly noted in those cases that the larger the SEP, the longer the duration of the induced EMG silent period or the more prominent the induced negative myoclonus. Moreover, the EMG silent period also was elicited in the opposite (nonstimulated) hand only when the giant SEP was recognized also at the hemisphere ipsilateral to the stimulus. This may be explained by postulating, as in the case of positive myoclonus, the interhemispheric spread of the silent period–related cortical activity through the corpus callosum (36). Thus, this stimulus-sensitive negative myoclonus seems to be mediated by the transcortical reflex mechanism, probably based on the abnormal hyperexcitability of inhibitory components of the motor cortex (55).

As regards the stimulus-sensitive negative myoclonus, Gambardella et al. (56) reported a patient with photosensitive epilepsy in whom photo-paroxysmal EEG response was sometimes accompanied by loss of postural tone in both arms. This is considered to be an example of photic cortical reflex negative myoclonus.

As for the generating mechanism of cortical negative myoclonus, a possible role of the frontal cortex anterior to the motor cortex has been proposed. Rubbolli et al. (57) in 1995 reported a patient with epileptic negative myoclonus. By using the spike-averaging technique, they demonstrated 1 negative EEG peak at the contralateral central region and the following negative peak at the contralateral frontal region. The latter of the 2 negative peaks preceded the onset of the EMG flattening by 30 ms and was always associated with the epileptic negative myoclonus, but the earlier peak was not necessarily so. Baumgartner et al. (58) in 1996 reported a patient manifesting brief repetitive lapses in postural tone of the right upper extremity while the ictal EEG showed repetitive left frontal spikes that were located much more anterior to the central sulcus as determined by the N20 component of the median nerve SEP. The EEG transient preceded the onset of the EMG silent period by 20 to 40 ms. Baumgartner et al. further demonstrated a marked regional hyperperfusion in the left middle frontal gyrus by single-photon emission computed tomography (SPECT) during the epileptic negative myoclonus. These findings were interpreted to suggest that the epileptic negative myoclonus might be generated by epileptic activity in the premotor area (58). Lüders et al. (59) found that 2 cortical areas, 1 on the mesial frontal cortex and 1 on the lateral frontal convexity just in front of the face motor area, interrupt the ongoing muscle contraction or repetitive movements when stimulated with a train of high-frequency (50 Hz) electric shocks. However, the relation between these negative motor areas and negative myoclonus has not been clarified.

Negative motor area also might exist in the primary sensorimotor cortex. Noachtar et al. (60) in 1997 reported a patient with focal epileptic negative myoclonus who was studied with subdurally placed electrodes. In that study, repetitive spikes in the postcentral gyrus were consistently followed by an EMG silent period in the contralateral arm with a latency of about 20 ms to 30 ms. In patients with medically intractable epilepsy who underwent presurgical evaluation with subdural electrodes, Ikeda et al. (61) in 2000 found that some areas of the sensorimotor cortex elicit a pure silent period without associated positive motor response when stimulated with a single electric shock.

STARTLE SYNDROME

Startle syndrome is a group of diseases characterized by exaggerated startle responses to sudden unexpected stimuli. Familial startle disease, or hyperekplexia, is mostly an autosomal dominant disorder characterized by muscular rigidity in the neonatal period and exaggerated startle response to sudden, unexpected acoustic or tactile stimuli. Recently, this condition has drawn the particular attention of many investigators, especially in relation to its genetic pathogenesis (62).

Ryan et al. (63) in 1992 performed systematic linkage analysis in a large family with hyperekplexia and found the polymorphic genetic marker locus mapped to chromosome 5q33-q35. The same authors further identified point mutations in the gene encoding the α_1 subunit of the inhibitory glycine receptor (GLRA1) in hyperekplexia patients from 4 families (64). All mutations occurred in the same base pair of exon 6 and resulted in the substitution of an uncharged amino acid (leucine or glutamine) for arginine in codon 271. A group of neurologists in Leiden made a linkage analysis in 44 Dutch patients with hyperekplexia. Patients were divided into 2 groups: 28 patients with the major form, associated with stiffness, and 16 patients with the minor form, unassociated with stiffness. The point mutation of the gene encoding GLRA1 was found exclusively in the major form, indicating that the minor form is not a different expression of the same genetic defect but may be merely an excessive form of normal startle response (65). Shiang et al. (66) in 1995 reported families with hyperekplexia showing a different mutation that changed tyrosine at amino acid 279 to cysteine, and also patients with atypical clinical features or absent family history of hyperekplexia who did not have mutation in the gene encoding GLRA1. Rajendra et al. (67) in 1994 showed that the mutation in hyperekplexia profoundly reduces the sensitivity of receptor currents activated by agonist glycine as well as the binding affinity of glycine to the mutant glycine receptors, thus reducing the efficacy of glycinergic inhibitory neurotransmission. In 1999, Saul et al. (68) reported a pedigree showing dominant transmission of hyperekplexia that was found to have another point mutation of GLRA1 with the substitution of P250, which was located in the intracellular M1-M2 loop. They showed that recombinant $\alpha 1P^{250T}$ receptors displayed dramatic alterations in chloride conductance, suggesting an important role of glycine receptor channel gating in the pathogenesis of this syndrome (68).

Recently, the recessive form of hyperekplexia also was shown to have gene mutation encoding the inhibitory glycine receptor (69).

With regard to the site of action of inhibitory glycine receptors, blockade of the inhibitory glycine receptors in the caudal pontine reticular formation did not affect the acoustic startle response in rats, suggesting that deficiency of glycine receptors in the pontine reticular nucleus might not be involved in the human startle disease (70). Pierce et al. (71) in 2001 found mutations of glycine receptor gene in calves showing stimulus-sensitive myoclonus with autosomal recessive inheritance. Immunohistochemically, by using monoclonal antibody to α and β subunits of the glycine receptors, Pierce et al. demonstrated a loss of cell surface immunoreactivity in spinal neurons of the myoclonic animals (71).

Physiologically, the startle responses in hyperekplexia have been shown to involve the same structures as the physiological startle responses seen in normal subjects. The only difference is the excessive response and subnormal habituation resulting in widespread elevated gain of vestigial withdrawal reflexes in the patients (13,72,73). The pattern of the startle EMG responses starting from the sternocleidomastoid muscles and spreading both rostrally and caudally suggests the medulla oblongata as the most likely reflex center (13). At the spinal level, Floeter et al. (74) in 1996 demonstrated diminished reciprocal inhibition between flexor and extensor muscles of the forearm, but normal recurrent inhibition of the soleus H reflex, in patients with hereditary hyperekplexia with mutation in GLRA1. Based on these findings, Floeter et al. postulated that disynaptic reciprocal inhibition in humans is mediated through glycinergic interneurons.

SUMMARY

Myoclonus has been extensively studied by using various electrophysiological techniques. Among others, the recent application of MEG to the investigation of the generator source of giant SEP and pre-myoclonus cortical activity in cortical reflex myoclonus elucidated the complex involvement of precentral and postcentral gyri in this condition. As in other fields of clinical neurology, there have been remarkable advances in the genetic and molecular aspects of myoclonus, especially with regard to hyperekplexia, or hereditary startle syndrome. Hyperekplexia was found to be caused mainly by the point mutation of the gene encoding GLRA1, although there seem to be different mutations depending on families. Abnormalities of channel gating in GLRA1 have been studied extensively. Although electrophysiologically the startle response seen in hyperekplexia is an exaggerated form of the physiological startle response present in normal subjects, the precise site of dysfunction remains to be elucidated.

REFERENCES

1. Shibasaki H. Pathophysiology of negative myoclonus and asterixis. *Adv Neurol* 1995;67:199–209.
2. Caveness JN, Brown P. Myoclonus: current concepts and recent advances. *Lancet Neurol* 2004;3:598–607.
3. Shibasaki H, Hallett M. AAEE monograph #30: electrophysiological studies of myoclonus. *Muscle Nerve* 2005;31:157–174.
4. Lehesjoki A-E. Molecular background of progressive myoclonus epilepsy. *EMBO J* 2003;22:3473–3478.
5. Marseille Consensus Group. Classification of progressive myoclonus epilepsies and related disorders. *Ann Neurol* 1990;28:113–116.
6. Bhatia KP, Brown P, Gregory R, et al. Progressive myoclonic ataxia associated with coeliac disease: the myoclonus of cortical origin, but the pathology is in the cerebellum. *Brain* 1995;118:1087–1093.
7. Guerrini R, De Lorey TM, Bonanni P, et al. Cortical myoclonus in Angelman syndrome. *Ann Neurol* 1996;40:39–48.
8. Guerrini R, Bonanni P, Parmeggiani L, et al. Cortical reflex myoclonus in Rett syndrome. *Ann Neurol* 1998;43:472–479.
9. Quinn NP. Essential myoclonus and myoclonic dystonia. *Mov Disord* 1996;11:119–124.
10. Zimprich A, Grabowski M, Asmus F, et al. Mutations in the gene encoding ε-sarcoglycan cause myoclonus-dystonia syndrome. *Nat Gen* 2001;29:66–69.
11. Schuele B, Kock N, Svetel M, et al. Genetic heterogeneity in ten families with myoclonus-dystonia. *J Neurol Neurosurg Psychiatry* 2004;75:1181–1185.
12. O'Riordan S, Ozelius LJ, De Carvalho Aguiar P, et al. Inherited myoclonus-dystonia and epilepsy: further evidence of an association? *Mov Disord* 2004;19:1456–1459.
13. Brown P, Rothwell JC, Thompson PD, et al. The hyperekplexias and their relationship to the normal startle reflex. *Brain* 1991;114:1903–1928.
14. Brown P. The startle syndrome. *Mov Disord* 2002;17(suppl 2):S79–S82.
15. Jimenez-Jimenez FJ, Puertas I, De Toledo-Heras M. Drug-induced myoclonus: frequency, mechanisms and management. *CNS Drugs* 2004;18:93–104.
16. Gordon MF. Toxin and drug-induced myoclonus. *Adv Neurol* 2002;89:49–76.
17. Larner AJ. Antony van Leeuwenhoek and the description of diaphragmatic flutter respiratory myoclonus. *Mov Disord* 2005;20:917–918.
18. Shibasaki H, Yamashita Y, Kuroiwa Y. Electroencephalographic studies of myoclonus: myoclonus-related cortical spikes and high amplitude somatosensory evoked potentials. *Brain* 1978;101:447–460.
19. Hallett M, Chadwick D, Marsden CD. Cortical reflex myoclonus. *Neurology* 1979;29:1107–1125.
20. Shibasaki H, Yamashita Y, Neshige R, et al. Pathogenesis of giant somatosensory evoked potentials in progressive myoclonic epilepsy. *Brain* 1985;108:225–240.
21. Kakigi R, Shibasaki H. Generator mechanisms of giant somatosensory evoked potentials in cortical reflex myoclonus. *Brain* 1987;110:1359–1373.
22. Shibasaki H, Neshige R. Photic cortical reflex myoclonus. *Ann Neurol* 1987;22:252–257.
23. Kanouchi T, Yokota T, Kamata T, et al. Central pathway of photic reflex myoclonus. *J Neurol Neurosurg Psychiatry* 1997;62:414–417.
24. Shibasaki H, Nakamura M, Nishida S, et al. Wave form decomposition of "giant SEP" and its computer model for scalp topography. *Electroenceph Clin Neurophysiol* 1990,77.286–294.
25. Ikeda A, Shibasaki H, Nagamine T, et al. Peri-rolandic and fronto-parietal components of scalp-recorded giant SEPs in cortical myoclonus. *Electroenceph Clin Neurophysiol* 1995;96:300–309.
26. Mima T, Terada K, Ikeda A, et al. Afferent mechanism of cortical myoclonus studied by proprioception-related SEPs. *Electroenceph Clin Neurophysiol* 1997;104:51–59.
27. Kakigi R, Shibasaki H, Neshige R, et al. Pain-related somatosensory evoked potentials in cortical reflex myoclonus. *J Neurol Neurosurg Psychiatry* 1990;53:44–48.
28. Kanda M, Nagamine T, Ikeda A, et al. Primary somatosensory cortex is actively involved in pain processing in human. *Brain Res* 2000;853:282–289.
29. Shibasaki H, Kuroiwa Y. Electroencephalographic correlates of myoclonus. *Electroenceph Clin Neurophysiol* 1975;39:455–463.
30. Shibasaki H, Kakigi R, Ikeda A. Scalp topography of giant SEP and premyoclonus spike in cortical reflex myoclonus. *Electroenceph Clin Neurophysiol* 1991;81:31–37.
31. Mima T, Nagamine T, Nishitani, N, et al. Cortical myoclonus: sensorimotor hyperexcitability. *Neurology* 1998;50:933–942.
32. Uesaka Y, Terao Y, Ugawa Y, et al. Magnetoencephalographic analysis of cortical myoclonic jerks. *Electroenceph Clin Neurophysiol* 1996;99:141–148.
33. Mima T, Nagamine T, Ikeda A, et al. Pathogenesis of cortical myoclonus studied by magnetoencephalography. *Ann Neurol* 1998;43:598–607.
34. Silen T, Forss N, Jensen O, et al. Abnormal reactivity of the ~20-Hz motor cortex rhythm in Unverricht-Lundborg type progressive myoclonus epilepsy. *Neuroimage* 2000;12:707–712.
35. Mochizuki H, Machii K, Terao Y, et al. Recovery function of and effects of hyperventilation on somatosensory evoked high-frequency oscillation in Parkinson's disease and myoclonus epilepsy. *Neurosci Res* 2003;46:485–492.
36. Brown P, Day BL, Rothwell JC, et al. Intrahemispheric and interhemispheric spread of cerebral cortical myoclonic activity and its relevance to epilepsy. *Brain* 1991;114:2333–2351.
37. Brown P, Ridding MC, Werhahn KJ, et al. Abnormalities of the balance between inhibition and excitation in the motor cortex of patients with cortical myoclonus. *Brain* 1996;119:309–317.
38. Hanajima R, Ugawa Y, Okabe S, et al. Interhemispheric interaction between the hand motor areas in patients with cortical myoclonus. *Clin Neurophysiol* 2001;112:623–626.
39. Terada K, Ikeda A, Mima T, et al. Familial cortical myoclonic tremor as a unique form of cortical reflex myoclonus. *Mov Disord* 1997;12:370–377.
40. Van Rootselaar A, Aronica E, Steur ENHJ, et al. Familial cortical tremor with epilepsy and cerebellar pathological findings. *Mov Disord* 2004;19:213–217.
41. Plaster NM, Uyama E, Uchino M, et al. Genetic localization of the familial adult myoclonic epilepsy (FAME) gene to chromosome 8q24. *Neurology* 1999;53:1180–1183.
42. Mikami M, Yasuda T, Terao A, et al. Localization of a gene for benign adult familial myoclonic epilepsy to chromosome 8q23.3-q24.1. *Am J Hum Genet* 1999;65:745–751.
43. Shimizu A, Asakawa S, Sasaki T, et al. A novel giant gene CSMD3 encoding a protein with CUB and sushi multiple domains: a candidate gene for benign adult familial myoclonic epilepsy on human chromosome 8q23.3-q24.1. *Biochem Biophys Res Comm* 2003;309:143–154.
44. De Falco FA, Striano P, de Falco A, et al. Benign adult familial myoclonic epilepsy: genetic heterogeneity and allelism with ADCME. *Neurology* 2003;60:1381–1385.
45. Striano P, Chifari R, Striano S, et al. A new benign adult familial myoclonic epilepsy (BAFME) pedigree suggesting linkage to chromosome 2p11.1-q12.2. *Epilepsia* 2004;45:190–192.
46. Thompson PD, Day BL, Rothwell JC, et al. The myoclonus in corticobasal degeneration: evidence for two forms of cortical reflex myoclonus. *Brain* 1994;117:1197–1207.
47. Lu CS, Ikeda A, Terada K, et al. Electrophysiological studies of early stage corticobasal degeneration. *Mov Disord* 1998;13:140–146.
48. Canafoglia L, Panzica F, Franceschetti S, et al. Rhythmic cortical myoclonus in a case of HIV-related encephalopathy. *Mov Disord* 2003;18:1533–1538.
49. Valzania F, Strafella AP, Tropeani A, et al. Facilitation of rhythmic events in progressive myoclonus epilepsy: a transcranial magnetic stimulation study. *Clin Neurophysiol* 1999;110:152–157.
50. Manganotti P, Tamburin S, Zanette G, et al. Hyperexcitable cortical responses in progressive myoclonic epilepsy: a TMS study. *Neurology* 2001;57:1793–1799.
51. Brown P, Farmer SF, Halliday DM, et al. Coherent cortical and muscle discharge in cortical myoclonus. *Brain* 1999;122:461–472.
52. Grosse P, Kuhn A, Cordivari C, et al. Coherence analysis in the myoclonus of corticobasal degeneration. *Mov Disord* 2003;18:1345–1350.

53. Tatu L, Moulin T, Martin V, et al. Unilateral pure thalamic asterixis: clinical, electromyographic, and topographic patterns. *Neurology* 2000;54:2339–2342.
54. Lance JW, Adams RD. The syndrome of intention or action myoclonus as a sequel to hypoxic encephalopathy. *Brain* 1963;86:111–136.
55. Shibasaki H, Ikeda A, Nagamine T, et al. Cortical reflex negative myoclonus. *Brain* 1994;117:477–486.
56. Gambardella A, Aguglia U, Oliveri RL, et al. Photic-induced epileptic negative myoclonus: a case report. *Epilepsia* 1996; 37:492–494.
57. Rubboli G, Parmeggiani L, Tassinari CA. Frontal inhibitory spike component associated with epileptic negative myoclonus. *Electroenceph Clin Neurophysiol* 1995;95:201–205.
58. Baumgartner C, Podreka I, Olbrich A, et al. Epileptic negative myoclonus: an EEG-single-photon emission CT study indicating involvement of premotor cortex. *Neurology* 1996;46:753–758.
59. Lüders HO, Dinner DS, Morris HH, et al. Cortical electrical stimulation in humans: the negative motor areas. *Adv Neurol* 1995;67:115–129.
60. Noachtar S, Holthousen H, Lüders HO. Epileptic negative myoclonus: subdural EEG recordings indicate a postcentral generator. *Neurology* 1997;49:1534–1537.
61. Ikeda A, Ohara S, Matsumoto R, et al. Role of primary sensorimotor cortices in generating inhibitory motor response in humans. *Brain* 2000;123:1710–1721.
62. Rajendra S, Schofield PR. Molecular mechanisms of inherited startle syndromes. *Trends Neurosci* 1995;18:80–82.
63. Ryan SG, Sherman SL, Terry JC, et al. Startle disease, or hyperekplexia: response to clonazepam and assignment of the gene (STHE) to chromosome 5q by linkage analysis. *Ann Neurol* 1992;31:663–668.
64. Shiang R, Ryan SG, Zhu YZ, et al. Mutations in the alpha 1 subunit of the inhibitory glycine receptor cause the dominant neurologic disorder, hyperekplexia. *Nature Genet* 1993;5: 351–358.
65. Tijssen MA, Shiang R, van Deutekom J, et al. Molecular genetic reevaluation of the Dutch hyperekplexia family. *Arch Neurol* 1995;52:578–582.
66. Shiang R, Ryan SG, Zhu YZ, et al. Mutational analysis of familial and sporadic hyperekplexia. *Ann Neurol* 1995;38:85–91.
67. Rajendra S, Lynch JW, Pierce KD, et al. Startle disease mutations reduce the agonist sensitivity of the human inhibitory glycine receptor. *J Biol Chem* 1994;269:18,739–18,742.
68. Saul B, Kuner T, Sobetzko D, et al. Novel GLRA1 missense mutation (P250T) in dominant hyperekplexia defines an intracellular determinants of glycine receptor channel gating. *J Neurosci* 1999;19:869–877.
69. Humeny A, Bonk, T, Becker K, et al. A novel recessive hyperekplexia allele GLRA1 (S231R): genotyping by MALDI-TOF mass spectrometry and functional characterization as a determinant of cellular glycine receptor trafficking. *Eur J Hum Gen* 2002;10:188–196.
70. Koch M, Friauf E. Glycine receptors in the caudal pontine reticular formation: are they important for the inhibition of the acoustic startle response? *Brain Res* 1995;671:63–72.
71. Pierce KD, Handford CA, Morris R, et al. A nonsense mutation in the alpha1 subunit of the inhibitory glycine receptor associated with bovine myoclonus. *Mol Cell Neurosci* 2001;17:354–363.
72. Chokroverty S, Walczak T, Hening W. Human startle reflex: technique and criteria for abnormal response. *Electroenceph Clin Neurophysiol* 1992;85:236–242.
73. Matsumoto J, Fuhr P, Nigro M, et al. Physiological abnormalities in hereditary hyperekplexia. *Ann Neurol* 1992;32:41–50.
74. Floeter MK, Andermann F, Andermann E, et al. Physiological studies of spinal inhibitory pathways in patients with hereditary hyperekplexia. *Neurology* 1996;46:766–772.

Treatment

of Myoclonus

29

Michael R. Pranzatelli

The main tenet of treatment for myoclonus is reversing the underlying etiology, if possible (Fig. 29.1). If no reversible cause can be found, therapy will be focused on symptoms. Several other considerations then apply (Table 29.1). Does the myoclonus require any treatment? In patients with multiple neurologic problems or more than one dyskinesia, is myoclonus the most significant problem? What is the impact of myoclonus on the activities of daily living?

PHARMACOLOGIC THERAPY

The pharmacotherapy of myoclonus has been largely empiric. There are no FDA-approved therapies specifically for myoclonus, and the need for new, more effective treatments is clear. Most human myoclonic disorders are orphan diseases, so interest in research and development on the part of the pharmaceutical industry has been low. Many treatments have been found by serendipity (1).

The history of therapeutics for myoclonus is one of heavy reliance on antiepileptic drugs (AEDs), but attempts also have been made to utilize non-AED neuroreceptor-active drugs. In the case of benzodiazepine agonist AEDs, with their effects on $GABA_A$ receptor-gated chloride channels, the criteria for both antiepileptic and neuroreceptor drugs are met. Because the cellular and molecular pathophysiology of myoclonus is largely unknown, the antimyoclonic mechanism of action of most drugs used to treat myoclonus has not been established.

The greatest obstacle to treating myoclonus is the belief that monotherapy is the goal. In the more severe and progressive forms of myoclonus, monotherapy is seldom effective, and patients may require 3 or more medications (2). In progressive disorders, a 20% clinical improvement with each drug is considered a good response and may be functionally significant. Polytherapy still carries attendant risks for oversedation and drug–drug interactions, but it is a reality in myoclonus therapy.

Antiepileptic Drugs

AEDs remain the chief pharmacologic treatment for myoclonus (Table 29.2), probably because of the close neurophysiologic association of certain types of myoclonus and epilepsy (3). Newer AEDs, such as zonisamide (4,5) and levetiracetam (6,7), have contributed to the core armamentarium that once consisted only of clonazepam, primidone, and valproic acid. AEDs, especially those with different mechanisms of action (8), may have synergistic effects in myoclonus. Epileptic positive myoclonus and epileptic negative myoclonus respond to different AEDs (9). Some AEDs have applications to specific myoclonic disorders or syndromes (Table 29.3) (5,9,10).

Not all AEDs are antimyoclonic, however, and in some patients with epilepsy, especially those with intractable seizures, certain AEDs may be promyoclonic (11–14), even precipitating myoclonic status epilepticus (15). Others AEDs may contribute to the pathology, such as the toxic effects of phenytoin on the cerebellum, a presumed site of pathology in progressive myoclonus epilepsy (16).

When patients are being treated for concomitant epilepsy, they are often placed on AEDs that are not antimyoclonic. However, it is important to choose antiepileptic medications for their antimyoclonic potential. This usually means removing phenytoin and carbamazepine-like drugs (17) and replacing them with clonazepam, valproate, primidone, or other antimyoclonic drugs. Occasionally, a patient will need to remain on nonantimyoclonic AEDs for seizure control.

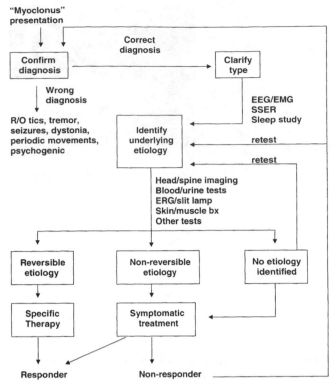

Figure 29.1 Schema for the evaluation and treatment of a patient with myoclonus. After the differential diagnosis of myoclonus has been considered and the diagnosis is confirmed, the underlying etiology must be established. Associated features and the presence of other organ system involvement guide the extent and type of diagnostic testing. When myoclonus is part of a larger neurological syndrome and no etiology is found, retesting the patient at a later time may be necessary. Symptomatic therapy does not replace specific therapy when a reversible etiology has been found.

Reduction in efficacy or development of tolerance is a significant problem in the treatment of myoclonus, regardless of the specific agent being used. The period of responsiveness may be months to years. Caution is indicated when the dose of clonazepam is increased due to tolerance in progressive myoclonus epilepsy, as choking on secretions may result at higher doses.

TABLE 29.1
CONSIDERATIONS IN CHOOSING A TREATMENT STRATEGY

Anticipated future needs	Major limitations
Cognitive abilities	Need for rehabilitation
Contributing factors	Patient/parental attitudes
Current therapy	Physician attitudes
Etiologic diagnosis	Prior interventions
Functional assessment	Realistic goals
General health	Risk for aspiration and choking
Level of independence	Risk for pregnancy

Drug side effects are another management problem, but they can be anticipated. Weight gain on valproate, an important drug for Unverricht-Lundborg epilepsy (EPM1) can be massive in wheelchair-bound patients. Coadministration of a very small dose of topiramate may offset this effect in individuals who are susceptible to topiramate's effects on weight and appetite.

Nonantiepileptic Drugs

Nonantiepileptic drugs as a group are the second line of symptomatic therapy for myoclonus, and they are often reserved for special circumstances (Table 29.4). They may be combined with antiepileptic drugs.

Neuropsychotropic Drugs

Many centrally active non-AEDs are antimyoclonic. Although gamma-aminobutyric acid (GABA), glycine, and serotonin seem to be the primary neurotransmitters in the mechanism of human myoclonus (18), few direct manipulations of neurotransmitter pathways or receptors have been applied or are available in the treatment of myoclonus. Some were subsumed under the heading of AEDs. Neuropsychotropic agents are active at a wide variety of neurotransmitter receptors or their exact mechanism of action remains unknown.

Agents that modify serotonergic neurotransmission can be helpful as adjunctive treatments for certain myoclonic disorders (19), such as posthypoxic myoclonus (20) and levodopa-induced myoclonus in Parkinson's disease (PD) (21), but they have a spotty performance in other types of myoclonus (22–24). Drugs active at dopamine, acetylcholine, beta-adrenergic, and opiate receptors have limited applicability (25). Piracetam, in contrast to levetiracetam, is not an AED but possesses stronger antimyoclonic properties (6,26). Although piracetam use is restricted to cortical myoclonus (27,28), a number of different etiologic disorders respond well to it, as least for a time (7,29,30). Chloral hydrate is a useful stopgap measure for progressive myoclonus epilepsy (31).

Immunotherapy

The pharmacologic treatment of autoimmune myoclonus serves as an example of therapy unrelated to AEDs or other neuropsychotropic drugs. Opsoclonus–myoclonus syndrome, a paraneoplastic syndrome (32) associated with B- and T-cell recruitment into the brain (33), is best treated with immunotherapy, such as corticosteroids (preferred in adults) or corticotropin (preferred in children). Tumor-directed therapy usually has little effect on the myoclonus. Symptomatic treatments, such as trazodone, can be coadministered for sleep disorder and rage attacks. Biologicals, such as intravenous immunoglobulins, and use

TABLE 29.2

EFFECTS OF ANTIEPILEPTIC DRUGS ON MYOCLONUS

Antimyoclonic	Sometimes Promyoclonic[a]	Often Promyoclonic[a]	Unstudied
Clonazepam	Gabapentin	Carbamazepine	Clobazam[b]
Ethosuximide	Lamotrigine	Oxcarbazepine	Eterobarb[b]
Felbamate	Lorazepam	Phenytoin	Remacemide[b]
Levetiracetam		Pregabalin[b]	Stiripentol[b]
Phenobarbital		Vigabatrin[b]	Tiagabine
Primidone			Topiramate
Valproic acid			
Zonisamide			

[a]In epileptic patients.
[b]Not available in the United States.

TABLE 29.3

ANTIEPILEPTIC DRUGS FOR SPECIFIC MYOCLONIC DISORDERS

Diaphragmatic Myoclonus	Epileptic Negative Myoclonus	Essential Myoclonus
Phenytoin	Ethosuximide	Primidone
Valproate		Gabapentin
Post-hypoxic		

Myoclonus	Progressive Myoclonus Epilepsy	Opioid-Induced Myoclonus
Clonazepam	Valproate	Clonazepam
Valproate	Clonazepam	Gabapentin
Levetiracetam	Zonisamide	
Felbamate[a]	Levetiracetam	

Status Myoclonus		
Phenobarbital		
Lorazepam		

[a]Should not be used in older children or as a first choice for any pediatric population.

of plasmapheresis, with or without immunoadsorption (34), are usually added to immunotherapeutic drugs (35).

NONPHARMACOLOGIC THERAPY

Metabolism-Related Therapy

Vitamins, cofactors, dietary restrictions, and chelation for metabolic disorders are examples of treating myoclonus by reversing the underlying disorder (36). Together they constitute the most important category of nonpharmacologic therapy. Reflex-sensitive segmental spinal myoclonus may be associated with vitamin B12 deficiency (37). Biotin can reverse the symptoms of biotinidase or biotin deficiency (38). Implementation of the ketogenic diet early in the course of Lafora's disease (EPM2A) may bypass a metabolic defect in carbohydrate metabolism (39).

Botulinum Toxin

Intramuscular injection of botulinum toxin temporarily alleviates painful segmental myoclonus (40,41). In preventing the release of acetylcholine at the neuromuscular junction, botulinum toxin may block involuntary movement but will preserve strength. The effects last from weeks to months, but the injections can be repeated for years (42). Both botulinum toxins A (Botox; Dysport) and B (NeuroBloc) are used clinically. The current trend is toward lower doses than those recommended initially to help avoid development of antibodies against botulinum toxin that can nullify the therapeutic benefit (43).

Hormones

Estrogen receptors on neurons provide the physiologic explanation for changes in myoclonus associated with the menstrual cycle or hysterectomy/oophorectomy (44).

TABLE 29.4
NON-AED NEUROPSYCHOTROPIC DRUGS FOR MYOCLONIC DISORDERS

Drug	Mechanism	Indication
Acetazolamide	Carbonic anhydrase inhibitor	Progressive myoclonus ataxia
Apomorphine	Dopamine agonist	Cortical reflex myoclonus
Baclofen	GABA$_B$ receptor blocker	Progressive myoclonus, epilepsy, spinal myoclonus
Chloral hydrate	Unknown	Progressive myoclonus epilepsy
5-hydroxytryptophan[a]/carbidopa	Indirect serotonin agonist	Post-hypoxic myoclonus
Lisuride[b]	Antiserotonergic, dopaminergic	Photosensitive myoclonus
Methysergide	Antiserotonergic	L-dopa induced myoclonus in Parkinson's disease
Metoprolol, propranolol	Beta-adrenergic blocker	Essential myoclonus
Midazolam	Benzodiazepine	Opiate-induced myoclonus in cancer patients
Piracetam[b]	Unknown	Cortical myoclonus (progressive myoclonus epilepsy, posthypoxic myoclonus)
Sodium oxybate[c]	GABA$_B$ receptor activation	Myoclonus-dystonia
Tetrabenazine[b]	Antidopaminergic	Spinal myoclonus
Trihexyphenidyl	Anticholinergic	Myoclonus-dystonia

[a]A physician may prescribe under the manufacturer's IND in the United States for this specific indication only.
[b]Not available in the United States.
[c]Gamma-hydroxybutyrate (GHB), a Schedule I drug.
[d]Interactions with excitatory and inhibitory amino acid neurotransmitter-operated ion channels.

Perimenstrual exacerbation of myoclonus often responds to oral contraceptives or depo-estrogen (45). Patients with mitochondrial encephalomyopathies often have gonadal dysfunction (46).

Transcranial Magnetic Stimulation

Transcranial magnetic stimulation (TMS) is a noninvasive, safe, and painless way to stimulate the human motor cortex in humans (47). Repetitive TMS (rTMS) can be used to transiently inactivate different cortical areas to study their functions. Modulation of cortical excitability by rTMS has therapeutic potential in myoclonic disorders, because low-frequency stimulation (1 Hz) reduces cortical excitability (48). High-frequency stimulation is avoided because of the risk of inducing a seizure (49,50). Currently, rTMS is investigational and not widely available; however, the equipment is not extremely costly and may well find its way into the clinical setting. The patient sits in a chair and a coil is lowered over the head. Although only cortical structures are currently accessible, rTMS seems capable of affecting activity in cortically linked deep-brain structures (51).

Deep-Brain Stimulation

Deep-brain stimulation certainly is not a first-line therapy for myoclonus and should be reserved for drug-refractory progressive disorders. There is a paucity of data, especially in the pediatric population, with experiences being largely anecdotal (52).

REASONS FOR TREATMENT FAILURE

Myoclonus may fail to respond or may increase as a result of misdiagnosis, mistreatment, noncompliance, or a refractory or progressive condition (Fig. 29.2). Persistence is the key to accurate diagnosis and treatment. It may be necessary to revisit the initial diagnosis, assess for overlooked factors, and verify that the drug regimen is being followed.

Exacerbating factors—dietary, hormonal, lifestyle, and psychosocial—are frequently overlooked or not mentioned. Comorbid illnesses, such as anxiety, depression, or other affective disorders, may compromise myoclonus treatment. An undiagnosed sleep disorder is common in some of the more severe myoclonic disorders, and poor sleep may increase myoclonus. Poor physical health is caused by inactivity, obesity, or injuries from falls. A good general physical examination is a simple necessity.

Pharmacotherapy may be inadequate for many reasons. The drug may be ineffective or used at the wrong doses. Several weeks are required to properly evaluate treatment successes or failures; avoid sudden changes. Further dose increases beyond the typical ceiling dose may be indicated in individuals with a partial drug response without side effects. Many different pharmacokinetic factors may be at play.

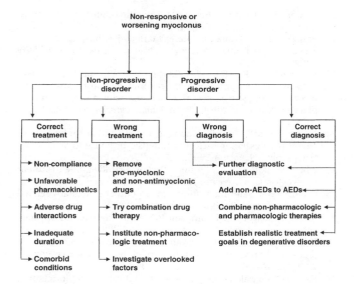

Figure 29.2 Troubleshooting flowchart. Lack of treatment response or worsening myoclonus should prompt reevaluation of the diagnosis and a search for exacerbating factors.

As a general rule, subcortical and segmental myoclonus are difficult to treat. The same is true for negative myoclonus. It also should be remembered that the neural substrate for drug responsiveness may be lost in progressive disorders, so medications do not work as expected. In that situation, it is important to set realistic treatment endpoints.

QUALITY-OF-LIFE ISSUES

It is easy to lose sight of quality-of-life issues (Table 29.5) in our focus on the medical aspects of myoclonus. However, patients and their families carry a burden of living with a chronic disease, whether or not it is progressive, often without prospects for significant improvement (53). Severe myoclonus may rob adolescents of the necessary "breaking away" from parents, which leads to maladaptive behaviors and habitual family conflicts. Isolation, inactivity, and a decline in physical strength result in marginalization and reduced quality of life. Perhaps confidence is the most essential element to reinforce because it carries over so prominently into activities of daily living. When we cannot cure myoclonus, we must at least help improve the way individuals with myoclonus feel about themselves. With gene therapy on the forefront, we must keep them in the best possible mental and physical shape. Different approaches should be taken at the same time.

SUMMARY

The approach to a patient with myoclonus should focus on identifying the underlying etiology in the hope that the disorder can be reversed. Restoring activities of everyday living should be a fundamental therapeutic goal. A regimen of multiple drugs is the rule in severe myoclonus and

---

TABLE 29.5

IMPROVING QUALITY OF LIFE IN PATIENTS WITH SEVERE MYOCLONUS

Goal	Means
Continue education	Tutors
Counter depression	Pharmacologic and nonpharmacologic
Decrease strife	Counselor/psychiatrist, individual and family
Encourage independent living	Assisted living; visiting health aide
Establish medical contingencies for travel	Take emergency drugs on vacations
Increase safety in wheelchair	Wheelchair seat belt
Improve quality of sleep	Sleep study; treat depression
Maintain strength	Physical therapy; regular exercise program
Diet and exercise	Offset drugs that cause hyperphagia
Maintain peer contact	School, church, community
Make home more accessible	Wheelchair ramps, move downstairs, make bathrooms handicapped-accessible
Prevent loneliness	Companion dog
Prevent pulmonary infections	Immunize
Reduce myoclonus when patient most needs to	Rearrange dosing schedule
Reduce stress	Modify school or work schedule
Set practical goals	Educational and vocational counseling

in progressive disorders. Responses to an agent are sometimes dramatic, but more often the improvements are incremental. In patients with substantial myoclonus, the combination of pharmacologic and nonpharmacologic measures can be effective. Therapeutic failure should prompt reevaluation of the diagnosis and treatment plan and a search for exacerbating factors. In the end, sensitivity to quality-of-life issues can be the most important contribution a clinician can make.

REFERENCES

1. Wong CG, Chan KF, Gibson KM, Snead OC. Gamma-hydroxybutyric acid: neurobiology and toxicology of a recreational drug. *Toxicol Rev* 2004;23:3–20.
2. Agarwal P, Frucht SJ. Myoclonus. *Curr Opin Neurol* 2003;16: 515–521.
3. Hallett M. Myoclonus: relation to epilepsy. *Epilepsia* 1985;26: 567–577.
4. Yagi K. Overview of Japanese experience-controlled and uncontrolled trials. *Seizure* 2004;13(suppl 1):S11–S15.
5. Yoshimura I, Kaneko S, Yoshimura N, et al. Long-term observations of two siblings with Lafora disease treated with zonisamide. *Epilepsy Res* 2001;46:283–287.
6. Genton P, Van Vleymen B. Piracetam and levetiracetam: close structural similarities but different pharmacological and clinical profiles. *Epileptic Disord* 2000;2:99–105.
7. Krauss GL, Bergin A, Kramer RE, et al. Suppression of post-hypoxic and post-encephalitic myoclonus with levetiracetam. *Neurology* 2001;56:411–412.
8. Wallace SJ. Newer antiepileptic drugs: advantages and disadvantages. *Brain Dev* 2001;23:277–283.
9. Capovilla G, Beccaria F, Veggiotti P, et al. Ethosuximide is effective in the treatment of epileptic negative myoclonus in childhood partial epilepsy. *J Child Neurol* 1999;14:395–400.
10. Mercadante S, Villari P, Fulfaro F. Gabapentin for opioid-related myoclonus in cancer patients. *Support Care Center* 2001;9:205–206.
11. Huppertz HJ, Feuerstein TJ, Schulze-Bonhage A. Myoclonus in epilepsy patients with anticonvulsive add-on therapy with pregabalin. *Epilepsia* 2001;42:790–792.
12. Janszky J, Rasonyi G, Halasz P, et al. Disabling erratic myoclonus during lamotrigine therapy with high serum level—report of two cases. *Clin Neuropharmacol* 2000;23:86–89.
13. Marciani MG, Maschio M, Spanedda F, et al. Development of myoclonus in patients with partial epilepsy during treatment with vigabatrin: an electroencephalographic study. *Acta Neurol Scand* 1995;91:1–5.
14. Asconape J, Diedrich A, DellaBadia J. Myoclonus associated with the use of gabapentin. *Epilepsia* 2000;41:479–481.
15. Guerrini R, Belmonte A, Parmeggiani L, et al. Myoclonus status epilepticus following high-dosage lamotrigine therapy. *Brain Dev* 1999;21:420–424.
16. Eldridge R, Iivanainen M, Stern R, et al. "Baltic" myoclonus epilepsy: hereditary disorder of childhood made worse by phenytoin. *Lancet* 1983;9:838–842.
17. Namba Y, Maegaki Y. Epileptic negative myoclonus induced by carbamazepine in a child with BECTS: benign childhood epilepsy with centrotemporal spikes. *Pediatr Neurol* 1999;21:664–667.
18. Pranzatelli MR, Nadi NS. Mechanism of action of antiepileptic and antimyoclonic drugs. *Adv Neurol* 1995;67:329–360.
19. Pranzatelli MR. Serotonin and human myoclonus: rationale for the use of serotonin receptor agonists and antagonists. *Arch Neurol* 1994;51:605–617.
20. Chadwick D, Hallett M, Harris R, et al. Clinical, biochemical and physiological features distinguishing myoclonus responsive to 5-hydroxy-tryptophan, tryptophan with a monoamine oxidase inhibitor and clonazepam. *Brain* 1977;100:455–487.
21. Klawans HL, Goetz C, Bergen D. Levodopa-induced myoclonus. *Arch Neurol* 1975;32:330–334.
22. Pranzatelli MR, Franz D, Tate E, Martens JM. Buspirone in progressive myoclonus epilepsy. *J Neurol Neurosurg Psychiatry* 1993;56:114–115.
23. Pranzatelli MR, Tate E, Baldwin M. Clinical responses to 5-hydroxy-L-tryptophan in chronic pediatric opsoclonus-myoclonus suggest biochemical heterogeneity: a double-blinded placebo crossover pilot study. *Clin Neuropharmacol* 1994;17: 103–116.
24. Pranzatelli MR, Tate E, Huang Y, et al. The neuropharmacology of progressive myoclonus epilepsy: response to 5-hydroxy-L-tryptophan. *Epilepsia* 1995;36:783–791.
25. Obeso JA, Rothwell JC, Quinn NP, et al. Lisuride in the treatment of myoclonus. *Adv Neurol* 1986;43:191–196.
26. Gouliaev AH, Senning A. Piracetam and other structurally related nootropics. *Brain Res Rev* 1994;19:180–222.
27. Brown P, Steiger MJ, Thompson PD, et al. Effectiveness of piracetam in cortical myoclonus. *Mov Disord* 1993;8:63–68.
28. Pranzatelli MR, Tate ED, Galvan I, et al. Controlled pilot study of piracetam for pediatric opsoclonus-myoclonus. *Clin Neuropharmacol* 2001;24:352–357.
29. Ikeda A, Shibasaki H, Tashiro K, et al. Clinical trial of piracetam in patients with myoclonus: nationwide multiinstitution study in Japan. *Mov Disord* 1996;11:691–700.
30. Feddi M, Reutens D, Dubeau F, et al. Long-term efficacy and safety of piracetam in the treatment of progressive myoclonus epilepsy. *Arch Neurol* 2001;58:781–786.
31. Pranzatelli MR, Tate ED. Chloral hydrate for progressive myoclonus epilepsy: a new look at an old drug. *Pediatr Neurol* 2001;25:385–389.
32. Pranzatelli MR. Paraneoplastic syndromes: an unsolved murder. *Semin Pediatr Neurol* 2000;7:118–130.
33. Pranzatelli MR, Travelstead AL, Tate ED, et al. B- and T-cell markers in opsoclonus-myoclonus syndrome: immunophenotyping of CSF lymphocytes. *Neurology* 2004;62:1526–1532.
34. Nitschke M, Hochberg F, Dropcho E. Improvement of paraneoplastic opsoclonus-myoclonus after protein A column therapy. *N Engl J Med* 1995;332:192.
35. Yiu VW, Kovithavongs T, McGonigle LF, et al. Plasmapheresis as an effective treatment for opsoclonus-myoclonus syndrome. *Pediatr Neurol* 2001;24,72–74.
36. Gascon GG, Ozand PT, Brismar J. Movement disorders in childhood organic acidurias: clinical, neuroimaging, and biochemical correlations. *Brain Dev* 1994;16(suppl):94–103.
37. Tsao JW, Cooper EC. Reflex-sensitive spinal segmental myoclonus associated with vitamin B12 deficiency. *Neurology* 2003;61: 867–868.
38. Colamaria V, Burlina AB, Gaburro D, et al. Biotin-responsive infantile encephalopathy: EEG-polygraphic study of a case. *Epilepsia* 1989;30:573–578.
39. Bara-Jimenez W, Pagan F, Boudreau E, et al. Therapeutic benefits of ketogenic diet in Lafora disease. *Neurology* 2003;60(suppl 1): A472.
40. Awaad Y, Tayem H, Elgamal A, et al. Treatment of childhood myoclonus with botulinum toxin type A. *J Child Neurol* 1999;14: 781–786.
41. Lagueny A, Tison F, Burbaud P, Le Masson G, Kien P. Stimulus-sensitive spinal segmental myoclonus improved with injections of botulinum toxin type A. *Mov Disord* 1999;14:182–185.
42. Mejia NI, Vuong KD, Jankovic J. Long-term botulinum toxin efficacy, safety, and immunogenicity. *Mov Disord* 2005;20:592–597.
43. Dressler D, Bigalke H. Antibody-induced failure of botulinum toxin type B therapy in de novo patients. *Eur Neurol* 2004;52:132–135.
44. Kompoliti K. Estrogen and movement disorders. *Clin Neuropharmacol* 1999;22:318–326.
45. Fahn S. Newer drugs for post hypoxic action myoclonus: observations from a well-studied case. *Adv Neurol* 1986;43:197–199.
46. Chen CM, Huang CC. Gonadal dysfunction in mitochondrial encephalomyopathies. *Eur Neurol* 1995;35:281–286.
47. Chen R. Studies of human motor physiology with transcranial magnetic stimulation. *Muscle Nerve Suppl* 2000;9:S26–S32.
48. Amassian VE, Cracco RQ, Maccabee PS, et al. Some positive effects of transcranial magnetic stimulation. *Adv Neurol* 1995;67: 79–104.

49. Lisanby SH, Luber B, Sackeim HA, et al. Deliberate seizure induction with negative transcranial magnetic stimulation in nonhuman primates. *Arch Gen Psychiatry* 2001;58:199–200.

50. McDonald WM, Greenberg BD. Electroconvulsive therapy in the treatment of neuropsychiatric conditions and transcranial magnetic stimulation as a pathophysiological probe in neuropsychiatry. *Depress Anxiety* 2000;12:135–143.

51. Triggs WJ, Kirshner HS. Improving brain function with transcranial magnetic stimulation. *Neurology* 2001;56:429–430.

52. Cif L, Valente EM, Hemm S, et al. Deep brain stimulation in myoclonus-dystonia syndrome. *Mov Disord* 2004;19:724–727.

53. Tate ED. The clinical challenge of progressive myoclonus epilepsy. *Nurse Pract* 1993;18:25–28.

Drug-Induced Movement Disorders

30

Kapil D. Sethi   John C. Morgan

Movement disorders are frequently due to prescribed drugs and to illicit drug use. In this chapter we focus on prescribed drugs but briefly mention drugs of abuse. The main emphasis is on movement disorders due to dopamine receptor–blocking agents (DBAs). However, movement disorders due to other drugs will be briefly reviewed as well.

MOVEMENT DISORDERS DUE TO DOPAMINE RECEPTOR–BLOCKING AGENTS

Unfortunately, even with the availability of atypical antipsychotic drugs, movement disorders due to dopamine receptor–blocking agents (DBA) continue to be a significant clinical problem. Chlorpromazine was first developed in France in 1952 and was introduced in the United States in 1954. It was heralded as a major advance in the treatment of psychosis (1). However, there were significant acute side effects, such as akathisia, drug-induced parkinsonism, and acute dystonia. A more disturbing persistent dyskinesia was first recognized in the late 1950s (2). In the past 40 years or so, significant clinical experience has accumulated with the use of DBA, and today the movement disorders caused by these drugs can be classified (see Table 30.1.)

Acute Movement Disorders due to Dopamine Receptor-Blocking Agents

Acute Dystonia

Background and Phenomenology
Acute dystonia occurs shortly after the introduction of DBA and occasionally after a dose increase. This reaction is particularly common with injectable high-potency DBA.

There is usually a delay between the administration of the drug and the appearance of dystonia. About 50% of patients experience the first signs of dystonia within 48 hours of drug intake, and 90% show signs within 5 days of drug treatment (3). Acute dystonia is more likely to occur with typical DBA; however, the newer atypical drugs, including clozapine, are also associated with a small risk of inducing acute dystonia (4).

Dystonic reactions are variable in location and can be painful. The usual manifestations are orofacial dystonia, back arching, and neck extension. Laryngospasm may occur and may be life threatening (5). Repeated acute dystonic reactions, even with a single dose of DBA, have been observed but are uncommon.

A form of acute dystonic reaction appearing 3 to 10 days after starting dopamine-blocking agents is called the *Pisa syndrome*. It is characterized by tonic lateroflexion of the trunk (6). However, Pisa syndrome also may be seen as a manifestation of tardive dystonia (7).

An oculogyric crisis (OGC) is characterized by tonic conjugate ocular deviation that may last minutes to hours, and OGCs can occur in both acute and tardive dystonia (8).

Frequency and Risk Factors
The frequency of acute drug-induced dystonic reactions varies widely from 2.3% (9) to 94% (10,11). Risk factors for dystonia include male gender, young age (under 30), potency and dose of neuroleptics used, familial predisposition, underlying psychiatric illness, mental retardation, and a history of electroconvulsive therapy (12). There is a 2:1 risk of drug-induced dystonia in men compared to women. The same ratio holds true for young adults and children. Cocaine abuse may predispose to acute dystonic reactions (13). AIDS also has been associated with increased risk (14).

TABLE 30.1

MOVEMENT DISORDERS INDUCED BY DOPAMINE BLOCKING AGENTS

I. Acute
   Acute Dystonia
   Acute Akathisia
   Drug-Induced Parkinsonism

II. Chronic

Common:	Tardive Dyskinesia
	Tardive Dystonia
	Tardive Akathisia
Uncommon:	Tardive Myoclonus
	Tardive Tics
	Tardive Tremor

III. Miscellaneous
   Neuroleptic Malignant Syndrome

Mechanism

The mechanism of acute dystonia is unclear, but two opposing hypotheses have been proposed. One hypothesis is that dopaminergic hypofunction results in a relative over-activity of cholinergic mechanisms (15). This hypothesis is supported by a consistent response of acute dystonia to anticholinergic drugs. Also supporting this hypothesis is the fact that acute dystonia can be suppressed in primates by the preadministration of dopaminergic drugs such as levodopa or apomorphine. Further support for this hypothesis comes from a marmoset model. In this model, acute administration of haloperidol results in a syndrome of excitation with sustained retrocollis, climbing upside down, biting the perch, repetitive turnings, and frequent backward movements. These dystonic movements are ameliorated by administration of the anticholinergic drug biperiden (16).

The other hypothesis proposes that there is paradoxical dopaminergic hyperfunction induced by DBA through blockade of presynaptic dopamine receptors. Moreover, as the level of the DBA decreases, postsynaptic receptors are exposed to the natural release of dopamine from presynaptic terminals (17).

The possible contribution of other neurotransmitter systems, such as gamma-aminobutyric acid (GABA), is unknown. Recently, the role of sigma receptors has been explored. It has been reported that the unilateral microinjection of sigma ligands into the red nucleus induces torticollis in rats (18). In animal models, the anticholinergic drug biperiden dose dependently ameliorates dystonia induced by two sigma ligands.

Management

Some evidence suggests that acute dystonic reactions may be prevented by the use of anticholinergic drugs (3). It is recommended by some that patients at high risk for acute dystonia (young patients, cocaine abusers, and AIDS patients) requiring DBA receive prophylactic anticholinergics.

Acute dystonia responds well to injectable anticholinergic drugs (19) or diphenhydramine (20). The response to anticholinergics is so consistent that if a patient with suspected DBA-induced acute dystonia fails to respond, clinicians should suspect phencyclidine (PCP)-induced dystonia (21). Occasionally, diazepam has been used with success. At times, acute dystonic reactions, such as laryngeal dystonia, are severe enough to warrant life-saving measures (tracheostomy).

Acute Akathisia

Background and Phenomenology

The term *akathisia* (from Greek, literally "not to sit") was introduced by Haskovec (22) in 1901, some time before the development of neuroleptics. The phenomenon of akathisia is somewhat paradoxical given that the same drugs that are supposed to calm patients actually result in restlessness.

There are two aspects of akathisia: (1) a subjective report of restlessness or inner tension, particularly referable to the legs, with a consequent inability to maintain a posture for several minutes, and (2) the objective manifestations of restlessness in the form of movements of the limbs, a tendency to shift body position in the chair while sitting or marching while standing.

The temporal association with drug administration is an important feature in the diagnosis of akathisia. The most recognized form of akathisia usually starts within hours or days after the initiation or increase in DBA dosage or change in the type of DBA, and even a single exposure to the drug is sufficient for the diagnosis (23); acute akathisia usually starts within the first 2 weeks (24,25) and almost always within the first 6 weeks (9). The term *pseudoakathisia* applies to patients with the objective features of akathisia without subjective complaints (26). As such, pseudoakathisia is a true akathisia but with limited manifestations. Psychotic patients may have trouble reporting subjective feelings, and it may be difficult to distinguish akathisia from dyskinetic movements.

The incidence of akathisia ranges from 21%–31% in psychotic patients treated with DBA (24,25). The risk with some of the atypical neuroleptics may be lower, but the published evidence for this is inconsistent because of the problems of carryover effects and equivalent doses not being used. The reported rates of akathisia with clozapine vary (27), but the Sandoz Pharmaceutical Corporation reported a rate of 3% in 842 treated patients (28).

It is important to distinguish akathisia from psychotic agitation, which is more generalized and is often chaotic, disorganized, and even frenzied. Another disorder that must be distinguished from akathisia is restless legs syndrome (RLS). RLS symptoms display a circadian pattern, being worse in the evening, and unlike RLS, periodic limb movements in sleep are not a characteristic finding in patients with akathisia.

Mechanism

DBA causes akathisia by blocking dopamine receptors, especially D2 receptors. This is supported by the observations that high-potency D2 antagonists are more likely to cause akathisia, and akathisia is related to drug dose and may occur after the administration of a single dose. Two studies using positron emission tomography (PET) (29,30) demonstrated an association between D2 occupancy in the striatum and the development of akathisia, with the latter authors suggesting a threshold between 74%–82% D2 receptor occupancy for the production of extrapyramidal effects including akathisia. The D2 antagonism hypothesis does not explain why cholinergic and β-adrenergic antagonists are effective in some cases of akathisia, however.

An alternative hypothesis was proposed by Marsden and Jenner (17), who proposed that DBA antagonism of mesocortical and mesolimbic dopaminergic projections leads to akathisia. This is supported by the observation that lesions of mesocortical dopaminergic neurons lead to increased locomotor activity in rodents.

Management

Two classes of drugs most commonly used in the treatment of akathisia are anticholinergic and antiadrenergic. Some literature supports the efficacy of these drugs in a proportion of patients; however, a recent Cochrane Database Review concluded that there was insufficient evidence to support their use (31,32).

Anticholinergics employed have included benztropine (dosage range 0.5–8 mg/day), trihexyphenidyl (1–15 mg/day), procyclidine (7.5–20 mg/day), biperiden (2–8 mg/day), and orphenadrine (100–400 mg/day). The optimal dosage should be titrated, starting with a small initial dose. Peripheral anticholinergic side effects (constipation, dry mouth, etc.) and central anticholinergic side effects (confusion, memory disturbance) should be monitored, especially in the elderly.

Of the antiadrenergic drugs, propranolol—a lipophilic, nonspecific beta-blocker—has been used most extensively. The suggestion from the literature is that lower doses of propranolol are sufficient, with most researchers using doses on the order of 60 mg/day and rarely above 120 mg/day. Propranolol seems to be well tolerated in this population, and the possible side effects of hypotension, bradycardia, sedation, and depression are not usually reported by appropriately selected individuals. Clonidine, an alpha2 agonist that reduces central noradrenergic activity, has been beneficial, but side effects limit its practical use.

Miller et al. (33) reported a single-blind open-label study of ritanserin, a specific $5HT_2$ antagonist, with overall improvement in patients with treatment-resistant neuroleptic-induced akathisia. Benzodiazepines have also been used with some benefit in small studies.

TABLE 30.2

MEDICATIONS LIKELY TO INDUCE OR EXACERBATE PARKINSONISM

Neuroleptics
Phenothiazines: chlorpromazine, promethazine, levopromazine, triflupromazine, thioridazine, trifluoperazine, prochlorperazine, perphenazine, fluphenazine, mesoridazine, piperazine, acetophenazine, trimeprazine, thiethylperazine
Butyrophenones: haloperidol, droperidol, triperidol
Diphenylbutylpiperidine: pimozide
Indolines: molindone
Substituted Benzamides: metoclopramide, cisapride, sulpiride, clebopride, domperidone, veralipride, alizapride, remoxipride, tiapride, veralipride
Benzoquinolizine: tetrabenazine
Rauwolfia derivate: reserpine
Dibenzazepine: loxapine
Thioxanthenes: flupentixhol, chlorprothiexene, thiothixene
Atypicals: risperidone, olanzapine, clozapine, quetiapine
Calcium channel blockers: flunarizine, cinnarizine

Drug-Induced Parkinsonism

Drug-induced parkinsonism (DIP) may result from a variety of prescribed medications. The most common offending drugs are DBAs. Other nonneuroleptic drugs, such as metoclopramide. also may cause DIP (34). Table 30.2 and Table 30.3 list drugs that are likely to occasionally cause or exacerbate parkinsonism.

Prevalance of Drug-Induced Parkinsonism

DIP is a common complication of antipsychotic drug use, occurring in 15%–60% of patients treated with DBA (9). In one study, 51% of 95 patients referred to a geriatric medicine service for evaluation had parkinsonism associated with prescribed drugs (35). Another study found that in a general neurology practice, 56.8% of the 306 cases of parkinsonism were either induced by or aggravated by drugs (36). Frequently, these patients are misdiagnosed

---

TABLE 30.3

MEDICATIONS THAT OCCASIONALLY INDUCE OR EXACERBATE PARKINSONISM

Amphotericin B
Amiodarone
Calcium channel blockers: verapamil, diltiazem, nifedipine, amlodipine
Cyclophosphamide
Cyclosporine
Cytosine arabinoside
Disulfiram
Lithium
Meperidine
Methyldopa
Selective Serotonin Reuptake Inhibitors (SSRIs): citalopram, fluoxetine, paroxetine, sertraline
Valproate

with idiopathic Parkinson's disease (PD) and treated with dopaminergic drugs without benefit. In a community study, 18% of all cases initially thought to be PD were subsequently diagnosed as DIP (37). Older patients may develop DIP after relatively small doses of a DBA. One study found that 32% of older patients met the criteria for DIP even while they were on low doses of DBA (chlorpromazine equivalent of 43 mg/day) (38).

Individual susceptibility to DIP has been postulated based on case reports indicating a familial predisposition to DIP and a bias toward the female gender (39–41) Family history also may be relevant, as Gartmann and colleagues (41) reported 6 patients with family history of PD who developed DIP on neuroleptics, whereas others without family history of PD tolerated neuroleptics without side effects. The dose and the potency of DBA therapy are of obvious importance.

Clinical Features

The symptoms of DIP are frequently indistinguishable from PD. Traditionally, DIP was characterized as symmetrical; however, asymmetry of signs and symptoms may occur in 30% of cases (42,43). Subgroups exist within DIP; some patients primarily experience bradykinesia, whereas others have tremor. In some patients, the symptoms are mixed. Postural reflexes are impaired in some patients, and many patients have an abnormal gait. Festination is uncommon, and sudden transient freezing, a symptom of PD, is rare (42,44). The coexistence of a hyperkinetic movement disorder, such as orobuccolingual dyskinesia in the absence of levodopa treatment, will support a diagnosis of DIP rather than idiopathic Parkinson's disease (IPD).

Time Course

In patients who develop DIP, the condition typically develops between 2 weeks and 1 month following introduction of a neuroleptic or an increase in dose. It also tends to coincide with clinical improvement of schizophrenia (45). In one series, 50%–70% of cases appeared within 1 month and 90% within 3 months (46).

The term *rabbit syndrome* refers to a perioral tremor that may develop in some patients at any time during neuroleptic treatment (47,48). The tremor has the typical characteristics of parkinsonian tremor and tends to respond to antiparkinsonian agents. The term adds nothing to our understanding of DIP and should be avoided.

DIP may resolve despite continuing DBA therapy, suggesting tolerance, but prospective studies to address this issue are lacking. Most cases resolve quickly after discontinuing DBA; however, in some patients, symptoms persist for months (49).

The Problem of Underrecognition

Early in the era of DBA therapy, it was thought that extrapyramidal side effects and antipsychotic efficacy were tightly linked, and DIP was ignored or thought to be essential for efficacy. In one series, residents recognized DIP in less than half the patients afflicted with it (50). Metoclopramide-induced DIP is also frequently unrecognized, as suggested by Miller (51).

Metoclopramide-induced parkinsonism is not uncommon. This nonneuroleptic DBA is frequently prescribed for the treatment of gastroesophageal reflux and gastroparesis. We have observed that metoclopramide is a frequent offender in elderly diabetic patients with renal insufficiency (34). Parkinsonism typically develops when these patients are taking a prescribed dose of 40 mg/day. Metoclopramide is renally cleared, and in renal failure the dose has to be reduced by 50%.

Drug-Induced Parkinsonism Due to Vestibular Sedatives

In countries other than the United States, a common cause of DIP is the use of the vestibular sedatives cinnarizine and its derivative, flunarizine (52,53). In one study of 172 cases of DIP over 15 years, 74 cases were due to cinnarizine (52). Cinnarizine-induced parkinsonism is more common in women, as is the case with neuroleptic-induced DIP. Complete recovery usually occurs after drug withdrawal, but in some cases signs persist (54). Drug dose is important, and the risk appears to be low in those taking less than 150 mg of cinnarizine. The mechanism of DIP induced by these drugs is unknown and may involve presynaptic dopamine depletion, postsynaptic dopamine receptor blockade, and effects on nondopaminergic neurons. These drugs also have marked antihistaminergic and calcium channel–blocking activity.

Pathophysiology

Superficially, DIP is the most easily understood side effect of DBAs and relates to their D2 receptor–blocking activity (17). DIP appears to develop in almost everyone given high doses of high-potency DBA, thereby achieving concentrations that would block about 80% of central dopamine receptors (55). However, the reasons why some individuals develop parkinsonism in the usual therapeutic dose range are unclear. Another unexplained aspect is the delay between the pharmacological action of the drugs and the onset of DIP. While neuroleptics block dopamine receptors within minutes to hours, DIP typically appears many days or weeks following drug exposure. This suggests that there is a complex relationship between exposure to neuroleptic drugs and the development of DIP.

Risk factors for DIP include the potency and dose of the neuroleptic and individual susceptibility. A high ratio between serotonin ($5HT_2$) and D2 dopamine receptor antagonism will produces less in the way of extrapyramidal effects, including DIP (56). Also, a rapid dissociation of the drug from the receptor may have a role to play in reducing the motor side effects (57).

Individual risk factors include older age, female sex, and the presence of cerebral atrophy. Genetic susceptibility to DIP has been postulated based on case reports indicating a familial predisposition to DIP. Genetic differences in drug metabolism are postulated to be important in some patients (58,59).

It has been suggested that DIP may merely be unmasking subclinical PD. DIP in treated patients is more prevalent than PD in the general population. However, the frequency of older patients with incidental Lewy bodies at autopsy is approximately 15 times the frequency of patients with clinically apparent PD (60). Therefore, DIP may represent an unmasking of subclinical PD. The evidence for DBA unmasking PD comes from both clinical (61) and pathological observations (62). In some cases of DIP, the condition may persist after discontinuing DBA, and some patients may go on to develop PD. A retrospective study done at the Mayo Clinic in Rochester, Minnesota, showed that IPD emerged over time in 2 out of 24 patients (8%) followed for DIP. A comparison with the expected number of IPD patients in the general population yielded a relative risk of 24.3 (63). Rajput et al. (62) reported pathological evidence of nigral Lewy body disease in 2 patients who developed DIP while on neuroleptic treatment but had a complete recovery on withdrawal of neuroleptics. After death from unrelated causes, autopsy revealed slight to moderate loss of nigral dopaminergic cells and Lewy bodies.

More recently, functional neuroimaging has been employed to study this problem (64–66). The first study examined [^{18}F]-fluorodopa PET scans in 13 DIP patients (64). In 4 of those 13, there was evidence of significant reduction of 18F-fluordopa uptake in the putamen within the PD range, and in 3 of these 4 patients, there was continuing or worsening parkinsonism (64). All 9 patients with normal scans recovered. Booij et al. imaged striatal dopamine transporter binding in patients with parkinsonism using (^{123}I) FP-CIT SPECT (65). Among 19 patients with normal scans and parkinsonism, 3 were eventually diagnosed with DIP. None of the 22 patients with abnormal scans were diagnosed with DIP. In this study, there was no evidence that DIP unmasks PD. (For a detailed review of SPECT imaging in DIP, see 66.)

Management

Prevention of DIP should be the goal. DBA should be administered only when absolutely necessary, and atypical antipsychotics should be used when possible. The use of anticholinergic drugs in prophylaxis is debatable. Anticholinergics may worsen psychiatric problems and cause confusion and memory difficulties. A reasonable approach may be to treat prophylactically patients who are at a higher risk (e.g., AIDS patients) with anticholinergics. This would be particularly useful if a high-dose, high-potency DBA is used. However, there is little prospective data to support this approach.

The treatment of clinically manifest DIP is difficult. An obvious choice is to reevaluate the need for DBA and to withdraw the drug whenever possible. This is done with a risk of reemergent psychosis. In most cases, the condition is reversible once the offending agent is withdrawn. In cases where DBA cannot be withdrawn, substitution with an atypical agent should be attempted. Clozapine, an atypical neuroleptic, has a low acute extrapyramidal symptom profile, but it may cause agranulocytosis in approximately 1% of patients. The risk of DIP is also low with quetiapine, but higher doses of olanzapine and risperidone may cause DIP.

Mild DIP may be left untreated. Where necessary, the symptoms can be managed with anticholinergic agents, antihistaminic agents, or amantadine. Amantadine is a useful drug and may be superior to anticholinergics, as shown in two studies (67,68).

There are limited data on the use of levodopa or dopamine agonists in the treatment of DIP. In one study, dopaminergic drugs seemed to worsen psychosis (69), but this approach has not been systematically studied.

Tardive Movement Disorders Due to Dopamine Receptor–Blocking Agents

DIP may occur in a delayed fashion, but the problems more frequently encountered in a tardive fashion include classic tardive dyskinesia and its variants and tardive akathisia.

Classic Tardive Dyskinesia

Tardive dyskinesia (TD) has been defined by the American Psychiatric Association Task Force as an abnormal involuntary movement following a minimum of 3 months of neuroleptic treatment in a patient with no other identifiable etiology for movement disorders (70). DSM-IV criteria, however, specify that the duration of exposure to neuroleptics may be only 1 month in individuals ages 60 and older (71).

Many of the writers in the preneuroleptic era described spontaneous abnormal movements in patients with schizophrenia. However, many motor phenomena seen in patients with schizophrenia are highly idiosyncratic and tend not to appear qualitatively different from normal movements in the way that dyskinesia, dystonia, and tremor do. Most of the reports from the preneuroleptic era suggest the presence of stereotypies and posturing (72). Some patients had orofacial dyskinesia, but it is unclear if they had other organic brain diseases, such as neurosyphilis. Patients with schizophrenia treated with antipsychotic agents exhibit relatively delineated, recognized syndromes of abnormal involuntary movement, which are abnormal in their nature and appear unrelated to the normal range of expressive gesture. Although motor problems such as tardive orobuccolingual dyskinesia are generally exacerbated by increased arousal and anxiety, they seem otherwise not to be directly driven by aberrant thought content, affect, or perception.

Epidemiology and Risk Factors

In a review of 56 studies that spanned from 1959 to 1979, Kane and Smith (73) reported point prevalence of TD ranging from 0.5% to 65%, with an average point prevalence of 20%. In a later review of 76 published studies, Yassa and Jeste (74) reported an overall TD prevalence of 24% among a total of 39,187 patients. The clinical significance of these figures is limited as they were derived from studies that differed in assessment criteria, methodology, and population characteristics.

Risk factors for development of TD most consistently defined by various epidemiologic studies include affective disorder, old age, female gender, total cumulative drug exposure, diabetes, alcohol, cocaine intake, persistence of neuroleptic drug use after the development of TD, and a history of electroconvulsive treatment (ECT). Advancing age is the most consistently established risk factor for TD, and there appears to be a linear correlation between age and both the prevalence and severity of TD. A number of studies have indicated a higher risk for women to develop TD (74). There is some evidence that diabetes increases the risk of TD. Woerner et al. (75) reported a risk ratio of 2.3 for diabetics exposed to neuroleptics compared to similarly treated nondiabetics, with the risk greater in aged diabetics. A number of investigators have commented on a higher incidence of TD in patients with affective disorder treated long term with neuroleptics, but this finding is inconsistent.

Clinical Features

Classic tardive dyskinesia manifests as repetitive, coordinated, seemingly purposeful movements affecting mainly the orofacial area. Some prefer to use the term *tardive stereotypy* to describe these movements. True chorea may occur but usually in the setting of withdrawal dyskinesia (see the following).

Many patients with TD exhibit a combination of movement disorders. Most frequently, stereotypy of classic TD is combined with choreic movements of the hands, fingers, arms, and feet or with dystonia. The diaphragm and chest muscles are frequently involved in respiratory dyskinesias, resulting in noisy and difficult breathing. The abdominal and pelvic muscles may also be involved, producing truncal or pelvic movements known as *copulatory dyskinesia*.

Orobuccolingual dyskinesia may occur in other clinical situations (Table 30.4) that should be considered in the differential diagnosis before blaming the DBA.

Withdrawal and Covert Dyskinesias

Sometimes dyskinesias first make their appearance when the DBA is discontinued or the dosage is reduced. This form of dyskinesia has been called *withdrawal or covert*

TABLE 30.4

DIFFERENTIAL DIAGNOSIS OF OROBUCCOLINGUAL DYSKINESIA

1. Spontaneous dyskinesia of elderly (usually dystonic)
2. Hereditary choreas
3. Basal ganglia strokes
4. Systemic lupus erythematosus
5. Edentulous dyskinesia
6. Other drugs causing dyskinesias: levodopa, amphetamines, cocaine, tricyclic antidepressants, cimetidine, flunarizine, antihistamines

---

dyskinesia (76). Withdrawal dyskinesia disappears within 3 months of drug withdrawal, whereas covert dyskinesia becomes apparent upon reduction of neuroleptic therapy and persists for longer periods. This distinction is arbitrary, however, because some of the covert dyskinesias will disappear after prolonged follow-up.

Tardive Tourettism

Tardive tourettism has been recognized as a complication of DBA (77–79). Patients may develop abnormal movements and vocalizations following chronic neuroleptic treatment. Further, the symptoms exhibited by the patients are indistinguishable from those of classic Tourette's syndrome. It is a requirement for the diagnosis of tardive tourettism that these patients had no tics as children. The neuropharmacology underlying tardive tourettism parallels that of TD and idiopathic Tourette's syndrome (80).

Tardive Myoclonus

Tardive myoclonus has been described as a late complication of prolonged neuroleptic therapy (81). Usually it is a postural myoclonus of the upper extremities, and associated movement disorders are common. Clonazepam pharmacotherapy ameliorates tardive myoclonus.

Tardive Tremor

Tardive tremor has only rarely been reported (82). It is said to be more of a postural and kinetic tremor, as compared to a resting tremor in DIP, and it is not usually associated with other signs of parkinsonism. Also, this tremor seems to respond to tetrabenazine, which suggests it is more related to tardive dyskinesia than to DIP. Tardive tremor is a rare complication, and more patients must be characterized before the phenomenon can be completely described.

Tardive Dystonia

Burke et al. reported a large series of 42 patients with tardive dystonia seen in 3 movement disorders centers in 1982 (83); however, scattered reports have existed since l962 (84). This variant of tardive dyskinesia is not uncommon, and in a study of veterans on chronic neuroleptic therapy, we found mild dystonic manifestations in 27 out of 125 patients (85). These most commonly involved the hands and the jaw. This is a prevalence of nearly 20%, approximately 10 times higher than a previous study on this subject (86). Recent studies have found an intermediate prevalence of about 9%–13% (87).

The reasons to differentiate classic tardive dyskinesia from tardive dystonia have been discussed by Kang et al. (88) and are as follows: The abnormal movements are distinct from classic tardive dyskinesia. Whereas tardive dyskinesia seems to occur more commonly in elderly women, tardive dystonia seems to be more common in younger patients showing no predilection for either sex. Moreover, anticholinergic drugs tend to worsen classic tardive dyskinesia but are beneficial in tardive dystonia. Tardive dystonia is said to be more persistent than classic tardive dyskinesia, but in our experience there is a significant incidence of remissions if the offending drug can be withdrawn. It should be noted that tardive dystonia may occur after a short exposure to neuroleptics, and in one large series at least 25% of patients were given neuroleptics for disorders other than psychosis (89).

The dystonic movements of patients with tardive dystonia are indistinguishable from those of idiopathic torsion dystonia. In contrast to idiopathic dystonia, however, other types of involuntary movements, such as orobuccolingual dyskinesia, may coexist. In general, the presence of multiple movement disorders in a patient should alert the physician to the possibility of a drug-induced movement disorder. The dystonia may be focal, segmental, and rarely generalized (88–90). In most patients, tardive dystonia is focal at onset, but, when fully developed, many patients have developed segmental dystonia (88–90) by the time of presentation. When the neck is involved, retrocollis is typical, and when the trunk is involved, truncal extension is the predominant abnormal posture. Rarely, truncal flexion may be seen. Lateral flexion of the trunk or the Pisa syndrome can occur in tardive dystonia and less commonly in idiopathic dystonia (91).

A rare variant is a *reverse obstructive sleep apnea syndrome* (92). These patients are completely obstructed during the day, but as soon as they sleep the tardive dystonia disappears and they sleep normally. This is the polar opposite of obstructive sleep apnea syndrome, where sleep actually brings on the abnormal breathing pattern. This could be life threatening, and one of our patients required tracheostomy; however, botulinum toxin treatment may obviate the need for such an invasive procedure. Another uncommon variant is recurrent oculogyric crises accompanied by obsessional thoughts and hallucinations (93).

When tardive dystonia appears in the setting of neuroleptic therapy, one should rule out other causes, such as Wilson's disease and symptomatic dystonia due to focal lesions in the basal ganglia. Obtaining a good family history is important to rule out inherited dystonias. *DYT1* gene mutations are not found in patients with tardive dystonia (94).

An earlier mean age of onset has been reported for tardive dystonia (mean 36 years) compared with classic TD (mean 61 years) (95). Children exposed to DBA are more likely to get tardive dystonia, and as children age they are less likely to develop generalized dystonia (83). Male predominance also has been a consistent finding in most studies (M:F ratio about 2:1).

Tardive Akathisia

Persistent akathisia may occur as a subtype of tardive dyskinesia, unlike acute akathisia, which is apparent shortly after starting DBA. Persistant akathisia is defined as being present for at least 1 month when the patient is on a constant dose of a DBA (96). If one considers both subjective and objective criteria to define akathisia, it is apparent the tardive akathisia (TA) is actually quite common. It occurs in about 20%–40% of DBA-treated schizophrenics (97). No case-control studies have been done to see if akathisia is more prevalent in neuroleptic-treated schizophrenics. However, other than restless leg syndrome and DIP, persistant akathisia is uncommon, and it appears that neuroleptics have a role to play in the genesis of TA.

As in classic TD, several types of TA have been described (i.e., covert and withdrawal akathisia) (98,99). In one report, the mean age of patients with TA was 58 years and women outnumbered men by 2 to 1 (96). Almost all classes of DBA have been responsible.

The time of onset of TA is difficult to establish retrospectively. In one study, the duration of neuroleptic treatment prior to the onset of TA ranged from 2 weeks to 22 years, with a mean 4.5 years (96). TA in this clinic population occurred in the first year of exposure in 15 of 45 patients. In another report (26), 12 of 23 chronic akathisia patients had an acute onset, with akathisia persisting for 7 months to 11 years. The remaining had an onset at withdrawal of the DBA.

The subjective experience of distress may be less in TA, but a longitudinal study to support this is lacking. Behavioral features seen in acute akathisia, such as an exacerbation of psychosis or aggressive/suicidal behavior, have not been described with TA. The motor phenomena of TA also are similar to those of acute akathisia, except many patients with TA tend to pump their legs up and down or abduct/adduct them in a stereotyped manner while sitting. TA patients also commonly exhibit truncal movements (rocking back and forth, or shifting while sitting) and respiratory irregularities (including panting, grunting, moaning, or even shouting). Since many TA patients also have TD, it is often difficult to be certain whether some of the movements described in TA are in fact part of TD. TA is commonly associated with TD or tardive dystonia. Barnes and Braude (26) reported a moderate to severe orofacial dyskinesia in 39% and choreoathetoid limb movements in 56% of their TA patients.

Pathophysiology of Tardive Dyskinesia

The pathophysiology of TD is poorly understood. The major antipsychotic activity of DBAs appears to be their inhibition of ventral tegmental dopaminergic projections to the mesolimbic/mesocortical areas. Likewise, the extrapyramidal side effects of DBAs appear to be from blockade of dopamine receptors in the striatum (100). However, TD is a paradoxical phenomenon distinct from DIP. Intuitively, TD, like chorea, would appear to be a manifestation of excessive dopaminergic activity in the basal ganglia (BG). There are several lines of clinical evidence to support a relative dopaminergic excess. First, reduction of DBA dose often can precipitate TD (withdrawal emergent syndrome or covert dyskinesia). Likewise, increasing the DBA dose can temporarily mask TD symptoms. Secondly, dyskinesias induced by levodopa in PD patients may closely resemble the movements seen in TD.

Animal studies have shown that DBA use results acutely in increased turnover of dopamine (100). This increased turnover may be stimulated by feedback mechanisms set off by postsynaptic blockade of dopamine receptors. This increased turnover, however, attenuates on chronic use. Furthermore, chronic dopamine blockade may precipitate dopamine receptor hypersensitivity by causing chemical denervation (101). TD is thought to result from an increased number and affinity of postsynaptic D2 dopamine receptors (102). This is based on the rodent models of TD where after 2 weeks of therapy with a conventional DBA, there is increased affinity and numbers of D2 dopamine receptors (103). This is a universal effect in animals; however, TD occurs in only about 20% of the human patients exposed to the DBA. Moreover, the role of other neurotransmitters, such as GABA and norepinephrine, may be important (104). Excitatory neurotransmission may play a role given that N-methyl-D-aspartate (NMDA) receptor–blocking agents reduce chewing movements in a rodent TD model (105).

Human studies investigating the mechanism of TD have been limited. In one human postmortem study of patients with TD who were neuroleptic free for 1 year prior to death, the dopamine D2 receptor density was diminished in the striatum but increased in the pallidum (106). A PET study using N-11c-methyl-spiperone failed to show a difference in D2 receptor density in patients with or without TD (107). Recently, however, another study found that D2 receptor density was increased in patients exposed both to typical and atypical antipsychotics (108). A PET study using 18F-fluorodeoxyglucose (FDG) uptake showed that the metabolic rates were increased in the motor cortex and the globus pallidus, suggesting overactivity of these regions (109).

An attempt has been made to study genetic polymorphisms for an association with TD in various ethnic populations. The Ser9Gly variant in the Msc I restriction site of the dopamine D3 receptor gene was reported to be associated with TD (110,111); however, others have failed to find such an association (112).

Cerebrospinal fluid (CSF) markers of oxidative stress were investigated in one study. TD patients had significantly higher concentrations of N-acetylaspartate, N-acetylaspartylglutamate, and aspartate in their CSF than did patients without TD when controlling for age and neuroleptic dose (113). TD symptoms correlated positively with markers of excitatory neurotransmission and protein carbonyl groups and negatively with CSF superoxide dismutase activity.

Thus, the role of dopamine receptor supersensitivity in the development of TD has not been conclusively established. Ideally, a model for TD would explain why only a minority of patients treated with DBA develop TD, why the onset requires long-term exposure, and why the movement disorder persists in many cases, even when the DBA is withdrawn.

Recently, research has focused on the idea that GABAergic changes occur in the BG of subjects exposed to chronic DBA, leading to an imbalance in BG output. In this scenario, the activity of the indirect pathway would be diminished in relation to the direct pathway, a possible explanation for the origin of this hyperkinetic disorder. Currently, it is thought that a complex interaction between dopaminergic, cholinergic, GABAergic, and glutamatergic systems may be important in the development of TD (101).

Neuroleptic Malignant Syndrome

This is perhaps the most severe reaction to DBA. A similar condition, known as *lethal catatonia*, was described in untreated psychiatric patients in the 19th century (114). According to the American Psychiatric Association, the diagnostic criteria include severe rigidity and fever along with 2 of 10 minor features, which include tremor, diaphoresis, altered mentation, dysphagia, incontinence, tachycardia, mutism, labile or elevated blood pressure, leukocytosis, and elevated creatinine phosphokinase (115). In a study conducted by Kurlan et al. (116), it was determined that most patients presumed to have this syndrome had a constellation of symptoms including fever, autonomic dysfunction, and a movement disorder. In another review it was found that 92% of 115 patients with a diagnosis of neuroleptic malignant syndrome (NMS) had temperatures above 100.4°F and 91% showed signs of rigidity (116).

Parkinsonism hyperpyrexia syndrome may occur in patients with PD where dopaminergic drugs are suddenly withdrawn (117). Tetrabenazine, a dopamine-depleting drug, may also cause an NMS-like syndrome (118).

Fortunately, NMS occurs in only about 0.1%–1.8% of patients exposed to DBA (119,120). NMS typically occurs 3 to 9 days following DBA administration (121), but it can occur acutely or even years after initiating DBA. NMS also appears to favor young adults and men compared to women in a 1.5–2:1 ratio. The presentation is usually subacute (24–72 hours), but it can occur precipitously over hours. NMS typically lasts 10 to 13 days when caused by oral neuroleptics and twice as long when depot agents are employed (122).

It is believed that a patient who has previously had NMS is at a higher risk of recurrence when reexposed to DBA. In one study involving 54 patients, it was found that 37% (20/54) had recurrent NMS after reexposure, but the authors did not mention which neuroleptics were involved (122). In another study, only 2 of 15 patients with a prior episode of NMS developed NMS again when rechallenged with various neuroleptics (123).

Mortality from NMS ranges from 4% to 22% (124). Death is often secondary to renal failure or pneumonia. Early recognition of a premalignant syndrome and withdrawal of DBA are of crucial importance.

Management of Tardive Syndromes

Orobuccolingual Dyskinesia

TD is, by definition, iatrogenic. Preventing development of TD is one of the most important principles in the utilization of DBA for psychiatric disease, and DBA should not be prescribed for anxiety and other neuroses. The only accepted indication for chronic DBA therapy is chronic schizophrenia. The need for DBA therapy should be reviewed periodically, even in patients showing no signs of TD. Some patients with acute psychosis may not require high levels of DBA that were prescribed initially. Every 3 to 6 months patients should be examined for early signs of TD. If signs are present, switching to clozapine or another atypical neuroleptic may prevent TD.

A variety of drugs have been used in the symptomatic treatment of TD, but none is uniformly effective. The most important step is, if possible, to stop the DBA. The mainstay of treatment is dopamine-depleting agents such as reserpine or tetrabenazine. The usual dose of reserpine is 0.25 mg/day, and the dose is increased gradually to 3–5 mg/day. Tetrabenazine is initiated at 25 mg/day and gradually increased to 150 mg/day (125,126). Another useful agent is α-methyl-p-tyrosine, which forms a false neurotransmitter. It has been employed alone or with reserpine (127). In general, anticholinergic drugs exacerbate orobuccolingual TD and should be discontinued (128). A number of cholinergic drugs, such as muscimol, have been used with variable results (129). Some patients with TD have been treated with low doses of bromocriptine (130). Baclofen has been used because of its GABA-agonist properties with some success (131). Clonazepam may be useful in some cases (132). Calcium channel blockers have produced varying results, with nifedipine and verapamil demonstrating efficacy (133) and diltiazem being ineffective (134). There has been a lot of interest in

vitamin E, but at best it produces a modest response (135,136) or may be ineffective (137). Risperidone was reported to improve TD in one retrospective review (138), but it may be associated with TD (139) and DIP. Clozapine has been used in patients with TD and tardive dystonia (see the following).

Tardive Toutrettism, Myoclonus, and Tremor

In general, the strategies to manage these variants closely resemble those for classic TD. Whenever possible, DBA should be withdrawn and dopamine-depleting drugs employed.

Tardive Dystonia

Tardive dystonia presents special challenges. The movement disorder is more severe and often more persistent than the other tardive syndromes. If the dystonia is focal (or segmental) botulinum toxin injections may be the most effective symptomatic treatment, particularly for craniocervical dystonia. Tarsy et al. reported moderate to marked improvement in 29 of 38 affected body parts injected with botulinum toxin in 34 patients with tardive dystonia, all of whom had an incomplete response to a variety of drugs (140).

For generalized dystonia, a number of drugs are available for symptomatic treatment. Drug response is variable, and often must switch between various agents or employ two or more drugs to help intractable dystonia (141). Whereas classic TD is often made worse by anticholinergic drugs, tardive dystonia is often ameliorated by them (88). Other medications commonly used are tetrabenazine, benzodiazepines, and baclofen. Less commonly used drugs are levodopa, amantadine, beta-blockers, and anticonvulsants. We try an anticholinergic (such as trihexyphenidyl) first and gradually increase the dose as tolerated. Next, tetrabenazine or reserpine is added to anticholinergic drugs. Oral baclofen in increasing doses can be helpful. Intrathecal baclofen for axial (truncal) dystonia can be very useful but may be tricky for long-term use due to pump or delivery problems and risk of infection (141).

Atypical Neuroleptics in the Treatment of Tardive Syndromes

Atypical neuroleptics are associated with a lower rate of TD than typical neuroleptics. Examples of atypical neuroleptics include clozapine, quetiapine, and, to a lesser degree, olanzapine. The reasons for atypicality are not clear. In general, these drugs have a lower affinity for the D2 receptor and have a high affinity for histamine, dopamine, and serotonin receptors (142). A high ratio between serotonin ($5HT_2$) and D2 dopamine receptor antagonism will produces less in the way of extrapyramidal effects, including TD (56). Also, the rapid dissociation of the drug from the receptor may have a role to play in reducing motor side effects (57).

Clozapine, a dibenzodiazepine, is an atypical neuroleptic that is currently approved for the treatment of neuroleptic-resistant schizophrenia (143). It has an extremely low propensity to cause extrapyramidal side effects. In fact, no convincing cases of TD secondary to clozapine have been reported. Several uncontrolled observations have suggested that clozapine benefits about 40% of patients with TD, particularly those with tardive dystonia (144,145). Long-term open-label follow-up of TD in a limited number of patients is available (146). It usually takes doses in the range of 500–900 mg/day, and the improvement may occur within days or may take months. The mechanism of this beneficial effect is unclear. Clozapine may have a passive effect by removal of the offending agent, allowing the underlying pathophysiological processes to reverse. It may only suppress TD like other neuroleptics; however, this appears unlikely as there is a delay in the improvement. Lastly, it may possess a specific antidyskinetic action. Clozapine has been reported to induce NMS and may cause positive and negative myoclonus (147–149). Other agents, such as olanzapine, have been studied in a limited fashion and may be effective in this setting (150,151).

Tardive Akathisia

Tardive akathisia does not consistently respond to any pharmacologic therapy, and patients afflicted with this syndrome often express symptoms of distress, violence, and even suicidal ideation. Burke et al., however, found that 87% of patients showed some improvement with reserpine and 58% with tetrabenazine (96). They reported complete resolution of symptoms in one-third of patients. Opioids and beta-blockers that help acute akathisia usually do not ameliorate tardive akathisia.

Neuroleptic Malignant Syndrome

This is a medical emergency, and patients with NMS should be admitted to the ICU and monitored closely. Supportive measures include intravenous fluids and control of elevated body temperature. Traditionally, dantrolene (152) or bromocriptine (153) alone, or in combination, have been used (154). Another alternative is electroconvulsive therapy (155). Some have raised doubts about the efficacy of drugs in the treatment of NMS. One review stated that the course of NMS was actually prolonged by the use of dantrolene and bromocriptine, as compared to supportive therapy alone (156).

Despite the uncertainty, most would agree that in addition to supportive measures, NMS should be treated initially with dopamine agonists. The drug most frequently used has been bromocriptine (at doses of 5–15 mg 3 times a day), but other dopaminergic drugs may be effective (157,158).

Clinical Course of Tardive Syndromes

TD was thought to be persistent in most cases, but several studies have shown that up to 40% of patients improve upon cessation of neuroleptic therapy (159). This is more likely to occur in younger patients and in patients with a shorter history of TD. If typical DBAs are continued, it is unlikely that TD will remit. The subtype of TD also may be important. Tardive dystonia is a rather persistent disorder, and remissions are relatively infrequent. The remission rate of tardive dystonia was low at 10% (21 of 231 patients) after a mean follow-up period of 6.6 years (83,88). These studies are from tertiary care centers, however, and it is possible that more cases of tardive dystonia remit than is generally realized.

MOVEMENT DISORDERS CAUSED BY OTHER DRUGS

A variety of other drugs produce movement disorders. When movement disorders are due to drugs that are not commonly perceived as causative agents, the diagnosis may be missed for extended periods of time, resulting in unnecessary diagnostic workup and inappropriate therapy. The diagnosis depends on a compulsive drug history not only from the patient but also from the patient's family, primary physician, and pharmacist. In general, the non–DBA-induced movement disorders remit upon discontinuation of the offending agent. Although drug-induced movement disorders can occur in previously "healthy" patients, patients with abnormal development or brain injury are more disposed to develop movements related to these drugs.

Given limited space, we have chosen to list the major drugs that can cause or exacerbate akathisia, chorea, myoclonus, restless legs syndrome, tics, and tremor in tabular form in Tables 30.5 through 30.10.

TABLE 30.5

DRUGS THAT MAY CAUSE OR EXACERBATE AKATHISIA

Antiepileptics: carbamazapine, ethosuximide
Buspirone
Calcium Channel Antagonists: diltiazem
Dopamine Antagonists/Depletors
Lithium
Methysergide
Selective Serotonin Reuptake Inhibitors (SSRIs)
Tricyclic Antidepressants (TCAs)
Vestibular sedatives: flunarizine, cinnarizine

Adapted from Sachdev PS. Acute and tardive drug-induced akathisia. In: Sethi KD, ed. *Drug-Induced Movement Disorders*. New York: Marcel Dekker; 2004:129–164.

TABLE 30.6

DRUGS THAT MAY CAUSE OR EXACERBATE CHOREA

Anticholinergics
Antidepressants: selective serotonin reuptake inhibitors (SSRIs), tricyclic antidepressants
Antiepileptics: carbamazepine, gabapentin, phenytoin, valproate
Antihistamines
Dopamine Antagonists
Dopaminergic Drugs: dopamine agonists, levodopa
Hormones: thyroid hormone, estrogen
Lithium
Stimulants: amphetamines, cocaine, methylpenidate
Miscellaneous: aminophylline, baclofen, cimetidine, digoxin

Adapted from Bhidayasiri R, Truong DD. Chorea and related disorders. *Postgrad Med J* 2004;80:527–534.

TABLE 30.8

DRUGS THAT MAY EXACERBATE RESTLESS LEGS SYNDROME

Antiepileptics: phenytoin
Antihistamines
β-Adrenergic Antagonists
Caffeine
Calcium Channel Antagonists
Dopamine Antagonists
Dopamine Depleters
Ethanol
Lithium
Selective Serotonin Reuptake Inhibitors (SSRIs)
Tricyclic antidepressants

Adapted from Chaudhuri KR, Forbes A, Grosset D, et al. Diagnosing restless legs syndrome (RLS) in primary care. *Curr Med Res Opin* 2004;20:1785–1795.

TABLE 30.7

DRUGS THAT MAY CAUSE OR EXACERBATE MYOCLONUS

Anesthetics: chloralose, etomidate, enflurane, propofol, spinal anesthetics
Antibiotics/Antimalarials: cephalosporins, fluoroquinolones, imipenem, mefloquine, penicillins
Antiepileptics: carbamazepine, gabapentin, lamotrigine, phenytoin, valproate, vigabatrin
Antidepressants: MAO inhibitors, selective serotonin reuptake inhibitors (SSRIs), tricyclics
Antineoplastic Drugs: chlorambucil, ifosfamide
Calcium Channel Antagonists: diltiazem, nifedipine, verapamil
Contrast Agents
    Dopaminergics: levodopa, dopamine agonists and antagonists
    Drugs of Abuse: MDMA (Ecstasy)
Gastrointestinal Drugs: bismuth salts
Narcotics: methadone, meperidine, morphine, oxycodone
Other Drugs: γ-hydroxybutyrate, tranexamic acid

Adapted from (1) Gordon MF. Toxin and drug-induced myoclonus. *Adv Neurol* 2002;89:49–76. (2) Lang AE. Miscellaneous drug-induced movement disorders. In: Lang AE, Weiner WJ, eds. *Drug-induced movement disorders.* New York: Futura Publishing, 1992:339–381. (3) Klawans HL, Carvey PM, Tanner CM, Goetz CG. Drug-induced myoclonus. In: Fahn S, Marsden CD, Van Woert MH, eds. *Myoclonus.* New York: Raven Press; 1986:251–264.

TABLE 30.9

DRUGS THAT MAY EXACERBATE OR CAUSE TICS

Antiepileptics: carbamazepine, lamotrigine
Drugs of Abuse: amphetamines, cocaine, heroin
Levodopa
Selective Serotonin Reuptake Inhibitors (SSRIs): fluoxetine, sertraline
Stimulants (controversial): methylphenidate

Adapted from (1) Kellett MW, Chadwick DW. Antiepileptic drug-induced movement disorders. In: Sethi KD, ed. *Drug-induced movement disorders.* New York: Marcel Dekker, 2004:309–356. (2) Sanchez-Ramos J. Stimulant-induced movement disorders. In: Sethi KD, ed. *Drug-induced movement disorders.* New York: Marcel Dekker, 2004:295–308. (3) Bharucha KJ, Sethi KD. Movement disorders induced by selective serotonin reuptake inhibitors and other antidepressants. In: Sethi KD, ed. *Drug-induced movement disorders.* New York: Marcel Dekker, 2004:233–257. (4) Tourette's Syndrome Study Group. Treatment of ADHD in children with tics: a randomized controlled trial. *Neurology* 2002;58:527–536.

TABLE 30.10
NON-NEUROLEPTIC DRUGS ASSOCIATED WITH TREMOR

Postural

Major Category	Typical Examples
Antiarrhythmics	amiodarone, mexiletine, procainamide
Antidepressants/Mood Stabilizers	amitriptyline, lithium, selective serotonin reuptake inhibitors (SSRIs)
Antiepileptics	valproate
Bronchodilators	albuterol, salmeterol
Chemotherapeutics	tamoxifen, Ara-C, ifosfamide
Drugs of Abuse	cocaine, ethanol, MDMA, nicotine
Gastrointestinal Drugs	metoclopramide, cimetidine
Hormones	thyroxine, calcitonin, medroxyprogesterone
Immunosuppressants	tacrolimus, cyclosporine, α-interferon
Methylxanthines	theophylline, caffeine

Intention

Major Category	Typical Examples
Antibiotics/Antivirals/Antifungals	Ara-A
Antidepressants/Mood Stabilizers	lithium
Bronchodilators	Albuterol, salmeterol
Chemotherapeutics	Ara-C, ifosfamide
Drugs of Abuse	ethanol
Hormones	epinephrine
Immunosuppressants	tacrolimus, cyclosporine

Resting

Major Category	Typical Examples
Antibiotics, Antivirals, Antifungals	trimethoprim/sulfa, amphotericin B
Antidepressants, Mood Stabilizers	selective serotonin reuptake inhibitors (SSRIs), lithium
Antiepileptics	valproate
Chemotherapeutics	thalidomide
Drugs of Abuse	cocaine, ethanol, MDMA
Gastrointestinal Drugs	metoclopramide
Hormones	medroxyprogesterone

Adapted from Morgan JC, Sethi KD. Drug- and toxin-induced tremor. In: Lyons KE, Pahwa R, eds. *Handbook of essential tremor and other tremor disorders.* London: Taylor & Francis, 2005:329–360.

REFERENCES

1. Delay J, Deniker P. Chlorpromazine and neuroleptic treatment in psychiatry. *J Clin & Exper Psychopath* 1956;17:19–24.
2. Uhrbrand L, Faurbye A. Reversible and irreversible dyskinesia after treatment with perphenazine, chlorpromazine, reserpine and electroconvulsive therapy. *Psychopharm* 1960;1:408–418.
3. Keepers GA, Clappison VJ, & Casey DE. Initial anticholinergic prophylaxis for neuroleptic-induced extrapyramidal syndromes. *Arch Gen Psychiatry* 1983;40:492–496.
4. Raja M Azzoni A. Novel antipsychotics and acute dystonic reactions. *Pharmacol Biochem Behav* 2000;67:497–500.
5. Flaherty JA, Lahmeyer HW. Laryngeal-pharyngeal dystonia as a possible cause of asphyxia with haloperidol treatment. *Am J Psychiatry* 1978;135:1414–1415.
6. Suzuki T, Koizumi J, Moroji T, Sakuma K, Hori M, Hori T. Clinical characteristics of the Pisa syndrome. *Acta Psych Scandinavica* 1990;82:454–457.
7. Suzuki T, Matsuzaka H. Drug-induced Pisa syndrome (pleurothotonus): epidemiology and management. *CNS Drugs* 2002;16:165–174.
8. Sachdev P. Tardive and chronically recurrent oculogyric crises. *Mov Disord* 1993;8:93–97.
9. Ayd FJ Jr. A survey of drug-induced extrapyramidal reactions. *J Am Med Assoc* 1961;175:1054–1060.
10. Chiles JA. Extrapyramidal reactions in adolescents treated with high-potency antipsychotics. *Am J Psychiatry* 1978;135:239–240.
11. Ayers JL, Dawson KP. Acute dystonic reactions in childhood to drugs. *N Z Med J.* 1980;92:464–465.
12. Priori A, Bertolasi L, Berardelli A, Manfredi M. Predictors of acute dystonia in first-episode psychotic patients. *Am J Psychiatry* 1994;151:1819–1821.
13. Van Harten PN, Trier Van JC, Horwitz EH, Matroos GE, Hoek HW. Cocaine as a risk factor for neurolepic-induced acute dystonia. *Am J Psychiatry* 1986;143:706–710.
14. Kleij Der Van FG, Vries De PA, Stassen PM, Sprenger HG, Gans RO. Acute dystonia due to metoclopramide: increased risk in AIDS. *Arch Intern Med.* 2002;162:358–359.
15. Neale R, Gerhardt S, Liebman JM. Effects of dopamine agonists, catecholamine depletors, and cholinergic and GABAergic drugs on acute dyskinesia in the squirrel monkeys. *Psychopharm* 1984;82:20–26.

16. Klintenberg R, Gunne L, Andren PE. Tardive dyskinesia model in the common marmoset. *Mov Disord* 2002;17:360–365.
17. Marsden CD, Jenner P. The pathophysiology of extrapyramidal side effects of neuroleptic drugs. *Psychol Med* 1980;10:55–72.
18. Matsumoto RR, Hemstreet MK, Lai NL, et al. Drug specificity of pharmacological dystonia. *Pharmacol Biochem Behav* 1990;36:151–155.
19. Keepers GA, Casey DE. Clinical management of acute neuroleptic-induced extrapyramidal syndromes. In: Masserman JH, ed. *Current psychiatric therapies*, New York: Grune & Stratton, 1986:139–157.
20. Waugh W H, Metts JC. Severe extrapyramidal motor activity induced by prochlorperazine: its relief by the intravenous injection of diphenhydramine. *N Engl J Med* 1960;262:353–354.
21. Piecuch S, Thomas U, Shah BR. Acute dystonic reactions that fail to respond to diphenhydramine: think of PCP. *J Emerg Med* 1999;17:527.
22. Haskovec L, *Akathisie. Arch Bohemes Med Clin* 1902;17:704–708.
23. Healy D, Farquhar G. Immediate effects of droperidol. *Human Psychopharmacol* 1998;13:113–120.
24. Braude WM, Barnes TR, Gore SM. Clinical characteristics of akathisia: a systematic investigation of acute psychiatric inpatient admissions. *Br J Psychiatry* 1983;143:139–150.
25. Sachdev P, Kruk J. Clinical characteristics and risk factors for acute neuroleptic-induced akathisia. *Arch Gen Psychiatry* 1994;51:963–974.
26. Barnes TR, Braude WM. Akathisia variants and tardive dyskinesia. *Arch Gen Psychiatry* 1985;42:874–878.
27. Pierre JM. Extrapyramidal symptoms with atypical antipsychotics: incidence, prevention and management. *Drug Saf* 2005;28:191–208.
28. Sandoz Pharmaceutical Corporation. *Hospital pharmacist's guide to the clozaril patient management system*. East Rutherford, NJ: Sandoz, 1991.
29. Nordstrom AL, Farde L, Halldin C. Time course of D2-dopamine receptor occupancy examined by PET after single oral doses of haloperidol. *Psychopharmacology Berl* 1992;106:433–438.
30. Farde L, Nordstrom A, Weisel F, et al. Positron emission tomographic analysis of central D1 and D2 dopamine receptor occupancy in patients treated with classical neuroleptics and clozapine. *Arch Gen Psychiatry* 1992;49:539–544.
31. Lima AR, Bacalcthuk J, Barnes TR, Soares-Weiser K. Central action beta-blockers versus placebo for neuroleptic-induced acute akathisia. *Cochrane Database Syst Rev* 2004;4:CD001946.
32. Lima AR, Weiser KV, Bacaltchuk J, Barnes TR. Anticholinergics for neuroleptic-induced acute akathisia. *Cochrane Database Syst Rev* 2004;1:CD003727.
33. Miller CH, Hummer M, Pycha R, et al. The effect of ritanserin on treatment-resistant neuroleptic induced akathisia: case reports. *Prog Neuropsychopharmacol Biol Psychiatry* 1992;16:247–251.
34. Sethi KD, Patel B, Meador KJ. Metoclopramide-induced parkinsonism. *South Med J* 1989;82:1581–1582.
35. Stephen PJ, Williams J. Drug-induced parkinsonism in the elderly. *Lancet* 1984;2:1082–1083.
36. Masso JF, Poza JJ. Druginduced or aggravated parkinsonism: clinical signs and the changing pattern of implicated drugs. *Neurologia.* 1996;11:10–15.
37. Mutch WJ, Dingwall-Fordyce I, Downie AW, et al. Parkinson's disease in a Scottish city. *Br Med J* 1986;292:534–536.
38. Caligiuri MP, Lacro JP, Jeste DP. Incidence and predictors of drug-induced parkinsonism in older psychiatric patients treated with very low doses of neuroloeptics. *J Clin Pharmacol* 1999;19:322–328.
39. Korczyn AD, Goldberg GJ. Extrapyramidal effects of neuroleptics. *J Neurol Neurosurg Psychiatry* 1976;39:866–869.
40. Myrianthopoulos NC, Waldrop FN, Vincent BL. A repeat study of hereditary predisposition in drug-induced parkinsonism. In: Barbeau A, Brunette JR, eds. *Progress in neurogenetics.* Amsterdam: Excerpta Medica International Congress Series, 1969:486–491.
41. Gartmann J, Hartmann K, Kuhn M. Sanz-Streitlicht Nr 14. *Schweiz Arzt Zeitung* 1993;29:1163–1164.
42. Sethi KD, Zamrini EY. Asymmetry in clinical features of drug-induced parkinsonism. *J Neuropsych Clin Neurosci* 1990;2:64–66.
43. Hardie RJ, Lees AJ. Neuroleptic-induced Parkinson's syndrome: clinical features and results of treatment with levodopa. *J Neurol Neurosurg Psychiatry* 1988;8:850–854.
44. Giladi N, Kao R, Fahn S. Freezing phenomenon in patients with parkinsonian syndromes. *Mov Disord* 1997;12:302–305.
45. Casey DE. Neuroleptic-induced acute extrapyramidal syndromes and tardive dyskinesia. *Psychiatr Clin North Am* 1993;16:589–610.
46. Marsden CD, Tarsy D, Baldessarani RJ. Spontaneous and drug-induced movement disorders. In: Benson DF, Blumer D, eds. *Psychiatric aspects of neurologic disease.* New York: Grune and Straton, 1975.
47. Villeneuve A. The rabbit syndrome: a peculiar extrapyramidal reaction. *Canadian Psychiatr Assoc J*1972;17:69–72.
48. Casey DE. The rabbit syndrome. In: Joseph AB, Young R, eds. *Disorders of movement in psychiatry and neurology.* Cambridge: Blackwell, 1992:139–142.
49. Klawans HL, Bergan D, Bruyn GW. Prolonged drug-induced parkinsonism. *Confin Neurol-* 1973;35:368–377.
50. Hansen TE, Brown WL, Weigel RM, et al. Underrecognition of tardive dyskinesia and drug-induced parkinsonism by psychiatric residents. *Gen Hosp Psychiatry* 1992;14:340–344.
51. Miller LG, Jankovic J. Metoclopramide-induced movement disorders. *Arch Intern Med* 1989;149:2486–2492.
52. Marti-Masso JF, Poza JJ. Cinnarizine-induced parkinsonism: ten years later. *Mov Disord* 1998;13:453–456.
53. Micheli FE, Pardal MM, Giannaula R, et al. Movement disorders and depression due to flunarizine and cinnarizine. *Mov Disord* 1989;4:139–146.
54. Negrotti A, Calzetti S. A long-term follow-up study of cinnarizine- and flunarizine-induced parkinsonism. *Mov Disord* 1997; 12:107–110.
55. Farde L, Wiessel FA, Halldin C, Sedvall G. Central D2 dopamine receptor occupancy in schizophrenic patients treated with antipsychotic drugs. *Arch Gen Psychiatry* 1988;45:71–76.
56. Meltzer HY, Matsubara S, Lee JC. Classification of typical and atypical antipsychotic drugs on the basis of dopamine D-1, D-2 and serotonin pKi values. *Pharmacol Exp Ther* 1989;251:238–246.
57. Kapur S, Seeman P. Does fast dissociation from the dopamine d(2) receptor explain the action of atypical antipsychotics? a new hypothesis. *Am J Psychiatry* 2001;158:360–369.
58. Eichelbaum M, Kroemer HK, Mikus G. Genetically determined differences in drug metabolism as a risk factor in drug toxicity. *Toxicol Lett* 1992;64:115–122.
59. Negrotti A, Calzetti S, Sasso E. Calcium-entry blockers-induced parkinsonism: possible role of inherited susceptibility. *Neurotoxicology* 1992;13:261–264.
60. Forno LS. Concentric hyaline intraneuronal inclusions of Lewy type in brains of elderly persons (50 incidental cases): relationship to parkinsonism, *J Am Geriatr Soc* 1969;17:557–575.
61. Goetz CG. Drug-induced parkinsonism and idiopathic Parkinson's disease. *Arch Neurol* 1983;40:325–326.
62. Rajput AH, Rozdilsky B, Hornykiewikcz O, Shannak K, et al. Reversible drug-induced parkinsonism: clinicopathologic study of two cases. *Arch Neurol* 1982;39:644–646.
63. Chabolla DR, Maraganore DM, Ahlskog JE, et al. Drug-induced parkinsonism as a risk factor for Parkinson's disease: a historical cohort study in Olmstead County, Minnesota. *Mayo Clin Proc* 1998;73:724–727.
64. Burn DJ, Brooks DJ. Nigral dysfunction in drug-induced parkinsonism: an [18]Fluorodopa PET study. *Neurology* 1993;43:552–556.
65. Booij J, Speelman JD, Horstink MW, Wolters EC. The clinical benefit of imaging striatal dopamine receptors with (^{123}I)FP-CIT SPECT in differentiating patients with presynaptic parkinsonism from those with other forms of parkinsonism. *Eur J Nucl Med* 2001;28:266–272.
66. Tolosa E, Coelho M, Gallardo M. DAT imaging in drug-induced and psychogenic parkinsonism. *Mov Disord* 2003;18(suppl 7): S28–S33.
67. Kelly JT, Zimmerman RL, Abuzzahab FS, Schiele BC. A double-blind study of amantidine hydrochloride versus benztropine mesylate in drug induced parkinsonism. *Pharmacology* 1974;12:65–73.
68. Fann WE, Lake CR. Amantidine versus trihexiphenidyl in the treatment of neuroleptic-induced parkinsonism. *Am J Psychiatry* 1976;133:940–943.
69. Shoulson I. Carbidopa/levodopa therapy of coexistent drug-induced parkinsonism and tardive dyskinesia. *Adv Neurol* 1983;37:259–265.

70. Baldessarini RJ, Cole JO, Davis JM, et al. Tardive dyskinesia: summary of a Task Force Report of the American Psychiatric Association. *Am J Psychiatry* 1980;137:1163–1172.

71. Jeste DV, Lacro JP, Palmer B, Rockwell E, Harris J, Calguri MP. Incidence of tardive dyskinesia in early stages of low-dose treatment with typical neuroleptics in older patients. *Am J Psychiatry* 1999;156:309–311.

72. Marsden CD. Is tardive dyskinesia a unique disorder? In: Casey DE, Chase TN, Christensen AV, Gerlach J, eds. *Dyskinesia: research and treatment*. Berlin: Springer-Verlag, 1985:64–71.

73. Kane JM, Smith J. Tardive dyskinesia: prevalence of risk factors, 1959–1979. *Arch Gen Psychiatry* 1982;39: 486–487.

74. Yassa R, Jeste DV. Gender differences in tardive dyskinesia: a critical review of the literature. *Schizophr Bull* 1992;18:701–715.

75. Woerner MG, Saltz BL, Kane JM, Lieberman JA, Alvir JMJ. Diabetes and development of tardive dyskinesia. *Am J Psychiatry* 1993;150:966–968.

76. Gardos G, Cole JO, Tarsy D. Withdrawal syndromes associated with antipsychotic drugs. *Am J Psychiatry* 1978;135:1321–1324.

77. Fog R, Pakkenberg H, Regeur L, et al. Tardive tourette syndrome in relation to long-term neuroleptic treatment of multiple tics. In: Friedhoff AJ, Chase TN, eds. *Advances in neurology: Gilles de la Tourette syndrome*, vol. 35. New York: Raven Press, 1982:419–421.

78. Sacks OW. Acquired tourettism in adult-life. In: Friedhoff AJ, Chase TN, eds. *Advances in neurology: Gilles de la Tourette syndrome*, vol. 35. New York: Raven Press, 1982:89–92.

79. Bharucha KJ, Sethi KD Tardive tourettism after exposure to neuroleptic therapy. *Mov Disord* 1995;10:791–793.

80. Stahl SM. Tardive Tourette's syndrome in an autistic patient after long-term neuroleptic administration. *Am J Psychiatry* 1980; 137:1267–1269.

81. Little JT, Jankovic J. Tardive myoclonus. *Mov Disord* 1987; 2:307–311.

82. Stacy MS, Jankovic J. Tardive tremor. *Mov Disord* 1992;1:53–57.

83. Burke RE, Fahn S, Jankovic J, et al. Tardive dystonia: late onset and persistent dystonia caused by antipsychotic drugs. *Neurology* 1982;32:1335–1346.

84. Keegan DL, Rajput AH. Drug-induced dystonia tarda: treatment with L-dopa. *Dis Nerv Sys* 1973;38:167–169.

85. Sethi KD, Hess DC, Harp RJ. Prevalence of dystonia in veterans on chronic antipsychotic therapy. *Mov Disord* 1990;5:4:319–321.

86. Yassa R, Nair V, Dimitor R. Prevalence of tardive dystonia. *Acta Psych Scand* 1986;73:629–633.

87. Van Harten PN, Matroos GE, Hoek HW, Kahn RS The prevalence of tardive dystonia, tardive dyskinesia, parkinsonism and akathisia: The Curacao Extrapyramidal Syndromes Study: I. *Schizophr Res* 1996;19:195–203.

88. Kang UJ, Burke RE, Fahn S. Natural history and treatment of tardive dystonia. *Mov Disord* 1986;1:193–208.

89. Kiriakakis V, Bhatia K, Quinn NP, Marsden CD. The natural history of tardive dystonia: a long-term follow-up study of 107 cases. *Brain* 1998;121:2053–2066.

90. Wojick JD, Falk WE, Fink JS, Cole JO, Gelenberg AJ. A review of 32 cases of tardive dystonia. *Am J Psychiatry* 1991;148:1055–1059.

91. Suzuki T, Matsuzaka H. Drug-induced Pisa syndrome (pleurothotonus): epidemiology and management. *CNS Drugs* 2002;16:165–74.

92. Sethi KD, Hess DC, Harmon D. Reverse obstructive sleep apnea syndrome. *Neurology* 1988;38(suppl 1):312.

93. Sachdev P. Tardive and chronically recurrent oculogyric crises. *Mov Disord* 1993;8:93–98.

94. Bressman SB, de Leon D, Raymond D, et al. Secondary dystonia and the DYT1 gene. *Neurology* 1997;48:1571–1577.

95. Gimenez-Roldan S, Mateo D, Bartolome P. Tardive dystonia and severe tardive dyskinesia: a comparison of risk factors and prognosis. *Acta Psychiatr Scand* 1985;71:488–494.

96. Burke RE, Kang UJ, Jankovic J, Miller LG, Fahn S. Tardive akathisia: an analysis of clinical features and response to open therapeutic trials. *Mov Disord* 1989;4:2:157–175.

97. Schilkrut R, Duran E, Haverbeck C, Katz I, Vidal P. Course of psychopathologic and extrapyramidal motor symptoms during long-term treatment of schizophrenic patients with psycholeptic drugs. *ArzneimittelForschung* 1978;28:1484–1495.

98. Lang AE. Withdrawal akathisia: case reports and a proposed classification of chronic akathisia. *Mov Disord* 1994;9:188–192.

99. Sachdev P. Research diagnostic criteria for drug-induced akathisia: a proposal. *Psychopharmacology* 1994;114:181–186.

100. Weiner WJ, Lang, AE. *Movement disorders: a comprehensive survey.* Mount Kisco, NY: Futura Publishing, 1989:645–684.

101. Calon F, Goulet M, Blanchet PJ, et al. L-dopa or D2 agonist-induced dyskinesias in MPTP monkeys: correlation with changes in dopamine and GABA-A receptors in the striatopallidal complex. *Brain Res* 1995;680:43–52.

102. Goetz, CG. Tardive dyskinesias. In: Watt RL, Koller WC, eds. *Movement disorders: neurologic principles and practice*. New York: McGraw-Hill, 1997:519–526.

103. Hitri A, Weiner W, Borison R, et al. Dopamine binding following prolonged haloperidol pretreatment. *Ann Neurol* 1978;3:134–140.

104. Jeste DV, Wyatt RJ. Dogma disputed: is tardive dyskinesia due to postsynaptic dopamine receptor supersensitivity? *J Clin Psychiatry* 1981;42:455–457.

105. Naidu PS, Kulkarni SK. Excitatory mechanisms in neuroleptic-induced vacuous chewing movements (VCMs): possible involvement of calcium and nitric oxide. *Behav Pharmacol* 2001;12:209–216.

106. Reynolds GP, Brown JE, McCall JC, Mackay AV. Dopamine receptor abnormalities in the striatum and pallidum in tardive dyskinesia: a post mortem study. *J Neural Transm Gen Sect* 1992;87:225–230.

107. Anderson U, Eckernas SA, Harting P, Ulin J, Langstrom B, Haggestrom JE. Striatal binding of 11C-NMSP studied with positron emission tomography in patients with persistent tardive dyskinesia: no evidence for altered dopamine D2 receptor binding. *J Neural Transm Gen Sect* 1990;79:215–226.

108. Silvestri S, Seeman MV, Negrete JC, et al. Increased dopamine D2 receptor binding after long-term treatment with antipsychotics in humans: a clinical PET study. *Psychopharmacology (Berl)* 2000;152:174–80.

109. Pahl JJ, Mazziotta JC, Bartzokis G, et al. Positron-emission tomography in tardive dyskinesia. *J Neuropsychiatry Clin Neurosci* 1995;7:457–465.

110. Lerer B, Segman RH, Fangerau H, et al. Pharmacogenetics of tardive dyskinesia: combined analysis of 780 patients supports association with dopamine D3 receptor gene Ser9Gly polymorphism. *Neuropsychopharmacology* 2002;27:105–119.

111. Woo SI, Kim JW, Rha E, et al. Association of the Ser9Gly polymorphism in the dopamine D3 receptor gene with tardive dyskinesia in Korean schizophrenics. *Psychiatry Clin Neurosci* 2002;56:469–474.

112. Hori H, Ohmori O, Shinkai T, Kojima H, Nakamura J. Association between three functional polymorphisms of dopamine D2 receptor gene and tardive dyskinesia in schizophrenia. *Am J Med Genet* 2001;105:774–778.

113. Tsai G, Goff DC, Chang RW, Flood J, Baer L, Coyle JT. Markers of glutamatergic neurotransmission and oxidative stress associated with tardive dyskinesia. *Am J Psychiatry* 1998;155:1207–1213.

114. Mann SC, Caroff SN, Belieer HR, Welz WK, Kling MA, Hayashida M. Lethal catatonia. *Am J Psychiatry* 1986;143:1374–1381.

115. American Psychiatric Association. Diagnostic and statistical manual for mental disorders, 4th ed. Washington, DC: American Psychiatric Association, 1994:739–742.

116. Kurlan R, Hamill R, Shoulson I. Neuroleptic malignant syndrome: review. *Clin Neuropharmacol* 1984;7:109–120.

117. Granner MA, Wooten GF. Neuroleptic malignant syndrome or parkinsonism hyperpyrexia syndrome. *Semin Neurol* 1991; 11:228–235.

118. Petzinger GM, Bressman SB. A case of tetrabenazine-induced neuroleptic malignant syndrome after prolonged treatment *Mov Disord* 1997;12:246–248.

119. Deng MZ, Chen GQ, Phillips MR. Neuroleptic malignant syndrome in 12 of 9,792 Chinese inpatients exposed to neuroleptics. *Am J Psychiatry* 1990;147:1149–1155.

120. Naganuma H, Fujii I. Incidence and risk factors in neuroleptic malignant syndrome. *Acta Psychiatr Scand* 1994;90:424–426.

121. `Pearlam CA. Neuroleptic malignant syndrome: a review of the literature. *J Clin Psychoparmacol* 1986;6:257–273.

122. Kellam AMP. The neuroleptic malignant syndrome, so-called: a survey of the world literature. *Br J Psychiatry* 1987;150:752–759.

123. Rosebush PI, Stewart TD, Gelenberg AJ. Twenty neuroleptic rechallenges after neuroleptic malignant syndrome in 15 patients. *J Clin Psychiatry* 1989;50:295–298.

124. Shalev A, Hermesh H, Munitz H. Mortality from neuroleptic malignant syndrome. *J Clin Psychiatry* 1989;50:18–25.

125. Jankovic J, Beach J. Longterm effects of tetrabenazine in hyperkinetic movement disorders. *Neurology.* 1997;48:358–362.

126. De Leon ML, Jankovic J. Clinical features and management of classic tardive dyskinesia, tardive myoclonus, tardive tremor and tardive tourettism. In: Sethi K, ed. *Drug-induced movement disorders.* New York: Marcel Dekker, 2004:77–109.

127. Fahn S. Long-term treatment of tardive dyskinesia with presynaptically acting dopamine-depleting agents. In: Fahn S, Calne DB, Shoulson I, eds. *Advances in neurology: experimental theraputics of movement disorders,* vol. 37. New York: Raven Press, 1983:267–276.

128. Klawans HL, Rubovits R. Effect of cholinergic and anticholinergic agents on tardive dyskinesia. *J Neurol Neurosurg Psychiatry* 1974;37:941–947.

129. Tamminga CA, Crayton J, Chase T. Improvement in tardive dyskinesia after muscimol therapy. *Arch Gen Psychiatry* 1979;36:595–598.

130. Lieberman JA, Alvin J, Mukherjee S, Kane JM. Treatment of tardive dyskinesia with bromocriptine: a test of the receptor modification strategy. *Arch Gen Psychiatry* 1989;46:908–913.

131. Stewart RM, Rollins J, et al. Baclofen in tardive dyskinesia patients maintained on neuroleptics. *Clin Neuropharm* 1982;5:365–373.

132. Thaker GK, Nguyen JA, Strauss ME, Jacobson R, Kaup BA, Tamminga CA. Clonazepam treatment of tardive dyskinesia: a practical GABAmimetic strategy. *Am J Psychiatry* 1990;147:445–451.

133. Duncan E, Adler L, Angrist B, Rotrosen J. Nifedipine in the treatment of tardive dyskinesia. *J Clin Pharm* 1990;10:414–416.

134. Loonen AJ, Verwey HA, Roels PR, Van Bavel LP, Doorschot CH. Is diltiazem effective in treating the symptoms of (tardive) dyskinesia in chronic psychiatric inpatients? *J Clin Psychopharmacol* 1992;12:39–42.

135. Elkashef AM, Ruskin PE, Bacher N, Barrett D. Vitamin E in the treatment of tardive dyskinesia. *Am J Psychiatry* 1990;147:4:505–506.

136. Lohr JB, Caligiuri MP. A double-blind placebo-controlled study of vitamin E treatment of tardive dyskinesia. *J Clin Psychiatry* 1996;57:167–173.

137. Shiriqui CL, Bradwejn J, Annable L, Jones BD. Vitamin E in the treatment of tardive dyskinesia: a double-blind placebo-controlled study. *Am J Psychiatry* 1992;149:391–393.

138. Chouinard G. Effects of risperidone in tardive dyskinesia: an analysis of the Canadian multicenter risperidone study. *J Clin Pharmacol* 1995;15(suppl 1):36S–44S.

139. Gwinn KA, Caviness JN. Risperidoneinduced tardive dyskinesia and parkinsonism. *Mov Disord* 1997;12:119–121.

140. Tarsy D, Kaufman D, Sethi KD, Rivner MH, Molho E, Factor S. An open-label study of botulinum toxin A for treatment of tardive dystonia. *Clin Neuropharmacol* 1997;20:90–93.

141. Bhatt M, Sethi KD, Bhatia K. Acute and tardive dystonia. In: Sethi KD, ed. Drug-induced movement disorders. New York: Marcel Dekker, 2004:111–128.

142. Littrell KH, Johnson CG, Littrell S, Peabody CD. Marked reduction of tardive dyskinesia with olanzapine. *Arch Gen Psych* 1998;55:279–280.

143. Meltzer HY. New drugs for the treatment of schizophrenia. *Schizophrenia* 1993;16:365–385.

144. Lieberman JA, Saltz BL, Johns CA, Borenstein M, Kane J. *Br J Psych* 1991;158,503– 510.

145. Factor SA, Friedman JH. The emerging role of clozapine in the treatment of movement disorders. *Mov Disord* 1997; 12:483–496.

146. Spivak B, Mester R, Abesgaus J, Wittenberg N, Adlersberg S, Gonen N, Weizman A. Clozapine treatment for neuroleptic-induced tardive dyskinesia, parkinsonism, and chronic akathisia in schizophrenic patients. *J Clin Psychiatry* 1997;58:318–322.

147. Miller DD, Shafruddin MJA, Kathol RG. A case of clozapine-induced neuroleptic malignant syndrome *J Clin Psychiatry* 1991;52:99–101.

148. Pierre, JM. Extrapyramidal symptoms with atypical antipsychotics: incidence, prevention and management. *Drug Saf* 2005;28:191–208.

149. Bharucha KJ, Zamrini E, Evans D, Durrell D, Sethi KD. Clozapine-induced asterixis. *Neurology* 1996;46:A262.

150. Strauss AJL, Bailey RK, Dralle PW, et al. Conventional psychotropic-induced tremor extinguished by olanzapine. *Am J Psychiatry* 1998;155:1132.

151. Sachdev PS. Neuroleptic-induced movement disorders: an overview. *Psychiatr Clin North Am* 2005;28:255–274.

152. Goulon M, de Rohan-Chabot P, Elkharrat D, Gajdos P, Bismuth C, Conso F. Beneficial effects of dantrolene in the treatment of the neuroleptic malignant syndrome. *Neurology* 1983;33:516–518.

153. Dhib-Jalbut S, Hesselbrook R, Mouradian MM, Means ED. Bromocriptine treatment of neuroleptic malignant syndrome. *J Clin Psychiatry* 1987;48:69–73.

154. Mueller PS. Neuroleptic malignant syndrome. *Psychosomatics* 1985;26:654–662.

155. Addonizio G, Susman VL. ECT as a treatment alternative for patients with symptoms of neuroleptic malignant syndrome. *J Clin Psychiatry* 1987;48:102–105.

156. Rosebush PI, Stewart TD, Mazurek MF. The treatment of neuroleptic malignant syndrome. Are dantrolene and bromocriptine useful adjuncts to supportive care? *Br J Psych* 1991;159:709–712.

157. Buckley PF, Hutchinson M. Neuroleptic malignant syndrome. *J Neurol Neurosurg Psychiatry* 1995;58:271–273.

158. Friedman JH, Fernandez HH. Neuroleptic malignant syndrome. In: Sethi KD, ed. *Drug induced movement disorders.* New York: Marcel Dekker, 2004:165–192.

159. Gardos G, Cole JO. Overview: public health issues in tardive dyskinesia. *Am J Psychiatry* 1980;137:776–781.

Restless Legs Syndrome

31

William G. Ondo

CLINICAL RESTLESS LEGS SYNDROME

In 1995, the International Restless Legs Syndrome Study Group described a set of minimal inclusion criteria for restless legs syndrome (RLS) consisting of four cardinal features: (1) desire to move the extremities, often associated with paresthesia/dysesthesia; (b) motor restlessness; (c) worsening of symptoms at rest and at least temporary relief with activity; and (d) worsening of symptoms in the evening or night (1). Most RLS studies through 2003 incorporated these inclusion criteria. More recently a National Institutes of Health (NIH) consensus panel modified these criteria to include (a) an urge to move the limbs with or without sensations; (b) worsening at rest; (c) improvement with activity; (d) worsening in the evening or night (2). The diagnosis of RLS is exclusively based on those criteria. A validated diagnostic phone interview (3), rating scale (4), and quality-of-life scale (5) have all been developed based on these features.

Patients, however, seldom quote the RLS inclusion criteria at presentation, and they often have difficulty describing the sensory component of their RLS. The descriptions are varied and tend to be suggestive and dependent on education. The sensation is always unpleasant but not necessarily painful. It is usually deep within the legs. In a study of RLS patients, the most common terms used, in descending order of frequency included "need to move," "crawling," "tingling," "restless," "cramping," "creeping," "pulling," "painful," "electric," "tension," "discomfort," and "itching" (6). Patients usually deny any "burning" or "pins and needles" sensations, commonly experienced in neuropathies or nerve entrapments, although neuropathic pain and RLS can coexist.

Essentially, all patients report transient symptomatic improvement by walking, although some employ stationary bike riding or kicking. Other therapeutic techniques reported by our patients include rubbing or pressure, stretching, and hot water. Symptom relief strategies all increase sensory stimulation to the legs and are generally alerting. Other clinical features typical for RLS include the tendency for symptoms to gradually worsen with age, improvement with dopaminergic treatments, a positive family history of RLS, and periodic limb movements in sleep (PLMS).

PLMS are defined by the Association of Sleep Disorders as "periodic episodes of repetitive and highly stereotyped limb movements that occur during sleep." The incidence in the general population increases with age and is reported to occur in as many as 57% of elderly people (7–9). Bixler reported that 29% of people over the age of 50 had PLMS, whereas only 5% of those aged 30 to 50 and almost none under 30 were affected (10). The largest single study, employing a cutoff of 5 PLMS/hour, reported that 81% of RLS patients showed pathologic PLMS (11). The prevalence increased to 87% if two nights were recorded. Therefore, most people with RLS have PLMS, but many patients with isolated PLMS do not have RLS. The exact relationship between the two phenotypes is unclear.

RLS in children can be difficult to diagnose. Although some children report classic RLS symptoms that meet inclusion criteria, other complain of "growing pains," (12,13), and some appear to present with an attention-deficit hyperactivity disorder (ADHD) phenotype. Kotagal et al. reported that children with RLS have lower than expected serum ferritin levels and in most cases appear to inherit the disorder from their mother (14). NIH diagnostic criteria for RLS in children is less well validated but emphasizes supportive criteria such as a family history of RLS, sleep disturbances, and the presence of PLMS, which is much less common in pediatric controls (15). The exact relationship between RLS and ADHD is not known. Children diagnosed with attention-deficit hyperactivity disorder, however, often have

PLMS (16–19) and meet criteria for RLS (16). Children with ADHD also have a higher prevalence of a parent with RLS (20), and children diagnosed with PLMS often have ADHD (21). Dopaminergic treatment of RLS/PLMS in children also improves ADHD symptoms (22.) Therefore, there is clearly some association between RLS and ADHD.

DIAGNOSTIC EVALUATION OF RESTLESS LEGS SYNDROME

In most cases, only a simple evaluation is justified for clinically typical RLS. Serum ferritin, and possibly iron-binding saturation, for serum iron deficiency, and electrolytes for renal failure should be obtained. Nerve conduction velocities (NCV) and electromyogram (EMG) should be performed in cases without a family history of RLS, atypical presentations (i.e., sensations beginning in the feet or superficial pain), in cases that have a predisposition for neuropathy (i.e., diabetes), or when physical symptoms and signs are consistent with a peripheral neuropathy. If EMG/NCV abnormalities are found, they should be further evaluated. Polysomnographic evaluation is usually reserved for patients in whom the diagnosis is in doubt, in cases where PLMS are suspected to be severe and result in arousals, or if other sleep disorders are suspected. A careful history and physical examination are generally sufficient to make a diagnosis of RLS; historically, however, diagnostic sensitivity has been low. One large survey reported that of the 357 patients with RLS who reported discussing RLS symptoms with their physicians, only 46 (12.9%) received a correct diagnosis of RLS (23). Upon reviewing the charts of this cohort, 52 of 209 patients (24%) who had a chart-documented complaint of RLS symptoms received a correct diagnosis. Clearly, awareness among physicians is still poor and may be obfuscated by the lack of objective measures (serologies, physical examination findings, etc.).

There are several potential diagnostic dilemmas. Akathisia represents an inner sense of restlessness accompanied by an intense desire to move. These subjects do not typically complain of limb paresthesia. The restlessness is usually generalized but may be most prominent in the legs. The condition is usually associated with the use of neuroleptic drugs. Akathisia patients generally have milder sleep complaints and less severe PLMS than that seen in RLS (24). Akathisia tends to be associated with whole-body rocking movements and marching in place and may concurrently show mild extrapyramidal features or tardive dyskinesias. Unlike RLS, the restlessness in akathisia is not necessarily worse in the evenings or at night.

Painful legs and moving toes present with neuropathic leg pain associated with persistent, semirhythmic toe movements that cannot easily be reproduced volitionally and may be only partially suppressed (25). The condition may be associated with peripheral nerve injury or minor leg trauma, but many patients have no identifiable etiology or pathology. This syndrome differs clinically from RLS in that the sensory symptoms are described as painful, are not worsened by immobility, are not necessarily worse at night, and are improved with movement.

Nocturnal leg cramps are a common, multifactorial disorder manifested by paroxysmal, disorganized spasms that usually involve the feet or calf muscles. The presentation is different from RLS, but patients may initially describe their RLS symptoms simply as "night cramps," which can lead to misdiagnosis if a more extensive history is not taken.

EPIDEMIOLOGY OF RESTLESS LEGS SYNDROME

Historically, epidemiologic studies of RLS were limited by the subjective nature of the disease, the lack of standardized diagnostic criteria, and the indolent onset of the condition. Ekbom initially estimated a 5% prevalence of RLS in the general population (26). Subsequent general population prevalence surveys varied from 1% to 29% (27–29).

Epidemiological studies have greatly improved since the publication and widespread acceptance of diagnostic criteria (Table 31.1). Rothdach et al. conducted a door-to-door personal interview of 369 people over the age of 65 in Augsburg, Germany (30). Employing International Restless Legs Study Group (IRLSSG) criteria, 13.9% of women and 6.1% of men reported RLS (9.8% total). Patients with RLS also reported a higher prevalence of depression and had lower self-reported mental health scores compared to normal controls.

Ulfberg et al. conducted two separate studies of RLS prevalence in Sweden (31). A written questionnaire, including IRLSSG criteria for RLS, was sent to 4,000 men aged 18–64 years. RLS was found in 5.8% and was correlated with greater age. RLS patients also reported more headaches, depressed mood, and decreased libido. A similar questionnaire sent to 200 women aged 18–64 demonstrated RLS in 11.4%. This concurs with others studies that suggest a higher prevalence in women.

A cross-sectional survey with face-to-face interviews and physical examination among 4310 participants (ages 20–79) in northeastern Germany found that 10.6% of the population reported RLS (32). Older age and female sex were risk factors for RLS. Interestingly, multiparity seemed to power the sex difference, as nulliparous women had a risk of RLS similar to that of men.

The largest epidemiological study of RLS involved more than 23,000 persons from 5 countries (23). As in smaller reports, 9.6% of all people met criteria for RLS. In general, northern European countries demonstrated a higher prevalence compared to Mediterranean countries. The vast majority of these subjects were not previously diagnosed, despite frequently reporting symptoms to their physicians.

RLS can occur in all ethnic backgrounds; however, most feel that Caucasians are most affected. Whereas most surveys of Caucasians demonstrate an approximate 10% prevalence, 2 surveys in Asian populations report much lower prevalences. Tan et al., in a door-to-door survey of 1000

TABLE 31.1

EPIDEMIOLOGY OF RESTLESS LEGS SYNDROME IN THE GENERAL POPULATION, SINCE 1995

Author/Reference/Year	N	RLS Diagnostic Criteria	Population	Location	%
Henning (23), 2004	23,052	NIH Written	Adults	Europe/United States	9.6
Garbarino (188), 2002	2,560	Written	Police Shift workers	Genoa, Italy	8.5: shift workers 4.2: day workers
Ohayan (189), 2002	18,980	ICSD Phone interview	15–100	Europe	5.5
Berger (32), 2004	4,310	IRLSSG Interview	20–79	Northeast Germany	10.6
Rothdach (30), 2000	369	IRLSSG Interview	65–83	Ausberg, Germany	9.8
Nichols (190), 2003	2,099	IRLSSG	Adult	Idaho, United States (single PCP)	24.0
Ulfberg (31), 2001	200	IRLSSG Written	Women 18–64 years of age	Sweden	11.4
Ulfberg (191), 2001	4,000	IRLSSG Written	Men 18–64 years of age	Sweden	5.8
Phillips (29), 2000	1,803	Single phone question	>18	Kentucky, United States	10.0
Lavigne (192), 1997	2,019	2 written questions	Adults	Quebec, Canada	10–15
Sevim (193), 2002	3,234	IRLSSG Interview	Adults, no secondary RLS	Turkey	3.2
Tan (33), 2001	1,000	IRLSSG Interview	>21	Singapore	0.1
Kageyama (34), 2000	3,600 females 1,012 males	Single written question	Adults	Japan	1.5

ICSD, International Classification of Sleep Disorders; IRLSSG, International Restless Legs Study Group diagnostic criteria; NIH, National Institutes of Health RLS diagnostic criteria.

people over age 21 in Singapore, found only 1 person (0.1%) who met IRLSSG criteria for RLS (33). Kageyama et al. distributed a written questionnaire asking "if you ever experience sleep disturbances due to creeping sensations or hot feeling in your legs" to 3600 women and 1012 men (34). They reported that approximately 5% responded affirmatively to that single question but that far fewer would meet all criteria for RLS. People from African descent have never been specifically studied, but anecdotally African-Americans only rarely present with RLS. It is unclear whether this represents a true lower prevalence or, rather, differences in medical sophistication and referral patterns.

GENETICS OF RESTLESS LEGS SYNDROME

In roughly 60% of RLS cases, a family history of RLS can be found, although this is often not initially reported by the patient (6). Twin studies also show a high concordance rate (35). Most pedigrees suggest an autosomal dominant pattern (36), although an autosomal recessive pattern with a high carrier rate is possible. A complex segregation analysis performed in German families revealed a single gene autosomal pattern in subjects with a young onset of RLS (<30 years) but no clear pattern in older onset subjects (36).

To date, several gene linkages have been demonstrated, although specific causative proteins remain elusive. Given the wide distribution of RLS, however, it is likely that additional specific genetic etiologies are yet to be discovered.

Desautels first reported a linkage using an autosomal recessive pattern with a high penetrance on chromosome 12q in a large French-Canadian family (37). Multipoint linkage calculations yielded a LOD score of 3.59. Haplotype analysis refined the genetic interval, positioning the RLS-predisposing gene in a 14.71-cM region between D12S1044 and D12S78. This linkage site has been corroborated in Iceland (David Rye, personal communication, 2006).

Bonati et al. next identified an autosomal dominant linkage in a single Italian family on chromosome 14q13-21 region. The maximum two-point log of odds ratio score value of 3.23 at theta = 0.0, was obtained for marker D14S288 (38).

Chen et al. characterized 15 large and extended multiplex pedigrees, consisting of 453 subjects (134 affected with RLS). Model-free linkage analysis identified 1 novel significant susceptibility locus for RLS on chromosome 9p24.2-22.3 with a multipoint nonparametric linkage (NPL) score of 3.22. Model-based linkage analysis assuming an autosomal dominant mode of inheritance validated the 9p24.2-22.3 linkage to RLS in 2 families (2-point LOD score of 3.77; multipoint LOD score of 3.91). This site has been independently corroborated in a separate German family (Juliana Winkelmann, personal communication, 2005).

Specific protein mutations have not been identified. The Montreal group did report that a specific allele of monoamine oxidase A conferred a modest risk for RLS (39). Numerous other candidate genes of dopaminergic and iron regulation, however, have not shown any association (40,41).

PATHOPHYSIOLOGY OF RESTLESS LEGS SYNDROME

Recent pathological research suggests that the pathophysiology of RLS involves central nervous system (CNS) iron homeostatic dysregulation. Cerebrospinal fluid (CSF) ferritin is lower in RLS cases (42), and specially sequenced MRI imaging studies show reduced iron stores in the striatum and red nucleus (Fig. 31.1) (43). Recently, RLS based on reduced iron echogenicity in the substantia nigra was identified with CNS ultrasonography (44). Using size cutoff of 0.2 cm^2 provided a sensitivity of 83% and a specificity of 95% to distinguish between RLS and controls. Most importantly, pathologic data for RLS in autopsied brains show reduced ferritin staining, iron staining, and increased transferrin stains, but they also show reduced transferrin receptors. Wang et al. also demonstrate reduced Thy-1 expression, which is regulated by iron levels (45). Substantia nigra dopaminergic cells are not reduced in number, nor are there markers associated with neurodegenerative diseases, such as tau or α-synuclein abnormalities (46,47). The reduced transferrin receptor finding is important because globally reduced iron stores would normally upregulate transferrin receptors. Therefore, it appears that primary RLS has reduced intracellular iron indices secondary to a perturbation of homeostatic mechanisms that regulate iron influx and/or efflux from the cell. Intracellular iron regulation is complex; however, subsequent staining of RLS brains has shown reduced levels of iron regulatory protein-type 1 (IRB-1) (48). This potentiates or inhibits (depending on the feedback mechanisms involving iron atoms themselves) the production of ferritin molecules, which are the main iron storage proteins in the CNS, as well as the periphery, and transferrin receptors, which facilitate intracellular iron transport. Reduced IRP-1 is consistent with the iron-staining data seen in RLS brains; however,

specific mutations of IRP-1 have not been identified. The mechanism by which low intracellular iron manifests RLS symptomatology, assuming iron underlies primary RLS pathology rather than epiphenomena, is not well understood and may involve other neurological systems.

CNS dopaminergic systems are strongly implicated in RLS. Most researchers agree that dopamine agonists (DA) most robustly treat RLS, dopaminergic functional brain imaging studies inconsistently show modest abnormalities (49–52), and normal circadian dopaminergic variation is also augmented in patients with RLS (53). There are several potential interactions between iron and dopamine systems. First, iron is a cofactor for tyrosine-hydroxylase, which is the rate-limiting step in the production of dopamine. Iron chelation reduces dopamine transporter (DAT) protein expression and activity in mice (54). Human CSF studies, however have failed to demonstrate reduced dopaminergic metabolites (55,56). Second, iron is a component of the dopamine type-2 (D2) receptor. Iron deprivation in rats results in a 40% to 60% reduction of D2 postsynaptic receptors (57,58). The effect is specific, as other neurotransmitter systems including D1 receptors are not affected. Third, iron is necessary for Thy-1 protein regulation. This cell adhesion molecule, which is robustly expressed on dopaminergic neurons, is reduced in brain homogenates in iron-deprived mice (59) and in brains of patients with RLS (45). Thy-1 regulates vesicular release of monoamines, including dopamine (60). It also stabilizes synapses and suppresses dendritic growth (61). This hypothesis, therefore, states that both presynaptic anatomy and postsynaptic dopaminergic anatomy are intact in RLS, but the actual junction itself is dysfunctional. In the author's opinion, this is most consistent with the functional imaging studies and clinical responses seen in RLS patients. This is also consistent with CSF studies that have failed to find any consistent abnormalities in levels or metabolites of dopaminergic, serotonin (55,56) or hypocretin (62).

Another puzzle remains: identification of a specific dopaminergic anatomy culpable for RLS. There are multiple dopaminergic systems in the brain, but RLS patients do not have symptoms consistent with the dysfunction seen in most known dopaminergic systems, such as parkinsonism or olfactory loss (63). Involvement of the seldom studied diencephalospinal dopaminergic tract, originating from the A11–A14 nuclei, might explain some

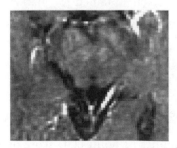 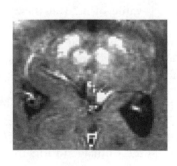

Figure 31.1 MRI sequenced to show iron as bright areas in normal control (*left*) and in patient with restless legs syndrome (*right*).

RLS features. It is involved in antinoscioception, is near circadian control centers, and would explain why legs are involved more than arms. A preliminary animal model with A11 lesions demonstrated increased standing episodes, which improved after the administration of ropinirole, a dopamine agonist (64). Subsequent studies of this model in mice, with and without dietary iron deprivation, also demonstrate increased movement, as measured in laser-marked cages, in the lesioned animals. This hyperkinesis is normalized by D2 agonists such as ropinirole and pramipexole but not by the D1 agonist SKF.

Several other CNS systems demonstrate abnormalities in RLS. Bucher et al., using functional MRI, demonstrated increased activity in the cerebellum and thalamus (65). During the motor component, activity increased in the red nucleus and brainstem. In contrast, voluntary mimicking of similar movements caused increased activity in the basal ganglia and cortex but no brainstem activity. Subcortical disinhibition likely resulting in enhanced spinal cord excitability was associated with PLMS in RLS patients using electrically stimulated spinal flexor reflexes (66). The lack of cortical Bereitschaftspotential during the motor component of both idiopathic and uremic RLS suggests that the movements are not planned or voluntary (67). In contrast, the cortex is indirectly implicated in RLS based upon abnormal transcranial magnetic stimulation experiments in some (68,69), but not all (70) studies of RLS and PLMS.

Pain thresholds in RLS patients may be abnormal. Stiasney-Kolster et al. found static mechanical hyperalgesia to pinprick stimuli, but they found no dynamic mechanical hyperalgesia (allodynia) in RLS patients, which improved with dopaminergic therapy (71). Schattschneider et al. postulated that central somatosensory processing is impaired in primary RLS, based on abnormal quantitative sensory testing assessing temperature perception despite normal quantitative nociceptor axon reflex tests (72). Recently (^{11}C) diprenorphine positron emission tomography (PET) demonstrated an inverse correlation between RLS severity and nonspecific opioid binding throughout the medial pain system (suggesting either increased endogenous opioid release or reduced receptor availability). There was, however, no overall difference between RLS subjects and controls.

SECONDARY RESTLESS LEGS SYNDROME

Despite the appropriate attention given to RLS genetics, 2% to 6% of the population probably suffer from RLS without any identifiable highly penetrant genetic pattern. It is not known whether some "genetic" forms of RLS could express low penetrance and mimic a sporadic pattern of onset. Currently, however, no evidence supports this pattern of penetrance (36). Therefore, patients without a positive family history are classified as either primary RLS, if no other explanation is found, or secondary RLS, if they concurrently possess a condition known to be associated with RLS.

Since the exact pathophysiology of RLS is unknown, the relationship between idiopathic RLS and secondary RLS is not elucidated in any case. It is not known why some persons with an associated medical condition develop RLS symptoms while others, usually most others, do not. Furthermore, it is not established whether persons with a genetic predisposition for RLS may be symptom free without an additional deficit caused by an associated condition, or if subclinical or mild genetic RLS is exacerbated by the coincidental occurrence of a secondary cause.

The most common causes of secondary RLS include renal failure, iron deficiency, neuropathy, myelinopathy, pregnancy, and possibly Parkinson's disease (PD) and essential tremor. There is some evidence to support an association of RLS with some genetic ataxias (73–75), fibromyalgia (76,77), and rheumatological diseases (78–80). A variety of other associations are at best tenuous. Finally, several medications are known to exacerbate existing RLS or possibly to precipitate RLS. The most notable of these include antihistamines, dopamine antagonists (including many antinausea medications), mirtazapine, and possibly tricyclic antidepressants and serotonergic reuptake inhibitors.

Numerous forms of neuropathy—including diabetes, alcoholism, amyloid disease, motor neuron disease, poliomyelitis, and radiculopathy—have been seen at higher-than-expected frequency in patients presenting with RLS (6,81–91). In contrast, series evaluating RLS in populations presenting with neuropathy have not shown a particularly high prevalence of RLS, usually ranging from 5% to 10%, which is similar to the general population (87,88).

For example, our series reported that 37 of 98 RLS patients (36.6%) demonstrated electrophysiologic evidence of neuropathy using standard EMG/NCV techniques. The exact etiologies varied. Many of these patients demonstrated no evidence of neuropathy on clinical examination. The presence of neuropathy was much higher in patients who did not have a family history of RLS, compared to those who did have a family history, 22 of 31 (71%) compared to 15 of 67 (24%), $p < 0.001$. Small fiber neuropathy, which is only detectable with biopsy, is also found in a large number of patients presenting with RLS (85).

Specific forms of neuropathy may incur different risks for the development of RLS. Gemignani et al. reported that 10 of 27 patients (37%) with Charcot-Marie-Tooth type II (CMT II), an axonal neuropathy, had RLS, whereas RLS was not seen in any of 17 patients with CMT I, a demyelinating neuropathy (81). The presence of RLS in CMT II correlated with other positive sensory symptoms such as pain. The same group has also suggested that symmetrical sensory neuropathies and female sex may predict RLS, at least in essential mixed cryoglobulinemia (82).The phenotype of neuropathic RLS may be slightly different from idiopathic RLS (6,85). In our population, neuropathic RLS symptoms initially presented more acutely and at an older age, and then progressed much more rapidly. A large number of patients with neuropathic RLS reached maximum symptom intensity within 1 year from the initial symptom onset, which is unusual in idiopathic cases. Neuropathic RLS may also have accompanying neuropathic pain, which is often burning and more superficial. The painful component and the urge to move, however, are seldom differentiated by the patient.

The spinal cord is implicated in the pathogenesis of RLS (64,66), and cases of RLS and PLMS are seen after transient or permanent spinal cord lesions. Traumatic spinal cord lesions (92, 93), neoplastic spinal lesions (94), demyelinating or post–infectious lesions (95-97), and syringomyelia (98) all can precipitate RLS and PLMS. Spinal cord blocks used for anesthesia also frequently cause or exacerbate RLS (99,100). Hogl et al. systematically evaluated RLS following spinal anesthesia (99). Of 161 subjects without any history of RLS, 8.7% developed RLS immediately after the procedure. Symptoms lasted for an average of 33±30 days and were associated with low mean corpuscular volume and mean corpuscular hemoglobin.

Uremia secondary to renal failure is strongly associated with RLS symptoms. Several series report a 20% to 57% prevalence of RLS in renal dialysis patients; however, only a minority of uremic patients volunteer RLS symptoms unless specifically queried (101–120) (Table 31.2). The prevalence of RLS in mild to moderate renal failure that does not require dialysis is unknown.

The RLS seen in dialysis patients is often severe. Wetter et al. compared clinical and polysomnographic features of idiopathic RLS and uremic RLS in a large clinical series (116). They reported no differences in sensory symptoms but noted increased wakeful leg movements (78% vs. 51%) and significantly greater numbers of PLMS in uremic RLS patients. In the most detailed study to evaluate this association, RLS was also strongly associated with sleep abnormalities (117). RLS in uremic patients is also clearly associated with insomnia and neuropsychiatric sequelae (121). Both RLS and PLMS have also been associated with increased mortality in the dialysis population (117,122).

Overall, dialysis does not improve RLS. In fact, one study suggested that RLS correlated with greater dialysis frequency (108). However, patients who receive a successful, but not unsuccessful, kidney transplant usually experience dramatic improvement in RLS within days to weeks (123,124). The degree of symptom alleviation appears to correlate with improved kidney function.

As previously discussed, reduced CNS iron is implicated in all cases of RLS. It is intuitive to suggest that reduced body stores of iron could also result in low CNS intracellular iron and also cause RLS symptoms. In fact, a possible association between RLS symptoms and systemic iron deficiency has long been recognized (26,125–128).

A series of recent reports have also associated low serum ferritin levels with RLS (42,43,129–133). Serum ferritin is the best indicator of low iron stores and the only serum measure to consistently correlate with RLS. Anemia has not been independently associated with RLS; however, blood donors do frequently develop RLS symptoms (131,134).

Low serum iron stores are only associated with certain demographics of RLS patients. We have reported that serum ferritin is lower in patients with RLS who lack a family history compared to those with familial RLS (129,135). Earley et al. have made the same general observation but segregated the groups based upon age of RLS onset (136). The patients with an older age of RLS onset had lower serum ferritin levels compared to patients with a younger age of onset. These groups, however, generally represent the same dichotomy as do genetic-based segregations since there is a strong correlation between a younger age of onset of RLS and the presence of a family history of RLS. An older age at onset and nonfamilial RLS appear to be strongly associated with low serum ferritin levels, whereas a younger age at onset and familial RLS generally are not associated with low serum ferritin levels.

The development of RLS during pregnancy has long been recognized (26,137,138). Manconi et al. recently evaluated risk factors for RLS in 606 pregnancies (139). They reported that 26% of these women suffered from RLS, usually in the last trimester. The authors could find no significant differences in age, pregnancy duration, mode of delivery, tobacco use, the woman's body mass index, baby weight, or iron/folate supplementation in those with RLS. Hemoglobin, however, was significantly lower in the RLS group, and plasmatic iron tended to be lower, compared to those without RLS. Lee et al. reported that 23% of 29 third-trimester women developed RLS during pregnancy (140). The RLS resolved shortly postpartum in all but 1 subject. Women with RLS in their population demonstrated lower preconception levels of ferritin but were similar to women without RLS during pregnancy.

RLS and PD both respond to dopaminergic treatments, both show dopaminergic abnormalities on functional imaging (51,141), and both are associated with periodic limb movements of sleep (142). We now know that the pathology of the two dopaminergically treated diseases are different and, in regard to iron accumulation, actually opposite (47). Historically, however, association studies between the conditions have been mixed (143–146).

In a survey of 303 consecutive PD patients, we found that 20.8% of all patients with PD met the diagnostic criteria for RLS. Only lower serum ferritin was associated with RLS (129). Similar epidemiological findings recently have been found by other groups evaluating Caucasian populations (147) (Ray Chaudhuri, personal communication, 2005) but not Asian populations (148,149). Despite this high number of cases, several caveats tend to lessen its the clinical significance. The RLS symptoms in PD patients are often ephemeral, usually not severe, and sometimes confused with other PD symptoms such as wearing-off dystonia, akathisia, or internal tremor. Furthermore, most patients in

TABLE 31.2

STUDIES EVALUATING RESTLESS LEGS SYNDROME IN RENAL FAILURE

Author/Reference/Year Author (year)	Cohort	RLS Diagnosis	# and % with RLS	RLS Predictors
Unruh (194), 2004	HD United States	Single question for "severe" RLS	15% of 894	Associated with increased mortality
Mucsi (195), 2004	HD/PD Hungary		15%	NR
Gigli (196), 2004	HD/PD Italy	Written IRLSSG	21.5% of 601	Greater duration of dialysis
Bhowmik (197), 2004	India		1.5% of 65	NR
Takaki (121), 2003	HD Japan	IRLSSG (4/4) IRLSSG (≥2/4)	60/490 (12.2%) 112/490 (22.9%)	Hyperphosphatemia Stress
Goffredo (198), 2003	HD Brazil	IRLSSG Interview	176 (14.8%)	Caucasian > Noncaucasian
Bhatia (102), 2003	HD India		6.6%	NR
Kutner (199), 2002	HD United States	IRLSSG Interview	308 68% Caucasian 48% African	Caucasian > African-American, no other significant predictors
Cirignotta (200), 2002	HD Italy	Written questionnaire IRLSSG Interview	127/50% 127/33.3%	NR
Sabbatini (112), 2002	HD Italy	RLS question	257/694 (37%)	None
Miranda (201), 2001	HD Chile	Interview	43/166 (26%)	None
Hui (106), 2000	PD Hong Kong	Written question	124/201 (62%)	Insomnia
Virga (115), 1998	HD	"RLS"[a]	(27.4%)	None
Collado-Seidel (103), 1998	HD Germany	IRLSSG (4/4) IRLSSG (≥3/4)	32/138 (23%) 44/138 (32%)	Including parathyroid hormone
Winkelmann (117), 1996	HD United States	IRLSSG (3/4)	204 (20%)	None Dec. Hct poor sleep
Walker (202), 1995	HD Canada	ICSD	31/54 (57%)	Inc. BUN, $p = 0.04$ Inc. Cr, $p = 0.08$
Stepanski (113), 1995	PD	Leg twitching	26/81 (32%)	NR
Holley (105), 1992	HD/PD	"RLS"[a]	30/70 (42%)	NR
Roger (111), 1991	HD/PD United Kingdom	"RLS"[a]	22/55 (40%)	Hct, $p = 0.03$ female
Bastani (203), 1987	HD	"RLS"[a]	6/42 (17%)	NR
Nielson (120), 1971	None	"RLS"[a]	43/109 (39%)	NR

[a] "RLS" means the diagnostic criteria were not otherwise defined.
HD, Huntington disease; ICSD, International Classification of Sleep Disorders; IRLSSG, International Restless Legs Study Group diagnostic criteria; NIH, National Institutes of Health; PD, Parkinson's disease; RLS, restless legs syndrome.

our group were not previously diagnosed with RLS and few recognized that this was separate from other PD symptoms.

We recently reported that 34 of 100 subjects presenting to a movement disorders clinic for essential tremor also had RLS, which was undiagnosed in the majority (150). Interestingly, these patients usually had a positive family history of RLS, suggesting a genetic association. In contrast only 1 of 68 consecutive patients presenting with RLS had any tremor of any severity, although many had a mild tremor more consistent with an enhanced physiological tremor.

TREATMENT OF RESTLESS LEGS SYNDROME

The development of validated rating scales and standardized diagnostic criteria have vastly improved the quality of RLS treatment trials in the past 5 years. Although multiple medications have demonstrated outstanding efficacy, all are felt to provide only symptomatic relief, rather than any "curative" effect. Therefore, treatment should be initiated only when the benefits are felt to justify any potential adverse effects and costs. Treatment decisions also need to consider the chronicity and general progressive course of RLS. Over time, both dosing and medication changes are often required to maximize benefit and minimize the risk of tolerance and adverse effects.

DA are clearly the best investigated and probably most effective treatments for RLS. The improvement is immediate and often very dramatic. Although no evidence favors any particular DA, ropinirole is currently the best studied. Three similar, large, multicenter, placebo-controlled trials done in Europe and North America (151–153) and a smaller polysomnogram based study (154) all evaluated ropinirole versus placebo in almost 1000 total subjects. These large studies titrated from 0.25 mg up to a maximum of 4 mg of ropinirole or placebo given as a single nightly dose over 8 weeks, but patients were allowed to stop titrating if necessary. The final dose was maintained for the final 4 weeks. The trials consistently demonstrated significant efficacy of ropinirole using the RLS rating scale and clinical global assessments. The polysomnogram study showed a marked reduction of PLMS and improved sleep architecture. Adverse events were similar but probably milder than those seen in PD, perhaps owing to the lower dose or differences in the disease state. Overall, 7% of subjects on ropinirole and 4% of subjects on placebo withdrew for adverse events. A smaller crossover trial employing 2 split doses showed even more robust efficacy (155).

Placebo-controlled trials also demonstrate efficacy of the DA pramipexole (156,157), pergolide (151,158–161), bromocriptine (162), apomorphine (163), cabergoline (164), and rotigotine (164), and of the dopamine precursor levodopa (165–169). Levodopa was inferior to pergolide in the only controlled comparative trial among dopaminergic medications (159). It is also felt that levodopa has greater potential for augmentation (170). There have been no comparative trials among the DA, but all are felt to provide similar efficacy. Several of these are petitioning for registration in North America and Europe.

Fewer data address the long-term use of DA for RLS. Although studies up to 1 year have shown that most patients on DA continue to benefit from the medications (171,172), some reports have raised specific concerns about both the development of tolerance and dopaminergic-induced augmentation. Augmentation is defined by an earlier phase shift of symptom onset, an increased intensity of symptoms, increased anatomic involvement, or less relief with movement. This was first noted and is still most problematic with levodopa, which has the shortest $T^{1/2}$ of any dopaminergic medication (170). The mechanisms behind augmentation, however, are not known, and it is also reported with pergolide (160,170,173), pramipexole (174–176), and ropinirole (177), but to date not with cabergoline (175,178,179). Winkelman et al. retrospectively assessed augmentation and tolerance in 59 patients treated for RLS with pramipexole for at least 6 months (mean duration = 21.2+/−11.4 months). Augmentation developed in 19 of 59 (32%), and tolerance occurred in

27 of 59 (46%) patients. These two complications were statistically related ($p<0.05$). The only clinical predictors of these complications were previous augmentation or tolerance to levodopa.

We evaluated for augmentation in 83 RLS patients initially started on a DA by us. Patients with at least 6 months of DA use were followed for a mean of 39.2 ± 20.9 months. Efficacy was maintained over time but at the expense of moderate but significant increases in dose ($p<0.01$). Adverse events were frequent but usually mild, and seldom resulted in discontinuation. Augmentation was frequent (48%) but usually modest, and predicted by a positive family history for RLS and especially the lack of any neuropathy on EMG/NCV (Fig. 31.2).

Opioid medications (narcotics) have long been known to successfully treat RLS. Open-label trials consistently demonstrate good initial and long-term results, without difficulty with tolerance, dependence, or addiction (180). There exist, however, only 2 controlled trials that demonstrate efficacy (168,181). We use opioids as second-line therapy and recently collated our experience with methadone (a μ specific opioid agonist) in RLS patients who had failed dopamine agonists due to lack of efficacy, adverse events, or severe augmentation (182). Overall, methadone at doses from 5–20 mg/day markedly benefits most refractory RLS patients without augmentation, tolerance, or evidence for dependency.

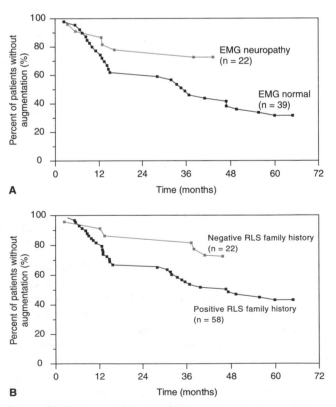

Figure 31.2 The lack of a family history of restless legs syndrome and the presence of neuropathy both protect against augmentation.

Gabapentin is an antiepileptic with multiple mechanisms of action, but a still unclear mechanism of action, which treats a variety of neurological conditions. Garcia-Borreguero et al. conducted a 24-patient, 6-week per arm, crossover study of gabapentin (mean dose 1,855 mg/day) or placebo. RLS Rating Scale, Clinical Global Impression, pain analogue scale, and the Pittsburgh Sleep Quality Index all improved on gabapentin. In addition, sleep studies showed significantly reduced PLMS and improved sleep architecture (increased total sleep time, sleep efficiency, and slow wave sleep, as well as decreased stage 1 sleep). The PLMS did not improve as robustly as seen in DA studies. Patients whose symptoms included pain benefit most from gabapentin. A single, small, open-label crossover trial reported similar efficacy and tolerability between gabapentin and ropinirole, but controlled trials are otherwise lacking (183).

Despite their past widespread use, few data support the use of benzodiazepines for RLS. In the opinion of most experts, benzodiazepines do help facilitate sleep but seldom improve RLS cardinal features. These can be used successfully in mild cases of RLS and as adjunct therapy for residual insomnia.

Although open-label oral iron supplementation has been reported to improve RLS (184), the only controlled study of oral iron supplementation failed to improve RLS symptoms (185). Oral iron, however, has numerous limitations related to absorption and tolerance. In contrast, the administration of intravenous iron can dramatically increase serum ferritin levels and an open-label study of intravenous iron demonstrated robust efficacy (186). Controlled trials of iron dextran with uremic RLS also show efficacy (187). Additional studies are ongoing.

Numerous other agents—including other antiepileptic medications, clonidine, baclofen, tramadol, and magnesium—been reported to help RLS but suffer from limited data and cannot be recommended as either first- or second-line therapy.

REFERENCES

1. Walters AS., The International Restless Legs Syndrome Study Group. Toward a better definition of the restless legs syndrome. *Mov Disord* 1995;10:634-642.
2. Allen RP, Picchietti D, Hening WA, et al. Restless legs syndrome: diagnostic criteria, special considerations, and epidemiology: a report from the Restless Legs Syndrome Diagnosis and Epidemiology Workshop at the National Institutes of Health. *Sleep Med* 2003;4:101-119.
3. Hening WA, et al. The Johns Hopkins telephone diagnostic interview for the restless legs syndrome: preliminary investigation for validation in a multi-center patient and control population. *Sleep Med* 2003;4:137-141.
4. Walters AS, et al. Validation of the International Restless Legs Syndrome Study Group rating scale for restless legs syndrome. *Sleep Med* 2003;4:121-132.
5. Atkinson, M.J., et al. Validation of the Restless Legs Syndrome Quality of Life Instrument (RLS-QLI): findings of a consortium of national experts and the RLS Foundation. *Qual Life Res* 2004;13:679-693.
6. Ondo W, and Jankovic J. Restless legs syndrome: clinicoetiologic correlates. *Neurology* 1996;47:1435-1441.
7. Ancoli-Israel S, et al. Periodic limb movements in sleep in community-dwelling elderly. *Sleep* 1991;14:496-500.
8. Mosko SS, et al. Sleep apnea and sleep-related periodic leg movements in community resident seniors. *J Am Geriatr Soc* 1988;36:502-508.
9. Roehrs T, et al. Age-related sleep-wake disorders at a sleep disorder center. *J Am Geriatr Soc* 1983;31:364-370.
10. Bixler EO, Kales A, Vela-Bueno A. Nocturnal myoclonus and nocturnal myoclonic activity in a normal population. *Res Commun Chem Pathol Pharmacol* 1982;36:129-140.
11. Montplaisir J, et al. Clinical, polysomnographic, and genetic characteristics of restless legs syndrome: a study of 133 patients diagnosed with new standard criteria. *Mov Disord* 1997;12:61-65.
12. Ekbom KA. Growing pains and restless legs. *Acta Paediatr Scand* 1975;64:264-266.
13. Rajaram SS, et al. Some children with growing pains may actually have restless legs syndrome. *Sleep* 2004;27:767-773.
14. Kotagal S, Silber MH. Childhood-onset restless legs syndrome. *Ann Neurol* 2004;56:803-807.
15. Allen RP, et al. Restless legs syndrome: diagnostic criteria, special considerations, and epidemiology: a report from the restless legs syndrome diagnosis and epidemiology workshop at the National Institutes of Health. *Sleep Med* 2003;4:101-119.
16. Chervin RD, et al. Associations between symptoms of inattention, hyperactivity, restless legs, and periodic leg movements. *Sleep* 2002;25:213-218.
17. Picchietti DL, et al. Periodic limb movement disorder and restless legs syndrome in children with attention-deficit hyperactivity disorder. *J Child Neurol* 1998;13:588-594.
18. Chervin RD, et al. Conduct problems and symptoms of sleep disorders in children. *J Am Acad Child Adolesc Psychiatry* 2003;42:201-208.
18a. Muller CM, de Vos RA, Maurage CA, et al. Staging of sporadic Parkinson disease-related alpha-synuclein pathology: inter- and intra-rater reliability. *J Neuropathol Exp Neurol* 2005;64:623-628.
18b. Klos KJ, Ahlskog JE, Josephs KA, et al. Alpha-synuclein pathology in the spinal cords of neurologically asymptomatic aged individuals. *Neurology* 2006;66:1100-1102.
19. Konofal E, et al. High levels of nocturnal activity in children with attention-deficit hyperactivity disorder: a video analysis. *Psychiatry Clin Neurosci* 2001;55:97-103.
20. Picchietti DL, et al. Further studies on periodic limb movement disorder and restless legs syndrome in children with attention deficit hyperactivity disorder. *Mov Disord* 1999;14:1000-1007.
21. Picchietti DL, Walters AS. Moderate to severe periodic limb movement disorder in childhood and adolescence. *Sleep* 1999;22:297-300.
22. Walters AS, et al. Dopaminergic therapy in children with restless legs/periodic limb movements in sleep and ADHD. Dopaminergic Therapy Study Group. *Pediatr Neurol* 2000; 22:182-186.
23. Hening W, et al. Impact, diagnosis and treatment of restless legs syndrome (RLS) in a primary care population: the REST (RLS Epidemiology, Symptoms, and Treatment) primary care study. *Sleep Med* 2004;5:237-246.
24. Sachdev P, Longragan P. The present status of akathisia [see comments]. *J Nerv Ment Dis* 1991;179:381-391.
25. Dressler D, et al. The syndrome of painful legs and moving toes. *Mov Disord* 1994; 9:13-21.
26. Ekbom KA. Restless legs syndrome. *Neurology* 1960;10:868-873.
27. Lavigne GJ, Montplaisir JY. Restless legs syndrome and sleep bruxism: prevalence and association among Canadians. *Sleep* 1994;17:739-743.
28. Oboler SK, Prochazka AV, Meyer TJ. Leg symptoms in outpatient veterans. *West J Med* 1991;155:256-259.
29. Phillips B, et al. Epidemiology of restless legs symptoms in adults. *Arch Int Med* 2000;160:2137-2141.
30. Rothdach AJ, Trenkwalder C, Haberstock J, et al. Prevalence and risk factors of RLS in an elderly population: the MEMO study. Memory and Morbidity in Augsburg Elderly. *Neurology* 2000;54:1064-1068.

31. Ulfberg J, et al. Restless legs syndrome among working-aged women. *Eur Neurol* 2001;46:17–19.
32. Berger K, et al. Sex and the risk of restless legs syndrome in the general population. *Arch Intern Med* 2004;164:196–202.
33. Tan EK, et al. Restless legs syndrome in an Asian population: a study in Singapore. *Mov Disord* 2001;16:577–579.
34. Kageyama T, et al. Prevalences of periodic limb movement-like and restless legs-like symptoms among Japanese adults. *Psychiatry Clin Neurosci*, 2000;54:296–298.
35. Ondo WG, Vuong KD, Wang Q. Restless legs syndrome in monozygotic twins: clinical correlates. *Neurology* 2000;55:1404–1406.
36. Winkelmann J, et al. Complex segregation analysis of restless legs syndrome provides evidence for an autosomal dominant mode of inheritance in early age at onset families. *Ann Neurol* 2002;52:297–302.
37. Desautels A, et al. Identification of a major susceptibility locus for restless legs syndrome on chromosome 12q [see comment]. *Am J Hum Genet* 2001;69:1266–1270.
38. Bonati MT, et al. Autosomal dominant restless legs syndrome maps on chromosome 14q. *Brain* 2003;126(pt 6:1485–1492).
39. Desautels A, et al. Evidence for a genetic association between monoamine oxidase A and restless legs syndrome. *Neurology* 2002;59:215–219.
40. Li J, Hu LD, Chen YG, Kong XY. Linkage analysis of the candidate genes of familial restless legs syndrome. *Yi Chuan Xue Bao* 2003;30:325–329.
41. Desautels A, et al. Dopaminergic neurotransmission and restless legs syndrome: a genetic association analysis [see comment]. *Neurology* 2001;57:1304–1306.
42. Earley CJ, et al. Abnormalities in CSF concentrations of ferritin and transferrin in restless legs syndrome. *Neurology* 2000;54:1698–1700.
43. Allen RP, et al. MRI measurement of brain iron in patients with restless legs syndrome. *Neurology* 2001;56:263–265.
44. Schmidauer C, et al. Brain parenchyma sonography differentiates RLS patients from normal controls and patients with Parkinson's disease. *Mov Disord* 2005;20(suppl10):S43.
45. Wang X, et al. Thy1 expression in the brain is affected by iron and is decreased in restless legs syndrome. *J Neurol Sci* 2004;220:59–66.
46. Pittock SJ, et al. Neuropathology of primary restless leg syndrome: absence of specific tau- and alpha-synuclein pathology. *Mov Disord* 2004;19:695–699.
47. Connor JR, et al. Neuropathological examination suggests impaired brain iron acquisition in restless legs syndrome. *Neurology* 2003;61:304–309.
48. Connor JR, et al. Decreased transferrin receptor expression by neuromelanin cells in restless legs syndrome. *Neurology* 2004;62:1563–1567.
49. Staedt J, et al. Nocturnal myoclonus syndrome (periodic movements in sleep) related to central dopamine D2-receptor alteration. *Eur Arch Psychiatry Clin Neurosci* 1995;245:8–10.
50. Trenkwalder C, et al. Positron emission tomographic studies in restless legs syndrome. *Mov Disord* 1999;14:141–145.
51. Turjanski N, Lees AJ, Brooks DJ. Striatal dopaminergic function in restless legs syndrome: 18F-dopa and 11C-raclopride PET studies. *Neurology* 1999;52:932–937.
52. Tribl GG, et al. Normal striatal D2 receptor binding in idiopathic restless legs syndrome with periodic leg movements in sleep. *Nucl Med Commun* 2004;25:55–60.
53. Garcia-Borreguero D, et al. Circadian variation in neuroendocrine response to L-dopa in patients with restless legs syndrome. *Sleep* 2004;27:669–673.
54. Nelson C, et al. In vivo dopamine metabolism is altered in iron-deficient anemic rats. *J Nutr* 1997;127:2282–2288.
55. Stiasny-Kolster K, et al. Normal dopaminergic and serotonergic metabolites in cerebrospinal fluid and blood of restless legs syndrome patients. *Mov Disord* 2004;19:192–196.
56. Earley CJ, Hyland K, Allen RP. CSF dopamine, serotonin, and biopterin metabolites in patients with restless legs syndrome. *Mov Disord* 2001;16:144–149.
57. Ben-Shachar C, Finberg JP, Youdim MB. Effect of iron chelators on dopamine D2 receptors. *J Neurochem* 1985;45:999–1005.
58. Ashkenazi R, Ben-Shachar D, Youdim MB. Nutritional iron and dopamine binding sites in the rat brain. *Pharmacol Biochem Behav* 1982;17(suppl 1):43–47.
59. Ye Z, Connor JR. Identification of iron responsive genes by screening cDNA libraries from suppression subtractive hybridization with antisense probes from three iron conditions. *Nucleic Acids Res* 2000;28:1802–1807.
60. Jeng CJ, et al. Thy-1 is a component common to multiple populations of synaptic vesicles. *J Cell Biol* 1998;140:685–698.
61. Shults, CW, Kimber TA. Thy-1 immunoreactivity distinguishes patches/striosomes from matrix in the early postnatal striatum of the rat. *Brain Res Dev Brain Res* 1993;75:136–140.
62. Stiasny-Kolster K, et al. CSF hypocretin-1 levels in restless legs syndrome. *Neurology* 2003;61:1426–1429.
63. Adler CH, Gwinn KA, Newman S. Olfactory function in restless legs syndrome. *Mov Disord* 1998;13:563–565.
64. Ondo WG, et al. Clinical correlates of 6-hydroxydopamine injections into A11 dopaminergic neurons in rats: a possible model for restless legs syndrome. *Mov Disord* 2000;15:154–158.
65. Bucher SF, et al. Cerebral generators involved in the pathogenesis of the restless legs syndrome. *Ann Neurol* 1997;41:639–645.
66. Bara-Jimenez W, et al. Periodic limb movements in sleep: state-dependent excitability of the spinal flexor reflex [comment]. *Neurology* 2000;54:1609–1616.
67. Trenkwalder C, et al. Bereitschaftspotential in idiopathic and symptomatic restless legs syndrome. *Electroencephalogr Clin Neurophysiol* 1993;89:95–103.
68. Rau C, Hummel F, Gerloff C. Cortical involvement in the generation of "involuntary" movements in restless legs syndrome. *Neurology* 2004;62:998–1000.
69. Scalise A, Cadore IP, Gigli GL. Motor cortex excitability in restless legs syndrome. *Sleep Med* 2004;5:393–396.
70. Provini F, et al. Motor pattern of periodic limb movements during sleep. *Neurology* 2001;57:300–304.
71. Stiasny-Kolster K, et al. Static mechanical hyperalgesia without dynamic tactile allodynia in patients with restless legs syndrome. *Brain* 2004;127(pt 4):773–782.
72. Schattschneider J, et al. Idiopathic restless legs syndrome: abnormalities in central somatosensory processing. *J Neurol* 2004;251:977–982.
73. Abele M, et al. Restless legs syndrome in spinocerebellar ataxia types 1, 2, and 3. *J Neurol* 2001;248:311–314.
74. Schols L, et al. Sleep disturbance in spinocerebellar ataxias: is the SCA3 mutation a cause of restless legs syndrome? *Neurology* 1998;51:1603–1607.
75. Van Alfen N, et al. Intermediate CAG repeat lengths (53,54) for MJD/SCA3 are associated with an abnormal phenotype. *Ann Neurol* 2001;49:805–807.
76. Yunus MB, Aldag JC. Restless legs syndrome and leg cramps in fibromyalgia syndrome: a controlled study. *BMJ* 1996;312:1339.
77. Moldofsky H. Management of sleep disorders in fibromyalgia. *Rheum Dis Clin North Am* 2002;28:353–365.
78. Reynolds G, Get al. Restless leg syndrome and rheumatoid arthritis. *BMJ* 1986;292:659–660.
79. Salih AM, et al. A clinical, serological and neurophysiological study of restless legs syndrome in rheumatoid arthritis. *Br J Rheumatol* 1994;33:60–63.
80. Gudbjornsson B, et al. Sleep disturbances in patients with primary Sjogren's syndrome. *Br J Rheumatol* 1993;32:1072–1076.
81. Gemignani F, et al. Charcot-Marie-Tooth disease type 2 with restless legs syndrome. *Neurology* 1999;52:1064–1066.
82. Gemignani F, et al. Cryoglobulinaemic neuropathy manifesting with restless legs syndrome. *J Neurol Sci* 1997;152:218–223.
83. Frankel BL, Patten BM, Gillin, JC. Restless legs syndrome: sleep-electroencephalographic and neurologic findings. *JAMA* 1974;230:1302–1303.
84. Iannaccone S, et al. Evidence of peripheral axonal neuropathy in primary restless legs syndrome. *Mov Disord* 1995;10:2–9.
85. Polydefkis M, et al. Subclinical sensory neuropathy in late-onset restless legs syndrome. *Neurology* 2000;55:1115–1121.
86. Salvi F, et al. Restless legs syndrome and nocturnal myoclonus: initial clinical manifestation of familial amyloid polyneuropathy. *J Neurol Neurosurg Psychiatry* 1990;53:522–525.
87. O'Hare JA, Abuaisha F, Geoghegan G. Prevalence and forms of neuropathic morbidity in 800 diabetics. *Ir J Med Sci* 1994;163:132–135.
88. Rutkove SB, Matheson JR, Logigian EL. Restless legs syndrome in patients with polyneuropathy. *Muscle Nerve* 1996;19:670–672.
89. Harriman DG, Taverner D, Woolf AL. Ekbom's syndrome and burning paresthesiae: a biopsy study by vital staining and electron

microscopy of the intramuscular innervation with a note on age changes in motor nerve endings. *Brain* 1970;93:393–406.

90. Gorman CA, Dyck PJ, Pearson JS. Symptom of restless legs. *Arch Intern Med* 1965;115:155–160.

91. Walters AS, Wagner M, Hening WA. Periodic limb movements as the initial manifestation of restless legs syndrome triggered by lumbosacral radiculopathy [letter]. *Sleep* 1996;19:825–826.

92. De Mello MT, et al. Incidence of periodic leg movements and of the restless legs syndrome during sleep following acute physical activity in spinal cord injury subjects. *Spinal Cord* 1996;34:294–296.

93. Hartmann M, Pfister R, Pfadenhauer K. Restless legs syndrome associated with spinal cord lesions [letter]. *J Neurol Neurosurg Psychiatry* 1999;66:688–689.

94. Lee MS, et al. Sleep-related periodic leg movements associated with spinal cord lesions. *Mov Disord* 1996;11:719–722.

95. Brown LK, Heffner JE, Obbens EA. Transverse myelitis associated with restless legs syndrome and periodic movements of sleep responsive to an oral dopaminergic agent but not to intrathecal baclofen. *Sleep* 2000;23:591–594.

96. Bruno RL. Abnormal movements in sleep as a post-polio sequelae. *Am J Phys Med Rehabil* 1998;77:339–343.

97. Hemmer B, et al. Restless legs syndrome after a borrelia-induced myelitis. *Mov Disord* 1995;10:521–522.

98. Winkelmann J, et al. Periodic limb movements in syringomyelia and syringobulbia. *Mov Disord* 2000;15:752–753.

99. Hogl B, et al. Transient restless legs syndrome after spinal anesthesia: a prospective study. *Neurology* 2002;59:1705–1707.

100. Moorthy SS, Dierdorf SF. Restless legs during recovery from spinal anesthesia [letter]. *Anesth Analg* 1990;70:337.

101. Bhatia M, Bhowmik D. Restless legs syndrome in maintenance haemodialysis patients. *Nephrol Dial Transplant* 2003;18:217.

102. Callaghan N. Restless legs syndrome in uremic neuropathy. *Neurology* 1966;16:359–361.

103. Collado-Seidel V, et al. Clinical and biochemical findings in uremic patients with and without restless legs syndrome. *Am J Kidney Dis* 1998;31:324–328.

104. Fukunishi I, et al. Facial paresthesias resembling restless legs syndrome in a patient on hemodialysis [letter]. *Nephron* 1998; 79:485.

105. Holley JL, Nespor S, Rault R. Characterizing sleep disorders in chronic hemodialysis patients. *ASAIO Trans* 1991;37:M456–457.

106. Hui DS, Wong DY, Ko FW, et al. Prevalence of sleep disturbances in chinese patients with end-stage renal failure on continuous ambulatory peritoneal dialysis. *Am J Kidney Dis* [computer file] 2000;36:783–788.

107. Hui DS, Wong TY, Li TS, et al. Prevalence of sleep disturbances in Chinese patients with end-stage renal failure on maintenance hemodialysis. *Med Sci Monit* 2002;8:CR331–336.

108. Huiqi Q, Shan L, Mingcai Q. Restless legs syndrome (RLS) in uremic patients is related to the frequency of hemodialysis sessions. *Nephron* 2000;86:540.

109. Parker KP. Sleep disturbances in dialysis patients. *Sleep Med Rev* 2003;7:131–143.

110. Pieta J, et al. Effect of pergolide on restless legs and leg movements in sleep in uremic patients. *Sleep* 1998;21:617–622.

111. Roger SD, Harris DC, Stewart JH. Possible relation between restless legs and anaemia in renal dialysis patients [letter]. *Lancet* 1991;337:1551.

112. Sabbatini M, et al. Insomnia in maintenance haemodialysis patients. *Nephrol Dial Transplant* 2002;17:852–856.

113. Stepanski E, et al. Sleep disorders in patients on continuous ambulatory peritoneal dialysis. *J Am Soc Nephrol* 1995;6:192–197.

114. Walker SL, Fine A, Kryger MH. L-dopa/carbidopa for nocturnal movement disorders in uremia. *Sleep* 1996;19:214–218.

115. Virga G, et al. Symptoms in hemodialysis patients and their relationship with biochemical and demographic parameters. *Int J Artif Organs* 1998;21:788–793.

116. Wetter TC, et al. Polysomnographic sleep measures in patients with uremic and idiopathic restless legs syndrome. *Mov Disord* 1998;13:820–824.

117. Winkelman JW, Chertow GM, Lazarus JM. Restless legs syndrome in end-stage renal disease. *Am J Kidney Dis* 1996;28:372–378.

118. Read DJ, Feest TG, Nassim MA. Clonazepam: effective treatment for restless legs syndrome in uraemia. *BMJ* 1981;283:885–886.

119. Tanaka K, et al. The features of psychological problems and their significance in patients on hemodialysis—with reference to social and somatic factors. *Clin Nephrol* 1999;51:161–176.

120. Nielsen V. The peripheral nerve function in chronic renal failure. I. Clinical symptoms and signs. 1971;190:105–111.

121. Takaki J, et al. Clinical and psychological aspects of restless legs syndrome in uremic patients on hemodialysis. *Am J Kidney Dis* 2003;41:833–839.

122. Benz RL, Pressman MR, Peterson DD. Periodic limb movements of sleep index (PLMSI): a sensitive predictor of mortality in dialysis patients. *J Am Soc Nephrol* 1994;5433.

123. Yasuda T, Nishimura A, Katsuki Y, Tsuji Y. Restless legs syndrome treated successfully by kidney transplantation: a case report. *Clin Transpl* 1986;138.

124. Winkelmann J, et al. Long-term course of restless legs syndrome in dialysis patients after kidney transplantation. *Mov Disord* 2002;17:1072–1076.

125. Norlander NB. Therapy in restless legs. *Acta Med Scand* 1953;143:453–457.

126. Apenstrom G. Pica och restless legs vid jardbist. 1964;61:1174–1177.

127. Matthews WB. Letter: iron deficiency and restless legs. *BMJ* 1976;1:898.

128. Ekbom KA. Restless legs: a report of 70 new cases. *Acta Med Scand Suppl* 1950;246:64–68.

129. Ondo, W.G., K.D. Vuong, and J. Jankovic, Exploring the relationship between Parkinson disease and restless legs syndrome. *Arch Neurol* 2002;59:421–424.

130. O'Keeffe ST, Gavin K, Lavan JN. Iron status and restless legs syndrome in the elderly. *Age Ageing* 1994;23:200–203.

131. Silber MH, Richardson JW. Multiple blood donations associated with iron deficiency in patients with restless legs syndrome. *Mayo Clin Proc* 2003;78:52–54.

132. Sun ER, et al. Iron and the restless legs syndrome. *Sleep* 1998;21:371–377.

133. Aul EA, Davis BJ, Rodnitzky RL. The importance of formal serum iron studies in the assessment of restless legs syndrome. *Neurology* 1998;51:912.

134. Ulfberg J, Nystrom B. Restless legs syndrome in blood donors. *Sleep Med* 2004;5:115–118.

135. Ondo W, Tan EK, Mansoor J. Rheumatologic serologies in secondary restless legs syndrome. *Mov Disord* 2000;15:321–323.

136. Earley CJ, et al. Insight into the pathophysiology of restless legs syndrome. *J Neurosci Res* 2000;62:623–628.

137. Goodman JD, Brodie C, Ayida GA. Restless leg syndrome in pregnancy. *BMJ* 1988;297:1101–1102.

138. Botez MI, Lambert B. Folate deficiency and restless-legs syndrome in pregnancy [letter]. *N Eng J Med* 1977;297:670.

139. Manconi M, et al. Epidemiology of restless legs syndrome in a population of 606 pregnant women. *Sleep* 2003;26(abstract suppl):A300–A301.

140. Lee KA, Zaffke ME, Baratte-Beebe K. Restless legs syndrome and sleep disturbance during pregnancy: the role of folate and iron. *J Womens Health Gend Based Med* 2001;10:335–341.

141. Ruottinen HM, et al. An FDOPA PET study in patients with periodic limb movement disorder and restless legs syndrome. *Neurology* 2000;54:502–504.

142. Wetter TC, et al. Sleep and periodic leg movement patterns in drug-free patients with Parkinson's disease and multiple system atrophy. *Sleep* 2000;23:361–337.

143. Horiguchi J, Inami Y, Nishimatsu O, et al. [Sleep-wake complaints in Parkinson's disease]. *Rinsho Shinkeigaku* 1990;30:214–216.

144. Banno K, et al. Restless legs syndrome in 218 patients: associated disorders. *Sleep Med* 2000;1:221–229.

145. Paulson G. Is restless legs a prodrome to Parkinson's disease? *Mov Disord* 1997;12(suppl 1):68.

146. Lang AE. Restless legs syndrome and Parkinson's disease: insights into pathophysiology. *Clin Neuropharmacol* 1987;10:476–478.

147. Braga-Neto P, et al. Snoring and excessive daytime sleepiness in Parkinson's disease. *J Neurol Sci* 2004;217:41–45.

148. Krishnan PR, Bhatia M, Behari M. Restless legs syndrome in Parkinson's disease: a case-controlled study. *Mov Disord* 2003;18:181–185.

149. Tan EK, Lum SY, Wong MC. Restless legs syndrome in Parkinson's disease. *J Neurol Sci* 2002;196:33–36.

150. Ondo W. The association of restless legs syndrome and essential tremor. *Mov Disord* 2005;20(suppl 10):S160.

151. Trenkwalder C, et al. Ropinirole in the treatment of restless legs syndrome: results from the TREAT RLS 1 study, a 12 week, randomised, placebo controlled study in 10 European countries. *J Neurol Neurosurg Psychiatry* 2004;75:92–97.

152. Walters AS, et al. Ropinirole is effective in the treatment of restless legs syndrome. TREAT RLS 2: a 12-week, double-blind, randomized, parallel-group, placebo-controlled study. *Mov Disord* 2004;19:1414–1423.

153. Bogan R, Connolly G, Rederich G. Ropinirole is effective, well-tolerated treatment for moderate-to-severe RLS: results of a U.S. study. *Mov Disord* 2005;20(suppl 10):S61.

154. Allen R, et al. Ropinirole decreases periodic leg movements and improves sleep parameters in patients with restless legs syndrome [see comment]. *Sleep* 2004;27:907–914.

155. Adler CH, et al. Ropinirole for restless legs syndrome: a placebo-controlled crossover trial. *Neurology* 2004;62:1405–1407.

156. Montplaisir J, et al. Restless legs syndrome improved by pramipexole: a double-blind randomized trial. *Neurology* 1999; 52:938–943.

157. Oertel W, Stiasney-Kolster K. Pramipexole is effective in the treatment of restless legs syndrome (RLS): results of a 6-week, multi-centre, double, and placebo controlled study. *Mov Disord* 2005;20(suppl 10):S58.

158. Earley CJ, Yaffee JB, Allen RP. Randomized, double-blind, placebo-controlled trial of pergolide in restless legs syndrome. *Neurology* 1998;51:1599–1602.

159. Staedt J, et al. Pergolide: treatment of choice in restless legs syndrome (RLS) and nocturnal myoclonus syndrome (NMS): a double-blind randomized crossover trial of pergolide versus L-dopa. *J Neural Transm (Budapest)* 1997;104:461–468.

160. Trenkwalder C, et al. A randomized long-term placebo controlled multicenter trial of pergolide in the treatment of restless legs syndrome with central evaluation of polysomnographic data. *Neurology* 2001;56(suppl 3):A5.

161. Wetter TC, et al. A randomized controlled study of pergolide in patients with restless legs syndrome. *Neurology* 1999;52:944–950.

162. Walters AS, et al. A double-blind randomized crossover trial of bromocriptine and placebo in restless legs syndrome. *Ann Neurol* 1988;24:455–458.

163. Reuter I, Ellis CM, and Ray Chaudhuri K. Nocturnal subcutaneous apomorphine infusion in Parkinson's disease and restless legs syndrome. *Acta Neurol Scand* 1999;100:163–167.

164. Happe S, Trenkwalder C. Role of dopamine receptor agonists in the treatment of restless legs syndrome. *CNS Drugs* 2004;18: 27–36.

165. Benes H, et al. Rapid onset of action of levodopa in restless legs syndrome: a double-blind, randomized, multicenter, crossover trial. *Sleep* 1999;22:1073–1081.

166. Brodeur C, et al. Treatment of restless legs syndrome and periodic movements during sleep with L-dopa: a double-blind, controlled study. *Neurology* 1988;38:1845–1848.

167. Collado-Seidel V, et al. A controlled study of additional sr-L-dopa in L-dopa-responsive restless legs syndrome with late-night symptoms. *Neurology* 1999;52:285–290.

168. Kaplan PW, et al. A double-blind, placebo-controlled study of the treatment of periodic limb movements in sleep using carbidopa/levodopa and propoxyphene. *Sleep* 1993;16:717–723.

169. Saletu M, et al. Acute double-blind, placebo-controlled sleep laboratory and clinical follow-up studies with a combination treatment of rr-L-dopa and sr-L-dopa in restless legs syndrome. *J Neural Transm* 2003;110:611–626.

170. Allen RP, Earley CJ. Augmentation of the restless legs syndrome with carbidopa/levodopa. *Sleep* 1996;19:205–213.

171. Stiasny K, et al. Long-term effects of pergolide in the treatment of restless legs syndrome. *Neurology* 2001;56:1399–1402.

172. Montplaisir J, Denesle R, Petit D. Pramipexole in the treatment of restless legs syndrome: a follow-up study. *Eur J Neurol* 2000;7(suppl 1):27–31.

173. Silber MH, Shepard Jr JW, Wisbey JA. Pergolide in the management of restless legs syndrome: an extended study. *Sleep* 1997;20:878–82.

174. Silber M, Girish M, Izurieta R. Pramipexole in the management of restless legs syndrome: an extended study. *Sleep* 2001;24 (abstract suppl):A18.

175. Ferini-Strambi L, et al. Augmentation of restless legs syndrome after long-term treatment with pramipexole and cabergoline. *Neurology* 2002;58(suppl 3):A515.

176. Winkelman JW, Johnston L. Augmentation and tolerance with long-term pramipexole treatment of restless legs syndrome (RLS). *Sleep Med* 2004;5:9–14.

177. Ondo W, et al. Long-term treatment of restless legs syndrome with dopamine agonists. *Arch Neurol* 2004;61:1393–1397.

178. Stiasny K, et al. Treatment of idiopathic restless legs syndrome (RLS) with the D2-agonist cabergoline—an open clinical trial. *Sleep* 2000;23:349–354.

179. Porter MC, Appiah-Kubf LS, Chaudhuri KR. Treatment of Parkinson's disease and restless legs syndrome with cabergoline, a long-acting dopamine agonist. *Int J Clin Pract* 2002;56: 468–474.

180. Walters AS, et al. Long-term follow-up on restless legs syndrome patients treated with opioids. *Mov Disord* 2001;16:1105–1109.

181. Walters AS, et al. Successful treatment of the idiopathic restless legs syndrome in a randomized double-blind trial of oxycodone versus placebo. *Sleep* 1993;16:327–332.

182. Ondo W. Methadone for refractory restless legs syndrome. *Mov Disord* 2005;20:345–348.

183. Happe S, et al. Gabapentin versus ropinirole in the treatment of idiopathic restless legs syndrome. *Neuropsychobiology* 2003;48: 82–86.

184. O'Keeffe ST, Noel J, Lavan JN. Restless legs syndrome in the elderly. *Postgrad Med J* 1993;69:701–703.

185. Davis BJ, et al. A randomized, double-blind placebo-controlled trial of iron in restless legs syndrome. *Eur Neurol* 2000;43:70–75.

186. Earley CJ, Heckler D, Allen RP. The treatment of restless legs syndrome with intravenous iron dextran. *Sleep Med* 2004;5: 231–235.

187. Sloand JA, et al. A double-blind, placebo-controlled trial of intravenous iron dextran therapy in patients with ESRD and restless legs syndrome. *Am J Kidney Dis* 2004;43:663–670.

188. Garbarino S, et al. Sleepiness and sleep disorders in shift workers: a study on a group of italian police officers. *Sleep* 2002;25:648–653.

189. Ohayon MM, Roth T. Prevalence of restless legs syndrome and periodic limb movement disorder in the general population. *J Psychosom Res* 2002;53:547–554.

190. Nichols DA, et al. Restless legs syndrome symptoms in primary care: a prevalence study. *Arch Int Med* 2003;163:2323–2329.

191. Ulfberg J, et al. Prevalence of restless legs syndrome among men aged 18 to 64 years: an association with somatic disease and neuropsychiatric symptoms. *Mov Disord* 2001;16:1159–1163.

192. Lavigne GL, et al. Cigarette smoking as a risk factor or an exacerbating factor for restless legs syndrome and sleep bruxism. *Sleep* 1997;20:290–293.

193. Sevim S, et al. Unexpectedly low prevalence and unusual characteristics of RLS in Mersin, Turkey. *Neurology* 2003;61:1562–1569.

194. Unruh ML, et al. Restless legs symptoms among incident dialysis patients: association with lower quality of life and shorter survival. *Am J Kidney Dis* 2004; 43:900-909.

195. Mucsi, I., et al. Sleep disorders and illness intrusiveness in patients on chronic dialysis. *Nephrol Dial Transplant* 2004;19: 1815–1822.

196. Gigli GL, et al. Restless legs syndrome in end-stage renal disease. *Sleep Med* 2004;5:309–315.

197. Bhowmik D, et al. Low prevalence of restless legs syndrome in patients with advanced chronic renal failure in the Indian population: a case controlled study. *Ren Fail* 2004;26:69–72.

198. Goffredo Filho GS, et al. Restless legs syndrome in patients on chronic hemodialysis in a Brazilian city: frequency, biochemical findings and comorbidities. *Arq Neuropsiquiatr* 2003;61:723–727.

199. Kutner NG, Bliwise DL. Restless legs complaint in African-American and Caucasian hemodialysis patients. *Sleep Med* 2002;3:497–500.

200. Cirignotta F, et al. Reliability of a questionnaire screening restless legs syndrome in patients on chronic dialysis. *Am J Kidney Dis* 2002;40:302–306.

201. Miranda M, et al. [Restless legs syndrome: a clinical study in adult general population and in uremic patients]. *Rev Med Chil* 2001;129:179–186.

202. Walker S, Fine A, Kryger MH. Sleep complaints are common in a dialysis unit. *Am J Kidney Dis* 1995;26:751–756.

203. Bastani B, Westervelt FB. Effectiveness of clonidine in alleviating the symptoms of "restless legs." *Am J Kidney Dis* 1987;10:326.

Hereditary Ataxias

32

Thomas Klockgether

INTRODUCTION

The hereditary ataxias comprise a wide spectrum of genetically determined disorders with progressive ataxia as the prominent symptom. In most of these disorders, ataxia is due to degeneration of the cerebellar cortex and the spinal cord. In many hereditary ataxias, the underlying gene mutations have been identified. Knowledge of the causative mutations allows a rational classification of hereditary ataxias (Table 32.1) as autosomal recessive or autosomal dominant. The autosomal dominant ataxias can be further subdivided into the progressive spinocerebellar ataxias (SCAs) and the episodic ataxias (EAs). In contrast to all other types of hereditary ataxias, the EAs are characterized by paroxysmal occurrence of ataxia. In addition, one disorder, fragile X tremor ataxia syndrome (FXTAS), has X-linked inheritance.

Improved understanding of the molecular events causing ataxia allows an alternative classification based on their pathogenesis. One group of disorders, including Friedreich's ataxia (FRDA), is due to mitochondrial dysfunction and oxidative stress; a second, including ataxia telangiectasia (AT), is due to defective DNA repair; a third, including a number of spinocerebellar ataxias (SCA), is due to protein aggregation; and a fourth group, including the episodic ataxias, is due to ion channel dysfunction (Table 32.2). Although pathogenetic classification is desirable with respect to the development of effective therapies, this classification is at best preliminary and cannot replace the genetic classification because the understanding of the pathogenesis of many hereditary ataxias is poor and a number of ataxias do not readily fit into one of the categories.

FRIEDREICH'S ATAXIA

FRDA Etiology and Pathogenesis

FRDA is the most common autosomal recessively inherited ataxia. In most cases of FRDA, the causative mutation is a homozygous, intronic GAA repeat expansion in a gene coding for the mitochondrial protein fraxatin. Less than 4% of FRDA patients are compound heterozygotes with 1 allele carrying the GAA repeat expansion and the other a point mutation [1,2]. A second FRDA locus was mapped to chromosome 9p [3].

The intronic GAA repeat expansion impedes normal transcription of the fraxatin gene, resulting in fraxatin tissue levels of less than 10% of normals. The degree of fraxatin reduction depends on GAA repeat length: Fraxatin deficiency is more pronounced in patients with long repeats than in those with only moderate expansions. Mice with a complete deletion of the fraxatin gene are embryonically lethal, showing that frataxin is an essential protein [4]. Conditional knockouts with fraxatin deficiency in the heart or nervous system reproduce relevant aspects of FRDA-related pathology [5].

The physiological function of fraxatin has been studied extensively in cellular models. Frataxin assembles to larger protein complexes that function as iron chaperones and iron storage proteins. Frataxin thereby protects DNA from iron-induced damage [6,7]. Frataxin deficiency results in reduced availability of iron for the synthesis of iron–sulphur clusters, which form essential parts of a number of cellular enzymes, including enzymes of the mitochondrial respiratory chain. Frataxin deficiency consequently leads to a decline of mitochondrial respiratory activity and increased production of free radicals [8].

TABLE 32.1

GENETIC CLASSIFICATION OF HEREDITARY ATAXIAS

Autosomal recessive ataxias with known gene mutation

Friedreich's ataxia (FRDA)
Ataxia telangiectasia (AT)
Autosomal recessive ataxia with oculomotor apraxia type 1 (AOA1)
Autosomal recessive ataxia with oculomotor apraxia type 2 (AOA2)
Spinocerebellar ataxia with neuropathy type 1 (SCAN1)
Autosomal recessive spastic ataxia of Charlevoix-Saguenay (ARSACS)
Ataxia with isolated vitamin E deficiency (AVED)
Abetalipoproteinemia
Refsum's disease
Cerebrotendinous xanthomatosis (CTX) with known gene locus
Autosomal recessive ataxia with hearing impairment
    and optic atrophy
Infantile onset spinocerebellar ataxia (IOSCA)
Marinesco-Sjögren syndrome (MSS)

Autosomal recessive ataxias with gene locus and mutation unknown

Early onset cerebellar ataxia (EOCA)

X-linked ataxias

Fragile X tremor ataxia syndrome (FXTAS)

Autosomal dominant ataxias

Spinocerebellar ataxias (SCA)
Episodic ataxias (EA)

TABLE 32.2

PATHOGENETIC CLASSIFICATION OF HEREDITARY ATAXIAS

Disorders due to mitochondrial dysfunction and oxidative stress

Friedreich's ataxia
Ataxia with isolated vitamin E deficiency (AVED)
Abetalipoproteinemia

Disorders due to defective DNA repair

Ataxia telangiectasia (AT)
Autosomal recessive ataxia with oculomotor apraxia
    type 1, 2 (AOA1, AOA2)
Spinocerebellar ataxia with neuropathy type 1 (SCAN1)

Disorders due to protein aggregation

Spinocerebellar ataxias type 1, 2, 3, 7, 17 (SCA1, SCA2, SCA3, SCA7, SCA17)

Disorders due to ion channel dysfunction

Spinocerebellar ataxia type 6
Episodic ataxias types 1, 2 (EA1, EA2)

FRDA Neuropathology

The first pathological changes in FRDA are thought to occur in the dorsal root ganglia with loss of large sensory neurons. In advanced cases, the neuropathological abnormalities comprise axonal sensory and motor neuropathies, degeneration of spinal tracts (spinocerebellar tracts, posterior columns, pyramidal tract), and concentric hypertrophic cardiomyopathy affecting all chambers and the septum. There is only occasional involvement of the cerebellum with loss of Purkinje cells and moderate cerebellar atrophy.

FRDA Epidemiology

Leone et al. found a prevalence of 1.7:100,000 in the Aosta valley in Italy (9). Another survey performed in Cantabria (Spain) yielded a prevalence of 4.7:100,000 (10).

FRDA Clinical Presentation

The most prominent sign of FRDA is progressive ataxia, initially affecting gait and stance, and later also arm movements. Muscle reflexes of the legs are absent in about 90% of the patients. Approximately 80% of the patients have extensor plantar responses. With progression of the disease, distal wasting of the lower and upper extremities develops. Due to pyramidal involvement and muscle wasting, FRDA patients may have considerable weakness. Approximately half of the patients have skeletal deformities (scoliosis, pes cavus), which are due to muscle wasting starting in early life. Almost all patients have sensory disturbances with reduced vibration and position sense (11).

All FRDA patients develop an ataxic speech disorder, usually within the first 5 years of the disease. Disorders of ocular motility are part of the clinical spectrum of FRDA. Oculomotor disorders include square wave jerks during fixation and reduced gain of vestibulo-ocular reflex. Oculomotor disturbances pointing to cerebellar dysfunction, such as gaze-evoked nystagmus or saccadic hypermetria, are usually absent in FRDA. Physical examination reveals pale discs in many FRDA patients. However, a loss of visual acuity is encountered in only 10%–20% of the patients. Similarly, 10%–20% develop sensorineural hearing problems.

In approximately 60% of FRDA patients, echocardiography reveals a hypertrophic cardiomyopathy. Diabetes mellitus is present in 10% to 30% of the patients (11).

FRDA Natural Course

Mean age at onset is 15 years, ranging from 2–51 years (11). FRDA is a progressive disease leading to disability and premature death. Median latency to become wheelchair-bound after disease onset is 11 years. Life expectancy after disease onset is estimated to be 35–40 years (12). Age of onset and progression rate are partly determined by the GAA repeat length of the shorter allele: In patients with longer expansions, disease onset is earlier and progression faster (11).

FRDA Diagnosis

A genetic test demonstrating the GAA repeat expansion is widely available and can be used to confirm a clinical diagnosis of FRDA. Genetic testing is particularly useful in atypical cases with preserved muscle reflexes and late disease onset.

MRI typically shows cervical spinal cord atrophy without major cerebellar atrophy (13). Nerve conduction studies reveal an axonal form of sensory neuropathy. Most patients have repolarization changes of the electrocardiogram. Hypertrophic cardiomyopathy is demonstrated by echocardiography.

FRDA Management

Idebenone (5 mg/kg per day), a short-chain quinone analogue improving mitochondrial electron transport, was found to decrease the left ventricular mass of FRDA patients in a number of open studies (14,15,16). This was recently confirmed in a randomized, placebo-controlled study of 29 FRDA patients. However, idebenone had no action on cardiac or neurological function (17). Antiataxic drugs, such as 5-hydroxytryptophan, buspirone, and amantadine, are ineffective or only marginally effective in FRDA. Physiotherapy and speech therapy are generally recommended. Patients with clinically relevant cardiomyopathy and diabetes mellitus should receive standard medical treatment.

ATAXIA TELANGIECTASIA

AT Etiology and Pathogenesis

Ataxia telangiectasia (AT) is an autosomal recessively inherited multisystem disorder caused by mutations of the ATM gene. The ATM gene encodes a member of the phosphoinositol-3 kinase family involved in cell cycle checkpoint control and DNA repair (18). Several hundred distinct mutations distributed over the entire gene have been reported. Rarely, a disorder similar to AT is caused by mutations in the double-strand break repair gene hMRE11 (19).

AT Neuropathology

There is atrophy of the cerebellum that mainly affects the cerebellar cortex of the vermis. The number of cerebellar Purkinje cells is reduced, and Purkinje cells show abnormal arborization and ectopic localization. In addition, there are degenerative changes of the spinal cord, including degeneration of the posterior and lateral columns and atrophy of the anterior horn. The peripheral nervous system may be involved with a demyelinating neuropathy.

AT Epidemiology

An Italian study found a prevalence of 1.2:100,000 (20).

AT Clinical Presentation

AT is clinically characterized by a combination of neurological and nonneurological symptoms. Cerebellar ataxia is the clinical hallmark of AT. Ataxia of gait and stance usually become apparent when the child has learned to walk. Other cerebellar symptoms, including dysarthria and ataxia of the upper extremities, develop in the further course of the disease. In addition, many patients have choreoathetosis and dystonia. Muscle reflexes are usually weak or absent. AT patients have a peculiar difficulty initiating saccades (oculomotor apraxia). In contrast to ophthalmoplegia, eye movements can be completed in the full range when given sufficient time. When AT patients intend gaze shifts, they move their head into the desired direction and cause a reflectory, tonic drift of the eyes away from the target. The target is then refixated with considerable delay. Intellectual abilities are normal in the beginning of the disease. Later, there may be mild impairments that are partly secondary to the physical disability. In late disease stages, patients develop sensory disturbances with impaired vibration and positional sense and distal muscle wasting.

Telangiectasias are the second hallmark of AT. They develop after the onset of ataxia and are most frequently found in the lateral angles of the conjunctivae and the external earlobes. Approximately 60% of AT patients have immunodeficiency. The most frequent clinical manifestations are recurrent sinopulmonary infections. AT patients have a considerably increased risk of malignancies. Overall, one-third of AT patients develop a malignant disease during their lives. Before the age of 20 years, malignancies are mainly lymphoid. In older patients, solid tumors are more frequent.

AT Natural Course

AT usually begins at 2–4 years after the child has learned to walk. Most patients need wheelchairs at the age of 10 years. Life expectancy is severely reduced due to recurrent infections and neoplasia. Most patients die in their third decade.

AT Diagnosis

A diagnosis of AT is probable in patients with a typical clinical phenotype and elevated serum levels of α-fetoprotein. In vitro demonstration of radiosensitivity of lymphocytes is used as a laboratory test to confirm the diagnosis. Genetic testing cannot be used routinely due to the size of the gene and the diversity of mutations causing AT.

AT Management

Although the gene defect causing AT has been found and the cellular pathogenesis is partly understood, effective therapies are not available. In particular, there is no way to improve ataxia.

Treatment of infections should be initiated early and maintained over a prolonged time. Usually, infections require intravenous or oral application of wide-spectrum antibiotics. Administration of immunoglobulins (IgA) can be considered in patients with repeated infections. However, standard IgA preparations are often poorly tolerated by AT patients owing to IgA deficiency. In these patients, a switch to preparations with low or absent IgA levels is required.

Treatment of malignant neoplasias is a particular problem because AT patients have increased sensitivity to radiation and chemotherapy. Therefore, conventional radiotherapy should be avoided, and chemotherapy should be administered only on an individual basis.

AUTOSOMAL RECESSIVE ATAXIA WITH OCULOMOTOR APRAXIA TYPE 1

Autosomal recessive ataxia with oculomotor apraxia type 1 (AOA1) is an autosomal recessively inherited ataxia that is caused by mutations of the aprataxin gene. AOA1 was initially described in Japan and Portugal but is also prevalent in other countries (21). In Portugal, AOA1 is the second most frequent recessive ataxia after FRDA (22).

Aprataxin is a protein of the histidine triad superfamily (23,24), and plays a role in repair of single-strand DNA breaks (25). It was recently shown that AOA1 patients have severe muscular coenzyme QO deficiency (26). The mechanisms leading to coenzyme QO deficiency have not been elucidated.

AOA1 starts in children with a mean age of onset of 7 years. Besides ataxia and oculomotor apraxia, the clinical spectrum of AOA1 involves chorea, neuropathy, and mental retardation (27). With progression of the disease, neuropathy becomes more and more disabling, whereas the oculomotor abnormalities may become less prominent. AOA1 patients survive in a severely disabled state into adulthood.

Characteristically, routine laboratory tests show hypoalbuminemia that increases with progression of the disease. A definite diagnosis of AOA1 can be made by genetic testing.

If the report on coenzyme QO deficiency is confirmed by other groups, AOA1 patients should be supplemented with coenzyme QO at a dose of at least 500 mg/day (26).

AUTOSOMAL RECESSIVE ATAXIA WITH OCULOMOTOR APRAXIA TYPE 2

Autosomal recessive ataxia with oculomotor apraxia type 2 (AOA2) is an autosomal recessively inherited ataxia caused by mutations of the senataxin gene. Senataxin is the human homologue ot the yeast gene Sen1p (28). It has been suggested that senataxin, like aprataxin, is involved in repair of single-strand DNA breaks. The prevalence of AOA2 is unknown, but it has been suggested that AOA2 is the second most frequent recessive ataxia in Europe after FRDA (29).

The mean age of onset of AOA2 is 15 years. Clinically, AOA2 is characterized by ataxia and neuropathy. Oculomotor apraxia is not present in all AOA2 patients (29,30).

All AOA2 patients have increased serum α-fetoprotein levels. To differentiate AOA2 from AT patients, who have also increased serum α-fetoprotein levels, a lymphocyte radiosensitivity assay should be performed. This test is normal in AOA2. Genetic testing for AOA2 is not routinely available.

SPINOCEREBELLAR ATAXIA WITH NEUROPATHY TYPE 1

Spinocerebellar ataxia with neuropathy type 1 (SCAN1) is an autosomal recessive disorder that was identified in a Saudi Arabian family. It is caused by a mutation in the conserved part of the tyrosyl-DNA phosphodiesterase 1 (TDP1) gene affecting the active enzymatic site (31). TDP1 is required for the repair of DNA single-strand breaks, which places SCAN1 in the group of recessive ataxias due to defects of DNA repair. Clinically, SCAN1 is characterized by ataxia in combination with sensory neuropathy.

AUTOSOMAL RECESSIVE SPASTIC ATAXIA OF CHARLEVOIX-SAGUENAY

Autosomal recessive spastic ataxia of Charlevoix-Saguenay (ARSACS) is an autosomal recessive ataxia with a distinctive phenotype that is prevalent in a restricted area in Quebec in Canada. ARSACS is due to mutations in a large, single exon gene encoding a novel protein named *sacsin*. The most frequent mutation, accounting for more than 90% of all mutations, is a deletion leading to protein truncation. Sacsin contains a heat-shock domain, which suggests that it subserves chaperone function (32). Autopsies of ARSACS patients showed cortical atrophy, pyramidal degeneration, atrophy of the upper cerebellar vermis, and loss of motoneurons. Immunocytochemical studies revealed abnormal accumulations of neurofilaments. The central nervous system abnormalities are accompanied by a mixed sensorimotor neuropathy.

The prevalence of ARSACS in the French-Canadian founder population in Quebec is 50:100,000. Outside Quebec, ARSACS is a rare cause of ataxia (33).

ARSACS is characterized by the combination of progressive cerebellar ataxia and spasticity. Muscle reflexes are exaggerated, and plantar responses are extensor. With progression of the disease, the ankle jerks disappear and distal wasting of foot muscles develops. A highly characteristic ocular sign is the presence of prominent myelinated fibers radiating from the optic disc at fundoscopy.

ARSACS typically starts at the age of 1–2 years. On average, patients become wheelchair bound around the age of 40 years.

The diagnosis of ARSACS can be confirmed by demonstration of the deletion in the sacsin gene (34). There is no effective therapy for ARSACS. A minority of patients with pronounced spasticity may benefit from antispastic drugs.

ABETALIPOPROTEINEMIA

Abetalipoproteinemia is a rare, autosomal recessively inherited disorder characterized by onset of diarrhea soon after birth and slow development of a neurological syndrome thereafter. The neurological syndrome consists of ataxia, weakness of the limbs with loss of tendon reflexes, disturbed sensation, and retinal degeneration. Abetalipoproteinemia is caused by mutations in the gene encoding a subunit of a microsomal triglyceride transfer protein (35). As a consequence, circulating apoprotein B-containing lipoproteins are almost completely missing, and patients are unable to absorb and transport fat and fat-soluble vitamins. The neurological symptoms are due to vitamin E deficiency. Management of abetalipoproteinemia consists of a diet with reduced fat intake and oral vitamin E supplementation (50–100 mg/kg per day).

ATAXIA WITH ISOLATED VITAMIN E DEFICIENCY

Ataxia with isolated vitamin E deficiency (AVED) is a rare, autosomal recessively inherited disorder with a phenotype resembling FRDA. AVED patients carry homozygous mutations of the gene encoding the α-tocopherol transport protein, a liver-specific protein that incorporates vitamin E into very low density lipoproteins (36). As a consequence, vitamin E is rapidly eliminated. AVED is a frequent cause of recessive ataxia in North African countries but is rarely encountered in other parts of the world. Since there is no absorption deficit, oral supplementation of vitamin E at a dose of 800–2000 mg/day is recommended.

REFSUM'S DISEASE

Refsum's disease is a rare, autosomal recessively inherited disorder due to mutations in the gene encoding phytanoyl-CoA hydroxylase that is involved in the α-oxidation of phytanic acid (37). The clinical phenotype of Refsum's disease is caused by accumulation of phytanic acid in body tissues. Clinically, Refsum's disease is characterized by ataxia, demyelinating sensorimotor neuropathy, pigmentary retinal degeneration, deafness, cardiac arrhythmias, and ichthyosis-like skin changes. Whereas ocular and hearing problems are usually slowly progressive, there may be acute exacerbations that are precipitated by low caloric intake and mobilization of phytanic acid from adipose tissue.

Refsum's disease is treated by dietary restriction of phytanic acid from the 50–100 mg/day contained in a normal Western diet to less than 10 mg/day. With good dietary supervision, ataxia and neuropathy may improve. In contrast, the progressive loss of vision and hearing cannot be prevented. In acute exacerbations, plasma exchange is effective in lowering phytanic acid levels and improving neurological and cardiac function.

CEREBROTENDINOUS XANTHOMATOSIS

Cerebrotendinous xanthomatosis (CTX) is a rare, autosomal recessively inherited lipid storage disorder with accumulation of cholestanol and cholesterol in various tissues. The disorder is due to mutations of the gene encoding sterol 27-hydroxylase (38). Sterol 27-hydroxylase is responsible for the degradation of 7a-hydroxy-cholesterol to bile acids. As a consequence of the enzymatic defect, there is reduced excretion of bile acids with feces, whereas the content of bile alcohols increases. In addition, cholesterol and 7a-hydroxy-cholesterol are increasingly degraded to cholestanol. It is assumed that CTX is caused by the accumulation of cholestanol.

CTX is a progressive multisystemic disorder. The neurologic syndrome includes ataxia, pyramidal signs, cognitive impairment, epilepsy, and peripheral neuropathy. In addition, patients have chronic diarrhea, xanthomatous tendon swelling, and catatracts. The tendon xanthomas that gave rise to the naming of the diosrder are not obligate, so their absence does not rule out a diagnosis of CTX.

CTX is treated by oral administration of chenodeoxycholate (750 mg/day). Treatment can be further improved by addition of HMG CoA reductase inhibitors, such as simvastatin or lovastatin.

AUTOSOMAL RECESSIVE ATAXIAS WITH KNOWN GENE LOCUS

In a number of recessive ataxias, the chromosomal locus has been found but the affected gene and mutations have not yet been identified.

Linkage to chromosome 6p was demonstrated in an Israeli family with early-onset recessive ataxia. Patients subsequently developed hearing impairment and optic atrophy (39).

Infantile onset spinocerebellar ataxia (IOSCA) is an early-onset recessive ataxia linked to a locus on chromosome 10q that has been described in Finnish families. The disease manifests around the age of 1 year as acute or subacute clumsiness, athetoid movements in hands and face, hypotonia, and loss of deep tendon reflexes in the legs. Ophthalmoplegia and a sensorineural hearing deficit are found by school age, sensory neuropathy and optic atrophy by the age of 10–15 years, and female hypogonadism and epilepsy by the age of 15–20 years. Most patients are wheelchair bound by the age of 20 years (40).

Marinesco-Sjögren syndrome (MSS) is an autosomal recessive condition characterized by cerebellar ataxia, mental retardation, and congenital cataracts. Linkage studies in two large consanguineous families of Turkish and Norwegian origin allowed to map MSS to a locus on chromosome 5q (41). MSS is genetically distinct from the congenital cataracts facial dysmorphism neuropathy (CCFDN) syndrome.

EARLY-ONSET CEREBELLAR ATAXIA

Early-onset cerebellar ataxia (EOCA) denotes those ataxias with an onset before the age of 20 years in which the etiology is unknown. It is assumed that most EOCAs are autosomal recessive disorders.

EOCA with retained tendon reflexes, the most frequent form of EOCA, is clinically distinguished from typical FRDA by the preservation of muscle reflexes. On MRI, these patients have cerebellar atrophy, and disease progression is slower than in FRDA (42).

A highly characteristic, clinically defined variant of EOCA is cerebellar ataxia with hypogonadism (43).

FRAGILE X AND FRAGILE X TREMOR ATAXIA SYNDROME

FXS, also known as *fragile X syndrome*, is the most common inherited form of mental retardation. It is an X-linked disorder caused by a CGG expansion (>200; normal: 6–44) in the 5' region of the FMR1 gene, resulting in hypermethylation of the FMR1 promotor, transcriptional silencing, and loss of FMR1 protein. FMR1 premutations (55–200) are frequent in the general population (females 386:100,000; males 123:100,000) and may give rise to full mutations. Female premutation carriers may have a number of health problems, including premature ovarian failure and emotional problems. Expansions ranging from 45–54 are outside the normal range but are not definite premutations. This range is therefore called *grey area*.

FXTAS is a unique form of clinical involvement in FMR1 older male premutation carriers characterized by progressive action tremor and cerebellar ataxia. These symptoms may be accompanied by cognitive decline, parkinsonism, neuropathy, and autonomic failure. Magnetic resonance imaging (MRI) of FXTAS patients show hyperintense signal changes lateral to the dentate nucleus extending into the middle cerebellar peduncles (44).

In contrast to FXS, FXTAS patients have increased levels of FMR1 mRNA and normal FMR1 protein levels. A recent neuropathological study showed the presence of neuronal intranuclear inclusions (45).

The prevalence and penetrance of FXTAS are unknown. Based on studies in FXS families it has been claimed that FXTAS has an age-dependent but complete penetrance (46). Given the high frequency of FMR1 premutations in the normal population, this would mean that FXTAS should be a frequent cause of ataxia and tremor in older male. On the other hand, screening for FMR1 premutations in male patients with unexplained ataxia yielded variable results. In most studies, including our own study in 390 ataxia patients, the frequency of the FMR1 premutation was less than 0.5%. However, one study reported a frequency of 5% (47).

SPINOCEREBELLAR ATAXIAS

SCA Genetics

The SCAs are a genetically heterogeneous group of autosomal dominant inherited progressive ataxia disorders. Up to now, more than 25 different gene loci have been found. Of the mutations that have been identified so far, SCA1, SCA2, SCA3, SCA6, SCA8, SCA10, SCA12, and SCA17 are expanded repeats. In six of those, SCA1, SCA2, SCA3, SCA6, SCA7, and SCA17, the mutation is a translated CAG repeat expansion coding for an elongated polyglutamine tract within the respective proteins. These disorders belong to a larger group of polyglutamine disorders that also include Huntington disease, dentatorubro-pallidoluysian atrophy (DRPLA), and spinobulbar muscular atrophy. It is assumed that the polyglutamine disorders share important pathogenetic features. In other SCAs, the repeat expansion is found in the 5'untranslated region (SCA12), in an intron (SCA10), or in the 3'untranslated region (SCA8). In two disorders, point mutations were found to cause the disease. SCA14 is due to mutations of the protein kinase Cγ (PKCγ), while another dominant ataxia is caused by mutations in fibroblast growth factor 14 (FGF14) gene (Table 32.3).

SCA Clinical Features

Although ataxia is the prominent symptom in all SCAs, their clinical presentation is diverse. Most SCAs are multisystemic disorders with a clinical syndrome suggesting widespread involvement of the central and peripheral nervous system going far beyond the cerebellum and spinal cord. In particular, the most common forms—SCA1, SCA2, and SCA3— usually present with progressive ataxia accompanied by a variety of additional symptoms. Correspondingly, neuropathological studies show neurodegeneration not only in the spinocerebellar system but also in the cortex, basal ganglia, and brainstem. Only a few mutations are characterized by an almost pure cerebellar syndrome and isolated degeneration of the cerebellar cortex. The most frequent disorder of this group is SCA6.

TABLE 32.3

MUTATIONS AND CLINICAL PHENOTYPES OF SPINOCEREBELLAR ATAXIAS WITH KNOWN MUTATION

SCA1	Translated CAG repeat expansion	Ataxin-1	Ataxia, pyramidal signs, neuropathy, dysphagia, restless legs syndrome
SCA2	Translated CAG repeat expansion	Ataxin-2	Ataxia, slow saccades, neuropathy, restless legs syndrome
SCA3 (Machado-Joseph disease)	Translated CAG repeat expansion	Ataxin-3	Ataxia, pyramidal signs, ophthalmoplegia, neuropathy, dystonia, restless legs syndrome
SCA6	Translated CAG repeat expansion	Calcium channel subunit (CACNA1A)	Almost pure cerebellar ataxia
SCA7	Translated CAG repeat expansion	Ataxin-7	Ataxia, ophthalmoplegia, visual loss
SCA10	Intronic ATTCT repeat expansion	Ataxin-10	Ataxia, epilepsy
SCA12	5′ untranslated CAG repeat expansion	Phosphatase subunit (PP2A-PR55β)	Ataxia, tremor
SCA14	Point mutation	Protein kinase C γ (PKCγ)	Ataxia, myoclonus, dystonia, sensory loss
SCA17	Translated CAG repeat expansion	TATA binding protein (TBP)	Ataxia, dystonia, chorea, dementia, psychiatric abnormalities
FGF14	Point mutation	Fibroblast growth factor 14	Ataxia, tremor, mental retardation

SCA, spinocerebellar ataxia.

SCA Epidemiology

An epidemiological study performed in the Netherlands found a prevalence of SCAs of 0.8–3.0:100,000 (48). Epidemiological data for specific SCA mutations are not available. However, there is some information on the distribution of specific SCA mutations among all dominant ataxias in different population.

SCA Management

Studies of the molecular pathogenesis of the SCAs have not yet resulted in development of therapies that are available for human use. Although it has been repeatedly claimed that a number of centrally acting drugs have antiataxic action, efficacy of these drugs has not been demonstrated convincingly (49). Patients should receive physiotherapy and speech therapy, if necessary.

Spinocerebellar Ataxia Type 1

SCA1 Etiology and Pathogenesis

The mutation causing SCA1 is a translated CAG repeat expansion in a gene coding for ataxin-1. While the repeat length in normals varies between 6–39 trinucleotides, SCA1 patients have one allele within a range of 40–81 repeat units (50). Normal alleles have a midstream CAT interruption and are stably transmitted to the next generation. In contrast, mutated SCA1 alleles contain uninterrupted CAG stretches and are unstable with a tendency to further expansion during meiosis.

Ataxin-1 is ubiquitously expressed within the central nervous system. Its physiological function is poorly understood. SCA1 knockout mice have mild learning disturbances but are otherwise normal. This observation makes it highly improbable that SCA1 is caused by a loss of ataxin-1 function. Rather, it is assumed that the pathogenesis of SCA1 is due to a novel deleterious function of the elongated ataxin-1 protein. To study the pathogenesis of SCA1, various transgenic mouse models have been created (51,52). Studies in these mice showed that nuclear localization of elongated ataxin-1, but not the occurrence of neuronal intranuclear inclusions, is a prerequisite for neurodegeneration (53). Another important finding of these animal studies was that SCA1 transgenic mice develop ataxia before onset of neuronal loss.

Phosphorylation of ataxin-1 at the serine 776 site allows binding of the 14-3-3 protein that stabilizes ataxin-1 by competing with factors mediating its degradation. Ataxin-1 phosphorylation thus contributes to its toxicity (54). There appear to exist several pathways through which elongated ataxin-1 causes neurodegeneration. One pathway is an abnormal interaction of elongated ataxin-1 with transcription factors causing transcriptional dysregulation. Indeed, a number of genes coding for proteins involved in intracellular calcium homeostasis and glutamate signaling are downregulated in Purkinje cells of transgenic SCA1 mice before the occurrence of ataxia (55).

SCA1 Epidemiology

The proportion of SCA1 among all dominant ataxias varies widely from population to population. In Germany, 27% of all families with dominant ataxia harbor the SCA1 mutation. In contrast, the proportion of SCA1 is much lower among Japanese and American families.

SCA1 Neuropathology

Neuropathological abnormalities involve degenerative changes with neuronal cell loss and gliosis in the cerebellar cortex, pontine nuclei, and inferior olives compatible with a neuropathological diagnosis of olivopontocerebellar atrophy. Often, there is additional cell loss in the caudal cranial nerve nuclei. Degeneration within the basal ganglia, thalamus, and cerebral cortex has been found less frequently. In the spinal cord, axonal loss and pallor of myelin are observed in the dorsal column pathways, spinocerebellar tracts, and, less frequently, in the pyramidal tracts (56). Recently, the presence of ubiquitin-positive nuclear inclusions containing ataxin-1 has been demonstrated in surviving neurons of the nucleus centralis pontis.

SCA1 Clinical Presentation

All SCA1 patients suffer from a progressive cerebellar syndrome with ataxia of gait and stance, ataxia of limb movements, dysarthria, and cerebellar oculomotor abnormalities. The oculomotor abnormalities include gaze-evoked nystagmus, saccade hypermetria, broken-up smooth pursuit, reduced optokinetic nystagmus, and impaired suppression of vestibulo-ocular reflex by fixation. In the majority of patients, there are additional noncerebellar symptoms. About half of the patients have supranuclear gaze paresis and/or saccade slowing. Pyramidal tract signs with spasticity, extensor plantar responses, and hyperreflexia are found in more than 50% of SCA1 patients. Decreased vibration sense is found in up to 80% of the SCA1 patients. Dysphagia is a frequent complaint of SCA1 patients and is a clinical problem in late disease stages. Disturbances of sphincter control, mainly bladder dysfunction, occur less frequently and are encountered in about 20% of patients. Basal ganglia symptoms with parkinsonism or dystonia are observed only occasionally. Mental disturbances are encountered in less than 10% of SCA1 patients (57,58).

SCA1 Natural Course

Disease onset in SCA1 varies between adolescence and late adulthood with an average around the age of 35 years. As in other polyglutamine disorders, there is an inverse correlation between CAG repeat length and age of onset. Anticipation has been observed in many SCA1 families. Median latency to become wheelchair bound after disease onset is 14 years, median survival after onset of symptoms 21 years, and median age at death is 56 years (12).

SCA1 Diagnosis

A genetic test demonstrating the CAG repeat expansion of the SCA1 gene is widely available. MRI typically shows cerebellar, brainstem, and spinal cord atrophy (59). Electrophysiological tests often provide evidence of both axonal polyneuropathy and pyramidal dysfunction.

Spinocerebellar Ataxia Type 2

SCA2 Etiology and Pathogenesis

The mutation causing spinocerebellar ataxia type 2 (SCA2) is a translated CAG repeat expansion in a gene coding for ataxin-2. The repeat length in normals varies between 6 and 31 trinucleotides with more than 90% of control alleles having 22 or 23 repeats. SCA2 patients have one allele within a range of 36–63 repeat units. Alleles with a length of 30–34 repeats represent an intermediate range that may give rise to expansion in the offspring. Normal alleles have CAA interruptions. Expanded alleles are unstable with a tendency to further expansion, particularly in father-to-child transmission (60).

Transgenic mice overexpressing an expanded SCA2 allele in cerebellar Purkinje cells show progressive incoordination and morphological alterations of Purkinje cells. In contrast to SCA1, nuclear localization of the abnormal protein is not necessary for the development of the disease (61). Ataxin-2 is a 140 kDa protein with a predominant intracellular localization in the Golgi apparatus. Overexpression of elongated ataxin-2 in cellular models results in disruption of the normal morphology of the Golgi apparatus and subsequent cell death (62).

SCA2 Neuropathology

Autopsy studies of SCA2 patients consistently show olivopontocerebellar atrophy with marked reduction of Purkinje cells, degeneration of the inferior olives, pontine nuclei, and pontocerebellar fibers. In most cases, there are additional degeneration of posterior columns and spinocerebellar pathways and cell loss in the substantia nigra. Ubiquitinated nuclear inclusions have not been observed in SCA2.

SCA2 Epidemiology

The proportion of SCA2 among all dominant ataxias varies from 4%–40%. In the Holguin province of Cuba, the prevalence of SCA2 is as high as 100:100,000 due to a founder effect.

SCA2 Clinical Presentation

All SCA2 patients suffer from a progressive cerebellar syndrome with ataxia of gait and stance, ataxia of limb movements, and dysarthria. Saccade slowing is a highly characteristic feature that is observed in the majority of SCA2 patients. About half of the patients have vertical or horizontal gaze palsy. Cerebellar oculomotor abnormalities are rarely found in SCA2. Typically, tendon reflexes are absent or decreased. Pyramidal tract signs are present in less than 20% of the patients. Vibration sense is decreased in most patients, whereas sensation is otherwise normal (58,63). Atypical SCA2 phenotypes with prominent dementia, an amyotrophic lateral sclerosis (ALS)-like presentation, and levodopa-responsive parkinsonism are also encountered. SCA2 patients usually have shorter expansions.

SCA2 Natural Course

Disease onset in SCA2 varies between childhood and adulthood with an average around the age of 30 years. As in other polyglutamine disorders, there is an inverse correlation between CAG repeat length and age of onset. Anticipation is present in many SCA2 families, in particular if the disease is inherited from the father. Median latency to become wheelchair-bound after disease onset is 15 years, median survival after onset of symptoms is 21 years, and median age at death is 68 years (12).

SCA2 Diagnosis

A genetic test demonstrating the CAG repeat expansion of the SCA2 gene is widely available. MRI typically shows cerebellar and brainstem atrophy suggestive of olivopontocerebellar atrophy (59). In addition, there is atrophy of the spinal cord. Electrophysiological tests often provide evidence of axonal polyneuropathy.

Spinocerebellar Ataxia Type 3

SCA3 Etiology and Pathogenesis

The mutation causing SCA3 is a translated CAG repeat expansion in a gene coding for ataxin-3 (64). The SCA3 mutation was initially found in families with the Machado-Joseph disease phenotype. Machado-Joseph disease denotes an autosomal dominant form of spinocerebellar ataxia with large phenotypical variation, first identified in inhabitants of the Azores Islands (65). After discovery of the gene mutation, it was found that this mutation is frequently found in ataxia families of non-Azorean origin.

Although the repeat length of the SCA3 gene in normals varies between 14 and 37 trinucleotides, SCA3 patients have one allele within a range of 55–84 repeat units. Both the normal and mutated SCA3 genes contain uninterrupted CAG stretches. Expanded SCA3 alleles display intergenerational instability with a tendency to further expansion. As shown by a worldwide haplotype analysis, the majority of abnormal alleles are derived from two founder mutations that originated in Portuguese families settling in the Azores (66).

Ataxin-3 is a 55 kDa protein that is ubiquitiously expressed in the central nervous system. It appears to be a multifunctional protein acting as a ubiquitin protease and a transcriptional repressor (67,68,69). A mouse knockout model has not yet been created, but observations in cellular models suggest that ataxin-3 may have an important cellular function. This raises the question whether a loss of function due to haploinsufficiency contributes to the pathogenesis. Although this is an unsettled question, it is undisputed that, as in other polyglutamine disorders, the elongated disease protein assumes a novel deleterious function and is mainly responsible for the neurodegeneration. Important initial steps of the pathogenesis are abnormal folding and aggregation of expanded ataxin-3. Ataxin-3 then undergoes interactions with a number of cellular proteins, including p97; two human homologues of the yeast DNA repair proteins RAD23, HHR23A, and HHR23B; and transcription factors (70).

SCA3 Neuropathology

SCA3 is a multisystemic disorder characterized by degeneration of spinocerebellar tracts, dentate nucleus, pontine and other brainstem nuclei, substantia nigra, and pallidum. In contrast to most other SCAs, the cerebellar cortex and the inferior olives are widely spared. Nuclear inclusions containing expanded ataxin-3 have been found in neurons of affected brain regions.

SCA3 Epidemiology

SCA3 is the most frequent mutation causing dominant ataxia worldwide. Among German families with dominant ataxia, the proportion of SCA3 is almost 40%. The corresponding figure for U.S. families is 21%. Due to a founder effect, SCA3 is endemic on the Azore islands of Flores and San Miguel, with a prevalence of 700:100,000.

SCA3 Clinical Presentation

The clinical picture of SCA3 is characterized by a wide range of clinical manifestations, the precise nature of which partly depends on repeat length. All SCA3 patients suffer from a progressive syndrome with ataxia of gait and stance, ataxia of limb movements, and dysarthria. Vertical or horizontal gaze palsy are frequent additional findings that occur independently of age of onset. At least 40% of SCA3 patients have a levodopa-responsive restless legs syndrome. Saccade velocity is usually normal. Patients with a repeat length of more than 74 have an early disease onset and clinical features of pyramidal tract and basal ganglia involvement. Most of these patients have increased tendon reflexes, extensor plantar responses, spasticity, and dystonia. Patients with an intermediate repeat length of 71–74 units have a disease onset in middle age and show mainly ataxia and gaze palsy. Patients with a repeat length of less than 71 have a later disease onset and show signs of peripheral neuropathy with loss of tendon reflexes, amyotrophy, and decreased vibration sense. However, the boundaries between these clinical syndromes are vague, and the clinical phenotype of an individual may change with progression of the disease (71).

SCA3 Natural Course

Disease onset in SCA3 varies between adolescence and late adulthood with an average around the age of 42 years. As in other polyglutamine disorders, there is an inverse correlation between CAG repeat length and age of onset. Median latency to become wheelchair bound after disease onset is 15 years, median survival after onset of symptoms is 25 years, and median age at death is 72 years (12).

SCA3 Diagnosis

A genetic test demonstrating the CAG repeat expansion of the SCA3 gene is widely available. MRI typically shows brainstem and spinal cord atrophy. In contrast to other SCAs, cerebellar atrophy is only mild (59). Nerve conduction studies show axonal polyneuropathy, the severity of which increases with age (72).

Spinocerebellar Ataxia Type 6

SCA6 Etiology and Pathogenesis

The mutation causing SCA6 is a CAG repeat expansion in the 3' translated region of the CACNA1A gene coding for the α_{1A} voltage-dependent calcium channel subunit (73). Calcium channels containing the α_{1A} subunit mediate P- and Q-type currents. The α_{1A} subunit is expressed throughout the brain, with the highest expression levels in cerebellar Purkinje cells. In contrast to other CAG repeat mutations, the expansions causing SCA6 are relatively short, ranging between 21 and 27, and do not undergo intergenerational length changes (74).

The pathogenesis of SCA6 is poorly understood. One hypothesis says that SCA6 is due to a gain-of-function mechanism resembling that of other polyglutamine disorders. On the other hand, altered calcium channel function might contribute to the pathogenesis of SCA6. The view that altered calcium channel function may be sufficient to cause progressive ataxia is supported by the observation that a missense mutation in the CACNA1A gene may cause progressive ataxia without episodic features (75). However, it is not clear whether the polyglutamine expansion results in increased or reduced influx of calcium into cerebellar Purkinje neurons (76,77).

SCA6 Neuropathology

Autopsy studies of SCA6 patients consistently show a pure cerebellar degeneration with prominent loss of cerebellar Purkinje neurons. In contrast to other polyglutamine diseases, neurons do not contain ubiquitinated nuclear inclusions but rather cytoplasmic inclusions containing channel protein (78).

SCA6 Epidemiology

The proportion of SCA6 among all dominant ataxias varies from 1%–30% in different populations. SCA6 is the most frequent cause of dominant ataxias with a pure cerebellar presentation.

SCA6 Clinical Presentation

SCA6 patients suffer from a progressive cerebellar syndrome with ataxia of gait and stance, ataxia of limb movements, and dysarthria. Horizontal gaze-evoked nystagmus is almost universally present, and downbeat nystagmus is found in more than half of SCA6 patients. Other cerebellar oculomotor findings are also common, such as impaired smooth pursuit and dysmetric saccades. With disease progression, some SCA6 patients have clinical evidence of noncerebellar involvement, including pyramidal signs and mild sensory disturbances (79).

SCA6 Natural Course

Disease onset in SCA6 is later than in other SCAs and varies between 30 and 75 years. Most patients become ataxic in their fifties. As in other polyglutamine disorders, there is an inverse correlation between CAG repeat length and age of onset. Disease progression in SCA6 is slower than in other SCAs. Although SCA6 is associated with considerable disability, life expectancy is almost normal.

SCA6 Diagnosis

A genetic test demonstrating the CAG repeat expansion of the SCA6 gene is widely available. MRI typically shows pure cerebellar atrophy without involvement of the brainstem. Electrophysiological tests only occasionally reveal abnormalities.

Spinocerebellar Ataxia Type 7

SCA7 Etiology and Pathogenesis

SCA7 is an autosomal dominant inherited ataxia that is distinct from all other SCAs in having the constant additional feature of retinal degeneration. The causative gene mutation is a translated CAG repeat expansion in a gene coding for ataxin-7. The normal range is 7–19 repeats, and the pathogenic alleles range from 37 to more than 300 repeats (80). Expanded alleles are unstable, with a strong tendency to further expansion, particularly in father-to-child transmission. SCA7 patients with childhood onset almost always have inherited the disease from their fathers.

Ataxin-7 is widely expressed through the brain and localized in the cytoplasm of neurons. In patients, ataxin-7 is redistributed to the nucleus to form ubiquitinated intranuclear inclusions. A transgenic mouse model of SCA7 has been created that replicates important features of the disease (81).

SCA7 Neuropathology

Neuropathological examinations of SCA7 patients consistently reveal olivopontocerebellar atrophy. All patients have primarily macular degeneration, which then spreads to involve the retina. There is often secondary atrophy of the optic nerve.

SCA7 Clinical Presentation

The clinical picture of SCA7 partly depends on the age of onset. In patients with late disease onset after the age of 40 years, cerebellar ataxia is the first symptom. There are some exceptional cases in which people never develop visual problems. In most patients, however, ataxia is followed by progressive loss of vision. In about half of the patients with late disease onset, there is no evidence of retinal degeneration or optic atrophy, suggesting that retinopathy only affects the macula. All patients with disease onset earlier than the age of 40 years have visual problems, starting either prior to or at the same time as cerebellar ataxia. The majority of these patients have retinal degeneration, some of them also optic atrophy. Tendon reflexes are usually absent. There are a number of additional symptoms that occur in less than half of the patients and that tend be more frequent in patients with long disease duration. These symptoms include gaze palsy, dysphagia, hearing loss, and muscle weakness. Dementia and basal ganglia symptoms are not typical features of SCA7 (82).

SCA7 Natural Course

Mean age of disease onset of SCA7 is 30 years, with a wide variation from 3 months to 70 years. As in other polyglutamine disorders, there is an inverse correlation between CAG repeat length and age of onset. Disease progression is more rapid in patients with early disease onset. On average, patients with juvenile disease onset die 5 years after disease onset, whereas patients with adult onset survive for about 15 years.

Other Rare Spinocerebellar Ataxias

Spinocerebellar Ataxia Type 4

Spinocerebellar ataxia type 4 (SCA4) is characterized by the combination of progressive ataxia and sensory axonal neuropathy. The SCA4 locus has been mapped to chromosome 16q, but the gene mutation has not yet been found (83). Japanese families with a cerebellar phenotpye have been linked to the same chromosomal region, suggesting that the disorder is an allelic variant of SCA4 (84).

Spinocerebellar Ataxia Type 5

Spinocerebellar ataxia type 5 (SCA5) is characterized by a pure cerebellar phenotype. Linkage with the SCA5 gene locus on the centromeric region of chromosome 11 was established in a family descended from the grandparents of President Abraham Lincoln (85). Another family was reported from Germany (86).

Spinocerebellar Ataxia Type 8

Spinocerebellar ataxia type 8 (SCA8) was defined in a large multigenerational family with incomplete penetrance. The mutation is a CTG repeat expansion in the 3' region of the gene located on chromosome 13q (87). Other families have not been identified, but the SCA8 mutation has been found in patients with sporadic ataxia. Nevertheless, there remains considerable doubt whether the CTG expansion at the SCA8 locus is causative because there is considerable overlap between the repeat lengths in normals, ataxia patients, and patients with other neuropsychiatric disorders (88).

Spinocerebellar Ataxia Type 10

Spinocerebellar ataxia type 10 (SCA10) is caused by massive expansions of an intronic ATTCT pentanucleotide repeat in the ataxin-10 gene located on chromosome 22q. Normal repeats range from 10–22 units, and the expanded repeats may have up to 4500 units (89). Ataxin-10 belongs to the family of armadillo repeat proteins and has an essential function for neuronal survival. All known SCA10 families are of either Mexican or Brazilian origin. In the Mexican families, SCA10 is frequently associated with epilepsy (90).

Spinocerebellar Ataxia Type 11

Two British families have been mapped to the spinocerebellar ataxia type 11 (SCA11) locus on chromosome 15q. Clinically, SCA11 is characterized by an almost pure cerebellar syndrome (91).

Spinocerebellar Ataxia Type 12

Spinocerebellar ataxia type 12 (SCA12) is caused by a CAG repeat expansion in the 5' untranslated region of a gene encoding a regulatory subunit of a phosphatase expressed in the brain (92). SCA12 accounts for 5%–10% of all dominant ataxias in India (93). The prominent clinical features of SCA12 are ataxia and tremor.

Spinocerebellar Ataxia Type 13

The spinocerebellar ataxia type 13 (SCA13) locus on chromosome 19q was established in a single, large French family characterized by slowly progressive ataxia with onset in childhood and moderate mental retardation (94).

Spinocerebellar Ataxia Type 14

Spinocerebellar ataxia type 14 (SCA14) is caused by missense mutations of the protein kinase Cγ (PKCγ) gene (95). The clinical phenotype includes late-onset cerebellar ataxia, axial myoclonus, hand dystonia, and mild sensory loss.

Spinocerebellar Ataxia Type 15

The spinocerebellar ataxia type 15 (SCA15) locus on chromosome 3p was found in a large Australian family with pure cerebellar ataxia (96). Linkage to the same region was recently demonstrated in two Japanese families (97).

Spinocerebellar Ataxia Type 16

The spinocerebellar ataxia type 16 (SCA16) locus was described in a four-generation Japanese family with an almost pure cerebellar phenotype. The locus was mapped to chromosome 8q (98).

Spinocerebellar Ataxia Type 17

Spinocerebellar ataxia type 17 (SCA17) is caused by a CAG repeat expansion in the coding region of the TATA binding protein (TBP) gene (99). SCA17 thus belongs to the group of polyglutamine disorders. Clinically, SCA17 is characterized by ataxia, dystonia, dementia, and other psychiatric abnormalities (100,101).

Spinocerebellar Ataxia Type 18

The spinocerebellar ataxia type 18 (SCA18) locus on chromosome 7q was established in a five-generation American family of Irish ancestry presenting with ataxia associated with peripheral neuropathy (102).

Spinocerebellar Ataxia Type 19

The spinocerebellar ataxia type 19 (SCA19) locus on chromosome 1p was identified in a four-generation Dutch family suffering from mild progressive ataxia associated with cognitive impairment, myoclonus, and postural tremor (103). The same locus was independently found in a Chinese family (104,105).

Spinocerebellar Ataxia Type 20

The spinocerebellar ataxia type 20 (SCA20) locus was identified in a family of Anglo-Celtic origin with an unusual clinical presentation, including dysarthria, dysphonia, and palatal tremor. MRIs showed calcification of the dentate nucleus. The SCA20 maps to the centromeric region of chromosome 11, overlapping with the SCA5 locus. Nevertheless, the SCA20 locus was provisionally assigned due to the unique phenotpye of the affected family (106).

Spinocerebellar Ataxia Type 21

Linkage analysis in a French family with slowly progressive ataxia variably associated with cognitive impairment, parkinsonian features, and hyporeflexia led to the definition of the spinocerebellar ataxia type 21 (SCA21) locus on chromosome 7p (107).

Spinocerebellar Ataxia Type 23

Spinocerebellar ataxia type 23 (SCA23) is another locus identified in a large Dutch family. It maps to chromosome 20p. Clinically, SCA23 is characterized by a relatively pure, slowly progressive cerebellar ataxia (108).

Spinocerebellar Ataxia Type 25

Spinocerebellar ataxia type 25 (SCA25) was defined in a French family with ataxia and sensory neuropathy. The locus lies on chromosome 2p (109).

Spinocerebellar Ataxia Type 26

Spinocerebellar ataxia type 26 (SCA26) is a new locus on chromosome 19p adjacent to SCA6 that was identified in a family of Norwegian origin with pure cerebellar ataxia (110).

Fibroblast Growth Factor 14

A missense mutation in the fibroblast growth factor 14 (FGF14) gene was found to be associated with slowly progressive ataxia, tremor, and mild mental retardation in a Dutch family (111). Subsequent studies showed that FGF14 mutations are no frequent causes of dominant ataxia (112).

Episodic Ataxia Type 1

EA1 Etiology and Pathogenesis

Episodic ataxia type 1 (EA1) is a rare disorder caused by point mutations in the KCNA1 gene encoding the pore-forming α subunit of the voltage-gated potassium channels Kv1.1 (113). Voltage-gated potassium channels consisting of Kv1.1 give rise to delayed-rectifier–type potassium currents. Mutations causing EA1 are found in highly conserved regions of the protein. Recently, a transgenic mouse model of EA1 displaying stress-induced incoordination was created (114).

EA1 Clinical Presentation

Clinically, EA1 is characterized by brief attacks of ataxia and dysarthria. The attacks last for seconds to minutes and may occur several times per day. They are often provoked by movements and startle. Apart from ataxia, the attacks may have dystonic or choreic features. EA1 is associated with interictal myokymia (i.e., twitching of small muscles around the eyes or in the hands). Ataxia or gaze-evoked nystagmus are absent between attacks.

EA1 Natural Course

EA1 starts in early childhood. It has a favorable prognosis and does not result in permanent disability. In most patients, attacks become milder with increasing age.

EA1 Diagnosis

Since a genetic test for EA1 is not routinely available, the diagnosis is based on a carefully taken history and clinical examination. In EA1, interictal electromyography (EMG) of muscles displaying myokymia shows spontaneous repetitive discharges that subside after nerve blockade. Imaging studies give normal results.

EA1 Management

Some patients learn to prevent attacks by avoiding sudden abrupt movements. If medical treatment is required, acetazolamide (500–700 mg/day) is used to prevent attacks (115). However, the action of acetazolamide is less reliable than in EA2. As a second-line treatment, carbamazepine and phenytoin can be tried.

Episodic Ataxia Type 2

EA2 Etiology and Pathogenesis

EA2 is a rare disorder caused by nonsense mutations causing truncation of the CACNA1A gene coding for the α_{1A} voltage-dependent calcium channel subunit (116). Missense mutations of the same gene are associated with familial hemiplegic migraine, whereas a CAG repeat expansion in the 3' end of the gene causes SCA6 (73,116). Expression of mutations causing EA2 in cell systems causes impairment of calcium channel function (117).

EA2 Clinical Presentation

Compared with EA1, attacks in EA2 last longer and are precipitated by emotional stress and exercise but not by startle. The episodes vary from pure ataxia to combinations of symptoms suggesting involvement of the cerebellum and brainstem and even occasionally the cortex. Vertigo, nausea, and vomiting are the most common associated symptoms, being present in more than 50% of patients. About half of the patients report headaches that meet criteria for migraine. Between attacks, many EA2 patients have a gaze-evoked nystagmus. With increasing age, some patients develop mild ataxia of gait and stance.

EA2 Natural Course

The age of onset in EA2 varies from 2–30 years. Although EA2 is principally an episodic disorder, some patients develop a persistent or slowly progressive ataxia.

EA2 Diagnosis

Since a genetic test for EA2 is not routinely available, the diagnosis is based on a carefully taken history and clinical examination. EA2 patients may have mild cerebellar atrophy.

EA2 Management

Acetazolamide (500–700 mg/day) is used to prevent attacks (118). Alternatively, 4-aminopyridine (10 mg/day), carbamazepine, or phenytoin may be used (119).

REFERENCES

1. Campuzano V, Montermini L, Moltò MD, et al. Friedreich's ataxia: autosomal recessive disease caused by an intronic GAA triplet repeat expansion. *Science* 1996;271:1423–1427.
2. Cossee M, Dürr A, Schmitt M, et al. Friedreich's ataxia: point mutations and clinical presentation of compound heterozygotes. *Ann Neurol* 1999;45:200–206.
3. Christodoulou K, Deymeer F, Serdaroglu P, et al. Mapping of the second Friedreich's ataxia (FRDA2) locus to chromosome 9p23-p11: evidence for further locus heterogeneity. *Neurogenetics* 2001;3:127–132.
4. Cossee M, Puccio H, Gansmuller A, et al. Inactivation of the Friedreich ataxia mouse gene leads to early embryonic lethality without iron accumulation. *Hum Mol Genet* 2000;9:1219–1226.
5. Puccio H, Simon D, Cossee M, et al. Mouse models for Friedreich ataxia exhibit cardiomyopathy, sensory nerve defect and Fe-S enzyme deficiency followed by intramitochondrial iron deposits. *Nat Genet* 2001;27:181–186.
6. Gakh O, Park S, Liu G, et al. Mitochondrial iron detoxification is a primary function of frataxin that limits oxidative damage and preserves cell longevity. *Hum Mol Genet* 2006;15:467–479.
7. O'Neill HA, Gakh O, Park S, et al. Assembly of human frataxin is a mechanism for detoxifying redox-active iron. *Biochemistry* 2005;44:537–545.
8. Rotig A, De Lonlay P, Chretien D, et al. Aconitase and mitochondrial iron-sulphur protein deficiency in Friedreich ataxia. *Nat Genet* 1997;17:215–217.
9. Leone M, Bottacchi E, D'Alessandro G, Kustermann S. Hereditary ataxias and paraplegias in Valle d'Aosta, Italy: a study of prevalence and disability. *Acta Neurol Scand* 1995;91:183–187.
10. Polo JM, Calleja J, Combarros O, Berciano J. Hereditary ataxias and paraplegias in Cantabria, Spain: an epidemiological and clinical study. *Brain* 1991;114:855–866.
11. Dürr A, Cossee M, Agid Y, et al. Clinical and genetic abnormalities in patients with Friedreich's ataxia. *N Engl J Med* 1996;335:1169–1175.
12. Klockgether T, Lüdtke R, Kramer B, et al. The natural history of degenerative ataxia: a retrospective study in 466 patients. *Brain* 1998;121:589–600.
13. Wüllner U, Klockgether T, Petersen D, Naegele T, Dichgans J. Magnetic resonance imaging in hereditary and idiopathic ataxia. *Neurology* 1993;43:318–325.
14. Rustin P, vonKleistRetzow JC, ChantrelGroussard K, Sidi D, Munnich A, Rotig A. Effect of idebenone on cardiomyopathy in Friedreich's ataxia: a preliminary study. *Lancet* 1999;354:477–479.
15. Hausse AO, Aggoun Y, Bonnet D, et al. Idebenone and reduced cardiac hypertrophy in Friedreich's ataxia. *Heart* 2002;87:346–349.
16. Buyse G, Mertens L, Di Salvo G, et al. Idebenone treatment in Friedreich's ataxia: neurological, cardiac, and biochemical monitoring. *Neurology* 2003;60:1679–1681.
17. Mariotti C, Solari A, Torta D, Marano L, Fiorentini C, Di Donato S. Idebenone treatment in Friedreich patients: one-year-long randomized placebo-controlled trial. *Neurology* 2003;60:1676–1679.
18. Savitsky K, Bar-Shira A, Gilad S, et al. A single ataxia telangiectasia gene with a product similar to PI-3 kinase. *Science* 1995;268:1749–1753.
19. Stewart GS, Maser RS, Stankovic T, et al. The DNA double-strand break repair gene hMRE11 is mutated in individuals with an ataxia-telangiectasia-like disorder. *Cell* 1999;99:577–587.
20. Filla A, De-Michele G, Marconi R, et al. Prevalence of hereditary ataxias and spastic paraplegias in Molise, a region of Italy. *J Neurol* 1992;239:351–353.
21. Habeck M, Zuhlke C, Bentele KH, et al. Aprataxin mutations are a rare cause of early onset ataxia in Germany. *J Neurol* 2004;251:591–594.
22. Barbot C, Coutinho P, Chorao R, et al. Recessive ataxia with ocular apraxia: review of 22 Portuguese patients. *Arch Neurol* 2001;58:201–205.
23. Moreira MC, Barbot C, Tachi N, et al. The gene mutated in ataxia-ocular apraxia 1 encodes the new HIT/Zn- finger protein aprataxin. *Nat Genet* 2001;29:189–193.
24. Date H, Onodera O, Tanaka H, et al. Early-onset ataxia with ocular motor apraxia and hypoalbuminemia is caused by mutations in a new HIT superfamily gene. *Nat Genet* 2001;29:184–188.
25. Sano Y, Date H, Igarashi S, et al. Aprataxin, the causative protein for EAOH is a nuclear protein with a potential role as a DNA repair protein. *Ann Neurol* 2004;55:241–249.
26. Quinzii CM, Kattah AG, Naini A, et al. Coenzyme Q deficiency and cerebellar ataxia associated with an aprataxin mutation. *Neurology* 2005;64:539–541.
27. Le Ber I, Moreira MC, Rivaud-Pechoux S, et al. Cerebellar ataxia with oculomotor apraxia type 1: clinical and genetic studies. *Brain* 2003;126:2761–2772.
28. Moreira MC, Klur S, Watanabe M, et al. Senataxin, the ortholog of a yeast RNA helicase, is mutant in ataxia-ocular apraxia 2. *Nat Genet* 2004;36:225–227.
29. Le Ber I, Bouslam N, Rivaud-Pechoux S, et al. Frequency and phenotypic spectrum of ataxia with oculomotor apraxia 2: a clinical and genetic study in 18 patients. *Brain* 2004;127:759–767.

30. Duquette A, Roddier K, McNabb-Baltar J, et al. Mutations in senataxin responsible for Quebec cluster of ataxia with neuropathy. *Ann Neurol* 2005;57:408–414.
31. Takashima H, Boerkoel CF, John J, et al. Mutation of TDP1, encoding a topoisomerase I-dependent DNA damage repair enzyme, in spinocerebellar ataxia with axonal neuropathy. *Nat Genet* 2002;32:267–272.
32. Engert JC, Berube P, Mercier J, et al. ARSACS, a spastic ataxia common in northeastern Quebec, is caused by mutations in a new gene encoding an 11.5-kb ORF. *Nat Genet* 2000;24:120–125.
33. Grieco GS, Malandrini A, Comanducci G, et al. Novel SACS mutations in autosomal recessive spastic ataxia of Charlevoix-Saguenay type. *Neurology* 2004;62:103–106.
34. Mercier J, Prevost C, Engert JC, Bouchard JP, Mathieu J, Richter A. Rapid detection of the sacsin mutations causing autosomal recessive spastic ataxia of Charlevoix-Saguenay. *Genet Test* 2001;5:255–259.
35. Sharp D, Blinderman L, Combs KA, et al. Cloning and gene defects in microsomal triglyceride transfer protein associated with abetalipoproteinaemia. *Nature* 1993;365:65–69.
36. Ouahchi K, Arita M, Kayden H, et al. Ataxia with isolated vitamin E deficiency is caused by mutations in the alpha-tocopherol transfer protein. *Nature Genet* 1995;9:141–145.
37. Jansen GA, Ofman R, Ferdinandusse S, et al. Refsum disease is caused by mutations in the phytanoyl-CoA hydroxylase gene. *Nat Genet* 1997;17:190–193.
38. Leitersdorf E, Reshef A, Meiner V, et al. Frameshift and splice-junction mutations in the sterol 27-hydroxylase gene cause cerebrotendinous xanthomatosis in Jews or Moroccan origin. *J Clin Invest* 1993;91:2488–2496.
39. Bomont P, Watanabe M, Gershoni-Barush R, et al. Homozygosity mapping of spinocerebellar ataxia with cerebellar atrophy and peripheral neuropathy to 9q33–34, and with hearing impairment and optic atrophy to 6p21–23. *Eur J Human Genet* 2000;8:986–990.
40. Lonnqvist T, Paetau A, Nikali K, von Boguslawski K, Pihko H. Infantile onset spinocerebellar ataxia with sensory neuropathy (IOSCA): neuropathological features. *J Neurol Sci* 1998;161:57–65.
41. Lagier-Tourenne C, Tranebaerg L, Chaigne D, et al. Homozygosity mapping of Marinesco-Sjogren syndrome to 5q31. *Eur J Hum Genet* 2003;11:770–778.
42. Klockgether T, Petersen D, Grodd W, Dichgans J. Early onset cerebellar ataxia with retained tendon reflexes: clinical, electrophysiological, and MRI observations in comparison with Friedreich's ataxia. *Brain* 1991;114:1559–1573.
43. Matthews WB, Rundle AT. Familial cerebellar ataxia and hypogonadism. *Brain* 1964;87:463–468.
44. Jacquemont S, Hagerman RJ, Leehey M, et al. Fragile X premutation tremor/ataxia syndrome: molecular, clinical, and neuro-imaging correlates. *Am J Hum Genet* 2003;72:869–878.
45. Moore CJ, Daly EM, Tassone F, et al. The effect of pre-mutation of X chromosome CGG trinucleotide repeats on brain anatomy. *Brain* 2004;127:2672–2681.
46. Jacquemont S, Hagerman RJ, Leehey MA, et al. Penetrance of the fragile X-associated tremor/ataxia syndrome in a premutation carrier population. *JAMA* 2004;291:460–469.
47. Macpherson J, Waghorn A, Hammans S, Jacobs P. Observation of an excess of fragile-X premutations in a population of males referred with spinocerebellar ataxia. *Hum Genet* 2003;112:619–620.
48. Van de Warrenburg BP, Sinke RJ, Verschuuren-Bemelmans CC, et al. Spinocerebellar ataxias in the Netherlands: prevalence and age at onset variance analysis. *Neurology* 2002;58:702–708.
49. Ogawa M. Pharmacological treatments of cerebellar ataxia. *Cerebellum* 2004;3:107–111.
50. Orr HT, Chung MY, Banfi S, et al. Expansion of an unstable trinucleotide CAG repeat in spinocerebellar ataxia type 1. *Nat Genet* 1993;4:221–226.
51. Burright EN, Clark HB, Servadio A, et al. SCA1 transgenic mice: a model for neurodegeneration caused by an expanded CAG trinucleotide repeat. *Cell* 1995;82:937–948.
52. Watase K, Weeber EJ, Xu B, et al. A long CAG repeat in the mouse Sca1 locus replicates SCA1 features and reveals the impact of protein solubility on selective neurodegeneration. *Neuron* 2002;34:905–919.
53. Klement IA, Skinner PJ, Kaytor MD, et al. Ataxin-1 nuclear localization and aggregation: role in polyglutamine-induced disease in SCA1 transgenic mice [see comments]. *Cell* 1998;95:41–53.
54. Chen HK, Fernandez-Funez P, Acevedo SF, et al. Interaction of Akt-phosphorylated ataxin-1 with 14-3-3 mediates neurodegeneration in spinocerebellar ataxia type 1. *Cell* 2003;113:457–468.
55. Lin X, Antalffy B, Kang D, Orr HT, Zoghbi HY. Polyglutamine expansion down-regulates specific neuronal genes before pathologic changes in SCA1. *Nat Neurosci* 2000;3:157–163.
56. Genis D, Matilla T, Volpini V, et al. Clinical, neuropathologic, and genetic studies of a large spinocerebellar ataxia type 1 (SCA1) kindred: (CAG)$_n$ expansion and early premonitory signs and symptoms. *Neurology* 1995;45:24–30.
57. Dubourg O, Dürr A, Cancel G, et al. Analysis of the SCA1 CAG repeat in a large number of families with dominant ataxia: clinical and molecular correlations. *Ann Neurol* 1995;37:176–180.
58. Bürk K, Abele M, Fetter M, et al. Autosomal dominant cerebellar ataxia type I: clinical features and MRI in families with SCA1, SCA2 and SCA3. *Brain* 1996;119:1497–1505.
59. Klockgether T, Skalej M, Wedekind D, et al. Autosomal dominant cerebellar ataxia type I. MRI-based volumetry of posterior fossa structures and basal ganglia in spinocerebellar ataxia types 1, 2 and 3. *Brain* 1998;121:1687–1693.
60. Pulst SM, Nechiporuk A, Nechiporuk T, et al. Moderate expansion of a normally biallelic trinucleotide repeat in spinocerebellar ataxia type 2. *Nature Genet* 1996;14:269–276.
61. Huynh DP, Figueroa K, Hoang N, Pulst SM. Nuclear localization or inclusion body formation of ataxin-2 are not necessary for SCA2 pathogenesis in mouse or human. *Nat Genet* 2000;26:44–50.
62. Huynh DP, Yang HT, Vakharia H, Nguyen D, Pulst SM. Expansion of the polyQ repeat in ataxin-2 alters its Golgi localization, disrupts the Golgi complex and causes cell death. *Hum Mol Genet* 2003;12:1485–1496.
63. Schöls L, Gispert S, Vorgerd M, et al. Spinocerebellar ataxia type 2: genotype and phenotype in German kindreds. *Arch Neurol* 1997;54:1073–1080.
64. Kawaguchi Y, Okamoto T, Taniwaki M, et al. CAG expansions in a novel gene for Machado-Joseph disease at chromosome 14q32.1. *Nature Genet* 1994;8:221–228.
65. Rosenberg RN. Machado-Joseph disease: an autosomal dominant motor system degeneration. *Mov Disord* 1992;7:193–203.
66. Gaspar C, LopesCendes I, Hayes S, et al. Ancestral origins of the Machado-Joseph disease mutation: a worldwide haplotype study. *Amer J Hum Genet* 2001;68:523–528.
67. Burnett B, Li F, Pittman RN. The polyglutamine neurodegenerative protein ataxin-3 binds polyubiquitylated proteins and has ubiquitin protease activity. *Hum Mol Genet* 2003;12:3195–3205.
68. Li F, Macfarlan T, Pittman RN, Chakravarti D. Ataxin-3 is a histone-binding protein with two independent transcriptional corepressor activities. *J Biol Chem* 2002;277:45,004–45,012.
69. Evert BO, Vogt IR, Vieira-Saecker AM, et al. Gene expression profiling in ataxin-3 expressing cell lines reveals distinct effects of normal and mutant ataxin-3. *J Neuropathol Exp Neurol* 2003;62:1006–1018.
70. Zhong X, Pittman RN. Ataxin-3 binds VCP/p97 and regulates retrotranslocation of ERAD substrates. *Hum Mol Genet* 2006; Jul 5:[Epub ahead of print].
71. Maciel P, Gaspar C, DeStefano AL, et al. Correlation between CAG repeat length and clinical features in Machado-Joseph disease. *Am J Hum Genet* 1995;57:54–61.
72. Klockgether T, Schols L, Abele M, et al. Age-related axonal neuropathy in spinocerebellar ataxia type 3/Machado-Joseph disease (SCA3/MJD). *J Neurol Neurosurg Psychiatry* 1999;66:222–224.
73. Zhuchenko O, Bailey J, Bonnen P, et al. Autosomal dominant cerebellar ataxia (SCA6) associated with small polyglutamine expansions in the alpha 1A voltage-dependent calcium channel. *Nature Genet* 1997;15:62–69.
74. Matsuyama Z, Kawakami H, Maruyama H, et al. Molecular features of the CAG repeats of spinocerebellar ataxia 6 (SCA6). *Hum Mol Genet* 1997;6:1283–1287.
75. Yue Q, Jen JC, Nelson SF, Baloh RW. Progressive ataxia due to a missense mutation in a calcium-channel gene. *Am J Hum Genet* 1997;61:1078–1087.

76. Matsuyama Z, Yanagisawa NK, Aoki Y, et al. Polyglutamine repeats of spinocerebellar ataxia 6 impair the cell-death-preventing effect of CaV2.1 Ca2+ channel–loss-of-function cellular model of SCA6. *Neurobiol Dis* 2004;17:198–204.

77. Restituito S, Thompson RM, Eliet J, et al. The polyglutamine expansion in spinocerebellar ataxia type 6 causes a beta subunit-specific enhanced activation of P/Q-type calcium channels in Xenopus oocytes. *J Neurosci* 2000;20:6394–6403.

78. Ishikawa K, Fujigasaki H, Saegusa H, et al. Abundant expression and cytoplasmic aggregations of [alpha]1A voltage-dependent calcium channel protein associated with neurodegeneration in spinocerebellar ataxia type 6. *Hum Mol Genet* 1999;8:1185–1193.

79. Geschwind DH, Perlman S, Figueroa KP, Karrim J, Baloh RW, Pulst SM. Spinocerebellar ataxia type 6: frequency of the mutation and genotype-phenotype correlations. *Neurology* 1997;49:1247–1251.

80. David G, Abbas N, Stevanin G, et al. Cloning of the SCA7 gene reveals a highly unstable CAG repeat expansion. *Nat Genet* 1997;17:65–70.

81. Yvert G, Lindenberg KS, Picaud S, Landwehrmeyer GB, Sahel JA, Mandel JL. Expanded polyglutamines induce neurodegeneration and trans-neuronal alterations in cerebellum and retina of SCA7 transgenic mice. *Hum Mol Genet* 2000;9:2491–2506.

82. Enevoldson TP, Sanders MD, Harding AE. Autosomal dominant cerebellar ataxia with pigmentary macular dystrophy: a clinical and genetic study of eight families. *Brain* 1994;117:445–460.

83. Flanigan K, Gardner K, Alderson K, et al. Autosomal dominant spinocerebellar ataxia with sensory axonal neuropathy (SCA4): clinical description and genetic localization to chromosome 16q22.1. *Am J Hum Genet* 1996;59:392–399.

84. Hirano R, Takashima H, Okubo R, et al. Fine mapping of 16q-linked autosomal dominant cerebellar ataxia type III in Japanese families. *Neurogenetics* 2004;5:215–221.

85. Ikeda Y, Dick KA, Weatherspoon MR, et al. Spectrin mutations cause spinocerebellar ataxia type 5. *Nat Genet* 2006;38:184–190.

86. Bürk K, Zuhlke C, Konig IR, et al. Spinocerebellar ataxia type 5: clinical and molecular genetic features of a German kindred. *Neurology* 2004;62:327–329.

87. Koob MD, Moseley ML, Schut LJ, et al. An untranslated CTG expansion causes a novel form of spinocerebellar ataxia (SCA8). *Nat Genet* 1999;21:379–384.

88. Schöls L, Bauer I, Zühlke C, et al. Do CTG expansions at the SCA8 locus cause ataxia? *Ann Neurol* 2003;54:110–115.

89. Matsuura T, Yamagata T, Burgess DL, et al. Large expansion of the ATTCT pentanucleotide repeat in spinocerebellar ataxia type 10. *Nat Genet* 2000;26:191–194.

90. Teive HA, Roa BB, Raskin S, et al. Clinical phenotype of Brazilian families with spinocerebellar ataxia 10. *Neurology* 2004;63:1509–1512.

91. Worth PF, Giunti P, Gardner TC, Dixon PH, Davis MB, Wood NW. Autosomal dominant cerebellar ataxia type III: linkage in a large British family to a 7.6-cM region on chromosome 15q14-21.3. *Am J Hum Genet* 1999;65:420–426.

92. Holmes SE, O'Hearn EE, McInnis MG, et al. Expansion of a novel CAG trinucleotide repeat in the 5′ region of PPP2R2B is associated with SCA12 [letter]. *Nat Genet* 1999;23:391–392.

93. Srivastava AK, Choudhry S, Gopinath MS, et al. Molecular and clinical correlation in five Indian families with spinocerebellar ataxia 12. *Ann Neurol* 2001;50:796–800.

94. HermanBert A, Stevanin G, Netter JC, et al. Mapping of spinocerebellar ataxia 13 to chromosome 19q13.3–q13.4 in a family with autosomal dominant cerebellar ataxia and mental retardation. *Amer J Hum Genet* 2000;67:229–235.

95. Yabe I, Sasaki H, Chen DH, et al. Spinocerebellar ataxia type 14 caused by a mutation in protein kinase C gamma. *Arch Neurol* 2003;60:1749–1751.

96. Knight MA, Kennerson ML, Anney RJ, et al. Spinocerebellar ataxia 15 (sca15) maps to 3p24.2-3pter: exclusion of the ITPR1 gene, the human orthologue of an ataxic mouse mutant. *Neurobiol Dis* 2003;13:147–157.

97. Hara K, Fukushima T, Suzuki T, et al. Japanese SCA families with an unusual phenotype linked to a locus overlapping with SCA15 locus. *Neurology* 2004;62:648–651.

98. Miyoshi Y, Yamada T, Tanimura M, et al. A novel autosomal dominant spinocerebellar ataxia (SCA16) linked to chromosome 8q22.1-24.1. *Neurology* 2001;57:96–100.

99. Nakamura K, Jeong SY, Uchihara T, et al. SCA17, a novel autosomal dominant cerebellar ataxia caused by an expanded polyglutamine in TATA-binding protein. *Hum Mol Genet* 2001;10:1441–1448.

100. Zühlke C, Hellenbroich Y, Dalski A, et al. Different types of repeat expansion in the TATA-binding protein gene are associated with a new form of inherited ataxia. *Eur J Hum Genet* 2001;9:160–164.

101. Rolfs A, Koeppen AH, Bauer I, et al. Clinical features and neuropathology of autosomal dominant spinocerebellar ataxia (SCA17). *Ann Neurol* 2003;54:367–375.

102. Brkanac Z, Fernandez M, Matsushita M, et al. Autosomal dominant sensory/motor neuropathy with ataxia (SMNA): linkage to chromosome 7q22-q32. *Am J Med Genet* 2002;114:450–457.

103. Verbeek DS, Schelhaas JH, Ippel EF, Beemer FA, Pearson PL, Sinke RJ. Identification of a novel SCA locus (SCA19) in a Dutch autosomal dominant cerebellar ataxia family on chromosome region 1p21-q21. *Hum Genet* 2002;111:388–393.

104. Schelhaas HJ, Verbeek DS, van de Warrenburg BP, Sinke RJ. SCA19 and SCA22: evidence for one locus with a worldwide distribution. *Brain* 2004;127:E6.

105. Chung MY, Lu YC, Cheng NC, Soong BW. A novel autosomal dominant spinocerebellar ataxia (SCA22) linked to chromosome 1p21-q23. *Brain* 2003;126(pt 6):1293–1299.

106. Knight MA, Gardner RJ, Bahlo M, et al. Dominantly inherited ataxia and dysphonia with dentate calcification: spinocerebellar ataxia type 20. *Brain* 2004;127:1172–1181.

107. Vuillaume I, Devos D, Schraen-Maschke S, et al. A new locus for spinocerebellar ataxia (SCA21) maps to chromosome 7p21.3–p15.1. *Ann Neurol* 2002;52:666–670.

108. Verbeek DS, van de Warrenburg BP, Wesseling P, Pearson PL, Kremer HP, Sinke RJ. Mapping of the SCA23 locus involved in autosomal dominant cerebellar ataxia to chromosome region 20p13-12.3. *Brain* 2004;127:2551–2557.

109. Stevanin G, Bouslam N, Thobois S, et al. Spinocerebellar ataxia with sensory neuropathy (SCA25) maps to chromosome 2p. *Ann Neurol* 2004;55:97–104.

110. Yu GY, Howell MJ, Roller MJ, Xie TD, Gomez CM. Spinocerebellar ataxia type 26 maps to chromosome 19p13.3 adjacent to SCA6. *Ann Neurol* 2005;57:349–354.

111. Van Swieten JC, Brusse E, de Graaf BM, et al. A mutation in the fibroblast growth factor 14 gene is associated with autosomal dominant cerebellar ataxia. *Am J Hum Genet* 2003;72:191–199.

112. Dalski A, Atici J, Kreuz FR, Hellenbroich Y, Schwinger E, Zühlke C. Mutation analysis in the fibroblast growth factor 14 gene: frameshift mutation and polymorphisms in patients with inherited ataxias. *Eur J Hum Genet* 2005;13:118–120.

113. Browne DL, Gancher ST, Nutt JG, et al. Episodic ataxia/myokymia syndrome is associated with point mutations in the human potassium channel gene, KCNA1. *Nature Genet* 1994;8:136–140.

114. Herson PS, Virk M, Rustay NR, et al. A mouse model of episodic ataxia type-1. *Nat Neurosci* 2003;6:378–383.

115. Griggs RC, Moxley RT, Lafrance RA, McQuillen J. Hereditary paroxysmal ataxia: response to acetazolamide. *Neurology* 1978;28:1259–1264.

116. Ophoff RA, Terwindt GM, Vergouwe MN, et al. Familial hemiplegic migraine and episodic ataxia type-2 are caused by mutations in the Ca2+ channel gene CACNL1A4. *Cell* 1996;87:543–552.

117. Spacey SD, Hildebrand ME, Materek LA, Bird TD, Snutch TP. Functional implications of a novel EA2 mutation in the P/Q-type calcium channel. *Ann Neurol* 2004;56:213–220.

118. Griggs RC, Nutt JG. Episodic ataxias as channelopathies [editorial; comment]. *Ann Neurol* 1995;37:285–287.

119. Strupp M, Kalla R, Dichgans M, Freilinger T, Glasauer S, Brandt T. Treatment of episodic ataxia type 2 with the potassium channel blocker 4-aminopyridine. *Neurology* 2004;62:1623–1625.

Disorders of Gait

Nir Giladi   Yacov Balash   Evžen Růžička   Joseph Jankovic

INTRODUCTION

The capacity to stand and walk upright is a fundamental homeostatic human mechanism. The ability to get up on one's feet and walk from one place to the other is learned at around 1 year of age and performed automatically throughout life. Gait is defined as a complex motor and mental skill that, when properly executed, requires the integration of mechanisms of locomotion with those of balance, motor control, cognition, and musculoskeletal function (1). The ability to walk freely is a basic component of quality of life, since gait is one of the most essential motor tasks required for independence and ambulation. The ability to walk freely is influenced by many disorders, as well as by normal aging (2).

Gait disorders are caused by many neurological and nonneurological diseases and often reflect a broad range of dysfunctions of the central and peripheral nervous systems, the musculoskeletal system, or all. In elderly patients, severity of gait disorders, postural reflex impairment, and the rate of their progression are associated with significant morbidity and mortality (3) and enhance the risk of death (4). The most severe consequence of gait disturbances is falls with risk for head trauma, bone fracture, or the development of fear of falling with loss of mobility and independence. Falls can lead to immediate and delayed mortality. According to Tinetti (5), 30% of elderly persons suffer at least one fall annually, with the figure being 40% among those older than 80 years and up to 50% or more among residents of nursing homes.

This chapter aims to provide a review of gait disorders that would be applicable to the medical practice of a clinical neurologist. Only a brief account of the motor physiology of gait will be given, as this topic is covered in a number of specialized reviews (6,7,8). An overview of clinical assessment and diagnostic approaches is followed by different possibilities of classifying gait disorders based on clinical characteristics. Therapeutic approaches will focus on physical, behavioral, medical, and surgical options that are currently available.

ANATOMIC AND PHYSIOLOGIC FOUNDATIONS OF GAIT

Mechanisms of Locomotion and Balance

Locomotion is affected by a continuous stream of integrated signals orchestrating the alternate advancing, loading, and unloading of lower extremities. Rather than being a consciously executed motor activity, this learned motor pattern is produced by complex coordinated spinal mechanisms that are triggered and modified by brainstem structures and supraspinal motor centers (9). The mechanism of locomotion depends on sensory input (visual, proprioceptive, and vestibular), cerebral central processing (identification, localization of a target, planning of the action), and execution of the movement (robust voluntary and involuntary muscular effectors' responses with prompt adjustments of the standing and stepping according to environmental or internal conditions) (10). Rhythmic walking movements evolve and persist even in decerebrated or "spinalized" cats and dogs. They arise from rhythmic activity in the network of spinal interneurons constituting the locomotor generator (an equivalent of the generator of the rhythmic movements of the wings in birds or flippers in fish). Unlike mammalian quadrupeds whose gait mainly depends on the motor pattern spinal generators (11), automatic gait in primates can be induced by electrical stimulation of the mesencephalic tegmentum (mesencephalic–locomotor center), the latero-dorsal portion of the pontomesencephalic junction (including the pedunculo-pontine nucleus, and the posterior subthalamus (12). The pedunculo-pontine nucleus (PPN) is a functionally defined area located in the lateral brainstem tegmentum where stimulation can elicit controlled locomotion of various rates (i.e., from stepping to running) in decerebrated animals and monkeys. PPN is a possible brainstem center of locomotion in humans. The PPN consists of cholinergic neurons that receive inputs from prefrontal motor cortex and subthalamic regions. It has dense GABAergic afferent projections from the medial globus pallidus (13). PPN axons project to pontomedullar motor reticular nuclei, which, in turn, provide bilateral outputs to the spinal cord. Selective lesions of PPN neurons in experiments produced contralateral akinesia and bradykinesia resembling parkinsonism with related gait disturbances (14,15).

The mesencephalic locomotor region is a hypothesized anatomical substrate for the development of hypokinetic gait. Severity of gait disturbance correlates with the diameter of the midbrain on magnetic resonance image (MRI) in patients with normal-pressure hydrocephalus (NPH) and related gait disorders (16). There are clinical observations of "midbrain ataxia" acutely developed after midbrain lacunar infraction (17,18,19), stressing the importance of this region for locomotion.

The cerebellum is also involved in the generation of rhythmic locomotor activity through its rubrospinal, pontomedullary, reticulo-spinal, olivary, and vestibulo-spinal centers. The cerebellar vermis was shown to be activated during gait, both in normal volunteers and in parkinsonian patients (20,21). Various kinds of cerebellar lesions produce postural instability and irregular stepping (22). Cerebellar damage in humans is associated with increased sway in quiet stance and hypermetric postural responses with overshooting of the initial posture accompanied by exaggerated and prolonged muscle activity (23). It also plays an integral role in the control of upright posture during walking (24).

One specific anatomic feature of the locomotion system specific to humans compared to other mammals is its considerably more significant contribution to the activation of the muscles through the direct monosynaptic projections from the motor cortex to the spinal motoneurons during locomotion (25). This anatomic feature could explain the tight connections between gait and various functional conditions of the cortical system, including cognitive and affective conditions in humans (see Gait and Mental Function in this chapter).

The posterior parietal cortex has been shown to play an important role in locomotion by providing perception of body posture, thus helping to maintain normal gait and balance (26). Single-photon emission computed tomography (SPECT)-detected, regional cerebral flow activation studies have shown that the cerebral cortex participates in the control of the normal volitional walking of healthy human subjects. The active brain areas include the foot and trunk regions of the primary sensorimotor cortex, as well as the supplementary motor area (SMA), lateral premotor cortex, and cingulated gyrus. Selected subcortical structures also exhibit walking-related activity, including the dorsal brainstem and cerebellum (27).

In healthy participants who were instructed to imagine normal gait, positron emission tomography (PET) revealed activations mainly of cortical areas: precuneus and dorsal premotor cortex (bilaterally), the left dorsolateral prefrontal cortex, the left inferior parietal lobule, and the right posterior cingulate cortex (28). During standing, activation patterns in functional MRI (fMRI) scans were seen in the thalamus, basal ganglia, and cerebellar vermis, as well as in the parahippocampal and fusiform gyri, which are the areas responsible for visuospatial navigation. Occipital visual areas and the cerebellum also were activated during walking (29).

Brain lesions have taught us much about the brain's role in normal locomotion. Bilateral damage of the inferiomedial parts of the frontal lobes due to infarction in the territory of the anterior cerebral artery resulted in an inability to initiate stepping, or "apraxia of gait" (30). In patients with unilateral lesions of the SMA, an impairment of posture or fall was seen when the weight was placed and then rapidly removed from the contralateral limbs (31). Interruptions of the frontopontocerebellar tract (Arnold's bundle), which originated in the frontal lobe in Brodmann's area 10 and carried information on intended movement to the contralateral cerebellum via the pontocerebellar peduncle deprived the brainstem cerebellum of this information, thereby inducing frontal lobe ataxia both in children and adults (32,33). Subcortical white matter lesions, such as periventricular ones, were associated with impaired balance, falls, and slowed gait speed (34). A variety of highest-level gait disorders were induced by cortical and subcortical lesions with or without cognitive decline (35,36).

A sudden inability to stand unsupported, marked balance impairment in attempts to walk, and recurrent falls despite good strength could be the manifestations of lacunar infarcts within the superior and/or posterior lateral thalamus with involvement of the vestibular thalamic subnuclei (37,38,39,40).

Bipedal Gait

The two essential prerequisites of erect bipedal gait are (a) *equilibrium*, the ability to keep the body upright and maintain balance, and (b) *locomotion*, the capacity for initiating and maintaining rhythmic stepping and for adjusting to environmental or internal conditions (35).

Erect posture is ensured by righting and antigravitational reflexes that keep the knees, hips, and back in extension that is continually adaptable to the head and neck position. This accounts, for example, for the ability to stand up into the erect position from lying or sitting. Postural reflexes depend on vestibular, somatosensory (proprioceptive and tactile), and visual inputs. Afferent stimuli are integrated at spinal, brainstem, and basal ganglia levels. The conventional model of decerebrated rigidity on brainstem transaction between the nucleus ruber and vestibular nuclei, which is marked by extreme extension, is an example of increased antigravitational reflexes.

Equilibrium is the ability to maintain balance under dynamic conditions in the plane of the direction of locomotion and in the plane at right angles to it. In walking, the mechanisms of equilibrium continually make up for shifts in the center of gravity associated with the forward direction of locomotion and with alternating leg movements. *Anticipatory postural reflexes* ensure adequate adjustment prior to intended voluntary movement. *Reactive postural responses* adapt the body attitude and posture to shifts of the center of gravity and sudden changes of external conditions. Appropriate reflex balancing function requires good *proprioceptive* (source of stretch reflexes) and *visual*, as well as *vestibular* (source of vestibulocerebellar reflexes), integration. At least 2 of the 3 afferent pathways must remain intact or the sense of balance fails.

Step initiation is a complex integration between postural and motor control. Initiating the first step requires a shift of the center of gravity over to the pivotal leg to raise the swinging leg and move it forward (41). "Start hesitation" is a specific disturbance in step initiation to demonstrate its complexity. *Stepping* is a basic, automatic motor function that appears to be programmed in the brainstem and spinal cord in early stages of development since it is present even before birth. The gait mechanisms of adults, however, are under the control of higher regulating centers (situated in the posterior subthalamus, caudal mesencephalon, and pons), which control spinal activity by means of reticulospinal, vestibulospinal, and tectospinal projections in the anterior funiculi of the spinal cord (12). Interaction with the environment is an important aspect of locomotion. To avoid tripping over an obstacle or bumping into other people, stepping has to be constantly controlled on-line by visual feedback, as well as by higher cortical functions, which will influence strategic planning of stepping and the way a person will interact with the expected and unexpected in the environment.

Normal Posture and Gait

Normal Gait

Characteristic features of a mature gait pattern include upright attitude of the trunk and neck; lower extremities resting on feet set slightly apart; hips, knees, and ankles flexing in coordinated forward locomotion with the pelvis tilting slightly at the corresponding moments, thus allowing the unloaded leg to pass forward without touching the floor; and upper extremities swinging freely along the sides in slight semiflexion and performing adequate synkinetic

movements relative to the strides of the contralateral legs while the chest also makes minor forward excursions toward the swinging arm side. The person's narrow-based walking proceeds straight ahead with the connecting line of the heel touchdown points on the floor running in a straight line while the strides of roughly equal length rhythmically follow one another.

Gait patterns are characteristic of each individual and provide useful information about individual personality and current psychic state. The walking body posture, the length and regularity of the strides, the touchdown impact, synkinetic movements of the upper extremities, and other consciously, as well as automatically, performed features of gait usually permit discrimination between male and female gait, between extroverts and introverts, and between persons feeling elated and those who are depressed. In addition, there are obvious cultural and ethnic differences among gait patterns, such as among those of Asian, European, Latin, or African origin, and among those living in urban rather than rural communities, which may influence the walking cycle parameters and gait characteristics (42,43). Running and jogging may be viewed as variants of accelerated walking wherein the double-support phase of gait cycle, which is a measure of instability, disappears and locomotion is affected by a series of jumps with greater amplitude and with intermittent contact with the ground. The running characteristics may also be genetically or ethnically determined and influenced by the need for optimal energy efficiency (44).

Changes in Old Age

Changes in the pattern of walking inevitably accompany aging without necessarily reflecting a pathologic involvement of the nervous system (45). According to Tinetti (46), 40%–50% of nursing home residents have difficulty walking and suffer from frequent falls. In the course of senescence, the elastic harmony of movements characteristic of young individuals wanes, walking becomes progressively slower, and the sense of balance deteriorates. There may be different degrees of bent posture, rigidity of the trunk and extremities, stride shortening, and widening of the leg support base. Gait changes associated with age are sometimes difficult to differentiate from disease-related gait disturbances because some of the functions that are significant for normal walking inevitably deteriorate over the years as part of the normal aging process. Aging-associated gait disturbances can be affected by deterioration of sight, proprioception, or vestibular function and may reflect weakening of skeletal muscles, as well as degenerative joints changes in the limbs or in the spinal column. In addition to deterioration in the motor system, cognitive changes with disturbances in executive functions, attention, visuospatial orientation, and reaction time all can lead to changes in locomotion, especially while asked to do 2 or more tasks at the same time (dual tasking). Awareness of deterioration in the quality of responses is a common cause for insecurity,

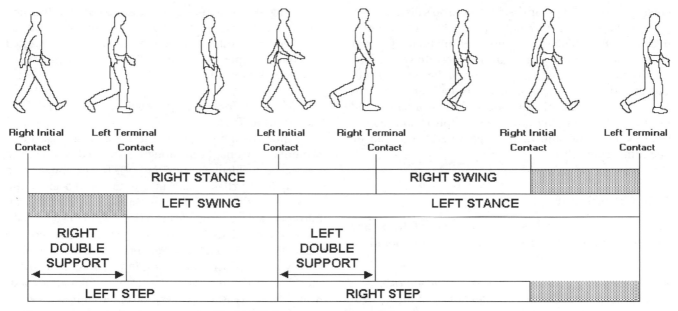

Figure 33.1 Normal gait cycle and its subphases

which is a characteristic of nonspecific gait disturbances in the elderly (cautious gait).

Overall, it is a good practice to look for a specific cause for any gait disturbance, even in an elderly person, and not to relate it to normal aging.

The Gait Cycle

Walking can be regarded as being a composite of numerous small and similar gait cycles, each based on an alternating single step carried out by both legs. A full cycle can be calculated from any given point because of the rhythmic and stereotypic manner of locomotion. Classically, a spatial description of the gait cycle starts when the right heel touches the ground while the right knee is stretched (locked) and the right foot is dorsiflexed. The foot rolls on the ground and carries most or all of the body mass as part of the *stance phase*. As the body mass moves forward, the heel leaves the ground. After a forced plantar flexion that pushes the center of body mass forward, the toes also leave the ground. When the right-foot toes leave the ground, the *swing phase* of the right leg starts. In the swing phase, the right leg swings forward after the right hip is pulled up (flexed) while the knee initially will be flexed and later extended to reach the ground in a locked position. During the swing phase, the foot is dorsiflexed to avoid any contact of the toes with the ground. The cycle ends when the right heel comes in contact with the ground again (Fig. 33.1).

The gait cycle also can be characterized temporally. The right foot normally touches the ground for about 60%–65% of the gait cycle. During 30%–40% of the cycle, only one leg is in contact with the ground (*single-support time*) and during one-third of that time, or 20%–25% of the whole cycle, both legs touch the ground (*double-support phase*). Based on the stated time frame, the *swing phase* of the right leg and the *stance phase* of the left leg (*single-support time* of the left leg*), which are equal in time by definition, take place during 35%–40% of the gait cycle. The proportion of each phase of the gait cycle is changed in relation to the speed of walking, as well as in relation to the individual's physical state, security, and equilibrium. Accelerated walk is associated with shortening of all phases but proportionally more of the double-limb support time is reduced. Aging, physical weakness, and disequilibrium lead to slower gait speed and increased double-limb support time.

Three additional spatiotemporal features of locomotion are stride length, cadence, and step width. *Stride length* is the distance between the places where the right heel first touches the ground at the initiation of one gait cycle to the place where it touches the ground again at the beginning of the next gait cycle. Stride length is also the summation of the distances of two steps (left + right). *Cadence* is the step rate or the number of steps in a given time (e.g., steps per minute), and *step width* describes the distance between the two feet at the perpendicular axis to the walking direction at a given step.

GAIT AND BALANCE EXAMINATION

Posture, balance, and gait assessment are fundamental parts of the physical and neurological examination. Locomotion should be evaluated in an open space, with the patient walking freely at his or her most comfortable pace for 7–10 meters, preferably with a turn at mid-distance. This is applicable even for cases when the etiology of some gait disturbances can be made the moment the patient enters the consulting room, as in Parkinson's disease (PD), progressive supranuclear palsy (PSP), hereditary motor neuropathy, muscular dystrophy, spastic hemiparesis or paraparesis, or psychogenic gait disorders. In spite of the important role of clinical observation in the assessment of gait disturbances, objective measures have an important role in the detection of early, subclinical disturbances and prior to surgical interventions. These tools include appropriate scales, gait, and balance parameters that can be quantified clinically (47).

Gait Assessment

Gait and posture should be assessed as part of the routine clinical examination. Several aspects of gait should be checked:

- *Assessment of the patient's ability to rise from a chair with his/her arms crossed*, which enables testing of the strength of the hip and knee extensor muscles, as well as general postural control.
- *Assessment of standing capacity*, looking at the base of support, the ability to stand with the feet together, in a tandem stand (up to 30 seconds), on one leg (up to 5 seconds), and standing with both feet together and eyes closed (Romberg test). These tests provide valuable information about postural control, balance, vestibular function, and sense of proprioception.
- *A challenge test allows a more fine assessment of postural control/responses*. Pulling backward (pull test) or pushing forward while keeping the patient from falling is a dynamic assessment that can provide significant functional information if performed correctly.
- *Assessment of normal walking in an open space* is informative with regard to locomotion, equilibrium, gross motor function, and interaction with the environment.
- *Assessment of turning in place* is another informative test in terms of general coordination, equilibrium, and gross motor function. Turning is best for provoking "freezing" (turning hesitation) and is significant because of its functional aspects.
- *Assessment of the ability to perform another cognitive or motor task while walking* (dual tasking) poses a challenge to the patient and is a form of functional testing that can provide important information on fall risk in daily activities.
- If the patient reports fear and insecurity or if it is suspected that these features might contribute to the clinical syndrome, the effect of support by a hand, rollator, or cane should be assessed.
- When testing gait, *other components of motor function should be assessed* (muscle strength, tone, coordination, and range of motion), as should cognition and affect. For cognition, it is important to assess specifically attention, working memory, cognitive slowing, reaction time, executive functions, and visuospatial orientation because of their importance to the performance of daily

walking. Depression can be assessed as part of the interview and the examination, but it will more frequently be picked up by validated tools, such as the self-reported Geriatric Depression Scale (48) or several interview-based questionnaires.

Bedside (Low Technology) Physical Examination Tools

The Timed Up and Go (TUaG) test is a gross measure of locomotion that has been strongly associated with fall risk in the general elderly population (49). The person is asked to get up from a chair, walk 3 meters, turn 180 degrees, and return to a sitting position in the same chair. Healthy volunteers are able to complete the test in less than 10 seconds. Needing more than 14 seconds to perform the test is a marker for increased fall risk. Patients who are independent in daily activities perform the test in no more than 20 seconds. Performing the TUaG test in more than 30 seconds means that there is a severe gait disorder and poor performance on the Barthel Activities of Daily Living Index (50).

The Tinetti Balance and Mobility scale was developed to screen for balance and mobility skills in the aged population and to determine the risk for falls (46). It consists of two parts for evaluating balance (16 points) and gait (12 points). A total score can be used to quantify gait and balance disturbances and to predict the risk for falls.

Morse (1998) developed the short and simpler validated Morse Falls Scale (MFS), which evaluates falls history, the presence of other disorders, the use of walking aids, mental status, and more. This scale has good inter-rater reliability ($r = 0.97$) and sensitivity to various medical disorders (51). It usually takes less than 3 minutes to rate a patient. A specific risk level carries with it recommended actions for fall prevention: e.g., a score of 0–24 = no interventions needed, 25–50 = standard fall prevention interventions, ≥ 51 = high-risk prevention interventions. In addition to the routine neurological examination, a study of orthostatic hypotension (blood pressure in the supine position and 3 minutes in the upright position) could be helpful in diagnosing gait disorders and falls.

Laboratory Methods

Many different systems of data acquisition are available to capture human movement, but most laboratories generally use three basic ones: (a) a motion capture system, (b) force plates, and (c) electromyography equipment. These three systems provide the necessary data to estimate kinematic and kinetic gait parameters (52). The choice of the system type depends upon the specific clinical or scientific task at hand.

Motion capture systems use camera-based equipment and track and record the trajectories of lightweight reflective markers located on the patient's skin, plus movements of the patient's body segments during walking. Using the three-dimensional position data that are obtained from a motion capture system, it is possible to compute joint angle, temporal-spatial, and kinematic data. Temporal data, such as the percentage of time in the swing phase or the walking velocity, can provide information about the patient's developmental stage and movement stability. Joint angle data provide information on the relative orientation of the body segments during the gait cycle. Angular parameters are also necessary for the calculation of joint moments and joint power.

A force plates system can simultaneously measure the interaction of the foot with the ground. The resultant force generated by this interaction is referred to as the ground reaction force (GRF). The GRF reflects the dynamic effects of the body (e.g., the external forces required to accelerate the center of mass of the body) and the foot's support of body weight. The examination of the characteristics of the force curves generated during the gait cycle can provide information about gait rhythmicity, stride-to-stride variability, gait asymmetry, and freezing of gait.

Electromyography (EMG) measures electrical activity produced during muscle contraction. The technology is used to determine the intensity of contraction and phasic activity of the lower extremity muscles during normal and pathological gait. Data from EMG provide insight into the underlying neuromuscular activity and aid in the interpretation of the kinematic and kinetic information.

The Role of Computerized Tomography and Magnetic Resonance Imaging

Brain imaging scans can be helpful in diagnosing gait disorders. There are at least six radiological signs relevant to gait disturbances.

1. MRI imaging evidences *precentral gyrus atrophy* in cases of primary lateral sclerosis manifested by spinobulbar spasticity, bradykinesia, frozen gait, and severe postural instability (53).
2. *Dilatation of the lateral ventricles on brain CT*, with or without cortical atrophy, may suggest the presence of hydrocephalus (normal or hyperpressure) with its related clinical symptoms. The key factor for the radiological diagnosing NPH is ventricular dilatation without cortical atrophy seen as sulci enlargement and bilateral widening of the Sylvian fissure.
3. *A broadening of the third ventricle* may be an additional sign of hydrocephalus accounting for the appearance of gait disorders (54). Idiopathic aqueduct stenosis may, however, be manifested clinically by festinations and freezing of gait (55). In patients with NPH, the diameter of the midbrain, as seen on MRI, was shown to inversely correlate with severity of gait disturbances (16).
4. *Multiple lacunar infarcts and/or white matter hyperintense lesions* on brain CT or MRI imaging, located in the centrum semiovale and basal ganglia, are well-known signs of Binswanger's disease. These changes have been shown to be connected with balance and gait dysfunction and falls in elderly people (56). Gradual worsening

of cerebral white matter disease was correlated with severity of locomotion disturbances observed in longitudinal MRI studies (mean time between MRIs of 4 years) (56).

5. *Leukoariosis* is another radiological sign of cerebral white matter disease, thought to be caused by small vessel disease and secondary ischemia that may be an independent predictor of gait disturbances (57). Reduction of the corpus callosum thickness, particularly in its anterior segment, had a significant association with severity of gait impairment and falls, as measured by the Nevitt gait scale's score (58).

Elderly patients with nonspecific or "highest level" gait disorders and disturbed gait dynamics can present with multiple white matter changes, mostly of vascular origin, or with a normal scan (59,60). In a subgroup of those elderly patients, however, q-space diffusion MRI revealed atrophy of the corpus callosum mostly in the genu area, further supporting the contribution of white matter changes to these symptoms (61).

6. *Cerebellar degeneration* (both vermis and/or hemispheric) is frequently found concomitant with ventriculomegaly, leukoariosis, and disseminated ischemic subcortical lesions. It may be seen in more than 80% of patients with various types of gait disorders and vascular dementia, and an ataxic component of gait disorder is usually present in those cases (62). In cases of prominent cerebellar atrophy, the differential diagnosis includes the spectrum of late onset of hereditary spinocerebellar ataxias (SCA) (63), gluten hypersensitivity- associated ataxia (64), multiple system atrophy, Tay-Sachs disease (65), and paraneoplastic cerebellar degenerations.

GAIT AND MENTAL FUNCTION

Gait is a complex motor and mental task involving all levels of the central and peripheral nervous systems. Only recently were the mental aspects of locomotion given the attention they deserve and mental disturbances were associated with gate disorders and vice versa. Dementia and depression have been shown to be associated with abnormal gait and stride-to-stride disrhythmicity, as well as with increased risk of falls (66). Patients with Alzheimer's disease are at higher risk to fall and, even if they might be classified by observation as walking normally, objective gait laboratory assessment can detect significant disturbances, mainly in timing (66). Moreover, recent prospective studies have demonstrated that abnormal walking is a very sensitive risk marker for the future development of non-Alzheimer's and Alzheimer's dementia (67,68).

Interestingly, walking regularly 4–5 times a week can delay the development of dementia, further supporting the relationships between cognition and locomotion (69).

Another aspect of cognition and gait is the ability to perform daily street walking while simultaneously paying attention to the traffic, talking on a mobile phone, or simply thinking of something else. Many studies were able to demonstrate that overloading the cognitive function, and especially the executive functions, is associated with decreased gait speed, increased stride-to-stride dysrhythmicity, and deterioration of postural control (70). It has recently been shown that the degree of dysrhythmicity is closely associated with the level of executive functions, demonstrating that locomotion requires the frontal lobe (71).

GAIT DISTURBANCES

Gait disturbances are among the most frequent symptoms in neurology. Taken together, the prevalence of this disorder is as high as 15% in the community dwelling elderly (over 65 years) population. The most common causes for abnormal gait in modern neurological clinics are stroke (21%), PD (17%), polyneuropathies (7%), multiple sclerosis (7%), spinal disorders (4%), and pain syndromes (4%) (72).

Classifications of Gait Disturbances

Gait disturbances can be classified according to the system affected, the phenomenology or objective signs, and the temporal aspects of the disturbance. The system-oriented

---

TABLE 33.1

SYSTEM-ORIENTED CLASSIFICATION OF GAIT SYNDROMES

Peripherally Originating Gait Syndromes

Musculoskeletal
Joints, bones, ligaments, tendons, muscles, peripheral nerves
Sensory
Proprioceptive, vestibular, visual

Centrally Originating Gait Syndromes

Spinal
Spastic paraparesis
Sensory ataxia
Pyramidal
Spastic
Paretic
Cerebellar
Ataxic
Extrapyramidal
Bradykinetic/hypokinetic
Rigid
Dyskinetic
Episodic
High Level
Disequilibrium
"Apraxic"
Unclassified
Cautious/fear of falling[a]

---

[a] The etiology of many gait syndromes is not always readily attributable to a single cause. For example, fear of falling may be due to changes in frontal, vestibular, visual, and/or extrapyramidal function.

---

classification (Table 33.1) helps in deciding at what level the disturbance originates. It is practical to work out the differential diagnosis of a person who does not walk well based on the level of the lesion. After a physical and neurological examination, it is usually not difficult to decide if the gait disturbance originates at the peripheral nerve, the spinal cord, or the pyramidal, cerebellar, or extrapyramidal systems. An experienced physician will differentiate between a cerebellar, spastic, and parkinsonian gait as the patient enters the counsultation room because of the typical appearance of each. It is more difficult to classify gait disturbances when multilevels and multisystems are involved, as is frequently the case in elderly people. The term *frontal gait disturbances* reflects the relatively recent observations that subcortical disequilibrium, "gait apraxia," and other more poorly characterized gait disorders are the result of dysfunction of the frontal lobe and its multiple connections. Previous classifications, such as the one by Nutt et al. (35), have coined the term *higher-level gait disorders* (HLGDs) for those poorly characterized gait disturbances, which stresses the involvement of cortical (frontal, mainly) and subcortical white matter structures in their pathophysiology. Some gait disturbances, however, cannot be classified based on the system-oriented classification. The most common among them is the "cautious gait" syndrome that was part of the HLGD subtypes, but its true origin is difficult to diagnose and thus difficult to classify. Cautious gait can be the earliest stage of the frontal disequilibrium gait disorder, as well as the result of a general anxiety state, visual or vestibular disturbances, or even secondary to peripheral problems such as pain, neuropathy, abnormal proprioception, or discomfort walking with high heels.

Gait is one of those tasks for which careful observation and physical/neurological examination can provide highly significant information, and it frequently leads to a system-oriented and etiologically based diagnosis.

Table 33.2 summarizes the main gait disorders, starting from the general category to the classical features observed while looking at the patient walking freely up to the classical physical or neurological finding on exam.

Paretic Gait

Paretic gait is associated with weakness of any reason as the main clinical feature. Weakness can be the result of muscle weakness (proximal or peripheral), peripheral motor neuropathy, or upper motor neuron lesion. As in other gait disorders, paretic gait is frequently characterized by the compensatory behavioral gait modifications, which sometimes become the main observed feature of a specific category. For example, paretic gait is frequently associated with locking of the knees during stance to avoid collapse at the level of the knee because of weakness at the quadriceps.

Paretic Gait Due to Muscular Weakness

Because of muscular weakness (in primary muscle diseases and peripheral nerve involvement), motion in the segment and intended direction are affected by reduced strength. Weakness severe enough to result in abnormalities of gait

TABLE 33.2

CLASSIFICATION OF GAIT DISTURBANCES ACCORDING TO CLINICAL CHARACTERISTICS

	General Category	Gait Characteristics	On Examination
I	Paretic gait (weakness of one or two legs or the pelvis girdle)	Symmetric/asymmetric Dropped foot with or without high pull-up of the knee while swinging Dragging one or two feet on the ground Exaggerated pelvic tilt or swing (waddling gait) Hyperextension or locking of the knee Short strides Weak "push off" (from the ground)	True leg(s) weakness, proximal or distal Reduced or absent tendon reflexes Decreased or normal muscle tone
II	Stiff gait (increased muscle tone in legs or trunk)	Symmetric or asymmetric Hyperadduction of thighs with or without scissoring Circumduction while swinging Plantar flexion on swinging Decreased knee flexion Stiffened spine Dragging feet on the ground Low swing of legs	Increased tone: rigidity, dystonia, spasticity Inability to fully relax the muscles Decreased joint range of motion Weakness of hip flexors and feet extensors Joints disease
III	Bradykinetic/ hypokinetic gait (mainly slow)	Symmetric/asymmetric Slow speed Short or normal stride Dragging feet on the ground Pain while walking Poor physical state (particularly poor cardiopulmonary function) Decreased arm swing Increased cadence with shorter strides Slow initiation or response	Parkinsonism Turning "en bloc" *Compensatory Exercise intolerance Fatigue Lack of motivation to walk Musculoskeletal pain Poor leg blood supply Visual disturbances Physiologic Disequilibrium

IV	Ataxic gait (unsteadiness, insecurity)	Wide base
		Short stride, slow speed
		Dragging feet on the ground (increased double support)
		Hesitancy, seeking support
		Constant deviation to one side (particularly with eyes closed)
		Aggravation of unsteadiness with closed eyes (in case of sensory ataxia or vestibular problems)
		Frequent tendency to lock the knees
			1. *Objective balance problems*
			   Abnormal sense of position
			   Abnormal cerebellar function
			   Disturbed postural responses
			   Severe visual disturbances
			   Vestibular disturbances
			   Fear of falling
			2. *Only subjective balance problems*

V	Dyskinetic gait (extra movements that affect gait)	*Extra movements of legs, trunk, or head while walking Can be task specific Dystonic gait Choreic gait Dysrhythmic locomotion	Continuous dyskinesia Only during walking Leg or general dystonia Chorea Compensatory movements to improve security or confidence or to decrease pain
VI	Episodic gait disturbances (freezing, festination, intermittent disequilibrium)	Normal locomotion between episodes Abnormal locomotion between episodes *Freezing* Feet get "glued" to the ground with transient akinesia or legs shake in place or forward motion with very small and fast steps; start hesitation, turning hesitation, hesitation in tight quarters, stressful situations or in an open runway	Parkinsonism Orthostatic hypotension Vestibulopathy Psychogenic syndrome

(continued)

TABLE 33.2
CONTINUED

General Category	Gait Characteristics	On Examination
	Festination Uncontrolled tendency to increase walking speed with small steps and a tendency to fall forward *Episodic disequilibrium* *Episodic weakness*	

is usually noticeable during the basic neurologic examination. Gait patterns are classified according to whether the proximal or distal muscles of the leg are affected, as discussed in the following sections.

Proximal Weakness: Waddling Gait, Duck Gait

Weakness affects pelvic girdle muscles and proximal muscles of the leg normally responsible for supporting hip abduction and for keeping the pelvis in a horizontal position while walking. Due to gluteal muscle weakness, the hip tends to tip toward the swing leg and lumbar hyperlordosis develops with the trunk flexing toward the support leg to compensate for this abnormality. The hip and trunk swing from side to side to compensate for the difficulties in lifting the leg. The alternate collapsing of the hip gives the impression of waddling, hence the term *duck gait*. Again because of muscle weakness, rising from a chair can often be accomplished only with the support of the upper extremities. The difficulties are even more conspicuous in getting up from a lying position or when sitting on the ground, with the patient forced to lean against the floor, surrounding objects, or his or her own lower extremities (*myopathic climb* or *Gower's sign*) (73). Walking upstairs and downstairs will also reveal proximal or distal weakness, respectively.

Distal Weakness: Cock Gait, Steppage, Foot Drop, Flail Foot, Slapping Gait

The most common pattern of gait disorder due to weakness of the anterolateral (peroneal) muscle group of the leg takes the form of foot drop as the patient lifts the foot to clear the ground. While walking, to keep the tip of the foot clear of the floor, the walker must flex the extremity excessively at the hip and lift the knee *(cock gait)*. In the touchdown phase, the foot first rubs against the floor with the great toe or with the anterolateral edge of the foot before putting down the entire sole of the foot *(steppage gait)*. Weakened dorsal flexion of the foot renders patients unable to walk on their heels because they cannot lift the tip of the foot on the affected side.

The involvement of the posterior group of crural muscles, especially of the triceps surae (separate or in combination with peroneal paresis), is characterized by weakened plantar flexion and leg adduction. While walking, the patient has problems rolling the sole of the foot off the floor and pushing off with the tip of the foot. Instead, the foot comes down flat like a flail (*slapping gait, flail foot*). In an effort to walk on tiptoe, the foot collapses on the affected side, or the patient is totally unable to assume the tiptoe position.

Hemiparetic (Hemiplegic) Gait

Hemiparetic gait is seen most frequently following a lesion in the upper motor neuron at any level above the foramen magnum. The paresis is at the contralateral side of the brain lesion. The weakness is classically at the extensors of the fingers, wrist, and elbow, which are held in flexion while the arm is abducted at the shoulder due to overactivity of the flexor muscles (spasticity). The lower extremity shows marked paresis of flexion and is held in extension of the hip and knee, with plantar flexion of the ankle and toes.

Patients with hemiparesis usually stand and walk with the paralyzed arm flexed and prone and the leg extended. If weakness is the main problem at the initial phase of upper motor neuron lesion, spasticity develops with time, and from a *paretic gait* the affected individual will develop the *stiffed gait*.

Stiffed-Legged Gait

Stiffed-legged gait is caused, classically, by an upper motor neuron lesion (pyramidal or extrapyramidal), but it also can be the end result of joint or muscle disease with secondary decreased range of limb motion. Circumduction is one classical compensatory behavioral response at the swing phase that improves ground clearance of the swinging foot.

Spastic Gait

Spastic gait is seen in the setting of diseases or dysfunctions of the motor cortex or corticospinal projections. Spastic hemiparesis and paraparesis lead to characteristic patterns of gait with reduced range of hip, knee, and ankle joint movements. The neurologic examination reveals common signs of upper motor neuron affection. Spastic hemiparesis typically produces the Wernicke-Mann attitude characterized by upper limb flexion and lower limb stretching with plantar flexion of the foot. On walking, the stiff leg circumducts, possibly in association with contralateral trunk flexion. Spastic paraparesis usually shows spasticity of hip adductors, as a result of which gait is stiff and associated with thigh scissoring, where each leg crosses in front of the other during the swing phase of walking.

Spasticity-based foot deformities later become fixed due to the development of contractures and articular changes. A detailed classification includes the following seven patterns that are likely to occur separately or in diverse combinations (74).

1. Equinovarus deformity is the most common pathologic position of the lower limb in central nervous system affections, with the foot and ankle turned downward and inward, mainly as a result of gastrocnemius and soleus hyperactivity. The foot touches down on the lateral edge where a tender bruise often develops. In the swing phase, the foot may rub against the floor and fail to provide stable support in the stance phase.
2. *Valgus foot* is bent outward as a result of peroneal muscle group hyperactivity. The foot touches the floor with the medial edge.
3. *Hyperextended great toe* tends to be a compensatory manifestation in paretically restricted dorsiflexion of the foot.
4. *Flexed knee* persists in all phases of the walking cycle, forcing the patient to assume a compensatory position in the support phase, and thus curtailing the stride length due to insufficient extension in the swing phase.
5. *Stiff (extended) knee* limits movement in the swing phase and leads to foot dragging, which, in turn, is compensated by circumduction (see the following).
6. *Adducted thigh* interferes, in particular, with the swing phase of gait, so that thigh scissoring curtails proper limb advancement (see Spastic Paraparetic Gait). The base is narrow in the support phase and balance may be impaired.
7. *Flexed hip* interferes with the support function of the extremity, resulting in a permanently flexed trunk and shortened stride.

Circumduction

The leg maintains a stiff posture in extension and rotates in a semicircle, first away from and then toward the trunk, in such a way that the proximal end of the leg is fixed while the distal end moves in a circle. The patient may be able to turn to the paralyzed side more easily than to the normal side. The hemiplegic/spastic gait tends to be quite slow, with decreased step length and increased stance phase. Compensatory changes include hip hiking from lack of knee flexion of the stance leg, a decreased lateral shift over the affected side, a lack of heel strike secondary to the plantar flexion of the ankle, and recurvatum of the affected knee. The extension moment at the knee is created by the plantar flexion moment occurring at the ankle. The swing phase is characterized by absent or markedly reduced knee flexion due to quadriceps spasticity. The flexor synergy gait occurs less commonly and consists of hip flexion, abduction and external rotation, knee flexion, and ankle dorsiflexion.

This synergy pattern does not allow the person to stand, thereby eliminating any ambulation potential.

Spastic Paraparetic Gait

Spastic paraparesis usually results from lesions of the thoracic portion of the spinal cord. The characteristics of the gait of these patients result from the combined effects of spasticity and weakness of the legs and consist of slow, stiff movements at the knees and hips with evidence of considerable effort. The legs are usually maintained extended or slightly flexed at the hips and knees and are often adducted at the hips. In some patients, particularly those with severe spasticity, each leg may cross in front of the other during the swing phase of walking, producing a scissors gait. The steps are short, and patients may move the trunk from side to side in attempts to compensate for the slow, stiff movements of the legs. The legs circumduct at the hips, and the feet scrape the floor so that the soles of the shoes become worn at the toes. There is associated tiptoeing to maintain balance, and great effort is exerted to swing the legs forward, all of which create an unsteady and tiring gait. In addition, isolated muscles or muscle groups may develop increased tone and spasticity. For example, spasticity of the tibialis posterior, a powerful plantar flexor and inverter of the foot, causes significant changes in gait during both the stance and swing phases of gait. During the stance phase, the initial contact will occur on the lateral aspect of the foot and plantar flexion at the ankle will result in an extension moment at the knee. Plantar flexion will also result in a relative lengthening of the limb, often causing dragging of the toes and requiring increased hip and knee flexion.

Spastic Gait in Cerebral Palsy

The term *cerebral palsy* is comprised of several different motor abnormalities that usually result from perinatal injury. Severe and extensive lesions often result in bilateral hemiparesis: Patients stand with legs adducted and internally rotated at the hips, extended or slightly flexed at the knees, with plantar flexion at the ankles. The arms are held adducted at the shoulders and flexed at the elbows and wrists. Patients walk slowly and stiffly with plantar flexion of the feet, causing them to walk on their toes. Bilateral adduction of the hips causes the knees to rub together or to cross, producing a scissors gait.

Bradykinetic Gait

Bradykinetic gait is the classic and early feature of parkinsonism. Walking slowly with a short stride and a stooped posture can, however, be the result of general physical weakness, depression, fear, or insecurity. It is an example of how careful one must be when diagnosing the etiology of gait disturbance based on observation alone.

Parkinsonian Gait

Parkinsonian gait is characterized by a paucity of movement of the facial, trunk, and upper and lower limb muscles, which results in a gait that is slow and shuffling with short rapid steps described as *festinating*. The trunk is flexed forward and the person may have difficulties with stops and turns, appearing to chase after his or her center of gravity. Joint motion is reduced due to rigidity, and there is usually little or no arm swing to help in balancing the individual. The gait in PD reflects a combination of akinesia (difficulty in initiating movement), impairment of postural reflexes, dystonia (relatively fixed abnormal postures), rigidity, and tremor. These patients stand in a posture of general flexion, with the spine bent forward, the head bent downward, the arms moderately flexed at the elbows, and the legs slightly flexed. They stand immobile and rigid, with a paucity of automatic movements of the limbs and a mask-like, fixed facial expression with infrequent blinking. Although the arms are held immobile, a rest tremor often involves the fingers and wrists at 4–5 cycles per second. When these patients walk, the trunk bends forward even more, while the arms remain immobile at the sides of the body or become further flexed and are carried somewhat ahead of the body. As the patient walk forward, the legs remain bent at the knees, hips, and ankles. The steps are short so that the feet barely clear the ground, and the soles of the feet shuffle and scrape the floor. Such a gait, with characteristically small steps, is termed *marche à petits pas*. Forward locomotion may lead to successively more rapid steps, and the patient may fall unless assisted; this tendency to shift from walking to a running pace with small steps as a result of an uncontrolled shift of the center of gravity forward, in front of the two feet, with an inability to bring it back is called *festination*. Parkinsonian patients can sometimes walk with surprising rapidity for brief intervals. They often have difficulty when they start to walk after standing still or sitting for a long time. They may take several very small steps that cover a short distance before taking longer strides. The walking movements may stop involuntarily, and the patient may freeze on attempts to pass through a doorway or into an elevator. Episodic gait disturbances (freezing or festination) are typical in parkinsonian gait and will be discussed in detail elsewhere in this chapter.

Ataxic Gait

Ataxic gait is mainly characterized by unsteadiness and insecurity causing a compensatory widening of the stride base. This normal compensatory response increases the ataxic patient's security and decreases the risk for falling. Unsteadiness can be the result of peripheral neuropathy or disturbance at the posterior column of the spinal cord with abnormal sense of position (sensory ataxia), vestibular disturbance (vestibular ataxia), cerebellar disorder, or frontal disturbance with frontal ataxia, which is the result of abnormal postural responses (reflexes). Ataxia can also be secondary to a psychological state of fear of falling but with no objective balance problem ("psychogenic ataxia"). The clinical diagnosis of ataxia is straightforward, based on observation of an unsecured walk and a compensatory wide base. Because most of what can be seen is

secondary to the imbalance, which can be the result of many etiologies, a thorough neurological exam by an experienced physician is required to understand the cause of the ataxia.

Widened Base with Directional Deviations: Veering Gait

Balance disorders and other conditions that aggravate lateral stability force the patient to compensate by widening the base while standing or walking. Typically, the etiologies include disorders of the balance and equilibrium system that is made up of the vestibular labyrinth in the inner ear and the eighth cranial nerve and its brainstem nuclei and connections. Deviations to one side also may be present in lesions of the nondominant parietal lobe associated with sensory neglect of the respective half of the space. Postural asymmetry and deviations in walking also may be due to unilateral leg weakness seen in peripheral or central paresis, except that base widening is not all that conspicuous in such cases.

The peripheral vestibular syndrome (reflecting disorders of the inner ear or seventh cranial nerve) is a typical cause of veering gait, with patients feeling propelled in some direction and having the illusion that their body or the environment is in motion (vertigo). In extreme cases, attempts to stand up are followed immediately by a fall. In less severe cases, patients will stand on a widened base to compensate for the lateral sway but will lose their balance and fall sideways in the dark or upon closing the eyes. Sometimes the head is held stiff in an obvious effort to control vestibular input. While walking, patients exhibit a widened base, instability, staggering with pronounced lateral sway, or falls. According to observations by Brandt et al. (75), lateral deviations affecting gait in the acute peripheral vestibular syndrome paradoxically abate while the person is running (75). One possible explanation is that running requires the activation of spinal locomotor mechanisms, inhibiting vestibular information. In less severe cases, the lateral sway will be revealed only upon closing the eyes (Romberg's sign) and in tandem gait. The sway to one side can likewise be elicited by stepping in place with the knees lifted high and with the eyes closed (Unterberger's stepping test). In the *central vestibular syndrome* (reflecting affections of the brainstem vestibular nuclei and their projections), there is usually no typical vertigo, and body and extremity deviations show none of the consistent unilateral tendency typical of the peripheral syndrome. There is, however, a tendency for the instability and unsteadiness of posture and gait to deteriorate in proportion to increased motor demands or in the setting of visual input restriction.

Widened Base with Cadence Alterations: Ataxic, Tottering, Wobbling Gait

Ataxic gait with the base widened or normal also may be part of a complex gait disorder in lesions of the cortex or white matter of frontal lobes (see Frontal Gait Disorder).

Disorders of Proprioception: Posterofunicular Spinal Ataxia, Tabes Gait

Sensory ataxia accompanies disorders of deep sensation from the lower extremities (as a rule, when the posterior spinal funiculi are affected). The patient complains of feeling unsteady when placing the foot down, which can be compared to walking over moss-covered ground or on cushions. This unsteadiness is more pronounced in situations characterized by decreased visual control (e.g., while walking at night in darkness to the toilet, or upon closing the eyes while washing one's face). Posterofunicular spinal ataxia is identified by a wide-based gait, strides of irregular length, and duration with the feet stepping down hard on the floor and arms held in abduction. Patients must keep looking at their feet and at the floor to avoid falling down. Apart from disordered vibration sensation and sense of position, there is usually areflexia of the lower extremities. Patients with disorders of proprioception stand on a wide base: Standing erect with the heels and toes close together (or in tandem gait) will increase their unsteadiness. Romberg's sign is markedly positive, although without lateral fall predilection and independent of head turns.

Cerebellar Ataxia: Drunken Gait

Ataxia is a major symptom of the *neocerebellar syndrome* in lesions of cerebellar hemispheres and their connections (76). In cases of unilateral involvement, ataxia and other symptoms of the cerebellar syndrome will become evident solely in the ipsilateral extremities. Cerebellar ataxia gait is marked by a wide base and irregular cadence of steps of unpredictable timing and unpredictable site of foot contact with the floor. Patients are incapable of walking straight ahead: Their deviations follow an irregular pattern, usually without unilateral bias. In less serious cases, difficulties become recognized only in situations that place increased demands on motor coordination (rising from a chair, turning around, walking downstairs, or walking in tandem). On examination, signs of a cerebellar syndrome predominate: dysmetria with overshoot of extremity movements, poor coordination, dyssynergy of muscles of the extremities and trunk, and rapid alternate movement irregularity (dysdiadochokinesia) (77). Equilibrium is unimpaired, and pull-test responses are hypermetric but otherwise normal (78). Although gait is markedly disordered, falls are relatively rare.

Persons with paleocerebellar syndrome in lesions of the anterior vermis or flocculonodular lobe have different symptoms, with severe postural and gait instability as a prominent sign, as well as a pronounced tendency toward toppling falls (see the following). As a rule, there are no signs of extremity ataxia or dysmetria (76).

Dyskinetic Gait

Dyskinetic gait is unique because extra involuntary movements appear while the person walks, making ordinary locomotion look bizarre. The involuntary movements can be caused by drugs/medications, metabolic disorders, or primary brain disturbances. Because of the involuntary nature, patients sometimes are not aware of the disturbance even if it might lead to tripping and falls. The immediate response of a patient who is aware of such movements is to suppress them voluntarily or incorporate them into the repertoire of normal gait. Ironically, gait might seem even more bizarre by the efforts made to suppress those extra movements. To observe the primary disturbance, patients should be instructed not to suppress any extra movements but to let them occur freely.

Choreic Gait: Dancing Gait

In choreic gait, lower limb chorea is superimposed on walking movements, thus giving rise to a peculiar ataxic gait pattern reminiscent of ballet dancing. Cadence is entirely irregular: The feet make accidental flat contact with the ground or, if they are turned, any part may touch down, and they purposelessly jump away from intended directions and the strides or jumps are of irregular length. When these involuntary movements simultaneously affect the trunk and upper extremities, there is a general impression of lack of control and direction. Although patients may sometimes assume highly unusual and unstable positions, falls are surprisingly rare. Spontaneous knee flexions with curtsying motions are common. Other clinical characteristics include wide-based station, lateral swaying, variable cadence, and sometimes bradykinesia. One biomechanical analysis illustrated that gait characteristics varied in each walk, with a mean decrease in velocity, stride length, and cadence (79). In addition, sudden forward or sideways thrusting movements of the pelvis and rapid twisting movements of the trunk and limbs result in a gait resembling a series of dancing steps. When walking, choreic patients speed up and slow down at unpredictable times, evoking a dystonic gait.

Dystonic Gait

Dystonic gait may take the form of a simple limp, inadequate stepping down from a higher level, or foot dragging due to dystonic inversion or eversion. Dystonic postures and motions are either constantly present or may appear only in the execution of some activities, such as walking. As a rule, these postures and motions propagate from the lower extremities to other muscle groups. A typical feature of dystonic gait disorder is its abatement in response to a variety of "tricks" or maneuvers, such as walking backward, trotting, or dancing. Even sensory tricks, such as putting one's hands in pockets, around the neck, or behind the back, may improve gait substantially. Bizarre pictures of dystonic gait are sometimes likened to animal gait. For instance, the so-called *dromedary gait* has been described in cases of progressive lordotic dysbasia (i.e., gradually increasing lordoscoliosis of the lumbar spine in walking, inducing bizarre position of the trunk with the hip bulging backward and sideways and compensatory turning of the shoulders and neck with the head held vertically). The major gait disorder in athetosis is classified as *mobile dystonia*. Characteristic features of these complex gait patterns include climbing movements of the legs or swinging flexion of the hips, often with contortion of the neck, trunk, and upper extremities, sometimes simulating wing-like movements (44).

Episodic Gait Disturbances

Episodic gait disturbances (EGD) are unique and most dangerous because of their association with falls (80). The unexpected and heterogeneous nature of the freezing or festination episodes can catch the patient unprepared, leading frequently to reckless responses and inevitable falls. Episodic gait disturbances are sometimes difficult to quantify because they appear more frequently at home and not in the examination room or the gait laboratory (81). The pathophysiology of episodic gait disturbances is complex and is associated with extrapyramidal disturbances and frontal gait disorders. Freezing of gait (FOG, mainly experienced in association with parkinsonism) can be defined as short (rarely exceeding 30 seconds), intermittent episodes of an inability to initiate or maintain locomotion or perform a turn. Most episodes are associated with a subjective feeling that the feet are "glued" to the ground. Patients either accept the situation and wait for its spontaneous disappearance or actively try to overcome the block, an effort that frequently causes tremor-like movements of both legs (82). Typically, most episodes can be overcome by motor, sensory, or mental tricks, but habituation has been described (83,84).

FOG episodes can be provoked most easily by asking the subject to turn around (turning hesitation) (81,85). In terms of everyday motor behavior, however, 360- or even 180-degree turns are rare and, as a result, start hesitation is experienced relatively more frequently in daily life (86). Our impression is that turning hesitation is important because of its possible contribution to falls during the act of turning. Other types of FOG occur while walking, passing through tight quarters, reaching the destination, or in stressful situations, such as crossing the street (open space) or entering an elevator (tight quarters) (85).

FOG can be associated with different degrees of motion during any given action. Phenomenologically, movement during FOG can be divided into three categories: small steps forward, trembling in place, or complete immobility (akinesia) (85,87). The three categories may be partially related to the amount of effort the patient expends to overcome the block. FOG appears to become more and more dynamic, less frequent, and of shorter duration as levodopa takes effect and parkinsonian symptoms improve (85).

Festination gait (FSG) is an intermittent episode that lasts a matter of seconds and involves disturbed locomotion characterized by uncontrolled propulsion associated with rapid small steps. Patients frequently report a feeling that they were "pushed from behind" (88). Both FOG and FSG are similar in their transient nature, but the latter is experienced mainly during free walking whereas the former is experienced more frequently during turning or initiation of walking. The two also differ in the unique subjective feeling that accompanies each: the feeling that the feet are "glued" to the ground in FOG and the feeling of being "pushed" by someone from behind in the FSG. Interestingly, tricks are much more effective in FOG and, when a trick is applied, it is inevitably used to overcome FOG and to avoid FSG, which is much more difficult to stop once it has started.

When FOG appears as part of PD, it is classically a hypodopaminergic symptom that is improved significantly with dopaminergic treatment (85). Not all FOGs, however, are levodopa responsive, especially when associated with PSP, vascular parkinsonism, or pure freezing syndrome (89). Festination is dangerous because it can lead to falls (86). Festinations are rarely improved by dopaminergic treatment. Both FOG and festination respond dramatically to cues and behavioral tricks (83). Episodic disequilibrium is another distressing gait disorder that leads to sudden feelings of instability. The pathophysiology can be of a vestibular, hemodynamic hypoperfusion, or psychogenic nature. Fear of falling and loss of self-confidence are frequent consequences of episodic gait disturbances. The psychological aspect of EGD is sometimes even more disabling than the physical difficulties. Patients may choose self-imposed home arrest to avoid the insecure, frustrated, and frequently embarrassing situations in which, without any warning, they suddenly become stuck (frozen) in place, become unstable (disequilibrium), or switch unintentionally to a running pace.

Not all gait disturbances can be classified according to the six major categories previously presented. The most difficult group to characterize is that of frontal and psychogenic gait disorders.

Frontal Gait: Apraxic, Disequilibrium, Normopressive Hydrocephalus

Frontal gait is often seen in normal elderly people. It is characterized by a slightly widened base, shortened stride, slowness of walking, and turning en bloc. There is no hesitancy in the initiation of gait and no freezing or shuffling, and the rhythm of walking and foot clearance is normal. There is mild disequilibrium in response to a push and difficulty in balancing on one foot.

Frontal Gait Disorder

Frontal gait disorder is a disturbance that is often seen with multi-infarct dementia or vascular (lower body) parkinsonism (90). Patients have a tendency to stand on a wide base and take short shuffling steps. Typical FOG may sometimes be present, especially turning and starting hesitations. Moderate-to-severe disequilibrium is the next characteristic feature, and the individual may experience almost constant severe uncertainty or real (up to panic) fear of falls. The patient usually feels considerable emotional relief and is able to walk better with external (sometimes altogether insignificant) help, like the arm of an assistant or rollator support. Associated findings could include cognitive decline, pseudobulbar palsy, asymmetry of tendon reflexes and frontal release signs, urinary urgency, or incontinence. Lumbar puncture, lumbar shunting, or ventricular shunting may improve gait in patients with NPH who have features of this gait disorder.

Subcortical Disequilibrium

This gait disorder is seen with PSP and multi-infarct dementia. Patients have marked difficulty maintaining the upright posture and show absent or poor postural adjustments in response to perturbations. Some patients hyperextend the trunk and neck and fall backward or forward, thus impairing locomotion. These patients commonly show ocular palsies, dysarthria, and the parkinsonian signs of rigidity, akinesia, and tremor.

Frontal Disequilibrium

Many patients with frontal disequilibrium cannot rise, stand, or walk; some cannot even sit without support. When they try to rise from a chair, they lean backward rather than forward, and they cannot bring their legs under their center of gravity. When they attempt to take a step, their feet frequently cross and move in a direction that is inappropriate to their center of gravity. Clinical examination usually reveals dementia, signs of frontal release (suck, snout, and grasp reflexes), motor perseveration, urinary incontinence, pseudobulbar palsy, exaggerated muscle stretch reflexes, and extensor plantar responses.

Psychogenic Gait Disorders

Psychogenic disorders of gait are a relatively rare finding among psychogenic movement disorders as a whole: They were encountered in 3.6% (530) of patients studied in a movement disorders clinic over a period of 16 years (91). There is a paucity of studies on this subject, and the available information permits only a few general diagnostic principles. The first is that not all kinds of gait that appear bizarre are psychogenic in origin (92). Diagnosis must be based not only on the signs generally accepted as being nonorganic during the clinical examination in real-time but also on data collected from video recordings (93).

There are seven major features characteristic of functional gait disorders, which were initially elaborated by Lempert et al. (94):

1. *Unilateral weakness of a leg, with it dragging behind the body as an alien object or a "log"*: The hip is either held in external or internal rotation so that the foot points inward or outward. This may be associated with a tendency to heave the leg onto an examination couch with both hands.
2. *Excessive slowness*: Exaggerated delay in gait initiation and subsequent "foot-sticking" without the subsequent improvement seen in the parkinsonism FOG.
3. *Falling toward or away from the doctor*: Falls were the most frequent posture disturbances in some studies (95).
4. *"Walking on ice" pattern*: This gait pattern is similar to the gait of a normal person walking on a slippery surface, i.e., cautious, broad-based steps with decreased stride length and height, and stiff knees and ankles.
5. *"Uneconomic" postures with waste of muscle energy*: A gait with an eccentric displacement of center of gravity, such as standing and walking with bent spine or flexion of hips and knees.
6. *Sudden knee buckling*: Patients usually prevent themselves from falling before they touch the ground. Knee buckling can also occur in Huntington chorea and neuroacanthocytosis.
7. *Pseudoataxia*: A gait characterized by crossed legs with a generally unsteady gait with sudden sidesteps.

In our experience, sudden attacks of the whole body trembling accompanied by anxiety or panic reactions during attempts to stand without support or during free walking are the most frequent manifestations of functional gait disorders. The patient usually calms down after clinging to the bed or other objects or after sitting down. Because of the severe emotional shock associated with the event, the patient rejects further attempts to stand and walk. Functional gait can present with hemiparesis, or paraparesis, but there are no signs of organic brain or spinal cord dysfunction: There is no spastic leg circumduction, clasp knife sign, hyperreflexia, or Babinski sign.

In some patients, however, functional gait disorders may be difficult to identify. An unusual and illusive presentation of hysterical gait is known as *astasia-abasia*. In this condition, the patient is unable to turn or walk but retains normal use of the legs while lying in bed. Atrophy of the vermis or epidermoid of the cerebellum can, however, result in frontal gait disorders with similar clinical manifestations (96). Another example is the mistaken diagnosis of psychogenic gait disorder in a man with status cataplecticus, whose gait was variably wide-based with sudden staggering to either side, accompanied by periodic buckling at the knees without falling. In that case, however, psychogenic-like gait disorders were associated with episodes of frequent naps during the daytime associated with vivid dreams and visual hallucinations, severe muscle weakness and hypotonia, and lack of deep tendon reflexes in all extremities. Genetic studies were positive for HLA DQB1*0602 (97). Thus, a full neurological examination is indicated despite compelling indications of nonorganic disease.

TREATMENT OF GAIT DISTURBANCES

Treatment Options in Paretic and Spastic Gait Disorders

Tizanidine Hydrochloride

Tizanidine is a centrally acting $\alpha 2$-adrenergic agonist, which is closely related chemically to clonidine. Tizanidine increases the presynaptic inhibition of excitatory spinal interneurons, which decreases the amount of excitatory neurotransmitter release and thus the excitatory input onto the postsynaptic α-motoneurons (98). In one uncontrolled study, tizanidine treatment produced an apparent improvement of mobility in patients with multiple sclerosis who had moderately marked paresis with legs spasticity (99). Patients with hemiplegic spasticity who were on tizanidine (8–24 mg) showed a statistically significant improvement in functional status, as assessed by walking distances on flat ground in a multicenter, double-blind study (100).

Intrathecal Baclofen Therapy

Another option in the treatment of disabling limb spasticity and walking improvement following stroke or spinal trauma is intrathecal baclofen therapy (ITB). ITB bolus injection consistently reduced spasticity in ambulatory patients with acquired brain injury. Gait velocity increased by an average of 12 cm/s, a mean gain of 33% over their baseline walking speed after a 50-c microgram ITB bolus injection (101). The Ashworth scores of the spastic upper and lower extremities diminished to a significantly larger extent in the baclofen group (102). Subsequently, a computer-controlled pump for continuous baclofen administration was implanted in 17 of the patients. This decreased the upper and lower limb Ashworth scores (0–5) by two levels over a follow-up period of 12 months (102). Acute ITB administration improved walking and reduced muscle stiffness at both the ankles and knees on the spastic hemiplegic side of seven subjects in another study (103). Francisco and Boake (104), using a case-series design with 10 subjects, examined functional gains following ITB administration. They found improved walking speed, functional mobility ratings, and spasticity while maintaining the muscle force in the uninvolved extremities. There were no significant adverse effects, and headaches due to cerebrospinal fluid (CSF) leak associated with catheter placement were transient (104).

Botulinum Toxin

For spastic drop foot, several open studies (105,106) have shown that intramuscular injection of botulinum toxin A into the plantar flexors reduces muscle tone and improves the mode of initial contact and the ankle range of motion with better advancement of the body, gait symmetry, and walking velocity for up to 4 months. Longer-lasting effects are rarely seen in adults with hemiparesis. There were no significant adverse effects except for a temporary bladder paresis that occurred with doses of botulinum toxin up to 400 IU of the Allergan product or 2000 IU of the Dysport product.

Botulinum toxin treatment of spastic equinovarus deformity after stroke resulted in a significant reduction in muscle tone, limb pain, and dependence on walking aids in a double-blind, placebo-controlled trial (107). The greatest benefits were in patients receiving 1500 units of

the product manufactured by Dysport, but 1000 units also had significant effects. Since few adverse events were reported, this therapy is considered safe and may be a useful treatment in poststroke rehabilitation of the leg (107).

Burbaud et al. (108) conducted a double blind, placebo-controlled study in 24 individuals with spastic drop foot (108). The authors injected EMG-guided 1000 IU of the Dysport product or placebo into the soleus, gastrocnemius, tibialis posterior, and flexor digitorum longus muscles. The patients reported a clear subjective improvement in foot spasticity after administration of botulinum toxin but not the placebo. Significant changes were noted in the Ashworth Scale values for ankle extensors and invertors and for active ankle dorsiflexion up to 3 months after injection. Gait velocity was slightly but not significantly improved after the injection of botulinum toxin.

Fernandez et al. conducted an open label study on the potential symptomatic effect of botulinum toxin type A injected into the calf muscles of patients with PD and significant FOG (109). A double blind, placebo-controlled study using botulinum toxin type A and type B could not confirm the initial observation (110,111).

Phenol

Obturator nerve block and tibial nerve block in the fossa poplitea induced by injection of 5%–7% phenol can be used for the treatment of adductors spasticity and equinovarus deformity. In the latter case, 5% phenol is injected close to the motor point of the plantar flexors. This treatment showed no statistical change in the walking velocity or step length, but there was improvement in the width of the base of support and in gait stability after injection (112). We are unaware of any double-blind studies on phenol efficacy for gait improvement.

Physiotherapeutic Methods of Gait Rehabilitation

Although it is possible for those with spastic gait disorders undergoing gait training to achieve normal gait during a therapy session, such patients revert to the previous pathological pattern once they lose concentration (113). There was no significant improvement in gait symmetry parameters after application of an intensive 4-week inpatient training program consisting, during sitting or standing, of typical physiotherapy sessions designed to normalize muscle tone, as well as inhibit tone and advanced postural reactions (114). Thus, spending much time and effort on normalizing gait may be inefficient, and it may be more effective to concentrate therapy on functional levels of locomotion.

Treadmill Training with Partial Body Weight Support

Treadmill therapy with partial body weight support (BWS) provides nonambulatory hemiparetic subjects the repetitive practice of complex gait cycles at a very early stage in their recovery. The theoretical background of treadmill therapy is the activation of spinal and supraspinal gait pattern generators. Within one session of 20 minutes, patients can perform up to 1000 steps, compared with 50–100 steps during a conventional physiotherapy session.

In an open study on treadmill therapy, the BWS group that consisted of 50 patients with acute stroke scored significantly better in mobility outcomes and walking velocity, endurance, and balance after a 6-week training period than did the group with no BWS. Three months later, the BWS group continued to have significantly higher scores for walking velocity and motor recovery (115).

In another study on ambulatory patients with hemiparesis, the subjects improved their walking speed and endurance more with treadmill training and harness support than with conventional therapy following 4 weeks of daily 20-minute sessions (116).

Automated Gait Rehabilitation

In the electromechanical gait trainer (117), the harness-secured patient is positioned on two foot plates, the movements of which simulate natural walking. A servo-controlled motor supports the patients according to their abilities, and the vertical and horizontal trunk movements are controlled in a phase-dependent manner by ropes attached to the harness. In a recent randomized study on subacute, nonambulatory subjects, 6 weeks of daily gait trainer therapy resulted in better gait outcome and less effort for the therapists compared with treadmill training with BWS (118).

Functional Electrical Stimulation

Shoulson et al. (119) conducted a randomized trial involving 32 chronic, ambulatory hemiparetic patients, each with a single dropfoot. The patients received either physiotherapy or matched functional electrical stimulation (FES) treatment sessions with a common peroneal stimulator. At the end of the study and at follow-up, the patients in the FES group walked significantly faster and more efficiently with the stimulator than patients in the usual physiotherapy group (120).

TREATMENT OF GAIT DISTURBANCES IN PARKINSON'S DISEASE

Symptomatic Medical Treatment in the Early Stages of Parkinsonism

Symptomatic medical treatment aimed specifically at gait disturbance in the early stages of PD should be given only if the gait difficulties result in significant disability. The main concern for considering the initiation of antiparkinsonian treatment is the risk of falls. Other reasons for weighing drug initiation are painful rigidity of one leg and dystonic posturing while walking. A mild-to-moderate slow gait or a decreased arm swing does not justify the use of drugs,

unlike a history of frequent falls or shuffling gait with low ground clearance for which drugs should be given. The four major groups of medications are amantadine, monoamineoxidase type-B inhibitors, dopamine agonists, and levodopa. The first two have mild to moderate symptomatic affects and are given mainly to patients with FOG or other episodic gait disturbances (e.g., festination). Selegiline has been shown to be possibly effective for the treatment of FOG in the DATATOP study (121). Similarly, rasagiline (a second generation MAO-B inhibitor) was shown to be of significant benefit over placebo for the treatment of FOG in PD (122). Amantadine has also been reported in open studies to be of some benefit for the treatment of FOG and general parkinsonian gait (123,124,125).

Both dopamine agonists (DAs) and levodopa were effective for the treatment of gait by improving gait stride, speed, and rhythmicity (126,127). It has been suggested in some prospective studies, however, that treatment with DAs might increase FOG (128,129,130).

Symptomatic, Nonmedical Treatment of Parkinsonian Gait

The role of physiotherapy in the early stages of PD is questionable. A daily walk for 30–45 minutes is probably the best recommendation one can give to a recently diagnosed parkinsonian patient. Special attention should be given to posture. Some patients develop a stooping posture at early stages, and their camptocormia (bent spine) is almost predictable. Those patients should receive specific instructions and physical treatment from the early stages of the disease and should pay strict attention to their posture. It is our experience that hydrotherapy has a specific beneficial effect on posture, and patients who tend to bend forward or to one side (Pisa syndrome) should try it. Patients with early postural instability as a major symptom can benefit from physical exercise by improving postural control and reflexes and by learning and practicing strategies for avoiding falls and identifying and responding appropriately to situations that pose some risk to them.

One common gait-related question concerns the need to intentionally swing the nonswinging arm while walking. No official study has ever looked into that question, but one of the undesirable outcomes of walking while intentionally swinging either one or both arms is the development of unnatural nonautomatic locomotion. We instruct our patients to walk as naturally as possible and practice an automatic stride, paying no attention to the arms.

Treatment of Gait Disturbances in the Advanced Stages of Parkinsonism

Disturbed gait and postural control represent major and very disabling aspects of advanced parkinsonism affecting all patients (131). Walking becomes difficult, and patients tend to fall, so they either suffer fractures or develop a fear of falling and implement avoidance strategies with loss of mobility and independence. Gait disturbances initially appear at the off state, when dopaminergic treatment is less effective. As the disease progresses, even the on state is associated with gait disturbances and postural instability that manifest as a very short stride with feet dragging on the ground, a conspicuously stooped posture, and frequent FOG or a tendency for propulsion and festination. In addition, significant gait dysrhythmicity with increased stride-to-stride variations can develop, and this itself becomes a significant risk factor for falls (132). Those symptoms can be improved initially up to the level of a normal gait during the on state when medications are effective. Other common problems of advanced parkinsonian stages are involuntary leg movements in the form of off dystonia and on dyskinesia. Those involuntary movements are the result of disease progression or long-term dopaminergic treatment. In the advanced stages of parkinsonism, cognitive disturbances play a major role in the fight for mobility and independence without falls. Dementia and psychosis can significantly influence the therapeutic options with regard to both drugs and nonmedical interventions. Other non-motor symptoms that can significantly affect gait are ortho-static hypotension, leg weakness, general fatigue, and leg or lower back pain. At the advanced stages, treatment is aimed at maintaining mobilization and avoiding falls. When insta-bility becomes a major risk for falls, walking aids can decrease the risk and preserve mobility. Use of a wheelchair is a practical and effective option when all others fail: It affords the patient much safer and easier mobilization.

Medical Treatment of Gait Disturbances

Gait disturbances are much more problematic during the off state. Fine-tuning of the medical regimen by decreasing the total daily off time while still decreasing the severity of on dyskinesia can significantly improve mobility and general stability. A combination of 4–8 daily doses of levodopa treatment in combination with dopamine agonist and amantadine can frequently achieve this goal. Subcutaneous injections of apomorphine (another dopamine agonist that acts within 2–3 minutes) can alleviate off periods and main-tain mobility even when offs are unpredictable. Controlled-release and long-acting drugs can contribute significantly to the goal of as many ons as possible throughout the day.

Aside from optimal control and balancing of off and on periods, specific treatments can improve localized prob-lems and nonmotor disturbances. Leg dystonia (painful or not), for example, can be treated with local injections of botulinum toxin, which has been reported to be of signifi-cant clinical benefit (133,134,135).

General fatigue, weakness, and apathy have been treated with methylphenidate with some benefit (136,137,138). Ritalin also has been reported to improve gait speed when added to levodopa (136).

Orthostatic hypotension is a common cause of disabil-ity, which can present as leg weakness, freezing episodes, or light-headedness and instability. The alpha agonist mido-drine and the mineralo-corticoid fludrocortisone are effec-tive in the treatment of orthostatic hypotension, in addition to such nonmedical treatments as elastic stock-ings and high fluid intake.

Medical treatment of depression and dementia can have a considerable symptomatic effect on confidence during mobility. It is our common clinical experience that treatment with antidepressants from the selective serotonin reuptake inhibitors (SSRIs) group can dramatically alleviate FOG for depressed PD patients who frequently experience it, but this has never been formally assessed. Dementia in PD has been shown to be improved by acetylcholine esterase inhibitors (AChE-I) (139,140,141). The main improvement with AChE-I concerns cognitive features associated with attention (140,142). Considering the importance of attention to the avoidance of falls (143), it stands to reason that gait and pos-ture can benefit from improved cognition and attention.

Lower back pain or referred radicular pain to one or both legs can frequently lead to loss of mobilization and severe stress. Uncontrolled pain can cause considerable stress and worsening of parkinsonian symptoms, including those involving gait and locomotion. Any pain should be treated aggressively by systemic medications or (preferably) locally. Pain can be caused centrally by parkinsonism (144,145,146). Better adjustment of medications and higher dosages of dopaminergic treatment can lead to sig-nificant amelioration of pain even if degenerative changes have been demonstrated on imaging studies of the spine or joints (147).

Surgical Treatment of Gait Disturbances in Parkinsonism

In the most advanced stages of PD, when drugs are no longer effective and side effects, such as dyskinesias, are causing major disability, functional neurosurgery at the level of the basal ganglia has been used successfully over the past 15 years (148). Pallidotomy was the first proce-dure to be carried out, and deep-brain stimulation (DBS) of the subthalamic nucleus (STN) and the internal globus pallidum (GPi) has been effective in avoiding motor response fluctuations with the elimination of off periods for the past 10 years. In addition, the ability to decrease medications in patients who have bilateral STN stimula-tion could stop dyskinesias dramatically (148). Similarly, bilateral GPi stimulation has stopped dyskinesias, but it did so with no decrease of dopaminergic drugs (148).

Both STN and GPi stimulations have been shown to improve spatio-temporal gait parameters in patients with advanced disease during the off medication state to a level of almost normal walking (149,150,151).

Other surgical interventions that should be considered on a case-to-case basis are laminectomy in lumbar spinal stenosis or disc hernia, hip or knee replacement in severe degenerative joint disease, and revascularization of the legs in severe peripheral vascular disease.

If a PD patient cannot walk and complains of pain, a differential diagnosis must be undertaken, taking into account that the disability could be caused by other non-parkinsonian causes.

Nonmedical Treatment of Gait Disturbances in the Advanced Stages of Parkinsonism

Antiparkinsonian medications can give moderate and transient improvement in locomotion in the more advanced stages of PD. The off periods are, however, much more difficult, characterized by severe freezing and akinesia. The nonmedical treatment should be focused on preservation of general physical fitness for maintaining good stride and walking speed and educating the patient how to overcome specific difficulties, such as walking in a crowd or avoiding or overcoming a freezing or festinating episode. Specific attention should be given to posture and postural reflexes to avoid falls and the development of a fear of falling.

General fitness can be maintained by daily exercise, which should be recommended to every patient but even more persuasively to those in the more advanced stages of PD. A daily walk for 30–45 minutes during the on period is highly recommended for general health and specific physical and mental needs. Patients should be encouraged to walk at their own most comfortable pace, although it is better to avoid frequent stops as much as possible to practice the automatic mode. Falling is the most serious complication of a daily walk. Patients should be instructed to walk with comfortable and closed shoes, in daylight, and in an open space and to avoid obstacles. Walking outdoors has the advantage of practicing locomotion and entails cognitive aspects, such as strategic planning, avoiding obstacles, and interacting with the environment. On the other hand, walking on a treadmill can be safer and has the advantage of introducing external rhythm (sensory cue), although balance is not practiced if the patient holds the bars and the upper body does not move. Still, walking either outdoors or on a treadmill is better than not walking at all. Daily exercise is of great importance to preserve the range of motion of joints, muscle strength, and an upright posture. A decreased range of ankle, knee, or hip motion, as well as a stooped posture with flexed shoulders, can significantly impede the ability to walk. Muscle strength, especially of the legs, plays a major role in maintaining stride length, walking speed, balance, and confidence. As a result, daily exercises should include both stretching and strengthening programs. Daily walking has been shown to improve stride length and walking speed with a carryover effect of several months, even when the exercise was stopped (151,152,153).

Much of the parkinsonian gait can be improved by the patient focusing attention on upright posture, stride length, and locomotion rhythm (154). Similarly, motor or sensory cues have been shown to be highly effective for the treatment of the parkinsonian gait (83). Stripes on the floor, marching, following external commands and external rhythms are commonly used cues (tricks) for maintaining mobility in difficult off periods (155). This improvement is maintained, however, only as long as attention is focused upon the act of walking and shortly thereafter (carryover effect), but not for a longer period of time (156). As a result, cues can be used to overcome difficult periods but are less effective for normal daily functioning. Since not all patients are aware of the dramatic and clinically significant effect of cueing on parkinsonian gait disturbances, it is important to teach them this skill and the application of cues in difficult situations. Having such an easy to use and always available solution on hand can improve the PD patient's confidence and, as a result, his or her mobility and independence.

Dysrhythmic locomotion with increased stride-to-stride variation in time is a primary disturbance of parkinsonian gait (157,158) and is associated with increased falls in patients with PD (132). Walking on a treadmill with a fixed speed can improve stride-to-stride variation with a short-term (15 minutes) carryover effect (159). Similarly, rhythmic auditory stimulation (RAS) has been shown to improve gait rhythmicity as another effective and easy-to-use mode of intervention (160–162). The long-term effect of RAS or treadmill exercise on locomotion has never been studied objectively, but there is good reason to speculate that it should have a positive effect.

Special attention should be given to the episodic gait disturbances of start hesitation and freezing in narrow places and in stressful situations, as well as those that occur while reaching the destination (89). These episodes can be the result of hypodopaminergic treatment but also of a hyperdopaminergic state. Most FOG episodes are caused by a hypodopaminergic state, and enhanced treatment of off periods will decrease their severity (132). When a patient can walk slowly but with no freezing before he or she takes the first morning dose of dopaminergic drugs, and FOG develops shortly after the first morning dose of medications has time to take effect, the patient is experiencing the relatively rare on freezing phenomenon and the levodopa dose—especially dopamine agonists—should be tapered down.

FOG can be avoided behaviorally or overcome by cues (85,156). Teaching the patient about FOG and its consequences is the first step to avoid it. Patients should be taught and should practice and use the cues at the right time and, more importantly, should deliberately relax during the freezing episode. Only by relaxing can the patient use cues effectively. Scientifically, RAS has been demonstrated to be effective in decreasing FOG frequency (160,161). Similarly, increased visual flow was shown to improve gait velocity and prevent or overcome FOG episodes (165).

Mobilization should be maintained for as long as possible, but not at the price of placing the individual at risk of dangerous falls. Walking aids should be considered if drugs and behavioral treatment failed in maintaining safe walking. Only rarely will the patient be the first to suggest the use of walking aids, so the obligation of raising this issue falls upon the doctor or the physical therapist. It is a process that has to be introduced tactfully and requires support and encouragement: This is what all patients fear and dread from the moment they learn that they are affected by PD, and it represents a turning point in the individual's process of coping with the development of the disease.

A rollator can improve security and balance while maintaining locomotion. Ambulation with a walker has recently been shown to improve internal rhythmicity of gait (159). A classical walker is the next step for maintaining short-distance mobilization, mainly at home. When walking becomes extremely difficult and dangerous and demands much effort and energy but does not substantially improve the patient's quality of life, it is time to switch the patient's mindset to regard walking as an exercise without any mobilization goal. This is the time to introduce the use of a wheelchair for mobilization and represents the end of the fight for ambulatory independence.

TREATMENT OPTIONS IN ATAXIC GAIT DISORDERS

Sporadic Cerebellar Degenerations

An important cause of sporadic cerebellar degeneration is gluten sensitivity in celiac disease. Cerebellar ataxia is the most common manifestation, and a diagnostic work up for antigliadin antibodies (immunoglobulin G or immunoglobulin A) should be performed in all cases of sporadic cerebellar syndrome (64). If the results are positive, a gluten-free diet, or, alternatively, treatment with intravenous immunoglobulin (IVIG) should be considered (166). Every patient with adult-onset ataxia should be checked routinely for nutritional deficiencies, such as vitamins B12 and E.

Hereditary Ataxias

Treatment options for hereditary ataxias are limited except for episodic ataxia and hereditary vitamin E deficiency (167). When episodic ataxia types 1 or 2 are suspected, a therapeutic trial with acetazolamide (250–500 mg) should be effective and may result in a decrease in the number of attacks (165).

Most current treatments include the use of amantadine, 5-hydroxytryptophan, or buspirone. Amantadine may be neuroprotective, blocking N-methyl-D-aspartate (NMDA) receptors, whereas 5-hydroxytryptophan acts as a precursor for serotonin (163). Clinical improvement of ataxia within

1 hour after ingestion of zolpidem (10 mg) was observed in a family of five patients with genetically confirmed spinocerebellar ataxia type 2 (SCA2) (168). Piracetam in daily doses of 60 g was demonstrated to be highly effective on tandem gait and gait ataxia (169).

Transcranial magnetic stimulation (TMS) in a single, controlled study was reported to be effective for improvement in posture and gait in 74 patients with inherited spinocerebellar degeneration (170).

A 6-month physical exercise program based on coordination, balance, and muscular conditioning exercises was impressively efficient in 82 patients with mild-stage SCA2. All neurological indices, both with open and closed eyes, significantly improved from pretest to posttest. Static balance, evaluated by the Romberg test, was also enhanced with training (171).

Paraneoplastic ataxias always should be included in the evaluation of adult-onset ataxia with gait dysfunction. Their treatment is routinely limited to cure the underlying malignancy, but there are anecdotal reports showing improvements in functional mobility and walking after sessions of plasma exchange (172) and courses of comprehensive inpatient rehabilitation (173,174). Although no definite therapy for autoimmune cerebellar ataxia has been established, plasma exchange should be considered as one of the main therapeutic choices.

TREATMENT OF DYSKINETIC GAIT

The primary goals in the treatment of dyskinetic gait is to avoid falls and then to decrease the dyskinesia. Avoiding falls should be achieved first by increased awareness of the risk, followed by taking precautions, such as using walking aids, having constant support, or—for the most severe cases—using a wheelchair. Such steps should be taken immediately upon diagnosing a dyskinetic gait, as part of the instructions at the end of the initial exam.

Dyskinesia can be primary—as in primary torsion dystonia, Huntington disease, or myoclonus—or secondary to drugs or metabolic disturbances. Treatment for the primary dyskinetic gait should be focused on decreasing dyskinesia with medications. The most effective drug to decrease chorea is tetrabenazine, a presynaptic dopamine depleter (175). Other drugs that have been effective for decreasing chorea are dopamine blockers (atypical neuroleptics), benzodiazepines, and amantadine (176). A drug-induced choreic gait (for example, tardive dyskinesia) should be treated by avoiding or decreasing (as in levodopa-induced chorea) the offending drug and using the same type of medications as those used for primary choreic gait for the remaining chorea.

Dystonic gait can be treated medically by drugs that decrease dystonia, such as anticholinergics, baclofen (orally or intrathecally), benzodiazepines, antiepileptics (valproic acid, topiramate, etc.), and atypical neuroleptics in severe cases (177). When dystonia is affecting gait in restricted areas, botulinum toxin can be of help and is mainly used for feet dystonia at the level of the calf muscles and the feet (178).

DBS of the GPi on both sides has recently been introduced for the most severe cases of dystonia and has been effective in improving primary dystonic gait, such as that seen in patients with DYT1 dystonia (179,180). In secondary dystonia, as in cerebral palsy or postanoxic brain damage, head trauma, or stroke, DBS has not shown similar clinical benefit (181).

REFERENCES

1. Dickson MH, Farley CT, Full RJ, et al. How animals move: an integrative view. *Science* 2000;288:100–106.
2. Baloh RW, Ying SH, Jacobson KM. A longitudinal study of gait and balance dysfunction in normal older people. *Arch Neurol* 2003;60:835–839.
3. Sudarsky L. Gait disorders: prevalence, morbidity, and etiology. *Adv Neurol* 2001;87:111–117.
4. Wilson RS, Schneider JA, Beckett LA, et al. Progression of gait disorder and rigidity and risk of death in older persons. *Neurology* 2002;58:1815–1819.
5. Tinetti ME, Speechley M, Ginter SF. Risk factors for falls among elderly persons living in the community. *N Engl J Med* 1988;319:1701–1707.
6. Pearson KG. Generating the walking gait: role of sensory feedback. *Prog Brain Res* 2004;143:123–129.
7. Chambers HG, Sutherland DH. A practical guide to gait analysis. *Am Acad Orthop Surg* 2002;10:222–231.
8. Dietz V. Do human bipeds use quadrupedal coordination? *Trends Neurosci* 2002;25:462–467.
9. Armstrong DM. The supraspinal control of mammalian locomotion. *J Physiol (Lond)* 1988;405:1–37.
10. Wolfson LI, Whipple R, Amerman P, et al. Gait and balance in the elderly: two functional capacities that link sensory and motor ability to falls. *Clin Geriatr Med* 1985;1:649–659.
11. Burke RE. The central pattern generator for locomotion in mammals. In: Ruzicka E, Hallett M, Jankovic J, eds. *Gait disorders.* Philadelphia: Lippincott Williams & Wilkins, 2001;11–24.
12. Eidelberg E, Walden JG, Nguyen LH. Locomotor control in macaque monkeys. *Brain* 1981;104:647–663.
13. Pahapill PA, Lozano AM. The pedunculopontine nucleus and Parkinson's disease. *Brain* 2000;123:1767–1783.
14. Kojima J, Yamaji Y, Matsumura et al. Excitotoxic lesions of the pedunculopontine tegmental nucleus produce contralateral hemiparkinsonism in the monkey. *Neurosci Lett* 1997;226:111–114.
15. Aziz TZ, Davies L, Stein J, et al. The role of descending basal ganglia connections to the brain stem in parkinsonian akinesia. *Br J Neurosurg* 1998;12:245–249.
16. Lee PH, Yong SW, Ahn YH, et al. Correlation of midbrain diameter and gait disturbance in patients with idiopathic normal pressure hydrocephalus. *J Neurol* 2005;252:958–963.
17. Masdeu JC, Gorelick PB. Thalamic astasia: inability to stand after unilateral thalamic lesions. *Ann Neurol* 1988;23:596–603.
18. Bhidayasiri R, Hathout G, Cohen SN, et al. Midbrain ataxia: possible role of the pedunculopontine nucleus in human locomotion. *Cerebrovasc Dis* 2003;16:95–96.
19. Hathout GM, Bhidayasiri R. Midbrain ataxia: an introduction to the mesencephalic locomotor region and the pedunculopontine nucleus. *AJR Am J Roentgenol* 2005;184:953–956.
20. Fukuyama H, Ouchi Y, Matsuzaki S, et al. Brain functional activity during gait in normal subjects: a SPECT study. *Neurosci Lett* 1997;228:183–186.
21. Hanakawa T, Katsumi Y, Fukuyama H, et al. Mechanisms underlying gait disturbance in Parkinson's disease: a single photon emission computed tomography study. *Brain* 1991;122:1271–1282.
22. Hallett M, Berardelli A, Matheson J, et al. Physiological analysis of simple rapid movements in patients with cerebellar deficits. *J Neurol Neurosurg Psychiatry* 1991;54:124–133.
23. Horak FB, Diener HC. Cerebellar control of postural scaling and central set in stance. *J Neurophysiol* 1994;72:479–493.
24. Morton SM, Bastian AJ. Cerebellar control of balance and locomotion. *Neuroscientist* 2004;10:247–259.
25. Nielsen JB. How we walk: central control of muscle activity during human walking. *Neuroscientist* 2003;9:195–204.
26. Schieppati M, Tacchini E, Nardone A, et al. Subjective perception of body sway. *J Neurol Neurosurg Psychiatry* 1999;66:313–322.
27. Shibasaki H, Fukuyama H, Hanakawa T. Neural control mechanisms for normal versus parkinsonian gait. *Prog Brain Res* 2004;143:199–205.
28. Malouin F, Richards CL, Jackson PL, et al. Brain activations during motor imagery of locomotor-related tasks: a PET study. *Hum Brain Mapp* 2003;19:47–62.
29. Jahn K, Deutschlander A, Stephan T, et al. Brain activation patterns during imagined stance and locomotion in functional magnetic resonance imaging. *Neuroimage* 2004;22:1722–1731.
30. Ueno E. Clinical and physiological study of apraxia of gait and frozen gait. *Rinsho Shinkeigaku* 1989;29:3275–3283.
31. Ghez C. Voluntary movement. In: Kandel ER., Schwartz JH, Jessel TM, eds. *Principles of neural science.* New York: Elsevier, 1991;609–625.
32. Terry JB, Rosenberg RN. Frontal lobe ataxia. *Surg Neurol* 1995;44:583–588.
33. Erasmus CE, Beems T, Rotteveel JJ. Frontal ataxia in childhood. *Neuropediatrics* 2004;35:368–370.
34. Starr JM, Leaper SA, Murray AD, et al. Brain white matter lesions detected by magnetic resonance [correction of resonance] imaging are associated with balance and gait speed. *J Neurol Neurosurg Psychiatry* 2003;74:94–98.
35. Nutt JG, Marsden CD, Thompson PD. Human walking and higher-level gait disorders, particularly in the elderly. *Neurology* 1993;43:268–279.
36. Elble RJ. *Gait disorders.* American Academy of Neurology 51st Annual Meeting, Toronto, Canada, *AAN.* 1999;8FS.96–122.
37. Masdeu JC, Gorelick PB. Thalamic astasia: inability to stand after unilateral thalamic lesions. *Ann Neurol* 1988;23:596–603.
38. Solomon DH, Barohn RJ, Bazan C, et al. The thalamic ataxia syndrome. *Neurology* 1994;44:810–814.
39. Saiki S, Yoshioka A, Yamaya Y, et al. Two cases of thalamic infarction presenting with "thalamic astasia". *Rinsho Shinkeigaku* 2000;40:383–387.
40. Lee PH, Lee JH, Joo US. Thalamic infarct presenting with thalamic astasia. *Eur J Neurol* 2005;12:317–319.
41. Maki BE, McIlroy WE. The role of limb movements in maintaining upright stance: the "change-in-support" strategy. *Phys Ther* 1997;77:488–507.
42. Davis JW, Nevitt MC, Wasnich RD, et al. A cross-cultural comparison of neuromuscular performance, functional status, and falls between Japanese and white women. *J Gerontol A Biol Sci Med Sci* 1999;54:M288–M292.
43. Ebersbach G, Sojer M, Muller J, et al. Sociocultural differences in gait. *Mov Disord* 2000;15:1145–1147.
44. Svehla F. *Introduction to the neurology of gait* (in Czech). Prague: Zdravotnické Nakladatelství, 1950.
45. Sudarsky L. Geriatrics: gait disorders in the elderly. *N Engl J Med* 1990;322:1441–1446.
46. Tinetti ME, Baker DI, McAvay G, et al. A multifactorial intervention to reduce the risk of falling among elderly people living in the community. *N Engl J Med* 1994;331:821–827.
47. Tinetti ME. Performance-oriented assessment of mobility problems in elderly patients. *J Am Geriatr Soc* 1986;34:119–126.
48. Lyness JM, Noel TK, Cox C, et al. Screening for depression in elderly primary care patients. *Arch Intern Med* 1997;157:449–454.
49. Podsiadlo D, Richardson S. The timed "Up & Go": a test of basic functional mobility for frail elderly persons. *J Am Geriatr Soc* 1991;39:142–148.
50. Mahoney FI, Barthel DW. Functional evaluation: the Barthel index. *Md State Med J* 1965;14:61–65.
51. Morse JM. Predicting fall risk. *Can J Nurs Res* 1998;30:11–12.

52. Chester VL, Biden EN, Tingley M. Gait analysis. *Biomed Instrum Technol* 2005;39:64–74.

53. Mabuchi N, Watanabe H, Atsuta N, et al. Primary lateral sclerosis presenting parkinsonian symptoms without nigrostriatal involvement. *J Neurol Neurosurg Psychiatry* 2004;75:1768–1771.

54. Sand T, Bovim G, Grimse R, et al. Idiopathic normal pressure hydrocephalus: the CSF tap-test may predict the clinical response to shunting. *Acta Neurol Scand* 1994;89:311–316.

55. Leheta O, Boschert J, Krauss JK, et al. Festination as the leading symptom of late onset idiopathic aqueductal stenosis. *J Neurol Neurosurg Psychiatry* 2002;73:599–600.

56. Whitman GT, Tang Y, Lin A, Baloh RW. A prospective study of cerebral white matter abnormalities in older people with gait dysfunction. *Neurology* 2001;57:990–994.

57. Briley DP, Wasay M, Sergent S, et al. Cerebral white matter changes (leukoaraiosis), stroke, and gait disturbance. *J Am Geriatr Soc* 1997;45:1434–1438.

58. Moretti M, Carlucci G, Di Carlo A, et al. Corpus callosum atrophy is associated with gait disorders in patients with leukoaraiosis. *Neurol Sci* 2005;26:61–66.

59. Hausdorff JM, Herman T, Baltadjieva R, et al. Balance and gait in older adults with systemic hypertension. *Am J Cardiol* 2003;91:643–645.

60. Giladi N, Herman T, Reider-Groswasser I, et al. Clinical characteristics of elderly patients with a cautious gait of unknown origin. *J Neurol* 2005;252:300–306.

61. Herman T, Giladi N, Gurevich T, et al. The non-specific gait disorders of the elderly: is it a disorder or a syndrome? In: *Research fair: book of abstracts*. Tel Aviv: Tel Aviv University Sackler Faculty of Medicine, 2003;183.

62. Thajeb P. Gait disorders of multi-infarct dementia: CT and clinical correlation. *Acta Neurol Scand* 1993;87:239–242.

63. Yu GY, Howell MJ, Roller MJ, et al. Spinocerebellar ataxia type 26 maps to chromosome 19p13.3 adjacent to SCA6. *Ann Neurol* 2005;57:349–354.

64. Hadjivassiliou M, Grunewald R, Sharrack B, et al. Gluten ataxia in perspective: epidemiology, genetic susceptibility and clinical characteristics. *Brain* 2003;126:685–691.

65. Neudorfer O, Pastores GM, Zeng BJ, et al. Late-onset Tay-Sachs disease: phenotypic characterization and genotypic correlations in 21 affected patients. *Genet Med* 2005;7:119–123.

66. Nakamura T, Meguro K, Sasaki H. Relationship between falls and stride length variability in senile dementia of the Alzheimer type. *Gerontology* 1996;42:108–113.

67. Verghese J, Lipton RB, Hall CB, et al. Abnormality of gait as a predictor of non-Alzheimer's dementia. *N Engl J Med* 2002;347:1761–1768.

68. Waite LM, Grayson DA, Piguet O, et al. Gait slowing as a predictor of incident dementia: 6-year longitudinal data from the Sydney Older Persons Study. *J Neurol Sci* 2005;229–230:89–93.

69. Verghese J, Lipton RB, Katz MJ, et al. Leisure activities and the risk of dementia in the elderly. *N Engl J Med* 2003;348:2508–2516.

70. Sheridan PL, Solomont J, Kowall N, et al. Influence of executive function on locomotor function: divided attention increases gait variability in Alzheimer's disease. *J Am Geriatr Soc* 2003;51:1633–1637.

71. Yogev G, Giladi N, Peretz C, et al. Dual tasking, gait rhythmicity, and Parkinson's disease: which aspects of gait are attention demanding? *Eur J Neurosci* 2005;22:1248–1256.

72. Stolze H, Klebe S, Baecker C, et al. Prevalence of gait disorders in hospitalized neurological patients. *Mov Disord* 2005;20:89–94.

73. Sutherland DH, Olshen R, Cooper L, et al. The pathomechanics of gait in Duchenne muscular dystrophy. *Dev Med Child Neurol* 1981;23:3–22.

74. Mayer NH, Esquenazi A, Childers MK. Common patterns of clinical motor dysfunction. *Muscle Nerve* 1997;6:S21–S35.

75. Brandt T, Strupp M, Benson J. You are better off running than walking with acute vestibulopathy. *Lancet* 1999;354:746.

76. Mauritz KH. Standing ataxia in cerebellar lesions. Differential diagnosis and pathophysiology of disorders of postural control. *Fortschr Med* 1980;98:1031–1035.

77. Hallett M. Cerebellar ataxic gait. In: Ruzicka E, Hallett M, Jankovic J, eds. *Gait disorders*. Philadelphia: Lippincott Williams & Wilkins, 2001;155–163.

78. Horak FB, Diener HC. Cerebellar control of postural scaling and central set in stance. *J Neurophysiol* 1994;72:479–493.

79. Koller WC, Trimble J. The gait abnormality of Huntington's disease. *Neurology* 1985;35:1450–1454.

80. Bloem BR, Hausdorff JM, Visser JE, et al. Falls and freezing of gait in Parkinson's disease: a review of two interconnected, episodic phenomena. *Mov Disord* 2004;19:871–884.

81. Giladi N, Hausdorff JM, Balash Y. Episodic and continuous gait disturbances in Parkinson's disease. In: Galvez-Jimenez N, ed. *The scientific basis for the treatment of Parkinson's disease*. Lancaster: Parthenon Publishing Group Ltd., 2004.

82. Yanagisawa N. Freezing gait. Pathophysiology. Prague: International Symposium on Gait Disorders, 1999(Abstr):45.

83. Rubinstein T, Giladi N, Hausdorff JM. The power of cueing to circumvent dopamine deficits: a review of physical therapy treatment of gait disturbances in Parkinson's disease. *Mov Disord* 2002;17:1148–1160.

84. Stern GM, Lander CM, Lees AJ. Akinetic freezing and trick movements in Parkinson's disease. *J Neural Transm* 1980:137–141.

85. Schaafsma JD, Balash Y, Gurevich T, et al. Characterization of freezing of gait subtypes and the response of each to levodopa in Parkinson's disease. *Eur J Neurol* 2003;10:391–398.

86. Giladi N, McDermott MP, Fahn S, et al. Parkinson Study Group freezing of gait in PD: prospective assessment in the DATATOP cohort. *Neurology* 2001;56:1712–1721.

87. Tompson PD, Marsden CD. Walking disorders. In: Bradley WG, Daroff RB, Fenichel GM, Marsden CD, eds. *Neurology in clinical practice: principles of diagnosis and management* Boston: Butterworth-Heinemann, 1999:341–354.

88. Bartels AL, Balash Y, Gurevich T, et al. Relationship between freezing of gait (FOG) and other features of Parkinson's disease: FOG is not correlated with bradikinesia. *J Clin Neurosci* 2003;10:584–588.

89. Giladi N, Kao R, Fahn S. Freezing phenomenon in patients with parkinsonian syndromes. *Mov Disord* 1997;12:302–305.

90. Winikates J, Jankovic J. Clinical correlates of vascular parkinsonism. *Arch Neurol* 1999;56:98–102.

91. Thomas M, Jancovic J. Psychogenic movement disorders: diagnosis and management. *CNS Drugs* 2004;18:437–452.

92. Stone J, Zeman A, Sharpe M. Functional weakness and sensory disturbance. *J Neurol Neurosurg Psychiatry* 2002;73:241–245.

93. Hayes MW, Graham S, Heldorf P, et al. A video review of the diagnosis of psychogenic gait: appendix and commentary. *Mov Disord* 1999;14:914–921.

94. Lempert T, Brandt T, Dieterich M, et al. How to identify psychogenic disorders of stance and gait: a video study in 37 patients. *J Neurol* 1991;238:140–146.

95. Diukova GM, Stoliarova AV. Psychogenic disorders of stance and gait as seen in videotaping. *Zh Nevrol Psikhiatr Im S S Korsakova* 2001;101:13–18.

96. Keane JR. Hysterical gait disorders: 60 cases. *Neurology* 1989;39:586–589.

97. Simon DK, Nishino S, Scammell TE. Mistaken diagnosis of psychogenic gait disorder in a man with status cataplecticus ("limp man syndrome"). *Mov Disord* 2004;19:838–840.

98. Milanov I, Georgiev D. Mechanisms of tizanidine action on spasticity. *Acta Neurol Scand* 1994;89:274–279.

99. Hoogstraten MC, van der Ploeg RJ, vd Burg W, et al. Tizanidine versus baclofen in the treatment of spasticity in multiple sclerosis patients. *Acta Neurol Scand* 1988;77:224–230.

100. Bes A, Eyssette M, Pierrot-Deseilligny E, et al. A multi-centre, double-blind trial of tizanidine, a new antispastic agent, in spasticity associated with hemiplegia. *Curr Med Res Opin* 1988;10:709–718.

101. Horn TS, Yablon SA, Stokic DS. Effect of intrathecal baclofen bolus injection on temporospatial gait characteristics in patients with acquired brain injury. *Arch Phys Med Rehabil* 2005;86:1127–1133.

102. Meythaler JM, Guin-Renfroe S, Brunner RC, et al. Intrathecal baclofen for spastic hypertonia from stroke. *Stroke* 2001;32:2099–2109.

103. Remy-Neris O, Tiffreau V, Bouilland S, Bussel B. Intrathecal baclofen in subjects with spastic hemiplegia: assessment of the antispastic effect during gait. *Arch Phys Med Rehabil* 2003;84:643–650.

104. Francisco GE, Boake C. Improvement in walking speed in post-stroke spastic hemiplegia after intrathecal baclofen therapy: a preliminary study. *Arch Phys Med Rehabil* 2003;84:1194–1199.

105. Dengler R, Neyer U, Wohlfarth K, et al. Local botulinum toxin in the treatment of spastic drop foot. *J Neurol* 1992;239: 375–378.

106. Johnson CA, Burridge JH, Strike PW, et al. The effect of combined use of botulinum toxin type A and functional electric stimulation in the treatment of spastic drop foot after stroke: a preliminary investigation. *Arch Phys Med Rehabil* 2004;85: 902–909.

107. Pittock SJ, Moore AP, Hardiman O, et al. A double-blind randomised placebo-controlled evaluation of three doses of botulinum toxin type A (Dysport) in the treatment of spastic equinovarus deformity after stroke. *Cerebrovasc Dis* 2003;15: 289–300.

108. Burbaud P, Wiart L, Dubos JL, et al. A randomised, double blind, placebo controlled trial of botulinum toxin in the treatment of spastic foot in hemiparetic patients. *J Neurol Neurosurg Psychiatry* 1996;61:265–269.

109. Giladi N, Gurevich T, Shabtai H, et al. The effect of botulinum toxin injections to the calf muscles on freezing of gait in parkinsonism: a pilot study. *J Neurol* 2001;248:572–576.

110. Fernandez HH, Lannon MC, Trieschmann ME, et al. Botulinum toxin type B for gait freezing in Parkinson's disease. *Med Sci Monit* 2004;10:CR282–CR284.

111. Giladi N, Gurevich T, Shabtai H, et al. The effect of botulinum toxin injections to the calf muscles on freezing of gait in parkinsonism: a pilot study. *J Neurol* 2001;248:572–576.

112. Ofluoglu D, Esquenazi A, Hirai B. Temporospatial parameters of gait after obturator neurolysis in patients with spasticity. *Am J Phys Med Rehabil* 2003;82:832–836.

113. Forssberg H, Hirschfeld H. *Movement Disorders in Children.* Basel, Switzerland: Karger Verlag, 1990.

114. Hesse SA, Jahnke MT, Bertelt CM, et al. Gait outcome in ambulatory hemiparetic patients after a 4-week comprehensive rehabilitation program and prognostic factors. *Stroke* 1994;25: 1999–2004.

115. Visintin M, Barbeau H, Korner-Bitensky N, et al. A new approach to retrain gait in stroke patients through body weight support and treadmill stimulation. *Stroke* 1998;29:1122–1128.

116. Pohl M, Mehrholz J, Ritschel C, et al. Speed-dependent treadmill training in ambulatory hemiparetic stroke patients: a randomized controlled trial. *Stroke* 2002;33:553–558.

117. Hesse S, Uhlenbrock D. A mechanized gait trainer for restoration of gait. *J Rehabil Res Dev* 2000;37:701–708.

118. Werner C, Von Frankenberg S, Treig T, et al. Treadmill training with partial body weight support and an electromechanical gait trainer for restoration of gait in subacute stroke patients: a randomized crossover study. *Stroke* 2002;33:2895–2901.

119. Shoulson I, Oakes D, Fahn S, et al. Impact of sustained deprenyl (selegiline) in levodopa-treated Parkinson's disease: a randomized placebo-controlled extension of the deprenyl and tocopherol antioxidative therapy of parkinsonism trial. *Ann Neurol* 2002;51:604–612.

120. Taylor PN, Burridge JH, Dunkerley AL, et al. Clinical use of the Odstock dropped foot stimulator: its effect on the speed and effort of walking. *Arch Phys Med Rehabil* 1999;80:1577–1583.

121. Giladi N, McDermott MP, Fahn S, et al. Parkinson Study Group. Freezing of gait in PD: prospective assessment in the DATATOP cohort. *Neurology* 2001;56:1712–1721.

122. Giladi N, Rascol O, Brooks DJ, et al. Rasagiline treatment can improve freezing of gait in advanced Parkinson's disease: a prospective, randomized, double blind, placebo- and entacapone-controlled study. *Neurology* 2004;62(suppl 5):A329–A330.

123. Yoritaka A, Hattori T, Hattori Y, et al. 85-year-old woman with the onset of progressive gait disturbance at 80 years of the age. *No To Shinkei* 1997;49:379–389.

125. Ahlskog JE. Medical treatment of later-stage motor problems of Parkinson disease. *Mayo Clin Proc* 1999;74:1239–1254.

125. Manek S, Lew MF. Gait and balance dysfunction in adults. *Curr Treat Options Neurol* 2003;5:177–185.

126. Kemoun G, Defebvre L. Gait disorders in Parkinson disease. Gait freezing and falls: therapeutic management. *Presse Med* 2001;30:460–468.

127. Shan DE, Lee SJ, Chao LY, Yeh SI. Gait analysis in advanced Parkinson's disease—effect of levodopa and tolcapone. *Can J Neurol Sci* 2001;28:70–75.

128. Ahlskog JE, Muenter MD, Bailey PA, et al. Dopamine agonist treatment of fluctuating parkinsonism. D-2 (controlled-release MK-458) vs combined D-1 and D-2 (pergolide). *Arch Neurol* 1992;49:560–568.

129. Rascol O, Brooks DJ, Korczyn AD, et al. A five-year study of the incidence of dyskinesia in patients with early Parkinson's disease who were treated with ropinirole or levodopa. *N Engl J Med* 2000;342:1484–1491.

130. Holloway R, Shoulson I, Kieburtz K et al. Pramipexole vs levodopa as initial treatment for Parkinson disease: a randomized controlled trial. *JAMA* 2000;284:1931–1938.

131. Hoehn MM, Yahr MD. Parkinsonism: onset, progression and mortality. *Neurology* 1967;17:427–442.

132. Schaafsma JD, Giladi N, Balash Y, et al. Gait dynamics in Parkinson's disease: relationship to Parkinsonian features, falls and response to levodopa. *J Neurol Sci* 2003;212:47–53.

133. Giladi N, Meer J, Kidan C, et al. Interventional neurology: botulinum toxin as a potent symptomatic treatment in neurology. *Isr J Med Sci* 1994;30:816–819.

134. Dowsey-Limousin P. Parkinsonian dystonia. *Rev Neurol* 2003; 159:928–931.

135. Tsui JK. Treatment of dystonia in Parkinson's disease. *Adv Neurol* 2003;91:361–364.

136. Nutt JG, Carter JH, Sexton GJ. The dopamine transporter: importance in Parkinson's disease. *Ann Neurol* 2004;55:766–773.

137. Camicioli R, Lea E, Nutt JG, et al. Methylphenidate increases the motor effects of L-dopa in Parkinson's disease: a pilot study. *Clin Neuropharmacol* 2001;24:208–213.

138. Chatterjee A, Fahn S. Methylphenidate treats apathy in Parkinson's disease. *J Neuropsychiatry Clin Neurosci* 2002;14:461–462.

139. Bullock R, Cameron A. Rivastigmine for the treatment of dementia and visual hallucinations associated with Parkinson's disease: a case series. *Curr Med Res Opin* 2002;18:258–264.

140. Giladi N, Shabtai H, Gurevich T, et al. Rivastigmine (Exelon) for dementia in patients with Parkinson's disease. *Acta Neurol Scand* 2003;108:368–373.

141. Fogelson N, Kogan E, Korczyn AD, et al. Effects of rivastigmine on the quantitative EEG in demented Parkinsonian patients. *Acta Neurol Scand* 2003;107:252–255.

142. Leitner Y, Barak R, Giladi N, et al. Attention: regulation of stride-to-stride variability of gait may require attention. *Mov Disord* 2004;19:S414.

143. Hausdorff JM, Balash J, Giladi N. Effects of cognitive challenge on gait variability in patients with Parkinson's disease. *J Geriatr Psychiatry Neurol* 2003;16:53–58.

144. Ford B. Pain in Parkinson's disease. *Clin Neurosci* 1998;5:63–72.

145. Waseem S, Gwinn-Hardy K. Pain in Parkinson's disease: common yet seldom-recognized symptom is treatable. *Postgrad Med* 2001;110:33–46.

146. Sage JI. Pain in Parkinson's disease. *Curr Treat Options Neurol* 2004;6:191–200.

147. Waters CH. Treatment of advanced stage patients with Parkinson's disease. *Parkinsonism Relat Disord* 2002;9:15–21.

148. Giladi N, Melamed E. The role of functional neurosurgery in Parkinson's disease. *Isr Med Assoc J* 2000;2:455–461.

149. Allert N, Volkmann J, Dotse S, et al. Effects of bilateral pallidal or subthalamic stimulation on gait in advanced Parkinson's disease. *Mov Disord* 2001;16:1076–1085.

150. Ferrarin M, Rizzone M, Lopiano L, et al. Effects of subthalamic nucleus stimulation and L-dopa in trunk kinematics of patients with Parkinson's disease. *Gait Posture* 2004;19:164–171.

151. Sunvisson H, Lokk J, Ericson K, et al. Changes in motor performance in persons with Parkinson's disease after exercise in a mountain area. *J Neurosci Nurs* 1997;29:255–260.

152. Lokk J. The effects of mountain exercise in Parkinsonian persons: a preliminary study. *Arch Gerontol Geriatr* 2000;31:19–25.

153. Scandalis TA, Bosak A, Berliner JC, et al. Resistance training and gait function in patients with Parkinson's disease. *Am J Phys Med Rehabil* 2001;80:38–43.

154. Morris ME, Huxham F, McGinley J, et al. The biomechanics and motor control of gait in Parkinson disease. *Clin Biomech* 2001;16:459–470.

155. Burleigh-Jacobs A, Horak FB, Nutt JG, et al. Step initiation in Parkinson's disease: influence of levodopa and external sensory triggers. *Mov Disord* 1997;12:206–215.

156. Nieuwboer A, Feys P, de Weerdt W, Dom R. Is using a cue the clue to the treatment of freezing in Parkinson's disease? *Physiother Res Int* 1997;2:125–132.

157. Baltadjieva R, Giladi N, Balash Y, et al. Gait changes in de novo Parkinson's disease patients: a force/rhythm dichotomy. *Mov Disord* 2004;19:S138.

158. Hausdorff JM, Cudkowicz ME, Firtion R, et al. Gait variability and basal ganglia disorders: stride-to-stride variations of gait cycle timing in Parkinson's disease and Huntington's disease. *Mov Disord* 1998;13:428–437.

159. Toledo-Frankel S, Giladi N, Gruendlinger L, et al. Treadmill walking as an external cue to improve gait rhythm and stability in Parkinson's disease. *Mov Disord* 2004;19:S138.

160. McIntosh GC, Brown SH, Rice RR, et al. Rhythmic auditory-motor facilitation of gait patterns in patients with Parkinson's disease. *J Neurol Neurosurg Psychiatry* 1997;62:22–26.

161. Freedland RL, Festa C, Sealy M, et al. The effects of pulsed auditory stimulation on various gait measurements in persons with Parkinson's disease. *Neuro Rehabilitation* 2002;17:81–87.

162. Lowenthal J, Gruedlinger L, Baltadjieva R, et al. Effects of rhythmic auditory stimulation on gait dynamics in Parkinson's disease. *Mov Disord* 2004;19:S139

163. Botez MI, Botez-Marquard T, Mayer P, Marchand L, Lalonde R, Reader TA. The treatment of spinocerebellar ataxias: facts and hypotheses. *Med Hypotheses* 1998;51:381–384.

164. Stern GM, Lander CM, Lees AJ. Akinetic freezing and trick movements in Parkinson's disease. *J Neural Transm Suppl* 1980;16:137–141.

165. Ferrarin M, Brambilla M, Garavello L, et al. Microprocessor-controlled optical stimulating device to improve the gait of patients with Parkinson's disease. *Med Biol Eng Comput* 2004;42:328–332.

166. Burk K, Bosch S, Muller CA, et al. Sporadic cerebellar ataxia associated with gluten sensitivity. *Brain* 2001;124:1013–1019.

167. Virgilio CH. Hereditaty ataxias. Mayo Clin Proc 2000, 75:475–490.

168. Clauss R, Sathekge M, Nel W. Transient improvement of spinocerebellar ataxia with zolpidem. *N Engl J Med* 2004;351:511–512.

169. Vural M, Ozekmekci S, Apaydin H, et al. High-dose piracetam is effective on cerebellar ataxia in patient with cerebellar cortical atrophy. *Mov Disord* 2003;18:457–459.

170. Shiga Y, Tsuda T, Itoyama Y, et al. Transcranial magnetic stimulation alleviates truncal ataxia in spinocerebellar degeneration. *J Neurol Neurosurg Psychiatry* 2002; 72:124–126.

171. Perez-Avila I, Fernandez-Vieitez JA, Martinez-Gongora E, et al. Effects of a physical training program on quantitative neurological indices in mild stage type 2 spino-cerebellar ataxia patients. *Rev Neurol* 2004;39:907–910.

172. Meloni C, Iani C, Dominijanni S, et al. A case report of plasma exchange therapy in non-paraneoplastic cerebellar ataxia associated with anti-Yo antibody. *Ther Apher Dial* 2004;8:500–502.

173. Sliwa JA, Thatcher S, Jet J. Paraneoplastic subacute cerebellar degeneration: functional improvement and the role of rehabilitation. *Arch Phys Med Rehabil* 1994;75:355–357.

174. Perlmutter E, Gregory PC. Rehabilitation treatment options for a patient with paraneoplastic cerebellar degeneration. *Am J Phys Med Rehabil* 2003;82:158–162.

175. Paleacu D, Giladi N, Moore O, et al. Tetrabenazine treatment in movement disorders. *Clin Neuropharmacol* 2004;27:230–232.

176. Bonelli RM, Hofmann P. A review of the treatment options for Huntington's disease. *Expert Opin Pharmacother* 2004;5:767–776.

177. Balash Y, Giladi N. Efficacy of pharmacological treatment of dystonia: evidence-based review including meta-analysis of the effect of botulinum toxin and other cure options. *Eur J Neurol* 2004;11:361–370.

178. Jacks LK, Michels DM, Smith BP, et al. Clinical usefulness of botulinum toxin in the lower extremity. *Foot Ankle Clin* 2004;9:339–348.

179. Coubes P, Cif L, El Fertit H, et al. Electrical stimulation of the globus pallidus internus in patients with primary generalized dystonia: long-term results. *J Neurosurg* 2004;101:189–194.

180. Krause M, Fogel W, Kloss M, et al. Pallidal stimulation for dystonia. *Neurosurgery* 2004;55:1361–1368.

181. Krauss JK. Deep brain stimulation for dystonia in adults: overview and developments. *Stereotact Funct Neurosurg* 2002;78:168–182.

Paroxysmal Dyskinesias: An Overview

34

Susanne A. Schneider   *Kailash P. Bhatia*

Paroxysmal movement disorders are defined as abnormal involuntary movements that are intermittent or episodic in nature, with sudden onset and with no change in consciousness. The episodic involuntary movements may be dystonia, chorea, ballismus, or a complex combination of these, hence referred to as paroxysmal dyskinesias (PxD) (1). Data on the prevalence are unclear, but these are rare disorders. For example, Blakeley and Jankovic identified only 92 cases among 12,063 patients (0.76 %) seen over 19 years (2). PxD episodes are often unwitnessed due to their short duration and, typically, no abnormal signs are exhibited between motor attacks. Thus, taking thorough history of the patient and witnesses is mandatory to make the right diagnosis and to offer the best treatment option.

Classifications to categorize this group of disorders have changed through the years. Subgroups can be distinct with regard to their duration (brief, intermediate, and prolonged), etiology (primary or idiopathic and secondary or acquired), and precipitating factors. With regard to the latter, Demirkiran and Jankovic's classification based on whether the attacks are induced by sudden movement—i.e., kinesigenic (PKD) or nonkinesigenic (PNKD) (3)—is widely accepted. Two other forms—exercise-induced dyskinesia (PED) and nocturnal hypnogenic dyskinesia (PHD)—are also recognized. Accordingly, four major forms of PxD can be distinguished and are discussed separately. It has been hypothesized that mutations in ion channel genes may be responsible for these disorders.

However, so far the pathomechanisms of episodic movement disorders are still not fully understood.

PAROXYSMAL KINESIGENIC DYSKINESIA

PKD is a condition in which brief episodes of involuntary movements are induced by a sudden movement.

Historical Aspects of PKD

In 1901, in his book on epilepsy, Gowers described attacks of an "unusual character" that could be induced by sudden movement (4). He noted that compared to typical epileptic seizures, consciousness was not lost during episodes and movements were tonic without a clonic component. However, he still regarded this as epileptic. *Extrapyramidal epilepsy, striatal epilepsy, tonic seizures, tonic motor attacks,* and *reflex epilepsy* were other terms used. It was also noted that some cases, reported under the heading of *"periodic dystonia,"* showed a good response to antiepileptics such as phenytoin (5). Furthermore, in 1963, Falconer et al. reported a case of possible PKD that was relieved by excision of a cortical scar from the left supplementary motor cortex (6). Detailed clinical features of the condition were first described by Kertesz in a seminal review of 31 cases from the literature and 10 new cases, including one that was autopsied (7). The autopsy was normal except for a slight loss of neurons from the nucleus ceruleus. In another case, a minor asymmetry of the substantia nigra was noted (8).

Clinical Aspects of PKD

The age of onset is variable between 6 months and 33 years but usually occurs between 7 and 15 years. Most studies show a higher prevalence in men than in women (4:1, even up to 8:1). Attacks are brought on by a sudden movement or increase in speed, amplitude, force strength, or sudden addition of new actions during ongoing steady movements (9). Startle, sound and photo stimulation, vestibular stimulation, hyperventilation, or stress also can induce attacks. Sometimes an abnormal sensation (historically referred to as *subliminal attacks*), such as numbness, pins and needles, or tautness, may occur in the affected limb or in the epigastric region (10) prior to the movement. An aura preceding the attack was reported by almost 70% of patients in one study (11). Some patients abort the attack by holding the affected limb tightly or crossing the legs.

The clinical manifestation is variable, and patients may present with dystonia, chorea, ballismus, or a combination of them. However, dystonia is the most common (2). Symptoms may affect limbs, usually hemibody, the face can be involved, and the attack may be generalized in some. Speech disturbance (dysarthria or anarthria, possibly from face involvement) was reported in 30.8% of patients (11). Unilateral distribution is seen in the majority of patients with the right and left sides equally affected (11). There may be a refractory period of about 20 minutes during which no further attacks can be induced (12). Most attacks (76%) are brief, lasting only seconds in most cases (11). The frequency of PKD episodes is variable. Climax of frequency is reached during puberty with as many as 30–100 attacks per day in both familial and sporadic cases (9). After the age of 20 years, the attack frequency may diminish and remissions can occur.

Pathophysiology of PKD

It is an issue of long disquisition whether paroxysmal dyskinesias are some form of epilepsy or a nonepileptic disorder. As mentioned, some authors consider PxD as reflex epilepsy given that episodes are brief, stereotyped motor events with a dramatic response to anticonvulsants. Usually, EEG studies in PxD patients do not show typical ictal or interictal changes and sleep electroencephelograms (EEGs) are also normal (13). However, some authors have reported abnormal EEGs in PxD. Hirata et al. demonstrated an abnormal EEG with rhythmic 5 Hz discharges during attacks (14), and another study showed transient epileptic discharges in 66% of cases (15). Lombroso showed ictal discharge arising focally from the supplementary sensory-motor cortex, with a concomitant discharge recorded from the ipsilateral caudate nucleus (16). Accordingly, some authors suspect an epileptogenic source of the paroxysmal attacks in the basal ganglia rather than in the cortex.

On the other hand, abnormalities of H reflex, contingent negative variation (CNV) and intracortical inhibition have been found in PxD, and these are similar to changes found in other such basal ganglia disorders as dystonia. In support of this basal ganglia theory are functional imaging studies, such as single-photon emission computed tomography (SPECT) scans showing increased perfusion of the basal ganglia contralateral to the side of attacks. However, another study showed decreased perfusion of basal ganglia, but this latter case was in a patient with hypoparathyroidism (17).

Etiology of PKD

Conditions of PxD can be inherited or acquired, and thus PKD can be classified into primary and secondary forms. Studies found 65%–72% of PKD cases to be familiar inherited in an autosomal dominant manner with variable penetrance (18). Complete penetrance occurred in more than half of the cases with familial occurrence, but in the other familial cases, inheritance was compatible with an autosomal dominant trait with incomplete penetrance (18).

Secondary Causes of PKD

An identifiable cause of PxD in general was reported in 22% of patients (2). Among the 76 identified patients suffering from secondary paroxysmal dyskinesias, only two had pure PKD (thus, 0.02% of the secondary forms) and another five (0.065%) exhibited mixed symptoms diagnosed as PKD/PNKD. Both patients presenting with mere PKD had short episodes lasting less than 5 minutes and occurring many times per day.

Characteristically, secondary forms of paroxysmal attacks are variable in the age at onset as a variety of etiologies can form the basis of PKD, some of them more common in younger patients, others more common in elderly patients. Secondary causes are shown in Table 34.1. Obviously, all secondary causes should be carefully ruled out before making the diagnosis of primary PKD.

Genetics of PKD

Some PKD families have been linked to the pericentromic region of chromosome 16 (19). However, there is clear genetic heterogeneity with at least two loci identified on chromosome 16 (20). Additionally, a third locus (21) must exist as some families with PKD do not link at all to chromosome 16.

Proximity or overlap with other syndromes, including infantile convulsions (ICCA; see the following), as well as rolandic epilepsy, paroxysmal exercise-induced dyskinesia, and writer's cramp (RE-PED-WC) in one family has been described (Table 34.2). The ICCA syndrome, defined by the combination of infantile convulsions and paroxysmal choreoathetosis, was mapped to a 10 cM interval around the

TABLE 34.1

SECONDARY CAUSES OF PKD, PNKD, PED, PHD

- Demyelination, such as multiple sclerosis
- Vasculopathy, such as ischemia, hemorrhage, moyamoya
- Infectious disease, such as encephalitis, HIV, CMV, after streptococcal pharyngitis
- Cerebral and peripheral trauma
- Neurodegenerative disease, such as Huntington's disease
- Hormonal and metabolic dysfunction, such as diabetes mellitus, hyperthyroidism, hypoparathyroidism, Albright pseudohypoparathyroidism, antiphospholipid syndrome, kernicterus
- Migraine
- Neoplasm (parsagittal meningioma)
- Chiari malformation, cervical syringomyelia
- Cerebral palsy after perinatal hypoxy
- Drug-induced (methylphenidate therapy)

PKD, paroxysmal kinesigenic dyskinesia; PNKD, paroxysmal nonkinesigenic dyskinesia; PED, exercise-induced dyskinesia; PHD, nocturnal hypnogenic dyskinesia.

centromere on chromosome 16 (22). The two regions of infantile convulsions and paroxysmal choreoathetosis overlapped by approximately 6 cM. In RE-PED-WC syndrome, both the seizures and paroxysmal dystonia have a strong age-related expression with a peak during childhood (23). Writer's cramp also appears in childhood but does not cease with age. Inheritance is as an autosomal recessive trait. Genome-wide linkage analysis identified a critical region spanning 6 cM on chromosome 16. In fact, ICCA syndrome entirely includes these 6 cM of the RE-PED-WC critical region. However, it remains unclear whether these conditions are caused by mutations of the same gene or two different genes.

Treatment of PKD

PKD attacks usually respond well to anticonvulsants, primarily carbamazepine, which is the drug of choice. Oxcarbazepine, phenytoin, hydantoin, and topiramate, as well as barbiturates, also can be beneficial. The dose of phenytoin needed to control PKD attacks in children is comparable to the dose used for epileptic seizures. In adults, a lower dosage is sufficient. Acetazolamide is a useful alternative or adjunct to carbamazepine in the treatment of PKD, especially due to demyelinating lesions. Benzodiazepines appeared beneficial in patients with HIV.

Prognosis for PKD

Attacks tend to diminish with age (9). Life expectancy is normal. However, if undiagnosed, this disorder can have a great impact on the quality of life, and suicide of patients suffering from PxD has been reported (7).

Differential Diagnosis for PKD

Differential diagnosis includes focal epilepsy with a tonic–clonic pattern in contrast to the tonic features of paroxysmal dyskinesias. In contrast to epileptic fits, consciousness is never lost in PKD, and attacks are not followed by amnesia (7).

TABLE 34.2

CLASSIFICATION OF PAROXYSMAL DYSKINESIAS

	PKD	PNKD	PED	PHD
Duration	Very brief	30 min–1 hr	2 min–2 hrs	30–60 sec
Triggering factors	Sudden movements, increase in speed, amplitude, force, strength	Alcohol, coffee, cola, tobacco, emotions, hunger, fatigue	Prolonged or sustained exercise	NREM sleep
Age at onset	7–15 yrs. (6 months–33 yrs)	2–79 yrs	2–30 yrs	Adolescence
Treatment	Carbamazepine	Benzodiazepines, anticonvulsants, acetazolamide, L-dopa	Gabapentin, L-dopa	Carbamazepine, phenytoin, acetazolamide
Gene	Chr. 16p11 (RE-PED-WC)	Chr 2q33–35 (MR-1)	Chr. 16p11 (RE-PED-WC)	15q24 , 20q 13.2–13.3 (CHRNA4, CHRNB2)

Summary of clinical and genetic characteristics of the four subgroups of Paroxysmal Dyskinesias, namely PKD, paroxysmal kinesigenic dyskinesia; PNKD, paroxysmal nonkinesigenic dyskinesia; PED, paroxysmal exercise-induced dyskinesia; PHD, paroxysmal hypnogenic (nocturnal) dyskinesia.

Other differentials are all other paroxysmal disorders. Historically, tetany (carpopedal spasm), drop seizures, myotonia congenita, cataplexy, Jumping Frenchmen of Maine syndrome, myriachit, paroxysmal hypertonia, and convulsive tics have been considered (7). Psychogenic origin and hysterical attacks should be ruled out.

PAROXYSMAL NONKINESIGENIC DYSKINESIA

Paroxysmal dyskinesias of the nonkinesigenic subtype (PNKD) are characterized by attacks of longer duration compared to PKD and are not induced by sudden movement. On the other hand, exacerbation factors, such as alcohol, coffee, etc., are present more commonly in PNKD.

Historical Aspects of PNKD

Mount and Reback (24) gave the first clear description, which they named *familial paroxysmal choreoathetosis* in a large family with 28 affected members in five generations. Typically, attacks were precipitated by alcohol, coffee, or fatigue, with improvement after rest and sleep. Scopolamine hydrobromide also had beneficial effects. Additional similar families were described, including one by Lance (25) 14 years later. In another report, Lance added a new family, reviewed 100 cases, and offered a classification of PxD into three groups (brief, intermediate, and prolonged attacks) (26).

Clinical Aspects of PNKD

Attacks occur both at rest spontaneously and after provocation by alcohol, coffee, cola, tobacco, emotional excitement, hunger, concentration, or fatigue (24). Attacks frequently can increase during menstruation or ovulation. Typically, an attack begins with a sensation of tightness or tugging in one limb or involuntary movements of the mouth and involuntary movements that begin on one side and tend to spread or even generalize (26). During severe episodes, patients may develop dysarthria or anarthria with full awareness (24). Episodes occur up to several times each week but typically only few times per year and last 30 minutes up to 4 hours (27). There is no consistent relationship between duration and frequency (2). Data about male–female ratio vary from 2:1 to 1:3. Onset of primary PNKD is in early childhood, with mean age approximately 8 years (24). Onset of symptoms of secondary paroxysms has a wider range (2.5–79 years), with a peak in the 20s when caused by trauma and mean age of 60 years when due to vascular factors (2).

A similar but distinct syndrome consistent of the co-occurrence with spastic paraparesis has been reported under the heading *choreoathetosis/spasticity (CSE)* by Aubuger and coworkers (28).

Pathophysiology of PNKD

EEGs are generally normal. An invasive video-electroencephalographic study by Lombroso and Fischman demonstrated discharge from the caudate nuclei (29). No cortical changes were recorded (29).

SPECT showed hyperperfusion on the right caudate and thalamus (30). PET studies based on ^{18}F-DOPA and [^{11}C]raclopride revealed reduced density of presynaptic dopa decarboxylase activity in the striatum and increased density of postsynaptic dopamine D2 receptors (29). The authors suggested a chronic upregulation of postsynaptic dopa receptors. ^{18}F-fluorodeoxyglucose (FDG) PET did not show metabolic abnormalities. Other PET studies using [^{11}C]dihydrotetrabenazine (DTBZ) as tracer did not reveal abnormal binding potential in the striatum (31). It was concluded that dopaminergic abnormalities, if present, may be due to altered regulation of dopamine release or to postsynaptic mechanisms, rather than to an altered density of nigrostriatal innervation.

Etiology of PNKD

Secondary Causes of PNKD

Similar to PKC, data on the prevalence and ratio of secondary causes in PNKD are rare. In the study by Blakeley and Jankovic cited previously, 52% of cases were diagnosed as pure PNKD (2). Bressman et al. (32) reviewed 25 patients, seven of whom (28%) were identified as secondary PNKD. Secondary causes are shown in Table 34.1.

Genetics of PNKD

PDC is transmitted in an autosomal dominant manner with high but incomplete penetrance of approximately 80% (33). Linkage to a locus termed *familial paroxysmal dyskinesia type 1 (FPD1)* was made to the distal chromosome 2q33-35 (34) in an area where there was a cluster of interesting candidate ion channel genes (35). Surprisingly, the abnormal gene is not an ion channel gene (36). Rainier et al. recently identified a missense mutation with substitution of valine for alanine at amino positions 7 and 9 in the myofibrillogenesis regulator gene MR-1 in two unrelated PDC kindreds (36). The mutation leads to alteration of the amino-terminal alpha helix. Lee et al. published data about the two isoforms MR-1L and MR-1S (37); although the MR-1L isoform is exclusively expressed in the cell membrane of the brain, the MR-1S isoform is ubiquitously expressed and shows diffuse cytoplasmic and nuclear localization (37). Data on gene function are still limited.

A distinct disorder termed *paroxysmal choreoathetosis/spasticity* combining PNKD and spasticity has been mapped to a region of 2 cM between D1S443 and D1S197 on chromosome 1p coding for a cluster of related potassium channel genes, but the gene is yet unknown (28).

Treatment of PNKD

First, triggering factors like caffeine, alcohol, or stress should be clarified and reduced or avoided. Pharmacologically, PNKD does not show such a dramatic response to antiepileptic treatment, in contrast to PKD. However, improvement is seen after treatment with benzodiazepines, including clonazepam, oxazepam, and sublingual lorazepam, sodium valproate, haloperidol, gabapentin, and acetazolamide, as well as L-dopa. Botulinum toxin improved PNKD symptoms secondary to stroke (2).

PAROXYSMAL EXERCISE-INDUCED DYSKINESIA

Historical Aspects

As previously mentioned, in 1977, Lance newly classified and delineated paroxysmal exercise-induced dyskinesias (PED) as an "intermediate type" of paroxysmal dystonic choreoathetosis distinct from classic PDC, because the attacks were shorter in duration, were not precipitated by alcohol, stress, or anxiety, and were never induced by movements (38). In the family described, attacks lasted 5 to 30 minutes, longer than the typically brief PKD attacks (less than 5 minutes, normally only seconds), but the attacks were not provoked by sudden movement. Instead, continuous exertion and physical exhaustion triggered attacks and an autosomal dominant inheritance was noted in the familial cases but sporadic cases have also been reported (3,39).

Clinical Aspects of PED

PED is a rare form of paroxysmal movement disorder with a male–female ratio of 2:3 (3). Mean age at onset of the autosomal dominant disease is approximately 5 years, ranging from 2–30 years. By definition, episodes are typically precipitated by prolonged or sustained exercise. However, in some cases, muscle vibration, passive movements, electric nerve stimulation, and cold exposure also can provoke attacks (40).

Although the episodes can be variable, the most common presentation is dystonia. In one report of eight patients, hemidystonic distribution was present in 50% of cases (39), but generalization did not normally occur. In a review of 19 patients (including the eight mentioned), feet were most commonly affected (79%) and hemidystonia was the next most common presentation (38).

Attacks normally last from 2–5 minutes up to 2 hours and cease in about 10 minutes after stopping the exercise. Frequency of attacks varies. Episodes occurred once or twice a month in a young girl described by Nardocci (41).

PED may be accompanied by migraine without aura (42) or a combination of alternating hemiplegia, epilepsy, and ataxia (43). A combination with rolandic epilepsy and writer's cramp (RE-PED-WC) has been reported (23). PED also may precede the onset of young-onset idiopathic Parkinson's disease (PD) (44).

Pathophysiology of PED

EEG recordings are typically normal. Other neurophysiological studies—including somatosensory-evoked potentials by stimulation of the median nerve (MN-SEPs), somatosensory-evoked potentials by posterior tibial nerve stimulation (PTN-SEPs), brainstem auditory-evoked potentials (BAEPs), visual-evoked potentials (VEPs), motor-evoked potentials (MEPs) by magnetic transcranial cortical stimulation (TCS), and electromyography (EMG)—suggested a hyperexcitability at the muscular and brain membrane levels (45).

Outside the attacks, cortical excitability and inhibitory neuronal mechanisms (response threshold and amplitudes, duration of the silent period ipsilaterally and contralaterally, corticocortical inhibition and facilitation) were normal (46), in contrast to task-dependent dystonia in which abnormal motor cortex inhibition is also detected during isometric muscle contraction (47). SPECT studies revealed decreased perfusion of the frontal cortex and basal ganglia during the motor attacks (48). Cerebellar perfusion was increased. This pattern was also described in both the idiopathic and the symptomatic forms of dystonia (48).

Two-fold increases compared to baseline of homovanillic acid and 5-hydroxyindoleacetic acid were measured in cerebrospinal fluid after motor attacks (49), supporting the hypothesis of dopamine involvement in the pathophysiology of PED.

Etiology of PED

Secondary Causes of PED

As in all the other subtypes of PxD, PED may be the symptomatic expression of a variety of injuries or insults that should be ruled out. Secondary causes are listed in Table 34.2.

Genetics of PED

The gene defect causing PED is unknown. Linkage analysis showed a common homozygous haplotype in the same region as PKD in an Italian pedigree in which three members in the same generation exhibited PED. They were additionally affected by rolandic epilepsy and writer's cramp (see above under "Genetics of PKD" and "RE-PED-WC syndrome") (50).

Treatment of PED

Generally, anticonvulsants are not useful in patients with PED. Gabapentin reduces frequency and severity of attacks. Levodopa had beneficial effects in one of five cases in which it was tried (3). Both trihexiphenidyl and acetazolamide showed some benefit in one case each (38). However, in another patient reported by Guimaraes, acetazolamide greatly worsened the condition (51). One case responded to pallidotomy (52).

PAROXYSMAL HYPNOGENIC DYSKINESIA/NOCTURNAL PAROXYSMAL DYSKINESIA

The syndrome of paroxysmal hypnogenic dyskinesia (PHD)/nocturnal paroxysmal dyskinesia is characterized by intermittent (sometimes complex) motor events like dystonic, choreoathetoid, and ballistic movements arising from nonrapid eye movement (NREM) sleep, in particular stages 2 to 3 (53). Together with paroxysmal arousals and episodic nocturnal wandering, PHD is thought to be part of the clinical spectrum of nocturnal frontal lobe epilepsy (NFLE)(53). Thus NFLE seizures can be divided into 3 main types: paroxysmal arousals (PA), lasting less than 20 seconds; nocturnal paroxysmal dystonia, lasting less than 2 minutes; and episodic nocturnal wandering, lasting up to 3 minutes. These seizures of different duration often overlap in the same patient (53). A genetic mutation is found to be responsible for some of these cases (see below under genetics).

Clinical Aspects of PHD

Attacks may occur up to several times per night over a period of years and consisting of tonic movements of the four limbs and the body axis, automatisms, affective mimicry, and vocalization and subsequent sleep fragmentation and insomnia (54). Often, attacks emerge in clusters of up to 20 spasms lasting about 30–60 seconds (55). Long-lasting variants are relatively rare. NFLE is more common in men (male–female ratio 7:3), and onset of symptoms is usually during adolescence.

Overall, intrafamilial and interfamilial variations in clinical features are not uncommon. Some patients may exhibit epileptic attacks during daytime.

Pathophysiology of PHD

No difference of classical sleep parameters is found although microstructure analysis shows sleep instability and arousal fluctuations (56). Electroencephalography is often normal but may show some evidence of epilepsy (53) resembling frontal-lobe seizures arising mesially or in depth. One polysomnographic study of 40 patients demonstrated ictal epileptiform abnormalities over frontal areas in 32% (57). Interictal EEGs are normal in 51% of NFLE cases (53). SPECT studies demonstrated hyperperfusion of anterior cingulate gyrus (58).

Etiology of PHD

Secondary Causes of PHD

As stated previously, different etiologies can form the basis of PHD, and a sound diagnostic workup should be done to confirm the correct diagnosis.

Among the group of patients with secondary paroxysmal movement disorders in general, 1 of 17 (6%) had episodes during sleep, secondary to stroke (2).

Genetics of PHD

About 40% of NFLE patients have a family history of nocturnal paroxysmal episodes (53). Provini reports autosomal dominant inheritance in 6% of documented cases (53). Penetrance is reduced to 80% (57). The autosomal dominant inherited disorder has been given the eponym *autosomal dominant nocturnal frontal lobe epilepsy* (ADNFLE) (55,56,57,58,59). Mutations on chromosomes 15q24 and 20q13.2-13.3 coding for the a4 and beta2 subunits of nicotinic acetylcholine receptors (CHRNA4 and CHRNB2) (59) are the underlying cause making the disorder a ligand gated channelopathy. Missense mutations (60) leading to the replacement of serine 248 by phenylalanine in the second transmembrane segment and a 3-base pair insertion in the CHRNA4 gene have been reported (61).

Treatment of PHD

Generally, short-lasting nocturnal dyskinesias respond well to low doses of carbamazepine. Phenytoin and acetazolamide also have beneficial effects.

Prognosis for PHD

Only a few data are published. However, it appears that NFLE does not show a tendency to spontaneous remission.

Differential Diagnosis of PHD

Video monitoring should be done to differentiate and delimit from parasomnias presenting with onset in early childhood, rare episodes of long duration, absence of stereotypy, and general disappearance after puberty. In contrast, NFLE occurs between the ages of 10 and 20, and it manifests frequent complex and repetitive behaviors of short duration—excluding rare prolonged seizures; nocturnal agitation; some daytime complaints, such as fatigue or sleepiness; and persistence into adulthood. Differentials include parasomnias, obstructive apneas, nocturnal myoclonus, and intensified hypnic jerks. Video monitoring can help to differentiate from PHD.

MISCELLANEOUS MOVEMENT DISORDERS: BURSTS OR PAROXYSMAL ATTACKS

Apart from the four classic paroxysms subsumed under the heading of *paroxysmal dyskinesias*, disorders occurring more intermittently have been described in the literature. Discussion of some of these hyperkinetic motor attacks follow. Major symptoms include dystonia, ataxia, and tremor.

Paroxysms with Dystonia as Major Symptom

Orthostatic Paroxysmal Dystonia
Recently, Sethi et al. coined the term *orthostatic paroxysmal dystonia* as attacks were provoked by assuming an upright position after sitting or lying (63). MRI showed vascular changes (correlative to the cerebrovascular history). There was decreased perfusion in the contralateral frontoparietal cortex during dystonic attacks in the PET scan.

Tonic Spasms of Multiple Sclerosis
Tonic spasms or tonic seizures are the most frequent movement disorder described in multiple sclerosis (MS). Attacks are of short duration (from 20 seconds to 1–2 minutes), frequent (up to 60 times per day), and stereotyped. Typically, one side of the body is affected. Spasms are often painful. Precipitating factors are voluntary movements, tactile stimulation, startling noise, or hyperventilation. These should be differentiated from typical PKD, which is not painful.

Transient Paroxysmal Dystonia/Torticollis in Infancy
In this disorder, intermittent head tilting or rotation, usually alternating from side to side, can be associated with irritability, vomiting, pallor, agitation, abnormal truncal posture, and gait disturbance (64). Less frequently, infantile migraine or other seizures may be associated. Age at onset is within the first 12 months of life. Duration varies between 10 minutes and 14 days, usually 2–3 days. There is no effective therapy. However, the disorder is of benign character and self-limiting, usually around 2 years of age. EMG studies revealed continuous electrical discharges over the sternocleidomastoid muscle on the same side as the torticollis. Secondary conditions, such as posterior fossa tumor, cervical dislocation, ocular palsy, dystonia due to side effects of drugs, and Sandifer's syndrome (65), referring to prolonged head tilting in children following eating due to hiatus hernia and gastroesophageal reflux, should be considered (66). In the latter, children or infants present with vomiting and feeding difficulties and occasionally with an iron-deficiency anemia. Bizarre posturing occurs immediately after feeding and subsides with fasting.

Paroxysmal Stereotypy Tic Dystonia Syndrome
Paroxysmal dyskinesias present as asymmetric bilateral dystonia of the upper limbs—mainly affecting the hands—and orofacial dyskinesias (67). Stereotypies (jumping and arm flapping) and tics (facial and sometimes vocal) may be associated. An autosomal, perhaps x-chromosome linked, trait has been suggested. As stereotypy and tics are classically recognized as a specific class of movement disorders, this condition should be separated from those labeled as paroxysmal (22).

Paroxysms with Ataxia as Major Symptom

Episodic ataxia (EA) is a rare, familial disorder producing brief attacks of generalized ataxia with normal or near-normal neurological function between attacks. Clinically, patients exhibit intermittent attacks of mere ataxia (EA-2) or ataxia associated with myokymia (rippling of muscles), also referred to as *neuromyotonia*, evident between attacks (EA-1). Inheritence is autosomal dominant. Attacks last seconds or minutes in EA-1 compared to minutes to days in EA-2. Episodes of EA-1 are provoked by physical and emotional stress, startle, or sudden movements. During episodes, dysarthria, tremor, and visual disturbances may occur (68). Continuous myokymia is present in EA-1 only. Vertigo is more commonly found in EA-2 (69). Drug treatment includes acetazolamide (EA-2) and the potassium channel blocker 4-aminopyridine (70). Both EA-1 and EA-2 have been identified as channelopathies. EA-2 typically results from nonsense mutations in the CACNA1A gene located on chromosome 19p13.2, which encodes the alpha1A subunit of the P/Q-type calcium channel. EA-1 was linked to missense mutations on chromosome 12p near the voltage gated K+ channel gene, KCNA1.

Paroxysms with Tremor as Major Symptom

Nardocci reported a case with MS exhibiting both paroxysmal dystonia and paroxysmal tremor (71). The brief unilateral dystonic posturings subsided after acetazolamide treatment. Tremor, particularly affecting the head as side-to-side tremor, was of high amplitude, slow rhythm, observed at rest, and increasing with movement.

Paroxysmal Superior Oblique Myokymia

Orbicularis myokymia frequently occurs in young, otherwise healthy individuals (3). The intermittent muscle fasciculations are transient and generally disappear with time (72). Muscle relaxants, botulinum-A toxin, and surgical myectomy are not needed in most cases.

Paroxysms with Tonic Conjugate Deviation of the Eyes

Major symptoms are sudden ocular movements with sustained upward deviation of the eyes beginning at around 9 months of age, disappearing spontaneously at about 2.5 years (73). Association of down-beating saccades in attempted downgaze, apparently preserved horizontal eye movements, and frequent association with mild ataxia or clumsiness at time of illness have been reported (74). Symptoms can be exacerbated by fatigue, illness, or vaccination and are relieved by sleep. A nocturnal polysomnographic study revealed focal or generalized paroxysmal discharges during NREM sleep in the form of polyspikewaves and spike-waves (75) and shortened rapid eye movement (REM) sleep latency. A long-term follow-up of 10 years concluded the good prognosis of this disorder with and without antiepileptic treatment (76). However, a conflictive study reported developmental delay in almost 70% of patients. Tics are an important differential diagnosis as the association of involuntary gaze deviation and tics is not uncommon (77).

Paroxysms of the Tongue

This disorder is characterized by a delayed onset of episodic, rhythmic, involuntary movements of the tongue after head and neck trauma (78). The 3-per-second waves begin as posterior midline focal tongue contractions, lasting approximately 10 seconds in each episode, persisting for 2–4 months. A similar disorder has been described as occurring mainly in sleep (79).

REFERENCES

1. Lotze T, Jankovic J. Paroxysmal kinesigenic dyskinesias. *Semin Pediatr Neurol* 2003;10:68–79.
2. Blakeley J, Jankovic J. Secondary paroxysmal dyskinesias. *Mov Disord* 2002;17:726–734.
3. Demirkiran M, Jankovic J. Paroxysmal dyskinesias: clinical features and classification. *Ann Neurol* 1995;38:571–579.
4. Gowers WR, ed. *Epilepsy and other convulsive diseases: their causes, symptoms and treatment*, 2nd ed. London: J & A Churchill, Ltd., 1901:109 ff.
5. Smith LA, Heersema PH. Periodic dystonia. *Proc Mayo Clin* 1941;16:842–846.
6. Falconer M, Driver M, Serafetinides E. Seizures induced by movement; report of a case relieved by operation. *J Neurol Neurosurg Psychiatry* 1963;26:300–307.
7. Kertesz A. Paroxysmal kinesigenic choreoathetosis, an entity within paroxysmal choreoathetosis syndrome: description of ten cases including one autopsied. *Neurology* 1967;17:680–690.
8. Stevens H. Parxysmal choreo-athetosis: A form of reflex epilepsy. *Arch Neurol* 1966;14:415–420.
9. Fahn S. The paroxysmal dyskinesias. In: Marsden CD, Fahn S, eds. *Movement disorders*. 3rd ed. Woburn, MA: Butterworth Heinemann, 1994:310–346.
10. Jung SS, Chen KM, Brody JA. Paroxysmal choreoathetosis: report of Chinese cases. *Neurology* 1973;23:749–755.
11. Houser MK, Soland VL, Bhatia KP, et al. Paroxysmal kinesigenic choreoathetosis: a report of 26 patients. *J Neurol* 1999;246:120–126.
12. Lishman WA, Symonds CP, Whitty CW, Willison RG. Seizures induced by movement. *Brain* 1962;85:93–108.
13. Sadamatsu M, Masui A, Sakai T, et al. Familial paroxysmal kinesigeneic choreoathetosis: an electrophysiologic and genotypic analysis. *Epilepsia* 1999;40:942–949.
14. Hirata K, Katayama S, Saito T, et al. Paroxysmal kinesigenic choreoathetosis with abnormal electroencephalogram during attacks. *Epilepsia* 1991;32:492–494.
15. Ohmori I, Ohtsuka Y, Ogino T, et al. The relationship between paroxysmal kinesigenic choreoathetosis and epilepsy. *Neuropediatrics* 2002;33:15–20.
16. Lombroso CT. Paroxysmal choreoathetosis: an epileptic or nonepileptic disorder? *Ital J Neurol Sci* 1995;16:271–277.
17. Volonté MA, Perani D, Lanzi R, et al. Regression of ventral striatum hypometabolism after calcium/calcitriol therapy in paroxysmal kinesigenic choreoathetosis due to idiopathic primary hypoparathyroidism. *J Neurol Neurosurg Psychiatry* 2001;71:691–695.
18. Nagamitsu S, Matsuishi T, Hashimoto K, et al. Multicenter study of paroxysmal dyskinesias in Japan: clinical and pedigree analysis. *Mov Disord* 1999;14:658–663.
19. Swoboda KJ, Soong B, McKenna C, et al. Paroxysmal kinesigenic dyskinesia and infantile convulsions: clinical and linkage studies. *Neurology* 2000;55:224–230.
20. Valente EM, Spacey SD, Wali GM, et al. A second paroxysmal kinesigenic choreoathetosis locus (EKD2) mapping on 16q13-q22.1 indicates a family of genes which give rise to paroxysmal disorders on human chromosome 16. *Brain* 2000;123:2040–2045.
21. Spacey SD, Valente EM, Wali GM, et al. Genetic and clinical heterogeneity in paroxysmal kinesigenic dyskinesia: evidence for a third EKD gene. *Mov Disord* 2002;17:717–725.
22. Szepetowski P, Rochette J, Berquin P, et al. Familial infantile convulsions and paroxysmal choreoathetosis: a new neurological syndrome linked to the pericentromeric region of human chromosome 16. *Am J Hum Genet* 1997;61:889–898.
23. Guerrini R, Bonanni P, Nardocci N, et al. Autosomal recessive rolandic epilepsy with paroxysmal exercise-induced dystonia and writer's cramp: delineation of the syndrome and gene mapping to chromosome 16p12-11.2. *Ann Neurol* 1999;45:344–352.
24. Mount L, Reback S. Familial paroxysmal choreoathetosis. *Arch Neurol Psychiatry* 1940;44:841–847.
25. Lance JW. Sporadic and familial varieties of tonic seizures. *J Neurol Neurosurg Psychiatry* 1963;26:51–59.
26. Lance JW. Familial paroxysmal dystonic choreoathetosis and its differentiation from related syndromes. *Ann Neurol* 1977;2:285–293.
27. Fink JK, Rainer S, Wilkowski J, et al. Paroxysmal dystonic choreoathetosis: tight linkage to chromosome 2q. *Am J Hum Genet* 1996;59:140–145.
28. Auburger G, Ratzlaff T, Lunkes A, et al. A gene for autosomal dominant paroxysmal choreoathetosis/spasticity (CSE) maps to the vicinity of a potassium channel gene cluster on chromosome 1p, probably within 2 cM between D1S443 and D1S197. *Genomics* 1996;3:90–94.
29. Lombroso CT, Fischman A. Paroxysmal non-kinesigenic dyskinesia: pathophysiological investigations. *Epileptic Disord* 1999;1:187–193.
30. Del Carmen Garcia M, Intruvini S, Vazquez S, et al. Ictal SPECT in paroxysmal non-kinesigenic dyskinesia: case report and review of the literature. *Parkinsonism Relat Disord* 2000;6:119–121.
31. Bohnen NI, Albin RL, Frey KA, et al. (+)-alpha-[11C] Dihydrotetrabenazine PET imaging in familial paroxysmal dystonic choreoathetosis. *Neurology* 1999;52:1067–1069.
32. Bressman SB, Fahn S, Burke RE. Paroxysmal non-kinesigenic dystonia. *Adv Neurol* 1988;50:403–413.
33. Zorzi G, Conti C, Erba A, et al. Paroxysmal dyskinesias in childhood. *Pediatr Neurol* 2003;28:168–172.
34. Hofele K, Benecke R, Auburger G. Gene locus FPD1 of the dystonic Mount-Reback type of autosomal-dominant paroxysmal choreoathetosis. *Neurology* 1997;49:1252–1257.
35. Jarman PR, Davis MB, Hodgson SV, et al. Paroxysmal dystonic choreoathetosis. Genetic linkage studies in a British family. *Brain* 1997;120:2125–2130.
36. Rainier S, Thomas D, Tokarz D, et al. Myofibrillogenesis regulator 1 gene mutations cause paroxysmal dystonic choreoathetosis. *Arch Neurol* 2004;61:1025–1029.
37. Lee HY, Xu Y, Huang Y, et al. The gene for paroxysmal non-kinesigenic dyskinesia encodes an enzyme in a stress response pathway. *Hum Mol Genet* 2004;13:3161–3170.
38. Bhatia KP. The paroxysmal dyskinesias. *J Neurol* 1999;246:149–155.
39. Bhatia KP, Soland VL, Bhatt MH, et al. Paroxysmal exercise-induced dystonia: eight new sporadic cases and a review of the literature. *Mov Disord* 1997;12:1007–1012.
40. Wali GM. Paroxysmal hemidystonia induced by prolonged exercise and cold. *J Neurol Neurosurg Psychiatry* 1992;55:236–237.

41. Nardocci N, Lamperti E, Rumi V, et al. Typical and atypical forms of paroxysmal choreoathetosis. *Dev Med Child Neurol* 1989;31: 670–674.
42. Munchau A, Valente EM, Shahidi GA, et al. A new family with paroxysmal exercise induced dystonia and migraine: a clinical and genetic study. *J Neurol Neurosurg Psychiatry* 2000;68: 609–614.
43. Neville BG, Besag FM, Marsden CD. Exercise induced steroid dependent dystonia, ataxia, and alternating hemiplegia associated with epilepsy. *J Neurol Neurosurg Psychiatry* 1998;65:241–244.
44. Bozi M, Bhatia KP. Paroxysmal exercise-induced dystonia as a presenting feature of young-onset Parkinson's disease. *Mov Disord* 2003;18:1545–1547.
45. Margari L, Perniola T, Illiceto G, et al. Familial paroxysmal exercise-induced dyskinesia and benign epilepsy: a clinical and neurophysiological study of an uncommon disorder. *Neurol Sci* 2000;21:165–172.
46. Meyer BU, Irlbacher K, Meierkord H. Analysis of stimuli triggering attacks of paroxysmal dystonia induced by exertion. *J Neurol Neurosurg Psychiatry* 2001;70:247–251.
47. Rona S, Berardelli A, Vacca L, et al. Alteration of motor cortical inhibition in patients with dystonia. *Mov Disord* 1998;13:118–124.
48. Kluge A, Kettner B, Zschenderlein R, et al. Changes in perfusion pattern using ECD-SPECT indicate frontal lobe and cerebellar involvement in exercise-induced paroxysmal dystonia. *Mov Disord* 1998;13:125–134.
49. Barnett MH, Jarman PR, Heales SJ, et al. Further case of paroxysmal exercise-induced dystonia and some insights into pathogenesis. *Mov Disord* 2002;17:1386–1387.
50. Guerrini R. Idiopathic epilepsy and paroxysmal dyskinesia. *Epilepsia* 2001;42(suppl3):36–41.
51. Guimaraes J, Vale Santos J. Paroxysmal dystonia induced by exercise and acetazolamide. *Eur J Neurol* 2000;7:237–240.
52. Bhatia KP, Marsden CD, Thomas DG. Posteroventral pallidotomy can ameliorate attacks of paroxysmal dystonia induced by exercise. *J Neurol Neurosurg Psychiatry* 1998;65:604–605.
53. Provini F, Plazzi G, Lugaresi E. From nocturnal paroxysmal dystonia to nocturnal frontal lobe epilepsy. *Clin Neurophysiol* 2000;111(Suppl2):S2–S8.
54. Hirsch E, Sellal F, Maton B, et al. Nocturnal paroxysmal dystonia: a clinical form of focal epilepsy. *Neurophysiol Clin* 1994;24:207–217.
55. Scheffer IE, Bhatia KP, Lopes-Cendes I, et al. Autosomal dominant nocturnal frontal lobe epilepsy: a distinctive clinical disorder. *Brain* 1995;118:61–73.
56. Zucconi M, Ferini-Strambi L. NREM parasomnias: arousal disorders and differentiation from nocturnal frontal lobe epilepsy. *Clin Neurophysiol* 2000;111(suppl2):S129–S135.
57. Oldani A, Zucconi M, Asselta R, et al. Autosomal dominant nocturnal frontal lobe epilepsy: a video-polysomnographic and genetic appraisal of 40 patients and delineation of the epileptic syndrome. *Brain* 1998;121:205–223.
58. Schindler K, Gast H, Bassetti C et al. Hyperperfusion of anterior cingulate gyrus in a case of paroxysmal nocturnal dystonia. *Neurology* 2001;57:917–920.
59. Bhatia KP. Familial (idiopathic) paroxysmal dyskinesias: an update. *Semin Neurol* 2001;21:69–74.
60. Weiland S, Witzemann V, Villarroel A, et al. An amino acid exchange in the second transmembrane segment of a neuronal nicotinic receptor causes partial epilepsy by altering its desensitization kinetics. *FEBS Lett* 1996;398:91–96.
61. Steinlein OK, Magnusson A, Stoodt J, et al. An insertion mutation of the CHRNA4 gene in a family with autosomal dominant nocturnal frontal lobe epilepsy. *Hum Mol Genet* 1997;6:943–947.
62. Montagna P, Sforza E, Tinuper P, et al. Paroxysmal arousals during sleep. *Neurology* 1990;40:1063–1066.
63. Sethi KD, Lee KH, Deuskar V, et al. Orthostatic paroxysmal dystonia. *Mov Disord* 2002;17:841–845.
64. Ishida T, Hattori S, Ueda T, et al. Benign paroxysmal torticollis in infancy: case report. *No To Hattatsu* 1990;22:274–278.
65. Menkes JH, Ament ME. Neurological disorders of gastroesophageal function. *Adv Neurol* 49;409–416.
66. Guerrero Vazquez J, de Paz Aparicio P, Luengo Casasola JL, et al. Benign infantile paroxysmal torticollis: apropos of 3 cases. *An Esp Pediatr* 1988;29:149–152.
67. Cabrera-Lopez JC, Marti-Herrero M, Fernandez-Burriel M, et al. Paroxysmal stereotypy-tic-dystonia syndrome. *Rev Neurol* 2003;26:729–734.
68. Klein A, Boltshauser E, Jen J, et al. Episodic ataxia type 1 with distal weakness: a novel manifestation of a potassium channelopathy. *Neuropediatrics* 2004;35:147–149.
69. Brandt T, Strupp M. Episodic ataxia type 1 and 2 (familial periodic ataxia/vertigo). *Audiol Neurootol* 1997;2:373–383.
70. Strupp M, Kalla R, Dichgans M, et al. Treatment of episodic ataxia type 2 with the potassium channel blocker 4-aminopyridine. *Neurology* 2004;62:1623–1625.
71. Nardocci N, Zorzi G, Savoldelli M, et al. Paroxysmal dystonia and paroxysmal tremor in a young patient with multiple sclerosis. *Ital J Neurol Sci* 1995;16:315–319.
72. Jordan DR, Anderson RL, Thiese SM. Intractable orbicularis myokymia: treatment alternatives. *Ophthalmic Surg* 1989;20: 280–283.
73. Ouvrier RA, Billson F. Benign paroxysmal tonic upgaze of childhood. *J Child Neurol* 1988;3:177–180.
74. Lispi ML, Vigevano F. Benign paroxysmal tonic upgaze of childhood with ataxia. *Epileptic Disord* 2001;3:203–206.
75. Merino-Andreu M, Arcas J, Ozal-Linares E, et al. Is benign childhood paroxysmal eye deviation a non-epileptic disorder? *Rev Neurol* 2004;39:129–132.
76. Verrotti A, Trotta D, Blasetti A, et al. Paroxysmal tonic upgaze of childhood: effect of age-of-onset on prognosis. *Acta Paediatr* 2001;90:1343–1345.
77. Frankel M, Cummings JL. Neuro-ophthalmic abnormalities in Tourette's syndrome:functional and anatomic implications. *Neurology* 1984;34:359–361.
78. Keane JR. Galloping tongue: post-traumatic, episodic, rhythmic movements. *Neurology* 1984;34:251–252.
79. Jabbari B, Coker SB. Paroxysmal, rhythmic lingual movements and chronic epilepsy. *Neurology* 1981;31:1364–1367.

Stereotypy and Catatonia

Joseph H. Friedman

Stereotypy and catatonia are distinct syndromes with some overlap, and they are discussed separately in this chapter. Both are most commonly seen as parts of more severe behavioral disorders (1). Stereotypy is an "involuntary or unvoluntary [unvoluntary defined as a physical response to an inner force] . . . coordinated, patterned, repetitive, rhythmic, purposeless but seemingly purposeful or ritualistic movement, posture or utterance" (1). It occurs in response to external or inner stimuli and is often perceived as a self-stimulatory behavior. Stereotypy refers to both motor and mental behaviors; this chapter focuses on motor stereotypy. Stereotypy was considered a core feature of schizophrenia until relatively recently. "The tendency to stereotype produces the inclination to cling to one idea to which the patient then returns again and again. This leads to repetitious motor and emotional behavior that is inescapable" (2). Catatonia, too, was generally considered a classic symptom complex of schizophrenia, but no longer is. Catatonia is by definition a syndrome complex that includes motor and behavioral abnormalities (3), although some authorities argue that it should be classified as a movement disorder in the *Diagnostic and Statistical Manual of Mental Disorders (DSM)* (4). Catatonia includes stereotypic behaviors, but most stereotypies are not part of catatonic syndromes. Their inclusion in a book on movement disorders underscores the acknowledgment of the increasing overlap between neurologic and psychiatric disorders. Catatonia was redefined in the *DSM*, 4th edition (DSM-IV), to be significantly different from earlier *DSM* definitions and is now thought to be considerably more prevalent than previously believed. Stereotypy has been suggested to be the most common motor manifestation of tardive dyskinesia.

CLINICAL ASPECTS OF STEREOTYPY

Phenomenology of Stereotypy

Stereotypy is variably defined. The American Psychiatric Association defines a stereotypy as a repetitive, nonfunctional motor behavior (3). The movements are generally repeated in a monotonous fashion without apparent conscious control, despite a normal level of consciousness. Although the definition provided in the introduction to this chapter includes an irresistible quality to the movement, this is not a universally accepted criterion. Some articles include repetitive movements that are easily suppressible without the tension buildup that accompanies suppression of a tic. Another definition for a pediatric population states that motor stereotypies are "clinically defined by their involuntary, patterned, coordinated, repetitive, rhythmic, and nonreflexive features; typically last for seconds to minutes; occur in clusters; appear many times per day; and are associated with periods of excitement, stress, fatigue, or boredom" (5). In addition, a stereotypy may simply be a habit or a self-stimulation in a manner that is not pathologic. For example, finger tapping, hair curling, and foot tapping are considered normal. All three are stereotypies, yet none is "pathologic" or involuntary. Among normal children, 20% exhibit stereotypies (6,7) at some time, and sterotypies are common in college students. Stereotypy also occurs in animals and has an agreed-on definition in farm animals as a repetitive action, fixed in form and orientation, that serves no obvious function.

Stereotypies may be simple or complex (1). Simple stereotypies are composed of a few simple maneuvers, such as rocking, tapping, clapping, clicking, hair twirling, and head banging. Complex stereotypies, such as running forward and backward with repeated gesticulations or vocalizations, repeated opening and closing of a door and then sitting down, and spitting into a hand then rubbing it in one's hair, are more clearly psychiatric and are not mistaken for tics, myoclonus, or other movement disorders. Either by the nature of the stereotypy or as a result of the repetitive nature of the act, self-mutilation may occur. Persistent hitting, rubbing, or licking, even lightly, may break down the skin. In other cases, the severity of each individual insult—such as hitting, biting, or scratching oneself; punching a wall; or head banging—may produce disfiguring wounds. Most cases of stereotypy are simple, with rocking, hugging, self-touching, patting, grunting, foot tapping, leg swinging, and hair pulling being the most common (1).

Differential Diagnosis of Stereotypy

Distinguishing a stereotypy from other movements is important and often difficult. Many of the people with stereotypies cannot describe their feeling states. Mannerisms, akathisia, tics, compulsions, restless legs syndrome, paroxysmal dyskinesias, epilepsy, and perseveration may be included in the differential diagnostic list, with tics and mannerisms being the most likely to cause confusion (Table 35.1). Mannerisms are movements performed in a highly idiosyncratic manner, such as grasping a pen with both hands to write or always holding a cup with the hand in a peculiar posture. "Mannerisms are a bizarre way of carrying out a purposeful act which usually occurs as the result of the incorporation of a stereotypy into a goal directed behavior" (8). On one end of the spectrum, the definition requires that these postures be grotesque and clearly abnormal to any untrained eye. On the other end of the spectrum, mannerisms may be simple gesticulations unique to that individual or a trait of a particular culture. For example,

TABLE 35.1

DIFFERENTIAL DIAGNOSIS OF STEREOTYPIC MOVEMENTS

Akathisia
Automatisms
Compulsions
Drug-induced dyskinesias
Epileptic seizures
Complex partial
Focal tonic
Petit mal
Mannerisms
Perseverations
Paroxysmal dyskinesias
Restless legs syndrome
Complex tics

hand gesticulation is particularly common among the Haitians. Unusual rituals, such as those that ballplayers may exhibit before batting or making a free throw, are accepted as mannerisms by some authorities (1).

Complex tics may be repetitive and thus appear stereotypic. Simple tics are sudden, brief movements that occur in isolation or in brief bursts. The movements are generally repeated and typically involve eye blinking, grimacing, or head jerking. Complex tics are a more elaborate sequence of movements that may be repeated at regular or irregular intervals. Examples include repetitive head shaking, abnormal posturing, throwing oneself on the ground, and complex gesturing (see videotape in reference 9). If the patient has Tourette's syndrome, these may be associated with vocalizations. Some authorities (10) distinguish between perseveration and stereotypy, with some limiting stereotypy to the motor components and perseveration to the mental components of repetitive purposeless activities. However, some investigators consider perseverations to be motor acts. Ridley (10) proposed that perseveration should refer to repetitive "but not excessive" actions, whereas stereotypy should refer to "excessive production of one type of motor act or mental state." Unlike a stereotypy, which is repeated endlessly, perseverations continue for a limited period. They do not become part of a fixed repertoire of movements. Perseverations generally occur at the end of a normal, purposeful movement and consist of repetitions of parts of the original movement, which fade out eventually. In clinical practice, neurologists often encounter verbal perseverations, usually in demented, encephalopathic, or aphasic patients. The subject answers one question and then repeats this answer when asked further questions, no matter how unrelated the questions are. Motor perseverations are less common.

Restless legs syndrome is defined as a syndrome induced by a desire to move the legs (see Chapter 31). Limb restlessness is associated with sensory discomfort, improvement with movement and worsening with rest, worsening of symptoms at night, and absence of akathisia (no history of dopamine antagonists and no sign of whole-body restlessness). Over time, the initially suppressible movements may become involuntary. The patients provide histories that clearly distinguish this from stereotypy. The patients generally need to move their legs, and their movements appear normal. They stop frequently upon relieving their symptoms.

Obsessive–compulsive spectrum disorders (OCSD) are "intrusive events with associated repetitive behaviors." These include tics, hair pulling, nail biting and the like, and they differ from obsessive–compulsive disorders (OCDs) in that they are not due to "cognitive intrusions" (11); they are due to "sensory intrusions." Compulsions are repetitive thoughts or activities, such as counting, touching, checking, tapping, gambling, risk taking, or avoiding (11). In contrast to obsessions, which are recurrent unwanted thoughts or ideas, compulsions ease anxiety, whereas obsessive thoughts increase them. OCSD and OCD have similar phenomenology, and factor analysis reveals them to fall into three categories: "checking, religious, and sexual; symmetry and ordering; washing and cleaning" (11). Common compulsions are repeated hand washing, checking, tapping, arranging items on a desk so that everything is perfectly lined up, and stereotyped rituals. These may occur as part of a primary psychiatric disorder (OCD), in association with Tourette's syndrome, as a result of encephalitis lethargica, or, rarely, in response to a focal brain lesion. The movements generally appear normal but rarely lead to a pattern of movements so restricted or odd in appearance that they become a stereotypy. For example, patients with obsessional slowness may move as if parkinsonian and get stuck attempting to walk or sit, thereby adopting a relatively fixed posture, or they may move one step back and forth, as if caged.

Rhythmic movement disorder refers to a benign syndrome of stereotyped movements that typically occur at sleep onset and during normal nighttime arousals, beginning in children under the age of 2. Primarily, these include head banging (jactatio capitis nocturna) and body rocking. They occur at sleep transitions, during naps, and during nocturnal arousals. Humming or chanting may accompany the movements. These are considered normal and resolve with development. They are seen as "soothing" behaviors that facilitate falling asleep. These are common in children under 1 year and decline from a prevalence of 67%–8% by age 4. Body rocking involves rocking to and fro, often on hands and knees. Head banging may be done in recumbent or sitting positions into soft or hard surfaces. Head rolling and body rolling side to side are less common. (7).

Paroxysmal dyskinesias fall into two major categories: kinesogenic and nonkinesogenic (see Chapter 34). These are episodic, lasting for minutes or hours, during which the patient has normal mentation but displays chorea or dystonia. As the movements are odd, they may be misinterpreted as stereotypic, but the episodic nature and the patient's normal mentation should clearly distinguish these movements from stereotypies.

Akathisia is the inability to remain still because of an inner sense of restlessness. The afflicted person is unable to sit in one place, feeling compelled to stand up frequently, march in place, or shift weight from one foot to the other. The person may perform jumping jacks or other calisthenics or walk briskly up and down a corridor. When the activity is repetitive, it is in fact a stereotypy, an unvoluntary act that relieves an inner sense of tension. Most cases of akathisia are induced by both dopamine receptor–blocking drugs (neuroleptics) and by dopaminergic drugs (levodopa). The syndrome may occur in both treated and untreated patients with Parkinson's disease (PD).

When a patient is noncommunicative, as is often the case in the psychotic or profoundly retarded, one cannot always categorize the movement pattern. For example, akathisia is a movement in response to an inner drive and

can manifest in a variety of behaviors, including worsened psychosis or stereotypy, yet the patient may not be able to explain the problem. Simply observing a behavior without obtaining a complete history, such as changes of medication, will lead to an incorrect diagnosis.

Epileptic seizures of various types also might be misconstrued as stereotypic behaviors. Children with petit mal seizures will look dazed and will blink, sometimes developing lip smacking if the spell lasts for several seconds. Complex partial seizures may induce stereotypic behaviors with an impaired consciousness, but if the patient has a mental impairment at baseline, a change may not be evident. In addition, focal tonic seizures may produce a stereotypy.

Many cases of repetitive movements are not easy to delineate clearly as a stereotypy in comparison to another type of movement disorder. The clinical context in which the movement is seen must be taken into account, perhaps more than in the assessment of other movement disorders.

In rare cases, the stereotypy is part of a neurodegenerative disorder, such as Rett's syndrome, Lesch-Nyhan syndrome, or neuroacanthocytosis.

Causation of Stereotypy

Certain stereotypies are normal (6,7), and others are virtually diagnostic of a specific disorder, so that the complete evaluation of the patient and the developmental history of the behavior are important (see Table 35.2). Thumb sucking is normal in children, and delayed onset or absence of this movement may indicate maturational dysfunction. Head banging, head rolling, and general rocking occur in about 20% of normal children at some point (6,7) and usually resolve spontaneously, so that even a behavior as dramatically upsetting as a baby purposefully banging its head on the floor may be deemed normal. Certainly, it is considered normal for adults to tap a foot or fingers, to pull on hair, and to cross and recross their legs, and thumb sucking in children is usually viewed as a normal and comforting stereotypy. The context of the movement and the culture of the patient help determine normality. Stress typically worsens stereotypies.

Stereotypy may be induced by alterations in perception. Probably the most common stereotypy is the self-stimulatory, vacuous chewing of edentulous adults. This may be considered normal, as it arises so commonly in otherwise completely normal individuals.

Stereotypies most commonly occur in the autistic, retarded, psychotic, congenitally blind, and congenitally deaf (1,12). The age of onset of the movements depends on the syndrome. In genetically determined disorders, the onset may be in late childhood. The incidence and phenomena of stereotypy vary to some degree with the syndrome and to a large degree with the severity of the underlying behavioral disorder. In studies of institutionalized nonhandicapped children, 59% exhibited one or more

TABLE 35.2
CAUSES OF STEREOTYPIES

Autism

Asperger's syndrome
Infantile autism
Kanner's syndrome

Drug Induced

Psychostimulants
Tardive dyskinesia

Inborn Errors of Metabolism

Lesch-Nyhan syndrome
Neuroacanthocytosis

Infectious

Encephalitis

Mental Retardation (all types)

Neurodegenerative Disorders

Physiologic Disorders

Psychiatric Disorders

Catatonia
Functional
Obsessive–compulsive disorder
Schizophrenia

Rett's Syndrome

Sensory Deprivation

Caging, constraint
Congenital blindness
Congenital deafness
Stroke

---

stereotypies (13). Thumb sucking declined and nail biting increased with age. In the retarded, the prevalence of stereotypy is higher and the movements more sustained (14).

Autism is a childhood-onset syndrome characterized by abnormal socialization with poor attachment and interaction with people, disordered cognitive and language skills, abnormal responses to stimulation, necessity for sameness in the environment, repetitive behavior, and a normal physical appearance. Autism is considered distinct from retardation, and although it is often thought that acquisition of motor skills and motor function is normal in autistic children, about 50% of autistic children are motor delayed, and many are clumsy. Autistic patients most often display "facial grimacing, staring at flickering lights, waving objects in front of the eyes, producing repetitive sounds, arm flapping, rhythmic body rocking, repetitive touching, feeling and smelling objects, jumping, walking on toes and unusual hand and body gesturing" (1). Clapping and tapping are also common. There are several variants of autism, which, with the exception of Rett's syndrome, affects boys considerably more often than girls. Fragile X syndrome, Kanner's syndrome (the original

describer of autism), and Asperger's syndrome are all causes or types of autism. Fragile X syndrome causes a wide variety of retardation syndromes and is the single most common cause of mental retardation in boys. Asperger's syndrome is a form of autism involving an isolated area of extreme, all-absorbing interest, such as astronomy or history. With good function in at least the one intellectual area, children with Asperger's syndrome have a mild form of autism. Those with Asperger's variant also have mild clumsiness, more so than those with the Kanner variant, but they are otherwise more mildly affected.

Rett's syndrome, a disorder restricted to female patients, causes persistent hand wringing or hand washing, which usually points to the correct diagnosis. In addition to these typical stereotypies, patients with Rett's syndrome manifest a variety of other movement disorders, including dystonia and parkinsonism.

Lesch-Nyhan syndrome is an X-linked disorder of boys that is attributable to a purine metabolism abnormality. Patients bite their lips, fingers, forearms, and nails. They may scratch their noses and mouths and draw blood. Unlike most other syndromes of self-injury, these children request restraints, an observation that contradicts the general hypothesis that stereotypy is a self-stimulatory behavior. The children also display a variety of movement disorders. They display aggressive behavior to other people and may hit objects, also sustaining injury.

Neuroacanthocytosis is a constellation of disorders that includes an increased percentage of acanthocytic red blood cells. One form of the syndrome includes tongue and lip biting.

Despite the different causes and ages of onset, the phenomena of most stereotypies tend to overlap, although certain ones tend to be more common in particular disorders. For example, the various sensory deprivation–induced stereotypies are relatively similar. Congenitally blind children rock, suck fingers, and display repetitive manipulation of objects (12). Blind adults rock and exhibit stereotypies as well, exemplified by the musician Stevie Wonder. Autistic and retarded children display eye poking as the most common stereotypy (12). Deaf children also have a high incidence of rocking behavior but do not seem to hit their ears as blind children hit their eyes. Generally, there is less self-injurious behavior (SIB) in these disorders than in the autistic and retarded (12). Intermittent stereotyped walking movements have been reported in a stuporous patient with medial frontoparietal cortical lesions in association with meningitis.

I once evaluated a rare case of focal stereotypy due to a parietal stroke. The patient developed right-sided numbness and a mild aphasia associated with a cortical infarct in the left parietal region seen on brain magnetic resonance imaging. Shortly after the stroke, the patient noted persistent movements of his tongue, pushing against the right side of his upper denture, and constant rubbing of his right index finger across his right thumbnail. He denied any feeling of compulsion or inner release of tension achieved by the movements, and he could stop them if he focused his attention on it. The movements continued to the point where he broke down the skin on his fingers and his dentures had to be replaced. Use of a thick glove that reduced sensory stimulation made it worse, but use of a thin silk glove made him feel better, although the movements persisted, suggesting that the loss of self-stimulation was bothersome despite his denial. Two other cases, both with more complex stereotypies, have been reported with strokes. One followed a series of brain insults in a child, including a right putaminal stroke, and the other followed a right lenticular infarction. I have also seen a stereotypy develop as part of an unidentified neurodegenerative disorder manifested by progressive aphasia, right hemiparesis, dementia, and an eye movement disorder. The patient, while seated, bent over every few seconds to touch her left foot or stocking with her left hand. Another patient, in his mid 70s, developed stereotypic bilateral finger rubbing in association with a gait disorder. A ventricular peritoneal shunt improved the gait, sustained for over 1 year, confirming the diagnosis of normal-pressure hydrocephalus, but the stereotypy was unaffected.

Stereotypies can be induced in adult humans and animals by imprisonment in close quarters (15). These caging stereotypies may occur at any age. Ritualistic behavior and extreme slowness are commonly seen in OCD. The rituals may be simple or complex and may be forms of stereotypy. Simple behaviors, such as repetitive touching, spitting, hair pulling, and hitting, are stereotypies. More complex behaviors, such as checking (repeated checks to confirm that the door is locked, the windows closed, the stove turned off, and so on) or persistent hand washing, may not be stereotypies in that the manner in which the repeated activity is carried out may vary and the behavior can be postponed. Obsessive slowness is a Parkinson's-like bradykinesia that may accompany OCD. This may result in a manneristic approach to routine activities, such as sitting, in which the movement may be arrested for a period followed by extreme slowness in completion of the action. Alternatively, a patient may get stuck as if frozen (mental block) and attempt to move but be unable to do so, causing a motor activity to be repeated, shifting weight as if about to take a step, and repeating this for long periods. These movements may thus fall into a gray zone between mannerism and stereotypy. In a psychotic individual, whether part of the primary diagnosis or induced by a neuroleptic, the disorder occurs in adulthood, sometimes quite late. The stereotypies of autism, retardation, and developmental sensory deprivation occur in childhood. Psychotic patients display a primary form of stereotypy, more often rocking back and forth than any other stereotypy, but may be catatonic (discussed elsewhere in this chapter). They also may have tardive stereotypy from treatment with neuroleptics.

Stereotypies as a central feature of tardive dyskinesia (TD) were highlighted in a study of patients with TD, most of whom were thought to have stereotypies as part of their syndrome. These affected the orolingual and facial regions most commonly, followed by the legs, arms, trunk, and pelvis, in that order. The orolingual movements were writhing with protrusion of the tongue, lip puckering, and chewing. Vocalization, with humming and belching most common, were also noted. Perhaps most typical of the stereotypies and least likely to cause disagreement over appropriate classification were leg crossing, leg swinging, finger or hand tapping, arm rubbing and grasping, picking, and thumb twiddling. These movements were described in patients already diagnosed as having TD, and the authors believe that tardive stereotypy may occur in isolation without other signs of TD, such as facial movements. Clearly, tardive stereotypy and tardive akathisia overlap, since akathisia frequently causes the patient to move about, rock, stand and sit, and fidget in general to relieve the urge to move.

Punding, a stereotypy typically induced by cocaine or amphetamines but also reported with levodopa (11), is a syndrome in which adults show intense fascination with repetitive handling of common objects or repeated picking to the point of self-injury. Cocaine and amphetamine may induce, under the spell of fascination, a desire to take apart (and rarely to rebuild) objects. In one PD patient, anti-Parkinson's drugs produced a need to tally strings of figures repetitively. This produced a feeling of great satisfaction in the patient, despite his knowledge that the work produced was of little value. He could reflect on this as a peculiar behavior that he felt as foreign but that was satisfying at the time. This is thought to reflect excessive sopamine stimulation (15) in PD, yet other compulsive behaviors have been linked to reduced dopamine, "off" states (16), or unrelated to increased or decreased dopamine (17).

Self-Injurious Behavior in Stereotypy

SIB is viewed by some as a continuum on the spectrum of stereotypic behavior (18). It most often occurs in the setting of autism and retardation but also with some genetic disorders. Body rocking has been associated with self-hitting (18) and other SIBs. Typical SIB includes nail biting, finger biting, punching objects and self, head banging, and lip biting. However, SIB is not specific for stereotypies and may be seen in Tourette's syndrome, neuroacanthocytosis, tuberous sclerosis, and in both psychotic and nonpsychotic psychiatric conditions. SIB in stereotypy tends to be the result of accumulated small injuries. Although this may be the case in psychiatric patients, more commonly, SIB in psychosis is a cataclysmic outpouring of emotion, perhaps as self-punishment or exorcism. Repeated self-inflicted cigarette burns and knife wounds also are seen in psychiatric patients but much less so in patients with retardation or autism. These injuries may occur in nonpsychotic states, such as personality disorder, or may represent disordered adjustment to an overwhelmingly bad social situation, as in the case of the physically abused wife who escapes beating by injuring herself first. Injuries in the psychiatric population may be a disguised plea for help. SIB occurs in 2%–20% of the institutionalized retarded (18), depending on the study, and 50% of autistic children (19). SIB has been classified into two major categories: social and nonsocial. Social SIB creates greater social consequences, being more "blatant and dramatic" (18) to watch, suggesting that the caregiver's response is an important instigator for the action. Social SIB includes head banging, biting, scratching, gouging, pinching, and hair pulling. Nonsocial SIB includes stuffing orifices, mouthing and sucking, ruminative vomiting, coprophagy, aerophagy, and polydipsia (18).

Biological Basis of Stereotypy

The basic mechanisms of stereotypy are unknown, although clear associations with causes, as previously discussed, are known. There is a general belief that stereotypy in higher animals is a form of self-stimulation (10). Support for this is based in part on these behaviors in children born blind or deaf (12). It occurs in animals deprived of their mothers (20) and in autistic and retarded children, who generally interact little with their environments. It is a biologically fascinating phenomenon because many of the behaviors are shared across causation and species, although the causative mechanisms are different (10,20). Animal data support deprivation as a cause for stereotypy. Animals raised alone develop deprivation stereotypy (10), which consists of repetitive movements, such as rocking, sucking, and head banging, that are seen in humans with impaired socialization (10). Once a critical period has passed, these behaviors are not reversible (10,20). An alternative theory holds that stereotypy reduces a state of chronic hyperarousal by channeling thought and action into the repeated movements, thus tempering environmental input rather than enhancing it. Stereotypies exist in animals as primitive as insects, which lack a brain. The foreleg and hindleg rubbing behavior of flies, or the stereotypic motor program by which some insects move their legs, indicates the genetic role for some repetitive motor programs that do not even require a brain.

The occurrence of particular stereotypies with certain drugs suggests common pharmacologic pathways for many of the behaviors. For example, both amphetamine and cocaine enhance catecholamine release and induce the same sniffing, picking, and repeated explorations in animals as in humans. Amphetamines given to rodents produce stereotypies that vary with the ratio of norepinephrine to dopamine. With a high ratio of norepinephrine to dopamine, amphetamine produces exploratory locomotor stereotypies, which are constrained by additional levodopa. Amphetamine-induced stereotypies are reduced when dopamine alone is depleted but are unaffected if both catecholamines are depleted. In rats, there is a correlation between D2 receptor density and apomorphine-induced stereotypy, although not with altered spontaneous behavior,

presumably because of decreased dopamine synthesis. Apomorphine and amphetamine given systemically or intrastriatally to rodents produce stereotypic licking, sniffing, gnawing behaviors that are blocked by D2 receptor–blocking drugs. Interestingly, apomorphine injected subcutaneously into humans produces yawning without sleepiness, yet the dopamine agonists bromocriptine, pergolide, and so forth do not. This implies that this one behavior is not specifically related to a pure dopamine effect or that the effect is extremely dependent on the ratio of the dopamine receptor activities of the drug, thus implying a need for caution in generalizing. Neuroleptics, which block dopamine receptors, cause TD and tardive stereotypy, possibly as the result of up-regulation of dopamine receptors. In Lesch-Nyhan syndrome, a deficiency in hypoxanthine guanylribosyltransferase leads to dopamine deficiency in all basal ganglia structures except the substantia nigra, probably due to a reduction in terminal arborization of dopamine-secreting neurons. However, the importance of dopamine in the behavior is unknown. Dopamine-blocking and enhancing drugs both have been helpful in isolated cases.

Biochemical interpretations are helpful in understanding certain stereotypies but may be specific to the behavior under evaluation, generalizing to a limited degree only. Catecholamine treatments that induce stereotypy in rodents fail to do so in mice bred to lack D1 receptors, implying a necessity for D1 activity. Hypotheses to explain drug-induced stereotypy involve imbalances in distinct basal ganglia circuits as measured by gene expression or by interruption of particular basal ganglia circuits (14). The same abnormal repetitive disorders in PD have been reported to result from dopamine excess and dopamine deficiency (17), suggesting multiple mechanisms mediating even a single behavior.

Inherited disorders, such as Tourette's syndrome and Lesch-Nyhan syndrome, cause different types of stereotypies. In some cases, as in Tourette's syndrome, the particular stereotypy varies considerably even between affected individuals in the same family who presumably share the same genes, whereas the behavior in Lesch-Nyhan syndrome is relatively similar in all families.

In Rett's syndrome, an X-chromosome genetic abnormality, girls begin to develop their movements in the first 2 years of life, and while hand wringing or hand washing is the major stereotypy, other self-mutilating behaviors occur (14). Some patients hit or bite themselves and, occasionally, others. Although the pathology is being defined, the explanation for this peculiar behavior remains a mystery.

It is increasingly accepted that stereotypic behaviors reflect basal ganglia disorders (14), although that does not indicate which neurotransmitter systems or circuits may be involved.

Treatment of Stereotypy

Patients with stereotypy may or may not require treatment. When stereotypy interferes with learning and socialization, treatment is necessary. SIB usually requires either treatment or restraint. This includes a minor segment of all people who display stereotypy but a significant fraction of the institutionalized population.

Treatment obviously depends on causation. In most cases, this means retardation and autism. Stereotypies in these conditions are most likely to interfere with education and socialization. Behavior modification using rewards or punishments, aversive therapy, or redirection to less intrusive behaviors is generally used. Results are mixed. Medications are sometimes effective. Naltrexone, an opiate antagonist, has been found to be helpful in reducing SIB in some studies but not in others. Selective serotonin reuptake inhibitors (SSRIs) also may be helpful. Risperidone has been shown to reduce both stereotypic behaviors and SIB in autistic and severely disturbed children (21).

Tardive stereotypy can be reduced with catecholamine-depleting drugs (22), such as tetrabenazine and reserpine. Using higher doses of the dopamine receptor–blocking drugs that caused the problems in the first place can mask the syndrome, but only temporarily, until the problem worsens.

Stereotypies associated with OCD respond to treatment for the OCD, usually with the SSRI types of antidepressant drugs.

PHENOMENOLOGY OF CATATONIA

Catatonia is a syndrome that occurs in many diseases (23). It is not a diagnosis. No single definition exists. Its association with psychiatric disorders has been and continues to be rethought, and its association with medical diseases continues to expand. In *DSM-IV*, catatonia is considered a subtype of schizophrenia, a syndrome due to a systemic medical disorder, and a descriptor for affective disorders (3) (Table 35.3). Johnson (24) described catatonia as "a neuropsychiatric syndrome in which an abnormal mental state is associated with cataleptic phenomena, namely akinesia, posturing, and mutism." *Catalepsy* is the term he reserved for akinesia, posturing, and mutism in the absence of "any psychiatric abnormality" (24). Bush et al. (25) described catatonia as "a neuropsychiatric syndrome in which the diagnosis does not depend upon individual interpretation of mental status abnormalities but these are severe," thus using the term as a syndrome seen in psychosis but independent of a particular diagnosis. A syndrome of *catatonia without psychosis* has been described (24), and the term *medical catatonia* has been accepted for the catatonic syndrome, including mental abnormalities, that is due to an organic illness (26).

Catalepsy, which was described at least as early as Galen's time, is derived from the Greek word meaning "a seizure of the body and soul." Catalepsy describes the development of fixed postures, either self or externally imposed. It was a phenomenon known for centuries and was associated with various mental disturbances. It could

TABLE 35.3
DSM-IV SUBTYPES OF CATATONIA

Motor Features

1. Motoric immobility
2. Excessive motor activity (purposeless and uninfluenced by external stimuli)
3. Extreme negativism or mutism
4. Peculiarities of voluntary movement
5. Echolalia or echopraxia

Catatonia Due to a Medical Condition (293.89)

Motor features (as above)
Evidence of a general medical condition
No better psychiatric explanation
Disturbance not exclusively part of delirium

Catatonic Schizophrenia (295.20)

Schizophrenia dominated by at least 2 of the 5 main motor features (as above)

Catatonic Features Specifier

Major affective disorder with 2 of the 5 major motor motor features (as above)

even be induced by psychosocial stressors, as occurred in epidemic fashion in response to religious preaching (24). Catatonia, however, was first coined in a famous monograph by Kahlbaum in 1874 (27). This term also is based on a Greek word meaning "to stretch tight." Kahlbaum's manuscript refers to catatonia as the "tension insanity." The disorder was recognized as a brain disease with a remarkably diverse panoply of signs that cycled between a hypoactive state in which catalepsy and bizarre stereotypies predominated and a hyperactive physical and emotional state often associated with abnormal, nonsensical speech production.

Catatonia was then "hijacked" (24) by Kraepelin and subsumed into the entity *dementia praecox*. Kraepelin interpreted the syndrome as a form of mental blocking, in contrast to Kahlbaum's conceptualization of it as an organic brain disease. Bleuler (2) later reinforced this notion in his famous text on schizophrenia, in which 26 pages of his chapter on the symptoms of schizophrenia are devoted to "the catatonic symptoms" (Table 35.4). Catatonia remained a syndrome of schizophrenia until *DSM-IV*. After *DSM-III-R* failed to include catatonia as a manifestation of mania, critics noted the frequent association of catatonia with both affective and medical disorders. This association was noted early in the 20th century, and recent criticism resulted in a modification of the *DSM* definition. Increased interest in the catatonic syndrome coincided with this change. Several published studies examine phenomenology, epidemiology, and etiology (23–37). Catatonia may be present in children (35,38) although standard diagnostic criteria do not exist. The associations among neuroleptic malignant syndrome, neuroleptic-induced catatonia,

TABLE 35.4
SIGNS OF CATATONIA

Bleuler, 1950 (2)

Catalepsy
Stupor
Hyperkinesis
Stereotypies, motor and behavioral, including speech
Mannerisms
Negativism
Command: automation and echopraxia
Automatisms, motor and speech
Impulsiveness

Johnson's Cataleptic Triad, Johnson, 1993 (24)

Immobility
Maintenance of imposed postures
Mutism

Bush et al., 1996 (29)

Excitement grimacing
Immobility, stupor echophenomena
Mutism stereotypy
Staring verbigeration
Posturing rigidity
Withdrawal waxy flexibility
Impulsivity, ambitendency
Automatic obedience grasp reflex
Mitgehen perseveration
Gegenhalten autonomic abnormality

Sadock and Sadock, 2000 (12)

Catalepsy posturing
Excitement waxy flexibility
Rigidity

Rosebush et al., 1990 (33)

Immobility negativism
Staring waxy flexibility
Mutism echolalia/echopraxia
Rigidity, stereotypy
Withdrawal verbigeration
Posturing, grimacing

TABLE 35.5
PROPOSED DIAGNOSTIC CRITERIA FOR CATATONIA

A. Immobility, mutism, or stupor of at least 1 hour in duration, associated with at least one of the following: catalepsy, automatic obedience, or posturing, observed or elicited on two or more occasions.
B. In the absence of immobility, mutism, or stupor, at least two of the following, which can be observed or elicited on two or more occasions: stereotypy, echophenomena, catalepsy, automatic obedience, posturing, negativism, gegenhalten, amitendency.

From Taylor MA, Fink M. Catatonia in psychiatric classification: a home of its own. *Am J Psychiatry* 2003;160:1233–1241. With permission.

catatonia, and lethal catatonia have been explored in the literature as well (39,40). Small series of open-label treatment have been reported, generally with excellent outcomes (37).

Clinical Signs of Catatonia

Signs considered part of the catatonic syndrome are wide ranging (2,23,24,25,37). The most important is catalepsy. Multiple distinct but overlapping criteria have been proposed for the diagnosis of catatonia since 1976 (23). Taylor and Fink believe that only two signs are required for the diagnosis (Table 35.5) and suggested that catatonia should be classified as a movement disorder in *DSM-IV* (23). Presumably *DSM-IV* (3) represents the closest to a consensus opinion. In an attempt to define objectively the likely diagnostic criteria, one study compared 32 catatonics to 155 noncatatonic psychiatric patients. Using receiver operating characteristic (ROC) analysis, any cluster of 3 of 11 "classic" signs discriminated between the two groups, giving equal weight to each sign: immobility/stupor, mutism, negativism, oppositionalism, posturing, catalepsy, automatic obedience, echophenomena, rigidity, verbigeration, and withdrawal (28). Bleuler (2) described patients maintaining postures for months at a time and considered this situation "not at all rare." Bleuler believed that this rigidity was psychologically produced and did not constitute an organic rigidity, a hypothesis that contrasts with some modern authors (37). Bleuler noted that the patients exerted precise control over muscular contractions so that movements could be made "like a piece of wood" or "as a lever" with exact compensation of other parts of the body. More common than whole-body rigidity was waxy flexibility (cerea flexibilities). Patients were akinetic but would maintain a posture imposed on them, apparently completely indifferent to discomfort. These imposed postures would persist for several minutes before resolving into more comfortable, albeit still bizarre, postures. In having a posture altered by an examiner, patients often participated, responding easily to mildly applied pressures, or they over-responded if moved quickly (mitgehen). At other times, however, displaying a negative approach, the patient might also resist alteration of a posture. The waxy flexibility or fixed posture might apply only to one part of the body, while another limb performed a variety of maneuvers. The catalepsy could sometimes be provoked or aborted by environmental changes, so that patients might suddenly become hyperactive after being stuporous if a particular person entered the room, or they would exhibit catalepsy only when observed and appear normal when thinking themselves unobserved.

Catatonic stupor is more difficult to define, as *stupor* has different meanings in the psychiatric and neurologic literature. *Psychiatric stupor* has been defined as "a temporary reduction or obliteration of both reactive and spontaneous relational functions" (29). Johnson (30) defined stupor as "a state of total psychomotor inhibition with retained normal or partial consciousness." This is obviously different from the standard neurologic definition. Yet it has been asserted that "stupor and catatonia have often been used interchangeably." Bleuler (2) considered it a form of "reduced psychic activity or of total blocking." He also merged states he considered "clouded" or "twilights" with conditions of complete alertness internally with external manifestations of stupor or coma. Examples would be the "comatose" patient who recalls complete details of events occurring during the apparent coma or the patient who rouses from lethargy upon receiving the appropriate cue, then lapses back into the torpid state. Catatonic stupor has been reported with organic brain diseases, including brain tumors, metabolic derangements such as diabetic ketoacidosis, and hepatic encephalopathy, implying the existence of "neurologic" or true stupor, a condition in the continuum to coma, rather than a psychogenic stupor or pseudocoma. One report describes a patient with catatonia resembling nonconvulsive status epilepticus, thus presenting the appearance of a clouded consciousness. The issues of stupor, coma, and pseudocoma are discussed elsewhere in this chapter, as they raise questions about the overlap between neurologic and psychiatric disorders.

Hyperkinetic states may punctuate the akinetic, plastic, unresponsive baseline. This hyperactive phenomenon, along with the frequently more benign prognosis that is typical for schizophrenia, supported the association between catatonia and affective states, particularly manic depression (24). These opposite poles of the catatonic syndromes, which were termed *catatonic stupor* and *catatonic excitement*, represented Kahlbaum's description of catatonia as having a cyclic alternating course (27). These hyperactive states involved outbursts of senseless activity such as running, jumping, exercising, and yelling.

Stereotypies of all types—motor, speech, and thought—were "one of the most striking external manifestations of schizophrenia" (2). The simple stereotypies, such as clapping, rocking, and tapping, appear similar to those seen in many other disorders. The complex behavioral routines, such as walking in a circle, bowing, and reciting a song, may be more diagnostic. Earlier authors (2) subsumed many of the features of catalepsy under the rubric of stereotypy, such as fixed bizarre postures, as well as features of immobility. Words, tunes, phrases, or rhymes may be repeated endlessly or for a precise number of times. In catatonia, the stereotypy may be linked to an obvious conscious effort that differs from that seen in retardation, autism, and sensory deprivation but that can be similar to the ritualistic behavior common in OCD. Some stereotypies, such as the rewriting of a phrase, are unlikely to be seen in organic disorders.

Mannerisms are a common feature of catatonia. Bleuler (2) noted that mannerisms may be always present but highly variable in certain individuals. For example, a patient may always grimace but may alter the facial expression each time or accompany it by a variety of body movements or sounds.

A core feature of catatonia is negativism, which can be divided into passive and active forms. In passive negativism, the patient fails to perform the requested activity, and in active negativism, the patient performs the opposite. The rigid postural abnormality may be interpreted as a form of negativism, with the patient in some cases resisting the movement of a limb to a new position, in contrast to the patient with waxy flexibility, who may assist the examiner in the repositioning.

As with catatonic stupor and catatonic excitement, catatonic negativism has its polar opposite, *command automatism*. In this condition, the patient obeys all commands like an automaton even when the request results in harm or in some other way goes against the patient's own externally perceived interest. *Echopraxia* is the syndrome in which patients repeat activities that they see. Thus, one patient who displays a bizarre stereotypy may be emulated by another with echopraxia. *Echolalia* is the repetition of sounds and phrases. Communicating with such a patient is, of course, extremely difficult. Patients may be echolalic, echopractic, or both.

Automatisms are activities carried out in response to inner commands. They are indistinguishable from activities displayed as part of a compulsion. The patient may in fact not want to perform the action and may find the impulse foreign, although it emerged from the patient's mind. Sometimes the automatism stands in contrast to other actions the patient is taking. For example, a patient may work at cleaning an area and then suddenly mess it up or break some object only to mend it.

Speech abnormalities, including echolalia (repetition of words and phrases), *palilalia* (repetition of syllables), and *verbigeration* (use of meaningless words and phrases), are sometimes present.

The remaining category of the catatonic symptom complex that Bleuler describes is *impulsivity*, which, he says, "often dominates the picture." The impulsivity, which may be explosive or less extreme, lasts from seconds to hours, rarely for days. The sudden discharge restores a sense of calm as if psychic tension has been temporarily relieved. The overlap among this form of impulse dyscontrol, automatic behavior responding to inner voices, and compulsive behavior in response perhaps to a perceived interruption of a mental or physical ritual can only be made in the context of the patient's diagnosis and other behavioral problems.

Patients may manifest only a single catatonic sign. The presence of "neurologic" motor manifestations in catatonia raises questions, addressed elsewhere in this chapter, regarding the diagnosis of catatonia in an organic disease. *Gegenhalten*, a tone abnormality in which patients seemingly increase their resistance to passive movements, transiently producing a go-and-stop, ratchety-type rigidity, is sometimes difficult to distinguish from the extrapyramidal rigidity of PD.

Catatonia has been described as a rare feature of multiple sclerosis, central pontine myelinolysis, antiretroviral therapy, the drug MDMA (also known as *ecstasy*), donepezil, malaria, and other organic disorders. It also has been precipitated by psychotropic drugs.

Epidemiology of Catatonia

The prevalence of catatonia and its relation to various psychiatric disorders is still being determined. In part, this is due to changing criteria for diagnosis (e.g., *DSM-III* versus *DSM-IV*). It is a function of the diligence of investigators and the criteria used in terms of both the absolute criteria applied and how significant the sign must be to be counted. Bleuler (2) reported that more than half of institutionalized patients displayed "catatonic symptoms either transitorily or permanently." Mahendra (31) noted that the decreasing incidence of catatonia had been recognized for years, and he speculated that many of the cases described in the previous literature may have had encephalitis lethargica, not primary schizophrenia. He also noted the association between catatonia and manic depression but agreed that the syndrome had become less common. Gelenberg (26), considering *catatonia* a generic term describing a syndrome found in organic and functional disorders, including nonpsychotic neurotic conditions, wrote that it "is not a rare phenomenon." In my own university's psychiatric hospital, a review of discharge diagnostic codes between July 1991 and July 1996 yielded only three patients with a principal diagnosis of catatonia out of 20,545 admissions. This survey would have ignored all patients with catatonic features but a principal diagnosis of other types of schizophrenia, affective disorder, organic diseases, and many other disorders. The rarity of the diagnosis supports the observation that catatonic schizophrenia, a common entity in the 19th and early 20th centuries (2,27), has undergone a dramatic decline, akin, perhaps, to the decline in hebephrenic schizophrenia. Northoff et al. (32) reported that the catatonia diagnosis constituted 2.5% of all admissions to a German psychiatric hospital.

Looking at catatonia as a syndrome, a collection of motor signs yields a vastly different result. In 140 consecutive admissions to an inpatient psychiatry service, 90% of which were emergency admissions, "catatonic syndrome" was diagnosed 15 times in 12 patients, constituting 9% of all admissions for the year. Among these patients, four had an affective disorder, two had paranoid schizophrenia, two had atypical psychoses, three had organic causes (two of these due to cocaine), and one had a nonpsychotic personality disorder (37). In one year, 65 patients admitted to a university hospital psychiatry service were catatonic, of whom 19 were schizophrenic, 16 were depressed, and 30 were "idiopathic." Other authors, using *DSM-IV* criteria, found "catatonic features," that is, any one of the five *DSM-IV* features of at least a moderate degree, in 49 (37.7%) of 130 consecutive drug-free

patients admitted to a university psychiatric hospital. Only five patients (4%) were diagnosed with catatonic schizophrenia. Note the difference between this incidence and the incidence of catatonic schizophrenia cited previously. There were no significant differences in psychiatric diagnoses between those admitted with catatonic features and those without; that is, catatonia did not cluster in one or two primary diagnostic categories. Patients with catatonic features suffered from various types of schizophrenia, affective disorder (depression and mania), OCD, and dementia. Bush et al. (25) found that 15 (7%) of 215 consecutive patients admitted to a university psychiatric hospital over a 6-month period met *DSM-IV* criteria for catatonia. In a review of 28 patients referred to a university psychiatric service meeting predetermined criteria for catatonia, regardless of underlying diagnosis, immobility or stupor was seen in all. Staring, mutism, and withdrawal were the next most common signs, present in more than 80%. Posturing and rigidity were present in more than 60%. Waxy flexibility was present in 40%, stereotypy in 30%, excitement and impulsivity in more than 40%. Grasp reflexes and gegenhalten were not present in any patients (25).

Some authors assert that catatonia can be readily distinguished from related syndromes (23). Starkstein et al. (34) used a modified Rogers scale to evaluate 79 consecutive outpatients referred to a psychiatric clinic for evaluation of depression and compared these with 41 consecutive nondepressed PD outpatients seen in routine follow-up. They found 16 depressed patients with catatonia. The PD patients (severity of illness not described) matched with the catatonics for rigidity, slowness, and immobility could be distinguished from the catatonia patients according to abnormal postures, persistence of imposed postures, mutism, underactivity, stereotypies, mannerisms, hyperactivity, and echolalia. I have diagnosed catatonia in a patient with advanced PD, illustrating the possibility of both being present simultaneously. The patient had a history of a mood disorder and had become unresponsive, but he kept his eyes forcibly shut and demonstrated waxy flexibility, maintaining postures he was put in. Bush et al. (25) assert that, using strict guidelines, catatonia patients are clearly distinguished from noncatatonic psychiatric patients, which confirms another report. Although the underlying psychiatric diagnoses varied considerably, the catatonic syndrome appeared in a variety of primary and secondary psychiatric disorders (37). It should be considered in patients with pseudocoma and unexplained akinetic mutism. It is possible that some positive sodium amytal ("truth serum") interviews in previously unresponsive patients were due to a transient response to an anticatatonic agent rather than a conversion disorder.

Thus, catatonic features, when looked for, are apparently common, even in unmedicated patients with a wide variety of psychiatric disorders. The term *catatonic syndrome*, denoting the presence of two or more motor signs meeting *DSM-IV* criteria, is also common, probably in the 5%–10% range of patients requiring psychiatric admission. The underlying psychiatric diagnoses in which the catatonic syndrome occurs fall into a broad spectrum, including schizophrenia, affective and organic psychoses, OCD, and, rarely, nonpsychiatric disorders. However, catatonic schizophrenia appears to be fairly rare, reflecting an epidemiologic change in schizophrenia, alterations in treatment, or alterations in diagnostic criteria, as reflected in the revisions of the *DSM*.

Catatonia is rare in children and adolescents and is not even defined in those age groups. Only 99 cases were reported as of 2003 (38), the date of the most recent review. Only one child younger than 10 years and four children younger than 13 years have been reported as catatonic. The gender distribution favors males among children, whereas women are more commonly catatonic than men. Electroconvulsive therapy (ECT) may be the treatment of choice in catatonic children with an underlying psychotic depression (35).

Lethal Catatonia

One particular variant of catatonia, not yet identified with an underlying disease, is lethal catatonia or malignant catatonia (39,40). This syndrome, initially described in the preneuroleptic era, appears to be similar to neuroleptic malignant syndrome, with obtundation, extreme rigidity, and autonomic dysfunction leading to death but without exposure to any neuroleptic. The few autopsies of such patients have not found uniform abnormalities. Some authors suggested that neuroleptic malignant syndrome (NMS) is a drug-induced variant of lethal catatonia; however, another syndrome mimicking NMS rarely occurs when levodopa or amantadine is abruptly discontinued in patients with PD who have no history of psychiatric dysfunction. This suggests that psychiatric dysfunction need not be present for dopamine-blocking or dopamine-depleting drugs to induce such a syndrome. The serotonin syndrome, which also resembles NMS, is another syndrome to consider in patients who are rigid, tremulous, and febrile; it is seen in patients typically taking serotonin-enhancing medications and a monoamine oxidase inhibitor.

As with catatonia in general, the response to ECT has been excellent (41).

Biological Basis of Catatonia

One can separate catatonia into organic and nonorganic categories. Using current terminology, the psychiatric, nonorganic, or functional catatonic disorders are schizophrenia or affective psychosis. Taylor and Fink suggest further refinements (23). The organic causes are numerous. Bush et al. (25) described cases brought on by neuroleptics

(NMS and neuroleptic catatonia), anticholinergics, valproic acid, and risperidone in combination, as well as seizures and steroid-induced stupor. Many other organic etiologies are also described (26,37). Encephalitis lethargica, which may induce both parkinsonism and psychiatric disorders, is one viral cause. Although the virus has never been identified and has not been seen in epidemic form in 60 years, it still may be a causative factor in some cases. Other viral syndromes may rarely cause catatonia. Among other causes of catatonia are structural brain lesions, including tumors, infarcts, and hemorrhages in a variety of locations (26,27), such as the thalamus, third ventricle, frontal lobes, and temporal lobes. Catatonia may be induced by metabolic conditions, including neuroleptic-induced disorders, aspirin intoxication, porphyria, hepatic encephalopathy, hypercalcemia, poisoning, and structural or metabolic disorders such as Wernicke's encephalopathy. Infectious causes include encephalitis lethargica, AIDS dementia complex, and typhoid fever. Certain uses of the term *catatonia*—including as a replacement for *akinetic mutism*—should be discouraged, as the two syndromes are different. It is unclear in many reports how the terms *stupor*, *coma*, and *immobility* are defined.

Perhaps the strongest support for a biological basis for catatonia comes from genetic advances. An identified missense mutation in a gene on chromosome 15 appears to cause an autosomal dominant form of schizophrenia with periodic catatonia (42). However, there also appear to be other causes for familial schizophrenic syndromes with catatonia. The identified gene on chromosome 15 is thought to code for a protein involved in neuronal cation channels.

Some authors have considered NMS and catatonia as variants of one disorder (43), regarding mental state distinct from motor state. The underlying mechanisms may involve dopamine dysfunction to account for akinesia, right posterior parietal lobe dysfunction for posturing, and medial and lateral orbitofrontal cortical abnormalities to account for behavior abnormalities (39). Supportive evidence for these theories is scant.

Animal models of catatonia should be viewed with skepticism, as the psychiatric aspects of catatonia are crucial to a meaningful concept. Simply rendering an animal or person an akinetic mute via reserpine, neuroleptics, or a brainstem lesion would hardly advance insight into this condition. One report has found computed tomographic evidence of brainstem and cerebellar vermis atrophy in five cases of catatonia, but these findings are nonspecific and small. To attempt to localize a clinicopathologic correlation to midbrain pathology (24) is probably premature. Physiologic imaging will be more useful when applied to a large series of similar subjects.

If one looks at psychodynamic explanations for some of the "functional" cases, the concept of *blocking* figures is quite large. When resistance to physical and emotional stimuli results in rigidity, negativism, muteness, and so on, leading to psychic tension, an eruption occurs (catatonic excitement), temporarily relieving the emotional pressure.

Treatment of Catatonia

Despite the apparent differences in causation, a significant number of reports indicate that catatonia, whether schizophrenic or affective, can be treated successfully with lorazepam or ECT (23,37,41). Reports on the successful treatment of neuroleptic malignant syndrome with ECT also have been published. Bush et al. (41) enrolled 28 catatonia patients in a trial of lorazepam for 5 days, followed by ECT if necessary. Of these, five patients experienced spontaneous remission, and 21 of 23 patients had a response to lorazepam. Improvements were seen in 16 of 21, with 11 having complete relief. Improvement varied inversely with the duration of signs prior to the treatment. ECT was successful in all four of the patients who were unresponsive to lorazepam. The fifth refused ECT. Success was defined as "catatonia no longer present." The authors noted that 2 out of 3 patients with neuroleptic-induced catatonia responded to a single dose of intravenous lorazepam. Some 32% of patients were not psychotic upon completion of the treatment protocol. Patients primarily had the excited variant of catatonia.

Rosebush et al. (33) prospectively treated all patients suffering from catatonia with intravenous lorazepam, documenting that of 15 patients "12 responded completely or dramatically within 2 hours." Of these 12 patients, eight had histories or evidence of coexisting neurologic disorders, such as old stroke, hydrocephalus, or alcohol abuse. One nonresponder had a personality disorder. Another responded to a ventricular peritoneal shunt. Of the lorazepam responders, four took other benzodiazepines prior to and during lorazepam treatment. Catatonia recurred if lorazepam was not maintained. Subjects in this series primarily had the depressed form of catatonia. Severity of the psychiatric disorder once the catatonia resolved was not discussed.

Ungvari et al. prospectively treated 18 catatonic patients, and those with the diagnosis of schizophrenia improved partially. The authors hypothesized that underlying diagnosis was important in outcome, unlike others (41) who noted no response differences among schizophrenic, affective, or organic patients. Several isolated reports also support the use of lorazepam and other benzodiazepines. One report describes a case of catatonia responsive within 50 minutes to one 2.5 mg dose of oral lorazepam, which reversed with a single dose of a benzodiazepine antagonist (see reference 45 for a videotape demonstrating a catatonic patient's response to intravenous lorazepam). In the only placebo-controlled, double-blind trial of lorazepam in catatonia, 12 patients with chronic schizophrenic catatonia were treated in a crossover trial. None had a beneficial response to lorazepam (46). Underlying diagnosis or

duration of the catatonia may be pertinent to treatment responsiveness. Antipsychotics, including the atypicals, have been reported to be effective (47).

ECT also has been shown in several open studies, both retrospective and prospective (34,42,48), to cure the catatonic aspect of the psychosis. Ungvari et al. reported that nine of 18 patients who failed lorazepam improved with ECT. Bush et al. (41) reported that four of five lorazepam failures responded promptly to ECT.

Few treatment reports have been published in the last 5 years.

CONCLUSION

The existence of a syndrome, seen in a variety of primary psychiatric disorders, as well as in organic disorders, all responsive by and large to lorazepam or ECT, raises the question of whether these signs have a similar mechanism. The one report of reversal of improvement with a benzodiazepine antagonist supports the concept of a single pharmacologic mechanism responsive to benzodiazepines, possibly via a gamma-aminobutyric acid (GABA) mechanism. However, the case reports (37) of patients already on benzodiazepines (42) responding to lorazepam suggests either that lorazepam has a special action different from that of other benzodiazepines or that these patients may have been only partially treated and required the extra boost of an intravenous infusion. More likely is the conclusion that catatonia is a heterogeneous syndrome. Some experts believe treatment must be designed with this in mind. Presumably, further studies will determine whether catatonia has a single common pathway manifest in a variety of disorders or, like stereotypy, represents a common collection of behaviors that simply overlap among the various conditions.

The term *medical catatonia* should be reserved for catatonic syndromes in which a psychosis or other behavioral disorder is precipitated by a systemic medical condition such as dementia, encephalitis, lupus cerebritis, or toxic encephalopathy, in which an organic psychosis occurs.

SUMMARY

Stereotypy and *catatonia* are general terms for complex behavioral patterns that appear in a wide variety of disorders. It is clear that stereotypies arise from multiple brain disorders with highly varied mechanisms, both structural and metabolic. It is unlikely that a unitary theory can be found to explain the variety of stereotypies. Catatonia, which can be conceived of in broad terms as a complex stereotypic disorder, with a fixed response to inner and external stimuli, also appears in a variety of syndromes: schizophrenia, affective psychoses, and medical diseases. The response of many of these patients to lorazepam suggests the possibility of a single, shared, biochemical lesion for the psychiatric cases. Further studies, especially those looking at biochemical and physiological changes will undoubtedly prove helpful.

REFERENCES

1. Jankovic J. Stereotypies. In: Marsden CD, Fahn S, eds. *Movement disorders 3*. London: Butterworth-Heinemann, 1994:503–517.
2. Bleuler E. Dementia praecox. New York: International University Press, 1950.
3. American Psychiatric Press. *Diagnostic and statistical manual of mental disorders*, 4th ed., *text revision (DSM IV-TR)*. Washington, DC: American Psychiatric Press, 1994.
4. Taylor MA, Fink M. Catatonia in psychiatric classification: a home of its own. *Am J Psychiatry* 2003;160:1233–1241.
5. Mahone EM, Bridges D, Prahme C, Singer HS. Repetitive arm and hand movements (complex motor steroetypies) in children. *J Pediatr* 1004;145:391–295.
6. Kravitz H, Boehm JJ. Rhythmic and habit patterns of infancy: their sequence, age of onset and frequency. *Child Dev* 1971;42:399–413.
7. Mindell JA, Owens JA. *A clinical guide to pediatric sleep: diagnosis and management of sleep problems*. Philadelphia: Lippincott Williams & Wilkins, 2003.
8. Lees AJ. Facial mannerisms and tics. *Adv Neurol* 1988;49:255–261.
9. Jankovic J. Phenomenology of tics. *Mov Disord* 1986;1:17–26.
10. Ridley RM. The psychology of perseverative and stereotyped behavior. *Prog Neurobiol* 1994;44:221–231.
11. Voon V. Repetition, repetition, and repetition: compulsive and punding behaviors in Parkinson's disease. *Mov Disord* 2004;19: 367–370.
12. Fazzi E, Lanners J, Danova S, et al. Stereotyped behaviors in blind children. *Brain Dev* 1999;21:522–528.
13. Troster H. Prevalence and functions of stereotyped behaviors in nonhandicapped children in residential care. *J Abnorm Child Psychol* 1994;22:79–97.
14. Baghdadlie A, Pascal C, Grisi S, Aussilloux C. Risk factors for self-injurious behaviors among 22 young children with autistic disorders. *J Intell Dis Res* 2003;47:622–627.
15. Rojahn J. Self injurious and stereotypic behavior of noninstitutionalized mentally retarded people: prevalence and classification. *Am J Ment Retard* 1986;91:268–276.
16. Burke K, Lombroso PJ. Animal models of Tourette syndrome in rodents. In: Ledoux M, ed. *Animal models of movement disorders*. Boston: Elsevier Academic Press, 2004:441–448.
17. Evans AH, Katzenschlager R, Paviour D, et al. Punding in Parkinson's disease: its relation to the dopamine dysregulation syndrome. *Mov Disord* 2004;19:397–405.
18. Kurlan R. Disabling repetitive behaviors in Parkinson's disease. *Mov Disord* 2004;19:433–437.
19. Friedman JH. More on repetitive behaviors in Parkinson's disease. *Mov Disord*. 2005;20:509.
20. Cross HA, Harlow HF. Prolonged and progressive effects of partial isolation on the behavior of macaque monkeys. *J Exp Res Person* 1965;1:39–44.
21. Research Units on Pediatric Psychopharmacology Autism Network. Risperidone in children with autism and serious behavioral problems. *N Eng J Med* 2002;347:314–321.
22. Jankovic J, Beach J. Long-term effects of tetrabenazine in hyperkinetic movement disorder. *Neurology* 1997;48:358–362.
23. Taylor MA, Fink M. Catatonia in psychiatric classification: a home of its own. *Am J Psychiatry* 2003;160:1233–1241.
24. Johnson J. Catatonia: the tension insanity. *Br J Psychiatr* 1993;162:733–738.
25. Bush G, Fink M, Petrides G, et al. Catatonia: 1. Rating scale and standardized examination. *Acta Psychiatr Scand* 1996;93: 129–136.
26. Gelenberg AJ. The catatonic syndrome. *Lancet* 1976;1:1339–1341.
27. Kahlbaum KL. *Catatonia*. Levi Y, Pridon T, trans. Baltimore: Johns Hopkins University Press, 1973.
28. Peralta V, Cuesta MJ. Motor features in psychotic disorders. II. Development of diagnostic criteria for catatonia. *Schizophr Res* 2001;47:117–126.
29. Berrios GE. Stupor revisited. *Comp Psychiatry* 1981;22:466–477.
30. Johnson J. Stupor: a review of 25 cases. *Acta Psychiatr Scand* 1984;70:370–377.
31. Mahendra B. Where have all the catatonics gone? *Psychol Med* 1981;11:669–671.
32. Northoff G, Koch A, Wenke J, et al. Catatonia as a psychomotor syndrome: a rating scale and extrapyramidal motor symptoms. *Mov Disord* 1999;14:404–416.
33. Rosebush P, Hildebrand AM, Furlong BG, et al. Catatonic syndrome in a general psychiatric inpatient population: frequency, clinical presentation, and response to lorazepam. *J Clin Psychiatr* 1990;51:357–362.
34. Starkstein S, Petracca G, Teson A, et al. Catatonia in depression: prevalence, clinical correlates, and validation of a scale. *J Neurol Neurosurg Psychiatry* 1996;60:326–332.
35. Cohen D, Flament M, Dubos PF, et al. Case series: catatonic syndrome in young people. *J Am Acad Child Adolesc Psychiatry* 1999;38:1040–1046.
36. Ungvari GS, Leung SK, Ng FS, et al. Schizophrenia with prominent catatonic features ("catatonic schizophrenia"): I. Demographic and clinical correlates in the chronic phase. *Prog Neuropsychopharmacol Biol Psychiatry* 2005;29:27–38.
37. Rosebush PI, Mazurek MF. Catatonia: clinical features, differential diagnosis and treatment. In: Jeste D, Friedman JH, eds. *Psychiatry for neurologists*. Boston: Humana Press, 2006.
38. Takaoka K, Takota T. Catatonia in childhood and adolescence. *Psychiatry Clin Neurosci* 2003;57:129–137.
39. Northoff G. Catatonia and neuroleptic malignant syndrome: psychopathology and pathophysiology. *J Neural Transm* 2002;109: 1453–1467.
40. Philbrick KL, Rummans TA. Malignant catatonia. *J Neuropsychiatry Clin Neurosci* 1994;6:1–13.
41. Bush G, Fink M, Petrides G, et al. Catatonia: 2. Treatment with lorazepam and electroconvulsive therapy. *Acta Psychiatr Scand* 1996;93:137–143.
42. Stober G, Szelow D, Ruschendorf F, et al. Periodic catatonia: a confirmation of linkage to chromosome 15 and further evidence for genetic heterogeneity. *Hum Genet* 2002;111:323–330.
43. Fink M. Catatonia: syndrome or schizophrenia subtype? *J Neural Transm* 2001;108:638–644.
44. Stauder KH. Die todliche Katatonie. *Arc Psychiatr Nerrvenkr* 1934;102:614–634.
45. Rosenfeld MJ, Friedman JH. Catatonia responsive to lorazepam: a case report. *Mov Disord* 1999;14:161–162.
46. Ungvari GS, Chiu HFK, Chow LY, et al. Lorazepam for chronic catatonia: a randomized, double-blind, placebo-controlled crossover study. *Psychopharmacology* 1999;142:393–398.
47. Valevski A, Loeb T, Keren T, et al. Response of catatonia to risperidone: two case reports. *Clin Neuropharmacol* 2001;24:228–231.
48. Stein D, Kurtsman L, Stier S, et al. Electroconvulsive therapy in adolescent and adult psychiatric inpatients: a retrospective chart design. *J Affect Disord* 2004;83:335–342.

Movement Disorders in Children

36

Harvey S. Singer

Movement disorders in childhood are both similar and distinct from those occurring in adulthood. The two overlap in their definitions of specific movements and provision of diagnostic and therapeutic challenges. In contrast, there are several prominent differences with motor abnormalities in the pediatric population having (a) an increased occurrence of hyperkinetic movements, rather than bradykinesia or rigidity; (b) a high frequency of transient motor phenomena in the first year of life; (c) a higher prevalence of paroxysmal movement disorders; (d) a major primary etiology for chronic motor dysfunction being residue of static encephalopathy; (e) a greater likelihood that symptoms are secondary to hereditary metabolic disorders; and (f) an evolving pattern of movements associated with metabolic disorders. Hence, in recognition of these major differences, this chapter is divided into four major sections: I. Transient Developmental Disorders; II. Paroxysmal Movement Disorders; III. Noninherited Secondary Causes of Movement Disorders; and IV. Hereditary/Metabolic Disorders Associated with Extrapyramidal Symptoms. To avoid overlap and redundancy, selected movement disorders, such as Tourette's syndrome (see Chapter 27), dystonia (see Chapters 25 and 26), and chorea (see Chapter 19), are dealt with in other chapters.

GENERAL APPROACH TO THE CHILD WITH A MOVEMENT DISORDER

Movement disorders require observation by a knowledgeable physician. Since children with paroxysmal disorders do not often have attacks while in a physician's office, documentation may require the family to provide a videotaped recording. From the history, one should determine whether the problem is acute or chronic, paroxysmal or continuous, static or associated with the loss of previously acquired skills (degenerative disorder) or whether there is evidence for multiple system involvement. The description of the symptoms should include age of onset, type of movement, course, focality, timing, triggers, patient's ability to control, progression, presence during sleep, affect on activities, associated difficulties, and other facts and observations. Historical details about the patient's gestation, delivery, early development, previous illnesses, drug history, exposure to potential toxins, and social and family histories are often essential for proper classification. Factors helpful in separating paroxysmal dyskinetic disorders from epilepsy include the identification of certain specific movement abnormalities (e.g., dystonia, choreoathetosis, tics, or stereotypies), maintenance of consciousness, a normal respiratory pattern, lack of a postical state, and absence of an electroencephalographic (EEG) abnormality during attacks. A comprehensive, general examination is essential for properly defining the movement and for identifying clues that indicate a systemic problem. As will be discussed in this chapter, especially in younger children, many unusual movements are transient and do not represent pathologic disorders.

TRANSIENT DEVELOPMENTAL DISORDERS

Transient developmental movement disorders typically occur in otherwise healthy infants or young children with no evidence of acquired lesions, toxic or metabolic etiologies, or structural brain abnormalities. They are characterized by a pattern of abnormal movements, a lack of

TABLE 36.1
TRANSIENT DEVELOPMENTAL DISORDERS

Chorea/dystonia: Physiologic chorea or dystonia, fever-induced, benign idiopathic dystonia of infancy
Myoclonus: Benign neonatal myoclonus, benign myoclonus of early infancy
Shuddering: Shuddering (shivering) attacks
Torticollis: Benign paroxysmal torticollis; Sandifer's syndrome; spasmus nutans
Head Nodding: Periodic head nodding; spasmus nutans
Paroxysmal Tonic Upgaze
Jitteriness
Tics: Transient tics

---

progression, minimal disability, the absence of specific laboratory markers, normal development and neurological function, and complete resolution (1). Whether these movements should even be labeled as "disorders" is controversial. Pathologically, they may be manifestations of an evolving neural system or transient dysfunction. Management should focus on parent education, since pharmacotherapy has little role. (See Table 36.1.)

Chorea/Dystonia

Physiologic

Many newborns and infants manifest a variety of dyskinetic movements that tend to be brief in duration and of no apparent pathological consequence. Pursing and sucking of the lips, head and neck extensions, body and extremity twists, turns, and postures are but a few of the myriad of movements labeled as *physiologic chorea* or *dystonia* (2,3). Dystonia, recognizable as hyperextension in low-risk preterm infants, did not correlate with motor function at age 2.5 years (4). Unfortunately, since little has been done to investigate these phenomena, their frequency and physiologic mechanisms remain undetermined. One speculation is that these movements may represent interplay between the development of voluntary movements in an evolving nervous system and the presence of primitive reflexive responses. Difficulties with early coordination are routinely part of the maturational process. For example, a broad-based, uncoordinated, ataxic gait is the norm in infants beginning to walk independently. Brief myoclonic jerks are also common in early development.

Fever-Induced Dystonia

Two children (aged 2.5 and 6 years) have been reported with a syndrome of fever-induced episodic dystonia. Both had episodes, beginning at age 2 years, of lower-extremity dystonia with inversion of the feet and dorsiflexion of the great toes. Movements were triggered by fever, lasted up to 24 hours, and diminished in frequency as the children aged. Parents had a history of similar events. Metabolic and imaging studies were normal (5).

Benign Idiopathic Dystonia of Infancy

Several normal children have been described with transient dystonic postures, usually shoulder abduction, forearm pronation, and wrist flexion, that appear in the first months of life, briefly progress, and then resolve after 3 months to 5 years (3,6). Posturing of the upper extremity, body, or trunk can be intermittent or persistent, occur at rest, and disappear with volitional movements. Neurological examination is normal and developmental outcome is good.

Myoclonus

Benign Neonatal Myoclonus

Myoclonic movements are largely confined to sleep, and they appear most frequently during quiet stages and least often during rapid eye movement (REM) sleep. Myoclonic jerks are repetitive, occur in brief clusters, and last up to several minutes before stopping spontaneously. Rarely, the jerks may be prolonged (7). They may be focal or generalized, rhythmic or nonrhythmic, and typically more frequent in distal rather than proximal limbs (8). Onset is usually in the first month of life with myoclonus persisting for several months, rarely into early childhood (9,10). Jerks may be triggered by noise, and awakening the infant causes the movements to cease. Neurological examination, EEG evaluation, and neuroimaging studies are normal, and there is no subsequent association with developmental delay or seizures (11,12). Treatment, other than education, is not necessary, and the use of benzodiazepines may exacerbate the myoclonus.

Benign Myoclonus of Early Infancy

Children with this disorder are frequently misdiagnosed as having infantile spasms. Ictal and interictal EEGs, however, are normal. Onset is usually between ages 3–9 months, and most resolve within 1–8 months after onset, although some have persisted for longer periods (13,14). In contrast to the benign neonatal form that occurs during sleep, these occur while the child is awake. No treatment is indicated, and outcome is good.

Shuddering (Shivering) Attacks

Shuddering or shivering attacks are a benign movement disorder (15,16,17,18) characterized by periods of rapid tremor of the head, shoulder, or arms. Attacks are brief (several seconds), occur up to hundreds of times per day, and have no associated loss of awareness. Episodes start in infancy or early childhood, tend to become less frequent, and often spontaneously remit during the first decade. Children studied with EEG monitoring during the attacks showed no alteration of the electrocerebral background (16,18). The cause of shuddering attacks is unknown. On the basis of a strong family history of essential tremor and EMG recordings, it has been hypothesized that shuddering attacks may be a precursor for essential tremor (15,18). One patient has been successfully treated with beta-blockers (17). Antiepileptic drugs do not suppress the movements.

Torticollis

Benign Paroxysmal Torticollis

Benign paroxysmal torticollis typically occurs within the first 12 months of life. Attacks comprising torticollis and slight head and neck movements occur without warning or specific trigger and last from minutes to weeks (range 10 minutes to 14 days) (19,20,21,22). Some attacks may be preceded by agitation, crying, pallor, and vomiting, but no precipitating factor has been identified. Patients may have several attacks within a month, and the torticollis may alternate from side to side. There is no diurnal fluctuation, and torticollis is not affected by sleep. The attacks typically cease spontaneously by age 5 years, and no treatment is effective. Children with paroxysmal torticollis often develop benign paroxysmal vertigo of childhood and later migraine. Studies in children with paroxysmal torticollis—including neuroimaging, cerebrospinal fluid (CSF) analysis and EEG monitoring—have been unremarkable. The precise etiology remains unknown, but some cases may be inherited. Although a dysfunction of the vestibular apparatus has been hypothesized (19,20,21,22,23), an association with paroxysmal vertigo, the subsequent development of migraine, and a strong family history for migraine has suggested a migraine equivalent or disruption of blood flow to the brainstem (24,25). Two patients with benign paroxysmal torticollis, identified in a kindred with familial hemiplegic migraine with ataxia associated with a CACNA1A mutation, have raised the possibility of a calcium channel dysfunction in this disorder (22).

Sandifer Syndrome (Dyspeptic Dystonia)

This syndrome is one of gastroesophageal reflux, with or without a hiatal hernia, associated with dystonic movements of the head and neck and, at times, abnormal posturing of the body, including opisthotonos. Recurrent paroxysmal posturings are typically associated with feedings, although they may persist postprandially. Barium swallow studies, esophagoscopy, and pH probes are used to document the reflux and hernia. Symptoms usually resolve after appropriate gastrointestinal intervention (26). One adult with Sandifer syndrome has been misdiagnosed as refractory partial seizures (27).

Spasmus Nutans

Spasmus nutans is characterized by the triad of head nodding (horizontal or vertical tremor of the head); rapid, asymmetric, low amplitude nystagmus, which may be binocular or monocular; and torticollis (28,29). The nystagmus, often dysconjugate, may increase on lateral gaze.

Spasmus nutans usually appears between 3 and 12 months of age and spontaneously resolves by 3–5 years of age. Long-term visual acuity is good. Since the clinical findings used to diagnose spasmus nutans can be simulated by retinal dystrophies, an electroretinogram is recommended (30). The cause is unknown, but a low socioeconomic status represents a risk factor (31). An optic chiasm or third-ventricle glioma has been identified in a few patients who also had a later onset, optic nerve pallor, and monocular nystagmus. Hence, an magnetic resonance imaging (MRI) study is often considered part of the evaluation, especially in atypical patients (32,33).

Head Nodding

Periodic head nodding, consisting of repetitive flexion of the neck, is seen in otherwise normal young children (34). Movements may be vertical (yes–yes), horizontal (no–no), or oblique and may occur in the seated or standing position. There is no associated loss of awareness. Many of these cases resolve in several months, whereas others may persist (see motor stereotypies). Some head nodding occurs in association with shuddering or other stereotypies and in individuals with a family history of essential tremor (35). Development and outcome are good. This entity should be differentiated from the more serious condition referred to as bobble-head doll syndrome. In the latter, infants and young children have intermittent jerky head movements, resembling those of a doll's head perched atop a spring, with a frequency ranging from 2–3 cycles per second. Brain imaging studies in the bobble-headed doll syndrome typically identify an underlying structural abnormality, usually a third ventricular cyst, tumor, or dilatation of the third ventricle secondary to either aqueductal stenosis or a suprasellar arachnoid cyst (36–38). Cases also have been described in individuals with normal third ventricles, including one with aqueductal and fourth-ventricle enlargement (39). Surgical treatment usually corrects the abnormal movement.

Paroxysmal Tonic Upgaze of Infancy

This disorder is characterized by repeated episodes of tonic, conjugate, sustained upward deviation of the eyes with episodes lasting for hours to days (40,41,42). During the event, horizontal eye movements are normal, but down-beating saccades can occur with attempted downgaze. Episodes are exaggerated by illness and fatigue, improve with sleep, and may be accompanied by ataxia or clumsiness. Laboratory investigations are generally normal, but a case with associated periventricular leukomalacia has been reported (40,43). Symptoms resolve spontaneously in 1–4 years. Improvement has been reported with the use of levodopa (43).

PAROXYSMAL MOVEMENT DISORDERS

Paroxysmal movement disorders are the most common movement abnormalities encountered by child neurologists. The list of nonepileptic paroxysmal movement disorders is extensive, and it is extremely helpful to separate the various conditions on the basis of the type of movement disorder observed, such as ataxia, choreoathetosis, dystonia, head bob, shudder, startle, stereotypy, tic, torticollis, and so forth (Table 36.2). Hence, the initial step is to have a clear definition and understanding of the abnormal movement. This frequently requires viewing a videotape recording of the child's attack, since patient/parent history may be vague and inconclusive. Diagnostic possibilities can then be considered and the likely disorder identified. Lastly, after fully assessing the child, the physician, in conjunction with the patient, family, and school personnel, must determine whether the episodic movements are having a negative functional or psychological impact. Medications should be targeted and reserved only for those problems that are disabling and not remediable by other interventions.

Associated with Ataxia

Several familial forms of episodic ataxia have been identified, each representing a different genetic disorder (see Chapter 32).

Associated with Choreoathetosis or Dystonia

One commonly used classification identifies four variants (see Chapter 34): paroxysmal kinesigenic dyskinesia (PKD), paroxysmal nonkinesigenic dyskinesia (PNKD), intermediate or exertional (exercise-induced) dyskinesia (PED), and paroxysmal hypnogenic dyskinesia (PHD) (44). Linkage analyses have identified several paroxysmal dyskinesia loci: PKD loci on chromosome 16 between p12.1-q21 and a PNKD locus on chromosome 2q35 (45). Secondary paroxysmal dyskinesias have been reported in association with a variety of calcium and metabolic problems, thyroid dysfunction, cerebral palsy (CP), head trauma, medullary hemorrhage, and spinal cord lesions (46). Several reports have described the association of paroxysmal dyskinesias and various types of seizures, including benign infantile seizures (47,48), generalized seizures (45,49), early-onset absence (50), and rolandic epilepsy (51).

Associated with Tics

Tic disorders represent the most common movement disorder seen by physicians caring for children. For example, in Monroe County, Rochester, New York, the weighted prevalence estimates for tics were 23.4% for students in special education and 18.5% in regular education classrooms (52). Tourette's syndrome (TS), once considered a rare disorder, now has an estimated prevalence of 1–10 per 1000 children and adolescents (52,53,54). TS is common in children with autism, Asperger's syndrome, and other autistic spectrum disorders, but its presence is unrelated to the severity of autistic symptoms (55). (See Chapter 27).

Associated with Stereotypies

Although often inaccurately assumed to be strictly associated with mental retardation, autism, schizophrenia, tardive dyskinesia, or neurodegenerative diseases, stereotypic movements can occur in otherwise normal children (56) (see Chapter 35). Physiologic stereotypies can be divided into three major subdivisions based on the type of movements observed: common (e.g., body rocking, thumb sucking, nail biting) (57), head nodding (34), and complex (56,58,59). Complex stereotypies should be differentiated from complex motor tics and compulsions. Complex tics, defined as abrupt movements that involve either a cluster of simple motor tics or a more coordinated sequence of movements, have several features in common with stereotypies (e.g., they are intermittent and precipitated by excitement). A variety of clinical characteristics, however, can assist in distinguishing the two disorders: stereotypies (a) have onset at an earlier age (<2 years) than do tics (mean onset 6–7 years); (b) are more constant and fixed in pattern compared to the more variable action of tics; (c) involve arms, hands, or the entire body rather than eye blinks, facial grimaces, head twists, or shoulder shrugs; (d) are more rhythmic, with flapping and waving, than tics, which tend to be rapid and random; (e) are generally more continuous and prolonged in duration; (f) are not associated with premonitory urges or desires to reduce an inner tension; (g) often occur when the child is engrossed in an activity

---

TABLE 36.2

PAROXYSMAL MOVEMENT DISORDERS

Ataxia: Episodic ataxia without myokymia; episodic ataxia with myokymia; episodic ataxia with paroxysmal choreoathetosis; paroxysmal tonic upgaze with ataxia; familial metabolic periodic ataxias; other

Choreoathetosis or dystonia: Paroxysmal dystonic choreoathetosis; paroxysmal kinesigenic choreoathetosis; intermediate or exertion-induced; paroxysmal hypnogenic dyskinesia; secondary paroxysmal dyskinesias

Tics: Transient; chronic (motor/vocal) tic disorder; Tourette's syndrome; tourettism

Motor stereotypies: Physiologic (nonautistic) and pathologic (autism, Rett's syndrome, etc.)

Posturing during masturbation

Startle: Hyperekplexia; startle epilepsy; brainstem reticular reflex myoclonus; others

Restless legs: alone or in association with another disorder

Chin quivering

(e.g., computer game, games arcade), although both may occur during periods of excitement or stress; (h) can be stopped by distraction, but the child rarely makes a conscious effort to control the movements, whereas tics can be voluntarily suppressed for brief periods. Compulsions are differentiated from stereotypies by their association with an attempt to prevent or reduce distress or some dreaded event or situation. They are also frequently driven by an obsessive thought or by intrinsic rules that must be applied rigidly.

Posturing During Masturbation

Masturbation, or self-stimulation of the genitalia, is a normal part of human sexual behavior that occurs in both males and females. In infants and young children, masturbating activity may present in a variety of patterns and has been mistaken for epilepsy (12,60), paroxysmal dystonia, or dyskinesia (61,62). Observation of movements on a video can often clarify the diagnosis and eliminate the need for unnecessary diagnostic tests (63).

Associated with Startle

A startle response is a brief motor response, usually a jerk, elicited by an unexpected auditory or, less commonly, tactile, visual, or vestibular stimulus. A normal startle response to auditory stimuli usually involves the upper half of the body and readily habituates. In contrast, in startle syndromes, movements are of greater amplitude, are more widely distributed, and habituate poorly. In most patients with startle disease (hyperekplexia), the startle is immediately followed by another movement abnormality. For example, several seconds after the initial startle, there may be a period of generalized stiffening lasting for seconds, termed *tonic spasms*. While these occur, the patient is unable to respond voluntarily and, if standing, will fall rigidly to the ground without losing consciousness. If prevented from falling to the ground, the patient appears stiff despite a loss of muscle tone. In addition to tonic spasms, patients with familial or symptomatic hyperekplexia may experience excessive repetitive flexion of the limbs, especially the legs, during sleep, termed *nocturnal myoclonic jerks*. Despite the name, the movements are not myoclonic, and jerks may occur after an unexpected stimulus or as a spontaneous event.

Hyperekplexia (Hyperexplexia, Startle Disease)
Although it has been suggested that hyperexplexia and hyperekplexia are different, the general consensus is that they probably represent similar disorders, with hyperekplexia being the preferred and correct Greek term (64). Startle disease is inherited as an autosomal dominant disorder associated with a variety of mutations in the α1-subunit of the glycine receptor (GLRA1) (65–68). A small number of cases with hyperekplexia also have been attributed to compound heterozygote mutations in the β-subunit of the glycine receptor (69) and to mutations in the gephyrin

gene (70). Autosomal recessive (71) and sporadic cases without the mutation (72) have been described. Defective glycinergic inhibition in the lower brainstem has been proposed as the mechanism for the exaggerated startle.

Hyperekplexia is characterized by the presence of hypertonia in the neonatal period that disappears in sleep: a nonhabituating, exaggerated startle response to auditory, visual, or tactile stimuli; hypokinesia; hyperactive brainstem reflexes (e.g., head retraction, palmomental reflex, snout); jerks on falling asleep; and frequently, feeding difficulties and apnea (73). The startle response can be elicited by tapping the forehead, glabella, vertex, or nose and is exaggerated by tension, cold, fatigue, and anxiety. Both tonic spasms and nocturnal myoclonic jerks may be part of hyperekplexia (74). Severe neonatal hypertonia may be associated with a marked reduction of spontaneous movements, and an increased incidence of congenitally dislocated hips and abdominal hernias (75). Unexpected stimuli, such as noises or handling, can precipitate massive generalized muscle spasms causing apnea, cyanosis, and even death (76). Patients are often mistakenly given the diagnosis of spastic quadriplegia. Abnormal intrauterine movements, consisting of sudden forceful jerks lasting for seconds to minutes, may occur in response to external stimuli (77). As muscle tone diminishes during the first year of life, normal spontaneous activity increases. Cognitive capabilities are not affected. Familial hyperekplexia is usually a benign disorder, but atypical cases have had problems with spastic paraparesis (78,79), mental retardation, or refractory status epilepticus (80). Startle patterns on surface electromyographic recordings elicited by auditory and trigeminal stimulation have been reported (81).

Hyperekplexia has been improved with clonazepam or diazepam (73,76). Other agents, such as valproic acid, 5-hydroxytryptophan (5-HTP), and piracetam, also have produced some benefit, but clobazam has not. In life-threatening situations, where prolonged stiffness impedes respiration and produces apnea and bradycardia, hypertonia can be manually relieved by forcible flexion of the head and legs toward the trunk (82).

Restless Legs

(See Chapter 31.)

Chin Quivering

Hereditary chin trembling (geniospasm) is a rare autosomal dominant condition characterized by paroxysmal movement of the chin and the lower lip. Movements last for seconds to hours, may be triggered by stressful or emotional situations, and have been observed during sleep (83–85). Onset is in infancy or early childhood, and trembling (myoclonus) tends to diminish with aging. A linkage to markers on the long arm of chromosome 9 (9q13-21) have been identified (86), but families without this linkage have been described (85). Botulinum toxin has been a useful treatment to control the quick jerks of the mentalis muscle (87).

NONINHERITED SECONDARY CAUSES OF MOVEMENT DISORDERS

Noninherited secondary causes of movement disorders can be due to numerous types of damage or injury to the nervous system (Table 36.3). In these cases, the movement disorder may occur at the time of the insult, while the patient is recovering from other neurologic deficits, or after a prolonged period of neurologic stability. Although a variety of brain insults can result in the delayed onset of symptoms, in infants and children they usually appear after prematurity, birth injury, encephalitis, trauma, and stroke. In some children, in whom the initial brain insult was at age 2 years or before, the onset of a progressive movement disorder (often dystonia) occurred more than 25 years later (88). Hence, static brain lesions can cause movement disorders after a long latency, and some even appear to have a progressive course. Since many of the etiologic factors listed in Table 36.3 are common to both pediatric and adult patients, the reader is referred to other chapters in

---

TABLE 36.3
SECONDARY NONINHERITED CAUSES OF EXTRAPYRAMIDAL SYMPTOMS IN CHILDHOOD

Perinatal cerebral injury: Cerebral palsy, hypoxic–ischemic encephalopathy, kernicterus

Structural: Tumors (mesencephalic), trauma, burns, shunt failure

Vascular: Stroke, intracranial hemorrhage

Infection/postinfectious/autoimmune: Encephalitis—influenza, polio, mumps, measles, varicella, St Louis encephalitis, coxsackie virus or carditis, HIV, subacute sclerosing panencephalitis (SSPE). Poststreptococcus infections—Sydenham's chorea, pediatric autoimmune neuropsychiatric disorder associated with streptococcus infection (PANDAS), acute disseminated encephalomyelitis

Hypoxic–Ischemic Encephalopathy

Drug/Toxin:
DA related—neuroleptics, metaclopramide, reserpine, α-methyldopa, L-dopa
Antieleptic drugs (AEDs)—valproate, phenytoin, vigabatrin
Chemotherapy—vincristine, ARA-C, adriamycin
Other—calcium channel blockers, captopril, lithium, selective serotonin uptake inhibitors (SSRIs), buspirone
Toxins—MPTP, manganese, CO, cyanide, methanol, disulfram

Hormonal disorders— thyroid disease, Addison's disease, hypoparathyroidism

Associated with general medical conditions— systemic lupus erythematosus, polycythemia, antiphospholipid syndrome, paraneoplastic syndromes

---

this text for additional discussion. An important significant exception is the diagnosis and treatment of CP and movement disorders after streptococcus infections.

Perinatal Cerebral Injury

Cerebral Palsy

Cerebral palsy (CP) is not a single disease entity but rather a broad term used to describe a heterogeneous group of syndromes that cause a nonprogressive disorder arising early in life, of cerebral origin, with abnormal control of movement and posture. Whether the age of onset should be restricted to insults occurring before age 2 or 5 years remains controversial. The spectrum of motor dysfunction in CP is broad (e.g., spasticity, plegias, choreoathetosis, dystonia, and ataxia), and despite an underlying static lesion, movement problems may vary over time. The incidence of CP worldwide is about 2 to 2.5 per 1000 live births, and the risk is higher in low-birth-weight infants and in twin pregnancies (3).

The neurobiological mechanisms for CP are extensive, ranging from pre- and perinatal injury to the developing brain (e.g., genetic diseases, cerebral dysgenesis, hypoxia–ischemia, stroke, intrauterine exposure to infection or inflammation), which account for about 85% of cases, to postnatal events (e.g., infection, trauma, stroke) (89,90). In the premature infant, periventricular leukomalacia (PVL), which affects the developing white matter, is the most common neuropathologic lesion associated with CP. The role of birth asphyxia as a prominent cause for CP has not been supported by current research, and elimination of this problem has not reduced its incidence (91,92). Potentially treatable causes, such as maternal infection, thyroid dysfunction, and hereditary and acquired thrombophilias, are currently being investigated.

The prevalence, identification of risk factors, and predictors of CP in very premature infants are notably different from those in term infants (93). Premature and very-low-birth-weight infants are at the greatest risk for developing CP. Improved survival rates in this population have led to an increased prevalence of significant neurodevelopmental impairment (94). MRI findings at 20 days of life, in infants with a mean gestational age of 31 weeks, predict the size and location of periventricular leukomalacia (PVL) and the outcome at age 1.5 years (95). Cerebellar injury in the extremely premature infant is relatively common (96,97). Single nucleotide polymorphisms on genes for endothelial nitric oxide synthase, factor 7, lymphotoxin A, and plasminogen activator inhibitor-1 have been associated with the development of CP in very premature infants (98). In contrast, measures of inflammatory cytokines and the independent factor of interuterine exposure to infection do not distinguish premature infants who will develop CP (98,99).

In term infants, the source of one-half of CP cases, there has been no recent decline in prevalence. In this group the best available predictor of CP is encephalopathy. It has been emphasized that hypoxic–ischemic encephalopathy represents only a small category within the neonatal encephalopathies and is an even smaller contributor to the etiology of CP. Essential criteria required to define an acute intrapartum hypoxic event sufficient to cause CP have been published (100). Additionally, therapeutic interventions directed at preventing interruption of oxygen supply have not reduced the occurrence of CP. In case-control studies, risk factors for neonatal encephalopathy include maternal thyroid disease, fever in labor, and congenital malformations (101–103). Lastly, although CP is defined by the presence of motor disabilities, individuals with CP have a variety of nonmovement problems, including mental retardation (>50%), strabismus (about 50%), epilepsy (about 30%), and disorders of vision or hearing (about 20%) (104).

Cerebral palsy is divided into four major types based on the predominant motor disability: spastic (about 50%); dyskinetic (about 20%); ataxic (about 10%); and mixed (about 20%). In actuality, most CP patients are mixed in type to some degree (e.g., mild dyskinetic signs are present in subtypes of spastic CP). Serial neurodevelopmental evaluations, especially in young children, are required for proper classification of the subtype because findings on examination may be affected by the state of alertness, emotional stress, and irritability. Other contributors to the motor deficit include sensory deficits and cognitive and perceptual impairments. Early indicators of significant motor disability include delay in the appearance of motor milestones and exaggerated or persistent primitive reflexes (105,106).

Laboratory tests are not needed to confirm the diagnosis of CP, since it is a clinical diagnosis based on the history and physical examination. Nevertheless, an accurate determination of the etiology can have implications regarding required testing, prognosis, medical management, recurrence risk, counseling, and the development of prevention programs. A practice parameter published in 2004 (107) has recommended that the evaluation of all children with CP include a head MRI (preferred to a CT), whereas metabolic and genetic testing should be obtained only on those individuals with additional and atypical features. An EEG is not recommended unless there are indications for a seizure disorder. Lastly, screening for associated deficits of mental retardation, ophthalmologic and hearing impairments, speech and language disorders, and oral-motor dysfunction should be part of the initial examination.

Spastic Type

The spastic type of CP is further divided into several subtypes, based on the distribution of impairment: hemiplegia, quadriplegia, and diplegia. All subtypes of spastic CP are associated with hypertonia, hyperreflexia, clonus, and abnormal plantar responses. Spastic hypertonia is defined by the presence of resistance to an externally imposed movement (a) that increases with increasing speed and varies with the direction of joint movement and (b) has

a "catch" that occurs above a threshold velocity. Many infants with CP, however, pass through an initial hypotonic phase. In general, neurological abnormalities indicating spasticity are present during quiet periods and sleep and do not change significantly with activity or emotional stress. Pseudobulbar palsy, indicated by expressionless facies and clonus may be seen in both spastic and dyskinetic forms. The child with spastic CP is typically prone to develop earlier contractures and have more frequent orthopedic problems than a child with choreoathetotic CP.

Hemiplegic Subtype. This is the most common subtype of spastic CP with findings localized to one extremity, usually with the upper extremity more involved than the lower. The appearance of hemiplegic CP in full-term infants is usually associated with prenatal circulatory disturbances or cerebral dysgenesis. The incidence of seizures approaches 70%, although cognitive capabilities are generally spared.

Diplegic Subtype. This subtype has involvement of all four extremities, with the upper extremities being minimally impaired and maintaining good functional abilities. This form typically appears in premature infants and is associated with the presence of periventricular leukomalacia.

Quadriplegic Subtype. This is the most severe form, with all four limbs significantly involved and with considerable compromise of motor function. Spastic quadriplegia in the full-term infant may be the result of prenatal insults, brain malformations, or perinatal asphyxia. These children typically have severe mental retardation, epilepsy, dysarthria, microcephaly, and strabismus.

Management. Medical management of spasticity includes the use of physical therapy, benzodiazepines, dantroline, baclofen, tizanidine, and neuromuscular blocking agents. In general, these approaches help to reduce spasticity but have little beneficial effect on signs of weakness and incoordination. Despite an early treatment program, some children require orthopedic surgical intervention. Orthopedic therapy is directed at reducing deformity and facilitating function, e.g., tendon lengthening/transfers, bony osteotomies, and joint fusion procedures. Intrathecal baclofen and selective functional dorsal (posterior) rhizotomy are being used in children with spastic diplegia.

Dyskinetic (Choreoathetoid, Extrapyramidal) Type

Dyskinetic CP syndromes are characterized by the presence of the involuntary movements of chorea, athetosis, and dystonia. These movements typically begin after age 2 years, may progress slowly for several years, and then persist into adulthood. Abnormal movements usually involve all four extremities, with the upper extremities usually being functionally more involved then the lower extremities. Dyskinetic CP is often misdiagnosed as a spastic form because of the misinterpretation of clinical signs (e.g., inaccurate separation of spastic, dystonic, and rigid hypertonias). Cogwheel rigidity is unusual in young children with CP, whereas oral motor dysfunction and tongue thrusting are common symptoms. Extrapyramidal movements show marked variability depending on the state of the individual; they are decreased during relaxation and sleep and increased by anxiety and stress. Dyskinetic forms of CP, especially those associated with athetosis, tend to occur in term infants with severe perinatal asphyxia. The etiology of dyskinetic CP includes hypoxic–ischemic injury, metabolic disorders (mitochondrial cytopathies, organic acidurias, creatine deficiency, dopa-responsive dystonia), and kernicterus. Pathophysiologically, extrapyramidal CP has been localized within the basal ganglia (neostriatum and/or globus pallidus) and/or thalamus, although more precise localization is lacking (108). MRI studies in children with athetoid CP showed that 37% were normal and the rest had high-intensity lesions in the ventrolateral nucleus of the thalamus or the dorsal putamen (109).

Management. The treatment of dyskinetic CP is complicated because most individuals have mixed degrees of chorea, athetosis, and dystonia. The general approach to therapy in the child with CP is to target the dyskinetic movement that is causing the greatest difficulty. Therapeutic trials are largely empiric and responses often individualized. When the symptom is primarily chorea or athetosis, benzodiazepines, valproate, tetrabenazine, and neuroleptics are often prescribed. In contrast, therapy for dystonic CP includes trials with anticholinergic medications (trihexyphenidyl), antiparkinsonian medications (levodopa/carbidopa), anticonvulsants (benzodiazepines, carbamazepine), baclofen (oral and intrathecal), botulinum toxin, and deep-brain stimulation.

Ataxic (Cerebellar) Form

The cerebellar or ataxic form represents a clinically and etiologically heterogeneous group (110). Classical associated findings include truncal titubation, dysmetria, and cerebellar eye movements. Children with ataxic syndromes usually have a prenatal etiology (e.g., developmental cerebellar abnormality) and are born after a full-term gestation. Neuroimaging may be normal or show either biparietal or infratentorial lesions (110).

Kernicterus

Kernicterus is a preventable neurologic syndrome caused by severe and untreated hyperbilirubinemia in the newborn period. High levels of bilirubin are toxic to the developing brain, especially the globus pallidus, subthalamic nucleus, cerebellum, and auditory and vestibular pathways, although the mechanism(s) of neuronal injury and cell death remain unclear. In full-term infants, symptoms of hyperbilirubinemia include severe jaundice, lethargy,

and poor feeding. Features of kernicterus include dystonia, choreoathetosis, tremor, rigidity, mental retardation, sensorineural hearing loss, and gaze paresis. Pathologic findings include yellow staining of the subthalamic nucleus, Ammon's horn, globus pallidus, dentate nucleus, and inferior olives. The precise role of neuroimaging in confirming the diagnosis and determining outcome is unclear (111). Eight of 13 infants with acute kernicterus had bilateral symmetric increased signal intensity in the globus pallidus on T1-weighted imaging (112). In patients with athetotic CP, MRI findings at the posteromedial border of the globus pallidus are suggestive evidence of brain damage caused by kernicterus (113). Guidelines for the management of hyperbilirubinemia in the newborn have been published (114).

Streptococcus Infections: Postinfectious Disorders

Group A β-hemolytic streptococcus (GABHS) infections are the etiology for several postinfectious movement disorders, including Sydenham's chorea (SC), pediatric autoimmune neuropsychiatric disorder associated with streptococcus infection (PANDAS), and acute disseminated encephalomyelitis.

Sydenham's Chorea

Sydenham's chorea is the prototype for an infectious agent (GABHS) triggering an autoimmune disorder that, in turn, causes a movement disorder. SC usually occurs between the ages of 5 and 15 years, and a female predominance has been observed in all large studies. Chorea can range in severity and is usually generalized, but hemichorea occurs in about 20% of individuals. Associated neurologic symptoms may include dysarthria (about one-third), gait disturbances that correlate with severity of chorea, hypometric saccades, hypotonia, weakness, and hemiballismus (115,116). Most patients have concomitant psychological dysfunction presenting as personality changes, obsessive–compulsive symptoms, emotional irritability, distractibility, and age-regressed behaviors (117,118). Affected individuals may present with behavioral or emotional difficulties that predate the motoric abnormalities by weeks to months. Motor or vocal tics and oculogyric crises also have been reported in patients with SC (115,119). Rheumatic valvular cardiac disease is seen in about one-third of patients, whereas arthritis is uncommon.

The diagnosis of SC is based on clinical observation and the lack of evidence for other disorders (120). No confirmatory test is available, although serological evidence of streptococcus infection is found in about 80% of patients. The outcome in SC is favorable, with most cases resolving in 1 to 6 months, although persistent chorea has been described (121) and neuropsychiatric problems may persist (117,118,122). About 20% to 42% of patients have recurrent episodes of chorea (123). Recurrence usually occurs within 1 to 2 years after the original event, but it has occurred up to 10 years later (123,124). Reactivation may occur in association with a streptococcus infection or pregnancy (chorea gravidarum) or secondary to factors that are unrelated to streptococcus infection or rheumatic fever activity (123,125,126). An MRI volumetric study evaluating the size of the basal ganglia in children with SC showed a 10% increase in size of the caudate and a 7% increase in size of both the putamen and globus pallidus (127). Focal areas of T2 hypersignal in the caudate, pallidum, putamen, and white matter have been noted in recurrent cases.

Treatment is symptomatic, and the decision to initiate therapy is based on the degree of disability, whether due to chorea or to behavioral or psychiatric symptoms. To date, there have been no adequate, randomized double-blind studies to evaluate the symptomatic treatment of SC. In limited trials, improvement of chorea occurred with anticonvulsants (valproate, carbamazepine), neuroleptics (haloperidol, pimozide), and immunomodulatory therapy (128–130).

An autoimmune hypothesis has been proposed as the underlying mechanism in SC—that is, after a streptococcus infection in susceptible individuals, antibodies directed against bacterial antigens cross-react (molecular mimicry) with epitopes on neurons of the basal ganglia, causing choreiform movement abnormalities and behavioral disturbances. Several lines of evidence support the involvement of immune mechanisms in this disorder: improvement of symptoms following immunomodulatory therapies (129–131); documentation of autoreactive antibodies against human basal ganglia (132–134); the modest up-regulation of cytokine production in CSF and serum (135); and the demonstration that monoclonal antibodies, obtained from B clones derived from a patient with acute SC, cross-react with mammalian lysoganglioside GM1 and N-acetyl-β-D-glucosamine, a dominant epitope of the group A streptococcus carbohydrate (136).

Pediatric Autoimmune Neuropsychiatric Disorder Associated with Streptococcus Infection

In 1998, Swedo and colleagues proposed the existence of a subset of children with tic disorders and/or obsessive–compulsive disorder (OCD) who have the abrupt onset/exacerbation of symptoms that are temporally associated with a streptococcus infection (137). Labeled *pediatric autoimmune neuropsychiatric disorders associated with streptococcus infection* (PANDAS), diagnostic criteria include the presence of OCD and/or tic disorder; prepubertal age at onset; sudden, explosive onset of symptoms and/or a course of sudden exacerbations and remissions; a temporal relationship between symptoms and GABHS; and the presence of neurological abnormalities, including hyperactivity and choreiform movements. In subsequent reports, proponents have clarified several requirements (138). For example, diagnosis necessitates at least two exacerbations of neuropsychiatric symptoms with distinct intervening periods of remission, during which throat cultures and

antistreptococcus antibody titers are negative. Explosive tic exacerbations are defined as the simultaneous appearance of several different motor and phonic tics with an intensity that causes parents to seek immediate medical attention. These acute recurrences must begin simultaneously with a positive throat culture or within 7 to 14 days after the infection. Lastly, choreiform movements are described as fine piano-playing finger movements.

The existence of PANDAS remains controversial, with advocates and opponents taking firm positions on either side of the clinical issue (138–142). Support for PANDAS is derived from the description of additional cohorts (143); familial studies showing that first-degree relatives of children with PANDAS have higher rates of tic disorders and OCD than do those in the general population (144); expanded expression of a trait marker for susceptibility in rheumatic fever (the monoclonal antibody D8/17) in individuals with PANDAS (145); and MRI volumetric analyses showing that the average size of the caudate, putamen, and globus pallidus, but not the thalamus or total cerebrum, was significantly greater in PANDAS than in healthy children (146). Despite these findings, concerns continue to be raised about the existence of PANDAS. For example, no prospective epidemiologic study has confirmed that an antecedent GABHS infection is specifically associated with either the onset or exacerbation of tic disorders or OCD. Diagnostic criteria established for PANDAS are potentially confounded by the phenotypic variability commonly associated with tic disorders, such as a normal fluctuation in the frequency and severity of symptoms; exacerbation of tics by stress, fatigue, and illness; occurrence of sudden, abrupt onset and/or recurrence of tics in non-PANDAS subjects (147); and lack of a precise definition for associated neurological conditions (141). Additionally, longitudinal laboratory data, rather than studies that use only a throat culture or only a single antistreptolysin O (ASO) or antideoxyribonuclease B titer, are necessary to confirm the presence of a previous GABHS infection. Lastly, two prospective longitudinal studies have shown no clear relationship between new GABHS infections and the development or exacerbation of tic/OCD symptoms (148,149).

Similar to Sydenham's chorea, an immune-mediated mechanism involving molecular mimicry has been proposed for PANDAS. Indirect support for an immune hypothesis is derived from a single study showing that a small number of patients with PANDAS responded to immunotherapy with intravenous immunoglobulin and plasmapheresis (150). Antineuronal antibodies have been assessed in patients with PANDAS with variable results. One group of investigators has suggested that this cohort can be differentiated from a variety of disease controls by enzyme-linked immunoassay (ELISA) and Western immunoblotting methods (e.g., reactivity against frozen basal ganglia at 60, 45, and 40 kDa) (151). In contrast, others using several different epitopes from fresh human postmortem caudate, putamen, globus pallidus, and prefrontal cortex were unable to distinguish PANDAS subjects from controls (152,153). Lastly, the microinfusion of sera from children with PANDAS into rodent striatum did not change the number of observed motor stereotypy behaviors (154,155).

Acute Disseminated Encephalomyelitis

After a clinical pharyngitis with laboratory evidence of GABHS, 10 children with a mean age of 6.8 years developed behavioral changes (emotional lability, inappropriate laughter), somnolence, stupor or coma, and an extrapyramidal movement disorder (rigidity, dystonic posturing, or hemidystonia, but no tics or chorea) (156). CSF was abnormal in 7 of 10 (pleocytosis and/or elevated protein), MRI demonstrated T2 hyperintense lesions in the basal ganglia in 8 of 10, and all 10 had elevated serum antibasal ganglia antibodies. Recovery was rapid and often complete, although 2 patients had relapses associated with further streptococcus infections.

HEREDITARY/METABOLIC DISORDERS ASSOCIATED WITH EXTRAPYRAMIDAL SYMPTOMS

Movement abnormalities in children are frequently associated with hereditary metabolic disorders (Table 36.4). Metabolic diseases, or inborn errors of metabolism, are individually rare but cumulatively they cause significant morbidity and mortality. Because these entities are often typified by an evolving and variable pattern of signs and symptoms, they are commonly multilisted under headings of chorea, dystonia, and parkinsonism. Recognizing that for the clinician this often leads to confusion, especially in an evolving disorder, a broader classification can provide a more comprehensible subdivision. Since in the allotted space, it is not possible to discuss all of the metabolic disorders that can cause movement disorders, selected examples have been chosen.

TABLE 36.4
CLASSIFICATION OF METABOLIC DISORDERS

Pediatric neurotransmitter disorders
The following disorders:
Mineral accumulation disorders
Lysosomal disorders
Organic acid disorders
Amino acid disorders
Mitochondrial disorders
Purine metabolism disorders
Creatine metabolism disorders
Cofactor disorders
Tricarboxylic acid cycle disorders
Other metabolic disorders

Pediatric Neurotransmitter Diseases

The term *pediatric neurotransmitter disease* has been applied to relatively uncommon genetic disorders that affect the synthesis, metabolism, and catabolism of neurotransmitters. The primary neurotransmitters involved in these diseases are the monoamines (MAs), which include serotonin and catecholamines (dopamine and norepinephrine) and gamma-aminobutyric acid (GABA).

Monoamine-related neurotransmitter diseases can be divided into separate categories based on the site of abnormality in the metabolic pathway—that is, those affecting cofactors (e.g., tetrahydrobiopterin, BH4), enzymes of monoamine biosynthesis (e.g., tyrosine hydroxylase, TH; aromatic amino acid decarboxylase, AADC), or enzymes involved in catabolism. Diagnostic studies for pediatric neurotransmitter disorders include CSF for analysis of monoamines (dopamine, serotonin, and norepinephrine), neurotransmitter metabolites (homovanillic acid, HVA; 5-hydroxyindoleacetic acid, 5-HIAA; 3-methoxy-4-hydroxylphenylglycol, MHPG; and pterin, biopterin, and neopterin), quantitative plasma and urine catecholamines, and phenylalanine loading profiles with and without BH4 (157). (See Fig. 36.1.)

Tetrahydrobiopterin Metabolism

Tetrahydrobiopterin is an essential cofactor for the neurotransmitter-synthesizing enzymes phenylalanine hydroxylase, tyrosine hydroxylase, and tryptophan hydroxylase. BH4 itself is synthesized in a multistep pathway starting from guanosine triphosphate (GTP) and, when formed, requires several enzymes to maintain it in its active state. Several enzymatic defects have been identified in BH4 metabolism, such as deficiencies in the first and rate-limiting synthesizing enzyme GTP-1 cyclohydrolase (GCHI); in the second and third enzymatic steps, namely, 6-pyruvotetrahydropterin synthase (6-PTS) and sepiapterin reductase, respectively; and in the maintenance enzyme dihydropteridine reductase (DHPR). Although one might expect that a defect in BH4 metabolism would be readily detectable based on the presence of hyperphenylalaninemia, due to a deficiency of phenylalanine hydroxylase activity, this laboratory finding is not always present. Hence, classification of BH4 metabolism defects can be based on presentations with or without hyperphenylalaninemia.

BH4 Defects with Hyperphenylalaninemia

1. Autosomal recessive forms of GTP-1 cyclohydrolase (GCHI) deficiency (158,159)
2. 6-Pyruvotetrahydropterin synthase (6-PTS) deficiency (160,161)
3. Dihydropteridine reductase (DHPR) deficiency (162,164)

Since each produces hyperphenylalaninemia and reduces synthesis of monoamines, clinical signs and symptoms tend to overlap. In the neonatal period, presumably due to hyperphenylalaninemia, hypotonia, poor suck, diminished

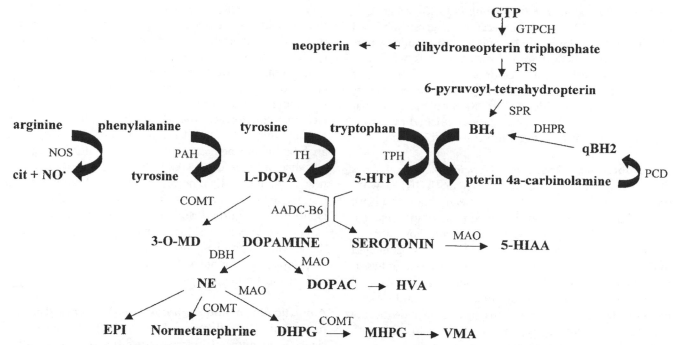

Figure 36.1 AADC, aromatic L-amino acid decarboxylase; B6, pyridoxine; COMT, catechol-o-methyltransferase; DBH, dopamine hydroxylase; DHPR, dihydropteridine reductase; GTPCH, GTP cyclohydrolase; MAO, monoamine oxidase; NOS, nitric oxide synthase; PAH, phenylalanine hydroxylase; PCD, pterin 4a-carbinolamine dehydratase; PTS, 6-pyruvoyl-tetrahydropterin synthase; SPR, sepiapterin reductase; TH, tyrosine hydroxylase; TPH, tryptophan hydroxylase. From Swoboda KJ, Hyland K. Diagnosis and treatment of neurotransmitter-related disorders. *Neurol Clin* 2002;20: 1143–1161. With permission.

movements, and microcephaly may be present. Generally, beginning several months later, more monoaminergic symptoms appear, including oculogyric crises, swallowing difficulties, hypersalivation, temperature instability, variable hypo- and hyperkinetic movements, seizures, and cognitive impairment (162,163). These patients can be detected by neonatal screening for phenylketonuria (PKU). In DHPR deficiency, a secondary reduction in central nervous system (CNS) folate has led to perivascular basal ganglia calcification and multifocal subcortical perivascular demyelination (164,165). Management of the hyperphenylalaninemia BH4 defects include the correction of phenylalanine metabolism, central monoamine deficits, and prevention of folate deficiency. Oral BH4 will correct the peripheral metabolism of phenylalanine when the defect is not due to a DHPR deficiency. Since BH4 does not readily cross the blood–brain barrier, management of central monoamine deficits is achieved by the use of levodopa and 5-hydroxytryptophan in combination with carbidopa. Therapy with folinic acid and monitoring of CSF folate is recommended.

BH4 Defects Without Hyperphenylalaninemia

Dopa-Responsive Dystonia. This group includes dopa-responsive dystonia (DRD), Segawa's disease, hereditary progressive dystonia, and DYT5. DRD is an autosomal dominantly inherited disorder caused by heterozygous mutations in the gene for GCHI located on chromosome 14 (166–169). New mutations are common, and there is an increased clinical penetrance in females. Although the spectrum of presentations is wide, patients typically present in midchildhood (ages 5 to 6 years) with dystonic posturing of the leg or foot, which affects the gait. Symptoms progressively worsen, and about one-fourth of patients develop hyperreflexia and spasticity, leading some to be inappropriately diagnosed with CP (170). A diurnal variation has been emphasized, with progressive worsening throughout the day and improvement in the morning after sleep. Cases without this variation, however, have been reported. Other presentations include arm dystonia (writer's cramp), features of parkinsonism (i.e., bradykinesia, rigidity, masked facies, hypophonic speech, and postural instability), and myoclonus–dystonia (i.e., myoclonic jerks beginning in childhood) (171–173).

Since patients respond dramatically and in a sustained fashion to low-dose levodopa, it is important to diagnose this disorder. Some DRD patients also have shown a good response to anticholinergics such as trihexyphenidyl (174). DRD has been distinguished from juvenile parkinsonism by use of fluorodopa positron emission tomography (PET); no abnormality shows in DRD. Dopamine uptake sites in DRD, measured by single-photon emission computed tomography (SPECT) with [123I]β-CIT, are normal, but PET of D2 dopamine receptors suggests increased binding in both symptomatic and asymptomatic carriers (175,176). The phenylalanine loading test has been advocated as a sensitive and specific study for detection of both affected and nonmanifesting GCHI gene carriers (177,178). Since individuals with PKU would show similar abnormalities, DRD carriers are distinguished by correction of the loading test after administering biopterin.

Dihydropteridine Reductase Deficiency. Several cases of dihydropteridine reductase deficiency (DHPR) without hyperphenylalaninemia have been reported (179). Neurologic symptoms have included psychomotor retardation, microcephaly, spasticity, dystonia, oculomotor apraxia, and hypersomnolence. The oral phenylalanine loading test in these patients was abnormal, despite the lack of hyperphenylalaninemia. CSF measurements show reduced monoamines and their metabolites but normal BH4 and neopterin levels. Treatment for this disorder includes the use of levodopa and 5-hydroxytryptophan in combination with carbidopa to correct central monoamine deficits.

Sepiapterin Reductase Deficiency. This inherited disorder of BH4 metabolism is characterized by signs and symptoms related to monoamine neurotransmitter deficiency, but without hyperphenylalaninemia. Sepiapterin reductase deficiency (SR) catalyzes the final two-step reduction of the intermediate pyruvoyltetrahydropterin (PTP) to BH4. The deficiency is an autosomal recessive disorder that has been reported in a small number of patients with progressive psychomotor retardation, dystonia, severe dopamine and serotonin deficiencies, and high levels of biopterin and dihydrobiopterin (BH2) in the CSF (180,181). Several mutations in the SR gene have been identified. It is speculated that alternative reductases, aldose reductase, and carbonyl reductase may be capable of replacing absent SR activity in peripheral tissues.

Primary Defects of Monoamine Biosynthesis

Defects of monoamine biosynthesis have been defined at three sequential enzymatic steps: (a) tyrosine hydroxylase (TH), the rate-limiting step in the formation of dopamine and norepinephrine, which catalyzes the conversion of tyrosine to L-dopa; (b) aromatic l-amino acid decarboxylase (AADC), which converts L-dopa to dopamine; and (c) dopamine β-hydroxylase (DBH), the enzyme that converts dopamine to norepinephrine.

Tyrosine Hydroxylase Deficiency. Tyrosine hydroxylase deficiency comprises a group of autosomal recessive disorders localized to chromosome 11p11.5 that respond partially to levodopa treatment. At least 8 different point mutations have been identified in the TH gene and, depending on the abnormality, syndromes have been extremely variable, ranging from severe presentations in infancy to

milder juvenile DRD or juvenile parkinsonism (182–187). In cases with a severe reduction of TH activity, onset occurs in infancy with symptoms of psychomotor retardation, rigidity, hypokinesia, axial hypotonia, and paroxysmal eye movements. In other presentations, cases have included parkinsonism, gait disorder and stiffness after exercise, dystonia, and ataxia. Neuroradiographic scans are normal, and electroencephalograms may show nonspecific background abnormalities (182,188). Diagnosis is confirmed by genetic analysis, but biochemical testing has been valuable (e.g., the presence of reduced levels of CSF dopamine, norepinephrine, HVA, and MHPG, normal 5-HIAA and pterins, and a normal phenylalanine load). Treatment involves the administration of low-dose levodopa, but responses have been variable and severe dyskinesias have occurred. Additional therapeutic recommendations include low-dose levodopa/carbidopa plus an monoamine oxidase B (MAO-B) inhibitor and an anticholinergic (189).

Aromatic Amino Acid Decarboxylase Deficiency. The aromatic amino acid decarboxylase (AADC) deficiency deficiency is an autosomal recessive disorder associated with a defect localized to chromosome 7p12.1-12.3 (190). Since AADC catalyzes both the formation of dopamine from L-dopa and serotonin from 5-HTP, a deficiency of this enzyme leads to a profound deficiency of CSF serotonin and catecholamines. Resultant clinical symptoms, therefore, tend to be more like a severe BH4 deficiency. Problems include paroxysmal movements with arm and leg extension and rolling eyes, orofacial dystonia, irritability, myoclonus, temperature instability, autonomic dysfunction, disordered sleep and feeding, and a diurnal variation of symptoms (162,191–193). If untreated, affected children develop a characteristic phenotype of extrapyramidal movements often preceded by oculogyric crises and convergence spasms (162). Magnetic resonance images may show mild cortical atrophy, and electroencephalograms show spike or polyspike bursts (194). CSF monoamines and their metabolites are reduced, but levels of the L-dopa metabolite 3-O-methyldopa are elevated. A mild form of AADC deficiency has been reported (195). Treatment with MAO inhibitors and dopamine agonists has improved some symptoms but not signs of developmental delay. Although L-dopa would not be expected to be beneficial, several patients did experience improvement of symptoms, possibly due to a mutation that alters the binding affinity of the protein for L-dopa (196). Others have suggested a trial of L-dopa without carbidopa and, since B6 is a cofactor for AADC, high-dose pyridoxal phosphate is also recommended.

GABA-Related Neurotransmitter Disease: Succinic Semialdehyde Dehydrogenase Deficiency (4-Hydroxybutyric Aciduria)

Succinic semialdehyde dehydrogenase (SSADH) works in conjunction with GABA transaminase to convert 4-aminobutyric acid (GABA) to succinic acid. SSADH deficiency, localized to chromosome 6, results in increased concentrations of GABA and 4-hydroxybutyric acid (GHB). Diagnosis is based on the detection of massive increases of GHB in the urine, plasma, and CSF. CSF levels of GABA and a GABA peptide—homocarnosine—are also elevated (197). Diagnosis is often delayed, and clinical findings include mental retardation, disproportionate language dysfunction, autistic traits, hypotonia, ataxia, aggression, anxiety, hallucinations, hyperactivity, and choreoathetosis, and about half have seizures (198). Atrophy of the cerebellum and T2 hyperintensities (especially in the white matter and globus pallidus) may be present on MRI. EEG may show diffuse background slowing and generalized or multifocal abnormalities. Proton MR spectroscopy has shown elevated GABA levels and traces of GHB in both the white and gray matter of the brain (199). Some patients have been improved by treatment with vigabatrin (gamma-vinyl GABA), which blocks GABA transaminase (200). Valproate is contraindicated because it may inhibit any residual SSADH activity. Prenatal diagnosis is possible (201).

Associated Metabolic Disorders

Mineral Accumulation

Wilson's Disease (Hepatolenticular Degeneration). Wilson's disease is inherited as an autosomal recessive trait; the gene, located on chromosome 13q14.3, encodes for an enzyme (copper-transporting P-type ATPase, ATP7B) that binds to copper and aids in its transport across the membrane (202). Mutations lead to failure to excrete copper in the bile and to subsequent accumulation in liver, brain, cornea, kidney, bones, and blood. Intestinal absorption of copper is normal and ceruloplasm, an α-globulin that binds and transports copper molecules, is frequently but not always reduced. Increased excretion of copper in the urine is insufficient to prevent copper accumulation.

In children, hepatic dysfunction (asymptomatic hepatomegaly, acute transient or fulminant hepatitis) is the most common clinical presentation; average age of onset is about 12 years (203). Since ceruloplasmin is an acute-phase reactant, its level may be increased in the presence of hepatitis, making this an unreliable diagnostic marker. The average age for the appearance of neurologic symptoms is about 19 years, although symptoms have been reported in a 6-year-old (204,205). Dysarthria or difficulties with gait are often an early manifestation. Several syndromes in this diagnosis have been described, including an akinetic-rigid and a generalized dystonic form (206). A resting, postural, or kinetic tremor occurs in about 50% of patients, and cerebellar symptoms (pseudosclerotic) also may be present. Psychiatric symptoms precede the neurologic abnormalities in 20% of cases, ranging from subtle changes in personality and behavior to frank psychosis. The Kaiser-Fleischer ring, a yellow-brown deposition of copper in Descemet's membrane of the cornea, is best observed by slit-lamp examination. The diagnosis is made through the use of a combination of studies, including measurement of serum ceruloplasmin, 24-hour urine copper, slit-lamp examination, and most definitively by liver biopsy with histologic assessment and determination of copper content.

Treatment strategies are reviewed in detail elsewhere (207–210). In brief, approaches include dietary therapy (avoidance of foods high in copper), therapy to reduce copper absorption (potassium, zinc, tetrathiomolybdate), treatment to increase copper chelation and elimination (d-penicillamine, trientine [triethylene tetramine dihydrochloride], dimercaprol [British anti-Lewisite, BAL]), and liver transplantation.

Neurodegeneration with Brain Iron Accumulation. The nosology of neurodegenerative disorders associated with the accumulation of iron has undergone revision based on recent genetic advances and revelations about the personal history of Julius Hallervorden. More specifically, pantothenate kinase–associated neurodegeneration (PKAN) is the new suggested terminology for a group of disorders previously known as Hallervorden-Spatz syndrome (HSS). However, it is likely that a group of phenotypically similar cases may be defined without this specific gene abnormality.

PKAN is a rare autosomal recessive disorder pathologically associated with abnormal iron deposition and high concentrations of lipofuscin and neuromelanin in the substantia nigra pars reticulata and the internal segment of the globus pallidus (211,212). The abnormality is mapped to chromosome 20p12.3-p13, and investigators have identified a mutation in the gene for pantothenate kinase 2 (PANK2), a regulatory enzyme in the synthetic pathway for coenzyme A, which catalyzes the cytosolic phosphorylation of pantothenate (vitamin B5), N-pantothenoylcysteine, and pantetheine (213). It has been hypothesized that the gene product results in an accumulation of cysteine, an iron chelator, and the combination, in turn, leads to oxidative stress and neurodegeneration. Other speculated mechanisms are based on PANK2 localization in mitochondria (214).

HSS has variable presentations (215) and has been divided into the more common early-onset form (diagnosis evident before age 10 years), a late-onset type (diagnosis evident between ages 10 and 18 years), and an adult variant (216,217). The classic presentation is characterized by onset between 5 and 8 years of age with progressive personality changes, cognitive decline, dysarthria, motor difficulties, and spasticity. Extrapyramidal dysfunction is usually present but may be delayed for several years. Dystonia is common, but rigidity, choreoathetosis, and a resting or action tremor also may be present. Ophthalmologic abnormalities include retinitis pigmentosa and optic atrophy. Seizures also can occur. Atypical presentations with onset in the second decade have included tourettism, hemiballism, and juvenile parkinsonism (218). The course of the disorder is variable. For example, the early-onset form is subdivided into rapidly and slowly progressive forms. The rapid-progressive early-onset type has a short transition from spasticity to severe movements with opisthotonos, and death within 1 to 2 years. In contrast, the more prevalent, slowly progressive, early-onset type can present with movement abnormalities but develop more slowly, with death occurring within 20 years. The late-onset childhood form is even slower in its progression than the early-onset types.

Diagnosis depends on the presence of obligate features: onset in the first two decades, progressive course, extrapyramidal symptoms, and classical magnetic resonance imaging (MRI) findings showing decreased T2-weighted and proton density signal in the globus pallidus and substantia nigra. Some patients also have a hyperintense area within the hypodense areas, named the "eye-of-the-tiger sign." Cranial MRI changes may predate the appearance of symptoms (211). Supportive diagnostic signs and symptoms include spasticity, extensor plantar signs, progressive intellectual impairment, ophthalmologic problems, abnormal cytosomes in lymphocytes, and sea-blue histiocytes in bone marrow (the latter findings being typical of ceroid–lipofuscin accumulation) (216). Cultured skin fibroblasts have been reported to accumulate 59Fe-transferrin. There is no specific treatment for HSS, although theoretically the downstream delivery of products in the coenzyme A pathway may be therapeutic. Iron chelation therapy with desferrioxamine has not been effective. Deep-brain stimulation has improved the painful spasms and dystonia (219).

HARP Syndrome. This term has been used to define a phenotype that includes hypoprebetalipoproteinemia, acanthocytosis, retinitis pigmentosa, and pallidal degeneration (220,221). Patients have had faciobuccolingual dyskinesias, eye-of-the-tiger sign, and some normal serum lipoproteins (221). This syndrome has been shown to be allelic with PKAN (222).

Lysosomal Disorders

Lysosomes are intracytoplasmic vesicles that contain a variety of degradative enzymes used to catabolize complex substrates, such as sphingolipids, gangliosides, cerebrosides, sulfatides, mucopolysaccharides, and glycoproteins. Levels of lysosomal enzyme activity are readily assayed in serum, white blood cells, or cultured fibroblasts. The inherited absence of a specific enzyme activity, in turn, results in the excessive deposition of the undegradable substance in the lysosome, with subsequent disruption of either neuronal or myelin function.

Neuronal Storage Diseases. The neuronal storage diseases, such as GM1 and GM2 gangliosidosis, Gaucher's disease, and Niemann-Pick disease, are generally characterized by the presence in infancy of progressive cognitive and motor deterioration, seizures, retinopathy, and, in some cases, hepatosplenomegaly. In general, the more slowly

progressive variants of these disorders, those that have only partial deficiencies of enzyme activity, are the ones that tend to have extrapyramidal signs. The older (adult, type 3) form of GM1 gangliosidosis typically presents during childhood or adolescence with a slowly progressive loss of cognitive function or abnormal gait. Generalized dystonia becomes a prominent feature, along with facial dystonia and severe speech difficulties (223). The adult form of GM1 gangliosidosis has higher residual GM1 β-galactosidase activity than the infantile or juvenile forms (224). Although older forms of GM2 gangliosidosis (deficiency of hexosaminidase A) typically have ataxia and progressive cerebellar atrophy (225), juvenile forms have presented with dystonia and rigidity, primarily involving the lower extremities (226,227). In the typical juvenile form of Niemann-Pick disease type C (NPC, due to a defect in intracellular cholesterol transport), patients present with hepatosplenomegaly, cognitive deterioration, dysarthria, supranuclear vertical gaze palsy, gait problems, cataplexy, dystonia, and cerebellar ataxia (228–230). In this disease, the abnormal esterification of exogenous cholesterol in fibroblasts and the accumulation of unesterified cholesterol and glycolipids in lysosomes (seen with filipin staining) provide the basis for biochemical diagnosis. The most common form of this disease results from mutations in the NPC1 gene (18q11-12) (231,232).

Neuronal Ceroid Lipofuscinoses. Among the most common neurodegenerative diseases in children are the neuronal ceroid lipofuscinoses (NCLs). In the pediatric population, they are autosomal recessive disorders characterized by the accumulation of autofluorescent material that resembles the lipopigments ceroid and lipofuscins that accumulate normally with age. Storage is present in brain tissue and various organs, but only the CNS and retina show damage with neuronal loss and gliosis (233,234). Historically, classifications of NCL were based on age of onset, clinical symptoms, and ultrastructural aspects of inclusions. The four classical variants are infantile (Santavuori-Haltia disease, CLN1), late-infantile (Jansky-Bielschowsky disease, CNL2), juvenile (Batten-Spielmeyer-Vogt disease, CLN3), and adult (Kufs, CLN4). CLN1 begins in the first year of life with regression of all psychomotor skills; CLN2 begins between ages 2 and 4 years with acute seizures that increase rapidly in frequency, myoclonus, and, later, retinopathy; CLN3 usually starts after age 5 years with visual failure due to pigmentary retinal degeneration and progresses to include behavioral, cerebellar, and extrapyramidal signs. A SPECT study in individuals with CLN3 and extrapyramidal findings has demonstrated a significant reduction of striatal dopamine transporter density, more prominent in the putamen than in the caudate (235).

More recently, clinicopathologic and genetic studies have shown that NCLs encompass a highly heterogeneous group with eight different forms, NCL1–8, based on mutations in specific genes (233,234). Juvenile NCL is caused by mutations in the CLN3 gene encoding a multi-transmembrane lysosomal protein of unknown function. The gene is located on chromosome 16p11.2-12.1, and more than 30 different mutations have been described. Diagnosis is based on clinical presentation, presence of vacuolated lymphocytes, pathological findings of autofluorescence, lysosomal storage with ultrastructural change (usually fingerprint profiles), and DNA testing. Treatment is supportive and bone marrow transplantation is ineffective (236).

White Matter (Dysmyelinating) Disorders.
White matter (dysmyelinating) disorders also can be associated with deficiencies of lysosomal enzymes: Krabbe's disease (has deficient galactocerebroside β-galactosidase) and metachromatic leukodystrophy (MLD, deficient arylsulfatase A). These disorders occur because both central and peripheral myelins contain cerebrosides and sulfatides, substances that require specific enzymes for degradation. Krabbe's disease and MLD typically present in infancy with symptoms and signs of progressive motor difficulties, spasticity, peripheral neuropathy, and optic atrophy. Extrapyramidal symptoms in these disorders are rare, although a dystonic phenotype has been reported in an individual with juvenile MLD (237).

Organic Acid Disorders
Organic acids are produced during the catabolism of amino acids in intermediary metabolism. They are compounds containing one or more carboxylic acid or acid phenolic groups without basic amino groups. If there is a defect in the metabolism of an organic acid, the organic acid level increases and causes an intoxication-type clinical presentation. There are multiple organic acidurias. Neurological manifestations are extremely common in organic acid disorders and frequently represent the presenting or primary feature.

Glutaric Aciduria Type 1.
Glutaric aciduria type 1 is an autosomal recessive disorder caused by a defect in the gene that codes for glutaryl-CoA dehydrogenase (GCDH, involved in lysine, hydroxylysine, and tryptophan metabolism) (238). Biochemically, deficiency of this enzyme results in the accumulation and excretion of glutaric acid and 3-hydroxyglutaric acid, detectable in the urine, blood, and CSF. The diagnosis is confirmed by documentation of deficient glutaryl-CoA dehydrogenase activity in cultured skin fibroblasts. Clinically, there are several forms of presentation, and phenotypic heterogeneity occurs within families (239–241). In about one-fourth of patients, development tends to be normal until the latter part of the first year of life, when progressive symptoms appear, including hypotonia, dystonia, choreoathetosis, and seizures. In the largest group, the patient is well for up to 2 years, until the abrupt onset of an acute deteriorating neurologic picture, typically associated with an infectious or encephalitic process. Residual symptoms include extrapyramidal movements and mental retardation. Repeated episodes of ketoacidosis, seizures, and loss of consciousness may occur throughout the course. A third form mimics the presentation of extrapyramidal CP. Clinical variability does not correlate with the extent of residual enzyme activity, more than 100 mutations in the GCDH gene have been identified, and no molecular basis differentiates the groups. Neuroradiographic studies show atrophy of the frontotemporal cortex and "bat-winged" dilatation of the sylvian fissures, hypodensity of the lenticular nuclei, and caudate degeneration (242). Bilateral temporal arachnoid cysts are common. Excitotoxic mechanisms involving 3-hydroxyglutaric acid as the major neurotoxin have been proposed (243). Bilateral pallidotomy has improved dystonic symptoms in a young child with this disorder (244).

Methylmalonic Aciduria.
In all genetic forms of methylmalonic aciduria (MMA), the conversion of methylmalonyl-CoA to succinyl-CoA is impaired secondary to a deficit of methylmalonyl-CoA mutase, a vitamin B12-dependent enzyme. Presenting disorders represent either a genetic abnormality in the mitochondrial apoenzyme, methylmalonyl-CoA mutase, or the latter's adenosylcobalamin cofactor. Infants with absence of the apoenzyme (classical form) become symptomatic in the first week of life with hypotonia, lethargy, vomiting, metabolic acidosis, and ketosis. Survivors typically have severe residual neurologic impairments, including dystonia (245). Less frequently, especially in those with cobalamin cofactor deficiencies, onset is delayed to the late infantile or juvenile period. In general, the vitamin B12–responsive group has a milder course and better outcome. MRI studies show alterations in myelination and changes in the basal ganglia. The clinical phenotype is less severe in late-onset cases and those with cofactor deficiencies. Diagnosis is made by analysis of urine organic acids that show elevated methylmalonic acid; proprionic acid may also be increased due to secondary inhibition of proprionyl-CoA carboxylase. Enzyme assays can be performed on leukocytes and all cases should be tested for responsiveness to vitamin B12. Therapy directed toward extrapyramidal symptoms generally has a limited effect.

Amino Acid Disorders
Amino acids can be used to synthesize proteins and specialized products, such as porphyrins, creatine, and neurotransmitters. Catabolism of amino acids also can be a source of energy. When amino acids are catabolized, the amino group is removed and enters the urea cycle. The remaining carbon skeletons undergo further catabolism, leading to the formation of glucose, lipid, or energy production via the Krebs cycle.

Phenylketonuria.
PKU is an autosomal recessive disorder caused by a deficiency of hepatic phenylalanine hydroxylase (chromosome 12q24.1). The disorder is detected on

routine neonatal screening, and the neurological consequences of the disease can be prevented by the early initiation of a phenylalanine-free diet. Seizures, developmental delay, and microcephaly are common early neurological features of untreated PKU. In older patients, frequent signs include increased tone, hyperreflexia, extensor plantar responses, and an irregular, rapid, small amplitude tremor of the hands (246). Bizarre twisting movements, repetitious movements of the fingers, stereotypies, dystonia, and overt parkinsonian features also may be present (247–250). In general, the level of disability remains stable after early childhood, but there are cases of neurological deterioration in adulthood (249). The phenylalanine-free diet is generally beneficial, but treated patients may be intellectually impaired when compared to unaffected siblings or controls (251). Other causes for hyperphenylalanemia include defects in the synthesis of dihydrobiopterin and dihydropteridine reductase deficiency (see Pediatric Neurotransmitter Diseases elsewhere in this chapter).

Mitochondrial Disorders

Multiple biochemical reactions in a variety of metabolic pathways occur within the mitochondria. Nevertheless, the terms *mitochondrial cytopathies* and *mitochondrial diseases* are typically reserved for disorders of oxidative phosphorylation (OXPHOS) in the respiratory chain. The respiratory chain is composed of 5 complexes and 2 electron carriers (ubiquinone or coenzyme Q10 and cytochrome C) that generate energy via ATP. The assembly and function of these complexes require 60 additional ancillary proteins.

Leigh's Syndrome. Leigh's syndrome (subacute necrotizing encephalomyelopathy) is a complex of progressive neurodegenerative disorders caused by several defects of energy metabolism, including the pyruvate dehydrogenase complex, pyruvate carboxylase, and respiratory complexes I, II, IV, and V (252–254). The most common defect, affecting about one-fourth of patients, involves cytochrome C oxidase deficiency (complex IV). In some cases the defect in cytochrome C oxidase-deficient Leigh's disease has been mapped to chromosome 9q34 with the putative candidate gene (SURF-1) shown to encode an assembly or maintenance factor (255). The disorder usually presents in infancy or early childhood with psychomotor delay and hypotonia. As the disease progresses, feeding and swallowing defects, nystagmus, ophthalmoplegia, optic atrophy, ataxia, pyramidal signs, and respiratory problems become apparent. Movement disorders, such as dystonia, choreoathetosis, and myoclonus, have been prominent in some cases and, at times, may be the initial sign (256–259). Pathologic findings include symmetric necrotic lesions (spongy degeneration) with demyelination, vascular proliferation, and gliosis affecting the basal ganglia, diencephalon, and brainstem. Diagnosis is based on the presence of elevated arterial or CSF lactate levels and T2-weighted magnetic resonance images that show symmetric areas of increased signal in the putamen, or occasionally the caudate, globus pallidus, and substantia nigra (260). White matter involvement is also common in mitochondrial disorders (261).

Disorders of Purine Metabolism

Lesch-Nyhan Disease. Lesch-Nyhan disease (LND) is an X-linked recessive disorder associated with heterogeneous mutations in the gene for the enzyme hypoxanthine-guanine phosphoribosyltransferase (HPRT) located on chromosome Xq26-27 (262). The biochemical defect is a deficiency of HPRT that converts the free purine bases hypoxanthine and guanine to their respective nucleotides. Purines are important intermediaries in energy-dependent reactions, cofactor-requiring reactions, and inter- and intracellular signaling. In the absence of HPRT, hypoxanthine and guanine cannot be recycled, are degraded, and then are excreted as uric acid.

Clinically, the overproduction of uric acid leads to hyperuricemia and, if not treated, to renal stones and gouty arthritis. Since hyperuricemia is not present in all patients, measures of 24-hour urinary uric acid excretion and genetic testing may be required for diagnosis. Self-injurious behavior (e.g., self-biting, head banging, eye poking) is a hallmark, but nondiagnostic, feature of this disorder. These behaviors typically appear at about ages 2 to 3 years, although they may not emerge until the late teenage years. The motor disorder of LND typically begins with delayed motor development and hypotonia within the first 6 months of life. Involuntary movements usually appear within the next 18 months. These latter abnormalities have been variably described in the literature. In three older series, the cardinal features were either described as choreoathetosis and spasticity or dystonia with hypotonia (263–265). In a study of 17 patients (age range: 8 to 38 years) with LND, performed with particular attention to neurological features (266), motor dysfunction was best described as severe dystonia superimposed on hypotonia. Dystonia, present in all subjects, was typically absent at rest and increased with excitement or attempted purposeful movements. Choreiform movements were present in about one-half and ballismus of the upper extremity in about one-third, but these symptoms were usually minor in comparison to the dystonia. Ocular motility is grossly abnormal (fixation interrupted by unwanted saccades and voluntary saccades preceded by head movement or eye blink) in patients with severe enzyme deficiency (267).

Elevated serum or urine uric acid values are suggestive but not diagnostic for LND (262). Total 24-hour urine uric acid provides strong evidence, but diagnosis should be confirmed by reduced HRPT enzyme activity in blood cells or fibroblasts and/or by demonstration of a mutation in the HPRT gene. Therapy includes generous hydration and allopurinol for hyperuricemia and protective measures, behavior modification therapy, and possibly pharmacotherapy (benzodiazepines, neuroleptics, gabapentin, carbamazepine) for self-injurious behavior. Although there have been no controlled trials focusing on the treatment of the motor disorder, extrapyramidal signs have not been significantly improved by neuroleptics, tetrabenazine, or levodopa.

Disorders of Creatine Metabolism

The creatine–phosphate system plays an important role in storage and transmission of phosphate-bound energy. It is synthesized in the liver and pancreas, and it is stored in the muscle and brain. Each day approximately 1.5% to 1.7% of creatine is nonenzymatically converted to creatinine. There are three creatine deficiency disorders: arginine:glycine amindinotransferase (AGAT) deficiency (268), guanidinoacetate methyltransferase (GAMT) deficiency (269), and the creatine transporter defect (270). All three cause mental retardation, significant language delay, and extrapyramidal symptoms. They all are associated with significantly decreased creatine and phosphocreatine peaks on brain spectroscopy (271).

Guanidinoacetate Methyltransferase Deficiency (Creatine Deficiency Syndrome). Guanidinoacetate methyltransferase converts guanidinoacetate to creatine. A deficiency of this enzyme represents a newly recognized inborn error of creatine biosynthesis. The disorder, transmitted in an autosomal recessive fashion, is localized to mutations on chromosome 19p13.3. It presents in infancy with progressive dystonia and dyskinesias, developmental delay, and drug-resistant epilepsy (269,272,273). The neurologic manifestations are believed to reflect a combination of cerebral energy deficiency due to a depletion of brain creatine/phosphocreatine and a neurotoxic effect of excess brain guanidinoacetate. T2-weighted images have shown high signal in the globus pallidus bilaterally. Clinical and biochemical abnormalities have responded to treatment with oral creatine supplementation.

The diagnosis is established by detection of creatine deficiency in the brain by magnetic resonance spectroscopy, the determination of guanidino compounds (decreased creatine and increased guanidinoacetate) in CSF and urine, low plasma and urine creatinine, and defective GAMT activity in fibroblasts or liver tissue. Biochemical and neuroradiological abnormalities respond to treatment with oral creatine supplementation, but clinical improvement may be incomplete. Dietary treatment with arginine restriction and ornithine supplementation has reduced EEG epileptogenic activity (274).

Cofactor Disorders

Molybdenum Cofactor (Sulfite Oxidase) Deficiency. Three mammalian enzymes require molybdenum as a cofactor for their function, including sulfite oxidase (essential for detoxifying sulfites), xanthine dehydrogenase (role in purine metabolism and formation of uric acid from xanthine and hypoxanthine), and aldehyde dehydrogenase (catalyzes conversion of aldehydes to acids). Molybdenum cofactor deficiency is a rare, autosomal recessive, neurodegenerative disease that affects the CNS primarily through sulfite oxidase deficiency. The cofactor is an unstable reduced pterin with a unique 4-carbon side chain, synthesized by a complex pathway that requires the products of at least 4 separate genes (275). The disorder often starts in the neonatal period with feeding difficulties and intractable seizures. A case has been reported with severe metabolic acidosis and intracranial hemorrhage (276). Other manifestations include axial hypotonia, hypomotility, limb rigidity, dislocated lenses, and profound developmental delay (277). Dystonia and bilateral basal ganglia changes have been reported early in the presentation (278), and survivors may develop a variety of extrapyramidal movements. Diagnosis is suspected by low levels of uric acid in serum and urine and increased urinary sulfite (detectable by dipstick), thiosulfate, S-sulfocysteine (detectable by anion exchange chromatography), taurine, xanthine, and hypoxanthine levels. Enzymatic diagnosis can be confirmed by absent sulfite oxidase activity in skin fibroblast culture. Brain imaging may show multiple cystic white matter cavities in basal ganglia, brainstem, and cerebellum, loss of brain volume, and cessation of myelination. A short-term response to dietary methionine restriction with cysteine supplementation has been reported (279).

Tricarboxylic Acid Cycle Disorders

The tricarboxylic acid (TCA or Krebs) cycle generates the reducing equivalents NADH2 and FADH, essential components for the maintenance of energy. Reoxidation of these compounds by the mitochondrial respiratory chain generates energy for ATP formation.

Fumarase Hydratase Deficiency. Fumarase hydratase deficiency is a rare autosomal recessive inborn error of the tricarboxylic acid cycle; fumarase catalyzes the reversible interconversion of fumarate and malate. There are two isoforms of fumarase (coded on the same region of chromosome 1q42), mitochondrial and cytosolic, with similar structures except for the amino-terminal residue. The former is involved in the TCA cycle in mitochondria, whereas the physiological function of the latter is less clear (280). Variable clinical presentations have been reported (281,282). Early-onset cases have a progressive encephalopathy with failure to thrive, microcephaly, developmental retardation, hypotonia, seizures, and fumaric aciduria (283,284). Several cases at age 1 year, in addition to severe muscular atrophy, seizures, and pyramidal syndromes, had dystonia and paralysis of upgaze (285). Structural brain malformations (polymicrogyria, decreased cerebral white matter, large ventricles, and open opercula) and dysmorphic facial features also have been reported (286).

REFERENCES

1. Fernandez-Alvarez E. Transient movement disorders in children. *J Neurol* 1998;245:1–5.
2. Rothfield K, Behr J, McBride M, Kurlan R, Shoulson I. Developmental chorea and dystonia of infancy. *Neurology* 1987;37(suppl 1):37.
3. Willemse J. Benign idiopathic dystonia with onset in the first year of life. *Dev Med Child Neurol* 1986;28:355–360.
4. De Vries AM, de Groot L. Transient dystonies revisited: a comparative study of preterm and term children at 2.5 years of age. *Dev Med Child Neurol* 2002;44:415–421.
5. Dooley JM, Furey S, Gordon KE, Wood EP. Fever-induced dystonia. *Pediatr Neurol* 2003;28:149–150.
6. Deonna TW, Ziegler AL, Nielsen J. Transient idiopathic dystonia in infancy. *Neuropediatrics* 1991;22:220–224.
7. Turanli G, Senbil N, Altunbasak S, Topcu M. Benign neonatal sleep myoclonus mimicking status epilepticus. *J Child Neurol* 2004;19:62–63.
8. Resnick TJ, Moshe SL, Perotta L, Chambers HJ. Benign neonatal sleep myoclonus: relationship to sleep states. *Arch Neurol* 1986;43:266–268.
9. Di Capua M, Fusco L, Ricci S, Vigevano F. Benign neonatal sleep myoclonus: clinical features and video-polygraphic recordings. *Mov Disord* 1993;8:191–194.
10. Egger J, Grossmann G, Auchterlonie IA. Benign sleep myoclonus in infancy mistaken for epilepsy. *BMJ* 2003;326:975–976.
11. Coulter DL, Allen RJ. Benign neonatal sleep myoclonus. *Arch Neurol* 1982;39:191–192.
12. Daoust-Roy J, Seshia SS. Benign neonatal sleep myoclonus: a differential diagnosis of neonatal seizures. *Am J Dis Child* 1992;146:1236–1241.
13. Maydell BV, Berenson F, Rothner AD, Wyllie E, Kotagal P. Benign myoclonus of early infancy: an imitator of West's syndrome. *J Child Neurol* 2001;16:109–112.
14. Lombroso CT. Early myoclonic encephalopathy, early infantile epileptic encephalopathy, and benign and severe infantile myoclonic epilepsies: a critical review and personal contributions. *J Clin Neurophysiol* 1990;7:380–408.
15. Vanasse M, Bedard P, Andermann F. Shuddering attacks in children: an early clinical manifestation of essential tremor. *Neurology* 1976;26:1027–1030.
16. Holmes GL, Russman BS. Shuddering attacks. Evaluation using electroencephalographic frequency modulation radiotelemetry and videotape monitoring. *Am J Dis Child* 1986;140:72–73.
17. Barron TF, Younkin DP. Propranolol therapy for shuddering attacks. *Neurology* 1992;42:258–259.
18. Kanazawa O. Shuddering attacks: report of four children. *Pediatr Neurol* 2000;23:421–424.
19. Snyder CH. Paroxysmal torticollis in infancy. A possible form of labyrinthitis. *Am J Dis Child* 1969;117:458–460.
20. Cohen HA, Nussinovitch M, Ashkenasi A, Straussberg R, Kauschanksy A, Frydman M. Benign paroxysmal torticollis in infancy. *Pediatr Neurol* 1993;9:488–490.
21. Drigo P, Carli G, Laverda AM. Benign paroxysmal torticollis of infancy. *Brain Dev* 2000;22:169–172.
22. Giffin NJ, Benton S, Goadsby PJ. Benign paroxysmal torticollis of infancy: four new cases and linkage to CACNA1A mutation. *Dev Med Child Neurol* 2002;44:490–493.
23. Eviatar L. Benign paroxysmal torticollis. *Pediatr Neurol* 1994;11:72.
24. Deonna T, Martin D. Benign paroxysmal torticollis in infancy. *Arch Dis Child* 1981;56:956–959.
25. Al-Twaijri WA, Shevell MI. Pediatric migraine equivalents: occurrence and clinical features in practice. *Pediatr Neurol* 2002;26:365–368.
26. Gorrotxategi P, Reguilon MJ, Arana J, et al. Gastroesophageal reflux in association with the Sandifer syndrome. *Eur J Pediatr Surg* 1995;5:203–205.
27. Somjit S, Lee Y, Berkovic SF, Harvey AS. Sandifer syndrome misdiagnosed as refractory partial seizures in an adult. *Epileptic Disord* 2004;6:49–50.
28. Gottlob I, Zubcov A, Catalano RA, et al. Signs distinguishing spasmus nutans (with and without central nervous system lesions) from infantile nystagmus. *Ophthalmology* 1990;97:1166–1175.
29. Doummar D, Roussat B, Beauvais P, Billette de Villemeur T, Richardet JM. Spasmus nutans: apropos of 16 cases. *Arch Pediatr* 1998;5:264–268.
30. Smith DE, Fitzgerald K, Stass-Isern M, Cibis GW. Electroretinography is necessary for spasmus nutans diagnosis. *Pediatr Neurol* 2000;23:33–36.
31. Wizov SS, Reinecke RD, Bocarnea M, Gottlob I. A comparative demographic and socioeconomic study of spasmus nutans and infantile nystagmus. *Am J Ophthalmol* 2002;133:256–262.
32. Albright AL, Sclabassi RJ, Slamovits TL, Bergman I. Spasmus nutans associated with optic gliomas in infants. *J Pediatr* 1984;105:778–780.
33. Arnoldi KA, Tychsen L. Prevalence of intracranial lesions in children initially diagnosed with disconjugate nystagmus (spasmus nutans). *J Pediatr Ophthalmol Strabismus* 1995;32:296–301.
34. Hottinger-Blanc PM, Ziegler AL, Deonna T. A special type of head stereotypies in children with developmental (cerebellar) disorder: description of 8 cases and literature review. *Eur J Paediatr Neurol* 2002;6:143–152.
35. DiMario FJ, Jr. Childhood head tremor. *J Child Neurol* 2000;15:22–25.
36. Wiese JA, Gentry LR, Menezes AH. Bobble-head doll syndrome: review of the pathophysiology and CSF dynamics. *Pediatr Neurol* 1985;1:361–366.
37. Pollack IF, Schor NF, Martinez AJ, Towbin R. Bobble-head doll syndrome and drop attacks in a child with a cystic choroid plexus papilloma of the third ventricle: case report. *J Neurosurg* 1995;83:729–732.
38. Zamponi N, Rychlicki F, Trignani R, Polonara G, Ruggiero M, Cesaroni E. Bobble head doll syndrome in a child with a third ventricular cyst and hydrocephalus. *Childs Nerv Syst* 2005;21:350–354.
39. Coker SB. Bobble-head doll syndrome due to trapped fourth ventricle and aqueduct. *Pediatr Neurol* 1986;2:115–116.
40. Ouvrier RA, Billson F. Benign paroxysmal tonic upgaze of childhood. *J Child Neurol* 1988;3:177–180.
41. Rouveyrol F, Stephan JL. Benign paroxysmal tonic upgaze of infancy: 2 additional cases. *Arch Pediatr* 2003;10:527–529.
42. Lispi ML, Vigevano F. Benign paroxysmal tonic upgaze of childhood with ataxia. *Epileptic Disord* 2001;3:203–206.
43. Campistol J, Prats JM, Garaizar C. Benign paroxysmal tonic upgaze of childhood with ataxia: a neuro-ophthalmological syndrome of familial origin? *Dev Med Child Neurol* 1993;35:436–439.
44. Demirkiran M, Jankovic J. Paroxysmal dyskinesias: clinical features and classification. *Ann Neurol* 1995;38:571–579.
45. Cuenca-Leon E, Cormand B, Thomson T, Macaya A. Paroxysmal kinesigenic dyskinesia and generalized seizures: clinical and genetic analysis in a Spanish pedigree. *Neuropediatrics* 2002;33:288–293.
46. Blakeley J, Jankovic J. Secondary paroxysmal dyskinesias. *Mov Disord* 2002;17:726–734.
47. Demir E, Prud'homme JF, Topcu M. Infantile convulsions and paroxysmal choreoathetosis in a consanguineous family. *Pediatr Neurol* 2004;30:349–353.
48. Swoboda KJ, Soong B, McKenna C, et al. Paroxysmal kinesigenic dyskinesia and infantile convulsions: clinical and linkage studies. *Neurology* 2000;55:224–230.
49. Perniola T, Margari L, de Iaco MG, et al. Familial paroxysmal exercise-induced dyskinesia, epilepsy, and mental retardation in a family with autosomal dominant inheritance. *Mov Disord* 2001;16:724–730.
50. Guerrini R, Sanchez-Carpintero R, Deonna T, et al. Early-onset absence epilepsy and paroxysmal dyskinesia. *Epilepsia* 2002;43:1224–1229.
51. Guerrini R, Bonanni P, Nardocci N, et al. Autosomal recessive rolandic epilepsy with paroxysmal exercise-induced dystonia and writer's cramp: delineation of the syndrome and gene mapping to chromosome 16p12-11.2. *Ann Neurol* 1999;45:344–352.
52. Kurlan R, McDermott MP, Deeley C, et al. Prevalence of tics in school children and association with placement in special education. *Neurology* 2001;57:1383–1388.
53. Robertson MM. Diagnosing Tourette syndrome: is it a common disorder? *J Psychosom Res* 2003;55:3–6.

54. Khalifa N, von Knorring AL. Prevalence of tic disorders and Tourette syndrome in a Swedish school population. *Dev Med Child Neurol* 2003;45:315–319.

55. Baron-Cohen S, Mortimore C, Moriarty J, Izaguirre J, Robertson M. The prevalence of Gilles de la Tourette's syndrome in children and adolescents with autism. *J Child Psychol Psychiatry* 1999;40: 213–218.

56. Mahone EM, Bridges D, Prahme C, Singer HS. Repetitive arm and hand movements (complex motor stereotypies) in children. *J Pediatr* 2004;145:391–395.

57. Sallustro F, Atwell CW. Body rocking, head banging, and head rolling in normal children. *J Pediatr* 1978;93:704–708.

58. Tan A, Salgado M, Fahn S. The characterization and outcome of stereotypical movements in nonautistic children. *Mov Disord* 1997;12:47–52.

59. Trinidad KS, Wang D, Kurlan R. Paroxysmal stereotypic dyskinesias in children. *Mov Disord* 1993;8:417.

60. Deda G, Caksen H, Suskan E, Gumus D. Masturbation mimicking seizure in an infant. *Indian J Pediatr* 2001;68:779–781.

61. Mink JW, Neil JJ. Masturbation mimicking paroxysmal dystonia or dyskinesia in a young girl. *Mov Disord* 1995;10:518–520.

62. Nechay A, Ross LM, Stephenson JB, O'Regan M. Gratification disorder ("infantile masturbation"): a review. *Arch Dis Child* 2004;89:225–226.

63. Casteels K, Wouters C, Van Geet C, Devlieger H. Video reveals self-stimulation in infancy. *Acta Paediatr* 2004;93:844–846.

64. Andermann F, Keene DL, Andermann E, Quesney LF. Startle disease or hyperekplexia: further delineation of the syndrome. *Brain* 1980;103:985–997.

65. Zhou L, Chillag KL, Nigro MA. Hyperekplexia: a treatable neurogenetic disease. *Brain Dev* 2002;24:669–674.

66. Tijssen MA, Voorkamp LM, Padberg GW, van Dijk JG. Startle responses in hereditary hyperekplexia. *Arch Neurol* 1997;54: 388–393.

67. Ryan SG, Sherman SL, Terry JC, Sparkes RS, Torres MC, Mackey RW. Startle disease, or hyperekplexia: response to clonazepam and assignment of the gene (STHE) to chromosome 5q by linkage analysis. *Ann Neurol* 1992;31:663–668.

68. Rees MI, Lewis TM, Vafa B, et al. Compound heterozygosity and nonsense mutations in the alpha(1)-subunit of the inhibitory glycine receptor in hyperekplexia. *Hum Genet* 2001;109:267–270.

69. Rees MI, Lewis TM, Kwok JB, et al. Hyperekplexia associated with compound heterozygote mutations in the beta-subunit of the human inhibitory glycine receptor (GLRB). *Hum Mol Genet* 2002;11:853–860.

70. Rees MI, Harvey K, Ward H, et al. Isoform heterogeneity of the human gephyrin gene (GPHN), binding domains to the glycine receptor, and mutation analysis in hyperekplexia. *J Biol Chem* 2003;278:24,688–24,696.

71. Rees MI, Andrew M, Jawad S, Owen MJ. Evidence for recessive as well as dominant forms of startle disease (hyperekplexia) caused by mutations in the alpha 1 subunit of the inhibitory glycine receptor. *Hum Mol Genet* 1994;3:2175–2179.

72. Brown P. Physiology of startle phenomena. *Adv Neurol* 1995;67: 273–287.

73. Gordon N. Startle disease or hyperekplexia. *Dev Med Child Neurol* 1993;35:1015–1018.

74. Andermann F, Andermann E. Excessive startle syndromes: startle disease, jumping, and startle epilepsy. *Adv Neurol* 1986;43: 321–338.

75. Morley DJ, Weaver DD, Garg BP, Markand O. Hyperexplexia: an inherited disorder of the startle response. *Clin Genet* 1982;21:388–396.

76. Nigro MA, Lim HC. Hyperekplexia and sudden neonatal death. *Pediatr Neurol* 1992;8:221–225.

77. Leventer RJ, Hopkins IJ, Shield LK. Hyperekplexia as cause of abnormal intrauterine movements. *Lancet* 1995;345:461.

78. Baxter P, Connolly S, Curtis A, et al. Co-dominant inheritance of hyperekplexia and spastic paraparesis. *Dev Med Child Neurol* 1996;38:739–743.

79. Crone C, Nielsen J, Petersen N, Tijssen MA, van Dijk JG. Patients with the major and minor form of hyperekplexia differ with regards to disynaptic reciprocal inhibition between ankle flexor and extensor muscles. *Exp Brain Res* 2001;140:190–197.

80. Lerman-Sagie T, Leshinsky-Silver E, Watemberg N, Lev D. Should autistic children be evaluated for mitochondrial disorders? *J Child Neurol* 2004;19:379–381.

81. Oguro K, Hirano K, Aiba H. Trigeminally induced startle in children with hyperekplexia. *Mov Disord* 2005;20:484–489.

82. Pascotto A, Coppola G. Neonatal hyperekplexia: a case report. *Epilepsia* 1992;33:817–820.

83. Soland VL, Bhatia KP, Volonte MA, Marsden CD. Focal task specific tremors. *Mov Disord* 1996;11:665–670.

84. Destee A, Cassim F, Defebvre L, Guieu JD. Hereditary chin trembling or hereditary chin myoclonus? *J Neurol Neurosurg Psychiatry* 1997;63:804–807.

85. Grimes DA, Han F, Bulman D, Nicolson ML, Suchowersky O. Hereditary chin trembling: a new family with exclusion of the chromosome 9q13-q21 locus. *Mov Disord* 2002;17:1390–1392.

86. Jarman PR, Wood NW, Davis MT, et al. Hereditary geniospasm: linkage to chromosome 9q13-q21 and evidence for genetic heterogeneity. *Am J Hum Genet* 1997;61:928–933.

87. Gordon K, Cadera W, Hinton G. Successful treatment of hereditary trembling chin with botulinum toxin. *J Child Neurol* 1993;8:154–156.

88. Scott BL, Jankovic J. Delayed-onset progressive movement disorders after static brain lesions. *Neurology* 1996;46:68–74.

89. Mutch L, Alberman E, Hagberg B, Kodama K, Perat MV. Cerebral palsy epidemiology: where are we now and where are we going? *Dev Med Child Neurol* 1992;34:547–551.

90. Nelson K. Epidemiology and etiology of cerebral palsy. In: Capute AJ, Accardo PJ, eds. *Developmental disabilities in infancy and childhood*, 2nd ed. Baltimore: Paul Brooks, 1996:73–79.

91. Bax M, Nelson KB. Birth asphyxia: a statement. World Federation of Neurology Group. *Dev Med Child Neurol* 1993;35:1022–1024.

92. Nelson KB, Emery ES 3rd. Birth asphyxia and the neonatal brain: what do we know and when do we know it? *Clin Perinatol* 1993;20:327–344.

93. Nelson KB. The epidemiology of cerebral palsy in term infants. *Ment Retard Dev Disabil Res Rev* 2002;8:146–150.

94. Wilson-Costello D, Friedman H, Minich N, Fanaroff AA, Hack M. Improved survival rates with increased neurodevelopmental disability for extremely low birth weight infants in the 1990s. *Pediatrics* 2005;115:997–1003.

95. Sie LT, Hart AA, van Hof J, et al. Predictive value of neonatal MRI with respect to late MRI findings and clinical outcome: a study in infants with periventricular densities on neonatal ultrasound. *Neuropediatrics* 2005;36:78–89.

96. Bodensteiner JB, Johnsen SD. Cerebellar injury in the extremely premature infant: newly recognized but relatively common outcome. *J Child Neurol* 2005;20:139–142.

97. Johnsen SD, Bodensteiner JB, Lotze TE. Frequency and nature of cerebellar injury in the extremely premature survivor with cerebral palsy. *J Child Neurol* 2005;20:60–64.

98. Nelson KB, Dambrosia JM, Iovannisci DM, Cheng S, Grether JK, Lammer E. Genetic polymorphisms and cerebral palsy in very preterm infants. *Pediatr Res* 2005;57:494–499.

99. Grether JK, Nelson KB, Walsh E, Willoughby RE, Redline RW. Intrauterine exposure to infection and risk of cerebral palsy in very preterm infants. *Arch Pediatr Adolesc Med* 2003;157: 26–32.

100. Adamo R. Neonatal encephalopathy and cerebral palsy: defining the pathogenesis and pathophysiology: a report. Washington, DC: American College of Obstetricians & Gynecologists; 2003.

101. Badawi N, Kurinczuk JJ, Keogh JM, et al. Intrapartum risk factors for newborn encephalopathy: the Western Australian case-control study. *BMJ* 1998;317:1554–1558.

102. Badawi N, Kurinczuk JJ, Keogh JM, et al. Antepartum risk factors for newborn encephalopathy: the Western Australian case-control study. *BMJ* 1998;317:1549–1453.

103. Felix JF, Badawi N, Kurinczuk JJ, Bower C, Keogh JM, Pemberton PJ. Birth defects in children with newborn encephalopathy. *Dev Med Child Neurol* 2000;42:803–808.

104. Evans P, Elliot M, Alberman E, Evans S. Prevalence and disabilities in 4- to 8-year-olds with cerebral palsy. *Arch Dis Child* 1985;60:940–945.

105. Capute AJ. Identifying cerebral palsy in infancy through study of primative reflex profiles. *Pediatr Ann* 1979;8:589–595.

106. Caputo AJ, Palmer FB, Shapiro BK, Wachtel RC, Ross A, Accardo PJ. Primitive reflex profile: a quantitation of primitive reflexes in infancy. *Dev Med Child Neurol* 1984;26:375–383.

107. Ashwal S, Russman BS, Blasco PA, et al. Practice parameter: diagnostic assessment of the child with cerebral palsy: report of the Quality Standards Subcommittee of the American Academy of Neurology and the Practice Committee of the Child Neurology Society. *Neurology* 2004;62:851–863.

108. Filloux FM. Neuropathophysiology of movement disorders in cerebral palsy. *J Child Neurol* 1996;11(suppl 1):S5–S12.

109. Yokochi K, Aiba K, Kodama M, Fujimoto S. Magnetic resonance imaging in athetotic cerebral palsied children. *Acta Paediatr Scand* 1991;80:818–823.

110. Miller G, Cala LA. Ataxic cerebral palsy: clinico-radiologic correlations. *Neuropediatrics* 1989;20:84–89.

111. Blackmon LR, Fanaroff AA, Raju TN. Research on prevention of bilirubin-induced brain injury and kernicterus: National Institute of Child Health and Human Development conference executive summary. 2003. *Pediatrics* 2004;114:229–233.

112. Coskun A, Yikilmaz A, Kumandas S, Karahan OI, Akcakus M, Manav A. Hyperintense globus pallidus on T1-weighted MR imaging in acute kernicterus: is it common or rare? *Eur Radiol* 2005;15:1263–1267.

113. Sugama S, Soeda A, Eto Y. Magnetic resonance imaging in three children with kernicterus. *Pediatr Neurol* 2001;25:328–331.

114. Management of hyperbilirubinemia in the newborn infant 35 or more weeks of gestation. *Pediatrics* 2004;114:297–316.

115. Cardoso F, Eduardo C, Silva AP, Mota CC. Chorea in fifty consecutive patients with rheumatic fever. *Mov Disord* 1997;12:701–703.

116. Vidakovic A, Dragasevic N, Kostic VS. Hemiballism: report of 25 cases. *J Neurol Neurosurg Psychiatry* 1994;57:945–949.

117. Freeman JM, Aron AM, Collard JE, Mackay MC. The emotional correlates of Sydenham's chorea. *Pediatrics* 1965;35:42–49.

118. Swedo SE, Leonard HL, Schapiro MB, Casey BJ, Mannheim GB, Lenane MC, et al. Sydenham's chorea: physical and psychological symptoms of St Vitus dance. *Pediatrics* 1993;91:706–713.

119. Mercadante MT, Campos MC, Marques-Dias MJ, Miguel EC, Leckman J. Vocal tics in Sydenham's chorea. *J Am Acad Child Adolesc Psychiatry* 1997;36:305–306.

120. Stollerman GH. Rheumatic fever. *Lancet* 1997;349:935–942.

121. Cardoso F, Vargas AP, Oliveira LD, Guerra AA, Amaral SV. Persistent Sydenham's chorea. *Mov Disord* 1999;14:805–807.

122. Swedo SE, Rapoport JL, Cheslow DL, et al. High prevalence of obsessive-compulsive symptoms in patients with Sydenham's chorea. *Am J Psychiatry* 1989;146:246–249.

123. Korn-Lubetzki I, Brand A, Steiner I. Recurrence of Sydenham chorea: implications for pathogenesis. *Arch Neurol* 2004;61: 1261–1264.

124. Nausieda PA, Grossman BJ, Koller WC, Weiner WJ, Klawans HL. Sydenham chorea: an update. *Neurology* 1980;30:331–334.

125. Taranta A. Relation of isolated recurrences of Sydenham's chorea to preceding streptococcal infections. *N Engl J Med* 1959;260:1204–1210.

126. Berrios X, Quesney F, Morales A, Blazquez J, Bisno AL. Are all recurrences of "pure" Sydenham chorea true recurrences of acute rheumatic fever? *J Pediatr* 1985;107:867–872.

127. Giedd JN, Rapoport JL, Kruesi MJ, et al. Sydenham's chorea: magnetic resonance imaging of the basal ganglia. *Neurology* 1995;45:2199–2202.

128. Jordan LC, Singer HS. Sydenham chorea in children. *Curr Treat Options Neurol* 2003;5:283–290.

129. Cardoso F, Maia D, Cunningham MC, Valenca G. Treatment of Sydenham chorea with corticosteroids. *Mov Disord* 2003;18: 1374–1377.

130. Barash J, Margalith D, Matitiau A. Corticosteroid treatment in patients with Sydenham's chorea. *Pediatr Neurol* 2005;32:205–207.

131. Garvey MA, Swedo SE. Sydenham's chorea: clinical and therapeutic update. *Adv Exp Med Biol* 1997;418:115–120.

132. Husby G, van de Rijn I, Zabriskie JB, Abdin ZH, Williams RC, Jr. Antibodies reacting with cytoplasm of subthalamic and caudate nuclei neurons in chorea and acute rheumatic fever. *J Exp Med* 1976;144:1094–1110.

133. Church AJ, Cardoso F, Dale RC, Lees AJ, Thompson EJ, Giovannoni G. Anti-basal ganglia antibodies in acute and persistent Sydenham's chorea. *Neurology* 2002;59:227–231.

134. Singer HS, Loiselle CR, Lee O, Garvey MA, Grus FH. Anti-basal ganglia antibody abnormalities in Sydenham chorea. *J Neuroimmunol* 2003;136:154–161.

135. Church AJ, Dale RC, Cardoso F, et al. CSF and serum immune parameters in Sydenham's chorea: evidence of an autoimmune syndrome? *J Neuroimmunol* 2003;136:149–153.

136. Kirvan CA, Swedo SE, Karahara D, et al. Streptococcal mimicry and antibody-mediated cell signaling in the pathogenesis of Sydenham's chorea. *Autoimmunity* 2006;39:21–29.

137. Swedo SE, Leonard HL, Garvey M, et al. Pediatric autoimmune neuropsychiatric disorders associated with streptococcal infections: clinical description of the first 50 cases. *Am J Psychiatry* 1998;155:264–271.

138. Swedo SE, Leonard HL, Rapoport JL. The pediatric autoimmune neuropsychiatric disorders associated with streptococcal infection (PANDAS) subgroup: separating fact from fiction. *Pediatrics* 2004;113:907–911.

139. Kurlan R, Kaplan EL. The pediatric autoimmune neuropsychiatric disorders associated with streptococcal infection (PANDAS) etiology for tics and obsessive-compulsive symptoms: hypothesis or entity? Practical considerations for the clinician. *Pediatrics* 2004;113:883–886.

140. Singer HS, Loiselle C. PANDAS: a commentary. *J Psychosom Res* 2003;55:31–39.

141. Singer HS. PANDAS—Pediatric autoimmune neuropsychiatric disorders associated with streptococcal infection: is it a specific clinical disorder? *Rev Bras Psiquiatr* 2004;26:220–221.

142. Snider LA, Swedo SE. Post-streptococcal autoimmune disorders of the central nervous system. *Curr Opin Neurol* 2003;16:359–365.

143. Murphy ML, Pichichero ME. Prospective identification and treatment of children with pediatric autoimmune neuropsychiatric disorder associated with group A streptococcal infection (PANDAS). *Arch Pediatr Adolesc Med* 2002;156:356–361.

144. Lougee L, Perlmutter SJ, Nicolson R, Garvey MA, Swedo SE. Psychiatric disorders in first-degree relatives of children with pediatric autoimmune neuropsychiatric disorders associated with streptococcal infections (PANDAS). *J Am Acad Child Adolesc Psychiatry* 2000;39:1120–1126.

145. Swedo SE, Leonard HL, Mittleman BB, et al. Identification of children with pediatric autoimmune neuropsychiatric disorders associated with streptococcal infections by a marker associated with rheumatic fever. *Am J Psychiatry* 1997;154:110–112.

146. Giedd JN, Rapoport JL, Garvey MA, Perlmutter S, Swedo SE. MRI assessment of children with obsessive-compulsive disorder or tics associated with streptococcal infection. *Am J Psychiatry* 2000;157:281–283.

147. Singer HS, Giuliano JD, Zimmerman AM, Walkup JT. Infection: a stimulus for tic disorders. *Pediatr Neurol* 2000;22:380–383.

148. Perrin EM, Murphy ML, Casey JR, et al. Does group A beta-hemolytic streptococcal infection increase risk for behavioral and neuropsychiatric symptoms in children? *Arch Pediatr Adolesc Med* 2004;158:848–856.

149. Luo F, Leckman JF, Katsovich L, et al. Prospective longitudinal study of children with tic disorders and/or obsessive-compulsive disorder: relationship of symptom exacerbations to newly acquired streptococcal infections. *Pediatrics* 2004;113: e578–e585.

150. Perlmutter SJ, Leitman SF, Garvey MA, et al. Therapeutic plasma exchange and intravenous immunoglobulin for obsessive-compulsive disorder and tic disorders in childhood. *Lancet* 1999;354:1153–1158.

151. Church AJ, Dale RC, Giovannoni G. Anti-basal ganglia antibodies: a possible diagnostic utility in idiopathic movement disorders? *Arch Dis Child* 2004;89:611–614.

152. Singer HS, Hong JJ, Yoon DY, et al. Serum antibodies do not differentiate RANDAS and Tourette Syndrome from controls. *Neurology* 2005;65:1701–1707.

153. Singer HS, Williams PN. Autoimmunity and pediatric movement disorders. *Adv Neurol* 2006;99:166–178.

154. Loiselle CR, Lee O, Moran TH, Singer HS. Striatal microinfusion of Tourette syndrome and PANDAS sera: failure to induce behavioral changes. *Mov Disord* 2004;19:390–396.

155. Singer H, Mink J, Loiselle C, et al. Microinfusion of antineuronal antibodies into rodent striatum: failure to differentiate between elevated and low titers. *J Neuroimmunol* 2005;163:8–14.

156. Dale RC, Church AJ, Cardoso F, et al. Poststreptococcal acute disseminated encephalomyelitis with basal ganglia involvement and auto-reactive antibasal ganglia antibodies. *Ann Neurol* 2001;50:588–595.

157. Saunders-Pullman R, Blau N, Hyland K, et al. Phenylalanine loading as a diagnostic test for DRD: interpreting the utility of the test. *Mol Genet Metab* 2004;83:207–212.

158. Hwu WL, Wang PJ, Hsiao KJ, Wang TR, Chiou YW, Lee YM. Dopa-responsive dystonia induced by a recessive GTP cyclohydrolase I mutation. *Hum Genet* 1999;105:226–230.

159. Garavaglia B, Invernizzi F, Carbone ML, et al. GTP-cyclohydrolase I gene mutations in patients with autosomal dominant and recessive GTP-CH1 deficiency: identification and functional characterization of four novel mutations. *J Inherit Metab Dis* 2004;27:455–463.

160. Hanihara T, Inoue K, Kawanishi C, et al. 6-Pyruvoyl-tetrahydropterin synthase deficiency with generalized dystonia and diurnal fluctuation of symptoms: a clinical and molecular study. *Mov Disord* 1997;12:408–411.

161. Chien YH, Chiang SC, Huang A, et al. Treatment and outcome of Taiwanese patients with 6-pyruvoyltetrahydropterin synthase gene mutations. *J Inherit Metab Dis* 2001;24:815–823.

162. Hyland K. Presentation, diagnosis, and treatment of the disorders of monoamine neurotransmitter metabolism. *Semin Perinatol* 1999;23:194–203.

163. Hyland K. Abnormalities of biogenic amine metabolism. *J Inherit Metab Dis* 1993;16:676–690.

164. Kaufman S, Holtzman NA, Milstien S, Butler LJ, Krumholz A. Phenylketonuria due to a deficiency of dihydropteridine reductase. *N Engl J Med* 1975;293:785–790.

165. Smith KJ, Hall SM, Schauf CL. Vesicular demyelination induced by raised intracellular calcium. *J Neurol Sci* 1985;71:19–37.

166. Ichinose H, Nagatsu T. Molecular genetics of DOPA-responsive dystonia. *Adv Neurol* 1999;80:195–198.

167. Ichinose H, Inagaki H, Suzuki T, Ohye T, Nagatsu T. Molecular mechanisms of hereditary progressive dystonia with marked diurnal fluctuation, Segawa's disease. *Brain Dev* 2000;22(suppl 1): S107–S110.

168. Furukawa Y. Update on dopa-responsive dystonia: locus heterogeneity and biochemical features. *Adv Neurol* 2004;94:127–138.

169. Uncini A, De Angelis MV, Di Fulvio P, et al. Wide expressivity variation and high but no gender-related penetrance in two dopa-responsive dystonia families with a novel GCH I mutation. *Mov Disord* 2004;19:1139–1145.

170. Steinberger D, Weber Y, Korinthenberg R, et al. High penetrance and pronounced variation in expressivity of GCH1 mutations in five families with dopa-responsive dystonia. *Ann Neurol* 1998;43:634–639.

171. Leuzzi V, Cardona F, Carducci C, Cardona F, Artiola C, Antonozzi I. Autosomal dominant GTP-CH presenting as inherited dopa-responsive myoclonus dystonia syndrome. *Neurology* 2002;59:1241–1243.

172. Deonna T, Ferreira A. Idiopathic fluctuating dystonia: a case of foot dystonia and writer's cramp responsive to L-dopa. *Dev Med Child Neurol* 1985;27:819–821.

173. Deonna T, Roulet E, Ghika J, Zesiger P. Dopa-responsive childhood dystonia: a forme fruste with writer's cramp, triggered by exercise. *Dev Med Child Neurol* 1997;39:49–53.

174. Jarman PR, Bandmann O, Marsden CD, Wood NW. GTP cyclohydrolase I mutations in patients with dystonia responsive to anticholinergic drugs. *J Neurol Neurosurg Psychiatry* 1997;63:304–308.

175. Naumann M, Pirker W, Reiners K, Lange K, Becker G, Brucke T. [123I]beta-CIT single-photon emission tomography in DOPA-responsive dystonia. *Mov Disord* 1997;12:448–451.

176. Kishore A, Nygaard TG, de la Fuente-Fernandez R, et al. Striatal D2 receptors in symptomatic and asymptomatic carriers of dopa-responsive dystonia measured with [11C]-raclopride and positron-emission tomography. *Neurology* 1998;50: 1028–1032.

177. Hyland K, Fryburg JS, Wilson WG, et al. Oral phenylalanine loading in dopa-responsive dystonia: a possible diagnostic test. *Neurology* 1997;48:1290–1297.

178. Hyland K, Arnold LA, Trugman JM. Defects of biopterin metabolism and biogenic amine biosynthesis: clinical diagnostic, and therapeutic aspects. *Adv Neurol* 1998;78:301–308.

179. Blau N, Thony B, Renneberg A, Arnold LA, Hyland K. Dihydropteridine reductase deficiency localized to the central nervous system. *J Inherit Metab Dis* 1998;21:433–434.

180. Blau N, Thony B, Renneberg A. Disorders of tetrahydrobiopterin and related biogenic amines. In: Scriver CR, Beaudet AL, Sly WS, eds. *The metabolic and molecular basis of inherited diseases*, 8th ed. New York: McGraw-Hill, 2001:1725–1776.

181. Bonafe L, Thony B, Penzien JM, Czarnecki B, Blau N. Mutations in the sepiapterin reductase gene cause a novel tetrahydrobiopterin-dependent monoamine-neurotransmitter deficiency without hyperphenylalaninemia. *Am J Hum Genet* 2001;69:269–277.

182. Ludecke B, Knappskog PM, Clayton PT, et al. Recessively inherited L-DOPA-responsive parkinsonism in infancy caused by a point mutation (L205P) in the tyrosine hydroxylase gene. *Hum Mol Genet* 1996;5:1023–1028.

183. Swaans RJ, Rondot P, Renier WO, Van Den Heuvel LP, Steenbergen-Spanjers GC, Wevers RA. Four novel mutations in the tyrosine hydroxylase gene in patients with infantile parkinsonism. *Ann Hum Genet* 2000;64(pt 1):25–31.

184. Furukawa Y, Nygaard TG, Gutlich M, et al. Striatal biopterin and tyrosine hydroxylase protein reduction in dopa-responsive dystonia. *Neurology* 1999;53:1032–1041.

185. Hoffmann GF, Assmann B, Brautigam C, et al. Tyrosine hydroxylase deficiency causes progressive encephalopathy and dopa-nonresponsive dystonia. *Ann Neurol* 2003;54(suppl 6):S56–S65.

186. Schiller A, Wevers RA, Steenbergen GC, Blau N, Jung HH. Long-term course of L-dopa-responsive dystonia caused by tyrosine hydroxylase deficiency. *Neurology* 2004;63:1524–1526.

187. Furukawa Y. Genetics and biochemistry of dopa-responsive dystonia: significance of striatal tyrosine hydroxylase protein loss. *Adv Neurol* 2003;91:401–410.

188. Van den Heuvel LP, Luiten B, Smeitink JA, et al. A common point mutation in the tyrosine hydroxylase gene in autosomal recessive L-DOPA-responsive dystonia in the Dutch population. *Hum Genet* 1998;102:644–646.

189. Swoboda KJ, Hyland K. Diagnosis and treatment of neurotransmitter-related disorders. *Neurol Clin* 2002;20:1143–1161.

190. Pons R, Ford B, Chiriboga CA, et al. Aromatic L-amino acid decarboxylase deficiency: clinical features, treatment, and prognosis. *Neurology* 2004;62:1058–1065.

191. Maller A, Hyland K, Milstien S, Biaggioni I, Butler IJ. Aromatic L-amino acid decarboxylase deficiency: clinical features, diagnosis, and treatment of a second family. *J Child Neurol* 1997;12: 349–354.

192. Korenke GC, Christen HJ, Hyland K, Hunneman DH, Hanefeld F. Aromatic L-amino acid decarboxylase deficiency: an extrapyramidal movement disorder with oculogyric crises. *Eur J Paediatr Neurol* 1997;1:67–71.

193. Swoboda KJ, Saul JP, McKenna CE, Speller NB, Hyland K. Aromatic L-amino acid decarboxylase deficiency: overview of clinical features and outcomes. *Ann Neurol* 2003;54(suppl 6):S49–S55.

194. Hyland K, Surtees RA, Rodeck C, Clayton PT. Aromatic L-amino acid decarboxylase deficiency: clinical features, diagnosis, and treatment of a new inborn error of neurotransmitter amine synthesis. *Neurology* 1992;42:1980–1988.

195. Yokochi M. Development of the nosological analysis of juvenile parkinsonism. *Brain Dev* 2000;22(suppl 1):S81–S86.

196. Chang YT, Sharma R, Marsh JL, et al. Levodopa-responsive aromatic L-amino acid decarboxylase deficiency. *Ann Neurol* 2004;55:435–438.

197. Gordon N. Succinic semialdehyde dehydrogenase deficiency (SSADH) (4-hydroxybutyric aciduria, gamma-hydroxybutyric aciduria). *Eur J Paediatr Neurol* 2004;8:261–265.

198. Pearl PL, Gibson KM. Clinical aspects of the disorders of GABA metabolism in children. *Curr Opin Neurol* 2004;17:107–113.

199. Ethofer T, Seeger U, Klose U, et al. Proton MR spectroscopy in succinic semialdehyde dehydrogenase deficiency. *Neurology* 2004;62:1016–1018.

200. Gropman A. Vigabatrin and newer interventions in succinic semialdehyde dehydrogenase deficiency. *Ann Neurol* 2003;54 (suppl 6):S66–S72.

201. Hogema BM, Akaboshi S, Taylor M, et al. Prenatal diagnosis of succinic semialdehyde dehydrogenase deficiency: increased accuracy employing DNA, enzyme, and metabolite analyses. *Mol Genet Metab* 2001;72:218–222.

202. Sarkar B. Copper transport and its defect in Wilson disease: characterization of the copper-binding domain of Wilson disease ATPase. *J Inorg Biochem* 2000;79:187–191.

203. Brewer GJ. Recognition, diagnosis, and management of Wilson's disease. *Proc Soc Exp Biol Med* 2000;223:39–46.

204. Walshe JM. The eye in Wilson disease. *Birth Defects Orig Artic Ser* 1976;12:187–194.

205. Strickland GT, Leu ML. Wilson's disease: clinical and laboratory manifestations in 40 patients. *Medicine (Baltimore)* 1975;54:113–137.

206. Svetel M, Kozic D, Stefanova E, Semnic R, Dragasevic N, Kostic VS. Dystonia in Wilson's disease. *Mov Disord* 2001;16:719–723.

207. Brewer GJ, Askari FK. Wilson's disease: clinical management and therapy. *J Hepatol* 2005;42(suppl):S13–S21.

208. Brewer GJ. Neurologically presenting Wilson's disease: epidemiology, pathophysiology and treatment. *CNS Drugs* 2005;19:185–192.

209. Leggio L, Addolorato G, Abenavoli L, Gasbarrini G. Wilson's disease: clinical, genetic and pharmacological findings. *Int J Immunopathol Pharmacol* 2005;18:7–14.

210. Walshe JM. Penicillamine: the treatment of first choice for patients with Wilson's disease. *Mov Disord* 1999;14:545–550.

211. Hayflick SJ. Unraveling the Hallervorden-Spatz syndrome: pantothenate kinase-associated neurodegeneration is the name. *Curr Opin Pediatr* 2003;15:572–577.

212. Hayflick SJ. Pantothenate kinase-associated neurodegeneration (formerly Hallervorden-Spatz syndrome). *J Neurol Sci* 2003;207:106–107.

213. Zhou B, Bae SK, Malone AC, et al. hGFRalpha-4: a new member of the GDNF receptor family and a candidate for NBIA. *Pediatr Neurol* 2001;25:156–161.

214. Johnson MA, Kuo YM, Westaway SK, et al. Mitochondrial localization of human PANK2 and hypotheses of secondary iron accumulation in pantothenate kinase-associated neurodegeneration. *Ann N Y Acad Sci* 2004;1012:282–298.

215. Thomas M, Hayflick SJ, Jankovic J. Clinical heterogeneity of neurodegeneration with brain iron accumulation (Hallervorden-Spatz syndrome) and pantothenate kinase-associated neurodegeneration. *Mov Disord* 2004;19:36–42.

216. Swaiman KF. Hallervorden-Spatz syndrome. *Pediatr Neurol* 2001;25:102–108.

217. Marelli C, Piacentini S, Garavaglia B, Girotti F, Albanese A. Clinical and neuropsychological correlates in two brothers with pantothenate kinase-associated neurodegeneration. *Mov Disord* 2005;20:208–212.

218. Carod-Artal FJ, Vargas AP, Marinho PB, Fernandes-Silva TV, Portugal D. Tourettism, hemiballism and juvenile Parkinsonism: expanding the clinical spectrum of the neurodegeneration associated to pantothenate kinase deficiency (Hallervorden Spatz syndrome). *Rev Neurol* 2004;38:327–331.

219. Castelnau P, Cif L, Valente EM, et al. Pallidal stimulation improves pantothenate kinase-associated neurodegeneration. *Ann Neurol* 2005;57:738–741.

220. Higgins JJ, Patterson MC, Papadopoulos NM, Brady RO, Pentchev PG, Barton NW. Hypoprebetalipoproteinemia, acanthocytosis, retinitis pigmentosa, and pallidal degeneration (HARP syndrome). *Neurology* 1992;42:194–198.

221. Malandrini A, Cesaretti S, Mulinari M, et al. Acanthocytosis, retinitis pigmentosa, pallidal degeneration: report of two cases without serum lipid abnormalities. *J Neurol Sci* 1996;140:129–131.

222. Ching KH, Westaway SK, Gitschier J, Higgins JJ, Hayflick SJ. HARP syndrome is allelic with pantothenate kinase-associated neurodegeneration. *Neurology* 2002;58:1673–1674.

223. Muthane U, Chickabasaviah Y, Kaneski C, et al. Clinical features of adult GM1 gangliosidosis: report of three Indian patients and review of 40 cases. *Mov Disord* 2004;19:1334–1341.

224. Yoshida K, Oshima A, Sakuraba H, et al. GM1 gangliosidosis in adults: clinical and molecular analysis of 16 Japanese patients. *Ann Neurol* 1992;31:328–332.

225. Grosso S, Farnetani MA, Berardi R, et al. GM2 gangliosidosis variant B1 neuroradiological findings. *J Neurol* 2003;250:17–21.

226. Meek D, Wolfe LS, Andermann E, Andermann F. Juvenile progressive dystonia: a new phenotype of GM2 gangliosidosis. *Ann Neurol* 1984;15:348–352.

227. Nardocci N, Bertagnolio B, Rumi V, Angelini L. Progressive dystonia symptomatic of juvenile GM2 gangliosidosis. *Mov Disord* 1992;7:64–67.

228. Uc EY, Wenger DA, Jankovic J. Niemann-Pick disease type C: two cases and an update. *Mov Disord* 2000;15:1199–1203.

229. Van de Vlasakker CJ, Gabreels FJ, Wijburg HC, Wevers RA. Clinical features of Niemann-Pick disease type C: an example of the delayed onset, slowly progressive phenotype and an overview of recent literature. *Clin Neurol Neurosurg* 1994;96:119–123.

230. Sturley SL, Patterson MC, Balch W, Liscum L. The pathophysiology and mechanisms of NP-C disease. *Biochim Biophys Acta* 2004;1685:83–87.

231. Chang TY, Reid PC, Sugii S, Ohgami N, Cruz JC, Chang CC. The NIEMANN-pick type C disease and intracellular cholesterol trafficking. *J Biol Chem* 2005;280:20,917–20,920.

232. Chikh K, Vey S, Simonot C, Vanier MT, Millat G. Niemann-Pick type C disease: importance of N-glycosylation sites for function and cellular location of the NPC2 protein. *Mol Genet Metab* 2004;83:220–230.

233. Goebel HH, Wisniewski KE. Current state of clinical and morphological features in human NCL. *Brain Pathol* 2004;14:61–69.

234. Mole SE. The genetic spectrum of human neuronal ceroid-lipofuscinoses. *Brain Pathol* 2004;14:70–76.

235. Aberg L, Liewendahl K, Nikkinen P, Autti T, Rinne JO, Santavuori P. Decreased striatal dopamine transporter density in JNCL patients with parkinsonian symptoms. *Neurology* 2000;54:1069–1074.

236. Lake BD, Steward CG, Oakhill A, Wilson J, Perham TG. Bone marrow transplantation in late infantile Batten disease and juvenile Batten disease. *Neuropediatrics* 1997;28:80–81.

237. Lang AE, Clarke JTR, Rosch L. Progressive longstanding "pure" dystonia: a new phenotype of juvenile metachromatic leukodystrophy. *Neurology* 1985;35(suppl 1):194.

238. Hoffmann GF, Zschocke J. Glutaric aciduria type I: from clinical, biochemical and molecular diversity to successful therapy. *J Inherit Metab Dis* 1999;22:381–391.

239. Hauser SE, Peters H. Glutaric aciduria type 1: an underdiagnosed cause of encephalopathy and dystonia-dyskinesia syndrome in children. *J Paediatr Child Health* 1998;34:302–304.

240. Zafeiriou DI, Zschocke J, Augoustidou-Savvopoulou P, et al. Atypical and variable clinical presentation of glutaric aciduria type I. *Neuropediatrics* 2000;31:303–306.

241. Strauss KA. Glutaric aciduria type 1: a clinician's view of progress. *Brain* 2005;128(pt 4):697–699.

242. Neumaier-Probst E, Harting I, Seitz A, Ding C, Kolker S. Neuroradiological findings in glutaric aciduria type I (glutaryl-CoA dehydrogenase deficiency). *J Inherit Metab Dis* 2004;27:869–876.

243. Kolker S, Koeller DM, Okun JG, Hoffmann GF. Pathomechanisms of neurodegeneration in glutaryl-CoA dehydrogenase deficiency. *Ann Neurol* 2004;55:7–12.

244. Rakocevic G, Lyons KE, Wilkinson SB, Overman JW, Pahwa R. Bilateral pallidotomy for severe dystonia in an 18-month-old child with glutaric aciduria. *Stereotact Funct Neurosurg* 2004;82:80–83.

245. Horster F, Hoffmann GF. Pathophysiology, diagnosis, and treatment of methylmalonic aciduria: recent advances and new challenges. *Pediatr Nephrol* 2004;19:1071–1074.

246. Brenton DP, Pietz J. Adult care in phenylketonuria and hyperphenylalaninaemia: the relevance of neurological abnormalities. *Eur J Pediatr* 2000;159(suppl 2):S114–S120.

247. Paine R. The variability in manifestation of untreated patients with phenylketonuria (phenylpyruvic aciduria). *Pediatrics* 1957;26:290.

248. French JH, Clark DB, Butler HG, Teasdall RD. Phenylketonuria: some observations on reflex activity. *J Pediatr* 1961;58:17–22.

249. Thompson AJ, Smith I, Brenton D, et al. Neurological deterioration in young adults with phenylketonuria. *Lancet* 1990;336:602–605.

250. Evans AH, Costa DC, Gacinovic S, et al. L-dopa-responsive Parkinson's syndrome in association with phenylketonuria: in vivo dopamine transporter and D2 receptor findings. *Mov Disord* 2004;19:1232–1236.

251. Michel U, Schmidt E, Batzler U. Results of psychological testing of patients aged 3–6 years. *Eur J Pediatr* 1990;149(suppl 1):S34–S38.

252. DiMauro S, De Vivo DC. Genetic heterogeneity in Leigh syndrome. *Ann Neurol* 1996;40:5–7.
253. De Vivo DC. Leigh syndrome: historical perspective and clinical variations. *Biofactors* 1998;7:269–271.
254. Longo N. Mitochondrial encephalopathy. *Neurol Clin* 2003;21: 817–831.
255. Zhu Z, Yao J, Johns T, et al. SURF1, encoding a factor involved in the biogenesis of cytochrome c oxidase, is mutated in Leigh syndrome. *Nat Genet* 1998;20:337–343.
256. Macaya A, Munell F, Burke RE, De Vivo DC. Disorders of movement in Leigh syndrome. *Neuropediatrics* 1993;24:60–67.
257. Campistol J, Cusi V, Vernet A, Fernandez-Alvarez E. Dystonia as a presenting sign of subacute necrotising encephalomyelopathy in infancy. *Eur J Pediatr* 1986;144:589–591.
258. Cacic M, Wilichowski E, Mejaski-Bosnjak V, et al. Cytochrome c oxidase partial deficiency-associated Leigh disease presenting as an extrapyramidal syndrome. *J Child Neurol* 2001;16:616–619.
259. Skladal D, Sudmeier C, Konstantopoulou V, et al. The clinical spectrum of mitochondrial disease in 75 pediatric patients. *Clin Pediatr (Phila)* 2003;42:703–710.
260. Barkovich AJ, Good WV, Koch TK, Berg BO. Mitochondrial disorders: analysis of their clinical and imaging characteristics. *AJNR Am J Neuroradiol* 1993;14:1119–1137.
261. Lerman-Sagie T, Leshinsky-Silver E, Watemberg N, Luckman Y, Lev D. White matter involvement in mitochondrial diseases. *Mol Genet Metab* 2005;84:127–136.
262. Jinnah HA, De Gregorio L, Harris JC, Nyhan WL, O'Neill JP. The spectrum of inherited mutations causing HPRT deficiency: 75 new cases and a review of 196 previously reported cases. *Mutat Res* 2000;463:309–326.
263. Christie R, Bay C, Kaufman IA, Bakay B, Borden M, Nyhan WL. Lesch-Nyhan disease: clinical experience with nineteen patients. *Dev Med Child Neurol* 1982;24:293–306.
264. Mizuno T. Long-term follow-up of ten patients with Lesch-Nyhan syndrome. *Neuropediatrics* 1986;17:158–161.
265. Watts RW, Spellacy E, Gibbs DA, Allsop J, McKeran RO, Slavin GE. Clinical, post-mortem, biochemical and therapeutic observations on the Lesch-Nyhan syndrome with particular reference to the Neurological manifestations. *Q J Med* 1982;51:43–78.
266. Jinnah HA, Harris JC, Reich SG, Visser JE, Garabas G, Eddey GE. The motor disorder of Lesch-Nyhan disease. *Mov Disord* 1998;13(suppl 2):98.
267. Jinnah HA, Lewis RF, Visser JE, Eddey GE, Barabas G, Harris JC. Ocular motor dysfunction in Lesch-Nyhan disease. *Pediatr Neurol* 2001;24:200–204.
268. Battini R, Leuzzi V, Carducci C, et al. Creatine depletion in a new case with AGAT deficiency: clinical and genetic study in a large pedigree. *Mol Genet Metab* 2002;77:326–331.
269. Stockler S, Holzbach U, Hanefeld F, et al. Creatine deficiency in the brain: a new, treatable inborn error of metabolism. *Pediatr Res* 1994;36:409–413.
270. Bizzi A, Bugiani M, Salomons GS, et al. X-linked creatine deficiency syndrome: a novel mutation in creatine transporter gene SLC6A8. *Ann Neurol* 2002;52:227–231.
271. Sykut-Cegielska J, Gradowska W, Mercimek-Mahmutoglu S, Stockler-Ipsiroglu S. Biochemical and clinical characteristics of creatine deficiency syndromes. *Acta Biochim Pol* 2004;51:875–882.
272. Leuzzi V, Bianchi MC, Tosetti M, et al. Brain creatine depletion: guanidinoacetate methyltransferase deficiency (improving with creatine supplementation). *Neurology* 2000;55:1407–1409.
273. Ganesan V, Johnson A, Connelly A, Eckhardt S, Surtees RA. Guanidinoacetate methyltransferase deficiency: new clinical features. *Pediatr Neurol* 1997;17:155–157.
274. Schulze A, Ebinger F, Rating D, Mayatepek E. Improving treatment of guanidinoacetate methyltransferase deficiency: reduction of guanidinoacetic acid in body fluids by arginine restriction and ornithine supplementation. *Mol Genet Metab* 2001;74:413–419.
275. Reiss J, Johnson JL. Mutations in the molybdenum cofactor biosynthetic genes MOCS1, MOCS2, and GEPH. *Hum Mutat* 2003;21:569–576.
276. Teksam O, Yurdakok M, Coskun T. Molybdenum cofactor deficiency presenting with severe metabolic acidosis and intracranial hemorrhage. *J Child Neurol* 2005;20:155–157.
277. Johnson JL, Rajagopalan KV, Wadman SK. Human molybdenum cofactor deficiency. *Adv Exp Med Biol* 1993;338:373–378.
278. Graf WD, Oleinik OE, Jack RM, Weiss AH, Johnson JL. Ahomocysteinemia in molybdenum cofactor deficiency. *Neurology* 1998;51:860–862.
279. Boles RG, Ment LR, Meyn MS, Horwich AL, Kratz LE, Rinaldo P. Short-term response to dietary therapy in molybdenum cofactor deficiency. *Ann Neurol* 1993;34:742–744.
280. Remes AM, Filppula SA, Rantala H, et al. A novel mutation of the fumarase gene in a family with autosomal recessive fumarase deficiency. *J Mol Med* 2004;82:550–554.
281. Elpeleg ON, Amir N, Christensen E. Variability of clinical presentation in fumarate hydratase deficiency. *J Pediatr* 1992;121(pt 1): 752–754.
282. Zeman J, Krijt J, Stratilova L, et al. Abnormalities in succinylpurines in fumarase deficiency: possible role in pathogenesis of CNS impairment. *J Inherit Metab Dis* 2000;23:371–374.
283. Gellera C, Uziel G, Rimoldi M, et al. Fumarase deficiency is an autosomal recessive encephalopathy affecting both the mitochondrial and the cytosolic enzymes. *Neurology* 1990;40(pt 1): 495–499.
284. Zinn AB, Kerr DS, Hoppel CL. Fumarase deficiency: a new cause of mitochondrial encephalomyopathy. *N Engl J Med* 1986; 315:469–475.
285. Lyon G, Adams RD, Kolodny EH. *Neurology of hereditary metabolic diseases of children*, 2nd ed. New York: McGraw-Hill, 1996.
286. Kerrigan JF, Aleck KA, Tarby TJ, Bird CR, Heidenreich RA. Fumaric aciduria: clinical and imaging features. *Ann Neurol* 2000;47:583–588.

Rigidity and Spasticity

37

Victor S.C. Fung   Philip D. Thompson

The clinical assessment of muscle tone is an integral part of the neurological evaluation of patients with movement disorders. *Rigidity* and *spasticity* are terms used to describe different patterns of increased resistance to passive joint movements (1). Rigidity implies pathology of the extrapyramidal system, and spasticity implies pathology of upper motoneurons or the corticospinal tracts (2). Increased resistance to passive movement can also arise from dystonia, peripheral nervous system disorders, and increased muscle activity due to failure to relax. Nonneural causes, such as joint stiffness or ankylosis, tendon shortening, and altered passive properties of muscle—for example, muscle shortening due to fibrosis with contracture—also may contribute to a clinical impression of increased muscle tone.

RIGIDITY

Rigidity is a continuous and uniform increase in muscle tone, felt as a smooth resistance throughout the range of passive movement (3). It is usually present in all directions of movement—for example, during both flexion and extension of the wrist and forearm. The relative uniformity of rigidity in all directions has given rise to the term *lead pipe rigidity*. Where there is tremor superimposed on the background increase in tone, a ratchet-like quality of resistance to limb manipulation called *cogwheel rigidity* is felt (1). This is commonly seen in Parkinson's disease (PD), when the cogwheeling has a frequency of 5 to 8 Hz, corresponding to the frequency of postural tremor (4). However, it is not diagnostic and may be encountered in any condition with rigidity and tremor. Incomplete relaxation and background voluntary contraction in patients with a postural or action tremor may also produce cogwheeling.

Rigidity is commonly assessed in the upper limbs at the wrist and elbow, in the neck and trunk, and at the ankle.

The patient is instructed to relax and not resist the passive movements. It is often useful to repeat this instruction during the course of the examination. In the upper limb, most examiners apply quasi-sinusoidal movements of around 0.5–2 cycles per second (5,6). Assessment of rigidity at the neck should be performed with the patient supine. Rigidity of the trunk and proximal muscles can be detected by assessing the ease of rotating the shoulders from side to side with the patient standing and, at the same time, rigidity of the shoulders is assessed by the freedom with which the proximal upper limbs and arms swing during trunk rotation. Rigidity in the legs is often difficult to assess because of the weight of the lower limb. Wartenberg's pendulum test may be useful if there is doubt. With the patient seated on the examination table, the relaxed lower legs are raised to the horizontal in the sagittal plane and then released simultaneously. On the more affected side, the leg can be observed to drop at a slowed but uniform rate when compared with the opposite side (7).

Rigidity can be attenuated with drowsiness or relaxation so that it may be absent or inconsistent at rest, even in advanced PD (8), but it is readily reinforced or activated by proximal voluntary movement of the opposite limb (Froment's maneuver). In basal ganglia (extrapyramidal) disease, rigidity is often more pronounced in proximal and axial muscles. Extensor rigidity of neck muscles is a striking feature of progressive supranuclear palsy (PD), and neck rigidity with anterocollis suggests the diagnosis of multiple system atrophy.

SPASTICITY

The increase in muscle tone in mild-to-moderate spasticity is velocity dependent (9). Hypertonia may be detected only following the application of fast muscle stretches to the affected limb, but it is not detected during slow movements. This characteristic should be sought specifically in the examination. Spasticity is commonly assessed at the elbows, knees, and ankles. At the elbow, fast flexion or extension movements may elicit a sudden increase in tone, whereas resistance to slow, passive movements is normal. There may be a supinator catch if the forearm is suddenly rotated. For the lower limb, the thigh is lifted quickly while the patient is supine, observing whether the heel is lifted from the bed, suggesting increased tone at the knee. Increased resistance to sinusoidal movements at the knee and ankle may be present, although this is often difficult to assess at the knee because of the weight of the lower leg. Wartenberg's pendulum test may demonstrate that the legs drop in a series of excursions with a catch between each movement, and they rotate about an axis instead of falling in a purely sagittal plane. A critical feature of the hypertonia of spasticity is the clasp-knife phenomenon (10,11), which is best seen in the lower limbs. As the knee is flexed from an extended posture, the resistance to passive movement is initially marked but then suddenly gives way. The clasp-knife phenomenon has a directional preponderance, owing to the tendency of spasticity to affect the extensors more that the flexors in the lower limbs, and the flexors more than the extensors in the upper limbs.

The basic clinical characteristics of the hypertonia following lesions of the descending motor pathways at the various sites from the cerebral hemispheres to the spinal cord are similar, with the exception of flexor spasms, which are a prominent feature of spinal lesions. Spasticity is usually accompanied by other signs that together comprise the upper motoneuron syndrome. Perhaps the most important of these is an increase in the tendon jerks, a phenomenon recognized by Charcot (12). Reflex threshold is lowered and irradiation of tendon reflexes throughout a limb or to the contralateral lower limb (as in the crossed adductor reflex) is caused by spread of the vibratory stimulus, transmitted through muscle and bone, recruiting distant reflexes. Other features include altered cutaneous reflexes with a Babinski's or extensor plantar response, loss of superficial abdominal reflexes, spontaneous and stimulus-induced flexor spasms, clonus, and paresis. *Clonus* refers to the repetitive movements of a limb elicited by rapid muscle stretch following a tendon tap or during manipulation of the limb and is caused by reverberating brisk spinal stretch reflexes. Paresis is usually in a pyramidal pattern and particularly affects the extensors in the upper limbs and flexors in the lower limbs. Even in the absence of weakness, there may be loss of the capacity to perform fractionated movements of the digits, evident as a slowness or clumsiness of sequential touching of the fingertips with the thumb, or rapid movements of the distal limb, such as foot tapping.

Spasticity typically evolves in the days and weeks after injury to upper motoneuron pathways. During the interval before the appearance of spasticity, muscle tone is often flaccid with depression of tendon reflexes. The duration of this interval varies according to the level of the lesion. For example, increased tone in the affected limbs may appear a few days after a capsular stroke, while flaccidity may persist after a spinal cord lesion for weeks or even months. The changes responsible for the generation of spasticity are poorly understood. Once spasticity is established, the chronically shortened muscle may develop physical changes, such as shortening and contracture, that further contribute to the muscle stiffness (13).

DIFFERENTIATING RIGIDITY FROM SPASTICITY

Although from the preceding discussion it may appear that differentiating rigidity from spasticity is a straightforward matter, the precise differences in the pathophysiology of *hypertonia* in the two conditions are poorly understood. The examination of tone is rarely undertaken without knowledge of the history, and this often influences the way in which muscle tone is evaluated in an individual. There are a number of other factors that potentially confound the distinction between rigidity and spasticity. Neither rigidity nor spasticity is associated with a single pathological entity. Hypertonia that accompanies cerebral lesions, such as ischemic brain infarction, or spinal lesions, such as cervical cord transection, are both termed *spasticity*, yet cerebral infarcts commonly involve the basal ganglia, which are an integral part of the extrapyramidal system. Conversely, diseases associated with hypertonia that have predominantly extrapyramidal pathology, such as Steele-Richardson-Olszewski syndrome (PSP) (14) or multiple system atrophy (15), may have varying degrees of pyramidal system involvement.

To further complicate the issue, *dystonia* also may be associated with hypertonia. Dystonia was first used by Oppenheim (16) to describe a motor disorder characterized by variable hyper- and hypotonia. Although dystonia is often present only with action in mild or early cases, in more advanced or secondary cases it can be associated with a sustained abnormality of resting posture with increased resistance to passive movement. Dystonia can be a prominent feature of juvenile or early-onset PD, and also advanced PD, especially as the effects of medication wear off (end of dose dystonia) (17). Separation of the rigid and dystonic components of hypertonia in parkinsonism is as much by convention as by science. There are no objective studies that can separate the two, and thus, the boundary between hypertonia in rigidity and dystonia is perhaps even more blurred than that between rigidity and spasticity.

OTHER CAUSES OF HYPERTONIA

Diseases of the frontal lobes and their connections may also produce a particular form of hypertonia. Frontal lobe hypertonia is characterized by increasing opposition and resistance to movement with increasing force of movement, called *gegenhalten* or *paratonia*. The examiner suspects the patient is not fully relaxed, and contrary to instructions to relax, manipulation of the limb leads to a progressive increase in tone. If gegenhalten is marked and there are associated frontal lobe release signs, such as grasp reflexes and mutism, or striatal signs, the distinction between hypertonia of frontal lobe origin and that associated with basal ganglia disease is straightforward. However, if the associated physical signs are minor, this distinction can be difficult. This raises the question of the mechanisms of hypertonia in different diseases whose primary pathologic change lies in the basal ganglia or the frontal lobes or both, as in corticobasal degeneration. It is not known how the mechanisms responsible for hypertonia in each of these situations differ, and in view of the rich interconnections between frontal lobe motor areas and the basal ganglia, there may be some similarities.

Hypertonia also may be seen in patients with disease of the spinal cord in which unrestrained anterior horn cell discharge leads to *alpha-rigidity*. Isolation of the anterior horn cells from normal interneuron inhibitory control is the presumed mechanism. Other signs of spinal cord disease are invariably present. Continuous motor unit activity leading to stiffness of axial muscles, particularly the thoracolumbar paraspinal muscles and muscles of the anterior abdominal wall, present a striking picture in the stiff person syndrome. A robust feature that aids identification of this rare syndrome is the board-like stiffness of the anterior abdominal wall and an exaggerated lumbar lordosis resulting from continuous contraction of the abdominal and paraspinal muscles. Stimulus-sensitive muscle spasms are usually present. Continuous muscle discharges due to peripheral nerve hyperexcitability in Isaacs' syndrome or acquired neuromyotonia causes muscle stiffness mimicking hypertonia. Clues to this include widespread fasciculations, myokymia, absent tendon reflexes, and, in some cases, other signs of a peripheral neuropathy. Finally, primary muscle disease can occasionally limit the range of limb motion, which suggests hypertonia. Myotonia may give rise to the complaint of stiffness during voluntary movement, usually due to delayed muscle relaxation, which may mimic hypertonia, though resistance to passive movement is normal. Rare congenital myopathies or muscular dystrophies with associated muscle contracture or hypertrophy also may limit the range of passive limb movement and be interpreted as hypertonia.

ANATOMICAL CORRELATES OF RIGIDITY AND SPASTICITY

Basal ganglia structures are clearly implicated in the pathophysiology of rigidity, since rigidity is a cardinal feature of nigrostriatal dopamine deficiency in PD. Moreover, rigidity is abolished following surgical lesions of the posteroventral globus pallidus, subthalamic nucleus, or ventrolateral thalamus in patients with PD. However, the changes in the basal ganglia are secondary rather than causal, since the structures named are structurally intact in PD and there are no reports of isolated rigidity following basal ganglia lesions. Bilateral lesions of the lentiform nucleus can cause parkinsonism, but this is rare and dystonia is more common (18). In contrast, unilateral lesions of the substantia nigra can cause typical parkinsonism with rigidity on the contralateral side. Rigidity with minimal other features of parkinsonism can develop in patients with a dopaminergic deficit due to exposure to neuroleptic medication or a metabolic defect in the production of dopamine. Therefore, loss of dopaminergic modulation of basal ganglia function appears to be the underlying basis of rigidity rather than loss of specific neural pathways.

Lesions of descending motor pathways at any level from the cerebral hemispheres to the spinal cord can result in spasticity and the upper motoneuron syndrome. However, there is surprisingly little certainty as to which neural pathways are responsible for generating spasticity. It is worth noting Hughlings Jackson's dictum that following a lesion of the nervous system, the *negative* features, or loss of function, inform us of the function of the structures that have been destroyed, whereas the *positive* abnormalities reflect the function of the structures that remain.

There are two striking and, at first, seemingly contradictory observations about spasticity that arise from lesion analysis:

1. *Spasticity does not develop following lesions restricted to the primary motor cortex or lesions of the corticospinal (pyramidal) tracts at the level of the medulla, but it does develop with combined lesions of the primary and premotor cortex or lesions of the corticospinal projections above the level of the medulla.* In subhuman primates, selective damage to area 4, the origin of a significant portion of the pyramidal tract, results in a contralateral flaccid paralysis, greatest in distal and least in proximal muscle groups (19). With the passage of time, strength is recovered, though it does not return to normal and fractionated movements of the digits remain significantly impaired. Increased muscle tone is not a prominent feature. Cortical lesions that involve the premotor cortex, area 6 anterior to area 4, result in impaired postural control of the contralateral limbs. Spasticity and paresis develop with combined lesions of areas 4 and 6. Whether these observations can be applied to humans has been the subject of debate over many years. The effect of selective lesions has rarely been reported in humans. Hemisphere lesions involving the corona radiata or internal capsule producing hemiplegia probably interrupt projections from both area 4 and area 6, since

descending motor pathways lie in close proximity at these sites. Flaccid paresis with loss of skilled and dexterous finger movements has been described after pure lesions of the medullary pyramid (20) or selective lesions of the spinal cord (21), apparently without major changes in muscle tone.

2. *Spasticity develops below the level of a spinal cord lesion.* These findings can be reconciled as follows: The first observation suggests that loss of the corticomotoneuronal projection to the spinal cord does not lead to the development of spasticity. Instead, loss of motor and premotor cortical input to the brainstem does lead to spasticity. The second observation—that loss of all descending inputs below the level of a spinal lesion also produces spasticity—suggests that spinal projections from these brainstem structures serve to inhibit the development of spasticity. It follows that innervation from the motor and premotor cortex facilitates activity in brainstem structures from which descending (for example, reticulospinal) motor pathways project to the spinal cord maintain normal tone. Thus, spasticity can also result from loss of this facilitation—for example, following interruption of cortical-brainstem pathways.

The typical flexed-limb posture after an upper motoneuron lesion is thought to reflect increased tone in flexor muscle groups and weakness of extensor muscles, although the latter has been questioned (22). This pattern of muscle activity does not appear to depend on reflexes driven by afferent feedback from sensory receptors in the affected limb, since dorsal root section has no effect on limb posture in the monkey (23). Voluntary mass movements of hemiplegic limbs and reflex mass movements—for example, yawning—indicate that descending inputs from brainstem motor centers gain access to spinal motoneurons in upper motoneuron lesions. The origin of these inputs is not known. Residual corticospinal fibers and vestibulospinal (24) and reticulospinal (25) pathways are all capable of influencing the posture and degree of spasticity of hemiplegic limbs.

PHYSIOLOGICAL CORRELATES OF RIGIDITY

There have been many studies of reflex activity in patients with rigidity. Many differ from the clinical assessment of rigidity in one or both of two crucial factors. First, rigidity is elicited by the application of relatively large, amplitude muscle stretches. Second, rigidity is assessed with the patient adopting a specific motor set, that of attempted relaxation of the limb or joint that is being manipulated. The relevance to the clinical phenomenon of rigidity of any abnormal reflex activity that is elicited under differing conditions must be questioned. With this caveat in mind, the physiology of rigidity will be reviewed.

The Reflex Origin of Parkinsonian Rigidity

Rigidity can be abolished by dorsal root section (26) and by the intramuscular injection of nonparalytic doses of local anesthetic (27). These studies provide strong evidence that rigidity is of reflex origin, with the afferent limb originating in muscle.

Tonic Stretch Reflex Activity

During passive movements of the wrist or elbow, patients with parkinsonian rigidity develop muscle bursting at the frequency of the perturbation rather than rigidity being due to unmodulated tonic muscle contraction (5,28). The timing of this bursting varies from subject to subject, but it is primarily the stretch-related activity that is responsible for rigidity (29). Enhanced tonic stretch reflex activity has also been noted following linear stretches (30,31).

Phasic Stretch Reflexes

The monosynaptic stretch reflex is not responsible for parkinsonian rigidity. Charcot (12) recognized that the tendon jerks are normal in PD. He wrote of the "essential distinction between rigidity and pyramidal or spinal hypertonicity—the absence of reflex accentuation in rigidity" (12). This dictum has subsequently been confirmed with quantitative studies (32,33). H reflexes also have generally been reported as being normal in PD.

Lee and Tatton (34,35) were the first to report enhanced long-latency stretch reflexes in parkinsonian patients, and they suggested this abnormality might correlate with rigidity. Although these studies did not control for background levels of muscle contraction, Tatton et al. (36) later showed that heightened reflex responsiveness could not be attributed merely to inadequate relaxation or increased supraspinal drive to α-motoneurons. However, the constancy of the relationship between long-latency stretch reflexes and rigidity has been questioned by a number of investigators (37,38,39,40).

One factor that rarely has been taken into account when interpreting studies of long-latency stretch reflexes in PD is that most recent studies have controlled for background EMG activity by asking subjects to maintain a low-level tonic contraction. As noted, clinical rigidity is tested with the subject attempting to relax the limb during passive movement. In normal subjects, long-latency stretch reflexes are modulated by alterations in motor set (41,42), and such modulation can be abnormal in PD (43). Therefore, the lack of a consistent correlation between long-latency stretch reflex amplitude and rigidity may be due merely to a failure to measure the two under comparable conditions.

Segmental and Supraspinal Influences

The tonic vibration reflex (TVR) is qualitatively normal in PD (44), although when the torque generated by this reflex is compared with controls, it is higher in patients and correlates with the degree of rigidity (33). However, it is unlikely to account for clinical rigidity, as the TVR is reduced following treatment with levodopa, even if rigidity persists (33). Inhibition of the H reflex by the TVR is normal in PD (45).

There are a number of segmental and supraspinal pathways that influence the excitability of the motoneurons pool. These can be studied by examining their effect on the amplitude of the H reflex. Following paired stimuli, the amplitude of the second H reflex varies in a characteristic fashion, showing periods of relative inhibition and excitation that depend on the interstimulus interval. In PD, the period of late facilitation is increased (46). Recurrent Renshaw inhibition is normal (47,48), but reciprocal Ia inhibition is increased, at least in the lower limbs (49,50).

Reflexes mediated by large-diameter afferents are not the only spinal pathways altered in PD. Following non-nociceptive cutaneous stimulation, both excitatory modulation and inhibitory modulation of tonic EMG activity in nearby muscles are observed (51). The first period of inhibition (I1), which is probably modulated at a spinal level, has been reported as being less marked in PD (52), although this has been disputed (53). It has subsequently been shown that I1 can be enhanced by the administration of apomorphine, which is a direct dopamine agonist (54).

One of the few reflex abnormalities demonstrated to correlate positively with parkinsonian rigidity is loss of short-latency autogenic Ib inhibition of the soleus H reflex (55). Corticospinal (56) and rubrospinal (57) projections augment Ib inhibition. However, the dorsal and noradrenergic reticulospinal tracts give rise to inhibitory inputs to Ib interneurons (55). Based on their findings and reports of increased Ia reciprocal inhibition in PD (49,50), Delwaide et al. (55) proposed that overactivity in the nucleus gigantocellularis of the dorsal reticulospinal system is responsible for rigidity in PD. This is consistent with previous suggestions that the Ib inhibitory system is concerned with the relation between muscle length and tension and, therefore, the control of muscle stiffness (58). Interestingly, inhibition in tonic activation of extensor digitorum communis by transcutaneous stimulation of Golgi tendon organ afferents is also less pronounced in PD (59), although the difference between patients and controls was more marked in patients with tremor than with rigidity. More recently, heteronymous group II excitation of quadriceps motoneurons as evidenced by facilitation of the quadriceps H reflex after peroneal nerve stimulation has been shown to be associated with asymmetrical lower-limb

rigidity in de novo patients with PD (60). However, patients with symmetrical lower-limb rigidity did not demonstrate this abnormality.

Finally, it has also been shown that α-motoneuron and possibly cortical excitability is enhanced in PD as tested by measuring resting cortical thresholds to transcranial magnetic stimulation, the duration of the cortical silent period, and F wave excitability (61). Each of these measures was found to correlate with clinical assessments of rigidity.

Voluntary Relaxation and Rigidity

Landau et al. (62) were the first to suggest that the primary abnormality in parkinsonian rigidity was "a continuous, excessive net excitatory drive to the final common path—a physiologically normal spinal cord," which challenged the popular belief of the time that there was a fundamental abnormality in gamma drive. This hypothesis was thought to be confirmed a decade later, when Burke et al. (63) reported that direct recordings of human spindle afferents in parkinsonian and incompletely relaxed, normal subjects showed similar characteristics. This led to the suggestion that "the most important cause of rigidity in PD is excessive and uncontrollable supraspinal drive to α-motoneurons, evident in the patient's inability to relax" (64). This hypothesis is further supported by the report of a correlation between clinical assessments of upper-limb rigidity and the amount of surface EMG activity recorded during attempted voluntary relaxation of an intrinsic hand muscle (65).

It is unlikely, however, that stretch reflex abnormalities in PD are entirely due to inadequate voluntary relaxation. Noth et al. (66) have shown that the short-latency stretch reflex recorded from the first dorsal interosseous muscle is attenuated following small stretches, but not when elicited by direct nerve stimulation in parkinsonian subjects when compared with controls. This was interpreted as consistent with enhanced static fusimotor drive in the patient group. Tatton et al. (36) demonstrated that long-latency stretch reflexes are enhanced in parkinsonian patients even when background levels of EMG activity and stretch velocity are matched with controls. These studies leave open the question of whether such changes are responsible for parkinsonian rigidity.

Shortening Reactions

Patients with PD can have a pronounced shortening reaction: the Westphal phenomenon. This is appreciated best in the biceps of the arm and tibialis anterior of the leg. Passive shortening of the muscle leads to muscle contraction at latencies consistent with a reflex. This behavior is the opposite of a stretch reflex. The mechanism and significance of the shortening reaction are not known. The presence of the shortening reaction does not correlate with changes in muscle tone (67).

Altered Passive Properties of Muscle

Two studies have purported to show evidence of increased nonneural stiffness in parkinsonian patients, possibly as a result of altered passive properties of muscle. Dietz et al. (13) found that during the swing phase of gait, EMG activity in the tibialis anterior was greater in parkinsonian patients as compared with controls, although similar angles of ankle dorsiflexion were present in the two groups. No evidence was found for increased cocontraction, alterations in joint properties, or the EMG-force relationship, and the authors concluded that increased EMG activity was necessary to overcome increased nonneural stiffness in the triceps surae muscles. No attempt was made to correlate these changes with clinical measures of ankle rigidity. Watts et al. (68) measured nonneural elastic stiffness at the elbow using an objective technique that eliminated coexistent EMG activity and found that it was increased in PD. However, no clear quantitative association with rigidity was demonstrated. These data suggest that PD can result in increased non-neural joint stiffness, possible due to altered passive properties of muscle, but the contribution of these changes to clinical measures of rigidity remain uncertain.

PHYSIOLOGICAL CORRELATES OF SPASTICITY

The Reflex Origin of Spasticity

Like parkinsonian rigidity, spasticity also can be abolished by dorsal root section (26) and intramuscular injection of local anesthetic (31). These studies provide strong evidence that spasticity is also of reflex origin, with the afferent limb originating in muscle. At the doses of local anesthetic that are required to abolish hypertonia, muscle strength is preserved or occasionally augmented, although exceptions may occur (31).

Enhanced Stretch Reflex Activity

A widely, although not universally, accepted definition of spasticity is that of "a motor disorder characterized by a velocity-dependent increase in tonic stretch reflexes (muscle tone') with exaggerated tendon jerks, resulting from hyperexcitability of the stretch reflex as one component of the upper motoneuron syndrome" (69).

Whereas rigidity is usually assessed with continuous sinusoidal stretches, spasticity is often assessed with a series of sudden, single movements corresponding to linear stretches. Short-latency reflex activity is elicited at much lower displacement velocities in spastic muscles than in normal muscles (70). This corresponds to the exaggerated tendon jerks. However, the critical abnormality that corresponds to spastic hypertonus is sustained stretch reflex activity following linear stretches. This sustained

reflex activity, which does not occur in normal subjects, persists as long as the muscle is undergoing an increase in length, ceases upon termination of movement even if the muscle is maintained in the lengthened state, and increases linearly with the velocity of stretch (10,71). Similar stretch reflex abnormalities have been reported in patients with both spasticity of predominantly cerebral (71) and spinal (10) origin. The ease with which this late muscle activity is elicited increases in the first month of spasticity; following that, the threshold remains stable, then declines after a year (71). These observations led Thilmann et al. (71) to conclude that the increase in muscle tone of spasticity was the result of enhanced stretch reflexes that reached a stable threshold about a month after the onset of spasticity. It is still debated whether such enhanced tonic stretch reflex activity arises from pathological increases in reflex gain or, alternatively, facilitation of normal reflex activity by involuntary increases in background muscle contraction in spastic limbs (see reference 72). The sustained late-onset stretch reflex activity in spasticity presumably arises from disinhibited segmental spinal pathways, since transcortical long-latency stretch reflexes can be abolished following lesions of the cortical and subcortical motor tracts that are associated with spasticity, as well as following lesions of the dorsal columns in the spinal cord.

Spinal and Segmental Reflex Behavior in Spasticity

At the level of the spinal cord, a number of alterations in reflex behavior have been described, some of which differ between spasticity of cerebral versus spinal origin. Subtle neurophysiologic changes in the excitability of motoneurons, interneuronal connections, and specific local reflex pathways have been demonstrated, though none can be held primarily responsible for the signs of spasticity. Many of these phenomena are secondary to changes in the descending control of the spinal circuits. These are discussed briefly in the following.

1. *α-Motoneuron excitability.* Enhanced H:M ratios (73) and F-wave amplitudes (74) suggest enhanced excitability of α-motoneurons. These changes most likely reflect changes in descending control of segmental spinal networks as the result of the lesion upstream from the motoneurons. It also has been reported that heteronymous group II excitation of quadriceps motoneurons, as evidenced by facilitation of the quadriceps H reflex after peroneal nerve stimulation, is also enhanced in spastic limbs, although this did not correlate with clinical assessment of the severity of spasticity (75).
2. *γ-Motoneuron excitability.* Fusimotor neurons innervate intrafusal muscle fibers and control primary spindle sensitivity. Hyperactivity of the fusimotor system increases spindle sensitivity to stretch, augmenting the Ia afferent response to stretch, and exaggerates

the stretch reflex. This may contribute to decerebrate rigidity in the cat, but there is no evidence that this is the case in humans. Local anesthesia injections into spastic muscles in humans can diminish spasticity by an effect on γ-motoneurons. This effect can be explained by reducing activity in the stretch reflex pathway without invoking a primary role in the mechanism of spasticity. Muscle spindle sensitivity is not enhanced in human spasticity, as judged by recordings from Ia spindle afferents (76).

3. *Recurrent inhibition.* Recurrent collateral axons from motoneurons activate Renshaw cells, which inhibit α-motoneurons. Renshaw cells receive inputs from descending motor pathways and are, therefore, subject to supraspinal control. Renshaw cell activity is not significantly reduced at rest in patients with cerebral spasticity (77) but may be increased in spinal spasticity (78).

4. *Reciprocal inhibition.* Reciprocal inhibition between agonist and antagonist muscles is mediated by the Ia inhibitory interneuron. Ia afferents make monosynaptic connections with homonymous motoneurons and project via the Ia inhibitory interneuron to antagonist muscles. The Ia inhibitory interneuron also receives synaptic input from descending pathways and other afferents. Altered activity in Ia inhibitory interneuronal pathways has been shown in upper motoneuron lesions and spasticity (79,80). Loss of Ia inhibitory reciprocal inhibition may interfere with voluntary activation of an agonist muscle by allowing the antagonist to develop a stretch reflex during agonist contraction that opposes the agonist effect. These effects are most likely to be evident during movement rather than influencing resting muscle tone. Again, such changes are most likely secondary to alterations in descending control of spinal interneurons.

5. *Presynaptic inhibition.* Inhibitory effects on α-motoneurons also are derived from inhibitory interneurons acting on primary afferent terminals of the α-motoneurons. Vibration-induced inhibition of the tendon reflex is one example of presynaptic inhibition of Ia synapses onto motoneurons. Interneurons mediating presynaptic inhibition also are influenced by descending motor projections. Accordingly, alterations in the balance of this descending control may change spinal neuron behavior. Presynaptic inhibition has been reported as being reduced in spasticity of spinal origin but preserved in spasticity of cerebral origin (81).

6. *Plasticity within the central nervous system.* A new consideration in mechanisms of spasticity is the role of axonal sprouting and the formation of new synapses. Previously, regeneration was not thought to occur within the central nervous system, and this is still the subject of debate. Nevertheless, the formation of new synapses and aberrant connections among motoneurons and interneurons is another theoretic explanation for some of the events in spasticity.

Clonus

Clonus, a common sign in spasticity, may be detected in any muscle group. It manifests as repetitive contraction and relaxation of an agonist–antagonist muscle pair. Electromyographic recordings show alternating contraction of muscle pairs. Clonus frequency varies inversely with reflex path length from the spinal cord, consistent with re-excitation within a peripheral reflex loop (82). Stretch of one muscle leads to an exaggerated reflex contraction, which in turn stretches the antagonist muscle, eliciting a further reflex contraction. Other authors have argued for oscillation within a central pacemaker, since the rhythm of clonus may be difficult to entrain and the frequency of clonus may be similar at different sites (83). This may explain why some patients with ankle clonus demonstrate synchronous rather than alternating bursts in the lower-limb antagonists (personal observation).

The Clasp-Knife Phenomenon

In human spasticity, the gradual increase in muscle tone with stretch of the knee extensor followed by an abrupt decline in resistance is called the *clasp-knife phenomenon.* Explanations for this reflex increase in muscle tone and its sudden abolition include activation of the Golgi tendon organ and autogenic inhibition of extensor motoneurons from group Ib afferents (10) and excitation of other muscle receptors and flexor reflex afferents. Nonspindle group II and III afferents from free endings in muscle also inhibit extensor muscles and facilitate flexor muscles in spasticity. Flexor reflex afferents exhibit similar effects. The spinal interneurons mediating these effects are subject to descending inhibitory input, particularly from dorsal reticulospinal tracts. Lesions of these descending reticulospinal pathways enhance these reflex effects and are, therefore, considered an important factor in spasticity.

Flexor Spasms

One of the most dramatic manifestations of spasticity is flexor spasms of the legs and trunk after spinal cord injury. Bilateral interruption of the corticospinal and dorsal reticulospinal projections releases activity in flexor reflex afferent systems. Various "natural" stimuli, ranging from cutaneous to bladder afferents, also engage the flexor reflex system to produce uninhibited activity in flexor muscles.

Babinski's Reflex and Flexor Reflexes

Babinski's reflex—extension of the great toe after stimulation of the sole of the foot—is one of the best known signs of an upper motoneuron lesion. Stimulation of the outer plantar surface of the foot evokes extension of the great toe (the extensor plantar response), fanning of the lateral toes, variable dorsiflexion of the ankle, and flexion of the hip and knee. It is closely related to impairment of foot movement and, therefore, to interruption of corticospinal projections to motoneurons innervating muscles of the distal leg and foot (84). The relation of the extensor plantar response to the triple flexion or withdrawal response of the leg has been the subject of much interest over the years. Walshe (85) emphasized that Babinski's reflex was one component of the flexion withdrawal response. Extension of the great toe was always accompanied by contraction of the proximal flexors of the leg and, in some cases, contraction of extensors of the contralateral leg: the crossed extensor response. This complex synergy added weight to the notion that Babinski's reflex was one part of a flexion withdrawal response of the lower limb in response to a noxious stimulus. In a study van Gijn (84) also noted that flexor reflex activity frequently accompanied Babinski's reflex, though this was not necessarily increased.

Nonneural Stiffness in Spasticity

The notion that hypertonia in spasticity is due predominantly to enhanced reflex activity has been challenged. Reduced ankle dorsiflexion was observed during walking in patients with lower-limb spasticity, despite enhanced activity in the ankle dorsiflexors and in the absence of co-contraction in antagonist muscles (13). Hypertonia at the elbow measured with mechanically driven, passive, low-amplitude sinusoidal movements was not found to correlate with stretch reflex activity in the biceps, but rather with the degree of contracture (86). There are increasing reports of structural alterations in the muscles of spastic limbs (see reference 87 for review). These observations have led to the suggestion that a significant contribution to hypertonia in spasticity arises from alterations in the intrinsic properties of muscle.

Treatment

A variety of strategies are available to reduce the muscle tone of spasticity and to lessen flexor spasms in patients who have upper motoneuron lesions. An important initial consideration is the indication for treatment and the expectations from such treatment. For example, loss of manual dexterity or weakness is not improved by treatments that reduce muscle tone. In a patient who can walk, a reduction of leg muscle tone may be detrimental to mobility if tone compensates for leg weakness and allows the patient to stand. Accordingly, the treatment of spasticity may not lead to an improvement in function. Physiotherapy is useful in maintaining limb mobility and preventing muscle contracture, in addition to maximizing functional capacity from residual movement. In patients with spinal cord lesions, management of cutaneous or bladder infections, maintenance of bladder function, and reduction of noxious stimuli may reduce painful flexor spasms and associated polysynaptic reflex activity.

Pharmacologic approaches entail the use of drugs that interfere with transmission in spinal reflexes and muscle contraction. Baclofen and diazepam increase presynaptic (GABAergic) inhibition of Ia afferents, depressing monosynaptic reflex activity. Baclofen also inhibits polysynaptic reflex activity. Gabapentin has recently been shown to be effective. Tizanidine and clonidine block α_2-adrenergic receptors in excitatory interneuronal pathways. Spasticity also can be lessened by inducing weakness of peripheral muscle by dantrolene, which reduces calcium release from sarcoplasmic reticulum, or injections of botulinum toxin, which create a presynaptic neuromuscular blockade. Good evidence of significant and sustained therapeutic benefit from such interventions is largely lacking (88) and, therefore, treatment should be carefully tailored to individual patients' circumstances.

REFERENCES

1. Holmes G. *Introduction to clinical neurology.* Edinburgh: E & S Livingstone, 1952.
2. Rothwell JC. *Control of human voluntary movement.* London: Chapman and Hall, 1994.
3. Fung VS, Burne JA, Morris JG. Objective quantification of resting and activated parkinsonian rigidity: a comparison of angular impulse and work scores. *Mov Disord* 2000;15:48–55.
4. Lance J, Schwab R, Peterson E. Action tremor and the cogwheel phenomenon in Parkinson's disease. *Brain* 1963;86:95–110.
5. Meara RJ, Cody FW. Relationship between electromyographic activity and clinically assessed rigidity studied at the wrist joint in Parkinson's disease. *Brain* 1992;115:1167–1180.
6. Prochazka A, Bennett DJ, Stephens MJ, et al. Measurement of rigidity in Parkinson's disease. *Mov Disord* 1997;12:24–32.
7. Wartenberg R. *Diagnostic tests in neurology.* Chicago: Year Book Publishers, 1953.
8. Webster DD. Dynamic measurement of rigidity, strength and tremor in Parkinson patients before and after destruction of mesial globus pallidus. *Neurology* 1960;10:157–163.
9. Burke D, Lance JW. Studies of the reflex effects of primary and secondary spindle endings in spasticity. In: Desmedt J, ed. *New developments in electromyography and clinical neurophysiology.* Basel, Switzerland: Karger, 1973:475–495.
10. Burke D, Gillies JD, Lance JW. The quadriceps stretch reflex in human spasticity. *J Neurol Neurosurg Psychiatry* 1970;33:216–223.
11. Lance JW. The control of muscle tone, reflexes, and movement. *Neurology* 1980;30:1303–1313.
12. Charcot JM. *Charcot, the clinician: the Tuesday Lessons.* New York: Raven Press, 1987.
13. Dietz V, Quintern J, Berger W. Electrophysiological studies of gait in spasticity and rigidity: evidence that altered mechanical properties of muscle contribute to hypertonia. *Brain* 1981;104:431–449.
14. Steele J, Richardson J, Olszewski J. Progressive supranuclear palsy. *Arch Neurol* 1964;10:333–359.
15. Wenning GK, Ben Shlomo Y, Magalhaes M, Daniel SE, Quinn NP. Clinical features and natural history of multiple system atrophy: an analysis of 100 cases. *Brain* 1994;117:835–845.
16. Oppenheim H. Uber eine eigenartige Krampfkrankheit des kindlichen und jugendlichen Alters (Dysbasia lordotica progressiva, Dystonia musculorum deformans). *Neurologie Centralblatt* 1911;30:1090–1107.
17. Marsden CD. Parkinson's disease. *J Neurol Neurosurg Psychiatry* 1994;57:672–681.
18. Bhatia KP, Marsden CD. The behavioural and motor consequences of focal lesions of the basal ganglia in man. *Brain* 1994;117(pt4):859–876.
19. Tower S. Pyramidal lesions in the monkey. *Brain* 1940;63:36–90.
20. Chokroverty S, Rubino FA, Haller C. Pure motor hemiplegia due to pyramidal infarction. *Arch Neurol* 1975;32:647–648.

21. Nathan PW. Effects on movement of surgical incisions into the human spinal cord. *Brain* 1994;117:337–346.

22. Colebatch JG, Gandevia SC. The distribution of muscular weakness in upper motor neuron lesions affecting the arm. *Brain* 1989;112:749–763.

23. Denny-Brown D. *The cerebral control of movement.* Liverpool: Liverpool University Press; 1966:142–143.

24. Walshe FMR. On the variations in the form of reflex movements, notably the Babinski plantar response, under different degrees of spasticity and under the influence of the Magnus an de Kleijn's tonic neck reflex. *Brain* 1923;46:281–300.

25. Burke D, Knowles L, Andrews C, Ashby P. Spasticity, decerebrate rigidity and the clasp-knife phenomenon: an experimental study in the cat. *Brain* 1972;95:31–48.

26. Foerster O. Analyse und Pathophysiologie der striaren Bewegungsstorungen. *Z Ges Neurol Psychiat* 1921;73:1–169.

27. Walshe FMR. Observations on the nature of the muscular rigidity of paralysis agitans and its relationship to tremor. *Brain* 1924;47:159–177.

28. Meyer M, Adorjani C. Quantification of the effects of muscle relaxant drugs in man by tonic stretch reflex. *Adv Neurol* 1983;39:997–1011.

29. Fung VS, Burne JA, Morris JG. Objective measurement of Parkinsonian rigidity II: Relationship with simultaneously acquired EMG activity. *Mov Disord* 13(suppl):1998.

30. Andrews CJ, Burke D, Lance JW. The response to muscle stretch and shortening in Parkinsonian rigidity. *Brain* 1972;95:795–812.

31. Rushworth G. Spasticity and rigidity: an experimental study and review. *J Neurol Neurosurg Psychiatry* 1960;23:99–118.

32. Dietrichson P. Phasic ankle reflex in spasticity and parkinsonian rigidity: the role of the fusimotor system. *Acta Neurol Scand* 1971;47:22–51.

33. McLellan DL. Dynamic spindle reflexes and the rigidity of Parkinsonism. *J Neurol Neurosurg Psychiatry* 1973;36:342–349.

34. Tatton WG, Lee RG. Evidence for abnormal long-loop reflexes in rigid Parkinsonian patients. *Brain Res* 1975;100:671–676.

35. Lee RG, Tatton WG. Motor responses to sudden limb displacements in primates with specific CNS lesions and in human patients with motor system disorders. *Can J Neurol Sci* 1975;2:285–293.

36. Tatton WG, Bedingham W, Verrier MC, Blair RD. Characteristic alterations in responses to imposed wrist displacements in parkinsonian rigidity and dystonia musculorum deformans. *Can J Neurol Sci* 1984;11:281–287.

37. Cody FW, MacDermott N, Matthews PB, Richardson HC. Observations on the genesis of the stretch reflex in Parkinson's disease. *Brain* 1986;109:229–249.

38. Marsden CD, Merton PA, Morton HB, Adam JER, Hallett M. Automatic and voluntary responses to muscle stretch in man. In: Desmedt JE, ed. *Cerebral motor control in man: long loop mechanisms.* Basel, Switzerland: Karger, 1978:334–341.

39. Meara RJ, Cody FW. Stretch reflexes of individual parkinsonian patients studied during changes in clinical rigidity following medication. *Electroencephalogr Clin Neurophysiol* 1993;89:261–268.

40. Rothwell JC, Obeso JA, Traub MM, Marsden CD. The behaviour of the long-latency stretch reflex in patients with Parkinson's disease. *J Neurol Neurosurg Psychiatry* 1983;46:35–44.

41. Bonnet M, Requin J, Stelmach GE. Changes in electromyographic responses to muscle stretch related to the programming of movement parameters. *Electroencephalogr Clin Neurophysiol* 1991;81:135–151.

42. Dietz V, Discher M, Trippel M. Task-dependent modulation of short- and long-latency electromyographic responses in upper limb muscles. *Electroencephalogr Clin Neurophysiol* 1994;93:49–56.

43. Johnson MT, Kipnis AN, Lee MC, Loewenson RB, Ebner TJ. Modulation of the stretch reflex during volitional sinusoidal tracking in Parkinson's disease. *Brain* 1991;114:443–460.

44. Lance JW, De Gail P, Neilson PD. Tonic and phasic spinal cord mechanisms in man. *J Neurol Neurosurg Psychiatry* 1966;29:535–544.

45. Delwaide P, Gonce M. Pathophysiology of Parkinson's signs. In: Jankovic J, Tolosa E, eds. *Parkinson's disease and movement disorders.* Baltimore, MD: Williams and Wilkins, 1993:77–92.

46. Sax DS, Johnson TL, Cooper IS. Reflex activity in extrapyramidal disorders. *Adv Neurol* 1976;14:285–296.

47. Delwaide PJ, Schoenen J. Clinical neurophysiology in the evaluation and physiopathology of Parkinson's disease. *Rev Neurol (Paris)* 1985;141:759–773.

48. Lelli S, Panizza M, Hallett M. Spinal cord inhibitory mechanisms in Parkinson's disease. *Neurology* 1991;41:553–556.

49. Bathien N, Rondot P. Reciprocal continuous inhibition in rigidity of Parkinsonism. *J Neurol Neurosurg Psychiatry* 1977;40:20–24.

50. Day BL, Marsden CD, Obeso JA, Rothwell JC. Peripheral and central mechanisms of reciprocal inhibition in the human forearm. *J Physiol (Lond)* 1981;317:59–60.

51. Caccia MR, McComas AJ, Upton AR, Blogg T. Cutaneous reflexes in small muscles of the hand. *J Neurol Neurosurg Psychiatry* 1973;36:960–967.

52. Fuhr P, Zeffiro T, Hallett M. Cutaneous reflexes in Parkinson's disease. *Muscle Nerve* 1992;15:733–739.

53. Chen R, Ashby P, Lang AE. Stimulus-sensitive myoclonus in akinetic-rigid syndromes. *Brain* 1992;115:1875–1888.

54. Clouston PD, Lim CL, Sue C, Morris JGL, Yiannikas C. Apomorphine can increase cutaneous inhibition of motor activity in Parkinson's disease. *Electroencephalog Clin Neurophysiol* 1996;101:8–15.

55. Delwaide PJ, Pepin JL, Maertens de Noordhout A. Short-latency autogenic inhibition in patients with Parkinsonian rigidity. *Ann Neurol* 1991;30:83–89.

56. Illert M, Lundberg A, Tanaka R. Integration in descending motor pathways controlling the forelimb in the cat. 2. Convergence on neurones mediating disynaptic cortico-motoneuronal excitation. *Exp Brain Res* 1976;26:521–540.

57. Hongo T, Jankowska E, Lundberg A. The rubrospinal tract. II. Facilitation of interneuronal transmission in reflex paths to motoneurones. *Exp Brain Res* 1969;7:365–391.

58. Houk J, Rymer WZ. Neural control of muscle length and tension. In: Brooks VB, ed. *Handbook of physiology.* Bethesda, MD: American Physiological Society, 1981:257–323.

59. Burne JA, Lippold OC. Loss of tendon organ inhibition in Parkinson's disease. *Brain* 1996;119:1115–1121.

60. Simonetta MM, Meunier S, Vidailhet M, Pol S, Galitzky M, Rascol O. Transmission of group II heteronymous pathways is enhanced in rigid lower limb of de novo patients with Parkinson's disease. *Brain* 2002;125:2125–2133.

61. Cantello R, Gianelli M, Bettucci D, Civardi C, De Angelis MS, Mutani R. Parkinson's disease rigidity: magnetic motor evoked potentials in a small hand muscle. *Neurology* 1991;41:1449–1456.

62. Landau WM, Struppler A, Mehls O. A comparative electromyographic study of the reactions to passive movement in parkinsonism and in normal subjects. *Neurology* 1966;16:34–48.

63. Burke D, Hagbarth KE, Wallin BG. Reflex mechanisms in Parkinsonian rigidity. *Scand J Rehabil Med* 1977;9:15–23.

64. Marsden CD. The mysterious motor function of the basal ganglia: the Robert Wartenberg Lecture. *Neurology* 1982;32:514–539.

65. Cantello R, Gianelli M, Civardi C, Mutani R. Parkinson's disease rigidity: EMG in a small hand muscle at "rest." *Electroencephalogr Clin Neurophysiol* 1995;97:215–222.

66. Noth J, Schurmann M, Podoll K, Schwarz M. Reconsideration of the concept of enhanced static fusimotor drive in rigidity in patients with Parkinson's disease. *Neurosci Lett* 1988;84:239–243.

67. Berardelli A, Hallett M. Shortening reaction of human tibialis anterior. *Neurology* 1984;34:242–245.

68. Watts RL, Wiegner AW, Young RR. Elastic properties of muscles measured at the elbow in man. II. Patients with parkinsonian rigidity. *J Neurol Neurosurg Psychiatry* 1986;49:1177–1181.

69. Lance JW. Symposium synopsis. In: Feldman R, Young RR, Koella W, eds. *Spasticity: disordered motor control.* Chicago: Year Book Medical, 1980:485–494.

70. Thilmann AF, Fellows SJ, Garms E. Pathological stretch reflexes on the "good" side of hemiparetic patients. *J Neurol Neurosurg Psychiatry* 1990;53:208–214.

71. Thilmann AF, Fellows SJ, Garms E. The mechanism of spastic muscle hypertonus. Variation in reflex gain over the time course of spasticity. *Brain* 1991;114:233–244.

72. Burne JA, Carleton VL, O'Dwyer NJ. The spasticity paradox: movement disorder or disorder of resting limbs? *J Neurol Neurosurg Psychiatry* 2005;76:47–54.

73. Angel RW. Muscular contractions elicited by passive shortening. *Adv Neurol* 1983;39:555–563.

74. Eisen A, Odusote K. Amplitude of the F wave: a potential means of documenting spasticity. *Neurology* 1979;29:1306–1309.
75. Marque P, Simonetta-Moreau M, Maupas E, Roques CF. Facilitation of transmission in heteronymous group II pathways in spastic hemiplegic patients. *J Neurol Neurosurg Psychiatry* 2001;70:36–42.
76. Hagbarth KE, Wallin G, Lofstedt L. Muscle spindle responses to stretch in normal and spastic subjects. *Scand J Rehabil Med* 1973;5:156–159.
77. Katz R, Pierrot-Deseilligny E. Recurrent inhibition of alpha-motoneurons in patients with upper motor neuron lesions. *Brain* 1982;105:103–124.
78. Shefner JM, Berman SA, Sarkarati M, Young RR. Recurrent inhibition is increased in patients with spinal cord injury. *Neurology* 1992;42:2162–2168.
79. Nakashima K, Rothwell JC, Day BL, Thompson PD, Shannon K, Marsden CD. Reciprocal inhibition between forearm muscles in patients with writer's cramp and other occupational cramps, symptomatic hemidystonia and hemiparesis due to stroke. *Brain* 1989;112:681–697.
80. Ashby P, Wiens M. Reciprocal inhibition following lesions of the spinal cord in man. *J Physiol* 1989;414:145–157.
81. Faist M, Mazevet D, Dietz V, Pierrot-Deseilligny E. A quantitative assessment of presynaptic inhibition of Ia afferents in spastics: differences in hemiplegics and paraplegics. *Brain* 1994;117:1449–1455.
82. Iansek R. The effects of reflex path length on clonus frequency in spastic muscles. *J Neurol Neurosurg Psychiatry* 1984;47:1122–1124.
83. Walsh EG, Wright GW. Patellar clonus: an autonomous central generator. *J Neurol Neurosurg Psychiatry* 1987;50:1225–1227.
84. Van Gijn J. The Babinski sign and the pyramidal syndrome. *J Neurol Neurosurg Psychiatry* 1978;41:865–873.
85. Walshe FMR. The physiological significance of the reflex phenomena in spastic paralysis of the lower limbs. *Brain* 1914;37:269–336.
86. O'Dwyer NJ, Ada L, Neilson PD. Spasticity and muscle contracture following stroke. *Brain* 1996;119:1737–1749.
87. Lieber RL, Steinman S, Barash IA, Chambers H. Structural and functional changes in spastic skeletal muscle. *Muscle Nerve* 2004;29:615–627.
88. Montane E, Vallano A, Laporte JR. Oral antispastic drugs in non-progressive neurologic diseases: a systematic review. *Neurology* 2004;63:1357–1363.

38

Muscle Cramps, Stiffness, and Myalgia

Yadollah Harati   *Justin Kwan*

Muscle cramps, stiffness, and myalgia are among the most common medical ailments (1,2). Many of the conditions causing these symptoms are benign, self-limited, and unlikely to cause confusion with typical movement disorders. Yet many uncommon disorders can result in postural abnormalities that simulate movement disorders. The main diagnostic confusion may be with the dystonic disorders (see Chapters 25 and 26). Also, the fasciculations or myokymia associated with several of these conditions may cause small-amplitude joint movements superficially resembling segmental myoclonus or choreiform movements. This chapter discusses these disorders in detail and briefly reviews other conditions associated with muscle cramps, stiffness, or myalgia. It focuses on advances that have helped to reveal the causation of specific cramp syndromes and attempts to classify these disorders according to their site of pathogenesis: (a) muscle, (b) motor neurons or peripheral nerves, or (c) central nervous system (CNS). When evaluating patients, applying this classification is useful in distinguishing among the various causes and provides the focus on recognizing specific disorders underlying the symptoms of muscle cramps (3).

MYOGENIC DISORDERS CAUSING MUSCLE CRAMP AND/OR CONTRACTURE

Muscle contraction is a complex process by which an electrical current, carried by the muscle membrane along T tubules, evokes calcium release from sarcoplasmic reticulum with subsequent contractile protein interaction and fiber shortening. This ATP- and calcium-dependent process is disrupted in several disorders with exercise-related cramps or muscle pain. The myopathic conditions causing cramps are listed in Table 38.1. Myogenic causes are often suspected for otherwise unexplained general myalgia. Muscle biopsies in various series have shown abnormalities, although not necessarily diagnostic, in up to 50% of such cases (4). Patients with persistent isolated myalgia and normal neurologic examination are among the most difficult to diagnose, and muscle biopsy has identified a specific muscle disease (polymyositis in 2, McArdle's disease in 2, mitochondrial myopathy in 1) in 5 of 100 patients reported by Pourmand (4).

Although many patients refer to the muscle discomfort caused by myogenic disorders as cramp or muscle ache, some simply have myalgia, and others have cramps, which should be differentiated, in a strict sense, from muscle contracture and myotonia (Table 38.2). The disorders discussed in this section include cramp, contracture, and myotonia.

A typical cramp may be defined as an involuntary, irregular, painful, usually brief and forceful skeletal muscle contraction whose muscle action potentials can be recorded on an electromyogram. Stretching or massaging the affected muscle often brings relief. On the other hand, a true contracture is usually defined as active muscle contraction without electrical activity. Unlike a typical cramp, stretching or massaging the contracted muscle will not relieve the symptoms. There are three types of contractures: antalgic contractures, painful contractures, and painless contractures (5).

Antalgic contracture is a compensating polysynaptic phenomenon lasting days to weeks. Painful contractures include various transient cramps and metabolic contractures. Painless contractures are painless, with fixed

TABLE 38.1

MYOGENIC DISORDERS CAUSING COMPLAINTS OF MUSCLE CRAMP AND PAIN

Disorders resulting from deficient muscle fuel use
  "Muscle cramp" resulting from glycogen metabolism abnormalities
    Myophosphorylase deficiency (type V glycogenosis)[a]
    Phosphofructokinase deficiency (type VII glycogenosis)[a]
    Phosphorylase b kinase deficiency (type VIII glycogenosis)[a]
    Phosphoglycerate kinase deficiency (type IX glycogenosis)[a]
    Muscle phosphoglycerate mutase deficiency (type X glycogenosis)[a]
    Lactate dehydrogenase deficiency (type XI glycogenosis)
  "Muscle cramp" resulting from lipid metabolism abnormalities
    Carnitine palmitoyltransferase II deficiency
  Myalgia resulting from purine nucleotide metabolism
    Myoadenylate deaminase deficiency

Disorders resulting from other muscle dysfunctions
  "Muscle cramp" resulting from dysfunction of sarcoplasmic reticulum
    Brody or Lambert-Brody syndrome
  Myalgia associated with other muscle dysfunctions
    Myalgia associated with tubular aggregates
    Myalgia with abnormal structure or function of mitochondria
    Myalgia with intracellular acidosis
    Myalgia with low myosin ATPase and phosphocreatine content
    Myalgia with type 2 muscle fiber predominance

Myotonic disorders
  Chloride channel diseases
    Myotonia congenita
      Thomsen's disease (autosomal dominant)
      Becker's disease (autosomal recessive)
    Sodium channel diseases
      Paramyotonia congenita (autosomal dominant)
        Normokalemic or hyperkalemic (adynamia episodica, autosomal dominant)
        other sodium channel myotonias
          ■ Acetazolamide-responsive myotonia
          ■ Myotonia fluctuans
          ■ Myotonia permanens
  Calcium channel diseases
    Hypokalemic periodic paralysis (autosomal dominant)
  Nondystrophic myotonias with unknown defect
    Myotonia congenita with painful cramps (autosomal dominant)
  Dystrophic myotonias (autosomal dominant)
    Myotonic dystrophy
    Proximal myotonic myopathy
  Schwartz-Jampel syndrome (autosomal recessive)
  Acquired myotonia
    Drug induced
    Associated with malignancy

[a]Disorders with documented electrically silent contracture.

limitation of joint movement, and include myostatic and myotactic contractures. Myostatic contractures result from prolonged immobility of a muscle, leading to irreversible contractures due to shortening of the sarcomeres. Myotactic contractures are due to hyperexcitable central reflexes, such as spasticity (5). Conditions known to cause such electrically silent contracture are listed in Table 38.1. Myotonia does not involve spontaneous and involuntary muscle contractions; rather, forceful muscle contraction is followed by delayed relaxation (action myotonia) caused by prolonged excitation of the muscle membrane. Myotonia can also be elicited by direct percussion of the muscle (percussion myotonia). Prolonged waxing and waning electrical discharges with gradually declining amplitude and the characteristic "dive bomber's sound" are induced by the insertion and subsequent manipulation of an electromyography needle (electrical myotonia).

TABLE 38.2

CRAMP, CONTRACTURE, AND MYOTONIA

Clinical Findings, Observations	Cramp	Contracture	Myotonia	Dystonia
EMG	Normal action potentials	Silent	Myotonic discharges	Normal action potentials
Duration	Minutes	Seconds to minutes	Seconds	500 ms, sustained
Physical activity at onset of symptoms	Rest (exacerbated by exercise)	Forceful exercise	Forceful exercise, direct muscle percussion	Often action task specific at onset; later occurs at rest
Pain	+	+/−[a]	−	+/−
Warm-up phenomenon	−	−	+	−
Second-wind phenomenon	−	+/−[a]	−	−
Alleviation by muscle massage	+	−	−	−
Effect of focal curare injection	+	−	−	+
Pathophysiology	Neurogenic diseases	Muscle metabolic abnormality	Muscle membrane ion conductance abnormality	Basal ganglia or brainstem dysfunction

[a]Present in glycogen metabolism defects.

+, present; −, absent; +/−, variable.

Disorders of Muscle Fuel Use

Disorders of Glycogen Metabolism

Muscle Phosphorylase Deficiency (McArdle's Disease, Type V Glycogenosis)

McArdle's disease is now considered the most common disorder of muscle carbohydrate metabolism. It was described by McArdle (1951), who correctly postulated that the illness resulted from an enzyme defect along the glycolytic pathway. Eight years later, the deficient enzyme was shown to be a muscle-specific phosphorylase, an enzyme responsible for initiating the breakdown of glycogen (Fig. 38.1) (6,7). This defect causes a deficiency in "energy" production that leads to exercise intolerance secondary to muscle fatigue, stiffness, and pain. Indirect effects of this defect, such as impaired oxidative metabolism (8), sarcolemmal dysfunction with reduced sodium–potassium pump (9), or impaired muscle tissue perfusion with exercise (10), may also contribute to symptoms. Moderate activities are well tolerated, even for long periods, and many affected patients learn their exercise threshold. With vigorous activity, symptoms usually develop within minutes and resolve with rest over minutes to hours. Exercise may involve intensive, brief, isometric contraction (pushing an object or carrying a heavy load) or sustained repetitive use of any muscle group (riding a bicycle, swimming, climbing stairs). Even unsuspected tonic seizure has been described as a provocative factor to trigger rhabdomyolysis and renal failure (11). Any skeletal muscle group can be affected, including the jaw and oropharynx (12). Patients often complain that they cannot fully extend the fingers after sustained gripping movements. Attempts to open the "clawed" fingers may result in increasing pain. This hand posture may superficially resemble that of myotonia or dystonia (Fig. 38.2). Severe spasms of large muscles may be followed by muscle necrosis, myoglobinuria, and renal failure. In most patients,

the performance improves after a warm-up period of nonstrenuous exercise. This "second-wind" phenomenon is attributed to two main factors: mobilization of plasma free fatty acids with the use of amino acids as alternative energy sources and increased blood flow to the exercising muscles, resulting in increased oxidative metabolism (13,14). This increased oxidative capacity, related to increased mobilization and utilization of alternative sources of fuel occurs in McArdle's disease and not in other disorders of glycolytic pathways, such as phosphofructokinase deficiency (Tarui's disease), which lack the ability to mount a second-wind phenomenon (15). When fasting, patients with McArdle's disease often demonstrate improved exercise capacity, a marked fall in creatine kinase (CK), and low serum free fatty acids at the end of the fast (16), again suggesting increased dependence on free fatty acids.

The biochemical basis of electrically silent muscle contractures in McArdle's disease and related glycolytic disorders is not understood. Logically, the unavailability of glycogen for anaerobic work should rapidly deplete adenosine triphosphate (ATP) stores in actively contracting muscles. Low ATP levels should in turn retard ATP-dependent calcium uptake by the sarcoplasmic reticulum, and the muscle should, therefore, shorten. However, neither biochemical studies of muscle biopsies (17) nor in vivo 31P-nuclear magnetic resonance (NMR) spectroscopy (18,19) has shown any drop of ATP levels in whole muscle. Whether ATP reduction affects only a specific subcellular component or involves a relatively small percentage of muscle fibers is not known. Other than limiting energy-dependent calcium uptake, increased sarcoplasmic calcium may result from an impaired sarcoplasmic reticulum calcium transport system. It has been hypothesized that such damage is mediated by the products of lipid peroxidation produced by increased reliance on fatty acid oxidation in this disorder (20).

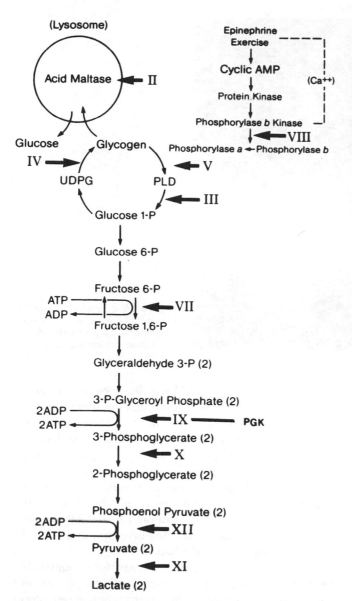

Figure 38.1 Glycogen metabolism and glycolysis. *Arrows,* enzyme defects that produce disease in the human; **II**, acid maltase; **III**, debranching enzyme; **IV**, branching enzyme; **V**, phosphorylase; **VII**, phosphofructokinase; **VIII**, phosphorylase *b* kinase; **IX**, phosphoglycerate kinase; **X**, phosphoglycerate mutase; **XI**, lactate dehydrogenase, and **XII**, β-enolase. *UDPG,* uridine diphosphate glucose; *PLD,* phosphorylase limit dextrin. (Courtesy Dr. S. DiMauro, College of Physicians and Surgeons, Columbia University, New York, NY.)

Most McArdle's disease patients have normal neurologic examinations between attacks. Thus, their complaints of effort intolerance and cramps may be considered psychogenic or indicative of malingering. A history of elevated CK levels or myoglobinuria ("Coca-Cola urine") distinguishes most cases. Forced exercise can precipitate severe myoglobinuria and renal failure. About one-third of patients develop a mild and permanent myopathy with weakness, rarely asymmetric (21), and atrophy as a late consequence of recurrent attacks (22).

McArdle's disease most commonly begins during the second decade of life, although milder unrecognized symptoms of easy fatigability without cramp or myalgia typically occur during childhood. Rarely do severe symptoms of cramps and myoglobinuria begin in childhood (23). Atypical presentations (22,24) include (a) mild forms with exercise induced fatigue; (b) fatal infantile form (25); (c) mild congenital myopathy in childhood (26); and (d) late-onset (fifth decade or later) of typical syndrome or pure myopathy (27,28). Patients with McArdle's disease, as well as patients with phosphofructokinase (PFK) deficiency, may have myogenic hyperuricemia (29).

The best-substantiated mode of inheritance is autosomal recessive. Reports of autosomal dominant inheritance (30) have yet to be supported by biochemical data. Heterozygotes demonstrate a partial decrease in enzyme activity (31) and are usually asymptomatic, although they may show a propensity to "cramp," especially during forearm exercise tests (32). Rarely, heterozygotes manifest overt symptoms when their enzyme activity falls below a critical threshold (33,34). This may explain the occasional reports of "autosomal dominant" inheritance as it may be a pseudoautosomal dominant inheritance. Male patients are affected 2.5 times as commonly as female patients (35). Gender-related differences in strenuous physical activity or metabolic control are probably responsible, but a sex-linked, sex-limited pattern of inheritance has not been excluded. The disorder is molecularly and genetically heterogeneous. Bartram et al. (35) summarize the molecular phenotypes, which include absent myophosphorylase protein (great majority of patients) with absent, normal, decreased, or truncated messenger RNA; decreased protein with normal messenger RNA; and, rarely, normal levels of inactive protein.

The dysfunctional muscle glycogen phosphorylase activity is caused by a genetic mutation in the PYGM, the gene encoding the muscle isoform of the enzyme located on chromosome 11q13 (36). More than 40 different mutations have been described, including missense, nonsense, insertion, inversion, and single base deletions (37). The most common among American and European patients appears to be a nonsense mutation (CGA to TGA) at arginine codon 49 (38), whereas a single codon 708/709 deletion is most common in Japanese patients (39). No clear genotype–phenotype correlation has emerged (40).

In mammals, there are liver and brain isozymes of glycogen phosphorylase, which are under the control of different genes present in other tissue not clinically involved in McArdle's disease. In humans, the liver isozyme predominates in most nonmuscular tissues, whereas the brain isozyme is the predominant form in brain and cardiac muscle (22) and is also probably the fetal form (35). The "fetal" isozyme is present in fetal and regenerating muscle cultures of patients with McArdle's disease (41), suggesting that the expression of this isozyme differs from that of the mature enzyme. The synthesis of the fetal form is repressed by the

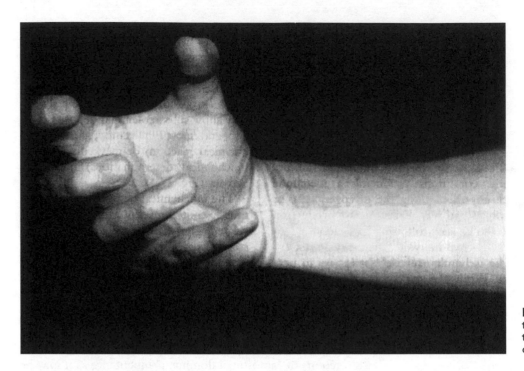

Figure 38.2 Forearm exercise test in McArdle's disease. Characteristic cramping posture developed after forearm exercise.

time of birth (42,43) and replaced during skeletal muscle maturation by the muscle isozyme (44).

Phosphorylase itself exists in two forms. The less active dimer, phosphorylase *b*, is converted to a more active tetramer, phosphorylase *a*, by phosphorylase *b* kinase (PBK). PBK is controlled by hormonal and neural factors via protein kinase and calcium-mediated activation. Epinephrine, by stimulating adenylate cyclase, increases cyclic adenosine monophosphate production, which activates protein kinase. This enzyme, in turn, activates PBK by phosphorylation. Neural control occurs through the events of muscle excitation. Calcium released from the sarcoplasmic reticulum activates PBK by binding to its calmodulin subunit. Thus, a defect in any of these cascade reactions theoretically can inhibit phosphorylase activity.

PBK is composed of four subunits: α, β, γ, and δ. The distinct genetic control of these subunits (45) and the existence of tissue-specific isoforms contribute to the clinical and genetic heterogeneity of PBK deficiency (type VIII glycogenosis). The clinical spectrum includes isolated involvement of liver, cardiac, or skeletal muscles (22,46,47), combined clinical involvement of liver and muscle, and possibly liver and renal diseases. Most myopathic cases have clinical features similar to those of McArdle's disease, including age of onset and symptoms of exercise intolerance, cramps, and myalgias (48–50). However, the forearm exercise test (discussion to follow) is less sensitive in this disorder. Other myopathic variants include infantile hypotonia (48–53) and possibly one infantile case of fetal arthrogryposis (54). Two cases of infantile hypotonia demonstrated a deficiency in one additional enzyme in glycogen metabolism: PFK in one (52) and debranching enzyme in

another (48). Another variant was described in one patient with progressive distal weakness beginning at age 46 (55).

Classically, a simple provocative test, the forearm exercise test for lactate production (56), is used to diagnose McArdle's disease (Figs. 38.2 and 38.3A, B). In McArdle's disease, lactic acid and pyruvate production are decreased. This test is not specific and may indicate any of several conditions producing a metabolic block along the glycogenolytic or glycolytic pathway. Failed lactate production also may be seen following ingestion of alcohol in normal individuals and alcoholics.

The forearm exercise test is easy to perform, but reliable results require preparation, cooperation of the patient, and good laboratory support. While the patient is at rest, blood is drawn for baseline levels of ammonia and lactate. The patient immediately begins repetitive rapid grip exercises. With strong encouragement, normal subjects are able to tolerate forearm exercise for 90 to 180 seconds before pain and fatigue force discontinuation of the test. Patients with disorders of glycogen metabolism seldom exercise for more than 60 seconds. When the patient fatigues, the exercise is terminated and blood ammonia and lactate levels are immediately drawn from the arm that has exercised. Similar samples are drawn again at 1, 2, 4, 6, and 10 minutes following the end of exercise. A flexible intravenous catheter (heparin lock) for phlebotomy and prelabeling of the test tubes enhance the ease of performing the test. Normal subjects exhibit a three- to fivefold increase in lactate level within 5 minutes after the end of the exercise, with a full return to baseline level in about 30 minutes. Submaximal exercise also results in an inadequate rise in venous lactate. The venous ammonia level also rises during forearm exercise; failure of the two to rise together suggests

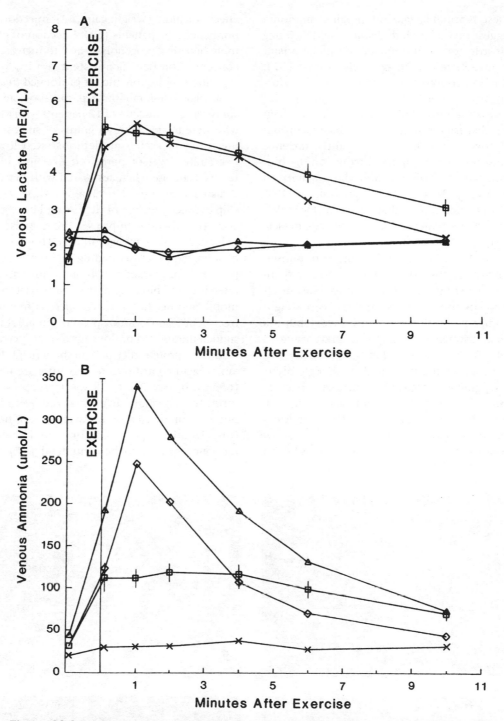

Figure 38.3 Forearm exercise test in McArdle's disease. Lactate and ammonia production after exercise. A venous blood sample was obtained from the antecubital vein at rest before the ischemic exercise. Then the patient was asked to repeat full extension and flexion of the fingers until muscle contracture developed. The venous blood samples were obtained 0, 1, 2, 4, 6, and 10 minutes later. **A:** Venous lactate levels. **B:** Venous ammonia levels. *Box line,* controls with a bar of standard error of mean (*n* = 21). *Diamond* and *triangle lines,* patients with McArdle's disease; *x line,* patient with myoadenylate deaminase deficiency. In McArdle's disease, lactate production is deficient but ammonia production shows a compensatory increase (Brooke MH, Patterson VH, Kaiser KK. Hypoxantine and McArdle's disease: a clue to metabolic stress in the working forearm. *Muscle and Nerve* 1983;6:204–206.). In myoadenylate deaminase deficiency, lactate production is normal but ammonia production is deficient (Fishbein WN, Armbrastmacher VW, Griffin JL. Mayoadenylate deaminase deficiency: a new disease of muscle. *Science* 1978;200:545–548.).

an inadequate test. Normal lactate but impaired ammonia production suggest myoadenylate deaminase deficiency or a related disorder of purine nucleotide metabolism. The two enzyme deficiencies may rarely coexist (57). In disorders of glycogenolysis, ammonia production during exercise may be excessive (58,59).

Muscle biopsy is the most definitive procedure to diagnose McArdle's disease. It may show subsarcolemmal deposits of glycogen and, most importantly, absence (by histochemical reaction) or marked reduction (by biochemical determinations) of phosphorylase activity in most fibers (60) (Fig. 38.4). Genetic analysis of DNA isolated from leukocytes can be diagnostic for McArdle's disease in up to 90% of patients and may obviate muscle biopsy in most cases (61).

The treatment of McArdle's disease begins with counseling the patient regarding the risks of exercise-induced rhabdomyolysis. Patients should be instructed to adjust their lifestyles to avoid strenuous exercise and excessive weight and to seek prompt medical evaluation if myoglobinuria develops. Minor adjustments in lifestyle can prevent attacks in some patients. Treatments aimed at bypassing the biochemical block by supplying the muscle with a glycolytic intermediate (i.e., glucose, fructose) or increasing alternative energy sources (e.g., plasma free fatty acids) improve exercise endurance in some patients (13). However, long-term oral glucose or fructose or high-fat diets usually show disappointing results and have potential deleterious health

effects, including weight gain (62). Injection of d-ribose did not benefit the patients (63). Injection of glucagon to promote hepatic glycogenolysis and to increase blood glucose concentration had inconsistent results, and its repeated injection is objectionable for prolonged treatment.

A single-blind, randomized, placebo-controlled crossover study reported in 2003 of 12 patients with McArdle's disease who were treated with 75 grams of sucrose 30 to 40 minutes prior to exercising demonstrated lower mean peak heart rate, level of perceived exertion in patients who received sucrose when compared with placebo (64). There is also a suggestion that there is a dose response relationship between the dose of sucrose and heart rate during exercise. This therapy improves the exercise tolerance and reduces the risk of myoglobinuria. However, the limitations of short-term sucrose loading include short-lived benefits, potential for marked weight gain further limiting exercise tolerance, and blunting of the compensatory mechanism to mobilize other fuel sources, such as free fatty acids. This treatment also does not prevent myoglobinuria due to a sudden unexpected prolongation of or increase in activity.

A high-protein diet may be beneficial; however, which amino acid contributes to this improvement is uncertain (65,66). In vivo 31P-NMR spectroscopy and exercise performance were partially normalized by a high-protein diet but were unaffected by intravenous amino acid infusion (66). Despite expectation, branched chain amino acids have not proven to be beneficial (67) although their

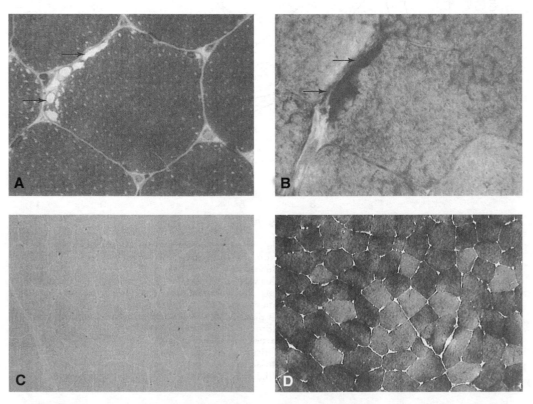

Figure 38.4 Muscle histopathology in McArdle's disease. Note subsarcolemmal blebs (**A**, hematoxylin and eosin) (*arrows*), which contain PAS-positive material (**B**, *arrows*). Phosphorylase activity is absent in muscle fibers (**C**) in contrast to the control (**D**).

oxoacid analogs, which delay ammonia production, may offer short-term benefit (68). These findings suggest that intramuscular protein stores provide an alternative energy substrate and partially correct the metabolic deficits. We have treated a patient experiencing mild proximal weakness secondary to late-onset McArdle's syndrome with a high-protein, low-carbohydrate diet, with nearly complete resolution of weakness within 3 months.

A derivative of vitamin B6 is bound to myophosphorylase and constitutes the body's major pool of this vitamin. Decreased phosphorylase protein in McArdle's disease causes a relative vitamin B6 deficiency. Preliminary data for an oral vitamin B6 supplement suggest benefit in reducing muscle fatigue, possibly by enhancing any one of a number of vitamin B6–dependent processes that increase energy production or use (69,70). The beneficial effect of daily creatine intake remains controversial. While improvement of symptoms was observed in one study, worsening clinical symptoms were reported in another (71).

The potential of gene therapy has been shown by studies with recombinant adenovirus capable of introducing myophosphorylase into differentiating myoblasts and mature myotubes (72). Sustained functional enzyme activity that can be regulated was demonstrated in myotubes. This offers the hope of restoring glycogenolytic function in patients with McArdle's disease by direct adenovirus-mediated enzyme delivery into skeletal muscle (73).

Phosphofructokinase Deficiency (Tarui's Disease, Type VII Glycogenosis)

Phosphofructokinase deficiency, described by Tarui in 1965 (74), is a rare familial disorder with clinical characteristics closely mimicking those of McArdle's disease. It is distinguished by histochemical and biochemical evidence of deficiency (usually absence) of PFK in muscle, resulting in blockage of glycolysis. The forearm exercise test and muscle biopsy results are otherwise similar to those of McArdle's disease. The diagnosis may be suggested by a mild anemia and elevated reticulocyte count resulting from a partial defect of the erythrocyte PFK enzyme with a resultant impaired erythrocyte Ca2+ homeostasis (75) leading to hemolysis (76). Other features of PFK deficiency include significant hemolysis, gouty arthritis, and possibly recurrent gastric ulcers (77). Like McArdle's disease, phosphofructokinase deficiency can show clinical heterogeneity, including the following: late-onset myopathy with (78,79) or without (80) preceding symptoms of exercise intolerance; (b) infantile or childhood severe myopathy without hemolysis and with multiple contractures and/or progressive weakness and respiratory failure (22), rare association with cerebral and cerebellar abnormalities (81), or intrauterine fetal akinesia (82); and (c) isolated hemolysis.

Three isozymes of human PFK have been described: muscle (M), liver (L), and platelets (P), which are variably expressed in tissues. This enzyme forms a polymer in physiologic conditions with the tetramer being minimally active. Human skeletal muscle PFK consists only of M subunits, which are usually absent in this disorder (83). Tissues that express both M subunit and another, such as the L subunit in erythrocytes, have a partial PFK deficiency. Demonstrating a partial deficiency in red blood cells may be useful in diagnosing cases in which histochemical or biochemical studies of muscle are not feasible (84). Muscle study is still needed in infantile variants because the erythrocyte PFK activity is usually normal.

Analysis with 11P-NMR spectroscopy can differentiate disorders of glycolysis, such as PFK deficiency, from those of glycogenolysis, such as McArdle's syndrome (85,86). The former disorders have accumulation of glycolytic intermediates during exercise as phosphorylated sugars with dephosphorylation occurring during recovery and resulting in a slow return to normal orthophosphate (Pi) level. In PFK deficiency, 11P-NMR spectroscopy shows decreased ATP levels at rest that continue to decline during exercise, a finding not present in McArdle's syndrome (85,87). The exact reason for this difference is unknown.

The inheritance pattern in most cases of PFK deficiency is autosomal recessive, and reduced erythrocyte PFK activity may be demonstrated in otherwise asymptomatic parents. Genetic studies have revealed several mutations in the PFK M-subunit gene on chromosome 12q13. Two common mutations involving a splicing defect and a nucleotide deletion with frameshift mutation have been recognized in Ashkenazi Jews (88). Several mutations of these types and missense mutations have been identified in patients from at least six other ethnic backgrounds (89,90).

No specific treatment for PFK deficiency is available. Since the metabolic block affects glycolysis rather than glycogenolysis, there is no rationale for giving glucose or hyperglycemic agents in this condition. In fact, glucose may induce exertional fatigue by inhibiting lipolysis and depriving the muscle of these fuel sources (91). Dietary supplementation with ketone bodies or fatty acids may be beneficial, and in theory, a high-protein diet may be helpful.

Phosphoglycerate Kinase Deficiency (Type IX Glycogenosis)

Phosphoglycerate kinase (PGK) deficiency is an X-linked recessive disorder of the second stage of glycolysis. Since the enzyme is a single ubiquitous polypeptide without tissue-specific isozymes, one might expect multisystem involvement. Nevertheless, primary muscle disorder with exercise-induced painful muscle cramps, myoglobinuria, and impaired lactate production (92–95) and one case with retinitis pigmentosa (96) have been reported. Besides muscle and myoblast cultures, tPGK activities in these cases are also reduced in red blood cells, leukocytes, platelets, and fibroblasts. Cases of PGK deficiency without muscle symptoms are associated with hemolytic anemia, mental retardation, behavioral abnormalities, tremor, and seizure. Combinations of myopathy with hemolytic anemia (97) or with mental retardation (98,99) also have been reported. The gene of PGK, a monomeric enzyme, is located on chromosome Xq13. Molecular genetics studies have shown most errors to be missense mutations with single amino acid substitutions and one splice-junction mutation. The genetic heterogeneity continues to expand (100), although explanation for clinical heterogeneity remains uncertain. The only effective treatment is to avoid intense exercise.

Phosphoglycerate Mutase Deficiency (Type X Glycogenosis)

Phosphoglycerate mutase (PGAM) deficiency, which also affects the second stage of glycolysis, has been recognized as a cause of recurrent episodes of exercise-induced muscle cramp and myoglobinuria in adults of African ancestry with no known family history of neuromuscular disorders (101–105) and in two siblings of an Italian family (106). In most of these studies, the rise of venous lactate after forearm exercise was found to be abnormally low, and the muscle biopsy showed increased glycogen content. PGAM activity was markedly reduced, and the residual activity represented by the brain (BB) isoenzyme suggested a genetic defect of the M subunit, which predominates in normal muscle. In muscle cultures, PGAM activity is normal, which is explained by the predominant or exclusive presence of PGAM-BB during earlier stages of muscle development. Findings with 11P-NMR spectroscopy have been described (107,108). The gene encoding the PGAM-M subunit has been mapped to chromosome 7 (109). So far, a common missense mutation at codon 78 has been identified in African-Americans, and another has been identified at codon 90 in the Italian kindred (106). No specific therapy other than exercise avoidance is available. In one patient with both PGAM deficiency and tubular aggregation, dantrolene was effective (110). This raises the possibility that cramps in muscle PGAM deficiency are caused by high calcium release from the sarcoplasmic reticulum relative to calcium reuptake capacity.

Lactate Dehydrogenase Deficiency (Type XI Glycogenosis)

Reduced levels of lactate dehydrogenase (LDH), the last enzyme involved in the second stage of glycolysis, were thought to cause exercise-induced pigmenturia, easy fatigability, and contracture during forearm exercise tests in an 18-year-old Japanese man. Absence of LDH impairs conversion of pyruvate to lactate, and the patient showed no rise in lactate despite a marked increase in venous pyruvate level (111). Since this original report, the same author and others have identified similarly affected Japanese families (112) and, rarely, Caucasian patients (113). One Japanese woman who was otherwise asymptomatic had skin lesions and childbirth difficulties with uterine stiffness (114). The significance of the typical scaly erythematous patches on extensor surfaces of extremities that worsens in the summer in these patients was later recognized (115), and nearly absent LDH activity in the skin lesions has been shown (116).

LDH is a tetrameric enzyme made up of subunits M (or A) and H (or B) with five different isozymes having been identified. The M subunit is deficient in type XI glycogenosis. This subunit predominates in skeletal muscle and is also abundant in other tissues, including skin and uterus. The biochemical mechanism that leads to marked reduction in muscle ATP and the presumed basis for symptoms has been demonstrated (117). Genetic analysis has shown a 20 base pair (bp) deletion in exon 6 of chromosome 11 (106,118), and additional mutations have been reported (107,119).

β-Enolase Deficiency (Type XII Glycogenosis)

β-Enolase is an enzyme that catalyzes the step interconverting 2-phosphoglycerate and phosphoenolpyruvate. Deficiency of this enzyme has been reported to cause episodic exercise intolerance, myalgia, and elevated creatine phosphokinase in a single adult patient (120).

Disorders of Lipid Metabolism

Use of free fatty acids is essential in prolonged exercise; 1 to 4 hours after uninterrupted exercise, muscle uptake of free fatty acid rises by 70% and the relative contribution of fatty acids to total oxygen use becomes twice that of carbohydrates. The free fatty acids taken up by a muscle are actively transported across the muscle mitochondrial membrane by a carrier, carnitine, with the help of the enzymes carnitine palmitoyltransferase (CPT) I and II (Fig. 38.5), located on separate mitochondrial membranes—CPT I on the outer and CPT II on the inner (121,122). There are three tissue-specific isoforms of CPT I (types A, B, and C), but the same CPT II exists throughout the body (123,124).

Initially it was believed that both CPT enzymes could cause a disorder of lipid metabolism in muscles. It is now recognized that CPT I deficiency causes hepatic disease and that no cases of isolated muscle involvement have been reported (125). CPT II deficiency can have different phenotypic expression, with the "adult" or muscle form being the most common (126). This presentation, in contrast to carnitine deficiency, is characterized by muscle ache and fatigability, with a feeling of muscle stiffness and observable contracture, followed by swelling, elevation of serum muscle enzymes, and sometimes progression to pigmenturia. The attacks are usually triggered by sustained, prolonged exertion, especially if exercise occurs during caloric deprivation (fasting), exposure to cold, or mild infection (127). Occasionally, symptoms are precipitated by the preceding factors even without exercise. Other reported triggers include emotional stress and general anesthesia, which has also been associated with rhabdomyolysis (128,129). Male predominance is reported in several series, but whether this is due to sex-related differences in activities, underlying modifier genes, or hormonal factors remains uncertain (128). Most patients develop symptoms in their first or second decades, although later onset has been reported. Symptoms can persist for hours to days, and the frequency of attacks during one's life can vary from a few to many. Any muscle group can be affected, including respiratory muscles. Progression to persistent muscle weakness is uncommon (130).

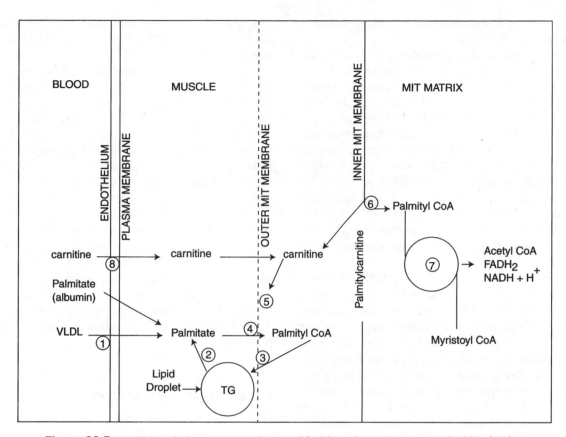

Figure 38.5 Lipid metabolism. Fatty acid (exemplified by palmitate) arrives in the blood either bound to albumin or as triglycerides in the very low-density lipoproteins (VLDLs). *TG*, endogenous lipid stores (triglycerides). The fatty acids pass through the mitochondrial membrane to the mitochondrial matrix, where they undergo β oxidation. Numbers indicate the enzymes or enzyme complexes involved in the process: **1**, lipoprotein; **2**, triglyceride, diglyceride, and monoglyceride lipase; **3**, synthesis of triglycerides from long-chain acyl-CoA involving glycerol-1-phosphate and the three enzymes glycerol phosphate acetyltransferase, phosphatidate phosphatase, and diglyceride acyltransferase; **4**, palmitoyl-CoA synthetase; **5**, carnitine palmitoyltransferase I; **6**, carnitine palmitoyltransferase II; **7**, modified β oxidation; **8**, active transport system of carnitine into muscle. (Courtesy Dr. D. C. DeVivo, Neurological Institute, New York, NY.)

Elevations in serum CK and myoglobinuria usually accompany the muscle symptoms. In a review of the metabolic causes of myoglobinuria, Tonin et al. (131) found CPT deficiency to be the most common cause. Between attacks, as well as during short-term exercise, patients usually are normal. Fasting at rest for 30 to 72 hours can increase the CK, triglyceride, and cholesterol levels or delay the rise of serum ketone bodies. The forearm exercise test is normal. Muscle biopsy between attacks is usually normal but may show variable lipid excess, especially in type 1 muscle fibers. During attacks, foci of muscle necrosis have been described; one report emphasized associated vascular lesions (132). Although CPT can be reduced in liver, leukocytes, platelets, and fibroblasts, biochemical determination of muscle CPT has been the standard for definitive diagnosis. However, a new biochemical technique using peripheral blood cells and fibroblasts may simplify diagnosis in the future (133).

CPT II deficiency is an autosomal recessive disorder (134), although autosomal dominant cases have been suggested, such as in a family with affected members over four generations (135). A study reported reported in 2005

noted impaired fatty acid oxidation in symptomatic carriers of CPT II gene mutation, suggesting that a single mutant allele may exert a dominant negative effect on the tetrameric CPT II protein (136). The gene encoding CPT II has been localized to chromosome 1p32 (137). The most common mutation in muscle CPT deficiency is a serine-to-leucine substitution at codon 113 (S131L) (138). Additional point mutations causing this disorder have been identified. These mutations have been shown to result in reduced catalytic activity and levels of the CPT II protein, the latter because of decreased stability. Zierz et al. (139) provide possible biochemical explanations for how various provocative factors cause intermittent symptoms in patients whose CPT II enzyme shows impaired regulation. Also, since ATP depletion does not fully explain why rhabdomyolysis occurs, other proposed mechanisms include the effects of increased substrates in muscle (e.g., long-chain fatty acylcarnitine) on sarcolemmal Na+,K+-ATPase, phospholipid membranes (140) and on the calcium release channel of muscle sarcoplasmic reticulum (141). There is poor phenotype–genotype correlation with CPT II deficiency (142,143), although the lethal neonatal phenotype is frequently associated with truncating mutations on both alleles (144).

Treatment includes avoiding situations likely to precipitate muscle damage (fasting, prolonged exercise, extreme cold, and infections) and encouraging moderation in exercise and consumption of a high-carbohydrate, high-protein diet with frequent snacks (145). Carbohydrate-rich diet with high polysaccharide content, but not monosaccharides such as glucose, has been shown to improve exercise tolerance (146). Since CPT catalyzes the transport of long-chain fatty acids into the mitochondria, a diet low in long-chain and high in medium-chain triglycerides (MCTs) may be beneficial (147). However, the benefit of MCTs may be limited, since evidence indicates that CPT is more involved in MCT transport than previously assumed (133).

Unusual nonmuscular presentations of CPT II deficiency involving liver, heart, brain, and kidney have been described. Rarely, muscular CPT deficiency has been associated with CNS manifestations, including seizures, infantile spasms (148,149), and athetotic quadriplegia (149). This latter report involving an 18-month-old Japanese boy is worth noting. At age 2 months he developed hypertonicity that gradually progressed to rigospastic quadriplegia; dystonic posture; athetotic movements of neck, trunk, and extremities; and signs of mental retardation. At approximately 1 year, he developed recurrent rhabdomyolysis provoked by mild viral infections. Ketone body production was delayed following long-chain triglyceride loading. Muscle histochemistry and biochemistry were consistent with CPT II deficiency. Treatment with a high-carbohydrate, low-fat (predominantly MCT) diet was successful in preventing myoglobinuria. Hypertonicity responded to diazepam and trihexyphenidyl, but the involuntary movements did not respond to any treatment, including levodopa.

Although true cramps are unusual in CPT deficiency, other defects of muscle lipid metabolism may be associated with repeated episodes of cramps and myalgia (150). They are probably responsible for many of the 51% of cases of myoglobinuria in which no enzyme deficiency is identified (131). In some cases a defect in long-chain acyl-coenzyme A dehydrogenase (LCAD) enzyme has been identified. However, the defect remains unknown in other cases, such as in a report by Engel et al. (151) of 18-year-old identical twin women who, following several hours of exercise, prolonged standing, or long car trips, developed myalgia and cramps, often accompanied by myoglobinuria. Fasting or a low-carbohydrate, high-fat diet precipitated attacks and was associated with sharply increased serum CK and no ketone body production. No CPT deficiency was identified in the muscle biopsy of 1 of the 2 patients. Administration of MCT resulted in normal ketone production, suggesting defective use of long-chain fatty acids. Other than MCT, oral carnitine has improved myopathic features in similar patients, and prednisone has reduced cramping and muscle membrane irritability

(152). In 2004, an immunohistochemical technique to identify LCAD deficiency in muscle biopsies has been reported (153).

We studied a similar case in an 18-year-old man who had two episodes of myoglobinuria following prolonged exercise while fasting. During the 25th hour of a diagnostic fast, he developed mild rhabdomyolysis and episodic vomiting without ketosis. Postfast urine and serum elevations of medium- and long-chain acylcarnitines suggest a deficiency in LCAD. Typically, patients with LCAD deficiency have fasting-induced infantile metabolic attacks (hypoketotic hypoglycemia with dicarboxylic aciduria) often resulting in coma. However, some who survive to adulthood develop a clinical picture with muscle involvement, as in the case just described. The human LCAD gene has been localized to chromosome 2q34-35 (154), and the molecular defects underlying LCAD deficiency are under investigation.

Another syndrome similar to CPT II deficiency, but associated with peripheral neuropathy, has been linked to a deficiency of the mitochondrial trifunctional enzyme of β oxidation (155).

Other Muscle Dysfunctions

Disorders with Contracture

Brody or Lambert-Brody Syndrome

Lambert and Goldstein (156) described a patient who exhibited impaired muscle relaxation that clinically, but not by electromyography, resembled myotonia ("silent myotonia"). Brody (157) described a similar patient and demonstrated that calcium ion (Ca2+) uptake by isolated sarcoplasmic reticulum was markedly reduced. Lambert-Brody syndrome develops during the first or second decade of life and consists of progressive exercise-induced pain, stiffness, and cramping in arm and leg muscles. After only 30 to 60 seconds of rapidly clenching and unclenching the fist, there is a transient, painless slowing of movements; when the fist is forcefully clenched for 10 seconds, the hand can be opened slowly only with initial flexion of the wrist; with excessive activity, pain develops. Similar but less severe impairment of relaxation is sometimes observed in craniobulbar (e.g., frontalis muscle during eye opening) or trunk muscles. The absence of impaired muscle relaxation in some cases (158) and the rare association with recurrent exertional rhabdomyolysis (159) challenge physicians to consider this diagnosis in the broader spectrum of patients with exercise-induced pain, stiffness, and myoglobinuria. There is no percussion or electrical myotonia, and immersion of the forearm in cold water does not influence the stiffness in typical cases. Electromyography shows no abnormalities, and there is electrical silence during the phase of delayed relaxation of strongly contracted muscles. Muscle biopsy usually shows mild, nonspecific, type 2 fiber atrophy and a normal ultrastructural appearance, although mild myopathic histology and swollen mitochondria with crystals were described in one atypical case (159). Although in vitro muscle response to halothane is normal, there is excessive sensitivity to caffeine, suggesting that precautionary anesthesia for malignant hyperthermia syndrome might be appropriate.

Sarcoplasmic reticulum calcium ATPase (SERCA) has been shown to be defective in this disorder. This enzyme exists in mammals as fiber type–specific isoforms (160) and is responsible for calcium reuptake, which allows for muscle relaxation. Cultured muscle cells of patients showing delayed restoration of calcium concentration following depolarization (161) and the distinct pattern of abnormal metabolic response to exercise with 11P-NMR spectroscopy (158) are both consistent with a defect that affects calcium homeostasis. Sarcoplasmic reticulum calcium ATPase is found in much higher concentrations in type 2 (fast-twitch) fibers (162), which helps to explain why impaired relaxation is noted only after phasic exercise, when primarily type 2 motor units are recruited. Earlier immunocytochemical analysis revealed severe reduction in both calcium ATPase content (163) and biologic activity (158). More recent studies on whole-muscle homogenates and muscle cultures using various methods to confirm their results (including monoclonal antibodies to fast-twitch muscle calcium ATPase isozyme) have shown a specific reduction in enzyme activity by about 50% but with normal enzyme concentration (161). This evidence supports the conclusion that this syndrome is due to a reduction in molecular activity of the type 2 muscle fiber sarcoplasmic reticulum calcium-ATPase isozyme, which Benders et al. (161) speculate is due to a structural modification of the protein.

Karpati et al. (163) reported 4 male patients who inherited the condition through an autosomal recessive or X-linked recessive mode. We have seen a female patient with this syndrome whose brother was similarly affected, supporting an autosomal recessive inheritance. Autosomal dominant inheritance has been suggested in one family (164). In about 59% of families with Brody's disease, different mutations of sarcoplasmic reticulum Ca2+ ATPase create stop codons that delete all or part of the Ca2+ binding and translocation domain, resulting in loss of SERCA1 function (165,166).

Studies on cultured muscle cells of patients showed that dantrolene sodium and calcium channel–blocking drugs improved calcium homeostasis (161). Despite such in vitro evidence of benefit, treatment with these drugs has been unsuccessful in some patients (163). However, other patients with less pronounced impairment of muscle relaxation had improvement of exertional myalgia with verapamil (158) or improvement of exercise intolerance with dantrolene sodium (159).

Rippling Muscle Disease

Rippling muscle disease (RMD) is a rare, usually hereditary, nonprogressive myopathy characterized by muscular hyperexcitability. The unusual finding of involuntary rolling muscle contractions or rippling movements are provoked by mechanical stimuli such as stretching or tapping the muscles (167–169). Other associated clinical signs and symptoms are muscle stiffness, often with initiation of physical activity after a period of rest, exercise-induced myalgia, and localized muscle mounding with percussion. There may be substantial phenotypic variability among members of families affected with this disease (170). A moderately elevated serum CPK level is commonly observed among affected individuals. An autosomal dominant inheritance with the gene localized to chromosome 1q41 was first reported in an Oregon family (171). Subsequent studies in families with autosomal dominant RMD could not confirm the same genetic defect and suggested other genetic loci. Mutations in the caveolin-3 gene on chromosome 3p25 were found in kindreds with RMD (172–174). Both heterozygote and homozygote mutations have been described in sporadically affected individuals, suggesting possible autosomal recessive inheritance (175). Caveolin-3 gene mutation is also responsible for limb girdle muscular dystrophy (type 1C LGMD) (176), but the modifying genetic and environmental factors responsible for the phenotypic variability of caveolinopathies remains unclear (173). The rippling movements and myoedema, which are electrically silent, usually occur in limb muscles, although involvement of extraocular muscles may be possible (177). The exact mechanism of these phenomenons is still not fully understood. However, the contraction observed may be the result of propagation of the action potential in the muscle tubular system without exciting the sarcolemma (178). Mild nonspecific myopathic features have been reported on muscle histology and electron microscopy (168,179), including abnormalities of sarcolemma and sarcoplasmic reticulum. Reduction of caveolin-3 and dysferlin in muscle membrane has been demonstrated by immunohistochemical techniques (180). In vitro muscle studies show sarcolemmal excitability and findings consistent with abnormal sensitivity of sarcoplasmic reticulum (calcium channel) to muscle distortion (169). An autoimmune mechanism has been hypothesized in sporadic cases associated with myasthenia gravis and thymoma (181–183).

Myotonia Congenita with Painful Cramps

Myotonia congenita with painful cramps is another rare muscle disorder with contracture, although it is more frequently included in discussions of autosomal dominant myotonic disorders (184–186). As opposed to most myotonic disorders, myotonia congenita has muscle contractions that are painful and are electrically silent after an initial period of electrical myotonia. The contractions that follow exercise are often prolonged. It is unclear whether this disease is a variant of typical autosomal dominant myotonia congenita (Thomsen's disease). A sporadic case resembling the recessive type (Becker's disease) also has been reported (187). Thomsen's and Becker's myotonia congenita are now known to be caused by mutations of the gene 7q32 encoding the skeletal muscle chloride channel protein (188,189). In familial myotonic disorder with painful myotonia and cramps, the symptom may be aggravated by injection of potassium (potassium-aggravated myotonia) (190). This condition was previously known as *myotonia fluctuans, myotonia permanens,* and *acetazolamide-sensitive myotonia.* This disease, like others in the adynamia–paramyotonia complex (191), now is known to be due to mutations of the skeletal muscle sodium channel gene (17q23) (192,193).

Hypothyroidism

Neuromuscular dysfunction is common in hypothyroidism (194,195). Three overlapping syndromes of hypothyroid myopathy have been identified. In infants and children, hypothyroidism often results in generalized muscular stiffness and hypertrophy, often most remarkable in the calf muscles, a condition known as Kocher-Debré-Sémélaigne syndrome. Adults with hypothyroid myopathy typically have mild shoulder and pelvic girdle weakness, with three-fourths of patients complaining of muscle pain, cramps, or stiffness (196). Muscular hypertrophy occasionally accompanies these symptoms in a constellation known as Hoffman's syndrome. Uncommonly, patients have exercise-induced myalgia with histologic (197) and clinical evidence of rhabdomyolysis (198). Myalgia and cramps with elevated serum CK also may accompany rapid reduction toward normal of serum thyroid hormone levels during treatment of hyperthyroidism, perhaps reflecting a relative hypothyroid state within muscle tissue (199).

Common to all forms of hypothyroid myopathy is slowness of muscle contraction and relaxation. When severe, this may result in muscle stiffness with slowed movements that suggest parkinsonism or dystonia. This is true especially of the intense stiffness that can accompany Kocher-Debré-Sémélaigne syndrome, and affected infants initially may be suspected of having tetany, dystonia, or spasticity. Hypothyroid-related prolongation of muscle contraction and relaxation is worsened by cold and can be detected clinically by the slowed return phase of the Achilles reflex ("hung up" reflex) and by myoedema following muscle percussion.

In all three conditions, serum CK levels may be elevated, and the electromyogram may reveal myopathic and polyphasic potentials, as well as hyperirritability with complex repetitive discharges (196,200). The delayed relaxation of grip combined with the "pseudomyotonia" that may be seen on electromyogram may produce diagnostic confusion with the myotonic disorders. However, the myotonia is not present except in patients believed to have an associated inherited myotonia (201), which may be unmasked by the hypothyroidism (202). Confusion also may arise between inflammatory myopathies and hypothyroid myopathy. Serum thyroid function tests reveal the proper diagnosis in most cases, although an associated inflammatory myopathy should be considered in patients

with evidence of autoimmune thyroid disease, particularly in those who do not respond to treatment.

Muscle pathology has revealed a host of nonspecific or inconsistent findings, including focal necrosis, variation in fiber size, vacuoles, increased numbers of central nuclei, type I fiber predominance, type II fiber atrophy, and central changes (196,203,204); it also reveals ultrastructural evidence of polysaccharide and glycogen accumulation, mitochondrial abnormalities and lipid droplets, dilated sarcoplasmic reticulum, and T-tubule proliferation (204). We also have observed muscle fibrosis and multiple ring fibers in a severely hypothyroid patient with a serum CK level 40 times normal. The mechanisms of hypothyroid-induced muscle pain, stiffness, cramps, hypertrophy, and delayed contraction and relaxation are uncertain. It is speculated that metabolic changes, particularly those affecting carbohydrate metabolism and mitochondrial function, may explain myalgias, cramps, and exercise intolerance (205). Forearm muscle exercise testing may reveal impaired lactate production, and 11P-NMR spectroscopy has shown delayed glycogen breakdown in muscle with exercise (206). Impaired muscle lysosomal acid maltase activity has been implicated (196,207). Glycogenolysis also may be diminished on the basis of decreased muscle β-adrenergic receptor density (208). Reduced mitochondrial oxidative capacity may be especially important (205). The delay in muscle contraction and relaxation may be related to the effects of reduced myosin ATPase activity (209) and decreased calcium uptake by the sarcoplasmic reticulum (210). Other abnormalities in muscle function include decreased muscle protein synthesis and diminished sodium–potassium pump activity.

The management of muscle dysfunction associated with hypothyroidism has not been studied objectively. In most cases, all signs and symptoms, as well as many pathologic and metabolic changes (198,207), resolve within 6 months of adequate thyroid hormone replacement. However, temporary worsening of the muscle pain and stiffness with the initiation of treatment has been reported (211).

Hyperparathyroidism

Muscle pain and cramps are common in hyperparathyroidism (212,213). The exact mechanisms responsible are unknown, and several explanations have been put forward. Elevated intracellular calcium concentrations, which result in prolonged muscle contraction, have been reported (214,215). Other researchers have demonstrated reductions in muscle energy production, transfer, and use induced by parathyroid hormone (216). The finding that the calcium channel blocker verapamil experimentally reverses most of these abnormalities suggests that calcium homeostasis plays a central role in hyperparathyroid-induced muscle dysfunction.

Myotonic Disorders

Myotonia is not difficult to diagnose once symptoms have been reported. However, except for the unusual myotonic disorders discussed previously (*see* Myotonia Congenita with Painful Cramps), this condition is painless, and many patients do not voluntarily complain of stiffness. It is usually relatively simple to differentiate the transient muscle stiffness of myotonia from muscle cramp and contracture (Table 38.2).

The myotonic disorders listed in Table 38.1 have been reviewed in detail elsewhere (217). We also direct interested readers to reviews of the advances in the understanding of the nondystrophic myotonias and periodic paralyses (218).

One condition in which muscle cramp and stiffness are prominent is Schwartz-Jampel syndrome (chondrodystrophic myotonia). This autosomal recessive illness (autosomal dominant inheritance has also been reported by Ferrannini et al. [219] and Pascuzzi et al. [220]) usually begins in infancy with myotonia, continuous muscle discharges, osteochondrodysplasia, respiratory distress, feeding difficulties, growth retardation, hypertrophic musculature, and a characteristic facies with blepharophimosis, micrognathia, pursed lips, and low-set ears (221; reviewed in 220) (Fig. 38.6). Patients are at risk for malignant hyperthermia (222). Cognitive impairment, estimated to occur in 25% of cases, may take the form of a developmental language disorder (223). Obstructive sleep apnea with hypoxia has been reported (224) and in patients with normal osteochondral development (225), including some without significant skeletal alterations (226) have been reported. It has been suggested that these patients develop mild skeletal dysplasia only as a consequence of myotonia and are distinct from the larger group of patients with heterogeneous forms of primary bone dysplasia (227). Muscle stiffness and osteochondrodysplasia often limit joint mobility, resulting in a rigid gait. This, combined with the masklike facies and paucity of movements observed in some cases, may suggest a movement disorder. Almost all patients have prominent action and percussion myotonia, and fine myokymic movements frequently are seen in resting muscle. On electromyogram, although true myotonic discharges have been noted, the electrical discharges often lack a waxing and waning pattern, and at rest there may be continuous, bizarre, high-frequency discharges. Although these discharges are not blocked by peripheral nerve block, the effect of curare has varied from one report to another (228). Thus, the origin of the discharges may be within the muscle in some cases but may be in the distal terminal of the nerve as well. In vitro studies of skeletal muscle fibers from a single patient showed an unstable resting membrane potential, decreased chloride conductance, and delayed sodium channel opening (229). These abnormalities were partially normalized by in vitro addition of the sodium channel blocker procainamide, which also resulted in reduced clinical myotonia and increased mobility. Further confirmation is needed regarding the efficacy of this treatment, as well as carbamazepine, the latter having been used successfully in improving myotonia, blepharospasm, stair climbing, height (230), and respiratory status. Early treatment may prevent features of skeletal dysplasia (231). The pathophysiology is probably distinct

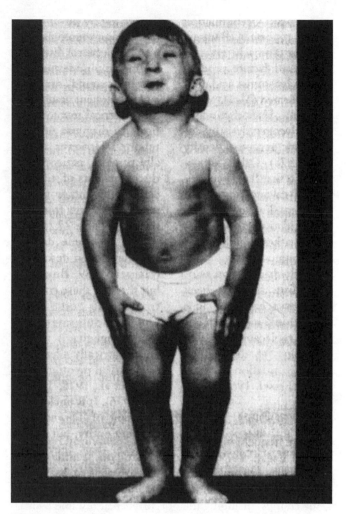

Figure 38.6 Schwartz-Jampel syndrome. Note blepharophimosis, low-set ears, hypertrophic muscles, and muscle stiffness with abnormal arm posture. (Reprinted with permission from Scriban N, Ionasescu V. Schwartz-Jampel syndrome: a case report—stimulatory effect of calcium and A 23187 calcium ionophore for propane synthesis in muscle cell cultures. *Eur Neurol* 1981;20:46–61.)

from known skeletal muscle channelopathies (229). This is supported by genetic studies that found linkage to chromosome 1p34-36.1 in several families with varying ethnicity (232), although there are reports that another locus may be responsible for the severe form (233).

Other Myogenic Conditions and Drug-Induced Myalgia and Cramps

A complete discussion of drug-induced myalgia and cramps and other myogenic conditions is beyond the scope of this chapter. For further information, see the reviews by Roy and Gutmann (234) and Simchak and Pascuzzi (235). Sufit and Peters (236) have reported exercise-induced myalgias in 2 patients with associated proximal muscle weakness of uncertain origin that responded to treatment with nifedipine. Other cases have been associated with abnormal components of skeletal muscle structure or function, such as mitochondrial alterations (237), intracellular acidosis (238), low myosin ATPase and phosphocreatine content (239), type 2 muscle fiber predominance (240), abnormal dystrophin (241,242), vascularized muscle fibers (243,244), and muscle tubular aggregates (245,246). Muscle pain and cramps also may be caused by local and diffuse myositis, polymyalgia rheumatica, endocrine myopathies, uremia, cirrhosis, gastrectomy, dehydration, and drugs. These drugs include clofibrate and other cholesterol-lowering agents, diuretics, ε-aminocaproic acid, vincristine, captopril, phencyclidine, ketoconazole, lithium, salbutamol, isoetharine, emetine, danazol, amphetamine, cimetidine, methoxyprogesterone, alcohol, amphotericin B, nifedipine, nicotinic acid, and cyclosporine (247,248). Muscle cramps also have been reported in cases of Becker's muscular dystrophy of later onset (241,242) and as an early manifestation of mild disease (249). Cramps also occur in the rare syndrome of insulin resistance, acanthosis nigricans, and acral hypertrophy (Flier's syndrome) (250). Sometimes myalgia and cramps occur with drug treatments or conditions in which myogenic and neurogenic causations overlap. In adults, the neuromuscular depolarizing blocking agent succinylcholine has a high association with postoperative myalgia and muscle damage. This is possibly due to the shearing forces of fasciculating muscle fibers induced by the drug's effect on neuromuscular junction and muscle spindles (251–253). Severe painful cramp is a major symptom of a rare probably autoimmune disease affecting local areas of muscle (interstitial myositis), skin, and subcutaneous fat (lipoatrophy) (254,255). This myogenic disorder has features, discussed in the next section, more commonly associated with neurogenic cramps, including their occurrence at rest and association with fasciculations.

Muscle pain and cramp also should be differentiated from disorders that affect bones, joints, and periarticular structures. Intermittent claudication secondary to atherosclerotic occlusion of leg arteries or vascular aneurysms should be considered in individuals with lower-extremity myalgia or cramp induced by effort. However, such ischemic pain typically subsides quickly with rest and does not cause residual muscle soreness unless the ischemia is severe.

Neurogenic Causes of Muscle Cramps

Most, but not all, disorders discussed in this section produce cramps at rest, which may worsen with exercise or repetitive use of the muscle. These conditions are thought to cause cramps or similar symptoms through a mechanism involving the portions of the motor unit proximal to the neuromuscular junction. Neurogenic cramps are common, affecting the majority of patients evaluated by the neurologist.

Common and Nocturnal Cramps

Spontaneous muscle cramps occurs commonly in the general population (256). Common muscle cramps typically entail a sudden involuntary and painful muscle shortening,

induced by movement, with visible and palpable contraction confined to one muscle or part of one muscle. Such cramps usually affect the gastrocnemius or the small intrinsic muscles of the soles of the feet, and they may cause abnormal posture of the affected joint. The individual may be aware of twitching (fasciculation) of the muscle before onset or at the end of the cramp; in some cases, fasciculations are widespread and continuous (257–259). The cramp usually is terminated by passive stretching of the affected muscle or by active contraction of antagonist muscles, but there may be residual soreness and swelling. Passive stretching before and after exercise tends to prevent such cramping during exercise.

Cramps occur frequently in two common circumstances: acute fluid or salt loss, such as with prolonged physical activity, and when muscles are maintained in shortened position, such as the feet and calves of swimmers (260). In a comparison between marathon runners who had a cramp during a marathon (18%) and those who were without cramps, there were no significant differences in degree of pretraining, performance, plasma electrolyte or bicarbonate concentrations, or changes in plasma volume (261). In a similar study, under conditions of more profuse sweating, magnesium loss correlated with cramping (262). Further studies of this common problem are needed, perhaps using 31P-NMR techniques to monitor intracellular electrolyte and pH changes.

Nocturnal leg cramps are extremely common, especially among the elderly (1,260). Exactly why this symptom is prevalent among the elderly is not known; speculation about such causal phenomena as progressive age-related loss of upper motor neurons, local tissue abnormalities of the leg, varicose veins, and muscle dehydration have remained unsubstantiated. Analysis of questionnaires completed by outpatients with general medical problems at a Veterans Affairs medical center revealed that nocturnal cramps were associated with peripheral vascular disease, hypokalemia, and coronary artery disease (1). A significant association with peripheral neurologic deficits was found in a retrospective study of male veterans (263). Evidence best supports a neurogenic origin for ordinary and nocturnal muscle cramps, and factors that cause cramping may have in common a hyperexcitable effect on intramuscular motor nerve terminals (264).

Prevention of ordinary and nocturnal muscle cramps is often difficult, as evidenced by the large number of proposed treatments (235). Patients should avoid the use of caffeine and adrenergic agonist medications. A simple set of exercises designed to gently stretch the gastrocnemius muscles should be discussed with all patients. The patient stands with feet flat on the floor, an arm's length away from and facing a wall, using the arms to support the body in a "standing push-up" as the upper torso is moved slowly toward the wall while the legs are held straight. This may result in a mild "burning" pain in the area behind the knees. The position is maintained for 10 seconds and repeated 9 times twice daily (265). Other stretching exercises also may be beneficial.

Nocturnal leg cramps also can be avoided by minimizing passive plantar flexion of the feet during sleep. Individuals who habitually sleep in a supine position should be advised to keep the bed covers loose or to use a foot cradle to keep the weight of the covers from exaggerating passive plantar flexion. Patients also can place a pillow against the sole of the feet as a footboard, a technique also used to prevent foot drop in unconscious or paralyzed patients. Prone sleepers can let their feet hang over the end of the mattress to maintain a more neutral foot position.

For patients whose symptoms do not respond to physical maneuvers, various medications have been found to be effective in the treatment of cramps, although most lack confirmation in well-designed studies. Quinine sulfate or its derivatives has been used for more than 50 years since its effectiveness in nocturnal leg cramps was initially reported (266). We and other physicians can attest to patient satisfaction with quinine. However, in August 1994 the U.S. Food and Drug Administration issued regulations that led to the removal of quinine from over-the-counter (OTC) use, and in early 1995 prescription quinine products no longer could be labeled for use in nocturnal leg cramps (267). Stopping OTC availability was mainly driven by potentially serious, although rare, idiosyncratic side effects of hypersensitivity reactions and thrombocytopenia or pancytopenia. Other side effects include cinchonism (nausea, vomiting, tinnitus, and deafness), visual toxicity, and cardiac effects (268), which occur at toxic drug levels not expected to result from usual low doses of quinine used in patients with common or nocturnal cramps. However, this may not be true in patients with hepatic or renal disease or those using drugs that decrease either clearance (cimetidine) or urinary excretion (alkalinizing agents) of quinine. The controversy over quinine's efficacy stems from placebo-controlled studies showing conflicting negative (269–271) and positive results (272,273) that have been questioned because of design flaws and/or small numbers of patients. The largest blinded placebo-controlled studies to date clearly have demonstrated in 4-week trials the efficacy with mild side effects of quinine sulfate 500 mg (274) and hydroquinine hydrobromide 300 mg (275) in reducing the frequency of ordinary muscle cramps. The latter study showed an almost threefold benefit over placebo. These studies, as well as their meta-analyses (276), support the short-term use of low-dose quinine products in the prevention of frequent common muscle cramps in otherwise healthy adults who are informed and monitored for adverse reactions. Since benefit from quinine can last weeks to months after discontinuation of treatment (277), short periods of treatment followed by periods without treatment may be advisable and effective (275). Questions for future studies include long-term safety, dose-related responses, and value of monitoring drug levels.

Since quinine is contraindicated in pregnancy, other treatments are needed. Under the guidance of the obstetrician, pregnancy-related cramps often can be relieved by an increase in dietary calcium and magnesium. Other medications that anecdotally or in uncontrolled studies have been found useful in managing neurogenic cramps include other membrane-stabilizing agents, such as phenytoin and carbamazepine; baclofen and clonazepam; verapamil 120 mg at bedtime (278); carisoprodol 350 mg 4 times daily (279); and nifedipine (236), which also can cause cramping (280). We have effectively used oral dantrolene sodium or mexiletine in patients with some forms of severe neurogenic cramps. Vitamin E has been reported effective in nocturnal leg cramps; however, in the only controlled study for this condition, benefit was not demonstrated (274).

Peripheral Nerve Injury, Nerve Root Compression, Radiculopathy, and Anterior Horn Cell Disease

Muscle cramps commonly are caused by dysfunction of peripheral nerves, nerve roots, and anterior horn cells. They are responsible for the majority of cramps in which a specific cause is determined. In a prospective study of 50 cancer patients referred for new complaints of muscle cramps, the problem originated in the peripheral nerve in 44%, in spinal roots in 26%, and in the plexus in 8%; no cause was found in 16% (281). Muscle cramps were the first symptom in 64% of these patients, which emphasizes the importance of a thorough diagnostic workup in patients with the new onset of cramps.

Localized motor unit hyperactivity, including myokymia and cramp, sometimes follows individual nerve or plexus injury (282,283), diffuse peripheral neuropathy (284), focal demyelinating neuropathy (285), and motor neuropathy with multifocal conduction block (286,287). It also may occur as a late effect of poliomyelitis (288). The persistent motor conduction block in many of these conditions, except the last, may be important to the pathogenesis of myokymia and cramp (286,289). The alpha motor neuron itself also has been proposed as the site of origin of cramping and myokymia, perhaps reflecting the dual property of its membrane, which can switch from a low- to a high-equilibrium potential capable of generating self-sustaining rhythmic firing (288). Central influences may affect these neural discharges, since in some patients these symptoms disappear during sleep and spinal anesthesia. In one case, back-averaging of the electroencephalogram revealed that severe cramps were preceded by a cortical potential (290).

Compression of a nerve root may cause fasciculation, myokymia, or cramp, with or without persistent muscle spasm, in muscles supplied by that root. Rish (291) estimated a 20% to 30% incidence of cramps in lumbar radiculopathy and noted that symptoms may persist after surgery. However, this may reflect the chronicity of the radiculopathy, since myokymia has been shown to cease immediately after decompression of a more acute nerve root lesion (292). On electromyogram, regular, rhythmic, and in some cases continuous discharges of motor unit potentials are often seen. Stretching the nerve increases spasm and muscle discharges (293).

A pseudomyotonic phenomenon consisting of difficulty opening the hand after holding an object has been reported in patients with chronic radiculopathy at the level of the seventh cervical nerve root (294). Electromyographic (EMG) examination revealed coactivation of finger flexors and finger extensors during voluntary contraction of the latter group of muscles. No electrical or percussion myotonia was present. This phenomenon is caused by misdirected reinnervation of the flexor muscles by nerve root fibers belonging to the extensor muscles. Local anesthetic block of the median nerve at the elbow level eliminates flexor muscle activity and temporarily abolishes the pseudomyotonic phenomena.

Muscle cramps are known to occur in motor neuron disease, and in the hereditary spinal muscular atrophies it can be the only clinical manifestation of early disease (295). It is a common, though seldom obtrusive, feature of amyotrophic lateral sclerosis (ALS) (296). As with fasciculation, it has been suspected that the cramps of ALS originate from dysfunction of the terminal branches of intramuscular nerves (297,298). The identification of presumed antibodies to voltage-gated calcium channels on nerve terminals and muscle fibers (299,300) suggests that some aspects of the pathogenesis of ALS are similar to those reported by Sinha et al. (301) in Isaacs' syndrome. Recommended treatments for the cramps of ALS include stretching exercises, baclofen, phenytoin, carbamazepine, and quinine (302).

Many patients who have had poliomyelitis have cramps and fasciculation (259). Following anterior horn cell damage, extensive sprouting of the remaining motor neurons allows for reinnervation of the muscle. These terminal nerve sprouts are less stable electrically and may discharge spontaneously or degenerate, presumably leading to fasciculation and cramps. Similar mechanisms may be active in ALS, chronic spinal muscular atrophies, and other disorders of motor neurons. Central mechanisms of cramp also may play a role in some of these disorders. Peripheral nerve stimulation distal to a nerve block could not induce cramps in a patient with ALS or bulbospinal neuronopathy (303). Cramps were suppressed selectively by gamma-aminobutyric acid (GABA) receptor agonists (diazepam and baclofen), suggesting that impairment of inhibitory GABAergic interneurons was involved in the pathogenesis of cramps in these patients.

Heat Cramps

Prolonged exertion in high temperatures can cause heat cramps, which are an occupational hazard among skilled mill workers, furnace stokers, boiler room workers, miners, and others who face high temperatures (304,305). They are more common among "acclimatized" workers, perhaps because of the increased volume and salt concentration of their sweat. Cramps are also a feature of the more severe syndrome of heat exhaustion; in both, the cause is probably sweat-induced hyponatremia or fluid replacement–induced osmotic shifts. However, a study reported in 2000 has deemphasized the role of hyponatremia and has indicated dehydration as the main pathogenic factor (306). The cramps may be delayed up to 24 hours following heat exposure. Although heat cramps have not been studied extensively, their clinical similarities to common and exertion-related cramps suggest that they are neurogenic and may share a common mechanism. The treatment of heat cramps consists of cessation of exertion, rest in a cool environment, and electrolyte and fluid replacement. A high-sodium diet or salt supplements with fluid intake may be helpful in preventing attacks.

Hemodialysis Cramps

Muscle cramps are prevalent in patients on hemodialysis, and they are the most common reason for early termination of treatment (307). They frequently appear toward the end of the dialysis sessions (associated with loss of 2 to 4 liters of body water), although they can occur earlier in dialysis when high rates of ultrafiltration are used (268). Hemodialysis-induced muscle cramps (308) are accompanied by high-voltage EMG activity and are considered to be neurogenic (309). Dialysis cramps are comparable to cramps induced by diuretics, diarrhea, vomiting, and profuse perspiration. Plasma volume contraction through an unknown mechanism is the most common explanation given for muscle cramps (310). Hypertonic solutions of dextrose, saline, and mannitol used to correct this volume change were all found to be equally safe and effective in relieving these muscle cramps (311). Plasma volume contraction leads to increased catecholamines, which may play a role in hemodialysis-induced muscle cramps (312). Medication that attenuates this sympathetic activation (low-dose prazosin) reduced cramp frequency, but it is limited for practical use because of hypotensive effects (313). Nifedipine, a vasodilator and calcium channel blocker, produced prompt relief of cramps and was three times as effective as placebo (314). Other treatments include quinine sulfate 325 mg and vitamin E 400 IU at bedtime, which proved to be equally effective in reducing cramp frequency and severity of pain in dialysis patients (315,316). Hemodialysis-induced cramps may be alleviated by oral quinine sulfate 300 mg given just before dialysis (317); and L-carnitine intravenous supplementation at the end of the dialysis session decreased cramp incidence (318).

Generalized Motor Unit Hyperactivity of Peripheral Nerve Origin

Motor unit hyperactivity arising in the peripheral nerves is a heterogeneous group of acquired and hereditary disorders that all have in common sustained, diffuse motor unit activity, probably of peripheral nerve origin with or without associated evidence of peripheral neuropathy (for review and classification, see 319). In Isaacs' (320) report of this syndrome, he used the term *continuous muscle fiber activity* (CMFA). A number of terms have been used to describe related syndromes, including *Isaacs-Mertens syndrome, neuromyotonia, generalized myokymia, pseudomyotonia, continuous motor unit activity, normocalcemic tetany, quantal squander, armadillo disease,* and *Morvan's chorea*. Broadly classified, these terms have limitations for accurate description of the spectrum of clinical and EMG findings in this group of disorders. Perhaps the most descriptive term, although cumbersome, is *sustained muscle activity of peripheral nerve origin* (321); even then the word *general* must be added to lend distinction from local conditions (*see* Peripheral Nerve Injury, Nerve Root Compression, Radiculopathy, and Anterior Horn Cell Disease). *Neuromyotonia*, the term favored by many (322), emphasizes the neurogenic origin of the myotonic-like clinical features. It also describes the most common EMG finding in Isaacs' form of this disorder: spontaneous (also induced by needle movement or voluntary contraction), irregularly occurring trains (usually a few seconds) of variably formed motor unit potentials firing at a frequency of 150 to 300 Hz (neuromyotonic discharge). Generalized myokymia emphasizes clinical myokymia (visible rippling movements from continuous muscle contractions) and one of its EMG correlates: the spontaneous, more regularly occurring grouped discharges (often brief bursts) of motor unit potentials (myokymic discharge). Other EMG findings include fasciculation or individual motor unit potentials spontaneously firing at fixed intervals of less than 20 ms, such as doublets, triplets, and multiplets (Fig. 38.7, which shows two doublets, triplets, and fasciculation). Cramp discharges with motor unit potentials firing at high frequency (up to 150 Hz) may occur in what is probably a related disorder at the mild end of the spectrum and a major feature in some hereditary conditions. These EMG patterns often occur in combination and do not provide a clear basis for pathogenic distinction. Since the predominant discharges are motor unit potentials, the term *continuous motor unit activity* (CMUA) (284) is more informative than CMFA because CMFA may imply spontaneous activity of individual muscle fibers. In this chapter, *CMUA* is used as an abbreviated term when referring in general to this syndrome. The word *continuous* is relative, applying variably to overall clinical muscle activity or EMG discharges, and it does not apply to lesser degrees of motor unit hyperactivity.

This section discusses generalized motor unit hyperactivity of peripheral nerve origin under the following main categories: idiopathic or autoimmune syndrome not associated with peripheral neuropathy, other acquired conditions, and hereditary disorders.

Idiopathic or Autoimmune (Isaacs') Syndrome Not Associated with Peripheral Neuropathy

The eponym *Isaacs' syndrome* is probably best applied to idiopathic cases without peripheral neuropathy. Current evidence indicates that at least some of these have an autoimmune basis. The onset is typically during the second or third decade of life, although onset up to the sixth decade also occurs (323). The sexes are affected equally. Complaints include muscle stiffness, intermittent cramping, and difficulty chewing, speaking, and even breathing. Ocular muscles and sphincters function normally, and sensation is not affected.

The most remarkable feature of Isaacs' syndrome is myokymia affecting limb (especially distally), trunk, jaw, face, and abdominal muscles. These widespread, continuous twitching movements resemble but usually are slower than fasciculation and have been described as having the appearance of a bag of worms. Repetitive passive limb movement leads to increasing resistance and pain. Voluntary movements are slow, resulting in gait difficulty, and fatigue sets in rapidly. However, repetitive voluntary activity tends to increase muscle mobility, although temporarily. There is no percussion or electrical myotonia. The cramps and myokymic movements persist during sleep. Some patients display marked hyperhidrosis, muscle hypertrophy, or elevated CK. Limited forms of the disease with facial myokymia and elevated voltage-gated potassium channel (VGKC) antibody (324) have also been reported. Some cases may be associated with thymoma (325). One case associated with malignant hyperthermia has been reported (326). Detailed laboratory and cerebrospinal fluid (CSF) evaluations are usually normal, although CSF oligoclonal bands were found in all 3 patients tested in one report (323), and mild elevations in CSF total protein can occur (327).

EMG studies typically show neuromyotonic and myokymic discharges; fasciculations, doublets, and multiplets are also seen. These discharges are abolished by curare, distinguishing them from myotonia, but persist during spinal and general anesthesia and sleep, indicating

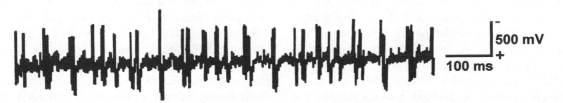

500 mV

100 ms

Figure 38.7   Continuous motor unit activity.

that they arise in the peripheral nerves. The site of origin along the nerve can be proximal or distal, as shown by variable response to nerve block. These discharges frequently persist after nerve block, and in some cases there is evidence that this activity arose distally and perhaps even in nerve terminals (328). Others have found that nerve block abolished these spontaneous discharges, indicating their source in proximal parts of nerves (329,330). In an isolated case, epidural block reduced the spontaneous discharges and led to a silent period after the H response, suggesting that the discharges arose in the ventral roots or spinal cord (331). The long trains of discharges can be difficult to distinguish from those of tetany. The clinical and electrophysiologic similarities of Isaacs' syndrome to hyperventilation-induced tetany (for more detail, *see* Tetany) raised some doubt about the authenticity of some reports (17). It is essential that calcium, phosphorus, and blood gas studies, as well as investigations of clinical and electrophysiologic effects of hyperventilation, be done for all patients suspected of having Isaacs' syndrome.

The cause of Isaacs' syndrome remains unknown, although evidence of autoimmunity is accumulating (332–335). Sinha et al. (301) reported an antibody-mediated mechanism in a man with a 7-year history of severe symptoms, serum thyroid microsomal antibodies, a poor clinical response to phenytoin and carbamazepine, but otherwise typical Isaacs' syndrome. Treatment with plasma exchange (PE) (5 to 10 exchanges) resulted in a transient but nearly complete subjective and objective improvement. Improvement was maximal at 7 to 14 days after the last exchange, and symptoms returned over the following few weeks. Attempts to passively transfer electrophysiologic or clinical signs of the disease to mice were unsuccessful. However, a phrenic nerve diaphragm preparation from mice pretreated with patient's plasma or gamma immunoglobulin (IgG) showed increased neuromuscular resistance to the effects of d-tubocurarine without altering postsynaptic ionic currents. These findings suggest that this patient's syndrome was caused by an IgG directed against a presynaptic ion channel that increases nerve terminal excitability, possibly a potassium channel. Since then, more similar patients, with no or partial control of symptoms from anticonvulsants, have responded to PE. Shillito et al. (336) studied 3 patients with Isaacs' syndrome and 3 patients with CMUA associated with peripheral neuropathy. Increased quantal release of acetylcholine (quantal content) was shown using a similar mouse nerve–muscle preparation, and the patient's IgG also caused increased repetitive electrical activity when applied to cultured dorsal root ganglion cells. Immunoglobulins from patients with Isaacs' syndrome suppress voltage-gated potassium currents but do not alter gating kinetics or significantly affect sodium currents (337). Antibodies against VGKCs were detected in half the patients, with the highest titers in 2 patients with classic Isaacs' syndrome and low titers in 1 patient with anti-GM1–associated neuropathy.

All 3 patients with Isaacs' syndrome and the 1 patient with neuropathy responded to PE. This response did not fully correlate with the presence of VGKC antibodies, although a decline in titers following therapy was demonstrated. Direct evidence that a humoral factor in patients with Isaacs' syndrome is indeed suppressing potassium channels from a neuronal cell line (PC12) has been demonstrated (338). Immune staining showed that these antibodies, particularly IgM, reacted to VGKC and/or a closely associated protein (confirmed by cross-linking studies) and human intramuscular nerve axons (339). Studies employing newer molecular immunohistochemical assay may increase the detection rate of VGKC antibodies (335).

Successful symptomatic treatment with phenytoin 300 to 400 mg/day or carbamazepine 200 mg 3 of 4 times a day has been reported frequently. In 1 patient with increased GABA in the CSF, dantrolene sodium was as effective as phenytoin or carbamazepine (331). Combined oral steroids and azathioprine (323) or azathioprine alone (340) have been effective for longer-term treatment and have given additional benefit to those showing response to PE. High-dose intravenous immunoglobulin (IVIG) has been reported both to improve (341) and to exacerbate symptoms (342), the latter possibly because of a direct effect of IVIG on muscle or nerve terminals (343). Patients often remain well on symptomatic therapy alone over many years, leading normal lives, as demonstrated by Isaacs' own 10-year follow-up report of his original cases (344). Diazepam, clonazepam, and baclofen usually offer no benefit, although partial response has been rarely noted (323,345).

Other Acquired Conditions

Other acquired conditions include those possibly related to or responsible for CMUA clinically similar to that of Isaacs' syndrome. Those conditions associated with tumor or other autoimmune disorders may prove to be indistinguishable from Isaacs' syndrome and may share an immune-mediated mechanism (325,333). A paraneoplastic syndrome has been implicated in conditions associated with bronchogenic carcinoma, with (346) and without (347,348) peripheral neuropathy; Hodgkin's lymphoma with resolution of cancer and CMUA following chemotherapy (349); and thymoma with (350,351) and without (350) peripheral neuropathy. The same association has occurred in patients who also had myasthenia gravis and peripheral neuropathy (351), and these two disorders with CMUA all improved dramatically with PE (352), implicating autoimmunity as a common pathogenetic factor. Patients with CMUA have been reported in association with immune-mediated neuropathy, including Guillain-Barré syndrome (353,354) and chronic inflammatory demyelinating polyneuropathy (CIDP) (355,356), including a nerve biopsy–proven case in which remission of the CIDP and motor unit hyperactivity followed treatment with prednisone and azathioprine (357,358). Le Gars et al. described a patient with antinuclear and anti-Gm antibodies and motor conduction block who responded to PE. Other autoimmune diseases associated with CMUA include juvenile rheumatoid arthritis (359).

An autoimmune pathogenesis even may play a role in some cases associated with drugs or toxins, such as penicillamine (360), which is also a known cause of myasthenia gravis. CMUA has been associated with exposure to other toxins—some with peripheral neuropathy, such as insecticides (361), and others without peripheral neuropathy, including gold therapy (362) and mercury (363). Some cases of mercury or gold intoxication may be the cause of Morvan's fibrillary chorea. This syndrome, mostly reported in the French literature, causes profuse fasciculations and can resemble Isaacs' syndrome, although it differs in the absence of muscle stiffness, presence of acrodynia, and signs of central disorder (350,364–367). It is now recognized that some cases of Morvan's syndrome may be of paraneoplastic origin or associated with other autoimmune disorders and increased VGKC antibody titers (368). Symptoms of some patients with CMUA may be exacerbated by other types of exposure, such as alcohol consumption, heat, and metrizamide myelography (the latter in 1 patient we observed). This syndrome also has been reported in association with peripheral neuropathy of known causation, such as diabetes (369) and nutritional (355) as well as idiopathic peripheral neuropathy (284,323,370,371). In a review of patients with CMUA and peripheral neuropathy, no significant difference from Isaacs' syndrome was found other than differences due to signs of neuropathy; splitting these disorders on this or any other basis has been questioned (372). However, there may be differences in pathogenesis. The electrophysiology may be more complicated in patients with peripheral neuropathy. For example, it has been suggested that the generator site for spontaneous activity in a patient with CMUA and an axonal motor neuropathy varies among discharges, perhaps affected by the location of a conduction block within an axon (373). In addition, response to treatment may differ, although more studies are needed before conclusions can be drawn. According to rare reports, immunosuppression and PE have been used without success in patients with this syndrome and idiopathic peripheral neuropathy (323), including a patient whose disease was refractory to multiple symptomatic medicines and oral steroids but who responded dramatically to valproic acid 200 mg 3 times a day (374). The only patients with peripheral neuropathy responding to immunotherapy have been those previously discussed who probably had immune-mediated neuropathy, suggesting that these patients have a disease closely related to Isaacs' syndrome and that patients with other acquired or idiopathic peripheral neuropathy may have had different pathogenetic factors.

Within the spectrum of this syndrome not associated with peripheral neuropathy are two disorders with mild and intermediate degrees of motor unit hyperactivity. Several similar cases of a mild phenotype of Isaacs' syndrome were characterized by cramps (whose discharges also may be captured on electromyograms) and occasionally myokymia, but with fasciculations as the only predominant EMG abnormality. This has been described by Tahmoush et al. (375) as the "cramp–fasciculation syndrome," which is effectively managed with carbamazepine. A similar syndrome has been reported as "muscular pain–fasciculation syndrome" (256,258). Intermediate in this spectrum is myokymia–cramp syndrome, which has both clinical and EMG evidence of myokymia (376). Symptomatic treatment is similar to that for Isaacs' syndrome; quinine sulfate also may be effective. Some of these cases also may have an autoimmune or paraneoplastic basis.

Hereditary Disorders

CMUA has been found in association with hereditary disorders with or without peripheral neuropathy. Those with peripheral neuropathy include hereditary motor neuropathy (377,378); hereditary motor sensory neuropathy (HMSN) type 2 (379,380); an interesting case of HMSN 1 whose predominant manifestation was incapacitating muscle cramps (381); and a case of autosomal dominant spinocerebellar ataxia type 1 (SCA2 linked) (382). The new type of hereditary motor and sensory neuropathy linked to chromosome 3 associated with painful muscle cramps and fasciculation has been reported from Japan (383). Those not associated with peripheral neuropathy are also commonly autosomal dominant. What follows is a brief review of these families, whose main features include (a) stiffness and continuous motor unit discharges or myokymia with cramps; (b) myokymia with paroxysmal movement disorders; and (c) persistent muscle cramps.

Persistent muscle twitching and episodic stiffness since early childhood were the predominant symptoms in an African-American family with the autosomal dominant form of CMUA (384). The continuous discharges appear to originate in the intrathecal portion of the nerve roots or motor neuron somata. Families with continuous discharges generated from distal portions of nerves also have been described (385). Generalized myokymia and mild calf cramps were the major manifestations in hereditary myokymia reported by Sheaff (386). Clinical variation within the same family can be seen with some of these inherited forms of CMUA. We have examined a patient with the Isaacs' syndrome phenotype whose daughter had myalgia, cramps, exercise intolerance, fasciculation, and electrical evidence of mild, distal denervation. Unlike her mother, she did not have myokymia and responded poorly to phenytoin and carbamazepine treatment. Rippling muscle disease, discussed previously, superficially resembles this group of hereditary disorders associated with CMUA. Schwartz-Jampel syndrome, described previously in the section on myotonic disorders, also can be classified under this section because its electrical discharges have muscle or neurogenic origin.

Myokymia is present in several rare familial paroxysmal movement disorders. These conditions display intrafamilial and interfamilial variations that often overlap and are traditionally named after the predominant clinical features. Several families with an autosomal dominant illness with paroxysmal (or episodic) ataxia (PA) and persistent myokymia (PA type 1, or PA-1) have been reported (387–390). Affected patients have attacks of sudden onset of stiffness or limpness, incoordination, trembling, and dysarthria that typically last for seconds to as long as 15 minutes. Associated congenital contractures of the distal extremities also have been described (388). The attacks are commonly precipitated by sudden, forceful movements (kinesigenic type) or by physical or emotional stress. Myokymia, present on the electromyogram and often clinically, helps distinguish these families from those with the more common illness, PA with interictal nystagmus (PA-2). PA-2 usually responds to treatment with carbonic anhydrase inhibitors, possibly because of normalization of intracellular pH with stabilization of neuronal membranes, normalization of transmitter release or ion channel function, or restoration of enzyme function (391). In contrast, it is usually stated that this treatment is ineffective in PA-1 (389,392). However, others have reported reduction in attacks, although the myokymia actually may worsen (390,393). Phenytoin may give partial control of symptoms, including myokymia. Potassium channels have been implicated, as in Isaacs' syndrome, in the pathogenesis of this disorder. Several point mutations in the VGKC gene have been reported (394,395).

Possibly related to PA-1 are some phenotypes of paroxysmal dyskinesia that rarely have been associated with myokymia. This is supported by some members of families with clinical and genetic features of PA-1 who also display clinical features of paroxysmal kinesigenic choreoathetosis (393,395). Paroxysmal dystonic choreoathetosis (PDC) with myokymia, an even more rare disorder, has been reported as affecting 5 generations in a single family whose members suffered from minute- to hour-long episodes of paroxysmal muscle stiffness, dystonic posturing, and choreoathetosis from childhood. These episodes were relieved rapidly by rest or sleep (396). Of the 7 affected family members, 2 had prominent myokymia. It remains to be seen whether this form is a variant of PDC without myokymia linked to chromosome 2q (397).

Also, a hereditary form of CMUA with persistent widespread or local cramps has been reported. Two families have been described with a dominantly inherited cramp syndrome affecting almost any muscle (especially thorax, abdomen, and neck) except those of the head (398,399). It begins in adolescence or young adulthood, is not associated with other neurologic abnormalities, and is neurogenic. A more localized dominantly inherited syndrome with persistent distal cramps also has been described

(400,401). This syndrome is characterized by painful distal cramps resulting in flexion or extension of toes, flexion of wrists and metacarpophalangeal joints, and extension of interphalangeal joints. The symptoms usually begin in childhood, initially only after exertion but later occurring at rest, especially after strenuous activity. Cramps also occur during sleep and are aggravated by exposure to cold. Episodes of muscle pain in the neck, chest, low back, and legs can be precipitated by infections, but alcohol ingestion, fasting, or excitement does not provoke cramping. Exercise-induced twitching of calf muscles without evidence of weakness and atrophy is sometimes present. The symptoms persist throughout life. Nerve conduction studies do not indicate a peripheral neuropathy, although mild abnormalities were noted in 1 case (401). Electromyogram shows signs of mild denervation with normal motor-unit potentials during cramps and electrical silence afterward. Neither spinal anesthesia nor nerve block modifies the cramp, but local infiltration of the hand muscles with lidocaine halts contraction, indicating a peripheral nerve origin. Carbamazepine, phenytoin, quinine, and various muscle relaxants offer no benefit.

Tetany

Tetany, commonly associated with hypocalcemia, is broadly characterized by distal nerve paresthesia, muscle cramps, involuntary carpopedal spasms, attacks of laryngeal stridor, and convulsions. Overt or subclinical hyperventilation with respiratory alkalosis and compression-induced ischemia are well-known triggering factors that can reveal "latent" tetany (402,403). The peripheral nerves of susceptible individuals also display hyperirritability to mechanical (Chvostek's sign) or electrical stimulation. Latent tetany also has been termed *spasmophilia* by French and German authors.

In tetany, paresthetic symptoms almost always precede spasm and cramp. In the hands, the intrinsic muscles are affected earliest, causing tonic adduction of the thumb and fingers, flexion of metacarpophalangeal joints, extension of interphalangeal joints, and flexion of wrist and elbow (Fig. 38.8). In susceptible individuals, these symptoms can be reproduced easily by application and inflation of a blood pressure cuff above the elbow (Trousseau's sign). If the sensory symptoms or signs appear within 3 minutes of ischemia, the test is interpreted as positive. In the feet, there is plantar flexion of the foot and toes followed by foot inversion. Rarely, trunk spasm occurs and causes opisthotonic posture. On EMG, tetanic spasms characteristically are accompanied by irregular repetitive action potentials resembling motor-unit potentials. As the disorder progresses, pairs or groups of potentials (double spikes, doublets, or multiplets) appear repeatedly at 5- to 15-ms intervals. In well-developed spasms, large, higher-frequency motor unit potentials, indistinguishable from one another, predominate (404,405). Tetanic potentials abate with infusion of curare but not with peripheral nerve block, suggesting that the spontaneous discharges occur at

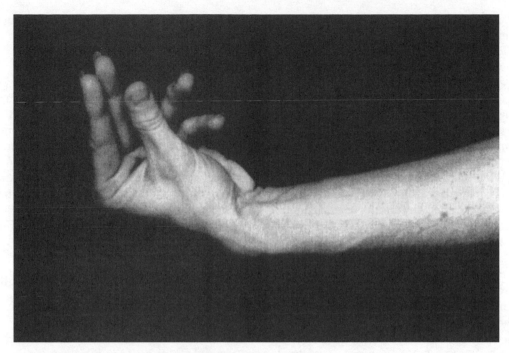

Figure 38.8 Tetany.

some point along the length of the peripheral nerve. Application of a blood pressure cuff below the nerve block induces carpopedal spasm. If the plasma level of ionized calcium is reduced (e.g., hypoparathyroidism, hyperventilation-induced alkalosis), decreased extracellular calcium results in increased sodium conductance, membrane depolarization, and spontaneous rhythmic action potentials (406). The largest nerves have the lowest thresholds, sensory nerves more than motor, and the proximal parts of nerves are more susceptible than distal portions to the effects of ischemia and hypocalcemia. If a subject hyperventilates with an inflated blood pressure cuff on one arm, the spasm occurs first in the free hand, implying that the alkalotic blood must reach the periphery to trigger the symptom. Ischemia of one arm leaves that hand more susceptible to spasm from hyperventilation. Other electrolyte abnormalities can cause tetany and carpopedal spasm. Hypocalcemia was probably the primary cause for tetany also associated with hyperphosphatemia resulting from routine bowel preparation with an oral phosphate–based laxative (407). Magnesium deficiency has also been associated with tetany (408), although levels of plasma-ionized calcium are seldom reported in these cases. Tetany has also been associated with drugs such as diltiazem (409) and alendronate (Fosamax) (410), and has occurred during thyroid surgery postoperative course (410,411). Even in patients diagnosed with panic disorder, concomitant latent tetany due to decreased intracellular magnesium responsive to magnesium salts can occur; therefore, it has been suggested that evaluation of such patients should include red blood cell magnesium levels (412). The alterations in potassium that can lead to tetany appear to be more complicated. While

potassium administration in hypocalcemic patients can exacerbate tetany, isolated hypokalemia also can paradoxically provoke tetany through an unknown mechanism (413). Occasional reports of *normocalcemic tetany* (414,415) are difficult to explain but emphasize that neuronal hyper-irritability may be related to any mechanism that brings the membrane potential nearer the firing threshold or delays repolarization.

Tetany is managed by correcting the underlying metabolic disorder or hyperventilation syndrome. In hyperventilation or anxiety states, patients usually are not aware of their overbreathing, although they sometimes admit to periods of sighing. It is, therefore, important to reproduce the tetanic symptom by encouraging the patient to overbreathe spontaneously and to demonstrate that they can hold their breath for a considerable period, even during an attack. An attack sometimes can be terminated by having the patient breathe in and out of a paper bag or inhale a 5% carbon dioxide mixture. However, attention to the underlying anxiety state is of utmost importance.

Other Mineral and Electrolyte Disorders

In addition to calcium, several other mineral and electrolyte disorders can induce cramps (416,417). Hypokalemia, commonly resulting from diuretic use, laxative abuse, diarrhea, hyperaldosteronism, or metabolic acidosis, is often associated with cramps. Cramps and fasciculation frequently are seen in acute hyponatremia. Hypomagnesemia—commonly resulting from inadequate dietary intake associated with alcoholism and malnutrition; malabsorption and increased intestinal losses associated with vomiting, diarrhea, or laxative abuse; or increased urinary excretion associated with renal dysfunction and diuretic use—can cause weakness, cramps, fasciculation, and tetany. A detailed history and appropriate laboratory studies readily reveal these reversible conditions.

Eosinophilia-Myalgia Syndrome

In 1989 and 1990 a transient epidemic known as eosinophilia–myalgia syndrome (EMS) affected more than 1500 users of L-tryptophan, with estimates of at least twice that number ultimately affected in the United States (418,419). The epidemic has been linked with the use of a single manufacturer's product containing several contaminants that appear to be chemically related to L-tryptophan. The exact toxin and its mechanism of action remain undefined. Theories include direct toxic effect from one or more contaminants, eosinophil products, or L-tryptophan metabolites, as well as effects mediated by activated T cells, macrophages, and fibroblasts, all possibly influenced by host factors such as genetic susceptibility (418). EMS shares many features with the Spanish toxic oil syndrome, including identification of a chemical link (420), and both appear to be chronic contaminant-induced immune-mediated disorders.

EMS is a clinically heterogeneous syndrome characterized by myalgia and fatigue with associated symptoms and signs that include eosinophilia, eosinophilic pneumonia, edema, fasciitis, alopecia, sclerodermatous skin changes, myopathy, arthralgia, and neuropathy (421,422). Severe disabling cramps and spasms, usually in axial muscles, can occur as a late sequela. Postural tremor and myokymia of suspected peripheral origin and myoclonus also have been reported as uncommon delayed manifestations of EMS (419). Although overall most signs and symptoms of EMS improve with time (423), it is common for patients to suffer from chronic myalgia and fatigue with variable presence of cardiac, neurologic, hematologic, dermatologic, and pulmonary complications (424,425). Some patients may show delayed neurocognitive deficits and have abnormalities of brain white matter (426). Muscle cramps are a common complaint among EMS patients. Among 19 EMS patients followed by us, severe cramps were noted by 4; moderate cramps by 6; and mild cramps by 5. The cramps typically have sudden onset precipitated by activity. They can occur in any muscle group, with the jaw, thorax, and legs particularly affected. The clinical features of the cramps suggest a neuropathic origin, but cramps also can occur in patients who do not have clinical or electrodiagnostic evidence of a neuropathy. When the cramps and spasms are severe and result in distortion of body posture, they bear some resemblance to those in Satoyoshi's syndrome (see Central Nervous System Causes of Cramps and Myalgia). In muscle biopsy specimens, inflammatory cells frequently surround the muscle spindles and small intramuscular nerves, and we suspect that immune-mediated damage to these structures leads to cramps. Most of the commonly used treatments for cramps are ineffective in EMS. Some patients have been treated successfully with oral dantrolene sodium.

Toxic Envenomation

Severe muscle spasm may accompany a variety of toxic envenomations and ingestions (427). In these conditions, the history and associated clinical findings are paramount in making the correct diagnosis. Muscle cramps are a significant clinical feature of stings by the stingray, scorpion, catfish's spike, and jellyfish. Timber rattlesnake venom can induce myokymia, and South American rattlesnake venom can cause myalgia, myonecrosis, and myoglobinuria. Cramps that follow the bite of the black widow spider can be relieved with intravenous calcium gluconate and intramuscular antivenin.

CNS Causes of Cramps and Myalgia

Satoyoshi's Syndrome (Progressive Muscle Spasm, Alopecia, and Diarrhea)

This distinctive progressive syndrome, first described by Satoyoshi and Yamada (428), has been reported mainly in several unrelated Japanese patients under the name *komura-gaeri* (calf spasm) disease. Additional cases in Chinese patients and non-Asian individuals have been described (429). The syndrome usually begins in childhood or adolescence and is marked by intermittent painful muscle spasms that are so severe that the limb, trunk, or other affected body part is twisted into a sustained abnormal posture (Fig. 38.9). Nonstimulus-sensitive myoclonus may be present at rest, giving the patient a twitchy appearance. Characteristically, patients are completely normal before the onset of cramps. Most patients are simultaneously or subsequently affected by additional abnormalities, including alopecia universalis, intestinal malabsorption with diarrhea, endocrinopathy with amenorrhea, and multiple secondary skeletal abnormalities mimicking metaphysial dysplasia (429). Patients are at risk for skeletal deformities, growth retardation, and general emaciation, which to some degree are preventable with early diagnosis and treatment.

In almost all cases, the initial symptom is muscle cramps. Alopecia appears simultaneously in about one-half of patients. Muscle spasms become progressively more severe and frequent; each painful spasm lasts up to a few minutes but may recur immediately with movement or stimulation of the affected area. The frequency of muscle spasms varies from several to hundreds per day. The spasms are readily precipitated by voluntary contraction and generally do not occur during rest or sleep. Factors such as exposure to cold, fever, dehydration, and emotional stress tend to lower the threshold for spasm. The spasms often displace and fix the limb (Fig. 38.9A), and with sustained contraction the muscle becomes boardlike to palpation and bulges prominently (Fig. 38.9B). The frequency, severity, and chronic course of cramps in this syndrome are far beyond the usual muscle spasm, may require emergency care for pain control, and are

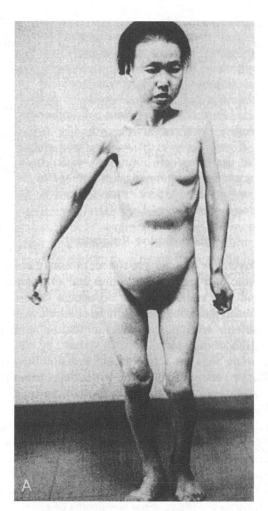
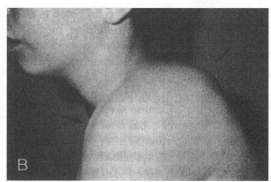

Figure 38.9 **A:** Satoyoshi's syndrome. Note the extreme emaciation, with distended abdomen; loss of scalp hair, eyebrows, and body hair; deformities of both knee joints and left elbow; and atrophy of the left biceps, deltoid, and triceps muscles. Muscle cramps continue to occur in the right arm and thigh muscles. Some muscles were hypertrophic when the subject was younger. **B:** Satoyoshi's syndrome. Note the severe pectoralis and trapezius cramps (arrows) induced by an attempt to lift the arm over the head. Severe neck extensor weakness is also present. (**A**, Courtesy of E. Satoyoshi, National Center of Neurology and Psychiatry, Kodaira-shi, Tokyo.)

appropriately described as *myospasm gravis* (430). The recurrent and severe nature of the cramps is probably responsible for traumatic injury to skeletal structures leading to the various skeletal abnormalities described in this syndrome (431).

During spasms, EMG recordings reveal synchronized motor unit discharges of 40 to 60 per second and of 4- to 10-mV amplitudes, similar to the rate of discharges in maximal voluntary contraction. Spasms also can be induced by repetitive nerve stimulation. There may be an afterdischarge following H reflex, suggesting an interruption of the inhibitory effect of Renshaw cells on motor neurons (430). This evidence, with the alleviation of cramp during sleep and general anesthesia and its elimination by nerve block and curare, supports a central origin for the cramp, presumably resulting from hyperexcitability of the anterior horn cells. Autopsy studies have not revealed structural abnormalities of the CNS. The pathogenesis of this syndrome remains unknown. Indirect evidence for

autoimmune mechanism includes beneficial response of muscle spasm, amenorrhea, and alopecia to glucocorticoids (429,432); association with other autoimmune disorders, such as myasthenia gravis (433), systemic lupus erythematosus, and idiopathic thrombocytopenia, 434); evidence of IgG production in the CSF (435); and presence of glutamic acid decarboxylase (GAD) antibodies (436). Malabsorption-related mechanisms, such as metabolic derangement, also have been suggested (430). However, with the exception of mild iron deficiency, a flat response to oral glucose loading, and mild hyperphosphatemia, metabolic measurements are usually normal.

We have followed a white patient with Satoyoshi's syndrome (Fig. 38.9B) in whom colonoscopy, esophagogastroduodenoscopy, intestinal biopsies, and laboratory tests for malabsorption are all normal. These findings make it unlikely that malabsorption is responsible for the syndrome. The patient, while keeping a daily log of cramp severity, was first treated with oral dantrolene sodium 200 mg/day, and later oral prednisone 1 mg/kg per day was added. Two months after starting prednisone, a significant, sustained reduction in cramp severity was noted. Attempts to taper prednisone below 0.5 mg/kg per day have resulted in worsening of cramps. Multiple studies of immune function were normal before treatment, including CSF (with oligoclonal banding), sedimentation rate, serum immunoelectrophoresis, C-reactive protein, C3, C4, CH100, antinuclear antibodies, rheumatoid factor, and antithyroid antibodies. A Raji cell assay for circulating immune complexes was elevated, and mild eosinophilia was present. The beneficial response to prednisone and the generally normal immunologic workup are consistent with reports from other investigators, although abnormalities in lymphocyte subpopulation studies have been noted (429). A similar patient from Thailand (437) also was treated successfully with corticosteroid. Improvements in the muscular and systemic symptoms have been reported to improve with oral tacrolimus in combination with steroids (438).

The need for adequate management of muscle spasms is particularly important when they are life threatening. Patients with severe and frequent spasm are at risk for death from respiratory arrest, and feeding difficulties from masticatory muscle spasm can lead to severe wasting. Some patients respond to calcium gluconate, quinine sulfate, procainamide, or phenytoin. Botulinum toxin may prove to be useful in the management of severe masticatory spasm (439). Dantrolene sodium 100 to 200 mg/day orally decreases or abolishes attacks of cramping, but neither controls spasms completely nor prevents muscle spasms precipitated by voluntary effort or by electrical stimulation. With dantrolene therapy, the long-term prognosis has improved, with patients surviving into adulthood and occasional remission of the illness. Immunosuppression shows promise in improving treatment, not only for the muscle spasms but also for other associated features. IVIG with frequent pulse therapy was effective in reducing muscle spasms and titers of serum autoantibodies in 1 patient and may prove to be a safer alternative to immunosuppressive agents in these young patients (434).

Strychnine Poisoning

Strychnine was previously used in rodent poisons and in some tonics and cathartics. Since it was removed from commercial use and from all medicinal products in the United States, strychnine poisoning has become rare (440). However, accidental and intentional poisonings continue as a result of its use as an adulterant for illicit drugs, presence in stored rodenticides and products from other countries, and use in home remedies. It acts by interfering with postsynaptic inhibition at all levels of the CNS via competition with the action of glycine. Its rapid absorption and distribution to neuronal tissues allow symptoms to develop within an hour after ingestion. The patient experiences heightened irritability and muscle twitching, followed by leg rigidity, facial tetanus, and apnea caused by

spasm of the respiratory muscles. Opisthotonos and general convulsions develop, but the patient remains alert. Excessive muscle activity may cause muscle injury and myoglobinuria; severe respiratory muscle involvement can result in anoxia and death. The clinical picture sometimes resembles that of tetanus or of stiff-man syndrome (SMS). Intravenous diazepam or short-acting barbiturates can control spasms effectively. Supportive care and close observation are essential. Gastric lavage should be performed only after the airway is secure and seizures controlled.

Tetanus

Tetanus is an acute fulminant disease with an improved but still significant mortality rate. It is caused by an exotoxin produced in a wound by *Clostridium tetani* (441). There are probably 300,000 to 500,000 cases of tetanus worldwide each year; improvement of treatment with intensive care has reduced mortality from 44% to 15% (442,443). In the United States, fewer than 100 cases per year are reported. Rarely, tetanus occurs in the fully immunized person (444).

The typical first symptoms of tetanus—muscle stiffness and pain—can begin 2 to 56 (usually 4 to 14) days after injury. Reflex spasm of the masseters on touching the posterior pharyngeal wall (spatula test) is highly specific for tetanus and can be useful in the evaluation of patients presenting during early stages of this illness (445). A short incubation period indicates severe disease. Jaw stiffness progressing to lockjaw (trismus), dysphagia, and rigidity of the back (opisthotonos), abdomen, and eventually all muscles are the cardinal symptoms of generalized tetanus. The intensity and severity of muscle involvement are variable. Within 24 to 72 hours of the first symptoms, reflex spasms (sudden intensification of a spasm triggered by sensory stimuli, emotion, or movement) develop. These severe spasms can be painful and can cause respiratory difficulties or muscle injury; they result from disinhibition of usual motor-neuron dampening mechanisms. Patients are almost invariably conscious and mentally alert. After about 10 days, spasms become less frequent. A hypersympathetic state often supervenes but disappears by the end of 2 weeks. A few patients have prolonged residual stiffness. Rare cases of chronic tetanus can closely resemble stiff-man syndrome, described in the next section (446); a primary differentiating factor is trismus, which is never seen in stiff-man syndrome, and the spasms seen in tetanus typically are more violent than in stiff-man syndrome.

A small proportion of patients develop yet another variety of tetanus—local tetanus—in which signs and symptoms develop only in the region of the injury. This disease is often mild and may persist for months. The symptoms of local tetanus usually resolve spontaneously but may develop into the general form. Rarely, local tetanus affects the facial and lower cranial musculature (cephalic tetanus), with a poor prognosis.

Electromyographic examination in tetanus reveals continuous motor unit discharges that disappear during sleep, during general or spinal anesthesia, and after peripheral nerve block. Masseter muscle reactions are usually abnormal in generalized tetanus. Specifically, there is no silent period following the elicitation of the masseter reflex by a jaw tap. Normally, this silent period lasts 50 to 100 ms and is mainly the result of recurrent inhibition of motor neuron excitability. The shortened or absent silent period in tetanus (446) probably results from failed Renshaw cell inhibition. This characteristic electrodiagnostic feature seldom occurs in other disorders of motor unit hyperactivity, including stiff-man syndrome.

The tetanus toxin is known to bypass retrograde axoplasmic transport to the CNS and to enter the presynaptic nerve terminal of inhibitory interneurons, blocking release of the inhibitory transmitter glycine and GABA (447). This results in the release of motor neurons from inhibitory controls, increasing motor neuron activity.

Strychnine poisoning and, superficially, the dystonic reactions resulting from phenothiazines and metoclopramide resemble tetanus. Doubt about the diagnosis usually is clarified by clinical observation over several hours. Treatment of tetanus is discussed in detail in standard textbooks and reviews (441,448). Spasms and rigidity are best treated with GABA agonists. A long-acting benzodiazepine (lorazepam) is recommended, but whenever high doses fail to control spasm, neuromuscular blocking agents should be used. Intravenous magnesium sulfate also has been used successfully in severe cases (449).

Stiff-Man Syndrome (Moersch-Woltman Syndrome)

Stiff-man syndrome, described by Moersch and Woltman (450) and critically reviewed by Gordon et al. (451), Whiteley et al. (452), Lorish et al. (453), McEvoy (454), and Pleitez and Harati (455), is characterized by the insidious onset of intermittent stiffness, usually symmetric, particularly of the axial muscles (thoracolumbar, abdominal, and cervical) and those of proximal limbs (Fig. 38.10). This syndrome usually occurs in adults, although it is seen in a wide

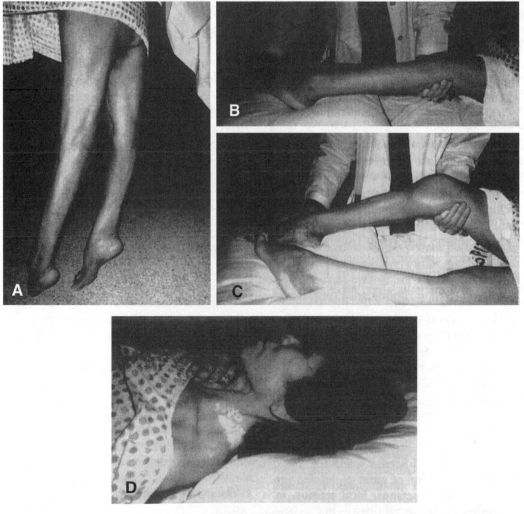

Figure 38.10 Stiff-man syndrome. **A:** Sustained hyperextension of the knees and plantar flexion of the feet. **B:** An examiner unsuccessfully attempts to flex the knees. **C:** After spinal anesthesia, the knees can be flexed. **D:** Vitiligo in a patient with stiff-man syndrome. (Courtesy of Joseph J. Jankovic, MD, Baylor College of Medicine, Houston, TX.)

range of ages, is slightly more common in women (456), and is usually sporadic. A congenital form also has been reported (457–459). As the disease slowly worsens, the fluctuating stiffness becomes persistent, and many patients develop painful and often violent spasms evoked by noise, fright, initiation of speech, strain at voiding, and other external stimuli. Active or passive movement aggravates the pain, and the extremities may be immobilized in unnatural positions, with simultaneous contractions of agonist and antagonist muscles. A lumbar hyperlordosis is common, and the neck may be held against the chest in a tonic posture of the fixed shrug. Paraspinal hypertrophy can be seen in later stages of disease. Stiffness produces a characteristic slow, stiff-legged gait with difficulties accentuated by attempts to turn. Generalized spasms show a pattern of opisthotonos and, if the patient is standing, can cause him or her to fall forward suddenly "like a wooden soldier" (454). The facial muscles usually are spared, although muscles of swallowing are occasionally affected (450). Attacks of muscle spasms have been associated with autonomic instability, which may explain some cases of sudden death (460). A focal form of SMS limited to one limb, with no or slow progression to other limbs, has been described (456,461,462).

Other than findings related to muscle rigidity, neurologic examination is normal, although there can be exaggeration of deep tendon reflexes and atrophy and weakness related to disuse. Myokymia or fasciculations are absent. In rare cases an unusual type of reflex myoclonus (spontaneous or triggered by muscle stretch or other sensory stimuli) can be superimposed on the rigidity in jerking SMS (463,464). SMS is typically a slowly progressive disease, but some cases remain stable for many years. Others may progress to total disability in a few years, and rare cases remit spontaneously.

The EMG in SMS shows continuous motor unit discharges (sustained interference pattern) similar to normal voluntary contractions, with simultaneous contractions in antagonist muscles despite the patient's attempts to relax. These findings are not pathognomonic for SMS, and it is the clinical setting that allows distinction from activity of unrelaxed muscles in otherwise normal patients or from abnormal muscle tone in patients with pyramidal or extrapyramidal disease. As expected from the clinical features, the motor unit discharges are more intense in axial and proximal limb muscles. Superimposed spontaneous and stimulus-evoked worsening of these discharges can be recorded in most patients. The clinical and electrical muscle activity disappears or decreases markedly during sleep, especially during rapid eye movement (REM) sleep; sedation; general anesthesia; nerve or ventral root block; or with administration of curare or diazepam. The silent period following elicitation of a stretch reflex (H reflex) has a normal duration, indicating no impairment of Renshaw cell inhibition. Meinck et al. (465), in a study of patients similar to those previously reported as having jerking SMS, described spasmodic reflex myoclonus and the unique characteristics of its burst potentials.

Routine laboratory testing and CSF analysis usually are normal. Nearly one-third of patients have evidence of insulin-dependent diabetes mellitus (IDDM); rare patients have oligoclonal bands in the CSF; and approximately 40% have organ-specific autoantibodies (454) related to associated autoimmune diseases (Hashimoto's thyroiditis, Graves' disease, myasthenia gravis vitiligo, pernicious anemia, and others). Autoantibodies to glutamic acid decarboxylase (GAD) (discussed in subsequent paragraphs) were found in the serum in up to 60% of patients (466) and in the CSF in 68% of patients from pooled data (455). A new immunoprecipitation assay is reported to make such autoantibody testing simpler and more readily available (467). Magnetic resonance imaging (MRI) of the brain in 1 patient revealed an inflammatory type of lesions first detected years after the onset of stiffness (454). Involvement of thoracic muscles results in a restrictive pattern on pulmonary function tests. Skeletal muscles are usually normal, although mild nonspecific changes of atrophic fibers, nuclear clumps, internal nuclei, and slight fibrosis (possibly due to spasm-induced prolonged ischemia) have been reported (468,469). In 2 cases, perimysial and perivascular inflammatory changes were observed (471).

Specific diagnostic criteria for SMS have been proposed by Gordon (451) and updated by Lorish et al. (453). They include (a) a prodrome of axial aching and stiffness; (b) slow progression of stiffness to include proximal limb muscles, with resultant difficulties in walking and other volitional movement; (c) a fixed lumbar lordosis or, less commonly, a permanent shrug of the shoulders; (d) superimposed episodic spasms precipitated by emotional or external stimuli; (e) abolition of rigidity during sleep; (f) normal findings on motor and sensory examinations; (g) normal intellect; and (h) typical EMG findings of continuous motor unit activity that is abolished or reduced by intravenous or oral diazepam. Meinck et al. (471) expanded the clinical features to include (a) spasmodic myoclonus with opisthotonos and stereotypic motor response in legs and feet, often preceded by (b) an auralike feeling of an impending attack; and (c) phobia associated with unaccompanied walking in open space. Supportive evidence includes the presence of anti-GAD antibodies (Abs) in the serum.

Since the spasms and rigidity of SMS abate or lessen during sleep and general anesthesia, abnormalities of the brain and/or spinal cord were investigated. In 1 autopsy case, a detailed count of neural perikarya in the spinal ventral horn confirmed that the disease selectively destroyed small and medium-sized neurons, most of which were spinal internuncial neurons. Damage to these inhibitory neurons theoretically allows for excessive and abnormal discharges by the motor neurons, producing stiffness and spasms (452). Pharmacologic "correction" of this deficient inhibition with diazepam has proved effective and provides support for this hypothesis. Several other autopsy studies have revealed normal or inconclusive findings (454). Histopathologic examinations of the CNS in SMS have shown in individual cases no pathologic changes (468); slightly decreased motor neurons in the lateral nuclei of the central horn in the cervical cord without gliosis (471); spinal neuronal atrophy, gliosis, and fibrosis, with a slight pallor of the dorsal columns (469); and cell loss in the medial motor nuclei of anterior horns that innervate the muscle attached to the axial skeleton (472,473).

Guilleminault et al. (474) suggested that a relative neurotransmitter imbalance, leading to a decreased GABA-mediated neuronal inhibition, was responsible for SMS. In this imbalance, either there is overactivity of the facilatatory descending catecholaminergic influences and/or underactivity of the inhibitory GABAergic influences. Drugs that increase the former (amine uptake inhibitors and levodopa) exacerbated stiffness and spasms, and drugs that either decreased the former (central adrenergic blockers, such as clonidine) or increased the latter (diazepam or baclofen) improved these symptoms (474,475). Catecholamine overactivity in SMS was supported in 2 case reports demonstrating increased urinary excretion of 3-methoxy-4-hydroxyphenylglycol (MHPG), which correlated with clinical status (476,477).

A deficiency of GABA, the main inhibitory neurotransmitter in the CNS, subsequently has become the focus of SMS research. Work by Solimena, De Camilli, and colleagues provided a link with the hypothesis of GABA deficiency and support for an autoimmune mechanism in SMS (478,479). Coexistence of other autoimmune diseases and other autoantibodies with SMS, as discussed, was the first indication that SMS may be an autoimmune disorder. In accordance with the association of SMS with IDDM and the knowledge that pancreatic β cells contain a high concentration of the enzyme GAD, which is responsible for the formation of GABA, they investigated the possibility that SMS was an autoimmune disease caused by autoantibodies directed against GAD (anti-GAD Abs). They postulated that anti-GAD Abs would result in a decrease in CNS GABA with resultant stiffness and spasms. Their initial report of a single SMS patient (who also had epilepsy, IDDM, oligoclonal IgG bands in the CSF, and serum antibodies to pancreatic β cells, parietal cells, thyroglobulin, and thyroid microsomes) provided support for this hypothesis. Antibodies in both the serum and CSF of this patient were immunocytochemically reactive to brain and β pancreatic cells in a pattern suggesting anti-GAD activity. The antibodies also reacted to a single protein that Western blot analysis revealed to be the same protein labeled by GAD antiserum. In subsequent studies, Western blot analysis and immunoprecipitation showed that 20 of 33 patients with SMS had anti-GAD Abs. Patients with anti-GAD activity had a much higher rate of associated autoimmune disease and serum autoantibodies to other antigens than did those without anti-GAD

activity but were otherwise clinically similar. This work subsequently has been confirmed by others, with Lennon and colleagues reporting anti-GAD antibodies in 45 of 46 patients diagnosed with SMS (454).

Interestingly, 4 patients without SMS who were studied by Solimena and colleagues also had anti-GAD Abs, and all had IDDM. This work has provided an exciting speculation that GAD may be the antigen in many cases of IDDM. Up to 80% of patients with newly diagnosed IDDM have serum antibodies to a 64-kd protein shown to be GAD (480). The degree of humoral response and the difference in target antigens are among the suggested explanations for few patients with IDDM developing SMS. Although anti-GAD Abs may arise as a secondary reaction to cellular destruction from other mechanisms, an autoimmune cause for many cases of SMS and IDDM appears likely (481).

More recent support for autoimmunity in SMS comes from human leukocyte antigen (HLA) studies that showed a twofold greater incidence in affected subjects than in controls of carrying a known susceptibility allele (DQB1*0201) for IDDM and other autoimmune diseases (482). SMS patients have an even greater frequency (61%) of circulating autoantibodies if nonorgan–specific types, such as anti-mitochondrial and antismooth muscle Abs, are included (483). Multiple organ-specific polyendocrine autoantibodies were reported in a patient with SMS and IDDM, and anti-GAD Abs were found to recognize a cerebellar protein when she later developed a pancerebellar syndrome (484). Additional organ-specific autoantibodies recognize antigens with tissue distribution similar to GAD. They include SMS cases that are anti-GAD Ab negative (485,486). Current research is focusing on the clues provided by the presence of anti-GAD Abs in SMS, IDDM, and other autoimmune diseases, which may help determine what pathogenic role, if any, this autoantibody has in SMS. In these diseases, antibodies to 1 of the 2 GAD isozymes (GAD65) appear to be most selective. Although there is overlap in the humoral response against GAD in SMS and IDDM, Daw et al. (487) found the titers 100- to 500-fold higher in SMS and, expounding on earlier studies (488), demonstrated that there were GAD65 epitopes uniquely recognized by SMS but not IDDM sera. This finding has been confirmed by a later study by Lohnmann, et al. (490) where distinct T-cell epitopes of GAD65 are observed in SMS and IDDM patients despite similar HLA background. However, the data also indicate that such disease-specific antibody differences probably do not solely determine whether SMS or IDDM develops. Differences in host factors and autoimmune response, including Th1- and Th2-biased immune responses (490), also may be important. Infants born to mothers with SMS and high GAD65 antibody titers may be completely asymptomatic despite the infants having high antibody titers, and this suggests that other coexisting factors are required to develop SMS (491). Other factors, such as hormones, though not causative may have a role in pathophysiology. For example, stiffness in a patient who also had deficiency of adrenocorticotropic hormone (ACTH), prolactin, and growth hormone, as well as SMS, was resolved with administration of ACTH (489). Stiffness of another patient with hyperthyroidism also decreased after the thyroid abnormality was corrected (492).

Several disorders may be confused with SMS. Tetanus, strychnine poisoning, and the tonic spasms of multiple sclerosis are discussed in other sections of this chapter. During early stages of this disease, when motor disturbances are intermittent and neurologic examination is entirely normal, it may be difficult to distinguish from psychogenic disorder. Trojaborg et al. (493) reported a patient whose spinal rigidity was later attributed to ankylosing spondylitis, and Drake (494) reported a patient with "SMS and dementia," which in our opinion was the result of a cerebral multi-infarct state.

The rare congenital myopathy known as *rigid-spine syndrome* is characterized by infantile or childhood onset of proximal limb weakness, followed by painless progressive severe limitations in spine flexion with associated myopathy of paraspinal muscles. Intramedullary spinal cord tumors, primarily cervical, have been associated with continuous motor unit discharges (alpha rigidity) (495). However, most of these patients have additional neurologic, laboratory, or imaging abnormalities.

Several disorders are closely related to SMS. A familial congenital form was mentioned in early discussions of this topic. An anti-GAD Ab negative stiff-man-like syndrome confined to the legs (stiff-leg syndrome) has been postulated to be due to a chronic spinal interneuronitis (496). A rapidly progressive stiff-man-like syndrome has been reported in some cases of encephalomyelitis (452,497–500). It is distinguished from SMS by its clinical course and abnormal neurologic findings, but idiopathic cases may be associated with anti-GAD Abs (501). Neuropathologic studies have shown findings of diffuse encephalomyelitis with perivascular inflammation (460,502) and dense mononuclear infiltrates with surrounding astrocytosis in the anterior horns of the lumbar spinal cord greater than in the cervical spinal cord with relative preservation of large motor neurons and axons (502). Several patients with SMS and malignancy, including some with signs of encephalomyelitis, have been reported (454). These paraneoplastic cases of SMS have anti-Ri antibody (503) and antibody directed against a synaptic vesicle–associated protein (amphiphysin) rather than GAD and may be pathogenically distinct from idiopathic SMS (455). The paraneoplastic SMS occurs most often with breast cancer (504), and SMS may precede the discovery of cancer (505).

The most effective symptomatic treatment for SMS is incremental high-dose diazepam or clonazepam. If these drugs have an unsatisfactory response or are not tolerated, other medications that potentiate the effect of GABA, such as baclofen or sodium valproate (506), and vigabatrin or tiagabine (507–509), may prove beneficial. Baclofen may be used intrathecally in severe cases (510). Phenytoin and carbamazepine are ineffective. Immunosuppression, including a dramatic response to corticosteroids, PE (455), and IVIG (511), has been reported in uncontrolled and controlled (512) studies. The role of anti-GAD Ab measurement in predicting response to immunosuppressive treatment is not known. In paraneoplastic SMS, management of underlying cancer may improve the symptoms.

Familial Nocturnal Cramps

In this unique familial condition, sleep-associated myoclonus is accompanied by sustained painful cramping of the legs, abdomen, and face. The severity of cramps often awakens the patient and causes children to cry (513). All-night polysomnographic recordings show nearly continuous or intermittent muscle EMG activity during sleep, abolished by peripheral nerve block. However, waking electromyography shows no evidence of peripheral neuropathy or radiculopathy. Although sleep normally attenuates muscle activity of central origin, the fact that the activity occurs only during sleep implicates a disturbance of sleep-related inhibitory influences on the lower motor neuron. These findings suggest a central origin (brainstem or spinal) for this syndrome. Treatment with clonazepam produces sustained improvement of symptoms. A similar autosomal dominant syndrome with cramps occurring during both exertion and at rest and during sleep has been reported in 4 generations of a Japanese family (514).

Tonic Spasm of Multiple Sclerosis

Paroxysmal dystonia, tonic spasm, or tonic seizures, first described by Matthews (515), involve brief, recurrent, often painful abnormal posturing of one or more extremities without alteration of consciousness, loss of sphincter control, or clonic movements. Episodes can occur at any time during the course of multiple sclerosis but also can be the initial symptoms of the disease (516–518). Episodes may be precipitated by voluntary movement, spinal flexion, tactile stimulation, hyperventilation, sudden noise, ingestion of alcohol, or sudden exposure to cold (519). Facial grimacing and paroxysmal dysarthria may be associated with dystonic posturing of an extremity. A few patients may have transient (only a few seconds in duration) sensory or autonomic disturbances in the involved limb preceding or during the attack. The entire phenomenon is brief, generally 30 to 45 seconds, and rarely longer than a few minutes in duration, but can recur as often as 30 times daily (520). The absence of electroencephalographic abnormalities and the high frequency of spinal cord abnormalities in these patients suggests that these paroxysms originate from the brainstem or spinal cord (521,522) and, in particular, within the corticospinal tract. This is supported by the findings of exacerbated upper motor neuron signs on the side of the tonic spasm immediately following an attack and by MRI evidence of demyelinating lesions affecting the contralateral corticospinal tract, which also shows electrophysiologic evidence of impairment (523). The most effective treatment is carbamazepine, although phenytoin occasionally is useful. The value of antispasmodic medications is uncertain, and future studies await newer and potentially more effective treatments for spasticity, such as tizanidine (524) and intrathecal baclofen (525).

REFERENCES

1. Oboler SK, Prochazka AV, Meyer TJ. Leg symptoms in outpatient veterans. *West J Med* 1991;155:256–259.
2. Riley JD, Antony SJ. Leg cramps: differential diagnosis and management. *Am Fam Physician* 1995;52:1794–1798.
3. Jansen PH, Joosten EM, Vingerhoets HM. Muscle cramp as a feature of neuromuscular disease: five neuromuscular disorders, accompanied by frequent muscle cramps. *Acta Neurol Belg* 1992;92:138–147.
4. Pourmand R. The value of muscle biopsy in myalgia. *Neurologist* 1997;3:173–177.
5. Serratrice G, Rowland LP. Muscle contractures: essay on a physiological approach to clarify the nomenclature. *Presse Med* 1999;28:1519–1521.
6. Mommaerts WFHM, Illingworth B, Pearson CM, et al. A functional disorder of muscle associated with the absence of phosphorylase. *Proc Natl Acad Sci USA* 1959;45:791–797.
7. Schmid R, Mahler R. Chronic progressive myopathy with myoglobinuria: demonstration of a glycogenolytic defect in the muscle. *J Clin Invest* 1959;38:2044–2058.
8. De Stefano N, Argov Z, Matthews PM, et al. Impairment of muscle mitochondrial oxidative metabolism in McArdle's disease. *Muscle Nerve* 1996;19:764–769.
9. Haller RG, Clausen T, Vissing J. Reduced levels of skeletal muscle Na^+-K^+-ATPase in McArdle disease. *Neurology* 1998;50:37–40.
10. Jehenson P, Leroy-Willig A, de Kerviler E, et al. Impairment of the exercise-induced increase in muscle perfusion in McArdle's disease. *Eur J Nucl Med* 1995;22:1256–1260.
11. Walker AR, Tschetter K, Matsuo F, Flanigan KM, McArdle's disease presenting as recurrent crytogenic renal failure due to occult seizures. *Muscle and Nerve* 2003, 28:640–643.
12. Thornhill MH. Masticatory muscle symptoms in a patient with McArdle's disease. *Oral Surg Oral Med Oral Pathol Oral Radiol Endodont* 1996;81:544–546.
13. Porte D, Crawford DW, Jennings DB, et al. Cardiovascular and metabolic response to exercise in a patient with McArdle's syndrome. *N Engl J Med* 1966;275:406–412.
14. Pernow BB, Havel RJ, Jennings DB. The second wind phenomenon in McArdle's syndrome. *Acta Med Scand* 1967;472(suppl): 294–307.
15. Haller RG, Vissing J. No spontaneous second wind in muscle phosphofructokinase deficiency. *Neurology* 2004,62:82–86.
16. Carroll JE, DeVivo DC, Brooke MH, et al. Fasting as a provocative test in neuromuscular diseases. *Metabolism* 1979;28:683–687.
17. Rowland LP, Araki S, Carmel P. Contracture in McArdle's disease. *Arch Neurol* 1965;13:541–544.
18. Ross BD, Radda GK, Gadian DG, et al. Examination of a case of suspected McArdle's syndrome by 11P nuclear magnetic resonance. *N Engl J Med* 1981;304:1338–1342.
19. Argov Z, Bank WJ, Maris J, et al. Muscle energy metabolism in McArdle's syndrome by in vivo phosphorus magnetic resonance spectroscopy (^{31}P NMR). *Neurology* 1987;37:1720–1724.
20. Russo PJ, Phillips JW, Seidler NW. The role of lipid peroxidation in McArdle's disease: applications for treatment of other myopathies. *Med Hypotheses* 1992;39:147–151.
21. Wolfe GI, Baker NS, Haller RG, et al. McArdle's disease presenting with asymmetric, late-onset arm weakness. *Muscle Nerve* 2000;23:641–645.
22. DiMauro S, Hays AP, Tsujino S. Nonlysosomal glycogenoses. In: Engel AG, Franzini-Armstrong C, eds. *Myology.* 3rd ed. New York: McGraw-Hill, 2004:1535–1558.
23. Kristjcinsson K, Tsujino S, DiMauro S. Myophosphorylase deficiency: an unusually severe form with myoglobinuria. *J Pediatr* 1994;125:409–410.
24. Chiadò-Piat L, Mongini T, Doriguzzi C, et al. Clinical spectrum of McArdle disease: three cases with unusual expression. *Eur Neurol* 1993;33:208–211.
25. DiMauro S, Hartlage PL. Fatal infantile form of muscle phosphorylase deficiency. *Neurology* 1978;28:1124–1129.
26. Cornelio F, Bresolin N, DiMauro S, et al. Congenital myopathy due to phosphorylase deficiency. *Neurology* 1983;33:1383–1385.
27. Engel WK, Eyerman EL, Williams HE. Late-onset type of skeletal muscle phosphorylase deficiency: a new familial variety with completely and partially affected subjects. *N Engl J Med* 1963;268:135–137.
28. Felice KI, Schneebaum AB, Jones HR. McArdle's disease with late-onset symptoms: case report and review of the literature. *J Neurol Neurosurg Psychiatry* 1992;55:407–408.
29. Mineo I, Kono N, Hara N, et al. Myogenic hyperuricemia: a common pathophysiologic feature of glycogenosis types III, V, and VII. *N Engl J Med* 1987;317:75–80.
30. Chui LA, Munsat TL. Dominant inheritance of McArdle syndrome. *Arch Neurol* 1976;33:636–644.
31. Servidei S, Shanske S, Zeviani M, et al. McArdle's disease: biochemical and molecular genetic studies. *Ann Neurol* 1988;24: 774–781.
32. Dawson DM, Spong LF, Harrington JF. McArdle's disease: lack of muscle phosphorylase. *Ann Intern Med* 1968;69:229–235.
33. Schmidt B, Servidei S, Gabbai AA, et al. McArdle's disease in two generations: autosomal recessive transmission with manifesting heterozygote. *Neurology* 1987;37:1558–1561.
34. Manfredi G, Silvestri G, Servidei S, et al. Manifesting heterozygotes in McArdle's disease: clinical, morphological, and biochemical studies in a family. *J Neurol Sci* 1993;115:91–94.
35. Bartram C, Edwards RH, Beynon RJ. McArdle's disease: muscle glycogen phosphorylase deficiency. *Biochim Biophys Acta* 1995;1272:1–13.
36. Lebo RV, Gorin F, Fletterick RJ, et al. High-resolution chromosome sorting and DNA spot-blot analysis assign McArdle's syndrome to chromosome 11. *Science* 1984;225:57–59.
37. DiMauro S, Andreu AL, Bruno C, Hadjigeorgiou GM. Myophosphoylase Deficiency. *Current Molecular Medicine* 2002,2:189–196
38. Tsujino S, Shanske S, DiMauro S. Molecular genetic heterogeneity of myophosphorylase deficiency (McArdle's disease). *N Engl J Med* 1993;329:241–245.
39. Sugie H, Sugie Y, Ito M, et al. Genetic analysis of Japanese patients with myophosphorylase deficiency (McArdle's disease): single-codon deletion in exon 17 is the predominant mutation. *Clin Chim Acta* 1995;236:81–86f.
40. Martin MA, Rubio JC, Buchbinder J, et al. Molecular heterogeneity of myophosphorylase deficiency (McArdle's disease): a genotype–phenotype correlation study. *Ann Neurol* 2001;50: 574–581.
41. Roelofs RI, Engel WK, Chauvin PB. Histochemical phosphorylase activity in regenerating muscle fibers from myophosphorylase-deficient patients. *Science* 1972;177:795–797.
42. Sato K, Imai F, Hatayama I, et al. Characterization of glycogen phosphorylase isoenzymes present in cultured skeletal muscle from patients with McArdle's disease. *Biochem Biophys Res Commun* 1977;78:663–668.
43. DiMauro S, Arnold S, Miranda AF, et al. McArdle disease: the mystery of reappearing phosphorylase activity in muscle culture: a fetal isoenzyme. *Ann Neurol* 1978;3:60–66.
44. Lockyer JM, McCracken JB. Identification of a tissue-specific regulatory element within the human muscle glycogen phosphorylase gene. *J Biol Chem* 1991;266:20,262–20,269.
45. Van den Berg IE, Berger R. Phosphorylase b kinase deficiency in man: a review. *J Inher Metab Dis* 1990;13:442–451.
46. Elleder M, Shin YS, Zuntova A, et al. Fatal infantile hypertrophic cardiomyopathy secondary to deficiency of heart specific

phosphorylase b kinase. *Virchows Arch A Pathol Anat Histopathol* 1993;423:303–307.

47. Kagalwalla AF, Kagalwalla YA, al Ajaj S, et al. Phosphorylase b kinase deficiency glycogenosis with cirrhosis of the liver. *J Pediatr* 1995;127:602–605.

48. Iwamasa T, Fukuda S, Tokumitsu S, et al. Myopathy due to glycogen storage disease. *Exp Mol Pathol* 1983;38:405–420.

49. Abarbanel JM, Bashan N, Potashnik R, et al. Adult muscle phosphorylase "b" kinase deficiency. *Neurology* 1986;36:560–562.

50. Wilkinson DA, Tonin P, Shanske S, et al. Clinical and biochemical features of 10 adult patients with muscle phosphorylase kinase deficiency. *Neurology* 1994;44:461–466.

51. Strugalska-Cynowska M. Disturbances in the activity of phosphorylase b kinase in a case of McArdle myopathy. *Folia Histochem Cytochem (Krakow)* 1967;5:151–156.

52. Danon MJ, Carpenter S, Manaligod JR, et al. Fatal infantile glycogen storage disease: deficiency of phosphofructokinase and phosphorylase b kinase. *Neurology* 1981;31:1303–1307.

53. Ohtani Y, Matsuda I, Iwamasa T, et al. Infantile glycogen storage myopathy in a girl with phosphorylase kinase deficiency. *Neurology* 1982;32:833–838.

54. Shin YS, Plochl E, Podskarbi T, et al. Fatal arthrogryposis with respiratory insufficiency: a possible case of muscle phosphorylase b-kinase deficiency. *J Inherit Metab Dis* 1994;17:153–155.

55. Clemens PR, Yamamoto M, Engel AG. Adult phosphorylase b kinase deficiency. *Ann Neurol* 1990;28:529–538.

56. Coleman RA, Stajich JM, Pact VW, et al. The ischemic exercise test in normal adults and in patients with weakness and cramps. *Muscle Nerve* 1986;9:216–221.

57. Heller SL, Kaiser KK, Planer GJ, et al. McArdle's disease with myoadenylate deaminase deficiency: observations in a combined enzyme deficiency. *Neurology* 1987;37:1039–1042.

58. Louboutin JP, Nataf S, Jardel-Bouissiere J, et al. Evidence for low production of lactate and pyruvate in alcoholic rhabdomyolysis. *Muscle Nerve* 1995;18:784–786.

59. Kanbe K, Nagase M, Udagawa E. Acute alcoholic rhabdomyolysis associated with abnormal ischemic exercise test. *Muscle Nerve* 1993;16:1269–1270.

60. Martinuzzi A, Schievano G, Nascimbeni A, et al. McArdle's disease: the unsolved mystery of the reappearing enzyme. *Am J Pathol* 1999;154:1893–1897.

61. El-Schahawi M, Tsujino S, Shanske S, et al. Diagnosis of McArdle's disease by molecular genetic analysis of blood. *Neurology* 1996;47:579–580.

62. Cochrane PR, Hughes R, Buxton PH, et al. Myophosphorylase deficiency (McArdle's disease) in two interrelated families. *J Neurol Neurosurg Psychiatry* 1973;36:217–224.

63. Steele IC, Patterson VH, Nicholls DP. A double-blind, placebo controlled, crossover trial of D-ribose in McArdle's disease. *J Neurolog Sci* 1996;136:174–177.

64. Vissing J, Haller RG. The effect of oral sucrose on exercise tolerance in patients with McArdle's Disease. *N Engl J Med* 2003;349:2503–2509.

65. Slonim AE, Goans PJ. Myopathy in McArdle's syndrome: improvement with a high-protein diet. *N Engl J Med* 1985;312:355–359.

66. Jansen PHP, Joosten EMG, Vingerhoots HM. Muscle cramp: main theories as to aetiology. *Eur Arch Psychiatr Neurol Sci* 1990;239:337–342.

67. MacLean D, Vissing J, Vissing SF, et al. Oral branched-chain amino acids do not improve exercise capacity in McArdle disease. *Neurology* 1998;51:1456–1459.

68. Coakley JH, Wagenmakers AJ, Edwards RH. Relationship between ammonia, heart rate, and exertion in McArdle's disease. *Am J Physiol* 1992;262:E167–E172.

69. Beynon RJ, Bartram C, Hopkins P, et al. McArdle's disease: molecular genetics and metabolic consequences of the phenotype. *Muscle Nerve* 1995;3(suppl 3):S18–S22.

70. Phoenix J, Hopkins P, Bartram C, et al. Effect of vitamin B6 supplementation in McArdle's disease: a strategic case study. *Neuromuscular Disord* 1998;8:210–212.

71. Vorgerd M, Grehl T, Jager M, et al. Creatine therapy in myophosphorylase deficiency (McArdle disease): a placebo-controlled crossover trial. *Arch Neurol* 2000;57:956–963.

72. Baqué S, Newgard CB, Gerard RD, et al. Adenovirus-mediated delivery into myocytes of muscle glycogen phosphorylase, the enzyme deficient in patients with glycogen-storage disease type V. *Biochem J* 1994;304:1009–1014.

73. Pari G, Crerar MM, Nalbantoglu J, et al. Myophosphorylase gene transfer in McArdle's disease myoblasts in vitro. *Neurology* 1999;53:1352–1354.

74. Tarui S, Okuno G, Ikura Y, et al. Phosphofructokinase deficiency in skeletal muscle: a new type of glycogenosis. *Biochem Biophys Res Commun* 1965;19:517–520.

75. Ronquist G, Rudolphi O, Engstrom I, et al. Familial phosphofructokinase deficiency is associated with a disturbed calcium homeostasis in erythrocytes. *J Intern Med* 2001;249:85–95.

76. Rowland LP, DiMauro S, Lazer RB. Phosphofructokinase deficiency. In: Engel AG, Banker BQ, eds. *Myology*. 1st ed. New York: McGraw-Hill, 1986:1603–1617.

77. Nakagawa C, Mineo I, Kaido M, et al. A new variant case of muscle phosphofructokinase deficiency, coexisting with gastric ulcer, gouty arthritis, and increased hemolysis. *Muscle Nerve* 1995;3(suppl 3):S39–S44.

78. Argov Z, Barash V, Soffer D, et al. Late-onset muscular weakness in phosphofructokinase deficiency due to exon 5/intron 5 junction point mutation: a unique disorder or the natural course of this glycolytic disorder? *Neurology* 1994;44:1097–1100.

79. Sivakumar K, Vasconcelos O, Goldfarb L, et al. Late-onset muscle weakness in partial phosphofructokinase deficiency: a unique myopathy with vacuoles, abnormal mitochondria, and absence of the common exon 5/intron 5 junction point mutation. *Neurology* 1996;46:1337–1342.

80. Massa R, Lodi R, Barbiroli B, et al. Partial block of glycolysis in late-onset phosphofructokinase deficiency myopathy. *Acta Neuropathol* 1996;91:322–329.

81. Pastoris O, Dossena M, Vercesi L, et al. Muscle phosphofructokinase deficiency in a myopathic child with severe mental retardation and aplasia of cerebellar vermis. *Childs Nerv Syst* 1992;8:237–241.

82. Moerman P, Lammens M, Fryns JP, et al. Fetal akinesia sequence caused by glycogenosis type VII. *Genet Couns* 1995;6:15–20.

83. Vora S, DiMauro S, Spear D, et al. Characterization of enzymatic defect in late onset muscle phosphofructokinase deficiency: new subtype of glycogen storage disease type VII. *J Clin Invest* 1987;80:1479–1485.

84. Buetler E. *Red cell metabolism: a manual of biochemical methods*, 3rd ed. New York: Grune & Stratton, 1984.

85. Argov Z, Bank WJ, Maris J, et al. Muscle energy metabolism in human phosphofructokinase deficiency as recorded by ^{31}P nuclear magnetic resonance spectroscopy. *Ann Neurol* 1987;22:46–51.

86. Grehl T, Muller K, Vorgerd M, et al. Impaired aerobic glycolysis in muscle phosphofructokinase deficiency results in biphasic post-exercise phosphocreatine recovery in ^{31}P magnetic resonance spectroscopy. *Neuromuscular Disord* 1998;8:480–488.

87. Bertocci LA, Haller RG, Lewis SF, et al. Abnormal high-energy phosphate metabolism in human muscle phosphofructokinase deficiency. *J Appl Physiol* 1991;70:1201–1207.

88. Raben N, Sherman JB, Adams E, et al. Various classes of mutations in patients with phosphofructokinase deficiency (Tarui's disease). *Muscle Nerve* 1995;3:S35–S38.

89. Nakajima H, Hamaguchi T, Yamasaki T, et al. Phosphofructokinase deficiency: recent advances in molecular biology. *Muscle Nerve* 1995;3(suppl 3):S28–S34.

90. Nichols RC, Rudolphi O, Ek B, et al. Glycogenosis type VII (Tarui disease) in a Swedish family: two novel mutations in muscle phosphofructokinase gene (PFK-M) resulting in intron retentions. *Am J Hum Genet* 1996;59:59–65.

91. Haller RG, Lewis SF. Glucose-induced exertional fatigue in muscle phosphofructokinase deficiency. *N Engl J Med* 1991;324:364–369.

92. DiMauro S, Dalakas M, Miranda AF. Phosphoglycerate kinase (PGK) deficiency: another cause of recurrent myoglobinuria. *Ann Neurol* 1983;13:11–19.

93. Rosa R, George C, Fardeau M, et al. A new case of phosphoglycerate kinase deficiency: PGK Creteil associated with rhabdomyolysis and lacking hemolytic anemia. *Blood* 1982;60:84–91.

94. Cohen-Solal M, Valentin C, Plassa F, et al. Identification of new mutations in two phosphoglycerate kinase (PGK) variants expressing different clinical syndromes: PGK Creteil and PGK Amiens. *Blood* 1994;84:898–903.

95. Ookawara T, Dave V, Willems P, et al. Retarded and aberrant splicings caused by single exon mutation in a phosphoglycerate kinase variant. *Arch Biochem Biophys* 1996;327:35–40.

96. Tonin P, Shanske S, Miranda AF, et al. Phosphoglycerate kinase deficiency: biochemical and molecular genetic studies in a new myopathic variant (PGK Alberta). *Neurology* 1993;43:387–391.

97. Fujii H, Kanno H, Hirono A, et al. A single amino acid substitution (157 Gly to Val) in a phosphoglycerate kinase variant (PGK Shizuoka) associated with chronic hemolysis and myoglobinuria. *Blood* 1992;79:1582–1585.

98. Sugie H, Sugie Y, Nishida M, et al. Recurrent myoglobinuria in a child with mental retardation: phosphoglycerate kinase deficiency. *J Child Neurol* 1989;4:95–99.

99. Tsujino S, Tonin P, Shanske S, et al. A splice junction mutation in a new myopathic variant of phosphoglycerate kinase deficiency (PGK North Carolina). *Ann Neurol* 1994;35:349–353.

100. Tsujino S, Nonaka I, Dimauro S. Glycogen storage myopathies. *Neurol Clin* 2000;18:125–150.

101. DiMauro S, Miranda AF, Khan S, et al. Human muscle phosphoglycerate mutase deficiency: a newly discovered metabolic myopathy. *Science* 1981;212:1277–1279.

102. DiMauro S, Miranda AF, Olarte M, et al. Muscle phosphoglycerate mutase deficiency. *Neurology* 1982;32:584–592.

103. Bresolin N, Ro YI, Reyes M, et al. Muscle phosphoglycerate mutase (PGAM) deficiency: a second case. *Neurology* 1983;33:1049–1053.

104. Kissel JT, Beam W, Bresolin N, et al. Physiologic assessment of phosphoglycerate mutase deficiency: incremental exercise test. *Neurology* 1985;35:828–833.

105. Tsujino S, Shanske S, Sakoda S, et al. The molecular genetic basis of muscle phosphoglycerate mutase (PGAM) deficiency. *Am J Hum Genet* 1993;52:472–477.

106. Toscano A, Tsujino S, Vita G, et al. Molecular basis of muscle phosphoglycerate mutase (PGAM-M) deficiency in the Italian kindred. *Muscle Nerve* 1996;19:1134–1137.

107. Argov Z, Bank WJ. Phosphorus magnetic resonance spectroscopy (^{31}P-MRS) in neuromuscular disorders. *Ann Neurol* 1991;30:90–97.

108. Vita G, Toscano A, Bresolin N, et al. Muscle phosphoglycerate mutase (PGAM) deficiency in the first Caucasian patient: biochemistry, muscle culture, and P-MR spectroscopy. *J Neurol* 1994;241:289–294.

109. Edwards YH, Sakoda S, Schon E, et al. The gene for human muscle-specific phosphoglycerate mutase, PGAM2, mapped to chromosome 7 by polymerase chain reaction. *Genomics* 1989;5:948–951.

110. Vissing J, Schmalbruch H, Haller RG, et al. Muscle phosphoglycerate mutase deficiency with tubular aggregates: effect of dantrolene. *Ann Neurol* 1999;46:274–277.

111. Kanno T, Sudo K, Takeuchi I, et al. Hereditary deficiency of lactate dehydrogenase M subunit. *Clin Chim Acta* 1980;108:267–276.

112. Miyajima H, Takahashi Y, Suzuki M, et al. Molecular characterization of gene expression in human lactate dehydrogenase-A deficiency. *Neurology* 1993;43:1414–1419.

113. Tsujino S, Shanske S, Brownell AK, et al. Molecular genetic studies of muscle lactate dehydrogenase deficiency in white patients. *Ann Neurol* 1994;36:661–665.

114. Maekawa M, Kanda S, Sudo K, et al. Estimation of the gene frequency of lactate dehydrogenase subunit deficiencies. *Am J Hum Genet* 1984;36:1204–1214.

115. Yoshikuni K, Tagami H, Yamada M, et al. Erythematosquamous skin lesions in hereditary lactate dehydrogenase M-subunit deficiency. *Arch Dermatol* 1986;122:1420–1424.

116. Takayasu S, Fujiwara S, Waki T. Hereditary lactate dehydrogenase M-subunit deficiency: lactate dehydrogenase activity in skin lesions and in hair follicles. *J Am Acad Dermatol* 1991;24:339–342.

117. Kanno T, Maekawa M. Lactate dehydrogenase M-subunit deficiencies: clinical features, metabolic background, and genetic heterogeneities. *Muscle Nerve* 1995;3(suppl 3):S54–S60.

118. Maekawa M, Sudo K, Li SSL, et al. Genotypic analysis of families with lactate dehydrogenase A(M) deficiency by selective DNA amplification. *Hum Genet* 1991;88:34–38.

119. Maekawa M, Sudo K, Li SSL, et al. Analysis of genetic mutations in human lactate dehydrogenase-A(M) deficiency using DNA conformation polymorphism in combination with polyacrylamide gradient gel and silver staining. *Biochem Biophys Res Commun* 1991;180:1083–1090.

120. Comi GP, et al. Beta-enolase deficiency: a new metabolic myopathy of distal glycolysis. *Ann Neurol* 2001;50:202–207.

121. Murthy MS, Pande SV. Some differences in the properties of carnitine palmitoyltransferase activities of the mitochondrial outer and inner membranes. *Biochem J* 1987;248:727–733.

122. McGarry JD, Brown NF. The mitochondrial carnitine palmitoyltransferase system: from concept to molecular analysis. *Eur J Biochem* 1997;244:1–14.

123. Murthy MS, Pande SV. Characterization of a solubilized malonyl-CoA-sensitive carnitine palmitoyltransferase from the mitochondrial outer membrane as a protein distinct from the malonyl-CoA-insensitive carnitine palmitoyltransferase of the inner membrane. *Biochem J* 1990;268:599–604.

124. Woeltje KF, Esser V, Weis BC, et al. Inter-tissue and inter-species characteristics of the mitochondrial carnitine palmitoyltransferase enzyme system. *J Biol Chem* 1990;265:10,714–10,719.

125. Bonnefont JP, Djouadi F, Prip-Buus C, et al. Carnitine palmitoyltransferases 1 and 2: biochemical, molecular and medical aspects. *Mol Aspects Med* 2004;25:495–520.

126. Demaugre F, Bonnefont JP, Mitchell G, et al. Hepatic and muscular presentations of carnitine palmitoyl transferase deficiency: two distinct entities. *Pediatr Res* 1988;24:308–311.

127. Villard J, Fischer A, Mandon G, et al. Recurrent myoglobinuria due to carnitine palmitoyltransferase II deficiency: expression of the molecular phenotype in cultured muscle cells. *J Neurolog Sci* 1996;136:178–181.

128. Deschauer M, Wiese T, Zierz S. Muscle carnitine palmitoyltransferase II deficiency. *Arch Neurol* 2005;62:37–41.

129. Katsuya H, Misumi M, Ohtani Y, et al. Postanesthetic acute renal failure due to carnitine palmityl transferase deficiency. *Anesthesiology* 1988;68:945–948.

130. Kieval RI, Sotrel A, Weinblatt ME. Chronic myopathy with a partial deficiency of the carnitine palmitoyltransferase enzyme. *Arch Neurol* 1989;46:575–576.

131. Tonin P, Lewis P, Servidei S, et al. Metabolic causes of myoglobinuria. *Ann Neurol* 1990;27:181–185.

132. Mantz J, Hindelang C, Mantz JM, et al. Vascular and myofibrillar lesions in acute myoglobinuria associated with carnitine-palmityl-transferase deficiency. *Virchows Arch A Pathol Anat Histopathol* 1992;421:57–64.

133. Schaefer J, Jackson S, Taroni F, et al. Characterization of carnitine palmitoyltransferases in patients with a carnitine palmitoyltransferase deficiency: implications for diagnosis and therapy. *J Neurol Neurosurg Psychiatry* 1997;62:169–176.

134. Angelini C, Freddo L, Battistella P, et al. Carnitine palmityl transferase deficiency: clinical variability, carrier detection, and autosomal recessive inheritance. *Neurology* 1981;31:883–886.

135. Ionasescu V, Hug G, Hoppel C. Combined partial deficiency of muscle carnitine palmitoyltransferase and carnitine with autosomal dominant inheritance. *J Neurol Neurosurg Psychiatry* 1980;43:679–682.

136. Orngreen MC, Duno M, Ejstrup BS, et al. Fuel utiliziation in subjects with carnitine palmitoyltransferase 2 gene mutations. *Ann Neurol* 2005;57:60–66.

137. Van der Leij FR, Huijkman NC, Boomsma C, et al. Genomics of the human carnitine acyltransferase genes. *Mol Genet Metab* 2000;71:139–153.

138. Taroni F, Verderio E. Willems PJ, et al. Identification of a common mutation in the carnitine palmitoyltransferase II gene in familial recurrent myoglobinuria patients. *Nat Genet* 1993;4:314–320.

139. Zierz S, Neumann-Schmidt S, Jerusalem F. Inhibition of carnitine palmitoyltransferase in normal human skeletal muscle and in muscle of patients with carnitine palmitoyltransferase deficiency by long- and short-chain acylcarnitine and acyl-coenzyme A. *Clin Invest* 1993;71:763–769.

140. Zierz S. Carnitine palmitoyltransferase deficiency. In: Engel AG, Franzini-Armstrong C, eds. *Myology*. 2nd ed. New York: McGraw-Hill, 1994:1577–1586.

141. El-Hayek R, Valdivia C, Valdivia HH, et al. Activation of the Ca^{2+} release channel of skeletal muscle sarcoplasmic reticulum by palmitoyl carnitine. *Biophys J* 1993;65:779–789.

142. Vladutiu GD, Bennett MJ, Fisher NM, et al. Phenotypic variability among first-degree relatives with carnitine palmitoyltransferase II deficiency. *Muscle Nerve* 2002;26:492–498.

143. Handig I, Dams E, Taroni F, et al. Inheritance of the S113L mutation within an inbred family with carnitine palmitoyltransferase enzyme deficiency. *Hum Genet* 1996;97:291–293.

144. Vladutiu GD, Quackenbush EJ, Hainline BE. Lethal neonatal and severe late infantile forms of carnitine palmitoyltransferase II deficiency associated with compound heterozygosity for different protein truncation mutations. *J Pediatr* 2002;141:734–736.

145. Carroll JE. Myopathies caused by disorders of lipid metabolism. *Neurol Clin* 1988;6:563–574.

146. Orngreen MC, Ejstrup R, Vissing J. Effect of diet on exercise tolerance in carnitine palmitoyltransferase II deficiency. *Neurology* 2003;61:559–561.

147. Przyrembel H. Therapy of mitochondrial disorders. *J Inherit Metab Dis* 1987;10:129–146.

148. Shintani S, Shiigai T, Sugiyama N. Atypical presentation of carnitine palmitoyltransferase (CPT) deficiency as status epilepticus. *J Neurol Sci* 1995;129:6973.

149. Ohtani Y, Tomoda A, Miike T, et al. Central nervous system disorders and possible brain type carnitine palmitoyltransferase II deficiency. *Brain Dev* 1994;16:139–145.

150. Stanley CA. New genetic defects in mitochondrial fatty acid oxidation and carnitine deficiency. *Adv Pediatr* 1987;34:59–88.

151. Engel WK, Vick NA, Glueck J, et al. A skeletal muscle disorder associated with intermittent symptoms and a possible defect in lipid metabolism. *N Engl J Med* 1970;282:697–704.

152. Snyder TM, Little BW, Roman-Campos G, et al. Successful treatment of familial idiopathic lipid storage myopathy with L-carnitine and modified lipid diet. *Neurology* 1982;32:1106–1115.

153. Ohashi Y, Hasegawa Y, Murayama K, et al. A new diagnostic test for VLCAD deficiency using immunohistochemistry. *Neurology* 2004;62:2209–2213.

154. Indo Y, Yang-Feng T, Glassberg R, et al. Molecular cloning and nucleotide sequence of cDNAs encoding human long-chain acyl-CoA dehydrogenase and assignment of the location of its gene (ACADL) to chromosome 2. *Genomics* 1991;11:609–620.

155. Schaefer J, Jackson S, Dick DJ, et al. Trifunctional enzyme deficiency: adult presentation of a usually fatal beta-oxidation defect. *Ann Neurol* 1996;40:597–602.

156. Lambert EH, Goldstein NP. Unusual form of "myotonia" (abstract). *Physiologist* 1957;1:51.

157. Brody I. Muscle contracture induced by exercise: a syndrome attributable to decreased relaxing factor. *N Engl J Med* 1969;281:187–192.

158. Taylor DJ, Brosnan MJ, Arnold DL, et al. Ca^{2+}-ATPase deficiency in a patient with an exertional muscle pain syndrome. *J Neurol Neurosurg Psychiatry* 1988;51:1425–1433.

159. Poels PJ, Wevers RA, Braakhekke JP, et al. Exertional rhabdomyolysis in a patient with calcium adenosine triphosphatase deficiency. *J Neurol Neurosurg Psychiatry* 1993;56:823–826.

160. Brandl CJ, Green NM, Korczak B, et al. Two Ca^{2+} ATPase genes: homologies and mechanistic implications of deduced amino acid sequences. *Cell* 1986;44:597–607.

161. Benders AA, Veerkamp JH, Oosterhof A, et al. Ca++ homeostasis in Brody's disease: a study in skeletal muscle and cultured muscle cells and the effects of dantrolene an verapamil. *J Clin Invest* 1994;94:741–748.

162. Benders AG, Van Kuppevelt TH, Oosterhof A, et al. Adenosine triphosphatases during maturation of cultured human muscle cells and in human muscle. *Biochim Biophys Acta* 1992;1112:89–98.

163. Karpati G, Charuk J, Carpenter S, et al. Myopathy caused by a deficiency of Ca++-adenosine triphosphatase in sarcoplasmic reticulum (Brody's disease). *Ann Neurol* 1986;20:38–49.

164. Danon MJ, Karpati G, Charuk J, et al. Sarcoplasmic reticulum adenosine triphosphatase deficiency with probably autosomal dominant inheritance. *Neurology* 1988;38:812–815.

165. Odermatt A, Barton K, Khanna VK, et al. The mutation of Pro789 to Leu reduces the activity of the fast-twitch skeletal muscle sarco(endo)plasmic reticulum Ca^{2+} ATPase (SERCA1) and is associated with Brody disease. *Hum Genet* 2000;106:482–491.

166. MacLennan DH, Rice WJ, Odermatt A, et al. Structure–function relationships in the Ca(2+)-binding and translocation domain of SERCA1: physiological correlates in Brody disease. *Acta Physiol Scand* 1998;643(suppl):55–67.

167. Torbergsen T. A family with dominant hereditary myotonia, muscular hypertrophy, and increased muscular irritability, distinct from myotonia congenita (Thomsen). *Acta Neurol Scand* 1975;51:225–232.

168. Ricker K, Moxley RT, Rohkamm R. Rippling muscle disease. *Arch Neurol* 1989;46:405–408.

169. Bums RJ, Bretag AH, Blumbergs PC, et al. Benign familial disease with muscle mounding and rippling. *J Neurol Neurosurg Psychiatry* 1994;57:344–347.

170. Vorgerd M, Bolz H, Patzold T, et al. Phenotypic variability in rippling muscle disease. *Neurology* 1999;52:1453–1459.

171. Stephan DA, Buist NR, Chittenden AB, et al. A rippling muscle disease gene is localized to 1q41: evidence for multiple genes. *Neurology* 1994;44:1915–1920.

172. Betz RC, Schoser BGH, Kasper D, et al. Caveolin-3 mutations cause mechanical hyperirritability of skeletal muscle in hereditary rippling muscle disease. *Nat Genet* 2001;28:218–219.

173. Fischer D, Schroers A, Blumcke I, et al. Consequences of a novel caveolin-3 mutation in a large German family. *Ann Neurol* 2003;53:233–241.

174. Yabe I, Kawashima A, Kikuchi S, et al. Caveolin-3 gene mutation in Japanese with rippling muscle disease. *Acta Neurol Scand* 2003;108:47–51.

175. Torbergensen T. Rippling muscle disease: a review. *Muscle Nerve* 2002;(suppl 11):S103–S107.

176. Minetti C, Sotgia F, Bruno C, et al. Mutations in the caveolin-3 gene cause autosomal dominant limb girdle muscular dystrophy. *Nat Genet* 1998;18:365–368.

177. Kosmorsky GS, Mehta N, Mitsumoto H, et al. Intermittent esotropia associated with rippling muscle disease. *J Neuroophthalmol* 1995;15:147–151.

178. Lamb GD. Rippling muscle disease may be caused by "silent" action potentials in the tubular system of skeletal muscle fibers. *Muscle Nerve* 2005;31:652–658.

179. Alberca R, Rafel E, Castilla JM, et al. Increased mechanical muscle irritability syndrome. *Acta Neurol Scand* 1980;62:250–256.

180. Schulte-Mattler WJ, Kley RA, Rothenfusser-Korber E, et al. Immune-mediated rippling muscle disease. *Neurology* 2005;64:364–367.

181. Ansevin CF, Agamanolis DP. Rippling muscles and myasthenia gravis with rippling muscles. *Arch Neurol* 1996;53:197–199.

182. Vernino S, Auger RG, Emslie-Smith AM, et al. Myasthenia, thymoma, presynaptic antibodies, and a continuum of neuromuscular hyperexcitability. *Neurology* 1999;53:1233–1239.

183. Greenberg SA. Acquired rippling muscle disease with myasthenia gravis. *Muscle Nerve* 2004;29:143–146.

184. Stohr M, Schlote W, Bundschu HD, et al. Myopathia myotonica. *J Neurol* 1975;210:41–46.

185. Sanders DB. Myotonia congenita with painful muscle contractions. *Arch Neurol* 1976;33:580–582.

186. Becker PE. Syndromes associated with myotonia. In: Rowland LP, ed. *Pathogenesis of the human muscular dystrophies*. Amsterdam: Excerpta Medica, 1977:699–703.

187. Sunohara N, Tomi H, Nakamura A, et al. Myotonia congenita with painful muscle cramps. *Intern Med* 1996;35:507–511.

188. Koch MC, Steinmeyer K, Lorenz C, et al. The skeletal muscle chloride channel in dominant and recessive human myotonia. *Science* 1992;257:797–800.

189. George AL Jr, Crackower MA, Abdalla JA, et al. Molecular basis of Thomsen's disease (autosomal dominant myotonia congenita). *Nat Genet* 1993;3:305–310.

190. Davies NP, Hanna MG. The skeletal muscle channelopathies: basic science, clinical genetics, and treatment. *Curr Opin Neurol* 2001;14:539–551.

191. Rüdel R, Ricker K, Lehmann-Horn F. Genotype–phenotype correlations in human skeletal muscle sodium channel diseases. *Arch Neurol* 1993;50:1241–1248.

192. Ptacek LJ, Tawil R, Griggs RC, et al. Linkage of atypical myotonia congenita to a sodium channel locus. *Neurology* 1992;42: 431–433.

193. Ptacek LJ, Tawil R, Griggs RC, et al. Sodium channel mutations in acetazolamide-responsive myotonia congenita, paramyotonia congenita, and hyperkalemic periodic paralysis. *Neurology* 1994;44:1500–1503.

194. Laycock MA, Pascuzzi RM. The neuromuscular effects of hypothyroidism. *Semin Neurol* 1991;11:288–294.

195. Duyff RF, Van den Bosch J, Laman DM, et al. Neuromuscular findings in thyroid dysfunction: a prospective clinical and electrodiagnostic study. *J Neurol Neurosurg Psychiatry* 2000;68:750–755.

196. Ramsey I. *Thyroid disease and muscle dysfunction.* Chicago: Year Book Medical, 1974.

197. Lochmiller H, Reimers CD, Fischer P, et al. Exercise-induced myalgia in hypothyroidism. *Clin Invest* 1993;71:999–1001.

198. Riggs JE. Acute exertional rhabdomyolysis in hypothyroidism: the result of a reversible defect in glycogenolysis? *Milit Med* 1990;155:171–172.

199. Suzuki S, Ichikawa K, Nagai M, et al. Elevation of serum creatine kinase during treatment with antithyroid drugs in patients with hyperthyroidism due to Graves' disease: a novel side effect of antithyroid drugs. *Arch Intern Med* 1997;157:693–696.

200. Pearce I, Aziz H. The neuromyopathy of hypothyroidism: some new observations. *J Neurol Sci* 1969;9:243–253.

201. Ubogu EE, Ruff RL, Kaminski HJ. Endocrine myopathies (hyper- and hypofunction of adrenal, thyroid, pituitary, and parathyroid glands and iatrogenic steroid myopathy). In: Engel AG, Banker BQ, eds. *Myology.* 1st ed. New York: McGraw-Hill, 1986:1713–1738.

202. Klostermann W, Wessel K, Moser A. Unmasking congenital myotonia by hypothyroidism (in German). *Nervenarzt* 1993;64:266–268.

203. Ho K. Basophilic degeneration of skeletal muscle in hypothyroid myopathy. *Arch Pathol Lab Med* 1984;108:239–245.

204. Evans RM, Watanabe I, Singer PA. Central changes in hypothyroid myopathy: a case report. *Muscle Nerve* 1990;13:952–956.

205. Kaminsky P, Klein M, Duc M. La myopathie hypothyroidienne: approche physiopathologyique. *Ann Endocrinol (Paris)* 1992;53: 125–132.

206. Taylor D, Rajagopalan B, Radda G. Cellular energetics in hypothyroid muscle. *Eur J Clin Invest* 1992;22:358–365.

207. McDaniel HG, Pittman CS, Oh SJ, et al. Carbohydrate metabolism in hypothyroid myopathy. *Metabolism* 1977;26:867–873.

208. Sharma VK, Banerjee SP. beta-Adrenergic receptors in rat skeletal muscle: effect of thyroidectomy. *Biochem Biophys Acta* 1978;539:538–542.

209. Wiles CM, Young A, Jones DA, et al. Muscle relaxation rate, fibre-type composition, and energy turnover in hyper- and hypothyroid patients. *Clin Sci* 1979;57:375–384.

210. Fanburg BL. Calcium transport by skeletal muscle sarcoplasmic reticulum in the hypothyroid rat. *J Clin Invest* 1968;47: 2499–2506.

211. Fessel WJ. Myopathy of hypothyroidism. *Ann Rheum Dis* 1968;27:590–595.

212. Stern LZ, Fagan JM. The endocrine myopathies. In: Vinken PJ, Bruyn GW, eds. *Handbook of clinical neurology,* vol 41. Amsterdam: Elsevier Science, 1979:235–258.

213. Turken SA, Cafferty M, Silverberg SJ, et al. Neuromuscular involvement in mild, asymptomatic primary hyperparathyroidism. *Am J Med* 1989;87:553–557.

214. Ritz E, Boland R, Krevsser W. Effects of vitamin D and parathyroid hormone on muscle. *Am J Clin Nutr* 1980;33:1522–1529.

215. Matthews C, Heimberg KW, Ritz E, et al. Effect on impaired calcium transport by the sarcoplasmic reticulum in experimental uremia. *Kidney Int* 1977;11:227–235.

216. Baczynski R, Massry SG, Magott M, et al. Effect of parathyroid hormone on energy metabolism of skeletal muscle. *Kidney Int* 1985;28:722–727.

217. Nagamitsu S, Ashizawa T. Myotonic dystrophies. *Neuromuscular disorders.* Advances in neurology, vol 88. Philadelphia: Lippincott Williams & Wilkins, 2002.

218. Renner DR, Ptacek LL. Periodic paralyses and nondystrophic myotonias. *Neuromuscular disorders.* Advances in neurology, vol 88. Philadelphia: Lippincott Williams & Wilkins, 2002.

219. Ferrannini E, Perniola T, Krajewska G, et al. Schwartz-Jampel syndrome with autosomal-dominant inheritance. *Eur Neurol* 1982;21:137–146.

220. Pascuzzi RM, Gratianne R, Azzarelli B, et al. Schwartz-Jampel syndrome with dominant inheritance. *Muscle Nerve* 1990;13:1152–1163.

221. Schwartz O, Jampel RS. Congenital blepharophimosis associated with a unique generalized myopathy. *Arch Ophthalmol* 1962;68:52–57.

222. Viljoen D, Beighton P. Schwartz-Jampel syndrome (chondrodystrophic myotonia). *J Med Genet* 1992;29:58–62.

223. Paradis CM, Gironda F, Bennett M. Cognitive impairment in Schwartz-Jampel syndrome: a case study. *Brain Lang* 1997; 56:301–305.

224. Cook SP. Borkowski WJ. Obstructive sleep apnea in Schwartz-Jampel syndrome. *Arch Otolaryngol Head Neck Surg* 1997;123: 1348–1350.

225. Spaans F, Theunissen P, Reekers AD, et al. Schwartz-Jampel syndrome: 1. Clinical, electromyographic, and histologic studies. *Muscle Nerve* 1990;13:516–527.

226. Figuera LE, Jimenez-Gil FJ, Garcia-Cruz MO, et al. Schwartz-Jampel syndrome: an atypical form? *Am J Med Genet* 1993;47: 526–528.

227. Giedion A, Boltshauser E, Briner J, et al. Heterogeneity in Schwartz-Jampel chondrodystrophic myotonia. *Eur J Pediatr* 1997;156:214–223.

228. Cao A, Cianchetti C, Calisti L, et al. Schwartz-Jampel syndrome: clinical, electrophysiological, and histopathological study of a severe variant. *J Neurol Sci* 1978;35:175–187.

229. Lehmann-Horn F, Iaizzo PA, Franke C, et al. Schwartz-Jampel syndrome: 2. Na$^+$ channel defect causes myotonia. *Muscle Nerve* 1990;13:528–535.

230. Topaloglu H, Serdaroglu A, Okan M, et al. Improvement of myotonia with carbamazepine in three cases with the Schwartz-Jampel syndrome. *Neuropediatrics* 1993;24:232–234.

231. Squires LA, Prangley J. Neonatal diagnosis of Schwartz-Jampel syndrome with dramatic response to carbamazepine. *Pediatr Neurol* 1996;15:172–174.

232. Nicole S, Ben Hamida C, Beighton P, et al. Localization of the Schwartz-Jampel syndrome (SJS) locus to chromosome 1p34-p36.1 by homozygosity mapping. *Hum Mol Genet* 1995;4: 1633–1636.

233. Brown KA, al-Gazali LI, Moynihan LM, et al. Genetic heterogeneity in Schwartz-Jampel syndrome: two families with neonatal Schwartz-Jampel syndrome do not map to human chromosome 1p34-p36.1. *J Med Genet* 1997;34:685–687.

234. Roy EP, Gutmann L. Myalgia. *Neurol Clin North Am* 1988;6: 621–636.

235. Simchak AC, Pascuzzi RM. Muscle cramps. *Semin Neurol* 1991;11:281–287.

236. Sufit RL, Peters HA. Nifedipine relieves exercise-exacerbated myalgias. *Muscle Nerve* 1984;7:647–649.

237. Morgan-Hughes JA. Defects of the energy pathways of skeletal muscle. In: Matthews WB, Glaser GH, eds. *Recent advances in clinical neurology,* vol 3. Edinburgh: Churchill-Livingstone, 1982:1–46.

238. Arnold DL, Radda GK, Bore PJ, et al. Excessive intracellular acidosis of skeletal muscle on exercise in a patient with a post-viral fatigue syndrome. *Lancet* 1984;1:1367–1369.

239. Sreter FA, Banman ML, Gergelo J, et al. Changes in muscle chemistry associated with stiffness and pain. *Neurology* 1972;22: 1172–1175.

240. Telerman-Toppet N, Bac QM, Khoubesserian P, et al. Type 2 fiber predominance in muscle cramp and exertional myalgia. *Muscle Nerve* 1985;8:563–567.

241. Gospe SM, Lazaro RP, Lava NS, et al. Familial X-linked myalgia and cramps: a nonprogressive myopathy associated with a deletion in the dystrophin gene (abstract). *Ann Neurol* 1989;26:466.

242. Kuhn E, Fiehn W, Schroder M, et al. Early myocardial disease and cramping myalgia in Becker-type muscular dystrophy: a kindred. *Neurology* 1979;29:1144–1149.

243. Sulaiman AR, Kinder DS. Vascularized muscle fibers: etiopathogenesis and clinical significance. *J Neurol Sci* 1989;82:37–54.

244. Isaacs H, Badenhorst ME. Internalized capillaries, neuromyopathy and myalgia. *J Neurol Neurosurg Psychiatry* 1992;55:921–924.

245. Niakan E, Harati Y, Danon MJ. Tubular aggregates: their association with myalgia. *J Neurol Neurosurg Psychiatry* 1985;48:882–886.

246. Brumback RA, Staton RD, Susaq ME. Exercise-induced pain, stiffness, and tubular aggregates in skeletal muscle. *J Neurol Neurosurg Psychiatry* 1981;44:250–254.

247. Eaton JM. Is this really a muscle cramp? *Postgrad Med* 1989;86:227–232.

248. Kunci RW, Wiggins WW. Toxic myopathies. *Neurol Clin North Am* 1988;6:593–619.

249. Ishigaki C, Patria SY, Wishio H, et al. A Japanese boy with myalgia and cramps has a novel in-frame deletion of the dystrophin gene. *Neurology* 1996;46:1347–1350.

250. Minaker KL, Flier JS, Landsberg L, et al. Phenytoin-induced improvement in muscle cramping and insulin action in three patients with the syndrome of insulin resistance, acanthosis nigricans, and acral hypertrophy. *Arch Neurol* 1989;46:981–985.

251. Waters DJ, Mapleson WW. Suxamethonium pains: hypothesis and observation. *Anaesthesia* 1971;26:127–141.

252. McLoughlin C, Leslie K, Caldwell JE. Influence of dose on suxamethonium-induced muscle damage. *Br J Anaesth* 1994;73:194–198.

253. Poon PW, Lui PW, Chow LH, et al. EMG spike trains of succinylcholine-induced fasciculations in myalgic patients. *Electroencephalogr Clin Neurophysiol* 1996;101:206–210.

254. Palliyath S, Garcia CA. Multifocal interstitial myositis associated with localized lipoatrophy: a benign course. *Arch Neurol* 1982;39:722–724.

255. Créange A, Renard JL, Millet P, et al. A patient with one limb interstitial myositis with localised lipoatrophy presenting with severe cramps and fasciculations. *J Neurol Neurosurg Psychiatry* 1994;57:1541–1543.

256. Miller TM, Layzer RB. Muscle cramps. *Muscle Nerve* 2005;32:431–442.

257. Denny-Brown D, Foley JM. Myokymia and the benign fasciculation of muscle cramp. *Trans Assoc Am Physicians* 1948;61:88–96.

258. Hudson AJ, Brown WF, Gilbert JJ. The muscular pain-fasciculation syndrome. *Neurology* 1978;28:1105–1109.

259. Fetell MR, Smallberg G, Lewis LD, et al. A benign motor neuron disorder: delayed cramps and fasciculation after poliomyelitis or myelitis. *Ann Neurol* 1982;11:423–427.

260. Weiner IH, Weiner HL. Nocturnal leg muscle cramps. *JAMA* 1980;244:2332–2333.

261. Maughan RJ. Exercise-induced muscle cramp: a prospective biochemical study in marathon runners. *J Sports Sci* 1986;4:31–34.

262. Williamson SL, Johnson RW, Hudkins PG, et al. Exertional cramps: a prospective study of biochemical and anthropometric variables in bicycle riders. *Cycling Sci* 1993;5:15–20.

263. Haskell SG, Fiebach NH. Clinical epidemiology of nocturnal leg cramps in male veterans. *Am J Med Sci* 1997;313:210–214.

264. Layzer RB. The origin of muscle fasciculations and cramps. *Muscle Nerve* 1994;17:1243–1249.

265. Daniel HW. Simple cure for nocturnal leg cramps. *N Engl J Med* 1979;301:216.

266. Moss HK, Herrmann LG. Use of quinine for relief of "night cramps" in the extremities. *JAMA* 1940;115:1358–1359.

267. Nightingale SL. Quinine for nocturnal leg cramps (letter). *ACP J Club* 1995;123:86–87.

268. Mandal AK, Abernathy T, Nelluri SN, et al. Is quinine effective and safe in leg cramps? *J Clin Pharmacol* 1995;35:588–593.

269. Lim SH. Randomised double-blind trial of quinine sulphate for nocturnal leg cramp. *Br J Clin Pract* 1986;40:462.

270. Warburton A, Royston JP, O'Neill Q, et al. A quinine a day keeps the leg cramps away? *Br J Clin Pharmacol* 1987;23:459–465.

271. Sidorov J. Quinine sulfate for leg cramps: does it work? *J Am Geriatr Soc* 1993;41:498–500.

272. Jones K, Castleden CM. A double-blind comparison of quinine sulphate and placebo in muscle cramps. *Age Ageing* 1983;12:155–158.

273. Fung MC, Holbrook JH. Placebo-controlled trial of quinine therapy for nocturnal leg cramps. *West J Med* 1989;151:42–44.

274. Connolly PS, Shirley DA, Wasson JH, et al. Treatment of nocturnal leg cramps: a crossover trial of quinine vs vitamin E. *Arch Intern Med* 1992;152:1877–1880.

275. Jansen PH, Veenhuizen KC, Wesseling AI, et al. Randomized controlled trial of hydroquinine in muscle cramps. *Lancet* 1997;349:528–532.

276. Man-Son-Hing M, Wells G. Meta-analysis of efficacy of quinine for treatment of nocturnal leg cramps in elderly people. *Br Med J* 1995;310:13–17.

277. Jansen PH, Veenhuizen KC, Verbeek AL, et al. Efficacy of hydroquinine in preventing frequent ordinary muscle cramp outlasts actual administration. *J Neurol Sci* 1994;122:157–161.

278. Baltodano N, Gallo BV, Weidler DJ. Verapamil vs quinine in recumbent nocturnal leg cramps in the elderly. *Arch Intern Med* 1988;148:1969–1970.

279. Stern FH. Value of carisoprodol (Soma) in relieving leg cramps. *J Am Geriatr Soc* 1963;11:1008–1013.

280. Keidar S, Binenboim C, Palant A. Muscle cramps during treatment with nifedipine. *Br Med J* 1982;85:1241–1242.

281. Steiner I, Siegal T. Muscle cramps in cancer patients. *Cancer* 1989;63:574–577.

282. Medina JL, Chokroverty S, Reyes M. Localized myokymia caused by peripheral nerve injury. *Arch Neurol* 1976;33:587–588.

283. Albers JW, Allen AA II, Bastron JA, et al. Limb myokymia. *Muscle Nerve* 1981;4:494–504.

284. Welch LK, Appenzeller O, Bicknell JM. Peripheral neuropathy with myokymia, sustained muscular contraction, and continuous motor unit activity. *Neurology* 1972;22:161–169.

285. Thomas PK, Claus D, Workman JM, et al. Focal upper limb demyelinating neuropathy. *Brain* 1996;119:765–774.

286. Roth G, Magistris MR. Neuropathies with prolonged conduction block, single and grouped fasciculation, localized limb myokymia. *Electroencephalogr Clin Neurophysiol* 1987;67:428–438.

287. O'Leary CP, Mann AC, Lough J, et al. Muscle hypertrophy in multifocal motor neuropathy is associated with continuous motor unit activity. *Muscle Nerve* 1997;20:479–485.

288. Baldissera F, Cavallari P, Dworzak F. Motor neuron "bistability": a pathogenetic mechanism for cramps and myokymia. *Brain* 1994;117:929–939.

289. Esteban A, Traba A. Fasciculation-myokymic activity and prolonged nerve conduction block: a physiopathologic relationship in radiation-induced brachial plexopathy. *Electroencephalogr Clin Neurophysiol* 1993;89:382–391.

290. Robberecht W, VanHees J, Adriaensen H, et al. Painful muscle spasms complicating algodystrophy: central or peripheral disease? *J Neurol Neurosurg Psychiatry* 1988;51:563–567.

291. Rish BL. Nerve root compression and night cramps. *JAMA* 1985;254:361.

292. Calancie B, Ayyar DR, Eismont FJ. Myokymic discharges: prompt cessation following nerve root decompression during spine surgery. *Electromyogr Clin Neurophysiol* 1992;32:443–447.

293. Denny-Brown D. Clinical problems in neuromuscular physiology. *Am J Med* 1953;15:368–390.

294. Satoyoshi E, Doi Y, Kinoshita M. Pseudomyotonia in cervical root lesions with myelopathy: a sign of the misdirection of regenerating nerve. *Arch Neurol* 1972;27:307–313.

295. Bussaglia E, Tizzano EF, Illa I, et al. Cramps and minimal EMG abnormalities as preclinical manifestations of spinal muscular atrophy patients with homozygous deletions of the SMN gene. *Neurology* 1997;48:1443–1445.

296. Forshew DA, Bromberg MB. A survey of clinicians' practice in symptomatic treatment of ALS. *Amyotroph Lateral Scler Other Motor Neuron Disord* 2003;4:258–263.

297. Roth G. The origin of fasciculations. *Ann Neurol* 1982;12:542–547.

298. Conradi S, Grimby L, Lundemo G. Pathophysiology of fasciculations in ALS as studied by electromyography of single motor units. *Muscle Nerve* 1982;5:202–208.

299. Smith RG, Hamilton S, Hofman F, et al. Serum antibodies to L-type calcium channels in patients with amyotrophic lateral sclerosis. *N Engl J Med* 1992;327:172–178.

300. Smith RG, Kimura F, McKinley K, et al. Alterations in dihydropyridine receptor binding kinetics in amyotrophic lateral sclerosis (ALS) skeletal muscle. *Soc Neurosci Abstr* 1991;17:1451.

301. Sinha S, Newsome-Davis J, Mills K, et al. Autoimmune aetiology for acquired neuromyotonia (Isaacs' syndrome). *Lancet* 1991;338:75–77.

302. Forshew DA, Bromberg, MB. A survey of clinicians' practice in the symptomatic treatment of ALS. *Amyotroph Lateral Scler Other Motor Neuron Disord* 2003;4:258–263.
303. Obi T, Mizoguchi K, Matsuoka H, et al. Muscle cramp as the result of impaired GABA function: an electrophysiological and pharmacological observation. *Muscle Nerve* 1993;16:1228–1231.
304. Talbott JH. Heat cramps. *Medicine* 1935;14:323–376.
305. Knochell JP. Environmental heat illness. *Arch Intern Med* 1974;133:841–864.
306. Donoghue AM, Sinclair MJ, Bates GP. Heat exhaustion in a deep underground metalliferous mine. *Occup Environ Med* 2000; 57:165–174.
307. Rocco MV, Burkart JM. Prevalence of missed treatments and early sign-offs in hemodialysis patients. *J Am Soc Nephrol* 1993;4: 1178–1183.
308. Neal CR, Resnikoff E, Unger AM. Treatment of dialysis-related muscle cramp with hypertonic dextrose. *Arch Intern Med* 1981;141:171–173.
309. Howe RC, Wombolt DG, Michil DD. Analysis of tonic muscle activity and muscle cramps during hemodialysis. *J Dialysis* 1978;2:85–99.
310. Mujais SK. Muscle cramps during hemodialysis (editorial). *Int J Artif Organs* 1994;17:570–572.
311. Canzanello VI, Hylander-Rossner B, Sands RE, et al. Comparison of 50% dextrose water, 25% mannitol, and 23.5% saline for the treatment of hemodialysis-associated muscle cramps. *ASAIO Trans* 1991;37:649–652.
312. Kaplan B, Wang T, Rammohan M, et al. Response to head-up tilt in cramping and noncramping hemodialysis patients. *Int J Clin Pharmacol Ther Toxicol* 1992;30:173–180.
313. Sidhom OA, Odoh YK, Krumlovsky FA, et al. Low-dose prazosin in patients with muscle cramps during hemodialysis. *Clin Pharmacol Ther* 1994;56:445–451.
314. Peer G, Blum M, Aviram A. Relief of hemodialysis-induced muscular cramps by nifedipine. *Dialysis Transplant* 1983;12:180–181.
315. Khajehdehi P, Mojerlou M, Behzadi S, et al. A randomized, double-blind, placebo-controlled trial of supplementary vitamins E, C, and their combination for treatment of haemodialysis cramps. *Nephrol Dial Transplant* 2001;16:1448–1451.
316. Roca AO, Jarjoura D, Blend D, et al. Dialysis leg cramps: efficacy of quinine versus vitamin E. *ASAIO J* 1992;38:M481–M485.
317. Panadero Sandoval J, Perez Garcia A, Martin Abad L, et al. Action of quinine sulphate on the incidence of muscle cramps during hemodialysis. *Med Clin* 1980;75:247–249.
318. Ahmad S, Robertson HT, Golper TA, et al. Multicenter trial of L-carnitine in maintenance hemodialysis patients: 2. Clinical and biochemical effects. *Kidney Int* 1990;38:912–918.
319. Auger RG. AAEM minimonograph #44: diseases associated with excess motor unit activity. *Muscle Nerve* 1994;17:1250–1263.
320. Isaacs H. A syndrome of continuous muscle-fiber activity. *J Neurol Neurosurg Psychiatry* 1961;24:319–325.
321. Auger RG, Daube JR, Gomez MR, et al. Hereditary form of sustained muscle activity of peripheral nerve origin causing generalized myokymia and muscle stiffness. *Ann Neurol* 1984;15:13–21.
322. Layzer RB. Neuromyotonia: a new autoimmune disease. *Ann Neurol* 1995;38:701–702.
323. Newsom-Davis J, Mills KR. Immunological associations of acquired neuromyotonia (Isaacs' syndrome). *Brain* 1993;116: 453–469.
324. Gutmann L, Tellers JG, Vernino S. Persistent facial myokymia associated with K(+) channel antibodies. *Neurology* 2001;57: 1707–1708.
325. Mygland A, Vincent A, Newsom-Davis J, et al. Autoantibodies in thymoma associated myasthenia gravis with myositis or neuromyotonia. *Arch Neurol* 2000;57:527–531.
326. Griffiths TD, Connolly S, Newman PK, et al. Neuromyotonia in association with malignant hyperpyrexia. *J Neurol Neurosurg Psychiatry* 1995;59:556–557.
327. Horikawa M, Yamaguchi Y, Katafuchi Y, et al. A case of Isaacs syndrome with high CSF protein and a large cisterna magna. *Brain Dev* 1993;15:129–132.
328. Kiernan MC, Hart IK, Bostock H. Excitability properties of motor axons in patients with spontaneous motor unit activity. *J Neurol Neurosurg Psychiatry* 2001;70:56–64

329. Irani PF, Porhout AV, Wadia NH. The syndrome of continuous muscle fiber activity: evidence to suggest proximal neurogenic causation. *Acta Neurol Scand* 1977;55:273–288.
330. Ochoa JJ, Castilla JM, Bautista J, et al. Neuromiotonia: origen periferico proximal de la actividad muscular continuua. *Arch Neurobiol (Madr)* 1979;42:309–320.
331. Sakai T, Hosokawa S, Shibisaki H, et al. Syndrome of continuous muscle fiber activity: increased C.S.F. GABA and effect of dantrolene. *Neurology* 1983;33:495–498.
332. Hart IK. Acquired neuromyotonia: a new autoantibody-mediated neuronal potassium channelopathy. *Am J Med Sci* 2000;319:209–216.
333. Vernino S, Auger RG, Emslie-Smith AM, et al. Myasthenia, thymoma, presynaptic antibodies, and a continuum of neuromuscular hyperexcitability. *Neurology* 1999;53:1233–1239.
334. Heidenreich F, Vincent A. Antibodies to ion-channel proteins in thymoma with myasthenia, neuromyotonia, and peripheral neuropathy. *Neurology* 1998;50:1483–1485.
335. Hart IK, Waters C, Vincent A, et al. Autoantibodies detected to expressed K+ channels are implicated in neuromyotonia. *Ann Neurol* 1997;41:238–246.
336. Shillito P, Molenaar PC, Vincent A, et al. Acquired neuromyotonia: evidence for autoantibodies directed against K+ channels of peripheral nerves. *Ann Neurol* 1995;38:714–722.
337. Nagado T, Arimura K, Sonada Y, et al. Potassium current suppression in patients with peripheral nerve hyperexcitibility. *Brain* 1999;122:2056–2066.
338. Sonoda Y, Arimura K, Kurono A, et al. Serum of Isaacs' syndrome suppresses potassium channels in PC12 cell lines. *Muscle Nerve* 1996;19:1439–1446.
339. Arimura K, Watanabe O, Kitajima I, et al. Antibodies to potassium channels of PC12 in serum of Isaacs' syndrome: Western blot and immunohistochemical studies. *Muscle Nerve* 1997; 20:299–305.
340. Riche G, Trouillas P, Bady B. Improvement of Isaacs' syndrome after treatment with azathioprine. *J Neurol Neurosurg Psychiatry* 1995;59:448.
341. Hayashi A, Ishii A, Ohkoshi N, et al. Reply (letter). *J Neurol Neurosurg Psychiatry* 1995;58:393.
342. Ishii A, Hayashi A, Ohkoshi N, et al. Clinical evaluation of plasma exchange and high dose intravenous immunoglobulin in a patient with Isaacs' syndrome. *J Neurol Neurosurg Psychiatry* 1994;57:840–842.
343. Van Engelen BG, Benders AA, Gabreels FJ, et al. Are muscle cramps in Isaacs' syndrome triggered by human immunoglobulin? *J Neurol Neurosurg Psychiatry* 1995;58:393.
344. Isaacs H, Heffron JJA. The syndrome of "continuous muscle fibre activity" cured: further studies. *J Neurol Neurosurg Psychiatry* 1974;37:1231–1235.
345. Koley KC, Roy AK, Sinho G. Neuromyotonia. *J Ind Med Assoc* 1992;90:131–132.
346. Waerness E. Neuromyotonia and bronchial carcinoma. *Electromyogr Clin Neurophysiol* 1974;14:527–535.
347. Walsh JC. Neuromyotonia: an unusual presentation of intrathoracic malignancy. *J Neurol Neurosurg Psychiatry* 1976;39: 1086–1091.
348. Partanen VSJ, Soinen H, Saksa M, et al. Electromyographic and nerve conduction findings in a patient with neuromyotonia, normocalcemic tetany and small-cell lung cancer. *Acta Neurol Scand* 1980;61:216–226.
349. Caress J, Preston DC, Abend WK, et al. A case of Hodgkin's lymphoma producing neuromyotonia (abstract). *Neurology* 1997;48(suppl 2):A147.
350. Halbach M, Homberg V, Freund HJ. Neuromuscular autonomic and central cholinergic hyperactivity associated with thymoma and acetylcholine receptor antibody. *J Neurol* 1987;234:433–436.
351. Garcia R, Boudene C, Cinsbourg M. Choree fibrillaire de Morvan et polyradiculonevrite d'etiologie mercurielle probable. *Rev Neurol* 1971;125:322–323.
352. Martinelli P, Patuelli A, Minardi C, et al. Neuromyotonia, peripheral neuropathy, and myasthenia gravis. *Muscle Nerve* 1996;19:505–510.
353. Vasilescu C, Florescu A. Peripheral neuropathy with a syndrome of continuous motor activity. *J Neurol* 1982;226:275–282.

354. Preston DC, Kelly JJ. "Pseudospasticity" in Guillain-Barré syndrome. *Neurology* 1991;41:131–134.

355. Valenstein E, Watson RT, Parker JL. Myokymial muscle hypertrophy and percussion "myotonia" in chronic recurrent polyneuropathy. *Neurology* 1978;28:1130–1134.

356. Joy JL, Allen RF, Sunwool N, et al. Isaacs' syndrome associated with chronic inflammatory demyelinating polyneuropathy. *Muscle Nerve* 1990;13:868.

357. Odabasi Z, Joy JL, Claussen GC, et al. Isaacs' syndrome associated with chronic inflammatory demyelinating polyneuropathy. *Muscle Nerve* 1996;19:210–215.

358. Bady B, Chauplannaz G, Vial C. Autoimmune aetiology for acquired neuromyotonia (letter). *Lancet* 1991;338:1330.

359. Le Gars L, Clerc D, Cariou D, et al. Systemic juvenile rheumatoid arthritis and associated Isaacs' syndrome. *J Rheumatol* 1997;24:178–180.

360. Reeback J, Benton JS, Swash M, et al. Penicillamine-induced neuromyotonia. *Br Med J* 1979;1:1464–1465.

361. Black JT, Garcia-Mullin R, Good E, et al. Muscle rigidity in a newborn due to continuous peripheral nerve hyperactivity. *Arch Neurol* 1972;27:413–425.

362. Mitsumoto H, Wilbourn AJ, Subramony SH. Generalized myokymia and gold therapy. *Arch Neurol* 1982;39:449–450.

363. Fraisse P, Sutter B, Tritschler JL, et al. Morvan's fibrillary chorea after gold therapy (letter). *Presse Med* 1985;14:1097.

364. Morvan A. De la choree fibrillaire. *Gaz Heb Med Chirurg* 1890;27:173–202.

365. Garcia-Merino A, Cabello A, Mora JS, et al. Continuous muscle fiber activity, peripheral neuropathy, and thymoma. *Ann Neurol* 1991;29:215–218.

366. Gil R, Lefevre JP, Neau JPH, et al. Choree fibrillaire de Morvan et syndrome acrodynique apres un troutement mercuriel. *Rev Neurol (Paris)* 1984;140:728–733.

367. Serratrice G, Azulay JP. What is left of Morvan's fibrillary chorea? (in French). *Rev Neurol* 1994;150:257–265.

368. Lee EK, Maselli RA, Ellis WG, et al. Morvan's fibrillary chorea: a paraneoplastic manifestation of thymoma. *J Neurol Neurosurg Psychiatry* 1998;65:857–862.

369. Hosokawa S, Shinoda H, Sakai T, et al. Electrophysiological study on limb myokymia in three women. *J Neurol Neurosurg Psychiatry* 1987;50:877–881.

370. Lublin FD, Tsairis P, Streletz LJ, et al. Myokymia and impaired muscular relaxation with continuous motor unit activity. *J Neurol Neurosurg Psychiatry* 1979;42:557–562.

371. Grassa C, Figa-Talamanca L, Lo Russo F, et al. Syndrome of continuous muscle fiber activity: case report. *Ital J Neurol Sci* 1981;4:415–418.

372. Jamieson PW, Katirji MB. Idiopathic generalized myokymia. *Muscle Nerve* 1994;17:42–51.

373. Torbergsen T, Stalberg E, Brautaset N. Generator sites for spontaneous activity: an EMG study. *Electroencephalogr Clin Neurophysiol* 1996;101:69–78.

374. O'Brien TJ, Gates P. Isaacs' syndrome: report of a case responding to valproic acid. *Clin Exp Neurol* 1994;31:52–60.

375. Tahmoush AJ, Alonso RJ, Tahmoush GP, et al. Cramp-fasciculation syndrome: a treatable hyperexcitable peripheral nerve disorder. *Neurology* 1991;41:1021–1024.

376. Smith KK, Claussen G, Fesenmeier JT, et al. Myokymia-cramp syndrome: evidence of hyperexcitable peripheral nerve. *Muscle Nerve* 1994;17:1065–1067.

377. Lance JW, Burke D, Pollard J. Neuromyotonia in the spinal form of Charcot-Marie-Tooth disease. *Clin Exp Neurol* 1979;16:49–56.

378. Hahn AF, Parkes AW, Bolton CF, et al. Neuromyotonia in hereditary motor neuropathy. *J Neurol Neurosurg Psychiatry* 1991;54:230–235.

379. Lance JW, Burke D, Pollard J. Hyperexcitability of motor and sensory neurons in neuromyotonia. *Ann Neurol* 1979;5:523–532.

380. Vasilescu C, Alexianu M, Dan A. Neuronal type of Charcot-Marie-Tooth disease with a syndrome of continuous motor activity. *J Neurol Sci* 1984;63:11–25.

381. Thomas PK, Marques W Jr, Davis MB, et al. The phenotypic manifestations of chromosome 17p11.2 duplication. *Brain* 1997;120:465–478.

382. Burk K, Stevanin G, Didierjean O, et al. Clinical and genetic analysis of three German kindreds with autosomal dominant cerebellar ataxia type I linked to the SCA2 locus. *J Neurol* 1997;244:256–261.

383. Takashima H, Nakagawa M, Nakahara K, et al. A new type of hereditary motor and sensory neuropathy linked to chromosome 3. *Ann Neurol* 1997;41:771–780.

384. Ashizawa T, Butler IJ, Harati Y, et al. A dominantly inherited syndrome with continuous motor discharges. *Ann Neurol* 1983;13:285–290.

385. McGuire SA, Tomasovic FF, Ackerman NJ R. Hereditary continuous muscle fiber activity. *Arch Neurol* 1984;41:395–396.

386. Sheaff HM. Hereditary myokymia. *Arch Neurol Psychiatry* 1952;68:236–247.

387. Van Dyke DH, Griggs RC, Murphy MJ, et al. Hereditary myokymia and periodic ataxia. *J Neurol Sci* 1975;25:109–118.

388. Hanson PA, Martinez LB, Cassidy R. Contractures, continuous muscle discharges, and titubation. *Ann Neurol* 1977;1:120–124.

389. Gancher ST, Nutt JG. Autosomal dominant episodic ataxia: a heterogeneous syndrome. *Mov Disord* 1986;1:239–253.

390. Brunt ER, VanWeerden W. Familial paroxysmal kinesigenic ataxia and continuous myokymia. *Brain* 1990;113:1361–1382.

391. Bain PG, O'Brien MD, Keevil SF, et al. Familial periodic cerebellar ataxia: a problem of cerebellar intracellular pH homeostasis. *Ann Neurol* 1992;31:147–154.

392. Vaamonde J, Artieda J, Obeso JA. Hereditary paroxysmal ataxia with neuromyotonia. *Mov Disord* 1991;6:180–182.

393. Lubbers WJ, Brunt ER, Scheffer H, et al. Hereditary myokymia and paroxysmal ataxia linked to chromosome 12 is responsive to acetazolamide. *J Neurol Neurosurg Psychiatry* 1995;59:400–405.

394. Browne DL, Gancher ST, Nutt JG, et al. Episodic ataxia/myokymia syndrome is associated with point mutations in the human potassium channel gene, KCNA1. *Nat Genet* 1994;8:136–140.

395. Browne DL, Brunt ER, Griggs RC, et al. Identification of two new KCNA1 mutations in episodic ataxia/myokymia families. *Hum Mol Genet* 1995;4:1671–1672.

396. Byme E, White O, Cook M. Familial dystonic choreoathetosis with myokymia: a sleep responsive disorder. *J Neurol Neurosurg Psychiatry* 1991;54:1090–1092.

397. Fink JK, Rainer S, Wilkowski J, et al. Paroxysmal dystonic choreoathetosis: tight linkage to chromosome 2q. *Am J Hum Genet* 1996;59:140–145.

398. Van den Bergh P, Bulcke JA, Dom R. Familial muscle cramps with autosomal dominant transmission. *Eur Neurol* 1980;19:207–212.

399. Ricker K, Moxley RT III. Autosomal dominant cramping disease. *Arch Neurol* 1990;47:810–812.

400. Jusic A, Dogan S, Stojanovic V. Hereditary persistent distal cramps. *J Neurol Neurosurg Psychiatry* 1972;35:379–384.

401. Lazaro PR, Rollinson RD, Fenichel GM. Familial cramps and muscle pain. *Arch Neurol* 1981;38:22–24.

402. Lun LC. Hyperventilation and anxiety state. *J Soc Med* 1981;74:1–4.

403. Magarian GJ. Hyperventilation syndromes: infrequently recognized common expressions of anxiety and stress. *Medicine* 1982;61:219–236.

404. Kugelberg E. Activation of human nerves by ischemia: Trousseau's phenomenon in tetany. *Arch Neurol Psychiatry* 1948;60:140–152.

405. Kugelberg E. Activation of human nerve by hyperventilation and hypocalcemia: neurologic mechanism of symptoms of irritation in tetany. *Arch Neurol Psychiatry* 1948;60:153–164.

406. Stein RB. *Nerve and muscles: membranes, cells, and systems.* New York: Plenum Press, 1980:56–59.

407. Vukasin P, Weston LA, Beart RW. Oral Fleet "Phospho-Soda" laxative-induced hyperphosphatemia and hypocalcemic tetany in an adult: report of a case. *Dis Colon Rectum* 1997;40:497–499.

408. Ramage IJ, Ray M, Paton RD, et al. Hypomagnesaemic tetany. *J Clin Pathol* 1996;49:343–344.

409. Shuster J. Methylprednisolone as a cause of anaphylaxis; diltiazem-induced tetany; NSAID-induced colonic stricture with ulceration and NSAID-induced erythema multiforme; lamotrigine and Tourette symptoms; anaphylactic reaction after dermal exposure to cephalexin. *Hosp Pharmacy* 2000;35:137,138,140,143.

410. Campisi P, Badhwar V, Morin S, et al. Postoperative hypocalcemic tetany caused by Fleet Phospho-Soda preparation in a patient taking alendronate sodium: report of a case. *Dis Colon Rectum* 1999;42:1499–1501.

411. Yamashita H, Noguchi S, Tahara K, et al. Postoperative tetany in patients with Graves' disease: a risk factor analysis. *Clin Endocrinol* 1997;47:71–77.

412. Taborska V. Incidence of latent tetany in patients with panic disorder. *Cesk Psychiatr* 1995;91:183–190.

413. Ault MJ, Geiderman J. Hypokalemia as a cause of tetany. *West J Med* 1992;157:65–67.

414. Isgreen WP. Normocalcemic tetany. *Neurology* 1976;26:825–834.

415. Day JW, Parry GJ. Normocalcemic tetany abolished by calcium infusion. *Ann Neurol* 1990;27:438–440.

416. Knochell JP. Neuromuscular manifestation of electrolyte disorders. *Am J Med* 1982;72:521–535.

417. Corbett AJ. Electrolyte disorders affecting muscle. *Semin Neurol* 1983;3:248–257.

418. Harati Y. Eosinophilia-myalgia syndrome and its relation to toxic oil syndrome. In: de Wolff FA, ed. *Handbook of clinical neurology: intoxications of the nervous system*, part 1, vol. 20. Amsterdam: Elsevier Science, 1994:249–271.

419. Kaufman LD, Kaufman MA, Krupp LB. Movement disorders in the eosinophilia-myalgia syndrome: tremor, myoclonus, and myokymia. *J Rheumatol* 1995;22:157–160.

420. Mayeno AN, Benson LM, Naylor S, et al. Biotransformation of 3-(phenylamino)-1,2-propanediol to 3(phenylamino)alanine: a chemical link between toxic oil syndrome and eosinophilia-myalgia syndrome. *Chem Res Toxicol* 1995;8:911–916.

421. Martin RW, Duffy J, Engel AG, et al. The clinical spectrum of the eosinophilia-myalgia syndrome associated with L-tryptophan ingestion. *Ann Intern Med* 1990;113:124–134.

422. Hertzman PA, Clauw DJ, Duffy JM, et al. Rigorous new approach to constructing a gold standard for validating new diagnostic criteria, as exemplified by the eosinophilia-myalgia syndrome. *Arch Intern Med* 2001;161:2301–2306.

423. Hertzman PA, Clauw DJ, Kaufman LD, et al. The eosinophilia-myalgia syndrome: status of 205 patients and results of treatment 2 years after onset. *Ann Intern Med* 1995;122:851–855.

424. Eosinophilia-myalgia syndrome: follow-up survey of patients—New York, 1990–1991. *MMWR* 1991;40:401–403.

425. Kaufman LD. Chronicity of the eosinophilia myalgia syndrome: a reassessment after three years. *Arthritis Rheum* 1994;37:84–87.

426. Armstrong C, Lewis T, D'Esposito M, et al. Eosinophilia-myalgia syndrome: selective cognitive impairment, longitudinal effects, and neuroimaging findings. *J Neurol Neurosurg Psychiatry* 1997;63:633–641.

427. White J. Bites and stings from venomous animals: a global overview. *Ther Drug Monit* 2000;22:65–68.

428. Satoyoshi E, Yamada K. Recurrent muscle spasms of central origin. *Arch Neurol* 1967;16:254–263.

429. Ehlayel MS, Lacassie Y. Satoyoshi syndrome: an unusual postnatal multisystemic disorder. *Am J Med Genet* 1995;57:620–625.

430. Satoyoshi E. A syndrome of progressive muscle spasms, alopecia, and diarrhea. *Neurology* 1978;28:458–461.

431. Ikegawa S, Nagano A, Satoyoshi E. Skeletal abnormalities in Satoyoshi's syndrome: a radiographic study of eight cases. *Skel Radiol* 1993;22:321–324.

432. Yamagata T, Miyao M, Momoi M, et al. A case of generalized komuragaeri disease (Satoyoshi disease) treated with glucocorticoid. *Rinsho Shinkeigaku* 1991;31:79–83.

433. Satoh AI, Tsujihata M, Yashimura T, et al. Myasthenia gravis associated with Satoyoshi syndrome: muscle cramps, alopecia, and diarrhea. *Neurology* 1983;33:1209–1211.

434. Arita J, Hamano S, Nara T, et al. Intravenous gamma-globulin therapy of Satoyoshi syndrome. *Brain Dev* 1996;18:409–411.

435. Takahashi J, Takahashi S, Kikuchi T, et al. The siblings of painful muscle cramps (generalized muscle cramp disease) with alopecia and endocrinological disorders (in Japanese). *Rinsho Shinkeigaku* 1994;34:152–156.

436. Drost G, Verrips A, Hooijkaas H, et al. Glutamic acid decarboxylase antibodies in Satoyoshi syndrome. *Ann Neurol* 2004;55:450.

437. Wisuthsarewong W, Likitmaskul S, Manonukul J. Satoyoshi syndrome. *Pediatric Dermatol* 2001;18:406–410.

438. Endo K, Yamamoto T, Nakamura K, et al. Improvement of Satoyoshi syndrome with tacrolimus and corticosteroids. *Neurology* 2003;60:2014–2015.

439. Merello M, Garcia H, Nogues M, et al. Masticatory muscle spasm in a non-Japanese patient with Satoyoshi syndrome successfully treated with botulinum toxin. *Mov Disord* 1994;9:104–105.

440. Katz J, Prescott K, Woolf AD. Strychnine poisoning from a Cambodian traditional remedy. *Am J Emerg Med* 1996;14: 475–477.

441. Roos KL. Tetanus. *Semin Neurol* 1991;11:206–214.

442. Trujillo MJ, Castillo A, Espana JV, et al. Tetanus in the adult: intensive care and management experience with 233 cases. *Crit Care Med* 1980;8:419–423.

443. Trujillo MJ, Castillo A, Espana J, et al. Impact of intensive care management on the prognosis of tetanus: analysis of 641 cases. *Chest* 1987;92:63–65.

444. Crone NE, Reder AT. Severe tetanus in immunized patients with high anti-tetanus titers. *Neurology* 1992;42:761–764.

445. Apte NM, Kamad DR. Short report: the spatula test—a simple bedside test to diagnose tetanus. *Am J Trop Med Hyg* 1995;53: 386–387.

446. Risk WS, Bosch EP, Kimura J, et al. Chronic tetanus: clinical report and histochemistry of muscle. *Muscle Nerve* 1981;4:363–366.

447. Melanby J, Green J. How does tetanus toxin act? *Neuroscience* 1981;6:281–300.

448. Bleck TP. Pharmacology of tetanus (review). *Clin Neuropharmacol* 1986;9:103–120.

449. Attygalle D, Rodrigo N. Magnesium sulphate for control of spasms in severe tetanus: can we avoid sedation and artificial ventilation? *Anaesthesia* 1997;52:956–962.

450. Moersch FP, Woltman HW. Progressive fluctuating muscular rigidity and spasm (stiffman syndrome): report of a case with some observations in 13 other cases. *Proc Staff Meet Mayo Clin* 1956;31:421–427.

451. Gordon EE, Janusko DM, Kaufman L. A critical survey of stiff-man syndrome. *Am J Med* 1967;42:589–599.

452. Whiteley AM, Swash M, Urish H. Progressive encephalomyelitis with rigidity: its relation to "subacute myoclonic spinal neuronitis" and to the "stiff-man syndrome." *Brain* 1976;99:27–42.

453. Lorish TR, Thorsteinsson G, Howard FM Jr. Stiff-man syndrome updated. *Mayo Clin Proc* 1989;64:629–636.

454. Walikonis JE, Lennon VA. Radioimmunoassay for glutamic acid decarboxylase (GAD65). Autoantibodies as a diagnostic aid for stiff-man syndrome and a correlate of susceptibility to type 1 diabetes mellitus. *Mayo Clinic Proc* 1998;73:1161–1166.

455. Pleitez MY, Harati Y. Stiff-person syndrome. In: Rolak LA, Harati Y, eds. *Neuroimmunology for the clinician.* Boston: Butterworth, 1997:253–262.

456. Dalakas MC, Fujii M, Li M, et al. The clinical spectrum of anti-GAD antibody-positive patients with stiff-person syndrome. *Neurology* 2000;55:1531–1535.

457. Klein R, Haddow JE, DeLuca C. Familial congenital disorder resembling stiff-man syndrome. *Am J Dis Child* 1972;124: 730–731.

458. Sander JE, Layzer RB, Goldsobel AB. Congenital stiffman syndrome. *Ann Neurol* 1980;8:195–197.

459. Lingam S, Wilson J, Hart EW. Hereditary stiff-baby syndrome. *Am J Dis Child* 1981;135:909–911.

460. Schwartzman MJ, Mitsumoto H, Chou M, et al. Sudden death in stiff-man syndrome with autonomic instability (abstract). *Ann Neurol* 1989;26:166.

461. Barker RA, Revesz T, Thom M, et al. Review of 23 patients affected by the stiff man syndrome: clinical subdivision into stiff trunk (man) syndrome, stiff limb syndrome, and progressive encephalomyelitis with rigidity. *J Neurol Neurosurg Psychiatry* 1998;65:633–640.

462. Saiz A, Graus F, Valldeoriola F, et al. Stiff-leg syndrome: a focal form of stiff-man syndrome. *Ann Neurol* 1998;43:400–403.

463. Leigh PN, Rothwell JC, Traub M, et al. A patient with reflex myoclonus and muscle rigidity: "jerking stiffman syndrome." *J Neurol Neurosurg Psychiatry* 1980;43:1125–1131.

464. Alberca R, Romero M, Chaparro J. Jerking-stiff-man syndrome. *J Neurol Neurosurg Psychiatry* 1982;45:1159–1160.

465. Meinck HM, Ricker K, Hulser PJ, et al. Stiff man syndrome: neurophysiological findings in eight patients. *J Neurol* 1995;242: 134–142.

466. Solimena M, Folli F, Aparisi R, et al. Autoantibodies to GABAergic neurons and pancreatic beta cells in stiff-man syndrome. *N Engl J Med* 1990;322:1555–1560.

467. Vincent A, Grimaldi LME, Martino G, et al. Antibodies to ^{125}I-glutamic acid decarboxylase in patients with stiff man syndrome. *J Neurol Neurosurg Psychiatry* 1997;62:395–397.

468. Asher R. A woman with the stiff-man syndrome. *Br Med J* 1958;1:265–266.

469. Trethowan WH, Allsop JL, Turner B. The "stiff-man" syndrome: a report of two further cases. *Arch Neurol* 1960;3:448–456.

470. Martinelli P, Pazzaglia P, Montagna P, et al. Stiff-man syndrome associated with nocturnal myoclonus and epilepsy. *J Neurol Neurosurg Psychiatry* 1978;41:463–465.

471. Meinck HM, Ricker K, Solimena M. Stiff-man syndrome: clinical and laboratory findings in eight patients. *J Neurol* 1994;241: 157–166.

472. Fujiya S, Yahara O, Kawakami Y, et al. Case of stiff-man syndrome with pathological changes in the spinal cord (article in Japanese). *Nippon Naika Gakkai Zasshi* 1982;71:1154–1163.

473. Nakamura N, Fujiya S, Yahara O, et al. Stiff-man syndrome with spinal cord lesion. *Clin Neuropathol* 1986;5:40–46.

474. Guilleminault C, Sigwald J, Castaigne P. Sleep studies and therapeutic trial with L-dopa in a case of Stiffman syndrome. *Eur Neurol* 1973;10:89–96.

475. Meinck HM, Ricker K, Conrad B. The stiff-man syndrome: new pathophysiologic aspects from abnormal exteroceptive reflexes and the response to clomipramine, clonidine, and tizanidine. *J Neurol Neurosurg Psychiatry* 1984;47:280–287.

476. Schmidt RT, Stahl SM, Spehlmann R. A pharmacologic study of the stiff-man syndrome: correlation of clinical symptoms with urinary 3-methoxy-4-hydroxyphenyl glycol excretion. *Neurology* 1975;25:622–626.

477. Isaacs H. Stiffman syndrome in a black girl. *J Neurol Neurosurg Psychiatry* 1979;42:988–994.

478. Solimena M, Folli F, Denis-Donini S, et al. Autoantibodies to glutamic acid decarboxylase in a patient with stiff-man syndrome, epilepsy, and type I diabetes mellitus. *N Engl J Med* 1988;318:1012–1020.

479. Solimena M, DeCamilli P. Autoimmunity to glutamic acid decarboxylase (GAD) in stiff-man syndrome and insulin-dependent diabetes mellitus. *Trends Neurosci* 1991;14:452–457.

480. Baekkeskov S, Aanstoot HJ, Chistgau S, et al. Identification of the 64K autoantigen in insulin-dependent diabetes as the GABA-synthesizing enzyme glutamic acid decarboxylase. *Nature* 1990;347:151–156.

481. Lohmann T, Hawa M, Leslie RD, et al. Immune reactivity to glutamic acid decarboxylase 65 in stiffman syndrome and type 1 diabetes mellitus. *Lancet* 2000;356:31–35.

482. Pugliese A, Solimena M, Awdeh ZL, et al. Association of HLA-DQBI*0201 with stiff-man syndrome. *J Clin Endocrinol Metab* 1993;77:1550–1553.

483. Grimaldi LM, Martino G, Braghi S, et al. Heterogeneity of autoantibodies in stiff-man syndrome. *Ann Neurol* 1993;34:57–64.

484. Giometto B, Miotto D, Faresin F, et al. Anti-gabaergic neuron autoantibodies in a patient with stiff-man syndrome and ataxia. *J Neurol Sci* 1996;143:57–59.

485. Bjork E, Velloso LA, Kampe O, et al. GAD autoantibodies in IDDM, stiff-man syndrome, and autoimmune polyendocrine syndrome type I recognize different epitopes. *Diabetes* 1994; 43:161–165.

486. Martino G, Grimaldi LM, Bazzigaluppi E, et al. The insulin-dependent diabetes mellitus–associated ICA 105 autoantigen in stiff-man syndrome patients. *J Immunol* 1996;156:818–825.

487. Daw K, Ujihara N, Atkinson M, et al. Glutamic acid decarboxylase autoantibodies in stiff-man syndrome and insulin-dependent diabetes mellitus exhibit similarities and differences in epitope recognition. *J Immunol* 1996;156:818–825.

488. Kim J, Namchuk M, Bugawan T, et al. Higher autoantibody levels and recognition of a linear NH_2-terminal epitope in the autoantigen GAD65, distinguish stiff-man syndrome from insulin-dependent diabetes mellitus. *J Exp Med* 1994;180:595–606.

489. George TM, Burke JM, Sobotka PA, et al. Resolution of stiff-man syndrome with cortisol replacement in a patient with deficiencies of ACTH, growth hormone, and prolactin. *N Engl J Med* 1984;310:1511–1513.

490. Lohnmann T, Londei M, Hawa M, Leslie DG. Humoral and cellular autoimmune responses in stiff person syndrome. *Ann NY Acad Sci* 2003;998:215–222.

491. Nemni R, Caniatti LM, Gironi M, et al. Stiff person syndrome does not always occur with maternal passive transfer of GAD65 antibodies. *Neurology* 2004;62:2101–2102.

492. Werk EE Jr, Sholiton LJ, Mamell RT. The "stiff-man" syndrome and hyperthyroidism. *Am J Med* 1961;31:647–653.

493. Trojaborg W, Rowland LP, Katz RI, et al. Stiff muscles and bony tendons. *Trans Am Neurol Assoc* 1970;95:169–171.

494. Drake ME Jr. Stiff-man syndrome and dementia. *Am J Med* 1983;74:1085–1987.

495. Rushworth G, Lishman WA, Hughes JT, et al. Intensive rigidity of the arms due to isolation of motoneurons by spinal tumor. *J Neurol Psychiatry* 1961;24:132–142.

496. Brown P, Rothwell JC, Marsden CD. The stiff leg syndrome. *J Neurol Neurosurg Psychiatry* 1997;62:31–37.

497. Kasperek S, Zebrowski S. Stiff-man syndrome and encephalomyelitis: report of a case. *Arch Neurol* 1971;24:22–30.

498. Lhermitte F, Chain F, Escouvolle R, et al. Un nouveau cas de contracture tetaniforme distinct du "stiffman syndrome." *Rev Neurol* 1973;128:321.

499. Howell DA, Lees AJ, Toghill PJ. Spinal internuncial neurones in progressive encephalomyelitis with rigidity. *J Neurol Neurosurg Psychiatry* 1979;42:773–785.

500. Watanabe K, Shimizu T, Mannen T, et al. An autopsy case with unusual muscle rigidity resembling the stiff-man syndrome. *Clin Neurol (Tokyo)* 1984;24:839–847.

501. Bum DJ, Ball J, Lees AJ, et al. A case of progressive encephalomyelitis with rigidity and positive antiglutamic acid decarboxylase antibodies. *J Neurol Neurosurg Psychiatry* 1991;54: 449–451.

502. Armon C, Swanson JW, McLean JM, et al. Subacute encephalomyelitis presenting as stiff-person syndrome: clinical, polygraphic, and pathologic correlations. *Mov Disord* 1996;11: 701–709.

503. McCabe DJ, Turner NC, Chao D, et al. Paraneoplastic "stiff person syndrome" with metastatic adenocarcinoma and anti-Ri antibodies. *Neurology* 2004;62:1402–1404.

504. Antoine JC, Absi L, Honnorat J, et al. Antiamphiphysin antibodies are associated with various paraneoplastic neurological syndromes and tumors. *Arch Neurol* 1999;56:172–177.

505. Schmierer K, Grosse P, De Camilli P, et al. Paraneoplastic stiff-person syndrome: no tumor progression over 5 years. *Neurology* 2002;58:148.

506. Miller F, Korsvik H. Baclofen in the treatment of stiffman syndrome. *Ann Neurol* 1981;9:511–512.

507. Vermeij FH, van Doom PA, Busch HF. Improvement of stiff-man syndrome with vigabatrin. *Lancet* 1996;348:612.

508. Prevett MC, Brown P, Duncan JS. Improvement of stiffman syndrome with vigabatrin. *Neurology* 1997;48:1133–1134.

509. Murinson BB, Rizzo M. Improvement of stiff-person syndrome with tiagabine. *Neurology* 2001;57:366.

510. Stayer C, Tronnier V, Dressnandt J, et al. Intrathecal baclofen therapy for stiff-man syndrome and progressive encephalomyelopathy with rigidity and myoclonus. *Neurology* 1997;49:1591–1597.

511. Barker RA, Marsden CD. Successful treatment of stiff man syndrome with intravenous immunoglobulin (letter). *J Neurol Neurosurg Psychiatry* 1997;62:426–427.

512. Dalakas MC, Fujii M, Li M, et al. High-dose intravenous immune globulin for stiff-person syndrome. *N Engl J Med* 2001;345: 1870–1876.

513. Jacobsen JH, Rosenberg RS, Huttenlocher PR, et al. Familial nocturnal cramping. *Sleep* 1986;9:54–60.

514. Chiba S, Saitoh M, Hatanaka Y, et al. Autosomal dominant muscle cramp syndrome in a Japanese family. *J Neurol Neurosurg Psychiatry* 1999;67:116–119.

515. Matthews WB. Tonic seizures in multiple sclerosis. *Brain* 1958;81:193–206.

516. Twomey JA, Espir MLE. Paroxysmal symptoms as the first manifestation of multiple sclerosis. *J Neurol Neurosurg Psychiatry* 1980;43:296–304.

517. Heath PD, Nightingale S. Clusters of tonic spasms as an initial manifestation of multiple sclerosis. *Ann Neurol* 1982;12: 494–495.

518. Berger JR, Sheremata WA, Melamed G. Paroxysmal dystonia as the initial manifestation of multiple sclerosis. *Arch Neurol* 1984;41:747–750.

519. Shibasaki H, Kuroiwa Y. Painful tonic seizure in multiple sclerosis. *Arch Neurol* 1974;30:47–51.

520. Matthews WB. Paroxysmal symptoms in multiple sclerosis. *J Neurol Neurosurg Psychiatry* 1975;38:617–623.

521. Osterman PO, Westberg CE. Paroxysmal attacks in multiple sclerosis. *Brain* 1975;98:198–202.

522. Watson CP, Chiu M. Painful tonic seizures in multiple sclerosis: localization of a lesion. *Can J Neurol Sci* 1979;6:359–361.

523. Rose MR, Ball JA, Thompson PD. Magnetic resonance imaging in tonic spasms of multiple sclerosis. *J Neurol* 1993;241:115–117.

524. Lataste X, Emre M, Davis C, et al. Comparative profile of tizanidine in the management of spasticity. *Neurology* 1994;44(suppl 9):S53–S59.

525. Penn RD. Intrathecal baclofen for spasticity of spinal origin: seven years of experience. *J Neurosurg* 1992;77:236–240.

Assessment of Behavior in Parkinsonian Disorders

Bernard Pillon   Bruno Dubois

Subtle but specific cognitive deficits can frequently be detected in patients with a variety of diseases accompanied by movement disorders. This is explained by the fact that the neuronal pathways connecting the basal ganglia to the cerebral cortex not only project to regions involved in the control of movements (motor, premotor, supplementary motor areas) but also to cortical areas contributing to cognitive functions (prefrontal cortex) and to emotional processing (cingulum and orbitofrontal cortex). Such lesions induce changes that resemble the consequences of frontal lobe damage and have been brought together under the term of *dysexecutive syndrome*. Indeed, each parkinsonian disorder is characterized by a specific pattern of neuronal lesions, within the basal ganglia, that is responsible for a characteristic motor syndrome with a specific pattern of response to L-dopa and also a recognizable profile of neuropsychological deficits. Together with the characterization of the motor features, the use of appropriate neuropsychological tests or questionnaires to detect the cognitive deficits and behavioral changes can, therefore, contribute to the diagnosis of such diseases.

This chapter will (a) define executive functions, (b) describe how to assess executive functions and other cognitive or behavioral disorders, and (c) show the influence of cognitive and behavioral changes in diagnostic decision trees.

WHAT ARE EXECUTIVE FUNCTIONS?

Executive functions are exhibited in novel or demanding situations that require the elaboration of goal-directed behaviors in opposition to more reflexive behavioral responses that can be activated easily in overlearned or routine situations. To be correctly realized, these goal-directed behaviors require (a) an anticipation of the goal, (b) the selection of appropriate pieces of information, (c) the maintenance and monitoring of information within the working memory buffer, (d) the elaboration and execution of the plan, and (e) the validation of its pertinence as a function of internal and external contingencies (1). The prefrontal cortex is involved in the control of these functions in closed but complementary relationship with the basal ganglia. The prefrontal cortex allows behavioral adaptation by inhibiting automatic activation of overlearned procedures and by elaborating new schemas of response based on two integrated processes: the programming of the response, whatever its input (cognitive, behavioral, social, etc.) and the evaluation of the affective valence that the response will have for the subject. In this framework, the role of the basal ganglia might be to translate these new programs in automatic procedures and, consequently, free the attention resources required by the prefrontal cortex for the elaboration of new programs (2).

ASSESSMENT OF EXECUTIVE FUNCTIONS

Given these interpretations, executive functions can be roughly conceptualized as including three classes of cognitive processes: (a) volition; (b) planning; (c) control of environmental autonomy and inhibition of automatic programs. Each may be assessed by distinctive questionnaires or tests (Table 39.1). Executive functions also may be evaluated more economically by global and composite but short scales.

Volition

Volition refers to intentional behavior and to all the processes that are necessary for a behavioral response to be activated (3). It includes *motivation* or the capacity to formulate a goal; *self-activation* or the capacity to initiate behavior to attain the goal; *control of impulsivity* or the capacity to maintain the goal; *self-awareness* or the capacity to perceive the congruence between the goal and the consequences of the projected behavior; and *sensitivity to reward* or the capacity to affectively appreciate the consequences of the action. The corresponding executive deficits (apathy, inertia, desinhibition, anosognosia, indifference to the consequences of action) have all been observed in

parkinsonian disorders (4,5), independently of the existence of depression (6). These deficits may be assessed by such questionnaires as the Apathy Scale (7) or the Neuropsychiatric Inventory (8) or by more objective tests such as the Gambling Task (9).

Planning

Planning includes the identification and organization of the steps needed to carry out an intention or to achieve a goal and involves strategic components of working and episodic memory, set activation, elaboration, maintenance, and shifting. The deficits are characterized by decreased attention resources, impaired encoding and retrieval strategies, cognitive slowing, decreased conceptualization, sensitivity to interferences, and perseverations (10). The required tools are now well-known and summarized in Table 39.1. In the Digit Ordering Test (DOT), the patient must remember series of 7 numbers randomly presented (for example,

TABLE 39.1

ASSESSMENT OF EXECUTIVE FUNCTIONS

Executive Functions	Executive Deficits	Neuropsychologial Tools
Volition		
Motivation	Apathy	Apathy Scale (7)
Self-activation	Inertia	NPI (8)
Control of impulsivity	Desinhibition	NPI (8)
Self-awareness	Anosognosia	NPI (8)
Reward sensitivity	Indifference to consequences of action	Gambling task (9)
Planning		
Working memory (strategic components)	Decreased attention	DOT[a]
Episodic memory (strategic components)	Impaired encoding and retrieval	CVLT[b] Grober and Buschke test[c]
Set activation	Cognitive slowing	Lexical fluency[d]
Set elaboration	Decreased conceptualization	WCST[e]
Set maintenance	Sensitivity to interferences	Stroop test[f]
Set shifting	Perseveration	TMT[g]
Behavioral autonomy		
Control of environmental stimulations	Environmental dependency	Search for prehension, utilization, and imitation behaviors (12)
Inhibition of automatic programs	Difficulty to stop an automatic program	Search for an applause sign[h]

[a] Cooper JA, Sagar HJ, Jordan N, et al. Cognitive impairment in early, untreated Parkinson's disease and its relationship to motor disability. *Brain* 1991;114:2095–2122.
[b] Delis DC, Kramer JH, Kaplan E, et al. *California Verbal Learning Test: research edition.* New York: Psychological Corporation, 1987.
[c] Grober E, Buschke H. Genuine memory deficits in dementia. *Dev Neuropsychol* 1987;3:13–36.
[d] Benton AL. Differential behavioral effects in frontal lobe disease. *Neuropsychologia* 1968;6:53–60.
[e] Nelson HE. A modified Card Sorting Test sensitive to frontal lobe defect. *Cortex* 1976;12:313–324.
[f] Golden CJ. *Stroop color and word test.* Chicago: Stoelting Company, 1978.
[g] Reitan RM. Validity of the Trail Making Test as an indication of organic brain damage. *Percept Mot Skills* 1958;8:271–276.
[h] Dubois B, Défontaines B, Deweer B, Malapani C, Pillon B. Cognitive and behavioral changes in patients with focal lesions of the basal ganglia. In: WJ Weiner, AE Lang, eds. *Behavioral neurology of movement disorders: Advances in Neurology,* vol 65. New York: Raven Press, 1995:29–41.

4-9-4-7-3-1-6) and reproduce them in serial order. The California Verbal Learning Test (CVLT) makes it possible to assess learning strategies and their effectiveness (the 16 words to memorize may be evoked randomly, in their order of presentation, or organized in four semantic categories: fruits, tools, spices, articles of clothing), whereas in the Grober and Buschke Test encoding and retrieval are controlled by the same semantic cues, allowing for assessment of more automatic aspects of memory. With this last procedure, it is therefore possible to isolate striatofrontal-related memory disorders (characterized by decreased free recall with a significant efficacy of cueing) from hippocampal-related memory disorders in which recall performance is only marginally improved by cueing. In lexical fluency tests, patients must evoke in a limited time (usually 60 sec) the maximum number of words pertaining to a semantic (e.g., animal names) or to a phonemic (e.g., words beginning with "m") category. The Wisconsin Card Sorting Test requires subjects to sort cards according to a single criterion (e.g., color, form, or number) that they must deduce from the feedback of the examiner, indicating if the response is correct or not; after a series of consecutive correct responses, the examiner shifts the rule without warning, requiring the subject to deduce a new criterion; it is therefore possible to determine several indices of performance: the number of categories achieved (a measure of the subject's concept or set formation ability), the number of perseverative errors (a measure of the patient's ability to move on from a previous category and to shift from one sorting principle to another), and the number of nonperseverative errors (a measure of attention deficits). Set maintenance may be investigated by the Stroop Test, where the subject must inhibit the strong tendency to read words in color to name the color of the ink they are printed with, whereas set shifting can be evaluated by the Trail Making Test, Part B, where the subject must connect alternatively numbered and lettered circles.

Behavioral Autonomy

Behavioral autonomy requires the capacity to inhibit the spontaneous activation of behavioral patterns in response to sensory stimuli or to stop automatic programs when they are no longer required. Dependency on physical environment is expressed by prehension and utilization behaviors. In the case of prehension behavior, the sight or sensory perception of the examiner's hands compels the patient to grasp them (11,12). Given the importance of the way these behaviors are assessed, a precise description of the testing situation is proposed. The examiner is seated in front of the patient and places the patient's hands, palms up, on the patient's knees. Without saying anything or looking at the patient's eyes, the examiner brings his or her hands close to the patient's hands and touches the palms of both of the patient's hands, to see if he or she will take them spontaneously. If the patient takes the hands, the examiner will try again later after explicitly stating "This time do not take my hands." The prehension behavior is

one of the subtests of the Frontal Assessment Battery (FAB). It is scored 3 if the patient does not take the examiner's hands, 2 if the patient hesitates and asks what to do, 1 if the patient takes the hands without hesitation, 0 if the patient takes the examiner's hand even after being explicitly told not to do so. In the case of utilization behavior, the sight of objects compels the patient to use them. To search for this behavior, the examiner is seated in front of the patient. Without saying anything or looking at the patient's eyes, the examiner brings objects (a candle and a semi-opened box of matches, a glass and a bottle of water, a pen and a sheet of paper) close to the patient's hands to see if he or she will take them spontaneously and use them. If the patient takes and uses the objects, the examiner will try again later after explicitly stating "This time do not take and use the objects." The score is 3 if the patient does not take the objects, 2 if the patient hesitates and asks what to do, 1 if the patient takes and uses the objects without hesitation, 0 if the patient takes and uses the objects even after being told explicitly not to do so.

Imitation behavior is related to dependency on social environment. The sight of the examiner's gestures compels the patient to imitate them. To test for this behavior, the examiner is seated in front of the patient. Without saying anything or looking at the patient's eyes, the examiner scratches his head, touches his chin, crosses his arms, and taps the legs with the hands to see if the patient will imitate him spontaneously. If the patient imitates, the examiner will try again later after explicitly stating "This time do not imitate what I am doing." The score is 3 if the patient does not imitate, 2 if the patient hesitates and asks what to do, 1 if the patient imitates without hesitation, 0 if the patient imitates even after being told explicitly not to do so.

Motor control can also be investigated by the "3 clap test." The patient is asked to clap 3 times, as quickly as possible, but only 3 times after demonstration by the examiner. The performance of the subject can be normal when he or she claps only 3 times (score = 3) or abnormal when he or she claps 4 times (score = 2), from 5 to 10 times (score = 1), or when he or she initiates a program of applause and cannot stop (score = 0). The *applause sign* refers to a tendency to initiate an automatic program of applause when one is asked to initiate a voluntary program of 3 claps. The environmental dependency syndrome has been observed in several parkinsonian disorders (10), whereas the applause sign would be relatively specific to progressive supranuclear palsy (PSP).

Global Evaluation of the Dysexecutive Syndrome

The severity of the dysexecutive syndrome may be assessed by global scales such as the Mattis Dementia Rating Scale (13) or the Frontal Assessment Battery (14). The Mattis Scale is more appropriate than the Mini Mental State Exam to evaluate the severity of cognitive deterioration in predominantly subcortical degenerative diseases, given the inclusion of tests evaluating attention and executive functions. It provides cutoff scores that allow a psychometric distinction between demented and nondemented patients (15). Dementia is usually not observed in Parkinson's disease (PD) with early onset or in the early stages of multiple system atrophy (MSA), but it may occur in patients with late-onset PD, PSP, or corticobasal degeneration (CBD). It is a major feature of diffuse Lewy body disease (DLBD), although there may be fluctuations of intellectual functioning from one day to another. The FAB is a battery that can be done in under 10 minutes at bedside and consists of 6 subtests exploring (a) conceptualization and abstract reasoning (similarities test), (b) mental flexibility (verbal fluency test), (c) motor programming and executive control of action (Luria's motor sequences), (d) resistance to interference (conflicting instructions), (e) inhibitory control (go–no go test), and (f) environmental autonomy (prehension behavior). The FAB has shown a good validity (correlation of $rho = 0.82$ with the Mattis Dementia Rating Scale) and inter-rater reliabilily ($k = 0.87$).

Assessment of Other Cognitive Disorders

Instrumental dysfunctions, suggestive of temporoparietal lesions, include aphasia, apraxia, and visuospatial deficits. Aphasia and apraxia may be investigated by clinical batteries, such as the Boston Diagnostic Aphasia Examination (16) or the Heilman and Gonzalez Rothi battery for apraxia (17), while the Clock Test can be used to assess visuospatial deficits (18). Impairment of instrumental activities is specific to neurodegenerative diseases with a cortical involvement. Aphasia may be observed in DLBD, whereas apraxia is more characteristic of CBD. In contrast, instrumental functions are mildly disturbed in PSP and PD with dementia (PDD) and are preserved in PD without dementia and MSA. A premotor syndrome may be observed in PSP and is characteristic of CBD: It can be investigated by test of bimanual coordination or opposition, manual dexterity, and finger selectivity and agility (19).

Assessment of Other Behavioral or Mood Disorders

Delusions and hallucinations are diagnosed in accordance with the *DSM-IV* criteria (20). They are common at early stages of DLBD and occur in PD, particularly in demented patients or as a result of treatment with anticholinergic or dopaminergic drugs, but they are not characteristic of MSA, PSP, or CBD. Mood disorders are considered to be frequent in basal ganglia diseases. They may be assessed by the Montgomery and Asberg (21) or the Beck (22) depression scales.

COGNITIVE AND BEHAVIORAL PATTERNS CHARACTERISTIC OF THE MAIN PARKINSONIAN DISORDERS

Well-characterized neuropsychological patterns can be drawn from the clustering of the cognitive and behavioral characteristics found in each parkinsonian disorder (Table 39.2).

TABLE 39.2
NEUROPSYCHOLOGICAL PATTERN OF PARKINSONIAN DISORDERS

	PD	MSA	PSP	PDD	CBD	DLBD
Dementia						
Mattis DRS (144)	−	−	+	+	+	+ +
Fluctuations	−	−	−	+	−	+
Dysexecutive syndrome						
FAB (18)	−	±	+ +	+ +	+ +	+ +
Envt dependency	−	±	+ +	+	±	+
Memory deficits						
Free recall (48)	±	±	+ +	+ +	+	+ +
Total recall (48)	−	−	−	+	+	+ +
Instrumental deficits						
Language	−	−	±	±	+	+
Gesture	−	−	±	±	+ +	±
Psychosis	−	−	−	+	−	+ +

−, normal; ±, impairment mild or discussed; +, impairment moderate or present in a proportion of patients; + +, impairment severe and present in a majority of patients; PD, Parkinson's disease; MSA, multiple system atrophy; PSP, progressive supranuclear palsy; PDD, Parkinson's disease with dementia; CBD, corticobasal degeneration; DLBD, diffuse Lewy body disease.

Parkinson's Disease

Cognitive changes in the majority of patients with PD are subtle and mainly restricted to attention and retrieval deficits. It is only by using appropriate neuropsychological tests that these cognitive changes can be detected. They mainly concern: (a) *executive functions*, namely, concept formation and problem solving, set-maintenance, and set-shifting; (b) *memory*: working memory, long-term memory, especially in tasks that involve self-organization of the to-be-remembered material, temporal ordering and conditional associative learning, and procedural learning; and (c) the *visuospatial domain*, in visuospatial paradigms that require self-elaboration of the response or forward planning capacity.

Mood and behavioral changes also are described in PD. Depression is encountered in about 30% of patients and has been the focus of a large number of studies (23). It is important to diagnose it because depression induces attention and memory disorders and, if sufficiently severe, impairs executive functions in relation to a significant decrease in frontal metabolism evidenced on PET-scan studies. Apathy is not infrequent in PD and has repercussions on cognitive functions, affect, and behavior (6). Unlike depression, anxiety symptoms almost always begin after the onset of the motor symptoms and in most of cases are related to medication-induced on–off fluctuations and wearing-off condition. Drug-induced psychiatric disorders are frequently found in PD and mainly consist of hallucinations and delusions. These disorders are, however, much more frequent in PDD or DLBD (24).

In late-onset PD, a subcortico-frontal dementia may occur after several years of evolution, which may result from the compounding effect of disease-related neuronal lesions and age-related neuronal changes. PDD is characterized by a marked dysexecutive syndrome, accompanied by a severe amnesic syndrome with a persistent response to cueing, in the absence of true aphasia, apraxia, or agnosia, and may be difficult to diagnose. *DSM-IV* criteria of dementia are well suited to Alzheimer's disease (AD) but less appropriate for PD because the severe motor deficits may themselves affect a patient's autonomy. Moreover, an overestimation of the severity of cognitive impairment may result from nonspecific factors (akinesia, hypophonia, depression, anxiety, marked cognitive slowing with delay in responses, uncontrolled dyskinesias) that interfere with the evaluation of cognitive functions.

Multiple System Atrophy

Cognitive changes are mild in the parkinsonian variant of multiple system atrophy (MSA) (or MSA-P, previously called *striatonigral degeneration*), at least in the early stage of the disease, before patients reach a severe akinetic state with dysarthria that may affect the cognitive evaluation. The few studies of cognition in MSA, including the MSA-P variant, display few differences from the neuropsychological pattern of nondemented PD: some more severe deficits in the Stroop test or in verbal fluency (25). Neuropsychological testing does not help to distinguish between the two disorders. In contrast, when faced with an axial parkinsonian syndrome poorly responsive to levodopa, the absence of a severe subcortico-frontal syndrome strongly favors the diagnosis of MSA-P and decreases the probability for PSP (26).

Psychiatric disorders have been poorly studied in MSA-P. Depression, anxiety, and emotional lability have been described, but psychosis has not (27).

Progressive Supranuclear Palsy

Cognitive and behavioral changes are consistent even in the early stages of the disease. Cognitive slowing and inertia occur in the first year in 52% of cases. As the disease progresses, these changes progressively worsen. From 24 patients who underwent 2 or more neuropsychological evaluations over time, 38% showed a global impairment at their first examination, and 70% showed it 15 months later. The changes may become severe enough to warrant the diagnosis of dementia, but the deficits still conform to the pattern of subcortico-frontal dementia. The dysexecutive syndrome of PSP is much more severe than that observed in any other subcortical disorders, and the memory deficit is dramatically improved in conditions that facilitate retrieval processing, such as cueing and recognition.

Cognitive slowing appears evident in patients with PSP, who answer questions and solve even the simplest problems with delay. It is a genuine slowing of central processing time unrelated to motor or affective disorders, as demonstrated experimentally using reaction time tasks and event-related brain potentials. Cognitive slowing may contribute to decreased lexical fluency that is more severely impaired in patients with PSP than in patients with PD or AD, although naming is more affected in the latter. A tendency to perseverate also may account for some of the deficits, particularly in tasks involving concept formation and shifting ability. In the Wisconsin Card Sorting Test, PSP patients complete fewer categories than patients with PD or MSA-P. This lack of flexibility affects both categorical and motor sequencing, as shown by the poor performance of patients with PSP in the Trail Making Test and in the motor series of Luria. Patients with PSP also experience difficulty in conceptualization and problem solving ability, which may account for their poor performance in similarities, interpretation of proverbs, comprehension of abstract concepts, arithmetic and lineage problems, tower tasks, and picture arrangement. This severe dysexecutive syndrome contributes to the memory deficits and instrumental disorders observed in PSP. Indeed, when encoding is controlled by using semantic category cues and when recall is performed with the same cues, as in the Grober and Buschke procedure, recall performance of the patients dramatically improves, confirming that there is no genuine amnesia in the disease (10). Various speech disorders have been described in PSP. A severe reduction of spontaneous speech resembling dynamic aphasia is usually observed, but abnormal loquacity also has been reported. Word-finding difficulty may occur, but it is generally less severe than in AD patients. Semantic or syntactic comprehension disorders are absent or mild. Dynamic apraxia may be found. Bilateral apraxic errors for transitive and intransitive movements have been reported, but they are much less severe than in corticobasal degeneration (28). Visual and auditory perception may be disturbed, but there is no evidence of object agnosia or alexia. Therefore, instrumental disorders of patients with PSP, when present, are rather considered to be a consequence of impaired executive and perceptual-motor functions or attention disorders.

Besides cognitive impairment, patients with PSP exhibit behavioral disorders. They show severe difficulty in self-guided behavior and are abnormally dependent on stimuli from the environment. They involuntarily grasp objects presented in front of them; they may imitate the examiner's gestures passively and use objects in the absence of any explicit verbal orders. PSP patients also have difficulty in inhibiting an automatic motor program once it is initiated. This can be evaluated easily with the applause sign: When asked to clap their hands 3 times consecutively, as quickly as possible, these patients have a tendency to clap more (4 or 5 times), sometimes initiating an automatic program of clapping that they are unable to stop, as if they had difficulty in programming voluntary acts that compete with overlearned motor skills. This sign seems to be specific to striatal dysfunction occurring in PSP.

Changes in mood, emotion, and personality also have been described: most frequently bluntness of affective expression and lack of concern about personal behavior or the behavior of others but sometimes obsessive disorders or disinhibition with bulimia, inappropriate sexual behavior, or aggressiveness. These changes are difficult to investigate, given the lack of insight and the transient nature of the emotions expressed. The testimony of caregivers is therefore required. Administering the Neuropsychiatric Inventory to patients' informants showed that patients with PSP exhibited apathy almost as a rule, since it was observed in 91% of the cases (4). Apathy was more frequent in PSP than in any other parkinsonian syndrome.

Corticobasal Degeneration

The cognitive profile of this disease is distinct from that of PSP, due to the presence of signs suggestive of cortical involvement. Many patients present only limb clumsiness and gesture disorders at the first examination, without any—or with few—cognitive or behavioral symptoms (29). In contrast, the disease may begin by other signs of cortical involvement, particularly nonfluent progressive aphasia (30). Also, a severe frontal cognitive and behavioral syndrome may initiate the disease in some patients (31).

CBD is typically defined by unilateral rigidity of one arm with apraxic features. Gesture disorders are so characteristic of the disease that the diagnosis can be suspected on the simple analysis of the motor disturbances. They consist, at first, of the patient experiencing difficulty or showing perplexity in the performance of delicate and fine movements of the fingers of one hand. At this stage, patients complain of clumsiness and loss of manual dexterity, reminiscent of "limb apraxia," variously described as *kinesthetic* in patients with lesions of the parietal cortex, or *kinetic* in patients with lesions of the premotor cortex. Systematic evaluation shows disorders of dynamic motor execution (impaired bimanual coordination, temporal organization, control, and inhibition). Asymmetric praxis disorders (difficulty in posture imitation, symbolic gesture execution, and object utilization) also are regularly observed, even at this stage. Ideomotor apraxia is frequent, especially in patients who have initial symptoms in the right limb, in agreement with the hypothesis of a predominant storage of "movement formulae" in the left hemisphere. In addition, central deficits in action knowledge and mechanical problem solving have been linked to parietal lobe pathology (32). *Alien limb phenomenon*, in which a limb behaves in an uncooperative or foreign way, has been attributed to lesions affecting the supplementary motor area. Its occurrence, in the absence of a known callosal lesion, would be highly suggestive of the diagnosis of CBD.

Other signs of cortical involvement have been observed in CBD. Linguistic disturbances are found, consisting of word-finding difficulties, decreased lexical fluency, transcortical motor aphasia, or progressive phonetic disintegration (33). These deficits resembling primary progressive nonfluent aphasia can even be an initial symptom of CBD. Neglect and visuospatial deficits also have been reported. Constructive apraxia is observed in patients with predominant right hemisphere lesions, in relation with the well-known influence of this hemisphere on visuospatial function.

Other cognitive changes resemble the subcortico-frontal dysfunction of PSP: a dysexecutive syndrome and a learning deficit that can be alleviated by semantic cueing. The environmental dependency syndrome, thought to be related to a release of the inhibition normally exerted by the frontal lobes on the activity of the parietal lobes, is less frequent, however, in CBD than in PSP, probably because of the parietal lobe dysfunction in this disease. Early subcortico-frontal syndrome in CBD would predict a shorter survival.

In most of the clinical studies performed on CBD patients, the level of intellectual deterioration was mild or moderate until an advanced stage of the disease. In some cases, however, patients with a severe dysexecutive syndrome associated with memory disorders and impaired instrumental activities may reach the threshold of dementia in which both cortical and subcortico-frontal components play a role. Thus, dementia is not infrequent in CBD and may even be observed from the onset in unusual clinical presentation. In 10 out of 13 cases with pathologically proven CBD, dementia was noticed within 3 years of onset of symptoms (34).

Besides frontal lobe–type behavioral alterations, patients with CBD may present with neuropsychiatric disorders. In a series of CBD patients, the Neuropsychiatric Inventory showed that depression, apathy, irritability. and agitation were the symptoms most commonly exhibited (35). The depression and irritability of patients with CBD were more frequent and severe than those of patients with PSP, whereas patients with PSP exhibited more apathy.

Dementia with Lewy Bodies

The diagnosis of DLBD can be suspected clinically on the basis of the early occurrence of a cognitive decline resembling a chronic confusional state with fluctuating cognitive signs and visual and/or auditory hallucinations in a patient with mild parkinsonism (36). The rapidly progressive dementia is accompanied by aphasia, dyspraxia, or spatial disorientation, suggestive of temporoparietal dysfunction. The neuropsychological profile differs from that of patients with AD: cognitive deficits are more acute, attentional fluctuations are more intense, and psychotic features appear earlier. Moreover, patients with DLBD present more severe dysexecutive impairment but less severe memory deficit than do patients with AD. The neuropsychological pattern of DLBD also can be distinguished from the subcortical dementia of PD on the basis of the early occurrence of cognitive deficits and psychotic features and the presence of linguistic and visuospatial disorders (18,24). It is, however, controversial whether DLBD constitutes a disorder different from or overlapping with PDD. By convention, DLBD is only considered when the cognitive changes appear before, with, or within one year after the occurrence of parkinsonism and cannot be proposed when they appear several years later. At a first glance, the clinical and cognitive profiles of both diseases are rather different with cortical signs only in DLBD. The profile of attentional impairments and fluctuating attention (37) and the cognitive pattern on the Mattis Dementia Rating Scale (38) would be, however, rather similar in PDD and DLBD, and postmortem examination revealed cortical Lewy bodies in both diseases, suggesting that their differential diagnosis may be more difficult than previously thought (39), in the absence of information about the occurrence of symptoms.

In conclusion, appropriate tests may help to differentiate among diseases associated with parkinsonism (Table 39.2). The absence of marked cognitive or behavioral changes makes more probable the diagnosis of PD or MSA, whereas a severe dysexecutive syndrome suggestive of a striatofrontal dysfunction reinforces the diagnosis of PSP and specific deficits related to a cortical involvement contribute to the diagnosis of CBD or DLBD. The differentiation of PDD and DLBD is an object of debate and further studies are required. Appropriate neuropsychological testing is, therefore, a useful technique for investigating the neuronal pathways affected in these diseases and can contribute not only to the diagnosis but also to our understanding of the underlying pathology.

REFERENCES

1. Dubois B, Levy R. Cognition, behaviour and the frontal lobes. *Int Psychogeriatr* 2004;16:379–387.
2. Pillon B, Boller F, Levy R, et al. Cognitive deficits and dementia in Parkinson's disease. In: Boller F, Cappa SF, eds. *Handbook of neuropsychology,* 2nd ed., vol 6. Amsterdam: Elsevier Science, 2001:307–367.
3. Lezak MD. *Neuropsychological assessment.* Oxford: Oxford University Press, 1995.
4. Litvan I, Paulsen JS, Mega MS, et al. Neuropsychiatric assessment of patients with hyperkinetic and hypokinetic movement disorders. *Arch Neurol* 1998;55:1313–1319.
5. Czernecki V, Pillon B, Houeto JL, et al. Motivation, reward and Parkinson's disease: influence of dopatherapy. *Neuropsychologia* 2002;40:2257–2267.
6. Brown RG, Pluck G. Negative symptoms: the "pathology" of motivation and goal-directed behavior. *Trends Neurosci* 2000;23 412–417.
7. Starkstein SE, Mayberg HS, Preziosi TJ, et al. Reliability, validity and clinical correlates of apathy in Parkinson's disease. *J Neuropsychiatry Clin Neurosci* 1992;4:134–139.
8. Cummings JL, Mega M, Gray K, et al. The Neuropsychiatric Inventory: comprehensive assessment of psychopathology in dementia. *Neurology* 1994;44:2308–2314.
9. Bechara A, Damasio H, Damasio AR. Emotion, decision making and the prefrontal cortex. *Cereb Cortex* 2000;10:295–307.
10. Pillon B, Dubois B, Agid Y. Testing cognition may contribute to the diagnosis of movement disorders. *Neurology* 1996;46:329–333.
11. Lhermitte F, Pillon B, Serdaru M. Human autonomy and the frontal lobes. Part I. Imitation and utilization behaviors: a neuropsychological study of 75 patients. *Ann Neurol* 1986;19:326–334.
12. Pillon B, Dubois B. From the grasping reflex to the environmental dependency syndrome. In: Freund HJ, Jeannerod M, Hallet M, Leiguarda R, eds. *Higher-order motor disorders: From neuroanatomy and neurobiology to clinical neurology.* Oxford, England: Oxford University Press, 2005;373–382.
13. Mattis S. *Dementia Rating Scale.* Odessa, FL: Psychological Assessment Resources Inc, 1988.
14. Dubois B, Slachevsky A, Litvan I, Pillon B. The FAB: A Frontal Assessment Battery at bedside. *Neurology* 2000;55:1621–1626.
15. Schmidt R, Freidl W, Fazekas F, et al. The Mattis Dementia Rating Scale: normative data from 1,001 healthy volunteers. *Neurology* 1994;44:964–966.
16. Goodglass H, Kaplan E. *The assessment of aphasia and related disorders.* Philadelphia: Lea & Febiger, 1976.
17. Heilman KM, Gonzalez Rothi LJ. Apraxia. In: Heilman KM, Valenstein E, eds. *Clinical neuropsychology,* 2nd ed. Oxford, England: Oxford University Press, 1985:131–150.
18. Gnanalingham K, Byrne E, Thornton A, et al. Motor and cognitive function in Lewy body dementia: comparison with Alzheimer's and Parkinson's disease. *J Neurol Neurosurg Psychiatry* 1997;62: 243–252.
19. Pillon B, Blin J, Vidailhet M, et al. The neuropsychological pattern of corticobasal degeneration: comparison with progressive supranuclear palsy and Alzheimer's disease. *Neurology* 1995;45: 1477–1483.
20. American Psychiatric Association. *Diagnostic and statistical manual of mental disorders,* 4th ed. DSM-IV™. Washington, DC: American Psychiatric Association, 1994.
21. Montgomery SA, Asberg MA. A new depression scale designed to be sensitive to change. *Br J Psychiatry* 1979;134:382–389.
22. Beck AT. *Beck depression inventory.* San Antonio, TX: The Psychological Corporation, 1987.
23. Slaughter JR, Slaughter KA, Nichols D, et al. Prevalence, clinical manifestations, etiology, and treatment of depression in Parkinson's disease. *J Neuropsychiatry Clin Neurosci* 2001;13:187–196.
24. Aarsland D, Ballard G, Larsen JP, et al. A comparative study of psychiatric symptoms in dementia with diffuse Lewy body disease and Parkinson's disease with and without dementia. *Int J Geriatr Psychiatry* 2001;16:528–536.
25. Soliveri P, Monza D, Paridi D, et al. Neuropsychological follow-up in patients with Parkinson's disease, striatonigral degeneration-type multisystem atrophy, and progressive supranuclear palsy. *J Neurol Neurosurg Psychiatry* 2000;69:313–318.
26. Brown RG, Pillon B, Uttner I, and Members of the Neuropsychology Working Group and NNIPPS Consortium, France, Germany, United

Kingdom. Cognitive function in patients with progressive supranuclear palsy and multiple system atrophy. The Movement Disorder Society, 7th International Congress of Parkinson's disease and Movement Disorders. Book of Abstracts, 2002, P706.

27. Ghika J. Mood and behavior in disorders of the basal ganglia. In: Bogousslavsky J, Cummings JL, eds. *Behavior and mood disorders in focal brain lesions.* Cambridge, England: Cambridge University Press, 2000:122–200.

28. Pharr V, Uttl B, Stark M, et al. Comparison of apraxia in corticobasal degeneration and progressive supranuclear palsy. *Neurology* 2001;56:957–963.

29. Wenning GK, Litvan I, Jankovic J, et al. Natural history and survival of 14 patients with corticobasal degeneration confirmed at postmortem examination. *J Neurol Neurosurg Psychiatry* 1998;64: 184–189.

30. Kertez A, Martinez-Lage P, Davidson W, et al. The corticobasal degeneration syndrome overlaps progressive aphasia and frontotemporal dementia. *Neurology* 2000;55:1368–1375.

31. Bergeron C, Davis A, Lang AE. Corticobasal ganglionic degeneration and progressive supranuclear palsy presenting with cognitive decline. *Brain Pathol* 1998;8:355–365.

32. Spatt J, Bak T, Bozeat S, et al. Apraxia, mechanical problem solving and semantic knowledge: contributions to object usage in corticobasal degeneration. *J Neurol* 2002;249:601–608.

33. Frattali CM, Grafman J, Patronas N, et al. Language disturbances in corticobasal degeneration. *Neurology* 2000;54:990–992.

34. Grimes DA, Lang AE, Bergeron C. Dementia is the most common presentation of corticobasal ganglionic degeneration. *Neurology* 1999;53:1969–1974.

35. Cummings JL, Litvan I. Neuropsychiatric aspects of corticobasal degeneration. In: Litvan I, Goetz CG, Lang AE, eds. *Corticobasal degeneration: Advances in neurology,* vol. 82. Philadelphia: Lippincott, Williams &Wilkins, 2000:147–152.

36. Barber R, Panikkar A, McKeith IG. Dementia with Lewy bodies: diagnosis and management. *Int J Geriatr Psychiatry* 2001;16 (suppl 1):12–18.

37. Ballard CG, Aarsland D, McKeith I, et al. Fluctuations in attention: PD dementia vs DLB with parkinsonism. *Neurology* 2002;59:1714–1720.

38. Aarsland D, Litvan I, Salmon D, et al. Performance on the dementia rating scale in Parkinson's disease with dementia and dementia with Lewy bodies: comparison with progressive supranuclear palsy and Alzheimer's disease. *J Neurol Neurosurg Psychiatry* 2003;74:1215–1220.

39. Apaydin H, Ahlskog JE, Parisi JE, et al. Parkinson disease neuropathology: later-developing dementia and loss of the levodopa response. *Arch Neurol* 2002;59:102–112.

Psychogenic Movement Disorders

40

Stanley Fahn

Like other psychogenic disorders, including hysteria, psychogenic movement disorders (PMDs) are caused by psychologic factors rather than by an organic etiology. Other terms, such as *functional, nonorganic,* and *medically unexplained symptoms,* have been used. Although the term *functional* might be easier to convey to patients and their families—because of existing stigmas—the term *psychogenic* best describes the condition related to psychologic disorder. This is much the same way neurologists label many disorders, such as postencephalitic parkinsonism, vascular parkinsonism, posttraumatic parkinsonism, drug-induced parkinsonism. Why not label *parkinsonism due to psychogenic etiology* as *psychogenic parkinsonism?* It places the emphasis on etiology and thereby guides the physician toward appropriate treatment. The term *functional* has been used in the past to denote organic diseases in which a specific cause was not determined, and it has been applied to chorea, epilepsy, and neuralgias (1), so it would be more ambiguous than *psychogenic.*

PMDs are not uncommon. In one large movement disorder clinic, such patients account for 10% of all nonparkinsonian new patient visits (2). Typically, patients are diagnosed by the predominant movement feature (e.g., psychogenic tremor, psychogenic dystonia, psychogenic myoclonus, etc.). When evaluated this way, tremor is the most common psychogenic phenomenology, followed by dystonia (Table 40.1).

NEUROLOGIC DIAGNOSIS

The diagnosis of PMD is a two-stage process (3). First, a positive diagnosis that the movements are psychogenic and are not due to an organic illness is made. Second, a psychiatric disorder is identified that could explain the etiology of the abnormal movements and prepare the way to deciding the best course for therapy of the individual patient. Deciding between abnormal movements due to a psychogenic cause or an organic cause can be extremely difficult. Therefore, never having seen strange movements before and pronouncing them to be psychogenic is not a satisfactory method because not even senior movement disorder specialists have seen the whole gamut of organic abnormal movements. An organic cause of the movements must be excluded (4,5). However, this is insufficient, and neurologists past and present advise that making a diagnosis of a psychogenic disorder is dependent on finding positive criteria and not simply failing to finding an organic cause (6,7).

The degree of certainty that the abnormal movements are psychogenic in origin was first proposed by Fahn and Williams (8), and was categorized into the following four categories.

Documented PMD. Movements are relieved by psychotherapy, by the clinician using psychological suggestion including physiotherapy, or by administration of placebos, or the patient must be witnessed as being free of symptoms when left alone, supposedly unobserved.

Clinically Established PMD. Movements are inconsistent over time (the features are different when the patient is observed at subsequent examinations) or are incongruent with a classic movement disorder. If only one of the following is witnessed, one or more additional features are needed: false weakness or sensory findings, self-inflicted injuries, multiple somatizations, or a definite psychiatric disturbance.

TABLE 40.1

PREDOMINANT MOVEMENT FEATURES IN PSYCHOGENIC MOVEMENT DISORDERS

Predominant Movement Feature	N	Percent
Tremor	467	37.5
Dystonia	365	29.3
Myoclonus	146	11.7
Gait disorder	114	9.2
Parkinsonism	60	4.8
Tics	29	2.3
Other	64	5.1
Total	1,245	100

A tabulation of psychogenic movement disorders seen at eight centers; most centers report their patients by a single primary motor feature, but some report multiple features if more than one is present.

Probable PMD. Movements are inconsistent over time or are incongruent, but the other features are lacking.

Possible PMD. It is suspected that the movements are psychogenic and a definite psychiatric disturbance is present.

PSYCHIATRIC DIAGNOSIS

In addition to the neurologist making the diagnosis of a PMD, the psychiatrist must evaluate the patient to explore psychodynamics and relevant environmental contingencies (3). PMDs can be due to one of the following three categories.

Somatoform Disorder. The physical symptoms are linked to psychological factors, yet the symptom production is *not under voluntary control* (i.e., not consciously produced). The two main types of somatoform disorders producing psychogenic neurologic problems are *conversion disorder* and *somatization disorder*, the latter also being known as *hysteria* or *Briquet's syndrome*. A somatization disorder involves recurrent and multiple complaints of several years' duration, for which medical care has been sought but which are apparently not due to any physical disorder. The dynamics are presumably the same as those of conversion disorder and the symptoms may emerge from chronic, recurrent, untreated conversion disorder.

Factitious Disorder. The physical symptoms are *intentionally produced* (hence, under voluntary control) due to psychological need. This group includes Munchausen's syndrome. Factitious disorders are due to mental disorders. They are generally associated with severe dependent, masochistic, or antisocial personality disorders.

TABLE 40.2

MOVEMENT DISORDERS WITHIN THE SYMPTOM COMPLEX OF SPECIFIC PSYCHIATRIC DISORDERS

Movement Disorder	Psychiatric Disorder
Psychomotor slowness	Depression
Obsessional slowness	Obsessive–compulsive disorder
Catatonia	Schizophrenia, depression
Stereotypies	Obsessive–compulsive disorder, autism, schizophrenia
Fear of falling	Anxiety, agoraphobia

Malingering. The physical symptoms are *voluntarily produced* in pursuit of a goal such as financial compensation, avoidance of school or work, evasion of criminal prosecution, or acquisition of drugs. Malingering is not considered to be a mental disorder. It is listed as a PMD not because of a psychologic cause but because it is not due to an organic cause, so this helps organize the clinician's thinking about diagnostic categories.

Somatoform disorders are the most easily treated, whereas malingering may be impossible to treat unless the patient's gain is obtained or the patient voluntarily gives up the symptoms. It should be noted that depression commonly accompanies somatoform disorders.

PMDs are not equivalent to abnormal movements that can be seen as part of some psychiatric conditions. Table 40.2 lists some of the movement difficulties seen as part of the psychiatric condition, such as stereotypies in schizophrenia or autism.

CLUES SUGGESTING THE PRESENCE OF A PSYCHOGENIC MOVEMENT DISORDER

There are often clues from the history and neurologic examination that lead the clinician to suspect a diagnosis of a PMD. If present, these clues should alert the observant clinician to consider the possibility that the abnormal movement could have a psychogenic etiology.

Historical Clues

1. Abrupt onset
2. Spontaneous remissions
3. Onset after minor trauma
4. Multiple somatizations of undiagnosed conditions
5. Obvious psychiatric disturbances
6. Employed in the health profession or in health insurance claims

7. Presence of secondary gain, including continuing care by a "devoted" spouse
8. Litigation or compensation pending

Clinical Clues

1. Inconsistent movements (changing characteristics over time; pattern, body distribution, rapidly varying severity).
2. Incongruous movements and postures (movements do not fit with recognized patterns or with normal physiological patterns.
3. Presence of certain types of abnormal movements that are fairly common among individuals with PMDs, such as rhythmical shaking, bizarre gait, deliberate slowness carrying out requested voluntary movement, bursts of verbal gibberish, excessive startle (bizarre movements in response to sudden, unexpected noise or threatening movements.
4. Presence of additional types of abnormal movements that are not known to be part of the primary or principal movement pattern that the patient manifests.
5. Manifesting exhaustion, excessive fatigue.
6. Delayed, often excessive, startle response to a stimulus.
7. Movements decrease or disappear with distraction.
8. Tremors disappears when handling treasured objects.
9. Entrainment of the tremor to the rate of the requested rapid successive movement the patient is asked to perform.
10. Dystonia beginning as a fixed posture.
11. Twisting facial movements that move the mouth to one side or the other. (*Note:* Organic dystonia of the facial muscles usually does not move the mouth sideways.)
12. False weakness.
13. False sensory complaints.
14. Response to placebo, suggestion, or psychotherapy.
15. Manifestation of a paroxysmal disorder.
16. Self-inflicted injuries.

GENERAL CLINICAL FEATURES

In addition to the specificities of the abnormal movements, some demographic features have been observed in patients with PMDs. In their review of 131 cases of documented or medically established PMDs, Williams et al. (9) observed that the mean age at onset was 36.9 years (range: 4–73 years), female gender predominates (87%), an organic component occurred in 13%, 75% of cases had previously received an organic diagnosis, 79% had more than a single type of abnormal movement, movements were paroxysmal in 55%, onset was abrupt in 60%, and symptoms spread from the original site to other sites in 43%. They also reported that the psychiatric diagnosis was conversion disorder in 75%, somatization disorder in 12.5%, factitious disorder in 8.3%,

and malingering in 4.2%. Depression was seen in 71% and anxiety in 17%.

PSYCHOGENIC TREMOR

Rhythmical shaking occurs in the majority of patients with PMDs. When tremor is the only abnormal movement or the predominant one, the patient is classified as having psychogenic tremor. This was the most common PMD diagnosis reported by Lang (10) and by Jankovic and Thomas (11). The tremor tends to be present equally at rest, with posture holding, and with action. Disappearance of the tremor when the patient is distracted is a helpful sign for determining that the tremor is psychogenic (12), but it is not specific enough. Many patients with organic tremor can temporarily suppress the tremor, as in parkinsonian tremor. Furthermore, distractibility is often difficult to observe. Many patients are sophisticated, and it is difficult to eliminate their tremor with distraction. Entrainment of the tremor to a new frequency may sometimes be observed by having the patient touch a thumb to different fingers in a dictated pattern.

Deuschl et al. (13) observed that finger tremor is usually absent in psychogenic tremors. They also reported the *coactivation sign* in which psychogenic tremors often show an increase of tremor amplitude when a weight is applied to the involved limb. This contrasts to a reduction in tremor amplitude with applied weights in organic tremors. Accelerometers applied to the affected body part can be helpful. Psychogenic tremors show larger tremor frequency changes and higher intraindividual variability while tapping (14). Motor control physiology can be useful for distinguishing psychogenic from organic tremor (15).

PSYCHOGENIC DYSTONIA

Psychogenic dystonia is the second most common type of PMD. Psychogenic dystonia is difficult to diagnose since no laboratory tests are available for establishing the diagnosis of organic primary idiopathic dystonia. For many years after dystonia was first described, many cases were considered psychogenic: 52% in the series by Eldridge et al. (16); 43% by Marsden and Harrison (17); 25% by Cooper et al. (18); and 44% by Lesser and Fahn (19). With the wider recognition of dystonia by neurologists, and with the knowledge that most cases are primary, not secondary, dystonia, it seems that psychogenic dystonia is currently underdiagnosed. The clinical clues previously listed and those reported by Fahn and Williams (8) should help the clinician suspect psychogenic dystonia when it is encountered.

Idiopathic torsion dystonia usually begins with action dystonia (20), but psychogenic dystonia often begins with a fixed posture. Fixed postures are sustained postures that resist passive movement, and the presence of such fixed postures are highly likely to be due to a psychogenic dystonia (9,21–23). Fixed posture dystonia is rare, and it is often psychogenic in origin when encountered; the evaluation of fixed postures requires the aid of anesthesia to see if contractures are present (24). The posture may manifest so much rigidity that it is extremely difficult to move the limb around a joint. Psychogenic dystonia may follow minor trauma and resembles reflex sympathetic dystrophy (complex regional pain syndrome), and there is debate as to whether such painful dystonia is psychogenic or due to reflex sympathetic dystrophy (21,22,25–27). To make matters confusing, sometimes organic dystonia of a body part can be preceded by an injury to that body part (28–32), so it can be difficult to distinguish between organic or psychogenic dystonia.

PSYCHOGENIC MYOCLONUS

Psychogenic myoclonus should be relatively easy to distinguish from organic myoclonus if access to a motor control physiology laboratory is available (33). The short duration of a myoclonic jerk (usually less than 100 ms) is almost impossible to duplicate voluntarily. The EMG pattern of voluntary jerks exhibits a triphasic pattern of activity between antagonistic muscles, whereas cortical myoclonus consists of short-duration 25–50 ms bursts of cocontracting antagonist muscles (34). Furthermore, the latency of reflex myoclonus is physiologically short (40–100 ms), whereas abnormal reactive voluntary jerks are much longer (34).

In the 18 patients with psychogenic myoclonus reported by Monday and Jankovic (35), the jerks were segmental in 10, generalized in 7, and focal in 1. Inconsistency with a continuously changing pattern, anatomically and temporally, were common. The movements often increased with stress, anxiety, and exposure to noise or light. A Bereitschaftspotential preceding muscle jerks was found in 5 of 6 patients with a diagnosis of psychogenic myoclonus (36).

PSYCHOGENIC GAIT DISORDER

Gait disorders are the next most common presentation of PMDs (Table 40.1). In Keane's report of 60 cases (37) with psychogenic gaits, the most common was ataxia. Others had trembling, knee buckling, dystonia, truncal myoclonus, and camptocormia (markedly stooped posture). In a video review of psychogenic gaits, Hayes et al. (38) emphasized certain features of the gait: exaggerated effort, extreme slowness, variability throughout the day, unusual or uneconomic postures, collapses, convulsive tremors, and distractibility. On the other hand, it is possible to misdiagnose as psychogenic an abnormal gait that is organic.

PSYCHOGENIC PARKINSONISM

Psychogenic parkinsonism is a rare cause of parkinsonism, but it does occur. Lang et al. (39) reported 14 patients with this disorder. Eleven had tremor at rest, but the tremor did not disappear with movement of the limb, and the frequency and rhythmicity varied. Rigidity was present in 6 patients, but without cogwheeling. All 14 patients had slowness of movement (bradykinesia) without the typical decrementing feature of organic bradykinesia.

TREATMENT OF PSYCHOGENIC MOVEMENT DISORDERS

Treatment depends on a team approach between neurologist, psychiatrist, and physiotherapist (40). Having the patient accept the diagnosis is a major hurdle. Most patients are reluctant to accept the diagnosis of PMD. This diagnosis should be explained in a tactful, positive, and gentle manner. The neurologist should do all necessary and reasonable tests to feel comfortable and secure that an organic basis for the symptoms has not been overlooked.

When explaining the diagnosis to the patient, it is usually helpful to name the movement disorder firmly (specifically identify the disorder, e.g., dystonia, tremor, etc.) and to make a general statement about such disorders—for example, "These disorders are caused by many different etiologies. Structural damage to the brain can be one cause, but that is not seen in your situation. The brain can react physiologically to stress to produce this type of movement, which is the cause in your case." The positive news also should be emphasized, specifically that the chance for reversing the abnormal physiology is great since the symptoms are not due to a structural lesion.

Treatment is a three-pronged approach. The first prong consists of the psychiatrist playing the major role with psychotherapy and exploring the psychodynamics, and a coexisting depression or anxiety being treated with appropriate pharmacotherapy. The second prong is intensive physiotherapy, such as retraining an abnormal posture to restore it to its proper alignment or overcoming any weakness. If there is excess startle, desensitization techniques should be used, with a gentle stimulus that does not trigger the abnormal jerk and a gradual increase in the strength of the stimulus until the jerks are no longer present. The third prong is facilitated by the neurologist, who makes the diagnosis and reinforces the benefits of the recommended treatments. After diagnosis, the neurologist explains to patients that they can get better only if they are willing to work hard with physiotherapy. The neurologist plays the role of a "bad cop" emphasizing to the patient that improvement must be seen each day of treatment. This gives the patient the added onus to work with the therapies to show such improvement. The psychiatrist takes the "good cop" role and reinforces the need for improvement to please the neurologist and keep the neurologist involved. Such an approach between the neurologist and psychiatrist can hasten improvement.

Admitting the patient to the hospital is the best way to provide intensive physiotherapy and psychotherapy, with the patient seen each day by the neurologist, who keeps emphasizing the treatment and providing encouragement. Such encouragement is important to keep the patient motivated.

After the patient has improved, maintaining improvement is not always easy because the patient returns to the same environment that led to causation of the movement disorder. Continual psychotherapy is necessary.

REFERENCES

1. Fahn S. The history of psychogenic movement disorders. In: Hallett M, Fahn S, Jankovic J, Lang JE, Cloninger CR, Yudofsky SC, eds. *Psychogenic movement disorders: Neurology and neuropsychiatry.* Philadelphia: Lippincott Williams & Wilkins, 2006:24–31.
2. Portera-Cailliau C, Victor D, Frucht SJ, Fahn S. Movement disorders fellowship training program at University Medical Center in 2001–2002. *Mov Disord* 2006;21:479–485.
3. Williams DT, Ford B, Fahn S. Treatment issues in psychogenic-neuropsychiatric movement disorders. *Adv Neurol* 2005;96:350–363.
4. Gowers WR. *A manual of diseases of the nervous system*, vol. II, 2nd ed. Philadelphia: Blakiston, 1893:984–1030.
5. Sachs B. *A treatise on the nervous diseases of children for physicians and students.* New York: William Wood and Company, 1895:85–108.
6. Stewart JP. *The diagnosis of nervous diseases.* London: Edward Arnold, 1920:358–399.
7. Fahn S. Psychogenic movement disorders. In: Marsden CD, Fahn S, eds. *Movement disorders 3*. Oxford, England: Butterworth-Heinemann, 1994:359–372.
8. Fahn S, Williams DT. Psychogenic dystonia. *Adv Neurol* 1988;50:431–455.
9. Williams DT, Ford B, Fahn S. Phenomenology and psychopathology related to psychogenic movement disorders. *Adv Neurol* 1995;65:231–257.
10. Lang AE. General overview of psychogenic movement disorders: epidemiology, diagnosis, and prognosis. In Hallett M, Fahn S, Jankovic J, Lang JE, Cloninger CR, Yudofsky SC, eds. *Psychogenic movement disorders:neurology and neuropsychiatry.* Philadelphia: Lippincott Williams & Wilkins, 2006:35–41.
11. Jankovic J, Thomas M. Psychogenic tremor and shaking. In: Hallett M, Fahn S, Jankovic J, Lang JE, Cloninger CR, Yudofsky SC, eds. *Psychogenic movement disorders: neurology and neuropsychiatry.* Philadelphia: Lippincott Williams & Wilkins, 2006:42–47.
12. Campbell J. The shortest paper. *Neurology* 1979;29:1633.
13. Deuschl G, Koster B, Lucking CH, Scheidt C. Diagnostic and pathophysiological aspects of psychogenic tremors. *Mov Disord* 1998;13:294–302.
14. Zeuner KE, Shoge RO, Goldstein SR, Dambrosia JM, Hallett M. Accelerometry to distinguish psychogenic from essential or parkinsonian tremor. *Neurology* 2003;61:548–550.
15. Deuschl G, Raethjen J, Kopper F, Govindan RB. The diagnosis and physiology of psychogenic tremor. In: Hallett M, Fahn S, Jankovic J, Lang JE, Cloninger CR, Yudofsky SC, eds. *Psychogenic movement disorders: Neurology and neuropsychiatry.* Philadelphia: Lippincott Williams & Wilkins, 2006:265–273.
16. Eldridge R, Riklan M, Cooper IS. The limited role of psychotherapy in torsion dystonia: experience with 44 cases. *JAMA* 1969;210:705–708.
17. Marsden CD, Harrison MJG. Idiopathic torsion dystonia. *Brain* 1974;97:793–810.
18. Cooper IS, Cullinan T, Riklan M. The natural history of dystonia. *Adv Neurol* 1976;14:157–169.
19. Lesser RP, Fahn S. Dystonia: a disorder often misdiagnosed as a conversion reaction. *Am J Psychiatry* 1978;153:349–452.
20. Fahn S, Marsden CD, Calne DB. Classification and investigation of dystonia. In: Marsden CD, Fahn S, eds. *Movement disorders 2.* London: Butterworths, 1987;332–358.
21. Lang A, Fahn S. Movement disorder of RSD. *Neurology* 1990;40: 1476–1477.
22. Schrag A, Trimble M, Quinn N, Bhatia K. The syndrome of fixed dystonia: an evaluation of 103 patients. *Brain* 2004;127: 2360–2372.
23. Schrag A. Psychogenic dystonia and reflex sympathetic dystrophy. In: Hallett M, Fahn S, Jankovic J, Lang JE, Cloninger CR, Yudofsky SC, eds. *Psychogenic movement disorders: Neurology and neuropsychiatry.* Philadelphia: Lippincott Williams & Wilkins, 2006:53–61.
24. Fahn S. The role of anesthesia in the diagnosis and treatment of psychogenic movement disorders. In: Hallett M, Fahn S, Jankovic J, Lang JE, Cloninger CR, Yudofsky SC, eds. *Psychogenic movement disorders: neurology and neuropsychiatry.* Philadelphia: Lippincott Williams & Wilkins, 2006:256–261.
25. Schwartzman RJ, Kerrigan J. The movement disorder of reflex sympathetic dystrophy. *Neurology* 1990;40:57–61.
26. Bhatia KP, Bhatt MH, Marsden CD. The causalgia–dystonia syndrome. *Brain* 1993;116:843–851.
27. Sa DS, MailisGagnon A, Nicholson K, Lang AE. Posttraumatic painful torticollis. *Mov Disord* 2003;18:1482–1491.
28. Schott GD. The relation of peripheral trauma and pain to dystonia. *J Neurol Neurosurg Psychiat* 1985;48:698–701.
29. Schott GD. Mechanisms of causalgia and related clinical conditions: the role of the central nervous and of the sympathetic nervous systems. *Brain* 1986;109:717–738.
30. Scherokman B, Husain F, Cuetter A, Jabbari B, Maniglia E. Peripheral dystonia. *Arch Neurol* 1986;43:830–832.
31. Gordon MF, Brin MF, Giladi N, Hunt A, Fahn S. Dystonia precipitated by peripheral trauma. *Mov Disord* 1990;5(suppl 1):67.
32. Goldman S, Ahlskog JE. Posttraumatic cervical dystonia. *Mayo Clin Proc* 1993;68:443–448.
33. Brown P. Clinical neurophysiology of myoclonus. In: Hallett M, Fahn S, Jankovic J, Lang JE, Cloninger CR, Yudofsky SC, eds. *Psychogenic movement disorders: neurology and neuropsychiatry.* Philadelphia: Lippincott Williams & Wilkins, 2006:262–264.
34. Thompson PD. The phenomenology of startle, latah, and related conditions. In: Hallett M, Fahn S, Jankovic J, Lang JE, Cloninger CR, Yudofsky SC, eds. *Psychogenic movement disorders: neurology and neuropsychiatry.* Philadelphia: Lippincott Williams & Wilkins, 2006:48–52.
35. Monday K, Jankovic J. Psychogenic myoclonus. *Neurology* 1993;43:349–352.
36. Terada K, Ikeda A, Van Ness PC, et al. Presence of Bereitschaftspotential preceding psychogenic myoclonus: clinical application of jerk-locked back averaging. *J Neurol Neurosurg Psychiatry* 1995;58:745–747.
37. Keane JR. Hysterical gait disorders: 60 cases. *Neurology* 1989;39:586–589.
38. Hayes MW, Graham S, Heldorf P, de Moore G, Morris JGL. A video review of the diagnosis of psychogenic gait: appendix and commentary. *Mov Disord* 1999;14:914–921.
39. Lang AE, Koller WG, Fahn S. Psychogenic parkinsonism. *Arch Neurol* 1995;52:802–810.
40. Jankovic J, Cloninger CR, Fahn S, Hallett M, Lang AE, Williams DT. Therapeutic approaches to psychogenic movement disorders. In: Hallett M, Fahn S, Jankovic J, Lang AE, Cloninger CR, Yudofsky S, eds. Psychogenic movement disorders: Neurology and neuropsychiatry. Philadelphia: AAN Enterprises and Lippincott Williams & Wilkins, 2006:323–328.

Neuroacanthocytosis

41

Shinji Saiki   Koichiro Sakai

INTRODUCTION

The term *acanthocytosis* derived from the Greek to describe "thorny" red blood cells. The actual process resulting in the formation of acanthocytes is not known. Echinocytes, which are found in several pathological conditions, such as uremia, liver failure, and splenectomy, may show a spicular appearance with uniform discontinuous projections that are usually larger at the base than in length, whereas the morphology of acanthocytes is characterized by a number of irregularly spaced thorny surface projections, often with a terminal bulb (Fig. 41.1). Although echinocytes can normally comprise up to 3% of red blood cells in healthy adults, true acanthocytes should never be present in normal blood. For the purpose of avoiding false positives, due to experimental artifacts or echinocytes, it is suggested that the limit to be considered pathological should be more than 3% crenated forms, and repeated sampling is required.

The term *neuroacanthocytosis* in the literature varies and is confusing because it has been referred to by at least four different names (Levine-Critchley syndrome, acanthocytosis with neurologic disorder, choreoacanthocytosis, amyotrophic choreoathetosis with acanthocytosis) and because it contains at least three hereditary neurologic disorders (chorea-acanthocytosis, ChAc: MIM200150); McLeod syndrome, MLS: MIM314850; abetalipoproteinemia, ABL: MIM200100). Furthermore, other hereditary disorders affecting central and/or peripheral nervous systems (Hallervorden-Spatz syndrome; mitochondrial myopathy, encephalopathy, lactacidosis, and stroke: MELAS; HARP syndrome, a variant form of Hallervorden-Spatz syndrome characterized by hypoprebetalipoproteinemia, acanthocytosis, retinitis pigmentosa, and pallidal degeneration; Huntington disease–like 2: HDL2) also can be associated with acanthocytosis in various degrees (1–4). The genes responsible for these hereditary disorders with involvement of the nervous system and erythrocytes have been identified; however, functions of the encoding proteins are not clear.

In this chapter, we focus on major neuroacanthocytosis (ChAc, MLS, and ABL).

CHOREA-ACANTHOCYTOSIS

ChAc (MIM200150) is a hereditary and devastating disease characterized by adult onset, progressive hyperkinetic movements, and an unusual spiny erythrocyte morphology. This condition, first described in detail in the late 1960s, is a rare neurodegenerative disorder associated with acanthocytosis, so there have been no available data on the prevalence or incidence of ChAc (5,6). Although the disorder seems to be particularly common in Japan, there have been numerous reports from various countries (7). Hardie et al. reviewed a series of 19 British cases and patients previously reported (8). Rampoldi et al. also reviewed clinical features and genotypes of the 20 genetically diagnosed ChAc patients (2).

Clinical Features

The clinical features of ChAc are listed in Table 41.1. The range of age at onset is between 6 and 62 years (mean around 35), although onset of symptoms is usually delayed until 25 to 45 years of age. Involuntary movement, such as orolingual/facial dyskinesias, chorea, and tics, are the most common symptoms, with chorea affecting the limbs, and sometimes the face, in almost all symptomatic patients (2,8). Choreic movements are enhanced by a command to stop the movements, mental calculations, or voluntary movements elsewhere in the body. Chorea is usually mild, and in some cases dystonia is the dominant movement disorder. Severe involuntary movements affect the orofacial region, which is often sufficient to cause tongue and lip biting and to interfere with speech and swallowing. Dystonia

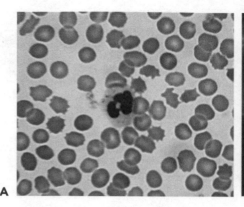 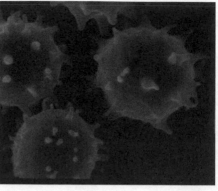

Figure 41.1 A: Wet blood smear shows many acanthocytes with spiky projections in peripheral blood. **B:** A scanning electron microscope study shows irregularly shaped acanthocytes with several spicules of variable length.

of the bulbar muscles often causes dysphagia and virtual anarthria, whereas abnormal palatal and pharyngeal contractions contribute to dysphagia. Coprolalia is rare. Dystonic protrusion of the tongue, induced by mastication, often forces food out of the mouth and exposes the tongue to being bitten. Persistent biting of the tongue, lips, or buccal mucosa is commonly found. Motor and vocal tics and

dystonia were observed in one-half of the patients reported by Hardie et al. (8). Vocal tics consist of involuntary vocalizations, including grunting, sucking, blowing, gasping, sighing, or monosyllabic utterances that are unrecognizable words and are often accompanied by belching, spitting, clicking, or sniffing. In addition to tics, ChAc patients often present with tourettism (6,9,10).

TABLE 41.1

CLINICAL FEATURES OF ChAc AND MLS PATIENTS WITH GENETIC DIAGNOSIS

Findings	% in ChAc[a]	% in MLS[b]
Weak Kell antigen	0	100
Acanthocytosis	88	100
Involuntary movements		
Hyperkinesia face	90	71
Chorea	94	64
Self-mutilation	40	7
Dystonia	50	31
Parkinsonian features	32	16
Cognitive and behavioral changes		
Cognitive changes	73	48
Other psychiatric symptoms	60	42
Dysarthria	88	63
Dysphagia	62	8
Elevation of serum creatine kinase	85	97
Cerebellar dysfunction	0	0
Neuromuscular manifestation		
Muscle weakness	54	61
Hypotonia	86	33
Muscle biopsy: myopathic/neuropathic	0/100	77/64
Hyporeflexia/areflexia	90	88
Sensory abnormality	13	33
Seizure	42	40

[a] Includes cases from Rampoldi L, Danek A, Monaco AP. Clinical features and molecular bases of neuroacanthocytosis. *J Mol Med* 2002;80:475–491.
[b] Includes cases from the following: (1) Ueyama H, Kumamoto T, Nagao S, et al. A novel mutation of the McLeod syndrome gene in a Japanese family. *J Neurol Sci* 2000;176:151–154. (2) Danek A, Rubio JP, Rampoldi L, et al. McLeod neuroacanthocytosis: genotype and phenotype. *Ann Neurol* 2001;50:755–764. (3) Jung HH, Russo D, Redman C, et al. Kell and XK immunohistochemistry in McLeod myopathy. *Muscle Nerve* 2001;24:1346–1351. (4) Barnett MH, Yang F, Iland H, et al. Unusual muscle pathology in McLeod syndrome. *J Neurol Neurosurg Psychiatry* 2000;69:655–657. (5) Hanaoka N, Yoshida K, Nakamura A, et al. A novel frameshift mutation in the McLeod syndrome gene in a Japanese family. *J Neurol Sci* 1999;165:6–9. ChAc, chorea-acanthocytosis; MLS, McLeod syndrome.

Parkinsonism is relatively rare and only present at a progressive stage (8). Although parkinsonism rather than chorea often can be the predominant movement disorder, progressive parkinsonism usually gradually replaces the hyperkinetic state (8). Masked faces, dysarthria, dysphagia, and postural instability are characteristic, although generalized bradykinesia is uncommon, progressive supranuclear palsy (PSP), and apraxia of eyelid opening may present.

Cognitive impairment and behavioral changes are observed in about half of the reported cases (2,8), with cognitive impairment and psychosis manifesting as dementia, paranoia, and personality changes (2,8,11). Psychiatric symptoms may include depression, anxiety, and obsessive–compulsive behaviors. Impulsive and distracted behaviors or apathy with loss of insight are shown in some patients. In a neuropsychological review of 10 patients, 7 showed psychiatric abnormalities similar to those of Huntington disease (HD) (12). A frontal lobe–like syndrome may appear, and patients exhibit inefficiencies in psychometric tests of attention and planning. Some patients have impaired executive skills, such as the ability to sustain concentration, or to plan or change their behavior to reach a particular goal. Patients also tend to neglect personal appearance and social skills.

Muscle weakness and atrophy are noted predominantly in the distal portion of the lower limbs in approximately one-half of cases. Amyotrophy precedes clinical recognition of involuntary movements. Deep tendon reflexes shown are areflexia or hyporeflexia, and muscle tone is hypotonic in one-fourth of ChAc patients. There is no consistent sensory change. Splenomegaly, hepatomegaly cardiomyopathy, pes cavus, and glove-and-stocking sensory loss are atypical.

Genetics

Both autosomal recessive and autosomal dominant inheritance have been proposed in familial cases, with the former seeming most likely (2,6,13,14). In families of diverse geographical origins, with ChAc having an autosomal recessive trait, the responsible gene for ChAc, VPS13A, has been identified on chromosome 9q21 and various mutations in autosomal recessive ChAc patients have been reported (15–17). This gene encodes a novel 3,096-amino acid protein chorein, a homologue of VPS13, which is a protein from *Saccaromyces cerevisiae* that is involved in trafficking of membrane protein between the trans-Golgi network and the prevacuolar compartment (18). The VPA13A gene is organized in 73 exons, and has 2 splicing variants, variant 1 (exons 1–68 and 70–73) and variant 2 (exons 1–69). Various mutations have been found in the VPS13A gene in the ChAc families with autosomal recessive inheritance, as well as those with autosomal dominant inheritance (17). By analyses of mutation in the VPS13A gene of 43 unrelated ChAc patients, 57 different mutations have been found. There are more than 60 different muta-

TABLE 41.2

MUTATION SPECTRUM OF THE VPS13A GENE IN ChAc PATIENTS

Mutation	N^a	Frequency(%)
Nonsense	17	28
Splice site	16	26
Missense	2	3
Small insertion/deletion	22	35
Gross deletion	5	8
Total	62	

[a] Includes mutation data from the following: (1) Saiki S, Sakai K, Kitagawa Y, et al. Mutation in the CHAC gene in a family of autosomal dominant chorea-acanthocytosis. *Neurology* 2003;61:1614–1616. (2) Ueno S, Maruki Y, Nakamura M, et al. The gene encoding a newly discovered protein, chorein, is mutated in chorea-acanthocytosis. *Nat Genet* 2001;28:121–122. (3) Dobson-Stone C, Danek A, Rampoldi L, et al. Mutational spectrum of the CHAC gene in patients with chorea-acanthocytosis. *Eur J Hum Genet* 2002;10:773–781. (4) Dobson-Stone C, Velayos-Baeza A, Jansen A, et al. Identification of a VPS13A founder mutation in French Canadian families with chorea-acanthocytosis. *Neurogenetics* 2005;6:151–158. (5) Lossos A, Dobson-Stone C, Monaco AP, et al. Early clinical heterogeneity in choreoacanthocytosis. *Arch Neurol* 2005;62:611–614.
ChAc, chorea-acanthocytosis; N, number of cases.

tions in VPS13A. The mutations that have been reported for the VPS13A gene of patients with ChAc are summarized in Table 41.2. Most mutations are nonsense or insertion/deletion mutations, some are changes affecting splicing, and a few are missense mutations. It is unclear how these VPS13A gene mutations lead to selective neuronal loss and the abnormal erythrocyte morphology in ChAc.

Neuropathology and Neurochemistry

Postmortem studies of ChAc patients have revealed severe and extensive neuronal loss and gliosis in the caudate and putamen, globus pallidus, and substantia nigra. The thalamus is mildly affected, but the subthalamic nuclei, cerebral cortex, pons, medulla, and cerebellum are spared (8,19). The spinal cord is spared in most cases, and anterior horn cells and anterior and posterior roots are preserved, although some reports have described losses of motor neurons in the spinal cord anterior horn area. In the substantia nigra, neuronal loss is greatest in the ventrolateral region (20). Histologically, both large and small neurons are depleted in the caudate. No amyloid or Lewy bodies have been reported.

Pathological studies with nerve biopsy specimens have indicated that the involvement affects primarily larger-diameter myelinated fibers with segmental de- and remyelination in both motor and sensory nerves (8). Unmyelinated fibers also are depleted. Some reports have suggested that demyelination is secondary to axonal degeneration (21–23).

In the studies using muscle biopsy specimens of ChAc patients, not only neuropathic changes but myopathic changes including nemaline rods and abnormal accumulation of tTGase product have been reported (2,24,25). Furthermore, Ishikawa et al. reported that computed tomography (CT) scans of lower legs of ChAc patients revealed primary myopathic changes, which were not consistent with peripheral nerve distribution (26).

Neurochemical studies have shown the depletions of dopamine and its metabolites in most brain areas, particularly in the striatum. Noradrenaline levels in the globus pallidus and putamen are elevated, whereas substance P levels are decreased in the striatum and substantia nigra (27).

Laboratory Findings

Acanthocytes are found in peripheral blood smears of ChAc patients, although the percentage of acanthocytes is highly variable, usually being between 5% and 50%. A high percentage of acanthocytes does not correlate with disease severity. Chorein expression in ChAc patients' erythrocytes is absent or reduced (28). The pathogenesis of acanthocyte formation remains unclear. Increased palmitic acid and decreased stearic acid in acanthocytes have been reported; however, these contributions of lipid components in erythrocytes to acanthocyte formation are still controversial (29,30). Freeze-fracture electron microscopic studies have revealed ultrastructural abnormalities of the erythrocyte membranous skeleton. Alteration in the degree of phosphorylation of membrane proteins (band 3 and beta-spectrin) and abnormal fluxes of chloride or sulphate anions have been reported.

Serum creatine kinase (CK) activity is commonly modestly elevated, although in some affected patients creatine kinase activity is within a normal range. Serum lipoprotein electrophoresis is normal in all subjects. Elevation in lactate dehydrogenase (LDH) and hepatic enzymes (aspartate aminotransferase, AST; and alanine aminotransferase, ALT) are frequently observed but are not invariable. There is no reduction of serum cholesterol or of beta-lipoprotein levels.

Nerve conduction velocity studies have shown a reduction of sensory nerve action potentials and prolongation of sensory conduction velocities in 25% to 50% of cases, but motor nerves are less affected. Electromyography studies have disclosed neurogenic changes with positive sharp waves and giant motor unit potentials, which are consistent with peripheral axonal pathology (23). Visual-evoked potentials, sensory-evoked potentials, and brainstem auditory-evoked potentials are normal.

Atrophy of the putamen and caudate nucleus with enlargement of lateral ventricles are typical findings of ChAc on CT and magnetic resonance imaging (MRI) (Fig. 41.2) (8,9,31). These findings closely resemble those seen in HD. In contrast to HD, CT bicaudate index and frontal horn/bicaudate ratio in ChAc patients have not been shown to correlate with age, duration of illness, or severity of hyperkinesia. T2-weighed MRI also revealed high signal changes in the putamen and caudate, although these changes are not specific findings of ChAc (8,32,33). Positron emission tomography (PET) with various isotopes has shown bilateral symmetrically decreased glucose and oxygen metabolism in the caudate, putamen, and frontal cortex (Fig. 41.3) (10,33,34). PET with [^{18}F]-fluorodopa has indicated decreased predopaminergic projection between the substantia nigra and the posterior putamen of affected patients, and PET with [^{11}C]-raclopride has revealed significant reduction of D_2 postsynaptic receptors in the putamen and caudate (20,35). Single-photon emission computed tomography (SPECT) has shown hypoperfusion in the frontal cortex and basal ganglia (Fig. 41.3) (24,36).

Differential Diagnosis

The clinical similarity of ChAc to HD and MLS has been reported. Axonal neuropathy depression of reflexes and muscle atrophy are shared by both ChAc and MLS. Walker et al. found that a family previously described as autosomal dominant chorea-acanthocytosis had the CTG trinucleotide repeat expansion mutation of the junctophilin-3 gene associated with Huntington disease–like 2 (HDL2) (37). One of the patients with HDL2 had acanthocytosis on a peripheral blood smear, suggesting that HDL2 should be considered in the differential diagnosis of chorea-acanthocytosis.

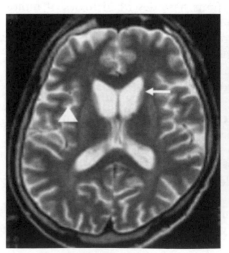
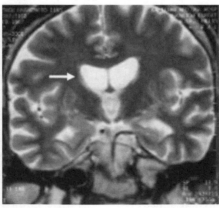

Figure 41.2 Axial and coronal T2-weighted imagings (1.5-T, Tr/TE=4500/9.6) show severe atrophy of the bilateral caudate nucleus (*arrows*) and heterogeneous intensity changes of the bilateral putamen (*arrowheads*).

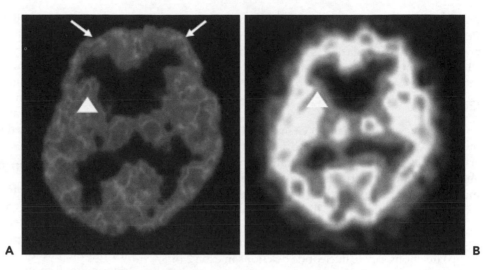

Figure 41.3 A: [^{18}F]-2-fluoro-deoxyglucose positron emission tomography shows marked hypometabolism of the bilateral striatum (*arrowheads*) and frontal cortices (*arrows*). **B:** [^{99m}Tc]-ethylcysteinate dimer single-photon emission computed tomography shows severe hypoperfusion of the bilateral striatum (*arrowheads*). (See color section.)

Treatment

There is no effective long-term treatment for ChAc. Symptomatic therapies largely focus on ameliorating the involuntary movements, psychological symptoms, and seizures. Verapamil is of temporary help. Seizures are usually easy to control with monotherapy including phenytoin, carbamazepine, or phenobarbital. Hyperkinetic movements may respond to benzodiazepines, phenothiazines, and dopamine depleters. Deep-brain stimulation of the motor thalamus is effective for reducing involuntary movements (38). Dysphagia may require a feeding gastrostomy. Disease follows a progressive course, and aspiration may cause death.

McLEOD SYNDROME

MLS (MIM314850) is an X-linked disorder characterized with weak expression of Kell blood-group antigens. Various clinical symptoms of McLeod phenomenon have been called *MLS*, first described by Marsh et al. (39), and are characterized by multiple organ disorders that include the central nervous system, erythrocytes, and skeletal muscles. The gene responsible for MLS was identified by Ho et al. (40); heterozygous mutations leading to amino cid changes in the Kell protein cause this disorder. Genotype–phenotype correlation in MLS has been analyzed extensively by Danek et al. (41).

Clinical Features

MLS is characterized by involuntary movements, especially limb chorea, primary myopathy, peripheral neuropathy, areflexia, cardiomyopathy, and elevation of serum creatinine kinase (41). Clinical features of MLS are similar to those of ChAc (Table 41.1). Limb chorea and dystonia are common in patients with McLeod syndrome, as are cognitive impairment and behavioral changes. Neuromuscular

manifestations include areflexia, neurogenic muscle atrophy, myopathy, and cardiomyopathy. Mild muscle weakness in the distal muscles, particularly of the lower limbs, is found in two-thirds of patients and becomes more common with increasing age. Facial and vocal tics are common. Coprolalia, habitual lip biting, involuntary tongue movements, and dysphagia also are found. Parkinsonian features are occasionally noted. General tonic–clonic seizures have been reported in MLS. Psychiatric abnormalities and such emotional disorders as lability, anxiety, and depression are noted. Abnormal behavior, socially inappropriate conduct, exhibitionism, hoarding compulsions, and paranoia occur, and memory and perspective functions are affected. Sleep apnea and peripheral components of breathing disorders are noted. The spleen and liver are enlarged in about 40% of patients.

Laboratory Findings

MLS is characterized by an absence of expression of Kx erythrocyte antigens, and weak expression of Kell blood group antigens. Acanthocytosis is noted in 3% to 40% of MLS. All patients show elevated resting levels of serum CK, and LDH is elevated in most patients (41). One-third of patients show increased activities of AST, ALT, and gamma-glutamyl transpeptidase.

Biopsy findings, neuropathic as well as myopathic, are mixed. Pathologically, decreased XK expression of the skeletal muscle has been reported, with no abnormalities in dystrophin of the sarcolemma (8,25,42). Sural nerve biopsies have demonstrated axonal loss and demyelination. Conduction velocities are normal, but sensory nerve action potentials and motor amplitudes are reduced. Electromyography has ascertained neuropathic but not myopathic components.

Neuroimaging has revealed caudate atrophy in the majority of MLS patients, with MRI disclosing abnormal signals in the basal ganglia on T2-weighted images. SPECT studies using [^{123}I]-iodobenzamide analysis have revealed decreased postsynaptic D2 receptors. On [¹⁸F]-2-fluoro-2deoxyglucose PET studies, glucose hypometabolism in the basal ganglia and frontal and parietal cortices have been shown to precede clinical symptoms (43).

Genetics

The XK gene, which contains 3 exons, is localized on chromosome Xp21. This gene encodes a protein of 444 amino acid residues predicted to have 10 transmembrane domains and structural characteristics of prokaryotic and eukaryotic membrane transport proteins. The XK protein contains the Kx antigen, missing in MLS, that forms a membrane complex with Kell protein. More than 20 different mutations in the gene have been reported, including minor (5 bp or 13 bp) deletions, single nucleotide deletions in exon 2 or 3, and dinucleotide deletion in exon 3 (2). All these mutations will cause shifts in the reading frame. Single nucleotide substitutions that occur in the coding region of XK and in some of these substitutions result in nonsense mutations. A few cases also show missense mutations.

Differential Diagnosis

Familial hemolytic anemia, undefined myopathy, spinal muscular atrophy, cardiomyopathy, familial neuropsychiatric disorders (HD, Tourette's syndrome, and autosomal recessive ChAc) should be ruled out.

Prognosis

This disease has a slowly progressive course in almost all patients, with most having manifested by the fifth decade of life, with a subclinical affection of muscles and peripheral nerves often appearing in the third decade. With advancing age, MLS can cause disabilities due to impaired cardiac function, chorea psychiatric symptoms, and dysautonomia.

Treatment

A causal therapy for MLS has not been determined. Patients have been treated symptomatically, as with cardiologic regimes of anticoagulation for the risk of cardiac embolism and as with psychopathology and epilepsy controlled with conventional treatments. Tiapride and sulpiride are beneficial for hyperkinesia.

ABETALIPOPROTEINEMIA

Clinical Features

ABL (MIM200100) is an autosomal recessive disorder characterized by fat malabsorption, retinitis pigmentosa, progressive cerebellar ataxia, peripheral neuropathy, and

acanthocytosis (44). Blephaloptosis, sometimes alternating ptosis, is seen. Retinal pigmentary abnormalities are present with nyctalopia. These clinical presentations result from malabsorption of vitamin E, and affected children develop malabsorption with abdominal bloating, steatorrhea, and failure to thrive (45,46). Valvular diseases, cardiac ventricular dilatation, and arrhythmia also are noted, and hemorrhagic complications are associated with vitamin K deficiency.

Laboratory Findings

Numerous acanthocytes and mild anemia are observed as prothrombin time is elevated. Serum betalipoprotein, very low-density lipoprotein, and low-density lipoprotein are absent. Fat malabsorption and inhibited transportation of fat from the intestinal mucosa lead to low serum triglyceride and total cholesterol. Mild elevations of AST and ALT, as well as CK, are found. Vitamin E and A levels are characteristically low, and apolipoprotein B, which is important for the absorption, transport, and delivery of Vitamin E to tissues, is absent. Electrophysiological findings are consistent with retinal degeneration, axonal neuropathy, and posterior column involvement.

Genetics

An autosomal recessive and an autosomal dominant mode of inheritance both have been reported. The main gene responsible for this disorder is the microsomal triglyceride transfer (MTP) protein gene, which is located on chromosome 4q and is organized in 18 exons. The function of MTP is associated with the translocation of apolipoprotein B across the endoplasmic reticulum and with its assembly with lipids. More than 20 mutations have been reported and are clustered in the middle and caroboxyl terminal region in the coding regions.

Treatment

Treatment with fat-soluble vitamins is essential (47). Clinical and electroretinographic improvements have been noted with supplemental vitamin A and vitamin E, which also play a role for maintaining normal retinal function.

ACKNOWLEDGMENT

We are grateful to Prof. Genjiro Hirose at the Department of Neurology, Kanazawa Medical University, for his innumerable clinical contributions on choreic disorders and for his helpful criticism.

REFERENCES

1. Higgins JJ, Patterson MC, Papadopoulos NM, et al. Hypoprebetalipoproteinemia, acanthocytosis, retinitis pigmentosa, and pallidal degeneration (HARP syndrome). *Neurology* 1992;42:194–198.

2. Rampoldi L, Danek A, Monaco AP. Clinical features and molecular bases of neuroacanthocytosis. *J Mol Med* 2002;80:475–491.

3. Walker RH, Rasmussen A, Rudnicki D, et al. Huntington's disease—like 2 can present as chorea-acanthocytosis. *Neurology* 2003;61:1002–1004.

4. Mukoyama M, Kazui H, Sunohara N, et al. Mitochondrial myopathy, encephalopathy, lactic acidosis, and stroke-like episodes with acanthocytosis: a clinicopathological study of a unique case. *J Neurol* 1986;233:228–232.

5. Levine IM, Estes JW, Looney JM. Hereditary neurological disease with acanthocytosis: a new syndrome. *Arch Neurol* 1968;19:403–409.

6. Critchley EM, Clark DB, Wikler A. Acanthocytosis and neurological disorder without betalipoproteinemia. *Arch Neurol* 1968;18:134–140.

7. Oshima M, Osawa Y, Asano K, et al. Erythrocyte membrane abnormalities in patients with amyotrophic chorea with acanthocytosis. Part 1. Spin labeling studies and lipid analyses. *J Neurol Sci* 1985;68:147–160.

8. Hardie RJ, Pullon HW, Harding AE, et al. Neuroacanthocytosis: a clinical, haematological and pathological study of 19 cases. *Brain* 1991;114(pt 1A):13–49.

9. Spitz MC, Jankovic J, Killian JM. Familial tic disorder, parkinsonism, motor neuron disease, and acanthocytosis: a new syndrome. *Neurology* 1985;35:366–370.

10. Saiki S, Hirose G, Sakai K, et al. Chorea-acanthocytosis associated with Tourettism. *Mov Disord* 2004;19:833–836.

11. Stevenson VL, Hardie RJ. Acanthocytosis and neurological disorders. *J Neurol* 2001;248:87–94.

12. Kartsounis LD, Hardie RJ. The pattern of cognitive impairments in neuroacanthocytosis: a frontosubcortical dementia. *Arch Neurol* 1996;53:77–80.

13. Saiki S, Sakai K, Kitagawa Y, et al. Mutation in the CHAC gene in a family of autosomal dominant chorea-acanthocytosis. *Neurology* 2003;61:1614–1616.

14. Vance JM, Pericak-Vance MA, Bowman MH, et al. Chorea-acanthocytosis: a report of three new families and implications for genetic counselling. *Am J Med Genet* 1987;28:403–410.

15. Rampoldi L, Dobson-Stone C, Rubio JP, et al. A conserved sorting-associated protein is mutant in chorea-acanthocytosis. *Nat Genet* 2001;28:119–120.

16. Ueno S, Maruki Y, Nakamura M, et al. The gene encoding a newly discovered protein, chorein, is mutated in chorea-acanthocytosis. *Nat Genet* 2001;28:121–122.

17. Dobson-Stone C, Danek A, Rampoldi L, et al. Mutational spectrum of the CHAC gene in patients with chorea-acanthocytosis. *Eur J Hum Genet* 2002;10:773–781.

18. Velayos-Baeza A, Vettori A, Copley RR, et al. Analysis of the human VPS13 gene family. *Genomics* 2004;84:536–549.

19. Rinne JO, Daniel SE, Scaravilli F, et al. The neuropathological features of neuroacanthocytosis. *Mov Disord* 1994;9:297–304.

20. Rinne JO, Daniel SE, Scaravilli F, et al. Nigral degeneration in neuroacanthocytosis. *Neurology* 1994;44:1629–1632.

21. Aminoff MJ. Acanthocytosis and neurological disease. *Brain* 1972;95:749–760.

22. Ohnishi A, Sato Y, Nagara H, et al. Neurogenic muscular atrophy and low density of large myelinated fibres of sural nerve in chorea-acanthocytosis. *J Neurol Neurosurg Psychiatry* 1981;44:645–648.

23. Sobue G, Mukai E, Fujii K, et al. Peripheral nerve involvement in familial chorea-acanthocytosis. *J Neurol Sci* 1986;76:347–356.

24. Tamura T, Matsui K, Yaguchi H, et al. Nemaline rods in chorea-acanthocytosis. *Muscle Nerve* 2005;31:516–519.

25. Melone MA, Di Fede G, Peluso G, et al. Abnormal accumulation of tTGase products in muscle and erythrocytes of chorea-acanthocytosis patients. *J Neuropathol Exp Neurol* 2002;61:841–848.

26. Ishikawa S, Tachibana N, Tabata KI, et al. Muscle CT scan findings in McLeod syndrome and chorea-acanthocytosis. *Muscle Nerve* 2000;23:1113–1116.

27. De Yebenes JG, Brin MF, Mena MA, et al. Neurochemical findings in neuroacanthocytosis. *Mov Disord* 1988;3:300–312.

28. Dobson-Stone C, Velayos-Baeza A, Filippone LA, et al. Chorein detection for the diagnosis of chorea-acanthocytosis. *Ann Neurol* 2004;56:299–302.

29. Sakai T, Antoku Y, Iwashita H, et al. Chorea-acanthocytosis: abnormal composition of covalently bound fatty acids of erythrocyte membrane proteins. *Ann Neurol* 1991;29:664–669.

30. Olivieri O, De Franceschi L, Bordin L, et al. Increased membrane protein phosphorylation and anion transport activity in chorea-acanthocytosis. *Haematologica* 1997;82:648–653.

31. Okamoto K, Ito J, Furusawa T, et al. CT and MR findings of neuroacanthocytosis. *J Comput Assist Tomogr* 1997;21:221–222.

32. Sorrentino G, De Renzo A, Miniello S, et al. Late appearance of acanthocytes during the course of chorea-acanthocytosis. *J Neurol Sci* 1999;163:175–178.

33. Tanaka M, Hirai S, Kondo S, et al. Cerebral hypoperfusion and hypometabolism with altered striatal signal intensity in chorea-acanthocytosis: a combined PET and MRI study. *Mov Disord* 1998;13:100–107.

34. Dubinsky RM, Hallett M, Levey R, et al. Regional brain glucose metabolism in neuroacanthocytosis. *Neurology* 1989;39:1253–1255.

35. Brooks DJ, Ibañez V, Playford ED, et al. Presynaptic and postsynaptic striatal dopaminergic function in neuroacanthocytosis: a positron emission tomographic study. *Ann Neurol* 1991;30:166–171.

36. Danek A, Uttner I, Vogl T, et al. Cerebral involvement in McLeod syndrome. *Neurology* 1994;44:117–120.

37. Walker RH, Morgello S, Davidoff-Feldman B, et al. Autosomal dominant chorea-acanthocytosis with polyglutamine-containing neuronal inclusions. *Neurology* 2002;58:1031–1037.

38. Burbaud P, Rougier A, Ferrer X, et al. Improvement of severe trunk spasms by bilateral high-frequency stimulation of the motor thalamus in a patient with chorea-acanthocytosis. *Mov Disord* 2002;17:204–207.

39. Marsh WL, Marsh NJ, Moore A, et al. Elevated serum creatine phosphokinase in subjects with McLeod syndrome. *Vox Sang* 1981;40:403–411.

40. Ho M, Chelly J, Carter N, et al. Isolation of the gene for McLeod syndrome that encodes a novel membrane transport protein. *Cell* 1994;77:869–880.

41. Danek A, Rubio JP, Rampoldi L, et al. McLeod neuroacanthocytosis: genotype and phenotype. *Ann Neurol* 2001;50:755–764.

42. Jung HH, Russo D, Redman C, et al. Kell and XK immunohistochemistry in McLeod myopathy. *Muscle Nerve* 2001;24:1346–1351.

43. Oechsner M, Buchert R, Beyer W, et al. Reduction of striatal glucose metabolism in McLeod choreoacanthocytosis. *J Neurol Neurosurg Psychiatry* 2001;70:517–520.

44. Bassen FA, Kornzweig AL. Malformation of the erythrocytes in a case of atypical retinitis pigmentosa. *Blood* 1950;5:381–387.

45. Kayden HJ, Hatam LJ, Traber MG. The measurement of nanograms of tocopherol from needle aspiration biopsies of adipose tissue: normal and abetalipoproteinemic subjects. *J Lipid Res* 1983;24:652–656.

46. Muller DP, Lloyd JK, Wolff OH. The role of vitamin E in the treatment of the neurological features of abetalipoproteinaemia and other disorders of fat absorption. *J Inherit Metab Dis* 1985;8(suppl 1):88–92.

47. Brin M. Acanthocytosis. In: Vinken PB, GW. Klawans, HL. ed. *Handbook of clinical neurology: Systemic diseases,* part I. Amsterdam: Elsevier, 1993:271–299.

48. Barnett MH, Yang F, Iland H, et al. Unusual muscle pathology in McLeod syndrome. *J Neurol Neurosurg Psychiatry* 2000;69:655–657.

49. Hanaoka N, Yoshida K, Nakamura A, et al. A novel frameshift mutation in the McLeod syndrome gene in a Japanese family. *J Neurol Sci* 1999;165:6–9.

Prion Diseases

42

Lev G. Goldfarb

Human transmissible spongiform encephalopathies (TSEs), or prion diseases, represent a unique group of fatal neurodegenerative disorders that may be infectious, hereditary, or sporadic. *Infectious forms* of TSE cause outbreaks, such as epidemics of kuru in New Guinea and variant Creutzfeldt-Jakob disease (CJD) in the United Kingdom. *Inherited forms* of TSE are associated with multiple missense, insertion, and deletion mutations in the prion protein (*PRNP*) gene. *Sporadic forms* have no apparent environmental or genetic source, and they occur around the world with an incidence rate of around 1 per million per year. Recent advances in cellular and molecular biology have yielded increasingly strong evidence that TSEs result from accumulation in the brain of a structurally modified host protein encoded by the *PRNP* gene. This conformational isoform, named *prion protein*, and its toxic fragments gradually accumulate in neurons, resulting in neuronal death and other pathogenic effects responsible for the TSE phenotypes. The pathogenesis of TSE is, therefore, similar to other neurodegenerative disorders such as Alzheimer's and Parkinson's diseases, which also are caused by accumulation of aberrant forms of constitutively expressed proteins. The ability of the prion protein to induce disease when transmitted to another host is the only feature that makes TSEs fundamentally different from other neurodegenerative diseases.

MOLECULAR PATHOGENESIS

The predominant view of TSE pathogenesis is based on the *protein-only hypothesis*. According to this hypothesis, the pathogenic prion protein (PrP-sc), a molecule with a predominantly beta-sheet structure, is derived from a normal functional prion protein (PrP-c), a largely alpha-helical 36 kD protein. The PrP-c function is unknown. Presumably, it may have a synaptic role since it regulates copper content of the synaptic cleft (1). The normal PrP-c is soluble in mild detergents and sensitive to protease digestion, whereas PrP-sc exhibits remarkable resistance to physical and chemical agents; its turnover is approximately 5 times slower than that of the wild-type PrP-c. With disease progression, PrP-sc tends to form insoluble fibrillar aggregates in cell compartments. After cell death, PrP-sc accumulates in the extracellular space forming amyloid plaques. These properties are directly related to the PrP-sc enhanced beta-sheet content (2). PrP-sc alone or in association with another as yet unidentified molecule has the capacity to initiate the conformational conversion of PrP-c into PrP-sc in a cyclic autocatalytic amplification requiring at least temporary dimerisation of the two isoforms (3).

Mutations in the *PRNP* gene promote the conversion from PrP-c to PrP-sc. Transgenic mice expressing PrP with introduced "human" mutations spontaneously developed ataxia, neurodegeneration, spongiform change, and astrogliosis (4,5). These experiments strongly suggest that *PRNP* mutations cause TSE. Strong evidence has been presented that Methionine/Valine (Met/Val) coding variation at codon 129 of the *PRNP* gene influences the disease phenotype and is responsible for susceptibility/resistance to kuru and to iatrogenic and sporadic forms of CJD (6). PrP-c and PrP-sc have identical amino acid composition; thus, they are antigenically indistinguishable by the infected host, accounting for the absence of inflammatory changes in TSE brains.

PrP-sc isolates originating from patients with various types of TSE have distinct biological characteristics. The strain *signature* is retained after experimental passage through a variety of intermediate species. The PrP-sc electrophoretic mobility pattern reflecting the size and abundance of its three major glycoforms is associated with protein conformation (7). The determination of the PrP-sc glycoform in combination with the *PRNP* codon 129 genotype has become a useful tool for classification of TSE strains and for establishing correlations with the disease phenotypes.

TABLE 42.1

CLASSIFICATION OF TRANSMISSIBLE SPONGIFORM ENCEPHALOPATHIES (PRION DISEASES)

Type of Transmissible Spongiform Encephalopathy	Subtype
Sporadic	Sporadic Creutzfeldt-Jakob disease (sCJD)
	Sporadic fatal familial insomnia (sFFI)
Infectious	Kuru
	Variant Creutzfeldt-Jakob disease (vCJD)
	Iatrogenic Creutzfeldt-Jakob disease (iCJD)
Hereditary	Familial Creutzfeldt-Jakob disease (fCJD)
	Fatal familial insomnia (FFI)
	Gerstmann-Sträussler-Scheinker disease (GSS)

CLINICAL CLASSIFICATION

The clinical and neuropathologic features of human TSEs are extremely diverse. The classification into sporadic, infectious, and hereditary forms is widely accepted (Table 42.1). The route of infection determines to a significant extent the features of the infectious forms, whereas the phenotype of the hereditary forms depends on the causative PRNP mutation. Most commonly, the presenting and leading feature is cognitive decline. Cerebellar ataxia expressed initially as unsteady gait, incoordination of fine movements, and dysarthria is part of the clinical spectrum of each TSE variant; in some, ataxia is the presenting sign that tends to dominate the clinical picture. Myoclonus is a sudden irregular jerking of an isolated muscle or a muscle group, most commonly in the limbs. Spongiform change and astrocytic gliosis are found in most but not all forms of TSE. The presence, morphology, localization, and the extent of spongiform change and amyloid plaques have become an important basis for classification. Cerebral cortex and subcortical ganglia are affected in all forms of Creutzfeldt-Jakob disease; the cerebellum is primarily affected in kuru and Gerstmann-Sträussler-Scheinker disease, and the thalamus is the major site of degeneration in fatal familial insomnia.

SPORADIC CREUTZFELDT-JAKOB DISEASE

Sporadic CJD is defined as a case of TSE lacking an apparent environmental source of infection or family history of disease. Sporadic CJD is believed to be a spontaneous neurodegenerative illness arising from either a somatic mutation in the PRNP gene or a stochastic change in the prion protein structure results in generation of misfolded PrP molecules. Sporadic forms constitute an absolute majority of TSEs varying between 83% and 93% in different countries and populations; they are evenly distributed throughout the world with an incidence of approximately 1 per million per year (8). The average age at disease onset is 60 years, with a range from 16 to 82 years. In contrast to Alzheimer's disease and Parkinson's disease, in which morbidity increases with age, sporadic CJD declines after age 70 years (9).

Nonspecific prodromal symptoms such as anxiety, insomnia, behavioral disturbance, anorexia, and weight loss occur in up to 26% of patients in the days or weeks prior to disease development. The onset of neurological disease is gradual, occurring over a period of several weeks, although abrupt (strokelike) presentations are also known in up to 13% of patients (10). Initial symptoms are usually cognitive impairment manifested by memory loss, confusion, and behavioral changes, followed by cerebellar ataxia and myoclonus (Table 42.2). Less common presentations include initial cortical blindness with visual hallucinations (Heidenhain variant) and pure cerebellar ataxia (Brownell-Oppenheimer variant), but even these unusual presentations are quickly followed by cognitive impairment, ataxia, and myoclonus. As the illness evolves, the patients develop deficits of higher cortical functions, progressive dementia, diplopia, nystagmus, dysarthria, gait ataxia, muscle rigidity, seizures, tremors, myoclonus, choreiform, or athetoid movements and pyramidal tract signs. Lower motor neuron signs are rare. The speed of progression is alarming. Typically, within 4 to 6 months patients become globally demented and physically incapacitated by motor dysfunction, including severe ataxia, myoclonus, and rigidity (10,11). The mean

TABLE 42.2

CLINICAL CHARACTERISTICS OF SPORADIC CREUTZFELDT-JAKOB DISEASE

Symptom/Sign	At Presentation (%)	In Advanced Disease (%)
Behavioral abnormalities	29	57
Memory deterioration	48	100
Dementia	0	100
Cortical blindness	19	42
Cerebellar ataxia	33	71
Myoclonus	0	78
Pyramidal	2	62
Extrapyramidal rigidity	0	56
Seizures	Rare	19
Lower motor neuron	—	12
Paresthesia	6	11
Akinetic mutism	0	58
EEG periodic discharge	?	80
MRI: pulvinar high signal	?	77
14-3-3 protein in the CSF	?	94

duration of illness is 7 months. Among these cases, 14% have illness durations of 1 year or more, and only 5% of 2 years or more.

The typical electroencephalogram (EEG) abnormality in advanced disease is 1–2 Hz bi/triphasic sharp waves superimposed on a depressed background. These periodic sharp-wave synchronous discharges are usually asymmetric, may occur in synchrony with myoclonic jerks, and tend to become slower with disease progression. Serial tracings reveal this characteristic pattern in up to 80% of patients. This pattern is particularly frequent in cases of rapidly progressive dementia and, if present, is considered to be diagnostic of sporadic CJD. MRI reveals enlargement of the ventricles and widening of the cortical sulci. A characteristic finding seen in 77% of patients is a symmetrical hyperintense signal in the basal ganglia (Fig. 42.1A) (12). Cerebrospinal fluid markers of neuronal injury provide the most useful tests for the diagnosis in a living patient. They include neuron-specific enolase and 14-3-3 proteins. In a large study, the 14-3-3 protein was detected in 94% of tested patients, and the test specificity was estimated at 84% (13). False-positive results may occur in patients with rapidly progressive substantial neuronal injury, such as herpes encephalitis, recent cerebral infarction, and paraneoplastic neurological disorders. Sporadic CJD patients do not show pathogenic mutations in the *PRNP* gene.

Homozygosity for 129Met is present in 71% of patients (as compared to 39% in the general population) (6). Analysis of the *PRNP* gene is recommended for exclusion of hereditary forms of CJD and determining the codon 129 genotype, which in combination with immunoblot analysis of brain extracts for PrP-sc allows delineation of 6 phenotypic subtypes of sporadic CJD (14,15).

The diagnosis of sporadic CJD should be considered in a middle-aged individual presenting with rapidly progressive dementia. The early presence of cerebellar ataxia, pyramidal signs, and extrapyramidal signs is diagnostically helpful, and the development of myoclonus is characteristic. Positive results of EEG, MRI, and 14-3-3 protein studies make the diagnosis highly probable. The distinction between sporadic CJD and other forms of dementia rests on rapid disease evolution and the presence of movement abnormalities. Stroke, encephalitis, and brain tumor should be considered in cases with abrupt onset. About 90% of sporadic CJD cases are recognized clinically, but definitive diagnosis requires neuropathologic confirmation (16).

Widespread spongiform change is the most characteristic histopathologic finding; the vacuoles are usually small, round, or oval and may become confluent. Spongiform degeneration is combined with the loss of neurons in the cerebral cortex, the striatum, and the molecular layer of the cerebellum. Reactive astrocytosis is a prominent

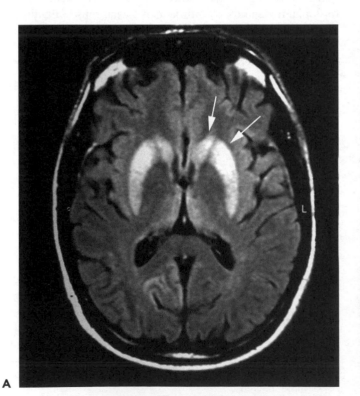

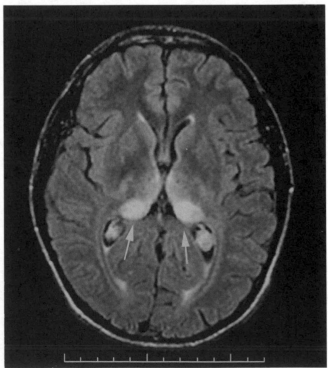

A   B

Figure 42.1 Magnetic resonance imaging in patients with sporadic Creutzfeldt-Jakob disease (CJD) and variant CJD. **A:** Sporadic CJD: axial FLAIR image at the level of the basal ganglia showing symmetrical high signal in the caudate head and anterior putamen *(arrows)*. **B:** Variant CJD: axial FLAIR image at the level of the basal ganglia showing symmetrical high signal in the pulvinar and dorsomedial nuclei of the thalamus *(arrows)*. (Photos courtesy of the National CJD Surveillance Unit, Western General Hospital, Edinburgh, United Kingdom.)

accompanying feature. An overt inflammatory response is not found, and the reaction of microglia and macrophages is minimal. The presence of spongiform change accompanied by neuronal loss and gliosis make the diagnosis definite (17).

KURU

Kuru has emerged in the beginning of the 20th century in a small indigenous population in the Eastern Highlands of New Guinea. The disease reached epidemic proportions in the mid-1950s and disappeared in the 1990s. The spread of kuru was associated with ritual cannibalistic consumption of deceased relatives (18). The youngest known kuru patient was diagnosed at age 4 and died at age 5. The mean age of disease onset is 19. Mean incubation time was assessed at between 10.3 and 13.2 years (19), with a range between 1 and 40 years. Kuru is a rapidly progressive fatal ataxia. Disequilibrium, clumsiness, and tremor are the initial signs of illness. Speech deteriorates as the disease advances (18). Dystonic movements and myoclonus-type jerks are present in the trunk, limbs, neck, and jaw. Emotional instability with inappropriate outbursts of laughter or crying is noted in some patients; others become depressed and withdrawn or paranoid and aggressive. Mental slowing is apparent, but severe dementia may not be evident. Mean duration of illness is 8 months, with a range from 4 to 24 months. Individuals homozygous for 129Met were preferentially affected during the kuru epidemic (20). Neuropathology is represented by the highly characteristic unicentric (kuru-type) amyloid plaques and perineuronal PrP deposits observed in large numbers in the cerebellum (21) and by neuronal loss, astrocytic gliosis, and some degree of spongiform change in the cerebral cortex and cerebellum (21,22). No significant inflammatory changes have been observed. Kuru was experimentally transmitted by intracerebral inoculation to chimpanzees and nonhuman primates after 12 to 31 months of incubation (23). The clinical features and neuropathology of experimental kuru were similar to human disease.

VARIANT CREUTZFELDT-JAKOB DISEASE

Variant CJD (vCJD) is a human disease linked to the consumption of contaminated meat products of animals incubating bovine spongiform encephalopathy (BSE, or mad cow disease). BSE was first identified in 1986 and spread throughout the United Kingdom to involve more than 180,000 animals (24). Close to 150 cases of human vCJD have so far occurred in Great Britain, 6 cases in France, and single cases in the United States, Canada, Italy, Republic of Ireland, and Hong Kong. A distinctive feature of vCJD is the early age of onset, mean 28 years, which is similar to kuru.

The calculated incubation time in humans is 6 to 12 years. Clinical presentation of vCJD has been determined as *psychiatric:* behavioral and personality change, dysphoria, withdrawal, anxiety, insomnia, apathy, and memory loss were observed in 63% of patients (25). Nonspecific and poorly localized limb pain, disesthesia, paresthesia, and feeling cold and numb are other distinctive features observed in 64% of patients, including 31% who had these symptoms from the onset (26). Ataxia was present in almost all patients. Dementia, chorea, dystonia, and myoclonus developed as the disease progressed. Associative signs of dysphasia, rigidity, hyperreflexia, and primitive reflexes may occur. Death in an akinetic mute state is a typical outcome. The mean duration of illness is about 14 months. EEG in patients with variant CJD does not show periodic sharp discharges; 14-3-3 protein is detected only in about 50% of cases, making this test less diagnostically valuable than it is in sporadic CJD (27), but a high T2 MRI signal in the pulvinar region (pulvinar sign) is present in about 75% to 90% of patients (Fig. 42.1B) (25).

In contrast to all other TSEs, variant CJD is characterized by the presence of large amounts of PrP-sc in lymphoreticular tissues such as the tonsils, spleen, and lymph nodes (28). This characteristic allows tonsil biopsy with PrP-immunostaining analysis to be used for diagnostic purposes (29). Tonsil biopsy has shown 100% sensitivity and specificity and secures the diagnosis at an early clinical stage; it also allows presymptomatic testing. The accumulation of infectious material in peripheral tissues increases the risk of human-to-human transmission through medical procedures, including general surgery, organ and tissue transplants, and blood transfusion. This concern has been reinforced following a report of vCJD developing in a patient who received a transfusion of packed red blood cells donated by an individual who subsequently died from vCJD (30). Patients with vCJD lack mutations in the *PRNP* gene, but all tested patients were homozygous for 129Met. The diagnosis of vCJD may be problematic in the early stages of illness because symptoms of anxiety, depression, and apathy are nonspecific. In addition, the disease atypically affects young people, and EEG and 14-3-3 protein testing are frequently negative. Bilateral pulvinar sign on MRI has acquired diagnostic significance, and tonsil biopsy, although invasive, helps to verify the diagnosis in difficult situations.

The defining neuropathologic feature of vCJD is an amyloid plaque composed of a central amyloid core with fibrillary periphery surrounded by a rim of spongiform vacuoles (*florid* plaque). Florid plaques and clusters of PrP-immunoreactive deposits not associated with spongiform change are abundant in the cerebrum and cerebellum (31). These features are distinct from all other types of human TSEs. Astrocytosis and neuronal loss characteristic of other CJD forms are also present. The thalamus exhibits severe neuronal loss and gliosis in the posterior nuclei, areas of high MRI signal.

IATROGENIC CREUTZFELDT-JAKOB DISEASE

The first report on transmission of CJD through corneal graft obtained from a donor with neuropathologically confirmed CJD was published in 1974 (32). Since then, about 300 cases of CJD have been caused by transmission of infection from person to person in the course of medical intervention and treatment. Neurosurgical procedures involving contaminated instruments, electrodes inserted into the brain for EEG studies, and corneal grafts are tragic but rare causes of CJD transmission (Table 42.3). Since 1985, CJD has been repeatedly recorded among young recipients of human pituitary growth hormone replacement therapy (6). The pituitary growth hormone inoculations and dura mater grafts account for most of the known cases of iatrogenic CJD (Table 42.3). Human pituitary hormones were produced by pooling many thousands of cadaveric pituitary glands with possible cross-contamination. Human dura mater grafts also were obtained from cadavers.

The length of the incubation time and clinical features of iatrogenic CJD are determined by the route of infection (Table 42.3). When the infectious agent is directly introduced into the brain, as with neurosurgical instruments or stereotactic EEG electrodes (*intracerebral route of infection*), the incubation time is only 16 to 28 months and the clinical features are similar to sporadic CJD, consisting of rapidly progressive dementia, myoclonus, and periodic discharges on EEG. The duration of illness is usually several months (6). However, when the contaminated material is applied to the surface of the brain, as with dura mater grafts (*intracranial route of infection*), the incubation time is on average 6 years and the clinical presentation is cerebellar ataxia (in about 70% of cases) or cortical blindness and mental deterioration with rapid progression of illness. In cases with *peripheral route of infection*, such as pituitary hormone replacement therapy, the mean incubation time is 12 years and the clinical presentation is invariably cerebellar dysfunction with limb and truncal ataxia, dysarthria, and nystagmus (6). Dementia occurs only rarely and in many cases meaningful communication is possible until the terminal stages. The patients

survive for about a year. Homozygosity for 129Met increases the risk of disease from intracerebral/intracranial infection.

The diagnosis of iatrogenic CJD requires knowledge of relevant risk factors and information about past medical conditions and medical procedures. Rapidly progressive cognitive decline or cerebellar ataxia should raise suspicion. The patient may be young. The usefulness of EEG, 14-3-3, and MRI exams vary with the clinical form, but these investigations should be performed in situations when the diagnosis is uncertain. Neuropathological examination reveals widespread spongiform change, marked astrocytic gliosis, and neuronal loss closely resembling the changes seen in sporadic CJD. Treatment of children of short stature with cadaveric pituitary growth hormone has in many countries been replaced with recombinant hormones. Guidelines have been established for sterilization techniques that significantly reduce infectivity.

FAMILIAL CREUTZFELDT-JAKOB DISEASE

Multiple mutations in the *PRNP* gene have been linked to various phenotypes of hereditary TSE. A total of 365 cases of hereditary TSE have been reported in the literature (33). Currently, 55 pathogenic mutations and 16 DNA polymorphisms have been identified, including 24 missense point mutations, 29 insertion/deletion mutations, and 2 nonsense mutations; there are 4 polymorphisms that alter the amino acid sequence, among these the Met/Val polymorphism at position 129 (34). Many of the pathogenic mutations are located within or near one of the PrP alpha-helix domains, which is in agreement with the view that mutations alter the protein secondary structure predisposing the PrP molecule to acquire a beta-sheet configuration.

Familial CJD Caused by the PRNP E200K Mutation

The *PRNP* E200K mutation is the most frequent cause of familial CJD, accounting for approximately 70% of the CJD-affected families worldwide. This mutation was identified in

TABLE 42.3
IATROGENIC CREUTZFELDT-JAKOB DISEASE WORLDWIDE

Route of Infection	Number of Cases	Mean Incubation Time (Years)	Presentation
Corneal transplant	3	1.5	Dementia
Stereotactic EEG	2	1.5	Dementia
Neurosurgery	5	1.5	Visual/dementia/ataxia
Dura matter transplant	114	6	Cerebellar ataxia/dementia
Human growth hormone	138	12	Cerebellar ataxia
Human gonadotrophin	4	13	Cerebellar ataxia

CJD clusters identified in Libyan Jews and in other isolated populations in Slovakia, Chile, Italy, and Japan (35). The clinical features of the E200K form are almost identical to sporadic CJD. The mean age at onset is 58 years, and the mean duration of illness is 6 months. Patients present with cognitive impairment, personality change, and cerebellar signs (Table 42.4). Limb and truncal ataxia and dysarthria are observed at the disease onset in approximately 50% of patients. During the course of illness, all patients developed dementia and incoordination, startle-induced or spontaneous myoclonic jerks were recorded in 73%, seizures in 40%, and sensory deficits in 24% (36). Periodic sharp wave discharge on EEG is characteristic of this form. The test for the 14-3-3 protein in the cerebrospinal fluid (CSF) has been reported positive in almost all examined cases of E200K CJD. Histopathology is characterized by spongiosis, astrogliosis, and neuronal loss; these lesions are most severe in the cerebral cortex. They also are present with decreasing severity in the striatum, diencephalon, and cerebellum.

Immunostaining is consistently positive throughout the brain with the punctate or synaptic pattern. No PrP-positive deposits either in the form of amyloid or nonamyloid plaques are observed. Intracerebral inoculation of brain homogenates from patients carrying the E200K mutation regularly transmitted the disease to primates (10).

Familial CJD Caused by the PRNP D178N Mutation

The *PRNP* D178N mutation has been linked to two separate familial disorders, a form of familial CJD and fatal familial insomnia. Considerable phenotypic distinction between them depends on coupling of the causative D178N mutation with the alternative residue at position 129: the D178N mutation located on allele with valine at position 129 (D178N/129Val) is responsible for a dementing form of familial CJD characterized by disease onset at age 45 years and mean duration of illness 22 months (37).

TABLE 42.4
GENOTYPE/PHENOTYPE RELATIONSHIPS IN HEREDITARY TSE

Genotype	Mean Age at Onset (years)	Mean Duration of Illness (months)	Signs and Symptoms at Presentation	Syndromes of Advanced Illness	Neuropathology
Familial CJD, *PRNP* E200K mutation	58	6	Cognitive decline/cerebellar ataxia	Dementia/ataxia/myoclonus	Spongiosis/astrogliosis/neuronal loss in the cerebral cortex
Familial CJD, *PRNP* D178N mutation	45	22	Severe memory loss	Dementia/ataxia/myoclonus	Spongiosis/astrogliosis/neuronal loss in the cerebral cortex
Familial CJD, *PRNP* 24-bp expansion, 1 to 4 extra repeats	67	4	Abnormal behavior/memory loss	Dementia/ataxia/myoclonus	Spongiosis/gliosis/neuronal loss in the cerebral cortex
Familial CJD, *PRNP* 24-bp expansion, 5 to 9 extra repeats	35	96	Abnormal behavior/cognitive decline	Dementia/ataxia/spasticity	Cortical atrophy/spongiosis/gliosis/neuronal loss/widespread multicentric amyloid plaques
Fatal familial insomnia, short duration	50	12	Insomnia/myoclonus	Insomnia/autonomic/ataxia/myoclonus	Neuronal loss/gliosis in thalamic nuclei and inferior olives
Fatal familial insomnia, long duration	44	26	Ataxia/insomnia	Ataxia/insomnia/autonomic/dementia	Spongiosis in the neocortex/neuronal loss and gliosis in thalamic nuclei
GSS, *PRNP* P102L mutation	48	72	Ataxia	Ataxia/dysarthria/spasticity/dementia	Uni- and multicentric amyloid plaques in the cerebellum/variable spongiform change in the neocortex
GSS, *PRNP* F198S and Q217R mutations	52	72	Cognitive decline	Dementia/ataxia/dysarthria/bradykinesia/rigidity	Uni- and multicentric amyloid plaques/neurofibrillary tangles in the cerebellum and the neocortex

bp, base pair; CJD, Creutzfeldt-Jakob disease; GSS, Gerstmann-Sträussler-Scheinker disease

More than 20 large pedigrees with this CJD variant have been reported. The characteristic presentation is cognitive impairment with early dramatic memory loss often associated with depression, irritability, and abnormal behavior. Ataxia, dysarthria and aphasia, tremor, and myoclonus appear during the course of illness. This type of familial CJD only rarely shows periodic sharp wave discharges on EEG (11). Neuropathologic changes consist of severe and widely spread spongiosis with prominent gliosis and neuronal loss; the frontal and temporal cortices are generally more severely affected than the occipital cortex. Among the subcortical structures, the putamen and the caudate nucleus show severe spongiosis with variable degrees of gliosis; the thalamus is minimally or moderately affected, the cerebellum is spared, and minimal or no pathology is seen in the brainstem. The immunostaining pattern is punctate. The disease has been transmitted to squirrel monkeys with brain tissue of 7 patients from 5 kindreds (10).

Familial CJD Caused by the PRNP 24-bp Repeat Expansion

The *PRNP* gene has 5 repeat sequences between codons 51 and 91. The 5′ sequence consists of 27 base pair (bp), whereas the 4 downstream sequences have each 24 bp. At least 32 families with more than 100 patients are now known to develop CJD due to insertion or deletion of 24-bp repeats in the repeat area of the *PRNP* gene (34). Each family carries a unique allele differing by the repeat number and the composition of the repeat elements. The mean age at disease onset in patients with *5 or more extra repeats* was 35, significantly earlier than in patients with other types of familial TSE, and the mean duration of illness in these patients was 8 years, much longer than in other forms. In patients with *1 to 4 extra repeats*, the mean age at onset was 67 years and the duration of illness 4 months. Thus, the age of disease onset correlates inversely with the repeat number, but the anticipation phenomenon observed in Huntington disease and other repeat-expansion disorders is not recognized in this type of CJD (38). Clinical features were determined to a significant extent by the number of repeats. Patients with *1 to 4 extra repeats* had rapidly progressive dementia often associated with ataxia and visual disturbances and marked with myoclonus and periodic sharp-wave discharges on EEG recordings. In patients with *5 or more extra repeats*, the illness is characterized as a slow, progressive mental deterioration preceded by a long, distinctive premorbid personality change. Premorbid symptoms commonly described are difficulty concentrating, excessive mood swings, irritability, lifelong depression, learning disability, social insensitivity, inability to keep a steady job, a history of long-time psychiatric care, clumsiness, and poor coordination. Such a long-lasting premorbid personality change was not observed in patients with point mutations. Slowly developing dementia is associated with cerebellar and extrapyramidal signs.

Periodic sharp-wave complexes on EEG or myoclonus are not frequently seen. Patients with low repeat numbers showed histopathologic changes consistent with those of sporadic TSE, including widespread spongiform degeneration, astrogliosis, and neuronal loss. In contrast, the autopsied patients with 7 or more 24-bp repeats show the presence of uni- or multicentric PrP amyloid plaques located in the molecular layer of the cerebellum and the cerebral gray matter, a phenomenon not seen in CJD and rather compatible with Gerstmann-Sträussler-Scheinker disease (34). Brain suspension from 3 studied patients with 5, 7, and 8 extra repeats transmitted the disease to primates after intracerebral inoculation (10).

FATAL FAMILIAL INSOMNIA

Fatal familial insomnia (FFI) is a unique hereditary disease characterized by insomnia, dysautonomia, and movement abnormalities. This syndrome is associated with the D178N/129Met haplotype. At least 25 families have been described. The disease starts between 20 and 72 years of age and may have either a relatively *short duration* (mean: 12 months in patients homozygous for 129Met) or *long duration* (mean: 26 months in heterozygous patients) course of illness (37,39). Sleep–wake and vigilance abnormalities are characterized by insomnia, episodes of hallucinations, and confusion. Polysomnographic recordings confirm strikingly reduced total sleep time and gross disorganization of sleep. Even such drugs as benzodiazepines and barbiturates may be unable to induce sleeplike EEG activity. Autonomic dysfunction is expressed as systemic hypertension, irregular breathing, diaphoresis, pyrexia, and impotence. Diplopia, dysarthria, dysphagia, ataxia/abasia, and dysmetria are common motor signs, and spontaneous and evoked myoclonus, spasticity, and occasional tonic–clonic seizures are observed. Patients with the *short-duration* FFI subtype present with prominent sleep–wake disturbances, myoclonus, and more evident autonomic alterations. In the *long-duration* subtype of FFI, these same features are seen at a more advanced stage, and the disease presents with ataxia and tends to have more prominent cognitive impairment. The periodic sharp waves on EEG and myoclonus may appear in cases of long duration. The test for 14-3-3 protein in the CSF, diagnostically useful in sporadic CJD, is usually negative in FFI. Conventional neuroimaging with MRI or CT scanning is usually normal or shows nonspecific cerebral or cerebellar atrophy. Positron emission tomography (PET) with radio-labeled fluorodeoxyglucose shows characteristic diminished metabolic activity in the thalamus (34).

The histopathologic hallmark of FFI is the loss of neurons and astrogliosis in the mediodorsal and anterior thalamic nuclei. Involvement of other thalamic nuclei varies. The inferior olives show neuronal loss and gliosis in most cases. The neocortex is spared in patients with *short-duration* FFI, focally affected by spongiosis and gliosis in patients with a course of illness between 12 and 20 month, while diffuse spongiform change is seen in patients with the *long-duration* subtype (40). The frontal, temporal, and parietal lobes are affected more severely than the occipital lobe. Brain suspension of FFI patients transmitted the disease to wild-type (41) and transgenic mice (42); transgenic mice showed degeneration and PrP accumulation in the thalamus.

GERSTMANN-STRÄUSSLER-SCHEINKER DISEASE

Gerstmann-Sträussler-Scheinker disease (GSS) is inherited with an autosomal dominant pattern and caused by mutations in the *PRNP* gene. The set of *PRNP* mutations responsible for GSS differs from familial CJD, suggesting that hereditary CJD and GSS are allelic variant disorders. To date, at least 56 families affected by GSS have been reported (34).

GSS Caused by the PRNP P102L Mutation

The P102L mutation is involved in about 80% of all studied GSS families (43). The disease onset is between the fourth and the seventh decades of life, mean 48 years, and the duration of illness is on average 6 years. The clinical phenotype is characterized by progressive dysarthria, incoordination of gait, and pyramidal and pseudobulbar signs. Mental and behavioral deterioration leading to dementia and akinetic mutism occur in the advanced stages of illness. In rare instances, the disease takes a rapid course of 5 to 9 months from onset to death, with a clinical picture indistinguishable from that of sporadic CJD. Myoclonic movements and periodic sharp-wave discharges on EEG are rarely observed. Cerebellar atrophy is usually visible on MRI. The distinctive neuropathologic feature is the presence of multicentric PrP amyloid plaques in the cerebellum and to a lesser extent in the cerebral cortex. The plaques appear as amorphous aggregates of spheroid bodies often consisting of a centrally located larger core encircled by several satellite plaques. Spongiform degeneration and astrogliosis are not frequently seen; they vary in severity even among members of the same kindred and are most pronounced when the course of illness is rapid (44). GSS was transmitted to nonhuman primates (10). The recipient primates developed a rapidly progressive disease with severe spongiform degeneration and no amyloid deposition.

GSS Caused by the PRNP F198S and Q217R Mutations

The large and well-studied Indiana kindred (43), another U.S. family segregating GSS with the *PRNP* F198S mutation, and 2 Swedish families in which GSS is associated with the *PRNP* Q217R mutation (45) are uniquely characterized by

severe dementia, progressive ataxia, and dysarthria in association with bradykinesia and rigidity. The age of onset is between 40 and 71 (mean: 52), and the duration of illness is between 2 and 12 years (mean: 6 years). Unicentric and multicentric PrP amyloid plaques are widely distributed in the cerebral, cerebellar, and midbrain parenchyma. A distinct feature of this GSS variant is PrP cerebral amyloid angiopathy. In the neocortex, the PrP amyloid cores are surrounded by abnormal tau-positive plaques similar to neuritic plaques in Alzheimer's disease (43). To increase the similarity, neurofibrillary tangles are present in the same areas of the neocortex. The diagnosis of GSS and other hereditary TSEs is helped by positive family history and detection of a pathogenic mutation in the *PRNP* gene.

TREATMENT AND MANAGEMENT

No effective treatment is currently available for TSE, but the progress of fundamental studies offers some hope. Prospective therapies most likely will be directed toward interruption of the conversion from normal prion protein to the abnormal PrP-sc isoform. Promising results were obtained in experimental studies of some compounds, such as polyanions, sulfonated dyes, tetrapyrroles, polyene antibiotics, branched polyamines, cysteine protease inhibitors, suramine, synthetic peptides (46), tricyclic derivatives of acridine and phenothiazine, quinacrine, and chlorpromazine (47). The antimalarial drug quinacrine showing inhibitory effect on PrP-sc in experiments was administered to CJD patients, but there was only transient benefit; several other compounds have been tested in patients with little success (48). Conformational transition from PrP-c to PrP-sc may be inhibited or prevented or even reversed by synthetic peptides homologous to PrP fragments implicated as transitional sites. These peptides, named *beta-sheet breakers*, reduced infectivity by 90% to 95% in mice with experimental TSE (49). Recent efforts at producing PrP-sc–specific antibodies that would block the production of PrP-sc by affecting the PrP-c→PrP-sc interactions resulted in a discovery that a repeat motif Tyr-Tyr-Arg is accessible to antibody binding in the misfolded PrP-sc isoform (50). Tyr-Tyr-Arg monoclonal antibodies reduce the cell content of PrP-sc. These findings may lead to the possibility of immunization with the Tyr-Tyr-Arg peptide and perhaps to immunotherapy (48).

Precautions are recommended in the general care and management of hospitalized TSE patients. The infectious agent is not present in any external secretion, but it may be present in the brain and spinal cord tissues, cerebrospinal fluid, eyeballs, pituitary gland, spleen, liver, kidneys, lymph nodes, and blood (17). Contaminated surgical instruments carry risk of infection. Accidental contamination of intact skin should be treated with application of fresh undiluted bleach or 1 N sodium hydroxide to the area for about 1 minute, followed by thorough washing with soap. Special precautions should be taken while handling pathology samples (51). There is an ongoing discussion on safety of blood and blood products. Contamination of blood with the vCJD agent is causing the most concern. Exclusion of at-risk donors may reduce or eliminate blood contamination. The identification of mutations in the *PRNP* gene opens a possibility of genetic counseling, as prenatal genetic testing can be done at the family's request. It is also expected that in the future the number of iatrogenic CJD cases will decrease as a result of the use of recombinant pituitary hormones replacing cadaveric hormones, and new highly efficient procedures are being introduced to sterilize dura mater grafts.

The infectious agents of TSE resist conventional sterilization and decontamination methods (52). Detergents, chlorine dioxide, alcohols, potassium permanganate, hydrogen peroxide, aldehydes, ultraviolet irradiation, and ethylene oxide are ineffective. Disposable instruments and other materials should be used whenever possible; if retained, instruments should be disinfected in 2 cycles of steam autoclaving at 134°C for 1 hour with subsequent soaking in 1 N sodium hydroxide for 2 hours to reduce infectivity.

REFERENCES

1. Lasmézas CI. Putative functions of PrPC. *Br Med Bull* 2003; 66:61–70.
2. Pan KM, Baldwin M, J Nguyen J, et al. Conversion of alpha-helices into beta-sheets features in the formation of the scrapie prion proteins. *Proc Natl Acad Sci USA* 1993;90:10,962–10,966.
3. Come JH, Fraser PE, Lansbury PT. A kinetic model for amyloid formation in the prion diseases: importance of seeding. *Proc Natl Acad Sci USA* 1993;90:5959–5963.
4. Hsiao KK, Groth D, Scott M, et al. Serial transmission in rodents of neurodegeneration from transgenic mice expressing mutant prion protein. *Proc Natl Acad Sci USA* 1994;91:9126–9130.
5. Chiesa R, Piccardo P, Ghetti B, Harris DA. Neurological illness in transgenic mice expressing a prion protein with an insertional mutation. *Neuron* 1998;21:1339–1351.
6. Brown P, Preece M, Brandel JP, et al. Iatrogenic Creutzfeldt-Jakob disease at the millennium. *Neurology* 2000;55:1075–1081.
7. Parchi P, Castellani R, Capellari S, et al. Molecular basis of phenotypic variability in sporadic Creutzfeldt-Jakob disease. *Ann Neurol* 1996;39:767–778.
8. Masters CL, Harris JO, Gajdusek DC, et al. Creutzfeldt-Jakob disease: patterns of worldwide occurrence and the significance of familial and sporadic clustering. *Ann Neurol* 1979; 5:177–188.
9. Cousens SN, Zeidler M, Esmonde TF, et al. Sporadic Creutzfeldt-Jakob disease in the United Kingdom: analysis of epidemiological surveillance data for 1970–96. *BMJ* 1997;315:389–395.
10. Brown P, Gibbs CJ Jr, Rodgers-Johnson P, et al. Human spongiform encephalopathy: the National Institutes of Health Series of 300 cases of experimentally transmitted disease. *Ann Neurol* 1994;35:513–529.
11. Brown P. Transmissible human spongiform encephalopathy (infectious cerebral amyloidosis): Creutzfeldt-Jakob disease, Gerstmann-Sträussler-Scheinker syndrome, and kuru. In: Calne DB, ed. *Neurodegenerative diseases*. Philadelphia: W.B. Saunders, 1994:839–876.
12. Collie DA, Sellar RJ, Zeidler M, et al. MRI of Creutzfeldt-Jakob disease: imaging features and recommended MRI protocol. *Clin Radiol* 2001;56:726–739.
13. Zerr I, Bodemer M, Gefeller O, et al. Detection of 14–3–3 protein in the cerebrospinal fluid supports the diagnosis of Creutzfeldt-Jakob disease. *Ann Neurol* 1998;43:32–40.
14. Parchi P, Giese A, Capellari S, et al. Classification of sporadic Creutzfeldt-Jakob disease based on molecular and phenotypic analysis of 300 subjects. *Ann Neurol* 1999;46:224–233.
15. Hill AF, Joiner S, Wadsworth JD, et al. Molecular classification of sporadic Creutzfeldt-Jakob disease. *Brain* 2003;126:1333-1346.
16. Knight RS, Will RG. Prion diseases. *J Neurol Neurosurg Psychiatry* 2004;75(suppl 1):i36–i42.
17. Budka H, Aguzzi A, Brown P, et al. Neuropathological diagnostic criteria for Creutzfeldt-Jakob disease (CJD) and other human spongiform encephalopathies (prion diseases). *Brain Pathol* 1995;5:459–466.
18. Gajdusek DC. Unconventional viruses and the origin and disappearance of kuru. *Science* 1977;197:943–960.
19. Huillard d'Aignaux JN, Cousens SN, Maccario J, et al. The incubation period of kuru. *Epidemiology* 2002;13:402–408.
20. Lee HS, Brown P, Cervenakova L, et al. Increased susceptibility to kuru of carriers of the PRNP 129 methionine/methionine genotype. *J Inf Dis* 2001;183:192–196.
21. McLean CA, Ironside JW, Alpers MP, et al. Comparative neuropathology of kuru with the new variant of Creutzfeldt-Jakob disease: evidence for strain of agent predominating over genotype of host. *Brain Pathol* 1998;8:429–437.
22. Hainfellner JA, Liberski PP, Guiroy DN, et al. Pathology and immunocytochemistry of a kuru brain. *Brain Pathol* 1997;7: 547–553.
23. Gajdusek DC, Gibbs CJ Jr, Alpers M. Experimental transmission of kuru-like syndrome to chimpanzees. *Nature* 1966;209:794–796.
24. Brown P, Will RG, Bradley R, et al. Bovine spongiform encephalopathy and variant Creutzfeldt-Jakob disease: background, evolution, and current concerns. *Emerg Infect Dis* 2001;7:6–16.
25. Will RG, Zeidler M, Stewart GE, et al. Diagnosis of new variant Creutzfeldt-Jakob disease. *Ann Neurol* 2000;47:575–582.
26. Spencer MD, Knight RS, Will RG. First hundred cases of variant Creutzfeldt-Jakob disease: retrospective case note review of early psychiatric and neurological features. *BMJ* 2002;324:1479–1482.
27. Green AJ, Thompson EJ, Stewart GE, et al. Use of 14-3-3 and other brain-specific proteins in CSF in the diagnosis of variant Creutzfeldt-Jakob disease. *J Neurol Neurosurg Psychiatry* 2001;70: 744–748.
28. Wadsworth JD, Joiner S, Hill AF, et al. Tissue distribution of protease resistant prion protein in variant Creutzfeldt-Jakob disease using a highly sensitive immunoblotting assay. *Lancet* 2001;358:171–180.
29. Hill AF, Butterworth RJ, Joiner S, et al. Investigation of variant Creutzfeldt-Jakob disease and other human prion diseases with tonsil biopsy samples. *Lancet* 1999;353:183–189.
30. Llewelyn CA, Hewitt PE, Knight RS, et al. Possible transmission of variant Creutzfeldt-Jakob disease by blood transfusion. *Lancet* 2004;363:417–421.
31. Ironside JW, Head MW. Neuropathology and molecular biology of variant Creutzfeldt-Jakob disease. *Curr Top Microbiol Immunol* 2004;284:133–159.
32. Duffy P, Wolf J, Collins G, et al. Possible person-to-person transmission of Creutzfeldt-Jakob disease. *New Engl J Med* 1974;290: 692–693.
33. Kovacs GG, Trabattoni G, Hainfellner JA, et al. Mutations of the prion protein gene: phenotypic spectrum. *J Neurol* 2002;249: 1567–1582.
34. Kong Q, Surewicz WK, Petersen RB, et al. Inherited prion diseases. In: Prusiner SB, ed. *Prion biology and diseases*, 2nd ed. New York: Cold Spring Habor Laboratory Press, 2003:673–775.
35. Lee HS, Sambuughin N, Cervenakova L, et al. Ancestral origins and worldwide distribution of the *PRNP* 200K mutation causing familial Creutzfeldt-Jakob disease. *Amer J Hum Genet* 1999; 64:1063–1070.
36. Brown P, Goldfarb LG, Gibbs CJ Jr, Gajdusek DC. The phenotypic expression of different mutations in transmissible familial Creutzfeldt-Jakob disease. *Eur J Epidemiol* 1991;7:469–476.
37. Goldfarb LG, Petersen RB, Tabaton M, et al. Fatal familial insomnia and familial Creutzfeldt-Jakob disease: disease phenotype determined by a DNA polymorphism. *Science* 1992;258: 806–808.
38. Goldfarb LG, Cervenakova L, Brown P, Gajdusek DC. Genotype-phenotype correlations in familial spongiform encephalopathies

associated with insert mutations. In: Court L, Dodet B, eds. *Transmissible subacute spongiform encephalopathies: erion diseases.* Paris: Elsevier, 1996:425–431.

39. Gambetti P, Parchi P, Petersen RB, et al. Fatal familial insomnia and familial Creutzfeldt-Jakob disease: clinical, pathological and molecular features. *Brain Pathol* 1995;5:43–51.
40. Lugaresi E, Tobler I, Gambetti P, Montagna P. The pathophysiology of fatal familial insomnia. *Brain Pathol* 1998;8:521–526.
41. Tateishi J, Brown P, Kitamoto T, et al. First experimental transmission of fatal familial insomnia. *Nature* 1995;376:434–435.
42. Telling GC, Parchi P, DeArmond SJ, et al. Evidence for the conformation of the pathologic isoform of the prion protein enciphering and propagating prion diversity. *Science* 1996;274: 2079–2082.
43. Ghetti B, Dlouhy SR, Giaccone G, et al. Gerstmann-Sträussler-Scheinker's disease and the Indiana kindred. *Brain Pathol* 1995;5:61–75.
44. Piccardo P, Dlouhy SR, Lievens PMJ, et al. Phenotypic variability of Gerstmann-Sträussler-Scheinker disease is associated with prion protein heterogeneity. *J Neuropath Exp Neurol* 1998;57: 979–988.

45. Hsiao K, Dlouhy SR, Farlow MR, et al. Mutant prion proteins in Gerstmann-Straussler-Scheinker disease with neurofibrillary tangles. *Nat Genet* 1992;1:68–71.
46. Brown P. Drug therapy in human and experimental transmissible spongiform encephalopathy. *Neurology* 2002;58:1720–1725.
47. Korth C, May BC, Cohen FE, Prusiner SB. Acridine and phenothiazine derivatives as pharmacotherapeutics for prion disease. *Proc Natl Acad Sci USA* 2001;98:9836–9841.
48. Cashman NR, Caughey B. Prion diseases: close to effective therapy? *Nat Rev Drug Discov* 2004;3:874–884.
49. Soto C, Kascsak RJ, Saborio GP, et al. Reversion of prion protein conformational changes by synthetic beta-sheet breaker peptides. *Lancet* 2000;355:192–197.
50. Paramithiotis E, Pinard M, Lawton T, et al. A prion protein epitope selective for the pathologically misfolded conformation. *Nature Med* 2003;9:893–899.
51. Budka H, Aguzzi A, Brown P, et al. Tissue handling in suspected Creutzfeldt-Jakob disease (CJD) and other human spongiform encephalopathies. *Brain Pathol* 1995;5:319–322.
52. Taylor DM. Inactivation of transmissible degenerative encephalopathy agents: a review. *Vet J* 2000;159:10–17.

Functional Neuroimaging in Movement Disorders

43

David J. Brooks

Functional imaging provides a sensitive means of detecting and characterizing the regional changes in brain metabolism and receptor binding associated with movement disorders. It can be of diagnostic value and may throw some light on the pathophysiology underlying parkinsonian syndromes and involuntary movements. Functional imaging also provides a means of detecting subclinical disease in subjects at risk for degenerative and genetic disorders and of objectively following disease progression.

The main approaches to functional imaging are either radiotracer or magnetic resonance based: positron emission tomography (PET) has the highest sensitivity, being able to detect femtomoles of radiotracer at a resolution of 3–5 mm after image reconstruction. It allows quantitative in vivo examination of alterations in regional cerebral blood flow (rCBF), glucose (rCMRGlc), oxygen (rCMRO$_2$), and dopa metabolism, neurotransmitter fluxes, and brain receptor availability. Single-photon emission computed tomography (SPECT) is less sensitive than PET but more widely available. It is limited in practice to [123]I- or ^{99m}Tc-based radiotracers, but commercial systems for human work provide measures of rCBF and receptor binding with a resolution up to 5 mm. Proton magnetic resonance spectroscopy (MRS) has lower sensitivity, providing measures of N-acetylaspartate (NAA), lactate, phospholipids, creatine, and ATP at a millimolar level and 1 cm resolution. Magnetic resonance imaging (MRI) can detect activation-induced changes in blood oxygenation to brain regions when subjects perform tasks: the so-called blood oxygenation level dependent (BOLD) technique. Although structural MRI has submillimeter resolution, functional MRI (fMRI) activation studies are usually smoothed to a spatial resolution of around 3 mm to improve signal-to-noise ratios.

The changes in regional cerebral function that characterize the different movement disorders can be examined in two main ways: First, focal changes in resting levels of regional cerebral metabolism, blood flow, and neuroreceptor availability can be measured. Second, abnormal patterns of activation-induced changes in brain blood flow and neurotransmitter release (reflected by altered receptor availability) can be demonstrated when patients with movement disorders perform motor and cognitive tasks.

PARKINSON'S DISEASE

The pathology of Parkinson's disease (PD) targets the dopamine cells in the substantia nigra in association with the formation of neuronal Lewy body inclusions. Serotonergic cells in the median raphe, cholinergic cells in the nucleus basalis and pedunculopontine nucleus, and noradrenergic cells in the locus ceruleus are also involved, as are other pigmented and brainstem nuclei. Loss of cells from the substantia nigra in PD results in profound dopamine depletion in the striatum, with the lateral nigral projections to the dorsal posterior putamen being most affected. While the pathology of PD targets subcortical nuclei and the brainstem, the anterior cingulate and association cortical areas also are involved, more so in demented patients. Currently it remains uncertain whether dementia with Lewy bodies (DLB) and PD represent ends of a spectrum. DLB has features that overlap with Alzheimer's disease (AD), though the former is associated with a higher prevalence of fluctuating confusion, hallucinations, early-onset rigidity, and gait difficulties.

The Presynaptic Dopaminergic System

The function of dopamine terminals in PD can be examined in vivo in several ways (1): First, terminal dopa decarboxylase (DDC) activity can be measured with ^{18}F-dopa or ^{11}C-dopa PET. Second, the availability of presynaptic dopamine transporters (DATs) can be assessed with tropane-based PET and SPECT tracers. Third, vesicle monoamine transporter (VMAT2) density in dopamine terminals can be examined with ^{11}C-dihydrotetrabenazine PET. Fourth, the ability of dopamine terminals to release dopamine after an amphetamine or L-dopa challenge can be studied by measuring changes in dopamine D2 receptor availability with ^{11}C-raclopride PET or ^{123}I-IBZM SPECT.

In early hemiparkinsonian cases ^{18}F-dopa PET shows normal caudate but bilaterally reduced putamen tracer uptake, with the signal being depressed approximately 50% in the posterior putamen contralateral to the clinically affected limbs and by 20% to 30% in the ipsilateral posterior putamen (2). Patients with more established disease show a 50% to 80% loss of specific putamen ^{18}F-dopa uptake, which is similar to the 60% to 80% loss of ventrolateral nigra compacta cells but less than the 95% loss of putamen dopamine reported at postmortem examinations (see Fig. 43.1). These findings suggest that striatal dopamine terminal DDC activity is up-regulated relative to dopamine levels in PD, presumably to boost dopamine turnover by remaining neurons. A 40% to 50% loss of posterior putamen DDC activity seems to coincide with the onset of symptoms in PD.

The pathology of PD is not uniform, with ventrolateral nigral dopaminergic projections to the dorsal putamen being more affected than dorsomedial projections to the head of caudate and tegmental projections to the ventral striatum (3). ^{18}F-dopa PET reveals that in the striatum contralateral to "asymptomatic" limbs in patients with unilateral PD (H&Y stage 1), dorsal posterior putamen dopamine storage is first reduced. As all limbs become clinically affected, dorsal posterior putamen ^{18}F-dopa uptake falls further while ventral and anterior putamen and dorsal caudate function now become involved. Only when the disease is well established does ventral head of caudate ^{18}F-dopa uptake start to fall.

More recently, it has become apparent that not all dopamine fibers degenerate in early PD. Along with the dense nigrostriatal dopamine pathway, there are lesser nigropallidal and more diffuse mesofrontal projections. The neostriatum is the main input and the globus pallidus pars interna (GPi), the main output nucleus of the basal ganglia, and dopaminergic fibers modulate the function of both these structures. Recent PET studies have established that GPi ^{18}F-dopa uptake initially increases by 50% in early PD but subsequently falls below normal levels as the disease advances (4). As pallidal dopamine storage falls below normal levels in PD, patients appear to enter an accelerated disease phase and develop treatment complications, such as fluctuating responses to levodopa. This suggests that both tonic striatal and pallidal dopamine release are required for fluent motor function. The mesofrontal dopamine fibers arise from the midbrain tegmentum and project to the orbitofrontal cortex, anterior cingulate, and amygdala. In early PD, all these areas can show increases in ^{18}F-dopa uptake, although these subsequently normalize in advanced disease. The functional consequences of raised frontal and anterior cingulate dopamine storage in early PD are unclear. Interestingly, levodopa treatment can worsen performance on some frontal executive tasks, such as reversal learning, which

^{18}F-Dopa PET

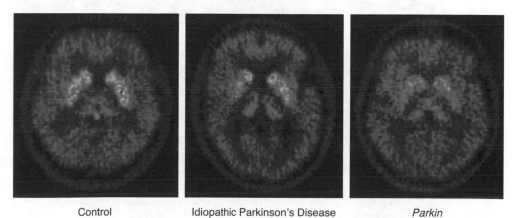

Figure 43.1 PET images of striatal ^{18}F-dopa uptake for a normal control, and patients with idiopathic PD and Parkinson's disease. (Images courtesy of P. Piccini and N. Khan.) (See color section.)

Control   Idiopathic Parkinson's Disease   *Parkin*

suggests that patients may be being overdosed (5). It is known that lesioning the mesofrontal dopaminergic fibers with 6-hydroxydopamine in nonhuman primates leads to a reciprocal increase in K+ evoked dopamine release from the caudate. It is, therefore, conceivable that, as the nigrostriatal dopaminergic system begins to degenerate in PD, there is an adaptive up-regulation of dopamine turnover in nigropallidal and mesofrontal dopaminergic pathways.

A wealth of tropane-based tracers are now available for measuring DAT binding on nigrostriatal terminals that can be used to provide a measure of integrity of dopaminergic function in PD (1). PET tracers include ^{11}C-CFT, ^{18}F-CFT, and ^{11}C-RTI-32 which bind to both dopamine and noradrenaline reuptake sites.

Available SPECT tracers include the tropane analogs ^{123}I-beta-CIT, ^{123}I-ioflupane (FP-CIT), ^{123}I-altropane, and ^{99m}Tc-TRODAT-1 (see Fig. 43.2). ^{123}I-beta-CIT gives the highest striatal:cerebellar uptake ratio of these SPECT tracers, although this reflects lower cerebellar rather than higher striatal uptake. ^{123}I-beta-CIT binds nonselectively to dopamine, noradrenaline, and serotonin transporters and has the disadvantage of requiring 24 hours to equilibrate throughout the brain following intravenous injection, so that scanning has to be delayed until the following day. In addition, the low cerebellar reference signal can be difficult to quantitate accurately. For these reasons, the SPECT tracers ^{123}I-ioflupane and ^{123}I-altropane, despite their lower and time-dependent striatal/cerebellar uptake ratios, have been developed as a diagnostic scan that can be performed within 2 to 3 hours of tracer injection. More recently, a technetium-based tropane tracer, ^{99m}Tc-TRODAT-1, has

been developed. This gives a lower striatal/cerebellar uptake ratio than the ^{123}I-based tracers and is less well extracted by the brain; however, it has the advantage of being readily available in kit form.

These PET and SPECT ligands, as well as the PET vesicle transporter marker ^{11}C-dihydrotetrabenazine, all have been shown to discriminate clinically probable PD patients from normal subjects and essential tremor cases with approximately 90% sensitivity and specificity. Given this, a positive PET or SPECT scan can be valuable for supporting a diagnosis of PD where there is diagnostic doubt. Three studies now have examined the role of DAT imaging in aiding the diagnosis of grey parkinsonian cases (6–8). All three concluded that management of these cases could be rationalized and improved by including SPECT in the workup, although clinical follow-up remains the gold standard as the pathology of these cases is still unknown. What is yet unclear is whether the finding of normal dopaminergic function with PET or SPECT fully excludes a diagnosis of PD. Long-term follow-up studies on patients clinically thought to have PD but with normal baseline ^{18}F-dopa PET or beta-CIT SPECT imaging have continued to show normal imaging findings, and none of these cases to date have clinically progressed (David J. Brooks, unpublished observations). This suggests that a finding of normal presynaptic dopaminergic function on imaging is associated with a good prognosis, whatever the ultimate diagnosis.

PET and SPECT measures of putamen dopamine terminal function show an inverse correlation with limb bradykinesia and rigidity in PD but correlate poorly with tremor severity (9,10). This suggests that parkinsonian

Imaging Dopamine Terminal Function

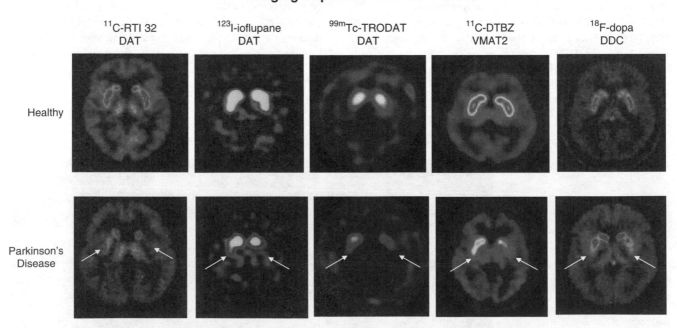

Figure 43.2   Striatal dopamine transporter and vesicular monoamine transporter binding and dopa decarboxylase activity in health and Parkinson's disease, measured with PET and SPECT. (See color section.)

tremors may derive from pathology outside the nigrostriatal pathway (see the following). Compared to putamen uptake of the monoamine vesicle transporter marker ^{11}C-dihydrotetrabenazine in PD, it has been shown that ^{18}F-dopa uptake is relatively up-regulated, whereas binding of the DAT marker ^{11}C-methylphenidate is relatively down-regulated (11). This finding makes physiologic sense, as increased turnover and decreased reuptake of dopamine in a deficiency syndrome would help to preserve synaptic transmitter levels.

Serotonergic, Noradrenergic, and Cholinergic Function in Parkinson's Disease

In PD there is loss not only of dopamine but also of serotonin, noradrenaline, and cholinergic projections. Median raphe serotonin HT_{1A} binding in the midbrain, measured with ^{11}C-WAY100635 PET, reflects the functional integity of serotonergic cell bodies. In PD a mean 25% loss of median raphe HT_{1A} binding has been reported, which, interestingly, correlated with severity of rest tremor but not rigidity or bradykinesia (12). This suggests that midbrain tegmentum pathology involving serotonin projections along with nigrostriatal projection loss may be relevant to the etiology of PD tremor.

There was no correlation with depressive symptoms and midbrain ^{11}C-WAY100635 uptake in PD, which argues against a direct role of serotonergic dysfunction. ^{123}I-beta-CIT binds to serotonergic transporters (SERT) in the midbrain and to DAT in the striatum. A recent beta-CIT SPECT study also reported no correlation between midbrain levels of tracer uptake and depressive symptoms in PD (13). ^{11}C-RTI 32 PET is a marker of both noradrenaline and dopamine terminal function. Patients with PD and depression compared to those equivalently disabled but without depression have been reported to show additional loss of thalamic and locus ceruleus ^{11}C-RTI 32 uptake, probably reflecting reduced noradrenergic input (14). The depressed cases also showed lower ^{11}C-RTI 32 signals in limbic areas (amygdala and ventral striatum). These findings would suggest that the presence of depression in PD is influenced more by the integrity of noradrenergic and limbic monoaminergic projections than by the serotonergic system.

Cholinergic function can be assessed presynaptically with the vesicular transporter marker ^{123}I-benzovesamicol SPECT, whereas ^{11}C-MP4A PET is a marker of postsynaptic muscarinic receptor availability. In nondemented PD cases, there is a significant reduction of parietal and occipital ^{123}I-vesamicol uptake (15), whereas ^{11}C-MP4A binding remains normal (16). PD patients with dementia, however, show more globally reduced ^{123}I-vesamicol binding and have raised frontal ^{11}C-MP4A binding. This would suggest that the presence of dementia is associated with a more severe loss of cholinergic projections, resulting in increased muscarinic receptor availability to the PET tracer.

Detection of Preclinical Disease

It has been estimated from postmortem studies that, for every patient who presents with clinical PD, in the community there may be 10 to 15 subclinical cases with incidental brainstem Lewy body disease. Surveys of the prevalence of PD will inevitably fail to recognize these cases with subclinical pathology. Subjects likely to be at risk of developing PD include carriers of genes known to be associated with parkinsonism, relatives of patients with the disorder, elderly subjects with idiopathic hyposmia, and patients suffering from REM sleep behavior disorders (RBD).

^{18}F-dopa PET has been used to study asymptomatic adult relatives in PD kindreds (17). Approximately one-quarter of asymptomatic adult relatives scanned show levels of putamen ^{18}F-dopa uptake reduced more than 2.5 standard deviations (SD) below the normal mean. One-third of these subsequently develop clinical parkinsonism over a 5-year follow-up period.

^{18}F-dopa PET findings for asymptomatic cotwins of idiopathic sporadic PD patients also have been reported (18). In one study, 10 (55%) of 18 monozygotic (MZ) and 3 (18%) of 16 dizygotic (DZ) cotwins showed reduced putamen ^{18}F-dopa uptake. The finding of a significantly higher concordance ($p = .03$) for dopaminergic dysfunction in MZ compared with DZ PD cotwins supports a genetic contribution toward this apparently sporadic disorder. Over 7 years of follow-up, 2 MZ and 1 DZ cotwins died without developing symptoms, while 4 MZ cotwins became clinically concordant for PD (14, 2, 9, and 20 years after the onset of PD in the cotwin), resulting in a clinical concordance of 22.2% at follow-up. None of the DZ twin pairs became clinically concordant.

It has been recognized for some time that elderly subjects with an impaired sense of smell (hyposmia) are more at risk for PD. It has been shown more recently that 4 of 40 (10%) elderly relatives of PD patients who had no overt parkinsonism but who manifested hyposmia on olfactory screening converted to clinical PD over a 2-year follow-up period (19). Of these, 7 of 40 showed reduced ^{123}I-beta-CIT uptake in 1 or more striatal subregions, and the 4 with the lowest DAT binding subsequently coverted to clinical PD. These findings suggest that, like ^{18}F-dopa PET, ^{123}I-beta-CIT SPECT is capable of detecting preclinical dopaminergic dysfunction when present in at-risk subjects for PD.

Neuroinflammation in Parkinson's Disease

Microglia constitute 10% to 20% of white cells in the brain and form its natural defense mechanism. They are normally in a resting state, but local injury causes them to activate and swell, expressing HLA antigens on the cell surface and releasing cytokines such as αTNF and interleukins. The mitochondria of activated but not resting microglia express peripheral benzodiazepine (BDZ) sites that may play a role in preventing cell apoptosis via membrane stabilization. ^{11}C-PK11195 is an isoquinoline that binds selectively to peripheral BDZ sites and so provides an in vivo PET marker of microglial activation.

Loss of substantia nigra neurons in PD has been shown to be associated with microglial activation and, more recently, histochemical studies have shown that microglial activation also can be seen in other basal ganglia, the cingulate, the hippocampus, and cortical areas (20). ^{11}C-PK11195 PET has been used to study microglial activation in PD vivo. In one series, increased midbrain signal in PD was reported, which correlated inversely with levels of posterior putamen DAT binding (21). A second series also has reported increased signal in the substantia nigra, though this was a less consistent finding, along with microglial activation in the striatum, pallidum, and frontal cortex (see Fig. 43.3) (22). Interestingly, these last workers found little change in the extent of microglial activation over a 2-year follow-up period, although the patients deteriorated clinically. This could imply that microglial activation is merely an epiphenomenon in PD; however, postmortem studies have suggested that these cells continue

to express cytokine mRNA, which implies that they are likely to be driving disease progression.

Monitoring Progression of Parkinson's Disease

Assessing the progression of PD with clinical rating scales can be problematic for several reasons: First, these scales are subjective, nonlinear, consider multiple aspects of the disorder, and are biased toward certain symptoms—bradykinesia in the case of the Unified Parkinson's Disease Rating Scale (UPDRS). Second, symptomatically effective therapy can mask disease progression. Functional imaging potentially provides a biological marker for objectively monitoring disease progression in vivo in PD alongside clinical evaluations (1,23). However, it is limited to providing information concerning one aspect of the condition—usually dopamine terminal function—and also may be subject to direct influence by treatment effects. In human subjects with an intact dopamine system, striatal ^{18}F-dopa uptake does not appear to be influenced by 2 years of exposure to clinical doses of levodopa (24); however, this

Microglial Activation in Parkinson's Disease

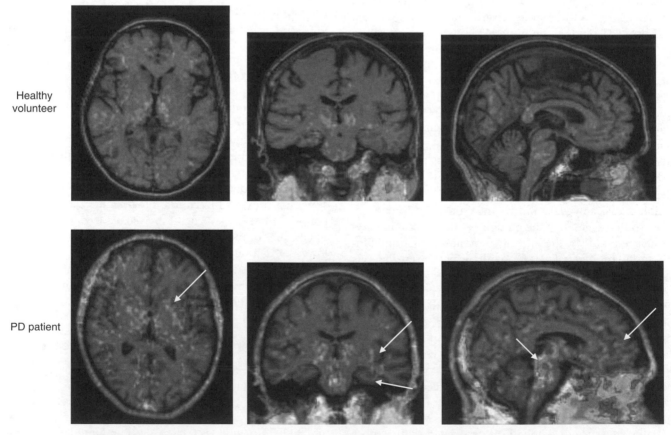

Figure 43.3   11C-PK11195 PET in a healthy elderly control and a Parkinson's disease patient. Increased microglial activation can be seen in the midbrain, basal ganglia, and frontal cortex in Parkinson's disease. (Images courtesy of A. Gerhard.) (See color section.)

may not be true in PD, where compensatory changes in dopamine terminal function occur following nigral cell loss. Striatal ^{123}I-beta-CIT uptake has been found in a small series not to be significantly altered in PD by several weeks of exposure to L-dopa and dopamine agonists (25).

Striatal ^{18}F-dopa uptake has been shown to correlate with subsequent postmortem dopaminergic cell densities in the substantia nigra and striatal dopamine levels of a small series of patients and of 1-methyl-4-phenyl-1,2, 3,6-tetrahydropyridine (MPTP)-lesioned monkeys (26,27). In principle, ^{18}F-dopa PET can be used as a marker of dopamine terminal function in PD, although it probably overestimates terminal density due to a relative up-regulation of DDC in remaining terminals as a response to nigral cell loss.

Several series now have reported that loss of striatal ^{18}F-dopa uptake occurs more rapidly in PD than in age-matched controls (1). In early L-dopa–treated PD putamen, ^{18}F-dopa uptake declines by 6% to 12% of its baseline value per annum. Parallel rates of loss of putamen dopamine transporter binding have been reported with ^{18}F-CFT PET and ^{123}I-beta-CIT, ^{123}I-FP-CIT, and ^{123}I-IPT SPECT. Annual loss of striatal ^{123}I-beta-CIT uptake in early PD correlates with initial levels of striatal transporter binding, suggesting an exponential disease process. Extrapolations assuming a linear disease progression have computed a preclinical disease window of only a few years in late-onset sporadic PD.

Despite the gradient of striatal involvement in early PD (dopamine terminal function is worse affected in posterior than in anterior putamen and head of caudate), longitudinal PET observations suggest a subsequent similar absolute rate of decline of function in all areas (28). This has led some workers to speculate that the mechanisms that trigger PD may not necessarily be the same as those mechanisms that subsequently lead to subsequent disease progression. For example, exposure to a toxic agent could initially lead to cell damage and then to progressive neuronal loss due to consequent oxidative stress and release of cytokines by activated glia.

Testing Possible Neuroprotective Agents

As functional imaging can objectively follow PD progression, it provides a potential means of monitoring the efficacy of putative neuroprotective agents such as dopamine agonists, monoamine oxidase B (MAO-B) inhibitors, free-radical scavengers, apoptosis inhibitors, and nerve growth factors/stimulators. It has been suggested that dopamine agonists have neuroprotective properties as they protect dopamine cells in culture and animals against the effects of nigral toxins (29). Dopamine agonists also suppress production of endogenous dopamine in vivo, thus attenuating its oxidative metabolism and reducing hydroxyl free radical formation. They are weak antioxidants and free radical scavengers in their own right, and some act as

mitochondrial membrane stabilizers, thereby blocking release of cytochrome c, a trigger of apoptosis via caspase activation.

Two different trials (see the following) have examined the relative rates of loss of dopamine terminal function in early PD in patients randomized to a dopamine agonist or levodopa.

The REAL PET trial was a 2-year double-blind multinational study where 186 de novo PD patients were randomized (1:1) to ropinirole or L-dopa (24). The primary endpoint was a change in putamen ^{18}F-dopa uptake (Ki) measured with PET. Interestingly, 11% of the untreated patients thought to have PD by referring clinicians were found to have normal caudate and putamen ^{18}F-dopa uptake at entry (identified by blinded review). This subgroup was analyzed separately. Reduction in mean putamen Ki was significantly slower over 2 years in the PD patient group taking ropinirole (-13.4%) than that taking L-dopa (-20.3%; $p = 0.022$). Clinically, the incidence of dyskinesia was 26.7% with L-dopa but only 3.4% with ropinirole ($p < 0.001$). Mean improvement in disability rated while taking medication was, however, superior (by 6.34 points) for the L-dopa cohort despite apparently faster disease progression.

The second trial comprised a subgroup of the CALM-PD study (30). A cohort of 82 early PD patients were randomized 1:1 to the dopamine agonist pramipexole (0.5 mg tds) or levodopa (100 mg tds) and had serial ^{123}I-beta-CIT SPECT over a 4-year period. Patients treated initially with pramipexole ($n = 42$) showed a significantly slower mean relative decline of striatal beta-CIT uptake compared to subjects treated initially with levodopa ($n = 40$) at 2 (47%), 3 (44%), and 4 (37%) years. Again, the incidence of complications was significantly reduced in the pramipexole cohort, but improvement in UPDRS score was greater in the L-dopa cohort.

These two imaging studies, therefore, produced parallel findings, both suggesting that treatment with an agonist in early PD relatively slows loss of dopamine terminal function by approximately one-third and delays treatment-associated complications. However, the functional imaging findings favoring use of agonists as early treatment for PD were not paralleled by a better clinical outcome in the PD agonist cohorts as judged by UPDRS motor scores, albeit rated while subjects were medicated. One possible confounder contributing toward the discordant imaging and clinical findings could be that the PET and SPECT signals were differentially influenced by the effects of L-dopa and agonist medications (31). Conceivably, administration of L-dopa could directly down-regulate dopa decarboxylase activity and DAT binding relative to agonist use, thus resulting in a more rapid loss of striatal ^{18}F-dopa and ^{123}I-beta-CIT uptake. Currently, there is no in vivo human evidence to support this viewpoint, but the findings of these two trials remain controversial. The real test will be whether early use of agonists delays the need for institutional care or deep-brain stimulation (DBS) in the longer term.

The ELLDOPA trial was designed to assess whether L-dopa is in fact toxic to PD patients (32). It compared rates of progression of 361 de novo PD patients randomized to 150 mg, 300 mg, 600 mg of levodopa or placebo. Subjects were followed for 9 months and then had a 2-week washout of their medication. Clinical disability was rated with the UPDRS. In a subgroup of 142, striatal DAT binding was measured with ^{123}I-beta-CIT SPECT at baseline before starting medication and then again at 9 months while receiving medication. Locomotor function improved most in those patients treated with 600 mg of levodopa daily and remained superior to placebo after 2 weeks of washout. SPECT imaging suggested, however, that loss of striatal DAT binding occurred most rapidly (−7%) in the high-dose levodopa arm of the trial compared with placebo (−1%). This, however, only reached statistical significance after exclusion of those 10% of subjects recruited who were found to have normal baseline ^{123}I-beta-CIT SPECT. Additionally, 30% of the high levodopa dosage cases developed fluctuating treatment responses and 17% developed dyskinesias, compared to 13% and 3%, respectively, in the placebo arm. These discordant clinical and imaging findings make it difficult to draw any firm conclusions about the toxicity of levodopa. A direct depressant effect of levodopa on striatal ^{123}I-beta-CIT uptake could have resulted in apparent disease acceleration, though this remains speculative. Conversely, a 2-week washout is unlikely to have been adequate to fully eliminate all symptomatic effects of levodopa, so the true clinical status of the PD patients after 9 months exposure to their treatment also remains uncertain.

[18]F-dopa PET has been used to study the possible neuroprotective action of the glutamate release inhibitor riluzole in PD. This agent was shown to slow disease progression and delay mortality of amyotrophic lateral sclerosis patients. De novo PD patients were blindly randomized to 50 mg of placebo and 100 mg of riluzole daily, and the clinical primary endpoint was time to requiring dopaminergic medication. No differences were found between the 3 PD cohorts, either in time to reaching the clinical endpoint or in reduction in putamen ^{18}F-dopa uptake over 2 years (David J. Brooks and Nicola Pavese, 2004).

Restorative Approaches to Parkinson's Disease

As well as providing a way of following natural disease progression, functional imaging provides a means for examining the function of striatal implants of dopaminergic cells in PD. Possible approaches include fetal mesencephalic cells; transformed cells engineered to secrete dopamine, nerve growth factors, or express anti-apoptotic genes; stem cells; xenografts; and direct striatal infusions of nerve growth factors.

Human Fetal Cell Implantation Trials

Early open series suggested that advanced PD patients showed a good clinical response to implantation of fetal mesencephalic cells or tissue into striatum (33). This was accompanied by increases in striatal ^{18}F-dopa uptake. An ^{11}C-raclopride PET study demonstrated that striatal grafts could release dopamine normally after a metamphetamine challenge (34). H_2[15]O PET revealed restored levels of frontal activation in 4 PD patients, although this only occurred 2 years after bilateral striatal grafts were implanted (Fig. 43.4) (35).

Given the encouraging findings of pilot open series, 2 major double-blind controlled trials on the efficacy of

[18]F-Dopa PET in Parkinson's Disease

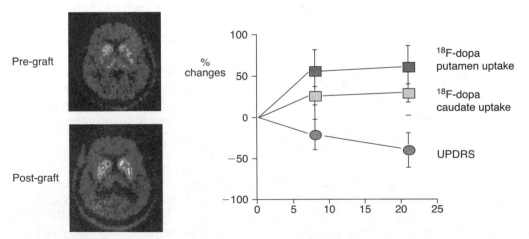

Figure 43.4   Serial PET images over 20 months of striatal ^{18}F-dopa uptake by a grafted PD patient alongside a graph showing putamen F-dopa uptake, motor United Parkinson's Disease Rating Scale (UPDRS) scores, and levels of activation-induced supplementary motor area and dorsal prefrontal cortex blood flow change. It can be seen that clinical recovery parallels improved cortical activation rather than graft dopamine storage capacity. (Images courtesy of P. Piccini.) (See color section.)

implantation of human fetal cells in PD were sponsored by the National Institutes of Health (NIH) in the United States. The first of these involved 40 patients who were 34 to 75 years of age and had severe PD (mean duration, 14 years) (36). They were randomized to receive either an implant of human fetal mesencephalic tissue or to undergo sham surgery and were followed for 1 year with a subsequent extension to 3 years. In the transplant recipients, mesencephalic tissue from 4 embryos cultured for up to 1 month was implanted into the putamen bilaterally (2 embryos per side) via a frontal approach. In the patients who underwent sham surgery, holes were drilled in the skull, but the dura was not penetrated. No immunotherapy was used.

The transplanted patients showed no significant improvement in the primary endpoint, clinical global impression, at 1 year, but there was a significant mean 18% improvement in mean UPDRS motor score, compared with the sham-surgery group when tested before receiving medication ($p = 0.04$). This improvement was more evident for patients under 60 years of age (34% improvement, $p = .005$). At 3 years, mean total UPDRS score was improved 38% in the younger and 14% in the older transplanted groups (both $p < .01$). Of 19 transplanted patients, 16 showed an increase in putamen ^{18}F-dopa uptake (group mean increase 40%), and increases were similar in the younger and older cohorts. A drawback was that off dystonia and dyskinesias developed in 15% of the patients who received transplants in this series, even after reduction or discontinuation of levodopa.

In the second NIH trial, 34 patients were randomized to receive (a) bilateral implants of fetal mesencephalic tissue from 4 fetuses per side or from 1 fetus per side into posterior putamen or (b) sham surgery (a partial burr hole without penetration of the dura) (37). Fetal tissue was cultured for less than 48 hours before transplantation, and all patients received immunosuppression for 6 months after surgery. The trial duration was 2 years, and the primary outcome variable was the UPDRS motor score and quality of life. Putamen ^{18}F-dopa uptake was assessed with PET in a subset of patients. Although 3 patients died subsequently from unrelated causes, 31 patients completed and 2 patients died during the trial. At postmortem, these 2 transplanted patients showed significantly higher tyrosine hydroxylase staining in the putamen relative to the sham-surgery patients, with graft innervation of the host evident. However, microglial activation surrounding the graft was also a feature. Putamen ^{18}F-dopa uptake was unchanged in the control patients, but in patients receiving tissue from 4 fetuses, uptake showed a one-third increase. Unfortunately, no significant differences in clinical rating scores were seen between the groups at 2 years, although there was a trend favoring the 4-fetus group, which had been significant at 6 months prior to withdrawal of immunosuppression. The mean UPDRS motor score off medication deteriorated by 9.4, 3.5, and −0.7 points over

2 years for the controls, 1 fetus, and 4 fetus groups (4 fetuses versus controls, $p = 0.096$). Off-period dyskinesias were evident in 13 (57%) of 23 implanted patients but were not seen in the control arm.

In conclusion, despite both histological and ^{18}F-dopa PET evidence of graft function, neither of these blinded controlled trials demonstrated significant clinical efficacy of grafts with their primary endpoints, and in both studies off period dyskinesias were problematic. There were indications, however, that grafts of human fetal dopamine cells could be efficacious in some younger, more severely affected patients.

Intraputaminal Glial-Derived Neurotrophic Factor Infusions

Glial-derived neurotrophic factor (GDNF) is a potent nerve growth factor known to protect dopamine neurons against nigral toxins in rodent and primate models of PD. The safety and efficacy of infusing GDNF directly into the posterior putamen was first tested in a small open pilot trial (38). In-dwelling catheters were inserted in 5 PD patients, and all tolerated continuous GDNF delivery at levels ranging from 14–40 μg/day (6 ml/hour) for more than 2 years, unilaterally in 1 and bilaterally in 4 patients, without serious side effects. Significant improvements were reported in UPDRS subscores: 39% and 61% improvements in the off-medication motor III and activities of daily living II subscales, respectively, at 12 months. There were 18% to 24% increases in putaminal ^{18}F-dopa Ki at the catheter tip. These clinical improvements were maintained at 2 years.

A more recent double-blind trial of GDNF efficacy in PD has studied 34 advanced patients who were randomized 1:1 to receive bilateral continuous intraputamen infusions of liatermin 15 μg/putamen/day or placebo. The primary endpoint was the change in UPDRS motor score in the practically defined off condition at 6 months. Secondary endpoints included posterior putamen ^{18}F-dopa uptake. At 6 months, there was no significant difference in mean percentage reductions in off UPDRS motor scores between the GDNF and placebo groups (10.0% and 4.5%, respectively). A 32% treatment difference favoring GDNF in mean posterior putamen ^{18}F-dopa influx constant ($p = .0061$) was present, equivalent to that seen in the open-label pilot study. It was concluded that GDNF infusions did not confer significant clinical benefit to patients with PD despite inducing local increases in ^{18}F-dopa uptake. Following completion of this clinical trial, 4 patients have developed persistent, high affinity, anti-GDNF antibodies, and 3 of these subsequently developed blocking antibodies.

The dissociated clinical and imaging outcomes in the double-blind controlled transplant and GDNF trials raise important issues about the information generated by imaging biomarkers. In these restorative trials, ^{18}F-dopa PET showed increased dopaminergic function after both grafting and GDNF infusion, although significant clinical efficacy was not evident. It must be remembered that ^{18}F-dopa PET is primarily a marker of dopa decarboxylase activity in striatal dopamine terminals and does not provide information about vesicular dopamine levels or effective release of dopamine during movement. It is also unable to reveal whether new dopamine terminals formed by grafts or under trophic influence are appropriately located next to postsynaptic receptors. The increased levels of dopamine storage seen after grafting and GDNF infusions may, therefore, fail to translate into physiologically effective dopamine release during motor function.

Fluctuations and Dyskinesias

PD patients with fluctuating responses to levodopa show 20% lower mean levels of putamen ^{18}F-dopa uptake than those with early disease and sustained therapeutic responses (39). There is, however, considerable overlap of fluctuator and nonfluctuator individual ranges. While loss of putamen dopamine terminal function predisposes PD patients toward development of levodopa-associated complications, it cannot be the only factor responsible for determining the timing of onset of fluctuations and involuntary movements.

The striatum contains mainly dopamine D1 and D2 receptors, both of which play a role in modulating movement. PET studies with spiperone-based tracers and ^{123}I-IBZM SPECT have reported normal levels of striatal D2 binding in untreated PD while ^{11}C-raclopride PET has revealed 10% to 20% increases in putamen D2 site availability (40). In treated PD, putamen D2 binding is normal, which explains the good locomotor response to levodopa. ^{11}C-SCH23390 PET, a marker of D1 site binding, reveals normal striatal uptake in de novo PD, while patients who have been exposed to levodopa for several years show a 20% reduction in striatal binding.

Cohorts of levodopa-exposed dyskinetic and nondyskinetic PD patients with equivalent clinical disease duration, disease severity, and daily levodopa dosage show similar levels of striatal dopamine D1 and D2 receptor availability (41,42). Putamen D1 and D2 binding are normal, while caudate D2 binding is mildly reduced. These findings, therefore, suggest that onset of motor complications in PD is not primarily associated with alterations in striatal dopamine receptor availability. PET and SPECT antagonist ligands bind with equal affinity to G-coupled receptors in high and low agonist affinity conformations. These findings, therefore, do not exclude a change in the proportions of D1 and D2 sites with a high agonist affinity conformation in dyskinetic PD patients or an exaggerated downstream response to receptor stimulation.

[11]C-raclopride PET is sensitive to changes in levels of dopamine in the synaptic cleft and so enables these to be monitored. The higher the extracellular dopamine level, the lower the dopamine D2 site availability to the tracer. When individuals in a group of early nonfluctuating PD patients were given 3 mg/kg of levodopa as an intravenous bolus, they showed a mean 10% fall in posterior putamen ^{11}C-raclopride

binding, while advanced cases with motor fluctuations showed a 23% fall (see Fig. 43.5) (43). These falls in receptor availability have been estimated to correspond to 4- and 10-fold rises in extracellular dopamine and indicate that, as loss of dopamine terminals in PD progresses, the ability of the striatum to buffer dopamine levels fails when clinical doses of exogenous levodopa are administered.

This regulation failure reflects a combination of increased striatal dopamine synthesis and release by the remaining terminals following administration of levodopa, along with a severe loss of dopamine transporters preventing its reuptake. It is this phenomenon, rather than changes in postsynaptic dopamine D1 and D2 receptor binding, that is likely to be the explanation for the more rapid response of advanced PD patients to oral levodopa. The failure to buffer dopamine levels by the striatum in advanced PD also will result in high nonphysiological swings in synaptic dopamine levels. This, in turn, may promote excessive dopamine receptor internalization leading to fluctuating and unpredictable treatment responses. In support of this viewpoint, de la Fuente-Fernández et al. have measured striatal ^{11}C-raclopride binding in PD at 1 and 4 hours after oral levodopa challenges (44). These workers found that (a) fluctuators show transiently raised synaptic dopamine levels after a levodopa challenge, while sustained responders generated a progressive rise in striatal dopamine and (b) off episodes could coincide with apparently adequate synaptic dopamine levels.

Medium spiny neurons in the caudate and putamen project to the external and internal pallidum where they release enkephalin (GPe) or dynorphin and substance P (GPi) in addition to gamma-aminobutyric acid (GABA). Enkephalin binds with high affinity to opioid sites and inhibits GABA release in the GPe. Dynorphin, binds to opioid sites and inhibits glutamate release from subthalamic projections to the GPi. It is thought that phasic firing of striatal projection neurons results primarily in GABA release in the pallidum, whereas sustained tonic firing causes additional modulatory opioid and substance P (SP) release. The caudate and putamen contain high densities of μ, κ, and δ opioid sites and also NK1 sites, which bind SP. Opioid receptors are located both presynaptically on dopamine terminals, where they regulate dopamine release, and postsynaptically on interneurons and medium spiny projection neurons.

There is now strong evidence supporting the presence of increased opioid and SP transmission in the basal ganglia of end-stage PD patients both from postmortem and animal lesion model studies. ^{11}C-diprenorphine PET is a nonselective marker of μ, κ, and δ opioid sites, and its binding is sensitive to levels of endogenous opioids. If raised basal ganglia levels of enkephalin and dynorphin are associated with levodopa induced dyskinesias (LIDs), then PD patients with motor complications would be expected to show reduced binding of ^{11}C-diprenorphine. Significant reductions in ^{11}C-diprenorphine binding in the caudate, putamen, thalamus, and anterior cingulate have been reported in dyskinetic patients compared with sustained responders (45).

[11]C-raclopride Binding at Baseline and Following 250 Mg Oral L-Dopa

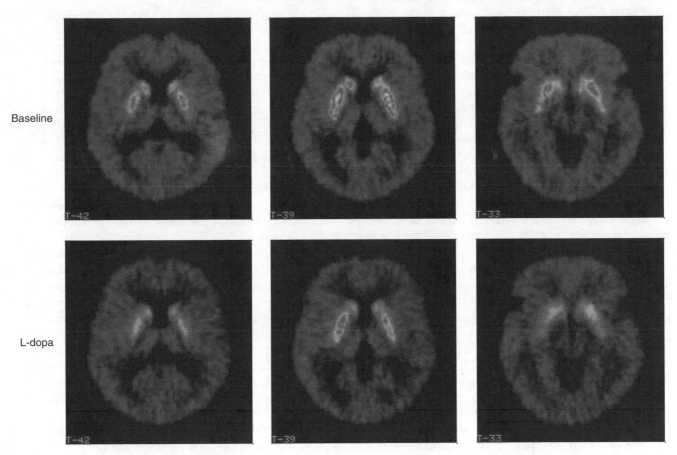

Figure 43.5 PET images of 11C-raclopride uptake in a Parkinson's disease patient before and after 250 mg of levodopa. It can be seen that after levodopa the striatum shows a fall in raclopride binding, indicating that increased levels of synaptic dopamine are present. (Images courtesy of P. Piccini.) (See color section.)

Individual levels of putamen ^{11}C-diprenorphine uptake correlated inversely with severity of dyskinesia. ^{18}F-L829165 PET is a selective marker of NK1 site availability. In a preliminary study, NK1 availability has been shown to be reduced in dyskinetic PD patients but normal in nondyskinetic cases (46). These in vivo findings support the presence of elevated levels of endogenous peptides in the basal ganglia of dyskinetic PD patients and suggest that this, rather than a primary alteration in dopamine receptor availability, leads to abnormal pallidal burst firing and may be responsible for the appearance of levodopa-induced involuntary movements.

Dementia and Parkinson's Disease

Resting Brain Metabolism

[18]FDG PET scans of frankly demented PD patients show an Alzheimer's pattern of impaired resting brain glucose utilization, posterior parietal and temporal association areas being most affected, frontal association areas less affected, and primary cortical regions, basal ganglia, and cerebellum being spared (47). Interestingly, up to one-third of nondemented

PD patients with established disease also show this pattern of reduced cortical metabolism, but to a lesser extent, suggesting that they may be at risk for later dementia (48).

Currently, it remains unclear whether this pattern of resting glucose hypometabolism in demented PD patients reflects coincidental AD, cortical Lewy body disease, loss of cholinergic projections, or some other degenerative process. Clinicopathological series suggest that there is considerable overlap in the cortical FDG PET findings of coincidental AD and cortical Lewy body disease but that cortical Lewy body disease cases show a greater reduction in resting glucose metabolism of the primary visual cortex (49,50). Some PET imaging agents are now capable of imaging beta amyloid plaque load in dementia patients. Using these markers it should be possible in the future to assess the contribution of amyloid pathology to PD dementia.

Dopaminergic Function

It has been estimated that one-fifth of cases with a clinical picture of AD show DLB at postmortem whereas other dementia cases have mixed pathology. Whether DLB and

PD represent opposite ends of a spectrum is unclear, but DLB patients show not only cerebral cortical neuronal loss, with Lewy bodies in surviving neurons, but also loss of nigrostriatal dopaminergic neurons. In contrast, nigral pathology is mild in AD.

[123]I-ioflupane SPECT studies have been performed on patients with clinically presumed DLB, AD, drug naive patients with PD, and healthy controls (51). The presumed DLB and PD patients both had significantly lower uptake of caudate and putamen ^{123}I-FP-CIT than patients with AD and controls. DLB cases showed greater involvement of caudate than equivalently disabled PD patients (52). These SPECT findings have subsequently been validated following postmortem examinations. Most DLB cases had parkinsonism in these series but, interestingly, even those nonrigid DLB cases show reduced striatal DAT binding uptake, suggesting that ^{123}I-ioflupane SPECT may be helpful in discriminating DLB from AD.

[18]F-dopa PET findings in PD patients with and without dementia but matched for locomotor disability also have been compared (53). The 2 PD cohorts showed equivalent levels of reduced putamen dopamine storage capacity, but cingulate and mesial prefrontal ^{18}F-dopa uptake were only reduced in the PD dementia group.

Brain Activation Studies in Parkinson's Disease

PET studies on resting brain function have shown relatively increased levels of both oxygen and glucose metabolism in the contralateral lentiform nucleus of hemiparkinsonian patients with early disease (54). PD patients with bilateral involvement generally have normal absolute levels of striatal glucose metabolism, but covariance analysis reveals an abnormal profile of relatively raised resting lentiform nucleus and lowered frontal metabolism (55,56). The degree of expression of this PD profile correlates with clinical disease severity rated when withdrawn from medication and the profile normalizes after administration of dopaminergic drugs or deep-brain stimulation (57,58).

Although studies of resting cerebral blood flow and metabolism provide insight into the basal cerebral dysfunction underlying movement disorders, measuring changes in regional cerebral blood flow (rCBF) with $H_2^{15}O$ PET or fMRI while patients perform motor or cognitive tasks or after pharmacological challenges are also revealing. When normal subjects perform freely selected limb movements, there are associated rCBF increases in the contralateral sensorimotor cortex (SMC) and the lentiform nucleus and bilaterally in the anterior cingulate, anterior supplementary motor area (SMA), lateral premotor cortex (PMC), and dorsolateral prefrontal cortex (DLPFC) (59–61). When PD patients, scanned after stopping levodopa for 12 hours, perform similar movements, there is impaired activation of the contralateral lentiform nucleus and the anterior cingulate, anterior SMA, and DLPFC—that is, of those frontal areas that receive direct input from the basal ganglia—while normal or increased activation of SMC, caudal SMA, PMC, and lateral parietal association areas is seen.

Although patients with PD can perform isolated limb movements efficiently, it is well recognized that attempts to perform repetitive or sequences of movements results in a fall in amplitude and motor arrest. Underactivity of mesial–frontal and deactivation of dorsolateral–prefrontal areas when patients perform prelearned, sequential, oppositional finger-thumb movements with one or both hands has been demonstrated (62,63). Lateral premotor and parietal cortex and cerebellum were relatively overactivated, suggesting adaptive recruitment of a network normally used to facilitate externally cued rather than freely chosen movements.

It has been proposed that dorsal prefrontal cortex plays a crucial role in motor decision making, whereas the anterior supplementary motor area prepares and optimizes volitional motor programs once selected and facilitates nonmirror bimanual movements. In contrast, the lateral premotor cortex has a primary role in facilitating motor responses to external visual and auditory stimuli. An inability to activate DLPFC and anterior SMA during freely selected and sequential limb movements could explain the difficulty that PD patients experience in initiating such actions. Their ability to overactivate lateral premotor and primary motor cortex, however, allows them to respond well to visual and auditory cues, such as stepping over lines on the floor or marching to a drumbeat to aid their walking.

If loss of dopamine is responsible for the impaired activation of striato-frontal projections in PD, it should be possible to restore it by administering dopaminergic medication. Administration of apomorphine, levodopa, and implants of fetal midbain dopamine cells all have been shown to increase activation of the anterior SMA and prefrontal cortex during arm and finger movements in association with a reduction of bradykinesia (35,62,64).

Lesions or high-frequency deep-brain electrical stimulation (DBS) of the motor GPi have been observed to improve bradykinesia and reduce dyskinesias in PD. DBS of the subthalamic nucleus (STN) may be even more effective in relieving parkinsonism. Regional cerebral activation has been studied in PD before and after these surgical interventions (65–67). DBS and pallidotomy both result in significantly increased activation of the SMA, lateral premotor cortex, and dorsal prefrontal cortex in PD patients off medication while performing volitional and paced limb movements.

ATYPICAL PARKINSONIAN SYNDROMES

Multiple System Atrophy

Multiple system atrophy (MSA), also known as Shy-Drager syndrome, includes striatonigral degeneration (SND), olivopontocerebellar atrophy (OPCA), and progressive autonomic failure (PAF) within its spectrum. It is characterized pathologically by argyrophilic, α-synuclein–positive inclusions in glia and neurons in the substantia nigra, striatum, brainstem, cerebellar nuclei, and intermediolateral columns of the spinal cord. The striatum appears normal on T2-weighted MRI in PD, but in striatonigral degeneration and multiple system atrophy (MSA) the lateral putamen can show reduced signal due to iron deposition, which may be bordered by a rim of increased signal due to gliosis (68). If concomitant pontocerebellar degeneration is also present, the lateral as well as longitudinal pontine fibers become evident as high signal on T2 MRI, manifesting as the "hot cross bun" sign. Cerebellar and pontine atrophy may be visually obvious with increased signal evident in the cerebellar peduncles. These changes are usually only evident in patients with well-established disease in whom putamen and brainstem atrophy can also be demonstrated with formal magnetic resonance (MR) volumetry.

More recently, the use of diffusion-weighted (DWI) and diffusion-tensor MRI have been developed for discriminating atypical from typical parkinsonian syndromes. DWI reflects the movement of water molecules along fiber tracts in the brain, the so-called *anisotropy of diffusion*. This anisotropy can be quantified as an apparent diffusion coefficient (ADC) by applying field gradients. In intact brain, the CNS is organized into bundles of fiber tracts along which water molecules move. Degenerative disease removes restrictions to water molecule movement, thereby reducing anisotropy and increasing the ADC. It has been reported that all cases with clinically probable parkinsonian multiple system atrophy (MSA-P) could be discriminated from typical PD patients as they showed significantly higher regional ADC values in the putamen (see Fig. 43.6) (69). How sensitive this approach is for classifying grey parkinsonian cases is currently being determined.

[18]FDG PET studies in levodopa-nonresponsive akinetic-rigid patients with clinically probable SND have reported reduced levels of striatal glucose metabolism in 80% to 100% of cases, in contrast to PD where striatal metabolism is preserved (70). Eidelberg et al. also noted that akinetic-rigid patients with low levels of striatal glucose metabolism, irrespective of their levodopa response, show little improvement after pallidotomy (71,72). Patients with the full syndrome of MSA show reduced mean levels of cerebellar and brainstem along with putamen and caudate glucose metabolism. [18]FDG PET, therefore, provides a sensitive means of detecting the presence of both striatal and cerebellar dysfunction where atypical parkinsonism is suspected. Proton magnetic resonance spectroscopy also provides a potential means of discriminating SND from PD. NAA is found in high concentrations in neurons and is believed to be a metabolic marker of neuronal integrity. Reduced NAA/creatine ratios in the proton MRS signal from the lentiform nucleus in 6 of 7 clinically probable SND cases have been reported, whereas 8 of 9 probable PD cases showed normal levels of putamen NAA (73).

In patients with clinically probable SND, the functions of both the pre- and postsynaptic dopaminergic systems are impaired. As in PD, putamen ^{18}F-dopa uptake is reduced to approximately 50% of normal levels in established SND and individual levels of putamen ^{18}F-dopa uptake correlate with locomotor status (74,75). In patients with the full syndrome of MSA, mean caudate ^{18}F-dopa uptake is significantly more depressed than in PD, although the individual ranges overlap. This finding suggests that the substantia nigra is more extensively involved by the pathology of SND than PD, and pathologic studies corroborate this conclusion. However, the pattern of caudate and putamen ^{18}F-dopa uptake only discriminates SND from PD with 70% specificity (76), so [18]FDG PET and DWI MRI provide more sensitive tools than ^{18}F-dopa PET for this purpose. When Pirker et al. examined ^{123}I-beta-CIT binding in 18 MSA patients, these workers concluded that, while ^{123}I-beta-CIT SPECT reliably discriminated PD and MSA from normal, it could not discriminate between the two parkinsonian conditions (77).

Striatal dopamine D1 and D2 binding has been studied with PET in SND. Mild but significant reductions in mean putamen ^{11}C-SCH23390 and ^{11}C-raclopride uptake have been reported, although an overlap between SND, normal, and PD ranges is evident (70). Striatal D1 and D2 binding, therefore, does not appear to provide sensitive discrimination of SND from PD. In support of this viewpoint, in their series of probable MSA-P compared with

Diffusion-Weighted MRI

Figure 43.6 Diffusion-weighted MRI of a Parkinson's disease and a multiple system atrophy (MSA) patient. It can be seen altered striatal signal is present in MSA. (Images courtesy of K. Seppi.) (See color section.)

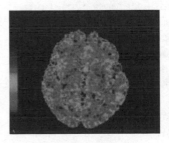

Normal   Parkinson's Disease

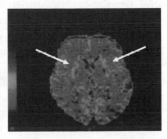

Multiple System Atrophy

PD cases, Seppi et al. (78) reported that the predictive value of ^{123}I-IBZM SPECT was 75% versus 97% for DWI MRI. Schwarz et al. (79) found reduced striatal D2 binding with ^{123}I-IBZM SPECT in only 8 of 12 de novo parkinsonian patients who showed a negative apomorphine response. As a significant number of parkinsonian patients who respond poorly to levodopa retain normal levels of striatal D2 binding, it seems likely that degeneration of downstream brainstem and pallidal rather than striatal projections is responsible for their poor response to levodopa.

Seppi et al. (80) have used ^{123}I-IBZM SPECT to objectively and longitudinally monitor striatal degeneration in a group of early MSA patients. They found an annual 10% loss of striatal D2 binding in their 18-month study and concluded that ^{123}I-IBZM SPECT provides a valid future approach for testing the efficacy of putative neuroprotective agents in MSA.

Druschky et al. have used ^{123}I-MIBG SPECT to study functional integrity of cardiac sympathetic innervation in PD and MSA (81). In PD there is a severe reduction in mediastinal ^{123}I-MIBG signal, even in cases where no clinical evidence of autonomic failure was present, while this is mild or absent in MSA. The authors interpreted this finding as demonstrating a greater involvement of postganglionic sympathetic innervation of the heart in PD, compared with MSA, and suggested normal cardiac ^{123}I-MIBG SPECT imaging excludes a diagnosis of PD.

[11]C-PK11195 PET, an in vivo marker of microglial activation, has been used to study neuroinflammatory changes in MSA (82). Widespread subcortical increases in ^{11}C-PK11195 uptake were seen, particularly in the substantia nigra, putamen, pallidum, thalamus, and brainstem. These changes were more extensive than those associated with PD, but again there was significant overlap in the findings for these two conditions.

PROGRESSIVE SUPRANUCLEAR PALSY

Progressive supranuclear palsy (PSP) is characterized pathologically by neurofibrillary tangle formation and neuronal loss in the substantia nigra, pallidum, superior colliculi, brainstem nuclei, and periaqueductal gray matter, with lesser cortical involvement. There have been a number of studies of resting regional cerebral glucose metabolism in patients with probable PSP, several of whom later had the diagnosis confirmed at autopsy (70). Cortical metabolism is globally depressed and frontal areas are particularly targeted, levels of metabolism correlating with disease duration and performance on psychometric tests of frontal function. Hypofrontality is not specific for PSP; it also can be seen in PD, SND, Pick's disease, Huntington disease (HD), and depression.

Basal ganglia, cerebellar, and thalamic glucose metabolism are also depressed in PSP, distinguishing it from PD where metabolism is preserved (see Fig. 43.7) (83). Proton

MRS studies have shown reduced lentiform nucleus NAA/Cr ratios in PSP in contrast to PD (84). Unfortunately, although [18]FDG PET and proton MRS are helpful in distinguishing PSP from PD, they are less useful for discriminating PSP from SND as striatal and frontal hypometabolism can be present in both of these disorders.

The pathology of PSP targets nigrostriatal dopaminergic projections so that, not surprisingly, striatal ^{18}F-dopa uptake in PSP is significantly reduced, the levels correlating with disease duration (74). However, unlike PD, putamen and caudate ^{18}F-dopa uptake appear to be affected equivalently in PSP, suggesting that the substantia nigra is uniformly involved by the pathology in agreement with postmortem studies. In practice, ^{18}F-dopa PET can discriminate 90% of PSP from PD cases on the basis of this uniform caudate and putamen involvement (76). There appears to be little correlation between levels of striatal ^{18}F-dopa uptake in PSP and the degree of disability. Unlike PD and SND, where locomotor impairment appears to result primarily from loss of dopaminergic fibers, loss of mobility in PSP is probably more determined by degeneration of pallidal and brainstem projections.

Loss of striatal DAT binding also has been studied in PSP with ^{123}I-beta-CIT SPECT. Messa et al. have reported a similar loss of putamen ^{123}I-beta-CIT uptake in PD and PSP but significantly greater caudate involvement in the latter (85). However, Pirker et al. were unable to discriminate between PD and PSP with ^{123}I-beta-CIT SPECT (77).

Caudate and putamen D2 binding in PSP has been studied with both PET and SPECT (70,86). Overall, groups of PSP patients consistently show reductions in mean caudate and putamen D2 binding, though only 50% to 70% of individual patients show significant receptor loss. It is likely that, as in SND, degeneration of downstream pallidal and brainstem projections is in part responsible for the poor L-dopa responsiveness of PSP, along with loss of dopamine receptors. Levels of acetylcholinesterase activity have been measured in PSP with ^{11}C-physostigmine and ^{11}C-MP4A PET. In the first series, striatal ^{11}C-physostigmine uptake was found to be significantly reduced and levels correlated with locomotor disability (87). The second study emphasized a one-third reduction of thalamic ^{11}C-MP4A uptake in PSP (16).

CORTICOBASAL DEGENERATION

Corticobasal degeneration (CBD) is also known as *corticobasal ganglionic degeneration, corticodentatonigral degeneration,* and *neuronal achromasia.* Patients classically present with an akinetic-rigid, apraxic limb that may exhibit alien behavior. Cortical sensory loss, dysphasia, myoclonus, supranuclear gaze problems, and bulbar dysfunction also are features, but intellect is spared until late. Eventually, all four limbs become involved and the condition is invariably poorly L-dopa responsive. The pathology consists of

^{18}FDG PET

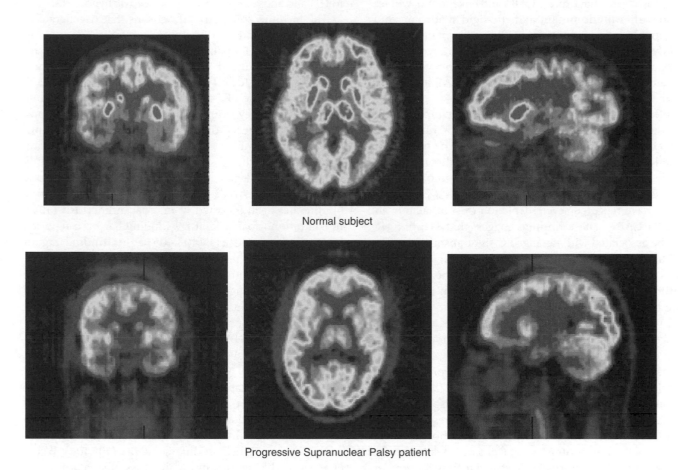

Normal subject

Progressive Supranuclear Palsy patient

Figure 43.7   18FDG PET images of a normal subject and a progressive supranuclear palsy (PSP) patient. Reduced striatal, thalamic, and frontal metabolism is evident in the PSP case. (Images courtesy of P. Piccini.) (See color section.)

collections of swollen, achromatic, tau-positive Pick cells in the absence of argyrophilic Pick bodies that target the posterior frontal, inferior parietal, and superior temporal lobes, the substantia nigra, and the cerebellar dentate nuclei.

PET and SPECT studies on patients with the clinical syndrome of CBD have predictably shown greatest reductions in resting cortical oxygen and glucose metabolism in posterior frontal, inferior parietal, and superior temporal regions (88). The thalamus and striatum also are involved, and the metabolic reductions are strikingly asymmetric, being most severe contralateral to the more affected limbs (89). This contrasts with PD patients, who have preserved and symmetric levels of striatal and thalamic glucose metabolism.

Striatal ^{18}F-dopa uptake is also asymmetrically reduced in CBD, again being most depressed contralateral to the more affected limbs (88). In contrast to PD, caudate and putamen ^{18}F-dopa uptake are similarly depressed in CBD. ^{123}I-beta-CIT SPECT also shows an asymmetric reduction

in striatal DAT binding in PSP, and ^{123}I-IBZM SPECT shows a severe asymmetric reduction of striatal D2 binding (90).

The preceding imaging findings help to discriminate CBD from Pick's disease, in which inferior frontal hypometabolism predominates; from PD, in which striatal metabolism is preserved and caudate ^{18}F-dopa uptake is relatively spared; and from PSP, in which frontal and striatal metabolism tend to be more symmetrically involved.

INVOLUNTARY MOVEMENT DISORDERS

Huntington Disease and Other Choreas

Huntington disease is an autosomal dominantly transmitted disorder associated with an excess of CAG triplet repeats (>38) in the *IT15* gene on chromosome 4. The function of this gene is still uncertain, but the pathology of HD results in intranuclear inclusion formation and targets medium spiny projection neurons in the striatum. Those patients with predominant chorea show a selective loss of striato-GPe projections that express GABA and enkephalin, whereas those with a predominant akinetic-rigid syndrome show additional severe loss of striato-GPi fibers containing GABA and dynorphin. A number of other degenerative disorders also can cause chorea, including neuroacanthocytosis (NA), dentatorubropallidoluysian atrophy (DRPLA), and benign familial chorea (BFC).

Inflammatory diseases, such as systemic lupus erythematosus (SLE) and Sydenham's chorea, also are associated with chorea, as is tardive dyskinesia (TD). The mechanism underlying TD is uncertain; postmortem studies have found low levels of subthalamic and pallidal glutamate decarboxylase, whereas neurochemical studies on a primate TD model have reported severe depletion of subthalamic and pallidal GABA. These findings suggest that TD, like HD, may be associated with deranged GABA transmission.

Clinically affected HD patients show severely reduced levels of glucose and oxygen metabolism of the caudate and lentiform nuclei. Levels of resting putamen metabolism have been reported to correlate with locomotor function (91) whereas caudate metabolism correlates with performance on tests sensitive to frontal lobe function (92).

In early HD, cortical metabolism is preserved but, as the disease progresses and dementia becomes prominent, it also declines, with the frontal cortex targeted (93). Caudate hypometabolism is not specific to HD; it is also seen in NA, DRPLA, and some cases of BFC, so that its presence cannot be used to discriminate these degenerative choreiform disorders (94–96). In contrast, striatal glucose metabolism has been reported to be normal or elevated it chorea secondary to SLE, Sydenham's chorea, and TD (97–99).

Regional cerebral metabolism in HD also has been studied with proton MRS. NAA levels in the basal ganglia are reduced in affected patients, whereas lactate levels in the basal ganglia and cortex are elevated, suggesting that mitochondrial dysfunction is a feature of this disorder (100). If the pathology of HD arises due to mitochondrial dysfunction, one might expect to find raised lactate levels in asymptomatic adult gene carriers. To date, lactate levels have been reported to be normal in asymptomatic gene carriers, which is more in favor of mitochondrial dysfunction representing an associated disease phenomenon than it being the cause of the degenerative process.

It also has been suggested that the pathology of HD may arise from abnormal sensitivity of striatal neurons to glutamate, a naturally occurring excitotoxic amino acid. This hypothesis has arisen from the observation that kainic acid, ibotenic acid, and quinolinic acid (all glutamate agonists) cause a loss of medium spiny neurons when injected into the striatum. A proton MRS study has reported that the glutamine plus glutamate (GLX) peak from the lentiform nuclei of affected HD patients is increased (101). As this peak contains proton resonances from both glutamate and glutamine moieties, the exact interpretation of this finding is not yet clear. However, it is compatible with abnormal compartmentalization of basal ganglia glutamate occurring in HD and adds support to the excitotoxic hypothesis.

The medium spiny striatal neurons that degenerate in HD express D1 and D2 dopamine receptors. Karlsson et al. studied affected HD patients with ^{11}C-SCH23390 PET and demonstrated reduced D1 binding in both striatum and temporal cortex (102). Turjanski et al. used ^{11}C-SCH23390 and ^{11}C-raclopride PET to study both D1 and D2 binding in HD (103). They found a parallel reduction in striatal binding to these receptor subtypes, with the levels of binding correlating with severity of rigidity rather than chorea. The finding of reduced striatal dopamine receptor binding in patients with degenerative chorea is, again, not specific for HD. A mean 70% reduction of striatal ^{11}C-raclopride binding has been reported in neuroacanthocytosis (104). In contrast, normal striatal D2 binding has been reported in SLE chorea and TD (103,105). This finding argues against the hypothesis that TD results from striatal D2 receptor supersensitivity following prolonged exposure to neuroleptics and suggests that the finding of downstream reductions in pallidal and subthalamic GABA levels may be of greater relevance.

Mildly affected HD patients show at least a 30% loss of striatal glucose metabolism and dopamine receptor binding, suggesting that [18]FDG, ^{11}C-SCH23390, and ^{11}C-raclopride PET should all be capable of detecting subclinical dysfunction when present in asymptomatic HD gene carriers (103,106). Reduced caudate glucose metabolism has been reported in one-third to three-quarters of asymptomatic adult HD gene carriers in different series (107,108). Weeks et al. showed a significant parallel loss of striatal D1 and D2 binding in 4 of 8 asymptomatic adults with the HD mutation (see Fig. 43.8) (109). The rate of progression of HD also has been followed with PET. Grafton et al. found that caudate glucose metabolism declined annually by 3.1% in their cohort of HD patients, whereas Antonini reported an annual 6% change in striatal D2 binding (110,111). Andrews et al. have reported an annual fall in striatal D1 and D2 binding of 3% to 4% in symptomatic *HD* gene carriers and 6% in asymptomatic *HD* gene carriers with active subclinical disease (112).

More recently, the role of striatal microglial activation in HD has been studied. Eleven HD patients were studied with ^{11}C-PK11195 PET, and 9 of them also underwent ^{11}C-raclopride PET (113). Mean ^{11}C-PK11195 binding in the striatum was increased, and D2 binding decreased in HD. Striatal ^{11}C-raclopride binding potentials (BPs) inversely correlated with striatal ^{11}C-PK11195 BPs ($r = -0.6809$, $p < 0.05$) in individual HD cases and clinical severity, rated with the UHDRS total motor score, correlated inversely with striatal ^{11}C-raclopride ($r = -0.84$, $p < 0.01$), and positively with striatal ^{11}C-PK11195 BP values ($r = 0.7495$, $p < 0.05$). These PET findings demonstrate that microglial activation accompanies striatal neuronal dysfunction in HD and are consistent with the view that microglial responses may contribute to the ongoing neuronal degeneration in HD.

^{11}C-raclopride PET: D2 Binding

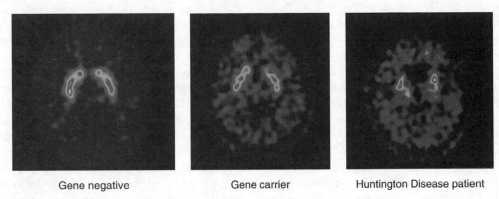

Gene negative   Gene carrier   Huntington Disease patient

Figure 43.8 PET images of ^{11}C-raclopride uptake in Huntington disease (HD) gene negative and positive subjects. It can be seen that significant loss of striatal dopamine D2 binding has occurred in the asymptomatic HD gene carrier. (Images courtesy of T. Andrews.) (See color section.)

TRANSPLANTATION OF HUNTINGTON DISEASE

Transplantation of embryonic striatal tissue into the degenerated striatum of rat and primate models of HD has been shown to be safe and has demonstrated good graft survival with differentiation and integration of striatal grafts into host striatum. Small-animal ^{11}C-raclopride PET has been able to detect recovery of striatal dopamine D2 binding in rats and marmosets lesioned with ibotenic acid after implantation of fetal striatal, but not fetal cortical, tissue (114). In primate models, recovery of skilled motor and cognitive performance has been reported within 2 months of grafting. No improvement in cognitive or motor function was seen in 3 sham-operated monkey controls. Physiologic, neurochemical, and anatomic studies have shown that partial restoration of striatal input and output circuitry by implanted striatal neurons does occur, but the time course of this in primates and humans remains unclear.

Bachoud-Levi et al. have reported the preliminary ^{18}FDG PET findings for 5 HD patients implanted with striatal cells from 8- to 9-week gestation fetuses (115). Three subjects were felt to have improved over the course of 12 months in this series, whereas 2 deteriorated. In those 3 who clinically improved, it was possible to detect striatal graft function, as evidenced by loci of increased glucose utilization seen with ^{18}FDG PET, but not in the 2 patients who subsequently deteriorated.

DYSTONIA

Dystonia is characterized by involuntary posturing and muscle spasms. The primary torsion dystonias (PTDs) range from severe, young-onset, generalized disorders to late-onset focal disease. The most common familial form of generalized PTD, *DYT1* dystonia, has early onset and is an autosomal dominant disorder with approximately 40% penetrance. Onset is usually in childhood and involves a limb, though onset in adulthood is seen occasionally. All cases of *DYT1* dystonia identified have a common mutation: a GAG deletion within the coding region of the *DYT1* gene on chromosome 9q34, which codes for torsin A, an ATP-binding protein of unknown function. A second generalized PTD locus has been mapped to chromosome 8p *(DYT6)*, and affected individuals have adult-onset generalized dystonia with craniocervical disease or focal dystonia. A third PTD gene *(DYT13)* has been mapped to chromosome 1p and has a phenotype of craniocervical and upper limb involvement with occasional generalization.

Postmortem studies have shown that *DYT1* mRNA is highly expressed in dopaminergic neurons of the substantia nigra pars compacta, suggesting possible abnormal dopaminergic neurotransmission in dystonia. However, pathologic studies have failed to identify consistent structural or neurotransmitter abnormalities in PTD. Inclusion bodies now have been described in the brainstem of *DYT1* gene carriers (116). Regions often affected by causes of secondary dystonia include the caudate, putamen, globus pallidus, and posterior thalamus (117). It has been suggested that PTD arises due to a reduced inhibitory output from the basal ganglia to the ventral thalamus and frontal association areas, causing these to become inappropriately overactive.

There have been a number of ^{18}FDG PET studies on resting levels of regional cerebral glucose metabolism in dystonia. A problem in interpreting the findings of earlier studies arises due to the heterogeneity of the patient groups recruited: Familial, sporadic, and acquired dystonia have all been considered together, and patients with focal or hemidystonia have been favored to provide side-to-side comparisons of basal ganglia function. As a consequence, the relevance to PTD of some of these PET findings is uncertain. In addition, some of these patients were clearly experiencing active muscular spasms while supposedly at rest. Resting lentiform nucleus metabolism in dystonia has been variously reported to be increased, normal, and decreased.

Covariance analysis of ^{18}FDG PET findings in *DYT1* carriers has produced more consistent and interpretable findings. In a series of reports, Eidelberg et al. have shown an abnormal inverse relationship in *DYT1* carriers between resting levels of lentiform nucleus and frontal metabolism, the former being relatively reduced and the latter raised (118,119). This pattern is seen whether gene carriers are clinically affected or asymptomatic and is a pattern opposite to that seen in PD. A study on dystonic patients during sleep also has shown preservation of this abnormal pattern of resting glucose metabolism and confirmed that it is not simply movement related. More recently, these workers have demonstrated a similar abnormal covariance pattern in DYT6 dystonia, suggesting that it represents a phenotypic manifestation of genetic dystonias irrespective of etiology (120). These findings would support the concept of hyperexcitable frontal circuitry in dystonic patients even in the absence of movement.

Initial cerebral activation studies in dystonia suggested an imbalance between sensorimotor and premotor cortex (PMC) function, the former being relatively underactive and the latter overactive. When dystonia patients performed paced joystick movements with their right hands in freely selected directions, they showed significantly increased levels of contralateral putamen, rostral SMA, lateral PMC, and dorsolateral prefrontal area activation as evidenced by $H_2^{15}O$ PET blood flow measurements (121). In contrast, there was impairment of activation of contralateral SMC and caudal SMA—that is, those cortical executive areas that send direct pyramidal tract projections to the spinal cord. Using a vibrotactile stimulator, Tempel and Perlmutter found impairment of SMC and caudal SMA activation in both PTD and focal dystonia with $H_2^{15}O$ PET (122). With fMRI, Butterworth et al. also found underactivation of sensory cortex on vibrotactile stimulation of individual fingers with abnormal cortical locations of digit representations (123). This pattern of activation in dystonia was, therefore, different from the pattern associated with PD where striatal, SMA, and prefrontal areas underfunction while primary motor cortex activation is normal or increased.

More recently, however, other workers have noted abnormal overactivation of motor areas when patients with task-induced dystonias (writer's cramp, guitar player's dystonia) perform the specific cramp-inducing tasks, and the premotor cortex has been reported to be underactive (124–126). The jury is out, therefore, as to whether dystonia is associated with relative premotor overactivity and sensorimotor underactivity or the reverse.

Patients with acquired hemi- or focal dystonia caused by basal ganglia and thalamic lesions show increased levels of mesial and lateral PMC and dorsolateral prefrontal area activation during arm movement and also show raised rather than reduced primary motor cortex activation (127). This finding would lend support to overactivity of motor and premotor areas being an associated feature of primary dystonia.

PET reports on dopaminergic function in dystonia also have suffered from inclusion of heterogeneous groups of patients. The only study to assess striatal ^{18}F-dopa uptake in purely familial PTD was by Playford et al. (128). These coworkers found that 8 of 11 PTD patients had normal striatal tracer uptake but that three with severe disease and taking high doses of anticholinergics showed mild impairment of putamen ^{18}F-dopa uptake. The authors concluded that dopamine terminal function was normal in the majority of PTD patients. Two asymptomatic obligate gene carriers were studied, and both had normal striatal ^{18}F-dopa uptake. Otsuka et al. have reported mildly raised levels of mean striatal ^{18}F-dopa uptake in 8 patients with idiopathic torsion dystonia (ITD) (129). More recently, a ^{123}I-beta-CIT SPECT study reported normal striatal uptake in 10 patients with torticollis (130). Combining the findings of these studies, it would appear likely that striatal dopamine terminal function is normal in the majority of ITD cases.

Striatal D2 binding also has been studied in dystonia. A recent ^{18}F-spiperone PET study reported a 25% reduction in mean putamen D2 binding in patients with Meige's syndrome and writer's cramp, but there was a wide overlap with the normal binding range (131). A similar finding was reported in a ^{123}I-epidepride SPECT study involving 10 torticollis cases (130). The authors speculated that reduced striatal D2 receptor availability could result in inappropriate activity of the indirect striatopallidal pathway similar to that seen in HD, resulting in involuntary movements.

DOPA-RESPONSIVE DYSTONIA AND DYSTONIA-PARKINSONISM

Dominantly inherited dopa-responsive dystonia (DRD) is related to GTP-cyclohydrolase 1 deficiency in the majority of cases, the genetic defect being located on chromosome 14. This enzyme constitutes part of the tetrahydrobiopterin synthetic pathway; tetrahydrobiopterin is the cofactor for tyrosine hydroxylase. Patients are unable to manufacture dopa, and hence dopamine, from endogenous tyrosine but can convert exogenous levodopa to dopamine. DRD patients generally present in childhood with diurnally fluctuating dystonia and later develop background parkinsonism. Occasionally, the condition presents as pure parkinsonism in adulthood. ^{18}F-dopa PET findings are normal in the majority of DRD patients, which can help to distinguish this condition from early-onset dystonia–parkinsonism, in which severely reduced putamen ^{18}F-dopa uptake is found (132,133). One might predict that striatal D2 availability would be raised in dopa-naive DRD patients in response to the chronically low levels of striatal dopamine present, and this has been reported to be the case (134). Treated DRD patients appear to have normal striatal D2 binding.

CONCLUSIONS

This chapter has detailed the ways in which functional imaging has been used to demonstrate and distinguish the characteristic patterns of derangement of regional resting cerebral metabolism and neuropharmacology in the different parkinsonian, choreiform, and dystonic syndromes. Both PET and SPECT provide an objective means for early detection and discrimination of parkinsonian syndromes. They also enable PD and HD progression to be objectively monitored and may have a role in evaluating the efficacy of putative neuroprotective and restorative agents, such as implants of fetal cells and infusions of nerve growth factors. In addition, PET has been able to detect subclinical functional abnormalities in at-risk subjects for PD and asymptomatic HD gene carriers and has provided strong support for a role of inheritance in the former.

More recently, ^{11}C-PK11195 PET has provided a means of detecting glial activation in PD, HD, and related disorders and so could be used to monitor the effects of anti-inflammatory agents. Amyloid load also can be measured in PD associated with dementia.

PET activation studies have helped to establish that the akinesia of PD is associated with selective underfunctioning of the SMA and dorsal prefrontal cortex, whereas inappropriate overactivity of these areas seems likely to be associated with dystonia. Ligand activation approaches can now be used to measure levels of synaptic dopamine release and have shown that (a) parkinsonian off periods and dyskinesias do not correlate well with basal ganglia synaptic dopamine levels, and (b) implants of fetal tissue can release normal amounts of dopamine after amphetamine challenge. In the future, it is likely that changes in release of other neurotransmitters during parkinsonism and involuntary movements will become measurable.

REFERENCES

1. Brooks DJ. Imaging end points for monitoring neuroprotection in Parkinson's disease. *Ann Neurol* 2003;53:S110–S119.
2. Morrish PK, Sawle GV, Brooks DJ. Regional changes in [18F]dopa metabolism in the striatum in Parkinson's disease. *Brain* 1996;119:2097–2103.
3. Kish SJ, Shannak K, Hornykiewicz O. Uneven pattern of dopamine loss in the striatum of patients with idiopathic Parkinson's disease. *N Engl J Med* 1988;318:876–880.
4. Whone AL, Moore RY, Piccini P, Brooks DJ. Plasticity in the nigropallidal pathway in Parkinson's disease: an 18F-dopa PET study. *Ann Neurol* 2003;53:206–213.
5. Cools R, Barker RA, Sahakian BJ, Robbins TW. Enhanced or impaired cognitive function in Parkinson's disease as a function of dopaminergic medication and task demands. *Cereb Cortex* 2001;11:1136–1143.
6. Booij J, Speelman JD, Horstink MW, Wolters EC. The clinical benefit of imaging striatal dopamine transporters with [123I]FP-CIT

7. SPECT in differentiating patients with presynaptic parkinsonism from those with other forms of parkinsonism. *Eur J Nucl Med* 2001;28:266–272.
7. Catafau AM, Tolosa E. Impact of dopamine transporter SPECT using 123I-Ioflupane on diagnosis and management of patients with clinically uncertain parkinsonian syndromes. *Mov Disord* 2004;19:1175–1182.
8. Jennings DL, Seibyl JP, Oakes D,, et al. (123I) beta-CIT and single-photon emission computed tomographic imaging vs clinical evaluation in parkinsonian syndrome: unmasking an early diagnosis. *Arch Neurol* 2004;61:1224–1229.
9. Vingerhoets FJG, Schulzer M, Calne DB, Snow BJ. Which clinical sign of Parkinson's disease best reflects the nigrostriatal lesion? *Ann Neurol* 1997;41:58–64.
10. Benamer HTS, Patterson J, Wyper DJ, et al. Correlation of Parkinson's disease severity and duration with I-123-FP-CIT SPECT striatal uptake. *Mov Disord* 2000;15:692–698.
11. Lee CS, Samii A, Sossi V, et al. In vivo positron emission tomographic evidence for compensatory changes in presynaptic dopaminergic nerve terminals in Parkinson's disease. *Ann Neurol* 2000;47:493–503.
12. Doder M, Rabiner EA, Turjanski N, et al. Tremor in Parkinson's disease and serotonergic dysfunction: an (11)C-WAY 100635 PET study. *Neurology* 2003;60:601–605.
13. Kim SE, Choi JY, Choe YS, et al. Serotonin transporters in the midbrain of Parkinson's disease patients: a study with 123I-beta-CIT SPECT. *J Nucl Med* 2003;44:870–876.
14. Remy P, Doder M, Lees AJ, Turjanski N, Brooks DJ. Depression in Parkinson's disease: loss of dopamine and noradrenaline innervation in the limbic system. *Brain* 2005;128:1314–1322.
15. Kuhl DE, Minoshima S, Fessler JA, et al. In vivo mapping of cholinergic terminals in normal aging, Alzheimer's disease, and Parkinson's disease. *Ann Neurol* 1996;40:399–410.
16. Shinotoh H, Namba H, Yamaguchi M, et al. Positron emission tomographic measurement of acetylcholine esterase activity reveals differential loss of ascending cholinergic systems in Parkinson's disease and progressive supranuclear palsy. *Ann Neurol* 1999;46:62–69.
17. Piccini P, Morrish PK, Turjanski N, et al. Dopaminergic function in familial Parkinson's disease: a clinical and 18F-dopa PET study. *Ann Neurol* 1997;41:222–229.
18. Piccini P, Burn DJ, Ceravalo R, et al. The role of inheritance in sporadic Parkinson's disease: evidence from a longitudinal study of dopaminergic function in twins. *Ann Neurol* 1999;45:577–582.
19. Ponsen MM, Stoffers D, Booij J, et al. Idiopathic hyposmia as a preclinical sign of Parkinson's disease. *Ann Neurol* 2004;56:173–181.
20. Imamura K, Hishikawa N, Sawada M, et al. Distribution of major histo-compatibility complex class II-positive microglia and cytokine profile of Parkinson's disease brains. *Acta Neuropathol (Berl)* 2003;106:518–526.
21. Ouchi Y, Yoshikawa E, Sekine Y, et al. Microglial activation and dopamine terminal loss in early Parkinson's disease. *Ann Neurol* 2005;57:168–175.
22. Gerhard A, Pavese N, Hotton GR, et al. In vivo imaging of microglial activation with [(11)c] (R)-PK11195 PET in idiopathic Parkinson's disease. *Neuro Biol Dis* 2006;21:404–412.
23. Ravina B, Eidelberg D, Ahlskog JE, et al. The role of radiotracer imaging in Parkinson's disease. *Neurology* 2005;64:208–215.
24. Whone AL, Watts RL, Stoessl J, et al. Slower progression of PD with ropinirol versus L-dopa: the REAL-PET study. *Ann Neurol* 2003;54:93–101.
25. Innis RB, Marek KL, Sheff K, et al. Effect of treatment with L-dopa/carbidopa or L-selegiline on striatal dopamine transporter SPECT imaging with [I-123]beta-CIT. *Mov Disord* 1999;14:436–442.
26. Snow BJ, Tooyama I, McGeer EG, et al. Human positron emission tomographic [18F]fluorodopa studies correlate with dopamine cell counts and levels. *Ann Neurol* 1993;34:324–330.
27. Pate BD, Kawamata T, Yamada T, et al. Correlation of striatal fluorodopa uptake in the MPTP monkey with dopaminergic indices. *Ann Neurol* 1993;34:331–338.

28. Lee CS, Schulzer M, de la Fuente-Fernández R, et al. Lack of regional selectivity during the progression of Parkinson disease: implications for pathogenesis. *Arch Neurol* 2004;61:1920–1925.

29. Schapira AH, Olanow CW. Neuroprotection in Parkinson disease: mysteries, myths, and misconceptions. *JAMA* 2004;291:358–364.

30. Parkinson Study Group. Dopamine transporter brain imaging to assess the effects of pramipexole vs levodopa on Parkinson disease progression. *JAMA* 2002;287:1653–1661.

31. Ahlskog JE. Slowing Parkinson's disease progression: recent dopamine agonist trials. *Neurology* 2003;60:381–389.

32. Fahn S, Oakes D, Shoulson I, et al. Levodopa and the progression of Parkinson's disease. *N Engl J Med* 2004;351:2498–2508.

33. Lindvall O. Cerebral implantation in movement disorders: state of the art. *Mov Disord* 1999;14:201–205.

34. Piccini P, Brooks DJ, Bjorklund A, et al. Dopamine release from nigral transplants visualised in vivo in a Parkinson's patient. *Nat Neurosci* 1999;2:1137–1140.

35. Piccini P, Lindvall O, Bjorklund A, et al. Delayed recovery of movement-related cortical function in Parkinson's disease after striatal dopaminergic grafts. *Ann Neurol* 2000;48:689–695.

36. Freed CR, Greene PE, Breeze RE, et al. Transplantation of embryonic dopamine neurons for severe Parkinson's disease. *N Eng J Med* 2001;344:710–719.

37. Olanow CW, Goetz CG, Kordower JH, et al. A double-blind controlled trial of bilateral fetal nigral transplantation in Parkinson's disease. *Ann Neurol* 2003;54:403–414.

38. Gill SS, Patel NK, Hotton GR, et al. Direct brain infusion of glial cell line-derived neurotrophic factor in Parkinson disease. *Nat Med* 2003;9:589–595.

39. De la Fuente-Fernández R, Pal PK, Vingerhoets FJG, et al. Evidence for impaired presynaptic dopamine function in parkinsonian patients with motor fluctuations. *J Neural Transm* 2000;107:49–57.

40. Playford ED, Brooks DJ. In vivo and in vitro studies of the dopaminergic system in movement disorders. *Cerobrovasc Brain Metab Rev* 1992;4:144–171.

41. Turjanski N, Lees AJ, Brooks DJ. PET studies on striatal dopaminergic receptor binding in drug naive and L-dopa treated Parkinson's disease patients with and without dyskinesia. *Neurology* 1997;49:717–723.

42. Kishore A, de la Fuente-Fernández R, Snow BJ, et al. Levodopa-induced dyskinesias in idiopathic parkinsonism (IP): a simultaneous PET study of dopamine D1 and D2 receptors. *Neurology* 1997;48:A327.

43. Torstenson R, Hartvig P, Långström B, et al. Differential effects of levodopa on dopaminergic function in early and advanced Parkinson's disease. *Ann Neurol* 1997;41:334–340.

44. De la Fuente-Fernández R, Lu JQ, Sossi V, et al. Biochemical variations in the synaptic level of dopamine precede motor fluctuations in Parkinson's disease: PET evidence of increased dopamine turnover. *Ann Neurol* 2001;49:298–303.

45. Piccini P, Weeks RA, Brooks DJ. Opioid receptor binding in Parkinson's patients with and without levodopa-induced dyskinesias. *Ann Neurol* 1997;42:720–726.

46. Whone AL, Rabiner EA, Arahata Y, et al. Reduced substance P binding in Parkinson's disease complicated by dyskinesias: an F-18-L829165 PET study. *Neurology* 2002;58(suppl 3:A488–A489.

47. Kuhl DE, Metter EJ, Benson DF, et al. Similarities of cerebral glucose metabolism in Alzheimer's and Parkinsonian dementia. *J Cereb Blood Flow Metab* 1985;5(suppl 1):S169–S170.

48. Hu MTM, Taylor-Robinson SD, Chaudhuri KR, et al. Cortical dysfunction in non-demented Parkinson's disease patients: a combined 31Phosphorus MRS and 18FDG PET study. *Brain* 2000;123:340–352.

49. Bohnen NI, Minoshima S, Giordani B, et al. Motor correlates of occipital glucose hypometabolism in Parkinson's disease without dementia. *Neurology* 1999;52:541–546.

50. Klunk WE, Engler H, Nordberg A, et al. Imaging brain amyloid in Alzheimer's disease with Pittsburgh compound-B. *Ann Neurol* 2004;55:306–319.

51. Walker Z, Costa DC, Walker RW, et al. Differentiation of dementia with Lewy bodies from Alzheimer's disease using a dopaminergic presynaptic ligand. *J Neurol Neurosurg Psychiatry* 2002;73:134–140.

52. Walker Z, Costa DC, Walker RW, et al. Striatal dopamine transporter in dementia with Lewy bodies and Parkinson disease: a comparison. *Neurology* 2004;62:1568–1572.

53. Ito K, Nagano-Saito A, Kato T, et al. Striatal and extrastriatal dysfunction in Parkinson's disease with dementia: a 6-[18F]fluoro-L-dopa PET study. *Brain* 2002;125:1358–1365.

54. Brooks DJ. PET studies on the function of dopamine in health and Parkinson's disease. *Ann N Y Acad Sci* 2003;991:22–35.

55. Eidelberg D, Moeller JR, Dhawan V, et al. The metabolic topography of parkinsonism. *J Cereb Blood Flow Metab* 1994;14:783–801.

56. Eidelberg D, Moeller JR, Ishikawa T, et al. Assessment of disease severity in parkinsonism with Fluorine-18-Fluorodeoxyglucose and PET. *J Nucl Med* 1995;36:378–383.

57. Feigin A, Fukuda M, Dhawan V, et al. Metabolic correlates of levodopa response in Parkinson's disease. *Neurology* 2001;57:2083–2088.

58. Fukuda M, Mentis MJ, Ma Y, et al. Networks mediating the clinical effects of pallidal brain stimulation for Parkinson's disease: a PET study of resting-state glucose metabolism. *Brain* 2001;124:1601–1609.

59. Playford ED, Jenkins IH, Passingham RE, et al. Impaired mesial frontal and putamen activation in Parkinson's disease: a PET study. *Ann Neurol* 1992;32:151–161.

60. Rascol O, Sabatini U, Brefel C, et al. Cortical motor overactivation in parkinsonian patients with L-dopa-induced peak-dose dyskinesia. *Brain* 1998;121:527–533.

61. Jahanshahi M, Jenkins IH, Brown RG, et al. Self-initiated versus externally triggered movements. I. An investigation of regional cerebral blood flow with PET and movement-related potentials in normals and Parkinson's disease subjects. *Brain* 1995;118:913–933.

62. Rascol O, Sabatini U, Chollet F, et al. Supplementary and primary sensory motor area activity in Parkinson's disease: regional cerebral blood flow changes during finger movements and effects of apomorphine. *Arch Neurol* 1992;49:144–148.

63. Rascol O, Sabatini U, Fabre N, et al. The ipsilateral cerebellar hemisphere is overactive during hand movements in akinetic parkinsonian patients. *Brain* 1997;120:103–110.

64. Jenkins IH, Fernández W, Playford ED, et al. Impaired activation of the supplementary motor area in Parkinson's disease is reversed when akinesia is treated with apomorphine. *Ann Neurol* 1992;32:749–757.

65. Limousin P, Greene J, Polak P, et al. Changes in cerebral activity pattern due to subthalamic nucleus or internal pallidum stimulation in Parkinson's disease. *Ann Neurol* 1997;42:283–291.

66. Ceballos-Baumann AO, Boecker H, Bartenstein P, et al. A positron emission tomographic study of subthalamic nucleus stimulation in Parkinson disease: enhanced movement-related activity of motor-association cortex and decreased motor cortex resting activity *Arch Neurol* 1999;56:997–1003.

67. Ceballos-Baumann AO, Obeso JA, Delong MR, et al. Functional reafferentation of striatal-frontal connections after posteroventral pallidotomy in Parkinson's disease. *Lancet* 1994;344:814.

68. Schrag A, Good CD, Miszkiel K, et al. Differentiation of atypical parkinsonian syndromes with routine MRI. *Neurology* 2000;54:697–702.

69. Seppi K, Schocke MF, Esterhammer R, et al. Diffusion-weighted imaging discriminates progressive supranuclear palsy from PD, but not from the parkinson variant of multiple system atrophy. *Neurology* 2003;60:922–927.

70. Brooks DJ. Diagnosis and management of atypical parkinsonian syndromes. *J Neurol Neurosurg Psychiatry.* 2002;72(suppl 1):I10–I16.

71. Eidelberg D, Takikawa S, Moeller JR, et al. Striatal hypometabolism distinguishes striatonigral degeneration from Parkinson's disease. *Ann Neurol* 1993;33:518–527.

72. Eidelberg D, Moeller JR, Kazumata K, et al. Metabolic correlates of pallidal neuronal activity in Parkinson's disease. *Brain* 1997;120:1315–1324.

73. Davie CA, Wenning GK, Barker GJ, et al. Differentiation of multiple system atrophy from idiopathic Parkinson's disease using proton magnetic resonance spectroscopy. *Ann Neurol* 1995;37:204–210.

74. Brooks DJ, Ibañez V, Sawle GV, et al. Differing patterns of striatal 18F-dopa uptake in Parkinson's disease, multiple system atrophy and progressive supranuclear palsy. *Ann Neurol* 1990;28:547–555.

75. Brooks DJ, Salmon EP, Mathias CJ, et al. The relationship between locomotor disability, autonomic dysfunction, and the integrity of

the striatal dopaminergic system, in patients with multiple system atrophy, pure autonomic failure, and Parkinson's disease, studied with PET. *Brain* 1990;113:1539–1552.

76. Burn DJ, Sawle GV, Brooks DJ. The differential diagnosis of Parkinson's disease, multiple system atrophy, and Steele-Richardson-Olszewski syndrome: discriminant analysis of striatal 18F-dopa PET data. *J Neurol Neurosurg Psychiatry* 1994;57:278–284.

77. Pirker W, Asenbaum S, Bencsits G, et al. [I-123]beta-CIT SPECT in multiple system atrophy, progressive supranuclear palsy, and corticobasal degeneration. *Mov Disord* 2000;15:1158–1167.

78. Seppi K, Schocke MF, Donnemiller E, et al. Comparison of diffusion-weighted imaging and [123I]IBZM-SPECT for the differentiation of patients with the Parkinson variant of multiple system atrophy from those with Parkinson's disease. *Mov Disord* 2004;19:1438–1445.

79. Schwarz J, Tatsch K, Arnold G, et al. 123I-iodobenzamide-SPECT predicts dopaminergic responsiveness in patients with de-novo parkinsonism. *Neurology* 1992;42:556–561.

80. Seppi K, Donnemiller E, Riccabona G, et al. Disease progression in PD vs MSA: a SPECT study using 123-I IBZM. *Parkinsonism Relat Disord* 2001;7:S24.

81. Druschky A, Hilz MJ, Platsch G, et al. Differentiation of Parkinson's disease and multiple system atrophy in early disease stages by means of I-123-MIBG-SPECT. *J Neurol Sci* 2000;175:3–12.

82. Gerhard A, Banati RB, Goerres GB, et al. [(11)C](R)-PK11195 PET imaging of microglial activation in multiple system atrophy. *Neurology* 2003;61:686–689.

83. Foster NL, Gilman S, Berent S, et al. Cerebral hypometabolism in progressive supranuclear palsy studied with positron emission tomography. *Ann Neurol* 1988;24:399–406.

84. Davie CA, Barker GJ, Machado C, et al. Proton magnetic resonance spectroscopy in Steele-Richardson-Olszewski syndrome. *Mov Disord* 1997;12:767–771.

85. Messa C, Volonte MA, Fazio F, et al. Differential distribution of striatal [123I]b-CIT in Parkinson's disease and progressive supranuclear palsy, evaluated with single-photon emission tomography. *Eur J Nucl Med* 1998;25:1270–1276.

86. Brooks DJ, Ibañez V, Sawle GV, et al. Striatal D2 receptor status in Parkinson's disease, striatonigral degeneration, and progressive supranuclear palsy, measured with 11C-raclopride and PET. *Ann Neurol* 1992;31:184–192.

87 Pappata S, Traykov L, Tavitian B, et al. Striatal reduction of acetylcholinesterase in patients with progressive supranuclear palsy (PSP) as measured in vivo by PET and 11C-physostigmine (11C-PHY). *J Cereb Blood Flow Metab.* 1997;17(suppl1): S687.

88. Sawle GV, Brooks DJ, Marsden CD, Frackowiak RSJ. Corticobasal degeneration: a unique pattern of regional cortical oxygen metabolism and striatal fluorodopa uptake demonstrated by positron emission tomography. *Brain* 1991;114:541–556.

89. Eidelberg D, Dhawan V, Moeller JR, et al. The metabolic landscape of cortico-basal ganglionic degeneration: regional asymmetries studied with positron emission tomography. *J Neurol Neurosurg Psychiatry* 1991;54:856–862.

90. Frisoni GB, Pizzolato G, Zanetti O, et al. Corticobasal degeneration: neuropsychological assessment and dopamine D-2 receptor SPECT analysis. *Eur Neurol* 1995;35:50–54.

91. Young AB, Penney JB, Starosta-Rubinstein S, et al. PET scan investigations of Huntington's disease: cerebral metabolic correlates of neurological features and functional decline. *Ann Neurol* 1986;20:296–303.

92. Berent S, Giordani B, Lehtinen S, et al. Positron emission tomographic scan investigations of Huntington's disease: cerebral metabolic correlates of cognitive function. *Ann Neurol* 1988;23: 541–546.

93. Kuwert T, Lange HW, Langen KJ, et al. Cortical and subcortical glucose consumption measured by PET in patients with Huntington's disease. *Brain* 1990;113:1405–1423.

94. Hosokawa S, Ichiya Y, Kuwabara Y, et al. Positron emission tomography in cases of chorea with different underlying diseases. *J Neurol Neurosurg Psychiatry* 1987;50:1284–1287.

95. Dubinsky RM, Hallett M, Levey R, Di Chiro G. Regional brain glucose metabolism in neuroacanthocytosis. *Neurology* 1989;39: 1253–1255.

96. Suchowersky O, Hayden MR, Martin WRW, et al. Cerebral metabolism of glucose in benign hereditary chorea. *Mov Disord* 1986;1:33–45.

97. Guttman M, Lang AE, Garnett ES, et al. Regional cerebral glucose metabolism in SLE chorea: further evidence that striatal hypometabolism is not a correlate of chorea. *Mov Disord* 1987;2:201–210.

98. Weindl A, Kuwert T, Leenders KL, et al. Increased striatal glucose consumption in Sydenham chorea. *Mov Disord* 1993;8:437–444.

99. Pahl JJ, Mazziotta JC, Cummings J,, et al. Positron emission tomography in tardive dyskinesia and Huntington's disease. *J Cereb Blood Flow Metab* 1987;7:1253–1255.

100. Jenkins BG, Koroshetz WJ, Beal MF, Rosen BR. Evidence for impairment of energy metabolism in vivo in Huntington's disease using localised 1H NMR spectroscopy. *Neurology* 1993;43:2689–2695.

101. Taylor-Robinson SD, Weeks RA, Sargentoni J, et al. Proton MRS in Huntington's disease: evidence in favour of the glutamate excitotoxic theory. *Mov Disord* 1996;11:167–173.

102. Karlsson P, Lundin A, Anvret M, et al. Dopamine D1 receptor number: a sensitive PET marker for early brain degeneration in Huntington's disease. *Eur Arch Psych Clin Neurosci.* 1994;243: 249–255.

103. Turjanski N, Weeks R, Dolan R, et al. Striatal D1 and D2 receptor binding in patients with Huntington's disease and other choreas: a PET study. *Brain* 1995;118:689–696.

104. Brooks DJ, Ibañez V, Playford ED, et al. Presynaptic and postsynaptic striatal dopaminergic function in neuroacanthocytosis: a positron emission tomographic study. *Ann Neurol* 1991; 30:166–171.

105. Andersson U, Eckernas SA, Hartvig P, et al. Striatal binding of 11C-NMSP studied with positron emission tomography in patients with persistent tardive dyskinesia: no evidence for altered dopamine receptor binding. *J Neural Transm* 1990;79: 215–226.

106. Hayden MR, Martin WRW, Stoessl AJ, et al. Positron emission tomography in the early diagnosis of Huntington's disease. *Neurology* 1986;36:888–894.

107. Hayden MR, Hewitt J, Martin WRW, et al. Studies in persons at risk for Huntington's disease. *N Engl J Med* 1987;317:382–383.

108. Grafton ST, Mazziotta JC, Pahl JJ, et al. A comparison of neurological, metabolic, structural, and genetic evaluations in persons at risk for Huntington's disease. *Ann Neurol* 1990; 28:614–621.

109. Weeks RA, Piccini P, Harding AE, Brooks DJ. Striatal D1 and D2 dopamine receptor loss in asymptomatic mutation carriers of Huntington's disease. *Ann Neurol* 1996;40:49–54.

110. Grafton ST, Mazziotta JC, Pahl JJ, et al. Serial changes of glucose cerebral metabolism and caudate size in persons at risk for Huntington's disease. *Arch Neurol* 1992;49:1161–1167.

111. Antonini A, Leenders KL, Feigin A, et al. PET studies of Huntington's disease rate of progression. *Neurology* 1997;48 (suppl 2):A120.

112. Andrews TC, Weeks RA, Turjanski N, et al. Huntington's disease progression PET and clinical observations. *Brain* 1999;122:2353–2363.

113. Pavese N, Gerhard A, TaiYF, et al. Microglial activation correlates with severity in Huntington disease: a clinical and PET study. *Nerology* 2006;66:1638–1643.

114. Torres EM, Fricker RA, Hume SP, et al. Assessment of striatal graft viability in the rat in vivo using a small diameter PET scanner. *Neuroreport* 1995;6:2017–2021.

115. Bachoud-Levi A, Remy P, Nguyen JP, et al. Motor and cognitive improvements in patients with Huntington's disease after neural transplantation. *Lancet* 2000;356:1975–1979.

116. McNaught KS, Kapustin A, Jackson T, et al. Brainstem pathology in DYT1 primary torsion dystonia. *Ann Neurol* 2004;56: 540–547.

117. Bhatia KP, Marsden CD. The behavioural and motor consequences of focal lesions of the basal ganglia in man. *Brain* 1994;117:859–876.

118. Eidelberg D, Moeller JR, Antonini A, et al. Abnormal metabolic brain networks in DYT-1 dystonia. *Neurology* 1997;48 (suppl 2):A62.

119. Eidelberg D, Moeller JR, Antonini A, et al. Functional brain networks in DYT1 dystonia. *Ann Neurol* 1998;44:303–312.

120. Trost M, Carbon M, Edwards C, et al. Primary dystonia: is abnormal functional brain architecture linked to genotype? *Ann Neurol* 2002;52:853–856.

121. Ceballos-Baumann AO, Passingham RE, Warner T, et al. Overactivity of rostral and underactivity of caudal frontal areas in idiopathic torsion dystonia: a PET activation study. *Ann Neurol* 1995;37:363–372.

122. Tempel LW, Perlmutter JS. Abnormal cortical responses in patients with writer's cramp. *Neurology* 1993;43: 2252–2257.

123. Butterworth S, Francis S, Kelly E, et al. Abnormal cortical sensory activation in dystonia: an fMRI study. *Mov Disord* 2003;18: 673–682.

124. Odergren T, Stone-Elander S, Ingvar M. Cerebral and cerebellar activation in correlation to the action-induced dystonia in writer's cramp. *Mov Disord* 1998;13:497–508.

125. Lerner A, Shill H, Hanakawa T, et al. Regional cerebral blood flow correlates of the severity of writer's cramp symptoms. *Neuroimage* 2004;21:904–913.

126. Pujol J, Roset-Llobet J, Rosines-Cubells D, et al. Brain cortical activation during guitar-induced hand dystonia studied by functional MRI. *Neuroimage* 2000;12:257–267.

127. Ceballos-Baumann AO, Passingham RE, Marsden CD, Brooks DJ. Overactivity of primary and accessory motor areas after motor reorganisation in acquired hemi-dystonia: a PET activation study. *Ann Neurol* 1995;37:746–757.

128. Playford ED, Fletcher NA, Sawle GV, et al. Integrity of the nigro-striatal dopaminergic system in familial dystonia: an 18F-dopa PET study. *Brain* 1993;116:1191–1199.

129. Otsuka M, Ichiya Y, Shima F, et al. Increased striatal 18F-dopa uptake and normal glucose metabolism in idiopathic dystonia syndrome. *J Neurol Sci* 1992;111:195–199.

130. Naumann M, Pirker W, Reiners K, et al. Imaging the pre- and postsynaptic side of striatal dopaminergic synapses in idiopathic cervical dystonia: a SPECT study using [123I]Epidepride and [123I]b-CIT. *Mov Disord* 1998;13:319–323.

131. Perlmutter JS, Stambuk MK, Markham J, et al. Decreased [F-18] spiperone binding in putamen in idiopathic focal dystonia. *J Neurosci* 1997;17:843–850.

132. Snow BJ, Nygaard TG, Takahashi H, Calne DB. Positron emission tomography studies of dopa-responsive dystonia and early-onset idiopathic parkinsonism. *Ann Neurol* 1993;34:733–738.

133. Turjanski N, Bhatia K, Burn DJ, et al. Comparison of striatal 18F-dopa uptake in adult-onset dystonia-parkinsonism, Parkinson's disease, and dopa-responsive dystonia. *Neurology* 1993;43: 1563–1568.

134. Kunig G, Leenders KL, Antonini A, et al. D-2 receptor binding in dopa-responsive dystonia. *Ann Neurol* 1998;44:758–762.

Botulinum Toxin in Movement Disorders

44

Alberto Albanese   *Anna Rita Bentivoglio*

INTRODUCTION

Clostridial neurotoxins encompass tetanus and botulinum neurotoxins (BoNTs), which have 7 different serotypes. Clinical observations of cases of botulism (systemic intoxication with BoNTs) have shown that the effects are widespread with paralysis of the neuromuscular junctions and blockade of neurosecretion and the autonomic nervous system (1). The availability of highly purified toxins raised the possibility of using BoNTs as therapeutic tools.

Type A BoNT (BoNT-A) has been introduced in clinical practice in 1980. Since then, it has proven to be the most flexible tool for medical treatment, with more than 50 indications that apply to many medical conditions (Fig. 44.1). With the notable exception of anal fissure, BoNTs do not provide a cure but constitute a symptomatic remedy producing topical chemodenervation. Following a reduction in the release of neurotransmitters in the injected area, BoNTs reduce the activity of striated or smooth muscles and the secretory function of glands. Thus, the general indication for their use is to reduce muscle overactivity, release sphincter spasm, and inhibit gland secretion (2). Since the injections are topical and the indications are so diverse, there are different modalities to deliver the toxin at its targets. BoNT injections can be intramuscular, subcutaneous, intradermic, or intraglandular and can be performed by direct inspection or with instrumental guidance (electromyography [EMG], endoscopy, ultrasonography, or computed tomography [CT] scan). Other factors affecting the clinical outcome are dilution and reconstitution, needle gauge, anatomical approach, muscle location and size. In addition, recently proposed alternative delivery techniques are iontophoresis or cream application. BoNT clinics are places where highly skilled artisans apply theoretical knowledge with hands-on expertise.

BOTULINUM NEUROTOXINS: MECHANISM OF ACTION

BoNTs produce a chemical denervation that is topical, reversible, and dose-dependent. They inhibit the docking and subsequent opening of synaptic vesicles containing acetylcholine in the presynaptic musculoskeletal terminal, thereby impeding neuromuscular transmission. In addition, BoNTs exert a similar action on neuroglandular and autonomic terminals. The limiting factor for the action of BoNTs is receptor-mediated endocytosis. At least three different groups of presynaptic BoNT receptors, with different serotype specificity, are present at nerve terminals. Their molecular identity is not known, nor is known their exact distribution on the different presynaptic terminals (Fig. 44.2).

Although the 7 BoNT serotypes (named from A to G) are antigenically distinct, they have a similar structure and molecular weight, consisting of a heavy chain and a light chain joined by a disulfide bond. BoNTs are zinc (Zn^{2+}) endopeptidases composed of 3 functional domains where the catalytic function is confined to the light chain, with proteolytic activity located at the N-terminal end; translocation activity is concentrated at the N-terminal half of the heavy chain, and receptor binding at the C-terminal half. Three steps are involved in BoNT-mediated paralysis: internalization, disulfide reduction and translocation, and inhibition of neurotransmitter release. BoNTs bind to the presynaptic nerve ending and enter by receptor-mediated selective and saturable

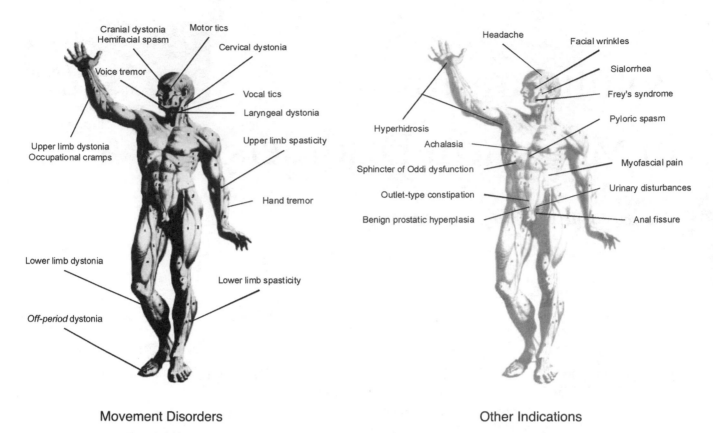

Movement Disorders

Other Indications

Figure 44.1 Synopsis of the main indications for clinical use of BoNT in movement disorders and other medical conditions.

endocytosis. The Zn-dependent catalytic domain of the toxin specifically cleaves different proteins essential for the fusion of synaptic vesicles containing the neurotransmitter. Table 44.1 lists the substrates cleaved by each BoNT serotype. Cleavage of any of these proteins interferes with the proper binding and fusion of a vesicle to the plasma membrane, and therefore impedes exocytosis-mediated neurotransmitter release.

Nerve terminals containing active BoNT do not degenerate; neurotransmitter release takes place again when the effect of BoNT wanes following degradation by proteolysis. Muscle denervation promotes a compensatory sprouting of nerve terminals and the formation of new synaptic contacts. This usually takes from 2 to 3 months and becomes a relevant phenomenon when repeated BoNT injections are performed in the same site. Following injection into a muscle or in the surroundings of nerve terminals, the main effect of BoNT is to produce a chemical denervation of neuromuscular junctions, resulting in weakness and atrophy of the striated muscle. BoNT diffuses from the injection site, depending on some physical variables; toxin spread is directly related to the total toxin dose injected and indirectly related to its concentration in the injection volume (3). Following injection into a muscle, BoNT diffuses locally and also may reach adjacent muscles and even

may trespass the muscle fascia. It also has been observed that BoNT can spread from the site of injection via the lymphatic system or bloodstream to reach distant sites, commonly producing subclinical effects (4). Clinical or subclinical BoNT-induced denervation can be detected by EMG, showing a reduction in the amplitude of compound motor action potentials (CMAP) following single or repetitive supramaximal nerve stimulation.

Although BoNT exerts its main action on the neuromuscular junction, some of the therapeutic responses observed in movement disorders appear not to be due only to peripheral effects. In most patients who receive treatment for dystonia or spasticity, the clinical benefit generally parallels muscle weakness; but other cases have been documented in whom the benefit is disproportionate, either because a significant improvement occurs without muscle weakness or, conversely, because there is little improvement notwithstanding marked weakness. In addition, BoNT-A also has been shown to inhibit release of mediators involved in nociception, such as substance P, calcitonin gene-related peptide (CGRP), and glutamate (5).

Some of the therapeutic responses observed in movement disorders are due to effects on the central nervous system (CNS). BoNTs do not cross the blood–brain barrier, and there is no in vivo convincing evidence that,

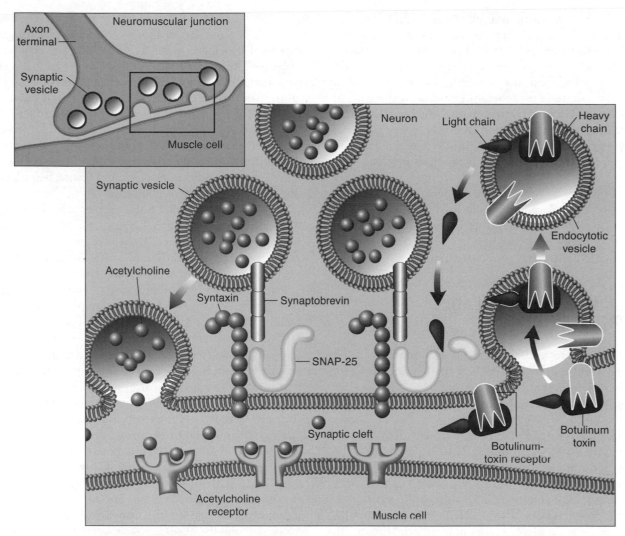

Figure 44.2 Sequence of action (*from right to left*) of botulinum neurotoxin type A (BoNT-A) at the neuromuscular junction: binding to the presynaptic terminal, entrance into the cell by endocytosis, and cleavage of SNAP-25 (25-kd synaptosomal-associated protein). The substrates of other BoNT serotypes are listed in Table 44.1. (From Hallett M. One man's poison: clinical applications of botulinum toxin. *N Engl J Med* 1999;341:118–120. With permission.)

TABLE 44.1
CLEAVAGE SITES OF BOTULINUM TOXINS

Serotype	Target
A	SNAP-25
B	Synaptobrevin
C	SNAP-25
	Syntaxin
D	Cellubrevin
	Synaptobrevin
E	SNAP-25
F	Cellubrevin
	Synaptobrevin
G	Synaptobrevin

SNAP-25, 25-kd synaptosomal-associated protein.

following injection in the periphery, they can reach the CNS and directly influence central sensory-motor integration. Notwithstanding, human and animal studies suggest that BoNT-A may indirectly influence the functional organization of the CNS by affecting the intrafusal terminals. Following BoNT denervation of gamma motor neurons, muscle spindle activity is decreased and inflow directed to the spinal alpha motor neurons is reduced (6). Since muscle activity is supported by afferent feedback, there may be a reduced alpha motor neuron drive. Furthermore, it has been postulated, but not demonstrated, that in humans BoNT may enter the CNS via retrograde axonal transport and may directly affect Renshaw cell activity by influencing the cholinergic recurrent motor neuron collateral (7). Many researchers have tried to elucidate the central effects of BoNT in patients with dystonia. In addition to the considerations mentioned, there is evidence to support that BoNT injections reverse a lack of inhibition that plays a pathogenetic role in dystonia, as demonstrated by the normalization of reciprocal inhibition and of intracortical inhibition. There is evidence of changes in the cortical organization, because cortical maps, which are distorted and extended in patients with dystonia, are normalized following peripheral injection of BoNT. Positron emission tomography (PET) studies on upper limb dystonia have demonstrated increased activation in the parietal cortex and in the caudal supplementary motor area, leaving unchanged the reduced activity of the primary motor cortex (8). The ultimate consequence of the reorganization of the human motor system induced by BoNT treatment may be long-term plastic changes in motor output.

COMMERCIALLY AVAILABLE NEUROTOXINS

Three BoNTs are available for clinical practice: 2 are serotype A and 1 is serotype B. These toxin brands differ for specific activity, packaging, constituents, excipients, and storage. Their main features are summarized in Table 44.2. Another BoNT-A, Xeomin produced by Merz Pharma (Germany), has been marketed in Germany. Furthermore, 3 additional BoNT-A products are to be released in the future: Linurase (Prollenium, Inc., Canada), CBTX-A (Lanzhou Biological Products Institute, China), and Neuronox (Medy-Tox Inc., South Korea). In addition to branded products, locally available BoNT-C and BoNT-F have been tested in blepharospasm, hemifacial spasm (9), and upper limb dystonia (10).

The 3 branded BoNTs are all marketed worldwide for cervical dystonia, which currently is the only approved indication for Myobloc/Neurobloc. In addition, Botox and Dysport have a number of approved indications, including other focal dystonias, spasticity, hyperhidrosis, hemifacial spasm, and facial wrinkles. Official approval has been granted with remarkable differences in different countries within these broad categories. For example, in Italy and in Spain, Botox is currently licensed only for upper limb spasticity, whereas Dysport is licensed for both upper and lower limb spasticity. Remarkably, there are a number of randomized controlled trials showing efficacy of BoNT brands for other indications (e.g., anal fissure, benign prostatic hyperplasia) for which approval has not been sought.

The potency of branded BoNTs is measured by using a mouse protection assay, as LD_{50} mouse units (U) that cannot be directly compared. Therefore, there is no formula to predict reliably which dose of a different toxin brand is to be used in a patient who already has received a standard treatment with another brand. A rough estimate is that 1 Botox U corresponds to 3–5 Dysport U and to 50 Myobloc/Neurobloc U. However, the equivalence varies based on the indication, the injected site, and the dilution. A gross equivalence ratio is required for practical reasons, particularly when it is necessary to shift a patient from one preparation to another. A critical revision of the available evidence on the comparability of Botox and Dysport has concluded that there are relevant intrinsic differences not allowing identification of a consistent bioequivalence (11). The two BoNT-A products differ in potency and tendency to diffuse, and their equivalence presumably varies according to the body part injected. Botox and Dysport must be reconstituted first; all the toxins are diluted before being loaded into a syringe for injection. The dilution ratio, the syringe size, and the needle gauge affect the immediate diffusion of the toxin into the injected tissue. Later diffusion depends on lymphatic drainage, blood supply, and local barriers (e.g., muscle fascia, connective tissue).

TABLE 44.2
MANUFACTURED BRANDS OF BOTULINUM TOXIN

Brand Names	Botox	Dysport	Myobloc/Neurobloc[a]	Xeomin
Manufacturer	Allergan Inc (USA)	IPSEN (France)	Solstice (United States)	Merz (Germany)
Serotype	A	A	B	A
Specific activity	20 U/ng	40 U/ng	70–130 U/ng	167 U/ng
Packaging	100 U/vial	500 U/vial	2500; 5000; 10,000 U/vial	100 U/vial
Constituents and excipients	Human albumin; sodium chloride	Hemagglutinin; human albumin 20% solution; lactose	Hemagglutinin and non-hemagglutinin proteins; human albumin solution 0.05%; sodium chloride; sodium succinate (pH 5.6)	Human albumin; sucrose
Preparation	Lyophilized	Lyophilized	Solution (5000 U/ml)	Lyophilized
Storage of packaged product	−5°C	Room temperature	Room temperature	Room temperature
Storage once reconstituted	2°C–8°C for several hours	2°C–8°C for several hours	2°C–8°C for several hours (if diluted)	2°C–8°C for several hours

[a] Myobloc is the brand name in the United States, Neurobloc is the brand name in Europe.

Based on the available evidence, BoNT-A provides the first choice treatment for all approved indications, because of the best combination of efficacy, duration of action, and tolerability. BoNT-B has a shorter duration of action and more side effects than BoNT-A (12,13).

PRIMARY AND SECONDARY FAILURE

The success rate of BoNT treatments depends on a number of variables, such as the affected body site and the usage of instrumental guidance. Failures may occur at the beginning of a treatment sequence or after a number of successful treatments.

Primary failure is defined as a lack of clinical response (less than 25%) following the first and, at least, the second consecutive treatments. Secondary failure is defined as a lack of clinical response following further treatment in a patient who previously had adequate clinical improvement. A rate of 9.1% primary nonresponders and of 7.5% secondary nonresponders was observed in a series of 235 patients (14); these data are in keeping with those reported by other investigators (15). The main causes for primary failure are an incorrect diagnosis, inappropriate choice of injection sites, insufficient dose, and decreased potency due to mishandling of toxin during storage and transport. The main causes of secondary failures are changes in the treated condition (worsening or changes of pattern of muscle involvement in dystonia); technical reasons (wrong or suboptimal target choice, muscle identification, or BoNT delivery); and development of antibodies against BoNT.

There is agreement that the development of neutralizing antibodies can cause secondary failure; this possibility is now considered much rarer than originally estimated. Toxin-neutralizing antibodies have been detected mostly in subjects who underwent repeated treatments with high doses of BoNT-A for long periods (16,17). Practical issues that are thought to increase the probability to develop neutralizing antibodies are injection of high BoNT doses, frequent and repeated treatments (less than 2 to 3 months since previous injections), and high total amount of BoNT injected. Studies have shown that the heavy-chain fragment of the BoNT protein contains epitopes that are recognized by anti–heavy chain antibodies and by heavy-chain–primed T lymphocytes. The antibodies directed against the 150 kDa neurotoxin complex are the only ones that block the toxic function, whereas those directed against the light-chain or the nontoxin protein components of the complex are ineffective (2). The occurrence of nonneutralizing antibodies explains why enzyme-linked immunosorbent assay (ELISA), which has been long used to detect antibodies, is no longer applied. The finding of antibodies does not allow the assertion that they are neutralizing or directly responsible for secondary failure. Several methods are currently used to detect BoNT antibodies; however, the mouse protection assay is considered the most useful in the clinic, as it detects blocking antibodies (18). An alternative

to the biologic assays is to test immunoresistance simply by performing a standard injection of BoNT, which is known to produce a focal paralysis, into a superficial muscle that is easy to inject and to test in terms of strength and EMG activity, such as the extensor digitorum brevis (19), the frontalis, or the sternocleidomastoid (20). The presence of blocking antibodies, as determined by the mouse protection assay or clinical test, means that the patient will no longer respond to the serotype that induced the antibodies but may respond to another serotype. However, because of epitope homology among the various serotypes, the cross-reactivity also may result in immunoresistance to other serotypes. In a single case, it has been shown that plasma exchange can deplete antibodies against BoNT and restore efficacy to subsequent treatments.

BOTULINUM NEUROTOXINS IN MOVEMENT DISORDERS

Dystonia

Dystonia has been the first movement disorder treated with BoNT (21); it is dominated by repetitive and patterned muscle contractions producing abnormal movements and postures. Localized injections of BoNT provide a symptomatic remedy for primary and nonprimary forms of dystonia, as demonstrated by some randomized controlled studies and by a much larger cohort of uncontrolled studies.

Local treatment with BoNT is considered the first choice for cranial, cervical, and laryngeal dystonia. The overactive muscles can be identified by direct inspection or by EMG-guided targeting. As mentioned, direct inspection is usually sufficient to target a superficial muscle, such as most facial and some cervical muscles. EMG is necessary to target the sublingual, laryngeal, and most limb muscles; EMG-guided targeting also provides a second-line approach whenever improvement of muscle selection is needed (e.g., in cervical dystonia).

Blepharospasm and Cervical Dystonia

Although there are no high-quality, randomized, controlled efficacy data to support the use of BoNT in blepharospasm (22), several open-label studies on large series indicate that it is efficacious and safe and support its use (23). In keeping with this, the recently set guidelines of the European Federation of Neurological Societies provide a class-A recommendation that BoNT-A (or BoNT-B if there is immunoresistance to serotype A) is a first-line treatment for primary cranial (excluding oromandibular) or cervical dystonia (24). The efficacy in blepharospasm has been confirmed by more than 50 open-label studies (that have recruited more than 2500 patients), and by few controlled studies. Typically, a total dose of 20–40 Botox U, of 75–175 Dysport U, or of 2500 Myobloc/Neurobloc U is injected. The average latency from the time of injection to the onset of improvement varies from 3 to 5 days; a benefit lasting for 2 to 3 months was observed in almost all patients. Side effects occur in less than 10% of treated patients and include ptosis, blurring of vision, diplopia, tearing, and local hematoma. The side effects normally resolve in fewer than 2 weeks. Blepharospasm may differentially affect the 3 concentric parts of the orbicularis oculi muscle; inadequate results are obtained if the toxin is injected in the orbital portion of a patient suffering from a predominant involvement of the pretarsal portion of the muscle (25). Furthermore, some patients with a predominant pretarsal involvement may have prevalent tonic eye closure and difficulty in voluntarily opening the eyelids (so-called *eyelid opening apraxia*) (26). EMG shows loss of the normal reciprocal inhibition between the levator palpebrae and the pretarsal portion of the orbicularis oculi, with co-contraction. BoNT-A is helpful in these cases if injected in the pretarsal portion and at doses lower than those used in the orbital part of the muscle (27). Secondary resistance to BoNT is exceedingly rare in patients who receive long-term treatment for blepharospasm (14); this is probably because the doses are lower and they are injected less often than in cervical dystonia or spasticity.

Cervical dystonia is the most common focal primary dystonia. BoNT is the first-choice treatment for this condition. As a result of early intervention with BoNT in patients with cervical dystonia, permanent neck contractures are now rare and surgical treatment, such as selective peripheral denervation, is seldom necessary (28). In a 12-week controlled trial, Dysport was found to be more efficacious than trihexyphenidyl, providing an obvious clinical advantage with fewer adverse events (29). Seven randomized controlled trials on cervical dystonia, encompassing a total of 233 patients, demonstrated beneficial effects (between 66% and 80% of subjective improvement) of repeated BoNT-A injections (30). The average total dose injected is 100–300 Botox U, 400–800 Dysport U, or 10,000–20,000 Myobloc/Neurobloc U; however, the doses can vary considerably based on individual variability. Most studies report that the average latency of clinical action is approximately 1 week; the average duration of efficacy is approximately 12 weeks or 3 months for BoNT-A and 12 to 16 weeks for BoNT-B. There is agreement that BoNT is more efficacious (and for longer) for pain reduction than it is for the control of involuntary movements. The most severe side effect and dose-limiting factor is dysphagia, which occurred in up to 36% of patients in a study. Open-label studies allow for greater flexibility than do randomized controlled trials in choosing BoNT doses and selecting the muscles to inject. These studies report efficacy of BoNT in cervical dystonia and point to a better outcome than randomized controlled trials. In keeping with this, it has been demonstrated that fixed BoNT doses and rigid muscle selection criteria provide less than optimal results (31). Two studies compared the efficacy of Botox and Dysport in cervical dystonia. In one study, Dysport proved to be more efficacious than

Botox in controlling pain and dystonic movements; however, there was a higher incidence of transient side effects (dysphagia, dysphonia, asthenia, neck weakness), probably because Dysport diffuses more than Botox (32). Dysphagia and dysphonia are thought to be caused by diffusion of BoNT injected in the sternocleidomastoid muscle to the underlying pharyngeal and laryngeal muscles. Particular care should be taken to avoid diffusion outside the sternocleidomastoid toward deeper structures.

The occurrence of primary or secondary failure is substantial in cervical dystonia. In a long-term study on 106 patients with cervical dystonia, 20 discontinued treatment for primary or secondary resistance and 13 were lost at follow-up (possibly due to inadequate improvement) (14). Controlled trials also have shown the efficacy of BoNT-B in cervical dystonia either in drug-naïve patients or in patients resistant to BoNT-A. Transient dysphagia and neck weakness are the most frequent complications. Compared to BoNT-A, BoNT-B is more likely to produce dryness of the mouth, presumably because it is more potent in blocking cholinergic release in postganglionic parasympathetic fibers to the salivary glands. BoNT-F also has been tested in cervical dystonia; the duration of efficacy, however, is much shorter and lasts for approximately 8 weeks (10).

Other Focal Dystonias

Several open studies, including more than 900 patients, have established the efficacy and safety of BoNT-A in the treatment of adductor and abductor laryngeal dystonia (also known as *spasmodic dysphonia*) (33). BoNT is considered the treatment of choice for this disorder despite the fact than no controlled studies have been performed. Most investigators report a 75% to 95% improvement in voice symptoms and a significant improvement in the quality of life. Adverse events include transient breathy hypophonia, hoarseness, and occasionally dysphagia with aspiration.

Other focal forms of dystonia (specifically oromandibular and upper limb dystonia) are improved by BoNT treatment, but the outcome is less satisfactory than that observed in cranial, cervical, or laryngeal dystonia. The main reason is that these forms usually have a complex combination of muscle involvement, making it difficult to find a therapeutic scheme with an acceptable side-effect profile. EMG-guided muscle selection and targeting are necessary in these cases. In addition, upper limb dystonia often occurs as an occupational cramp in people performing skilled fine movements with the hand or arm (e.g., musician's cramp, writer's cramp); in such cases, it remains difficult to ensure the requested quality of voluntary movement, without weakness, following BoNT treatment. A controlled trial on the efficacy of BoNT-A in oromandibular dystonia reported improvement in less than 40% of patients. The efficacy of BoNT-A treatment in writer's cramp has been the object of 2 placebo-controlled studies. In the first study, 5 patients (59%) had a nonsignificant improvement; in the second study, speed and accuracy of pen control improved in 7 patients (35%). Overall, BoNT-A treatment has provided variable efficacy in upper limb dystonia, with an average improvement of 60% to 70% observed in some, but not all, patients (estimated from 35% to 85%). Pain is the symptom that most frequently improves after treatment, often independently of motor function.

In addition, BoNT-A has been injected successfully into the masseter and temporalis muscles of patients with jaw closure dystonia or into the submental muscles and the lateral pterygoid muscles of patients with jaw opening dystonia. This treatment may markedly improve the symptoms of temporomandibular joint syndrome and other oral and dental problems, as well as dysarthria and chewing difficulties. Transient swallowing difficulties have been reported to occur after fewer than 20% of treatment sessions.

Hemifacial Spasm

Hemifacial spasm (HFS) is a unilateral, involuntary, intermittent, and irregular clonic (rarely tonic) contraction of the muscles supplied by the facial nerve. Usually the disorder starts with involvement of the orbicularis oculi muscle, which is eventually followed by a gradual ipsilateral spread to other muscles, such as the frontalis, procerus, zygomaticus, risorius, levator labii superioris, depressor labii inferioris, depressor anguli oris, and platysma. This movement disorder has been attributed most frequently to the occurrence of a direct contact between the facial nerve and an ectopic anatomical structure (e.g., the basilar artery) or a pathological process (e.g., neurinoma of the acoustic nerve). Familial HFS also has been described. The spasm is thought to be generated by an axono-axonal ephaptic transmission and a hyperexcitable facial motor nucleus. Peripheral facial nerve injury or prior Bell's palsy also can result in HFS, sometimes combined with mild ipsilateral facial weakness. Although not a life-threatening condition, HFS may cause unremitting social disability, sometimes making the patients unable to sleep. HFS rarely subsides spontaneously, and most patients must pursue treatment for many years, if not throughout life. Several symptomatic drugs have been tried. Carbamazepine is the most common oral medication that has been reported to alleviate HFS in approximately 50% of patients. Surgical vascular decompression of the facial nerve (Janetta's technique) is a potentially curative approach successfully performed in a high percentage of patients (from 80% to 97%). Surgery has a recurrence rate of up to 25% during 2 years of follow-up; these patients are candidates for a second surgical treatment or can be treated with BoNT. In addition, a significant proportion of the patients may have permanent complications such as unilateral deafness or facial palsy.

Local infiltrations of BoNT-A are currently recognized as the symptomatic treatment of choice for HFS. At variance with surgery, this treatment must be repeated to provide continued benefit. It has been suggested that BoNT also acts at the level of the nucleus of the facial nerve, following retrograde axonal transport to the cell body. This possibility has been confirmed by radionuclide studies in animals, but has not been further substantiated in humans. The efficacy and safety of BoNT-A in HFS are rated class A (34). In most cases it is sufficient to inject the periocular region to obtain improvement either in the upper or in the lower facial nerve territories. Therefore, a stepped approach is warranted with a progressive adjustment of the treatment scheme. A prudent dose choice is particularly advisable in cases of postparalytic HFS. In most studies, the average total dose injected is between 12.5 and 60 Botox U or between 10 and 120 Dysport U. It is considered that a minimum threshold BoNT dose is necessary to obtain benefit, particularly for the first treatment, and that the following doses must be titrated up or down according to the patient's response.

The average latency of clinical efficacy varies from 2 to 6 days, and the overall response to treatment is satisfactory with a successful outcome in 66% to 100% of patients. The mean duration of efficacy is reckoned to vary between 10 and 28 weeks. The duration of efficacy has been reported to increase with repeated treatments, more rarely to decrease or to remain unchanged. It also has been observed that the duration of benefit is shorter in severe cases than in those of moderate severity. The treatment is well tolerated. Facial weakness is the most commonly reported side effect, occurring in 75% to 95% of cases, particularly when injections are placed in the mid or lower face. In most patients who receive BoNT injections only in the orbicularis oculi region, marked benefit is also observed in mouth spasm, probably due to local diffusion of the toxin. Ptosis may occur following injections into the orbicularis oculi, with an incidence variably reported from 0% to 53% of cases. Primary or secondary failures are uncommon in patients with HFS. It has been reckoned that the incidence of primary failure varies from 0.02% to 1.4% of patients per year, and that secondary failure is as low as 0.9% of patients per year.

Spasticity

Spasticity is defined as a velocity-dependent increase in tonic stretch reflexes that arises from abnormal processing of sensory afferent inputs to the spinal cord. It is a central disorder of muscle tone characterized by increased resistance of an initially passive limb to externally imposed joint motion. Increase in tone is a reflection of the loss of descending inhibitory (reticulospinal) influences, resulting in increased excitability of dynamic gamma (fusimotor) and alpha neurons. In addition to the increase in tone, other frequently present features are increased muscle stretch reflexes, occurrence of muscle spasms and clonus, weakness (spastic paralysis), and impairment of voluntary movements. The goal of treatment is to reduce spasticity and the associated positive phenomena without worsening weakness (paresis). In addition, reducing antagonist muscle overactivity may uncover functional residual power. The therapeutic approach to spasticity requires a comprehensive and multidisciplinary judgment of functional goals. BoNT therapy is just one tool in a complex treatment plan (including physical therapy, orthosis, medication, etc.) that has to be progressively adjusted based on changing priorities. The simplest treatment paradigm is adult-onset focal spasticity, which customarily can be treated just with BoNT; at the other end of the spectrum, childhood-onset spasticity requires complex and gradually tuned medical decisions.

BoNT has been used to treat spasticity associated with juvenile cerebral palsy, stroke, brain trauma, amyotrophic lateral sclerosis, and multiple sclerosis, in which functional impairment includes difficulty in coping with activities of daily living and in obtaining adequate nursing care (dressing, hygiene). Often there are associated disabling limb and trunk postures, decreased range of motion of the joints, and excoriation of the palm caused by incoercible digit flexion. Severe or longstanding spasticity may lead to contractures and joint ankylosis. As a result, early treatment with BoNT may prevent musculoskeletal deformities and other orthopedic problems later in life, thus avoiding surgical interventions.

BoNT is injected into spastic muscles to balance muscle forces across joints. The approved indications in most countries are upper or lower limb spasticity, regardless of the etiology, and lower limb spasticity due to cerebral palsy. The amount of toxin injected into individual muscles depends on the toxin brand, the muscle size, the number of nerve terminals located in the muscle, and the patient's weight (Tables 44.3 and 44.4). As a rule, the doses of BoNT used in spasticity are higher than those used to treat other movement disorders. The dose limits for the use of BoNT in the treatment of spasticity, particularly in children, have been the object of evaluation. It is believed that a maximum of 6 Botox U/kg (body weight) in each muscle with a maximum total dose of 19 Botox U/kg should be injected (35); a safe upper limit for Dysport is 30 U/kg, with a maximum total dose of 1000 U in a child (36); a safe starting dose for children treated with Neurobloc/Myobloc is considered to be 400 U/kg weight, to be gradually up-titrated, with a maximum total dose of 10,000 U (37).

Observational and controlled studies have shown that BoNT-A improves function and symptoms in adult patients with poststroke upper or lower limb spasticity. Controlled studies on patients with increased flexor tone in the upper limbs, due to a previous stroke, have reported improvement of tone and of other features (dressing ability, hygiene, limb posture, and pain) 6 to 12 weeks following treatment with BoNT-A. Not as much evidence of efficacy has been

TABLE 44.3

RECOMMENDED DOSES OF BOTULINUM NEUROTOXINS IN CHILDREN WITH SPASTICITY

Injection Site	Botox Dose (U/kg)	Dysport Dose (U/kg)
Upper Limb		
Subscapularis	1–2	
Teres major	2	
Latissimus dorsi	2	
Pectoralis complex	2	
Triceps		
Biceps	2	
Brachialis	2	
Brachioradialis	1	
Pronator teres	1	
Pronator quadratus	0.5–1	
Flexor carpi radialis	1–2	
Flexor carpi ulnaris	1–2	
Flexor digitorum superficialis	1–2	
Flexor digitorum profundus	1–2	
Flexor pollicis longus	0.5–1	
Opponens pollicis		
Adductor pollicis		
Lumbricals	0.5–1	
Lower limb		
Quadriceps mechanism	3–6	
Hamstrings	3–6	6.5
Hip adductor group	3–6	
Gastrocnemius	3–6	10
Soleus	2–3	11
Tibialis posterior	1–2	
Tibialis anterior	1–3	
Extensor hallucis longus	1–2	
Flexor hallucis longus	1–2	
Flexor digitorum longus	1–2	
Flexor digitorum brevis	1–2	

collected for the lower limbs (spastic toe, in particular). The efficacy of BoNT-B on poststroke upper limb spasticity has been observed in open-label series but not confirmed by controlled trials.

Cerebral palsy is a disorder caused by perinatal brain injury that combines athetosis, dystonia, and spasticity in various degrees. Involvement of the lower limbs is responsible for early difficulties in gait and balance control. In children the most dynamic development can be observed during the first 6 years of life; accordingly, all therapeutic interventions on spasticity or movement disorders in this early period of life are evaluated against the background of a dramatically changing and developing motor system. To achieve an optimal therapeutic result, early intervention is required to tap into the developmental potential of the child. The trials of BoNT in children with cerebral palsy are limited by the small sample size

TABLE 44.4

RECOMMENDED DOSES OF BOTULINUM TOXIN IN ADULTS WITH SPASTICITY

Injection Site	Botox Dose (U)	Dysport Dose (U)	Myobloc/Neurobloc Dose (U)
Upper limb			
Subscapularis	50–100	150–200	1000–3000
Teres major	25–100	60–150	1000–3000
Latissimus dorsi	50–150	200–400	2500–5000
Pectoralis complex	75–150	300–500	2500–5000
Triceps	50–200	300–500	2500–5000
Biceps	50–200	100–400	2500–5000
Brachialis	40–100	200–300	1000–3000
Brachioradialis	25–75	150–200	1000–3000
Pronator teres	25–75	80–100	1000–2500
Pronator quadratus	10–50	80–100	1000–2500
Flexor carpi radialis	25–100	100–200	1000–3000
Flexor carpi ulnaris	20–70	100–150	1000–3000
Flexor digitorum superficialis	20–60	150–300	1000–3000
Flexor digitorum profundus	20–60	150–200	1000–3000
Flexor pollicis longus	10–30	30–60	1000–2500
Opponens pollicis	5–25	30–60	500–1500
Adductor pollicis	5–25	30–60	500–2500
Lumbricals	10–50 per hand	30–80 per hand	1500–4500 per hand
Lower limb			
Quadriceps mechanism	50–200	500–1000	5000–7500
Hamstrings	50–200	350–500	2500–7500
Hip adductor group	200–400	150–500	5000–10,000
Gastrocnemius	50–250	250–1000	3000–7500
Soleus	50–200	200–500	2500–5000
Tibialis posterior	50–150	200–500	3000–7500
Tibialis anterior	50–150	250–400	2500–5000
Extensor hallucis longus	50–100	150–250	2000–4000
Flexor hallucis longus	25–75	100–200	1500–3500
Flexor digitorum longus	25–100	150–300	2500–5000
Flexor digitorum brevis	20–40	100–200	2500–5000

and differ for methodology and outcome measures; this is probably the main reason why the available evidence has not been considered sufficient to prove efficacy by some recent meta-analyses. Notwithstanding the evident methodological difficulties, efficacy and safety of BoNT-A in the management of lower limb spasticity associated with cerebral palsy have been reported in controlled trials. This remains, notwithstanding, an open field for future research.

Common side effects observed in patients with adult spasticity or cerebral palsy include muscle soreness, pain at injection site, skin rash, fatigue, excessive weakness, influenzalike symptoms, infection, and allergic reaction. Autonomic side effects (especially dry mouth) are particularly common following treatment with BoNT-B and are dose dependent.

BoNT also has been used to treat spasticity in patients with motor neuron disease or multiple sclerosis. There is insufficient documentation to assess the efficacy and safety of BoNT treatment in these conditions.

Tics

BoNT-A has been used to treat motor or vocal tics in patients with chronic tic disorders. The first anecdotal observations were made in patients with Gilles de la Tourette's syndrome with dystonic tics (38). BoNT-A treatment reduced the frequency and the intensity of tics and ameliorated the associated premonitory sensory urge; this benefit lasted for several weeks. A trial of BoNT on vocal tics also yielded symptomatic improvement and ameliorated quality of life. A controlled trial has confirmed the efficacy of BoNT-A for the treatment of simple motor tics with a 39% reduction in the number of tics per minute on a videotape segment (compared to a 6% increase in the placebo group) and a significant reduction of the urge score. The patients, however, did not report a comparable subjective benefit from this treatment.

It is possible to try BoNT-A in patients who have simple and repetitive motor or vocal tics, particularly if there is no indication to prescribe a systemic medication. More studies are required to identify the long-term outcome of BoNT in patients with tic disorders.

Tremor

BoNT-A has been used to treat hand tremor of different origin with controversial results. Evidence of efficacy has been collected by a controlled study, showing improvement of postural, but not kinetic, hand tremor in patients with essential tremor (39). This study showed limited functional improvement and dose-dependent hand weakness as a side effect. Improvement of voice tremor was demonstrated using objective acoustic measures in 3 of the 10 patients who received bilateral BoNT-A injections (2.5 Botox U in each tyroarytenoid muscle).

The evidence collected is insufficient to indicate a primary role of BoNT in the symptomatic treatment of tremors; however, there may be an indication for some specific forms of tremor that cannot be adequately treated with systemic drugs or deep-brain stimulation. BoNT can be helpful, particularly with atypical presentations or when tremor is confined to a few muscles.

Other Movement Disorders

Some cases of myoclonus have been treated with BoNT injections. Tinnitus associated with palatal myoclonus has proven to be responsive to BoNT-A (4–10 Botox U or 30–60 Dysport U) injected in the tensor veli palatini muscle (or alternatively in the levator veli palatini). Other forms of myoclonus treated with BoNT-A are secondary to head trauma or spinal cord infarcts.

Tardive dyskinesias are a potentially persistent and disabling abnormal involuntary movement disorder secondary to the use of neuroleptic drugs. Tardive dyskinesias can be relieved by BoNT (40). Their clinical features are variable, but most often they present as orolingual and facial movements that usually are choreic or dystonic in nature. Tardive dystonia responds as well as primary dystonia to BoNT treatment, depending on the sites affected. It may present as blepharospasm, cervical dystonia, or orolingual dystonia. In a series of 300 patients with cervical dystonia, 6% were of tardive etiology. The range of doses overlaps with that used to treat primary dystonia.

Anecdotal reports indicate that akathisia and bruxism also can be treated with BoNT injections. Bruxism is grinding, gnashing, or clenching of the teeth during sleep or situations that evoke tension or anxiety. In some cases, bruxism may be associated with contractures of the temporalis muscle. It occurs most often in the early part of the night, and it may be idiopathic or a symptom of several neurological conditions. BoNT-A has been reported to be effective in bruxism, and it has been confirmed that satisfactory clinical control is achieved regardless of the etiology. The dose range is wide (25–100 Botox U).

Fixed Contractures

Patients with movement disorders may present fixed contractures that usually involve one or more limb joints and can be proximal or distal. Primary contractures occur in fixed dystonia or in spasticity; secondary contractures occur in Parkinson's disease (PD) or other parkinsonian syndromes. The use of BoNT to treat fixed contractures is a logical approach if there is no evidence of joint deformities or of tendon or muscle abnormalities that might impede an increase in range of motion following chemical denervation of the muscle. In some patients, the appropriate muscle selection can be performed by assessing passive joint mobility under general anesthesia.

Children who could not open the mouth due to focal spasticity of the masticatory muscles have been treated with BoNT-A bilaterally in the masseter and the temporalis (150 and 75 Dysport U, respectively, on each side) with satisfactory outcome lasting for 90 days. BoNT injections are also performed to reduce neck, jaw, or limb contractures in the advanced stages of parkinsonian syndromes (see the following). The problem with a clenched fist is hand hygiene. The hand becomes dirty and the nails cut the palm skin. Dirtiness and infections create a vicious circle that can be resolved by treatment with BoNT. Clenched fist can be relieved by injections to allow cleaning and drying the hand, and lockjaw (or trismus) can be treated to help feeding or to warrant mouth hygiene.

COMPREHENSIVE APPROACH TO PARKINSONIAN PATIENTS

Patients with parkinsonian syndromes can benefit from BoNT treatment for many symptoms associated with their conditions. Some indications are better established than others, but, in principle, a BoNT consultation should be available at every clinic devoted to parkinsonian syndromes (Table 44.5). Motor symptoms that are treatable with BoNT include dystonia, contractures, and possibly freezing of gait; nonmotor symptoms include sialorrhea, bladder hyperreflexia, constipation, and benign prostatic hyperplasia.

Off-Period Dyskinesias

Dyskinesias are a frequent finding in PD patients. Focal dystonia is the most common off-period dyskinesia observed in PD patients and in patients with Parkinson's-plus syndromes, such as corticobasal ganglionic degeneration. *Off-period* dystonia is often painful: It may occur in the morning (early morning dystonia) or during the daily off periods. In addition, *on-period* dystonia is also observed. Dystonia involves more frequently the limbs, the neck, or the face, mainly the periocular muscles, and can be painful, particularly off-period foot dystonia (41). BoNT-A is efficacious for treating off-period dystonia in limb muscles that must be

TABLE 44.5

INDICATIONS FOR BoNT TREATMENT IN PARKINSONIAN SYNDROMES

Motor Symptoms

Dystonia

- Painful foot dystonia
- Outlet-type constipation
- Laryngeal and cervical dystonia
- Cranial dystonia

Contractures

- Upper limb
- Trismus

Freezing of gait

Nonmotor Symptoms

Sialorrhea

Urinary symptoms

- Bladder hyperreflexia
- Prostate hyperplasia

---

selected based on the coincidence of a dystonic cramp and localized pain. Dystonia and pain respond as well, but off-period pain unrelated to dystonia does not respond adequately. EMG guidance may be required to inject deep muscles, particularly in the legs. Off-period cervical dystonia, blepharospasm, and oromandibular dystonia can be managed the same way as the corresponding forms of primary dystonia, by administering a relatively low starting dose to be gradually up-titrated.

Parkinsonian syndromes are often complicated in the advanced disease stages by neck or head contractures. The flexed PD posture (camptocormia) may give rise to fixed antecollis. A typical feature of multiple system atrophy, instead, is disproportionate antecollis, in which a flexed neck makes contact with a nonflexed trunk; in addition, there is often a certain degree of torsion. In progressive supranuclear palsy (PSP), there may be an extended neck with fixed retrocollis. In late stages, parkinsonian syndromes may be complicated by contractures of the masseters that impede oral hygiene and chewing. Swallowing also may become impaired in later stages of parkinsonian syndromes. Little experience has been reported abouthandling such late-stage complications with focal injections of BoNT, but we have successfully treated a few such patients.

It has been postulated that freezing of gait, a parkinsonian symptom poorly responsive to dopaminergic medication, improves following treatment with BoNT-A. A woman affected by hemiparkinsonism was treated for leg dystonia with injections in the gastrocnemius–soleus and in the extensor hallucis longus (42). An open-label trial with BoNT-A (total dose: 100–300 Botox U) produced some improvement of freezing of gait that lasted for 2 to 12 weeks.

This observation could not be confirmed by later open-label or controlled studies with BoNT-A and BoNT-B. The pathophysiology of freezing of gait in PD is poorly known, and there is no solid basis for understanding the principles by which BoNT should be helpful for this symptom.

Constipation

Chronic constipation occurs in more than one-half of PD patients and is caused mainly by a reduction of motility in the colon caused by peripheral dysautonomia and aggravated by antiparkinsonian medication. In 13% of PD patients, constipation also is caused by inability to evacuate stools at straining, associated with lack of relaxation of the puborectalis muscle (so-called *outlet-type constipation* or *pelvic floor dysfunction*) (43). Failure of the puborectalis muscle to relax (or its paradoxical contraction instead) during efforts to defecate have been considered a focal dystonia (44). With an effort to evacuate the rectum, the puborectalis muscle normally relaxes to straighten the anorectal canal. If this does not occur appropriately, patients are unable to defecate and stools accumulate in the rectum. The diagnosis of outlet-type constipation is supported by the observation of an abnormal anorectal angle during attempted evacuation of barium paste and by EMG of the puborectalis muscle during straining. BoNT-A injections into the puborectalis muscle improve defecation in patients with outlet-type constipation. A total of 30–100 Botox U or 90–300 Dysport U can be injected in the puborectalis muscle during transrectal ultrasonography. The procedure is simple and well tolerated. The effects last for less than 2 months, and the treatment can be repeated. Side effects are mild and consist mainly of transient incontinence.

Sialorrhea

Sialorrhea (or drooling) is commonly associated with PD or other parkinsonian syndromes, due to a reduction of automatic swallowing in patients with akinesia. Injections of BoNT into the salivary glands reduce the production of saliva, thereby reducing drooling. Reduced swallowing also occurs in other neurological conditions, such as motor neuron disease, cerebral palsy, encephalopathies, or stroke; by contrast, increased salivation can be caused by lesions or by foreign bodies introduced into the mouth, by rabies infection, by mercurial poisoning, or as a side effect of antiepileptic drugs or of atypical neuroleptics (e.g., clozapine). Traditional treatments of sialorrhea (e.g., anticholinergics, surgical gland resection, transposition of the excretory ducts, tympanic neurectomy, or local irradiation) are poorly efficacious and often irreversible. The advantage of using BoNT is that the total dose and the injection schedule can be modified according to the patient's needs and to variations of antiparkinsonian medication.

The idea of injecting the parotid glands with BoNT-A to treat sialorrhea was first developed in patients with motor neuron disease. Further open-label studies have investigated the possibility of controlling drooling by injecting the parotid glands (which are responsible for 20% of total saliva production, at the time of eating) or the submandibular glands (which are responsible for 70% of basal saliva production). Doses injected in the parotid gland varied from 5–40 Botox U and from 20–150 Dysport U; Neurobloc was injected at a dose of 1000 U. In the submandibuar gland, instead, the doses varied among 5–15 Botox U, 80 Disport U, or 250 Neurobloc U. Treatment of the submandibular gland alone is much less effective than is the combined treatment.

The reported duration of benefit of BoNTs varies from 3 to 30 weeks. No systemic side effects have been reported. Some patients experienced local side effects, such as excessive dryness of the mouth, worsening of dysphagia, chewing difficulties, jaw dislocation, weakness of nearby muscles, local pain at injection site, or hematomas.

In all studies, BoNT injections were placed percutaneously, with or without ultrasound guidance. In one pilot study, direct retrograde injections were placed through Stenon's duct and the lingual ducts using a small catheter; this technique was associated with serious side effects and was not tolerated by the patients. Ultrasound guidance improves the efficacy and safety of treatments and helps to avoid vascular and nervous structures, as well as the masseter muscle.

To prevent the potential side effects of BoNT treatment, it is appropriate to start with low doses only in the parotid gland, depending on the amount of drooling. There is an inverse relation between the extent of drooling before treatment and the duration and degree of clinical benefit. If the starting dose is ineffective, higher doses can be tested in the parotid glands; then the submandibular glands also may be injected. The reduction of saliva flow can increase dental caries and requires adequate dental supervision if the treatment is prolonged over time.

BoNT-A also has been used to treat sialorrhea in children and secondary sialorrhea caused by clozapine administration. Overall, BoNT is effective, especially when administered in more than just one salivary gland. Up to two-thirds of patients subjectively experience a marked to moderate improvement following treatment, resulting in amelioration in their quality of life. The reduction of drooling can be estimated with objective measures and is often substantial; the duration of clinical improvement lasts as long as for dystonia and spasticity.

Micturition Disturbances

PD patients typically present an overactive urinary bladder causing urgency and other urinary symptoms. In PD, urethral sphincter function is preserved and incontinence is an uncommon late occurrence. More severe symptoms may occur in other parkinsonian syndromes. Moderate-to-severe bladder dysfunction, consisting of urgency, hesitancy,

nycturia, incontinence, or retention requiring catheterization, is observed in up to 80% of patients with multiple system atrophy. Urinary symptoms of multiple system atrophy result from a combination of detrusor hyperreflexia and urethral sphincter weakness. These pathophysiological features account for the early appearance of incontinence after an initial period of urgency due to bladder hyperreflexia. In later stages of multiple system atrophy, the detrusor may become hypotonic, producing difficulty of voiding and incontinence due to the associated sphincter weakness.

Detrusor overactivity occurs in patients with neurogenic bladder. These patients can benefit from BoNT injections into the detrusor muscle, even if they respond inadequately to (or do not tolerate) anticholinergic medication. In patients with spinal cord injuries, it has been observed that BoNT-A injection (200–400 Botox U or 300 Dysport U) into the detrusor muscle increases the maximum cystometric bladder capacity and decreases the maximum detrusor voiding pressure. This improvement could still be detected 36 weeks after treatment. Anticholinergic medication could be reduced or abolished. Similar observations have been performed in children with neurogenic detrusor overactivity due to myelomeningocele. Experience with lower urinary tract dysfunction can be extrapolated to the micturition disturbances observed in parkinsonian syndromes. No study has specifically addressed parkinsonian patients, but unpublished evidence suggests that micturition disturbance in PD is amenable to treatment with BoNT (Brisinda et al., unpublished observation).

BoNT-A is effective in reducing urethral resistance and facilitating voiding efficiency in patients with urinary retention caused by cauda equina lesions, peripheral neuropathy, detrusor failure, or nonrelaxing urethral sphincter. The injections are made into the external urethral sphincter (100 Botox U, 300 Dysport U). Patients who used to void by means of Valsalva's maneuver improved after treatment and gave up using a catheter. Similar results were achieved in patients with dysuria or urinary retention due to detrusor underactivity and a nonrelaxing urethral sphincter. These results have not been confirmed by other series, indicating that further studies are necessary.

Benign prostatic hyperplasia is a nonmalignant enlargement of the prostate that involves both the stroma and the epithelium of the gland. Symptoms related to benign prostatic hyperplasia add up to other urinary symptoms associated with PD and lead to incomplete bladder emptying or complications, such as acute urinary retention. Benign prostatic hyperplasia is rarely detected before age 40 years, and its incidence increases with age. More than half of the men are symptomatic in their sixties and as many as 90% are symptomatic in their seventies or eighties. Prostate resection is the gold-standard treatment for symptomatic benign prostatic hyperplasia; however, approximately 25% percent of patients who undergo surgical treatment do not have a satisfactory long-term outcome. Patients with urinary symptoms due to neurogenic bladder dysfunction have a worse outcome after surgery. Direct BoNT-A injections into the prostate have been the object of a 2003 randomized controlled study (45). A dose of 200 Botox U was injected in 2 sites, 1 in each lobe. BoNT-A caused a reduction in prostate volume, inducing a decrease in the mean residual urinary volume.

OTHER INDICATIONS FOR BOTULINUM NEUROTOXINS

Secretory Disorders

Secretory disorders may be primary conditions but often are secondary to neurological diseases, such as sialorrhea in PD or in motor neuron disease, gustatory sweating after facial nerve injuries, or pathological tearing in blepharospasm. It has long been recognized that botulism has autonomic effects that are more pronounced following intoxication with BoNT-B (46). The denervation of peripheral cholinergic parasympathetic terminals, and possibly also of terminals containing other neurotransmitters, is responsible for the autonomic symptoms.

Hyperhidrosis is an idiopathic condition of exaggerated sweat production by the eccrine glands that affects approximately 1% of the population. Hyperhidrosis may be focal or generalized. Focal hyperhidrosis affects the axillae, palms or soles, and, less commonly, the face. The disease may be primary (caused by overactivity of sweat glands in specific areas) or secondary to spinal cord injuries or neuropathies. There is class-A evidence on the efficacy of BoNT-A in axillary hyperhidrosis and class-B evidence for the treatment of palmar and gustatory sweating (47). The doses used in each axilla are 50 Botox U or 100–200 Dysport U; more limited experience suggests that the dose of BoNT-B is as low as 250 Myobloc or Neurobloc U or by contrast much higher (2000–4000 U). The treatment is safe, and clinical efficacy lasts for 6 months or more, yielding a substantial improvement in quality of life. The doses used for palmar hyperhidrosis are between 50 and 100 Botox U in each hand or 200–400 Dysport U, or 5000 Myobloc/Neurobloc U. BoNT-A is effective in treating palmar hyperhidrosis in more than 70% of cases, yielding a substantial improvement for up to 6 months. The treatment is safe, although mild weakness of hand muscles repeatedly has been reported with all BoNT serotypes, and dry mouth has been noted with BoNT-B. The injection technique is based on the performance of multiple intradermic injections in the hyperhidrotic areas revealed by Minor's iodine test; direct injections are painful and usually require local anesthesia. As an alternative, iontophoretic delivery, not requiring anesthesia, has been used.

Gustatory sweating (Frey syndrome) is due to the aberrant sprouting of cholinergic secretomotor fibers after a parotid gland lesion; this condition also can be associated with diabetes and other neuropathies. Sweating occurs on the cheek in response to salivation or expectancy of food. Several uncontrolled studies have documented the efficacy and safety of BoNT-A injection into the affected skin areas detected by means of Minor's iodine test. The doses used are between 16 and 80 Botox U, 70–175 Dysport U, or 6000–7500 Myobloc/Neurobloc U. The procedure is well tolerated.

Pathological Tearing and Rhinorrhea

Secretomotor fibers of the facial nerve innervate the lacrimal gland through the greater superficial petrosal nerve. Following injuries to the proximal part of the facial nerve, the visceromotor fibers, originally innervating the salivary glands, aberrantly connect to the fibers of the lacrimal gland. This causes a hyperlacrimation whenever the patient salivates (crocodile tears). Local BoNT-A injections directly into the lacrimal gland or around the eye may correct this symptom. The doses used are 20–30 Botox U or 20–75 Dysport U.

A potential therapeutic role in treating rhinitis and rhinorrhea was postulated following experimental studies on animals. One controlled and several uncontrolled clinical trials have been performed. The submucosal injection into the turbinates of 20–30 Botox U on each side relieves rhinorrhea, nasal obstruction, sneezing, and itching.

Substitute for Avoidable Surgical Procedures

BoNT can be employed to avoid unnecessary surgery and general anesthesia in patients who have medical conditions, such as rectocele, anal fissure, or prostatic diseases.

Rectocele is a hernia of the anterior rectal wall into the lumen of the vagina. It has been suggested that in some instances the rectocele is caused by failure of relaxation or paradoxical contraction of the puborectalis muscle occurring during attempted evacuation, but the reason for its establishment is not clear. Injections are performed on either side of the puborectalis muscle and in the anterior third of the external anal sphincter. A total dose of 30–100 Botox U is employed.

A chronic fissure is a painful cut or crack in the anal canal or anal verge that can be seen as the buttocks are parted; it is associated with a spasm of the internal anal sphincter and has been treated traditionally with internal sphincterotomy. Controlled and uncontrolled studies have provided class-A evidence on the efficacy of BoNT-A injections into the internal anal sphincter, with doses ranging from 10–40 Botox U or 100–150 Dysport U. The external anal sphincter also can be targeted. The procedure is safe, and fissure healing is usually attained following a single or a few repeated treatment sessions.

BoNT-A has been used to treat some common situations confronting the practicing urologist: nonbacterial prostatitis and benign prostatic hyperplasia. The injections are made directly into the prostate by ultrasound guidance, as previously reported.

CHRONIC PAIN DISORDERS

BoNT improves chronic pain disorders, probably due to a direct antinociceptive effect. Although the mechanism of the analgesic action of BoNT remains obscure, there is a growing body of evidence of a direct influence on pain that is not mediated by muscle spasm (5,48). In keeping with this hypothesis, it has been observed repeatedly that pain relief precedes motor improvement in patients with dystonia or spasticity. The antinociceptive action of BoNT may be mediated by neurotransmitters other than acetylcholine.

REFERENCES

1. Davis LE. Botulism. *Curr Treat Options Neurol* 2003;5:23–31.
2. Jankovic J. Botulinum toxin in clinical practice. *J Neurol Neurosurg Psychiatry* 2004;75:951–957.
3. Borodic GE, Ferrante R, Pearce LB, Smith K. Histologic assessment of dose-related diffusion and muscle fiber response after therapeutic botulinum A toxin injections. *Mov Disord* 1994;9:31–39.
4. Lange DJ, Rubin M, Greene PE, et al. Distant effects of locally injected botulinum toxin: a double-blind study of single fiber EMG changes. *Muscle Nerve* 1991;14:672–675.
5. Cui M, Khanijou S, Rubino J, Aoki KR. Subcutaneous administration of botulinum toxin A reduces formalin-induced pain. *Pain* 2004;107:125–133.
6. Curra A, Trompetto C, Abbruzzese G, Berardelli A. Central effects of botulinum toxin type A: evidence and supposition. *Mov Disord* 2004;19(suppl 8):S60–S64.
7. Hallett M. How does botulinum toxin work? *Ann Neurol* 2000;48:7–8.
8. Ceballos-Baumann AO, Sheean G, Passingham RE, Marsden CD, Brooks DJ. Botulinum toxin does not reverse the cortical dysfunction associated with writer's cramp: a PET study. *Brain* 1997;120:571–582.
9. Eleopra R, Tugnoli V, Rossetto O, Montecucco C, De Grandis D. Botulinum neurotoxin serotype C: a novel effective botulinum toxin therapy in human. *Neurosci Lett* 1997;224:91–94.
10. Chen R, Karp BI, Hallett M. Botulinum toxin type F for treatment of dystonia: long-term experience. *Neurology* 1998;51:1494–1496.
11. Sampaio C, Costa J, Ferreira JJ. Clinical comparability of marketed formulations of botulinum toxin. *Mov Disord* 2004;19(suppl 8):S129–S136.
12. Eleopra R, Tugnoli V, Quatrale R, Rossetto O, Montecucco C. Different types of botulinum toxin in humans. *Mov Disord* 2004;19(suppl 8):S53–S59.
13. Dressler D, Benecke R. Autonomic side effects of botulinum toxin type B treatment of cervical dystonia and hyperhidrosis. *Eur Neurol* 2003;49:34–38.
14. Hsiung GY, Das SK, Ranawaya R, Lafontaine AL, Suchowersky O. Long-term efficacy of botulinum toxin A in treatment of various movement disorders over a 10-year period. *Mov Disord* 2002;17:1288–1293.
15. Mauriello JA, Leone T, Dhillon S, Pakeman B, Mostafavi R, Yepez MC. Treatment choices of 119 patients with hemifacial spasm over 11 years. *Clin Neurol Neurosurg* 1996;98:213–216.
16. Hanna PA, Jankovic J, Vincent A. Comparison of mouse bioassay and immunoprecipitation assay for botulinum toxin antibodies. *J Neurol Neurosurg Psychiatry* 1999;66:612–616.
17. Borodic G, Johnson E, Goodnough M, Schantz E. Botulinum toxin therapy, immunologic resistance, and problems with available materials. *Neurology* 1996;46:26–29.
18. Kessler KR, Skutta M, Benecke R, German Dystonia Study Group. Long-term treatment of cervical dystonia with botulinum toxin A: efficacy, safety, and antibody frequency. *J Neurol* 1999;246:265–274.
19. Kessler KR, Benecke R. The EBD test: a clinical test for the detection of antibodies to botulinum toxin type A. *Mov Disord* 1997;12:95–99.
20. Dressler D, Bigalke H, Rothwell JC. The sternocleidomastoid test: an in vivo assay to investigate botulinum toxin antibody formation in humans. *J Neurol* 2000;247:630–632.
21. Frueh BR, Felt TH, Wojno TH, Musch DC. Treatment of blepharospasm with botulinum toxin: a preliminary report. *Arch Ophthalmol* 1984;102:1464–1468.
22. Costa J, Espirito-Santo C, Borges A, et al. Botulinum toxin type A therapy for blepharospasm. *Cochrane Database Syst Rev* 2005; CD004900.
23. Balash Y, Giladi N. Efficacy of pharmacological treatment of dystonia: evidence-based review including meta-analysis of the effect of botulinum toxin and other cure options. *Eur J Neurol* 2004;11:361–370.
24. Albanese A, Barnes MP, Bhatia KP, et al. EFNS guideline on diagnosis and treatment of primary (idiopathic) dystonia and dystonia plus syndromes: report of an EFNS Task Force on Dystonia. *Eur J Neurol.* 2006;13:493–494.
25. Albanese A, Bentivoglio AR, Colosimo C, Galardi G, Maderna L, Tonali P. Pretarsal injections of botulinum toxin improve blepharospasm in previously unresponsive patients. *J Neurol Neurosurg Psychiatry* 1996;60:693–694.
26. Krack P, Marion MH. "Apraxia of lid opening," a focal eyelid dystonia: clinical study of 32 patients. *Mov Disord* 1994;9:610–615.
27. Aramideh M, Ongerboer de Visser B, Brans WM, Koelman HT, Speelman JD. Pretarsal application of botulinum toxin for treatment of blepharospasm. *J Neurol Neurosurg Psychiatry* 1995;59:309–311.
28. Krauss JK, Toups EG, Jankovic J, Grossman RG. Symptomatic and functional outcome of surgical treatment of cervical dystonia. *J Neurol Neurosurg Psychiatry* 1997;63:642–648.
29. Brans JW, Lindeboom R, Snoek JW, et al. Botulinum toxin versus trihexyphenidyl in cervical dystonia: a prospective, randomized, double-blind controlled trial. *Neurology* 1996;46:1066–1072.
30. Jankovic J. Treatment of cervical dystonia with botulinum toxin. *Mov Disord* 2004;19(suppl 8):S109–S115.
31. Koller W, Vetere-Overfield B, Gray C, Dubinsky R. Failure of fixed-dose, fixed muscle injection of botulinum toxin in torticollis. *Clin Neuropharmacol* 1990;13:355–358.
32. Ranoux D, Gury C, Fondarai J, Mas JL, Zuber M. Respective potencies of Botox and Dysport: a double blind, randomised, crossover study in cervical dystonia. *J Neurol Neurosurg Psychiatry* 2002;72:459–462.
33. Blitzer A, Brin MF, Stewart CF. Botulinum toxin management of spasmodic dysphonia (laryngeal dystonia): a 12-year experience in more than 900 patients. *Laryngoscope* 1998;108:1435–1441.
34. Jost WH, Kohl A. Botulinum toxin: evidence-based medicine criteria in blepharospasm and hemifacial spasm. *J Neurol* 2001;248(suppl 1):21–24.
35. Koman LA, Paterson SB, Balkrishnan R. Spasticity associated with cerebral palsy in children: guidelines for the use of botulinum A toxin. *Paediatr Drugs* 2003;5:11–23.
36. Bakheit AM, Severa S, Cosgrove A, et al. Safety profile and efficacy of botulinum toxin A (Dysport) in children with muscle spasticity. *Dev Med Child Neurol* 2001;43:234–238.
37. Schwerin A, Berweck S, Fietzek UM, Heinen F. Botulinum toxin B treatment in children with spastic movement disorders: a pilot study. *Pediatr Neurol* 2004;31:109–113.
38. Jankovic J. Botulinum toxin in the treatment of dystonic tics. *Mov Disord* 1994;9:347–349.
39. Brin MF, Lyons KE, Doucette J, et al. A randomized, double masked, controlled trial of botulinum toxin type A in essential hand tremor. *Neurology* 2001;56:1523–1528.
40. Truong DD, Hermanowicz N, Rontal M. Botulinum toxin in treatment of tardive dyskinetic syndrome. *J Clin Psychopharmacol* 1990;10:438–439.
41. Pacchetti C, Albani G, Martignoni E, Godi L, Alfonsi E, Nappi G. "Off" painful dystonia in Parkinson's disease treated with botulinum toxin. *Mov Disord* 1995;10:333–336.

42. Giladi N, Kao R, Fahn S. Freezing phenomenon in patients with parkinsonian syndromes. *Mov Disord* 1997;12:302–305.

43. Albanese A, Brisinda G, Bentivoglio AR, Maria G. Treatment of outlet obstruction constipation in Parkinson's disease with botulinum neurotoxin A. *Am J Gastroenterol* 2003;98:1439–1440.

44. Mathers SE, Kempster PA, Swash M, Lees AJ. Constipation and paradoxical puborectalis contraction in anismus and Parkinson's disease: a dystonic phenomenon? *J Neurol Neurosurg Psychiatry* 1988;51:1503–1507.

45. Maria G, Brisinda G, Civello IM, Bentivoglio AR, Sganga G, Albanese A. Relief by botulinum toxin of voiding dysfunction due to benign prostatic hyperplasia: results of a randomized, placebo-controlled study. *Urology* 2003;62:259–264.

46. Jenzer G, Mumenthaler M, Ludin HP, Robert F. Autonomic dysfunction in botulism B: a clinical report. *Neurology* 1975;25:150–153.

47. Naumann M, Jost W. Botulinum toxin treatment of secretory disorders. *Mov Disord* 2004;19(suppl 8):S137–S141.

48. Mense S. Neurobiological basis for the use of botulinum toxin in pain therapy. *J Neurol* 2004;251(suppl 1):I1–I7.

49. Hallett M. One man's poison: clinical applications of botulinum toxin. *N Engl J Med* 1999;341:118–120.

Surgery for Parkinson's Disease and Hyperkinetic Movement Disorders

45

Joachim K. Krauss   *Robert G. Grossman*

Neurosurgical treatment options for Parkinson's disease (PD) and other movement disorders have become an integral part of contemporary therapeutic concepts. The continuous progress in movement disorders surgery parallels the advances being made in neurophysiology, neurobiology, neurology, neurosurgery, neuroimaging, and medical technology. Symptomatic and functional benefit can be achieved today at a low risk in appropriately selected patients. Current models of functional basal ganglia organization allow better understanding of the pathophysiology underlying movement disorders and also of the effects of functional stereotactic surgery (1–3). New insights in functional anatomy have led to the introduction of such targets as the subthalamic nucleus (STN), which has become the most frequently used target for treatment of PD (4,5).

Various surgical procedures are available for the treatment of PD and hyperkinetic movement disorders. The goal of functional stereotactic surgery is to modulate the activity in the basal ganglia circuitry. Deep-brain stimulation (DBS) has replaced radiofrequency lesioning more and more. With regard to its adaptability and its reversibility, it allows explorations of new indications at a low risk. In particular, its risk profile is clearly more favorable when compared to the high incidence of side effects associated with bilateral ablative procedures. Neurotransplantation differs fundamentally from functional stereotactic neurosurgery, in the way that it attempts to repair the primary defect underlying the development of a movement disorder such as PD. Chronic DBS and neurotransplantation are dealt with elsewhere in this volume. This chapter surveys the basic principles of movement disorders surgery, the results of ablative functional stereotactic neurosurgery, central and peripheral denervation procedures, and intrathecal drug therapy.

DEVELOPMENT OF MOVEMENT DISORDERS SURGERY

Before the basal ganglia were recognized as a target for surgical treatment of movement disorders, various operations were performed on the peripheral and central nervous systems and on other organs (6,7). Lesions in the sensory systems were made by posterior rhizotomy, posterior or anterolateral cordotomy, sympathetic ramisectomy, and ganglionectomy. Most procedures, however, directly targeted the motor system and involved excision of the motor cortex, ablation or undercutting of the premotor cortex, and destruction of the pyramidal tract at various levels (e.g., by subcortical pyramidotomy, mesencephalic pedunculotomy, or high cervical cordotomy). In general, alleviation of the movement disorder was achieved only at the cost of hemiparesis. Other side effects, such as delayed appearance of spasticity, were frequent, and long-term relief was rare in patients with preserved motor function.

Surgery of the basal ganglia circuitry for treatment of movement disorders was not performed until Meyers, in 1939, pioneered his innovative techniques (8). Previously, it was generally thought that such an approach would be impossible because it might result in enduring coma. Among others, Dandy had hypothesized that vegetative centers and the center of consciousness were located in the basal ganglia. Meyers performed such techniques as transventricular section of pallidothalamic pathways, extirpation of the head of the caudate nucleus and the globus pallidus pars interna (GPi). Parkinsonian symptoms were improved in about 60% of patients; however, these procedures were burdened with high morbidity and a mortality rate of 12% (9). The next step in the development of functional neurosurgery for movement disorders included electrocoagulation of the pallidofugal pathways via subfrontal or transsylvian approaches (10).

The introduction of stereotactic neurosurgery revolutionized the surgical treatment of movement disorders. The first stereotactic frame was constructed in 1908 by the neurosurgeon Horsley and the mathematician Clarke for use in animal studies to investigate cerebellar physiology. It was not until 1947, however, that this technique was applied to humans. Spiegel and Wycis performed dorsomedial thalamotomies and pallidotomies with the goal to modify "afferent stimuli and emotional reactions" in patients with choreic and athetotic syndromes (11,12). Subsequently, the method also was used in PD patients by neurosurgeons and neuroscientists worldwide. The first ventrolateral thalamotomy for treatment of parkinsonian motor symptoms was performed in 1952 by Mundinger in Freiburg, Germany, in collaboration with Hassler and Riechert (13). Erroneously, the development of stereotactic pallidotomy and thalamotomy have been attributed to Cooper. In 1952, Cooper accidentally severed the anterior choroidal artery during pedunculotomy for parkinsonian tremor. Postoperative improvement of the tremor, however, which was thought to be related to pallidal infarction, led him to the use of anterior choroidal artery ligation and only later to pallidotomy. Likewise, when Cooper reported the unexpected striking improvement when a planned pallidal lesion was misdirected to the thalamus in the late 1950s, thalamotomies had already been done in many other centers.

In the early period of functional stereotactic surgery, lesions were created using leucotomes, injection of alcohol and procain oil, inflation of balloons, ultrasound, implantation of radioactive pellets, cryosurgery, and electrocoagulation. Later, all these techniques were almost completely replaced by radiofrequency lesioning. In the early 1960s and mid-1960s, most surgeons abandoned pallidotomy in favor of thalamotomy for the treatment of movement disorders. The subthalamic region was approached via campotomy and via lesions directed to the zona incerta (14). It was estimated that by 1965, more than 25,000 functional stereotactic procedures for parkinsonism had been performed worldwide. The number of functional stereotactic operations, however, dropped rapidly after the introduction of levodopa in clinical routine. Subsequently, in the late 1970s and 1980s only a few centers continued to perform thalamotomies, particularly for treatment of tremor and hyperkinetic movement disorders.

The interest in surgical therapy arose again when the limitations of levodopa therapy became apparent in PD, in particular the gradual loss of efficacy with development of motor fluctuations and dyskinesias. Increased attention was focussed on surgery for PD when the first results on autologous transplantation of adrenal medullary tissue to the striatum were reported in 1987. The rediscovery of pallidotomy by Laitinen had a major impact on the further development of functional stereotactic surgery for movement disorders (15). Scientific advancements have been made at a notably fast pace since the beginning of the 21st century. Although DBS has become a routine treatment for many conditions, few studies compare the different options available.

PRINCIPLES OF MOVEMENT DISORDERS SURGERY

Functional Anatomy and Targets

The current model of basal ganglia organization is based primarily on animal models of neurodegenerative diseases and is explained in detail elsewhere in this volume. The model allows for explanation of the occurrence of both parkinsonism and hyperkinetic movement disorders. A major principle of basal ganglia organization is that striatal projections are segregated into discrete pools on the basis of their projection targets. At present, it is thought that striatal output to the GPi involves both a direct pathway that is GABAergic and an indirect pathway via the globus pallidus pars externa (GPe) and the STN. The STN is thought to play a pivotal role by regulating the output of the GPi. Although this simplified model has been criticized often, it explains at least partially the effect of basal ganglia surgery. The GPi has an inhibitory GABAergic projection to the ventrolateral (VL) thalamic nucleus, which is also referred to as the *motor thalamus*. Until recently, Hassler's nomenclature subdividing the VL into the nucleus ventralis anterior (V.o.a) and nucleus ventralis posterior (V.o.p) was the terminology most commonly used (16,17). The nucleus ventralis intermedius (V.im) is located just posteriorly to the V.o.p. The pallidofugal fibers reach the thalamus via the ansa and the fasciculus lenticularis and are directed to the V.o.a, while the V.im receives afferents from dentatothalamic pathways. In 2001, a major reclassification of thalamic nuclei was proposed by Jones (18). This new terminology allows for unification of the different nomenclatures used thus far in monkeys and humans (Fig. 45.1). According to Jones, Hassler's V.o.p is a region in which islands and fingers of cells proper to the V.o.a and the V.im interdigitate. Therefore, it has been suggested that V.o.p has no standing as an independent nucleus, and an equivalent name in monkey and human would not be needed. On these grounds, it has been proposed to rename Hassler's V.o.a as the anterior ventrolateral nucleus (VLa) and to rename the V.im as the posterior ventrolateral nucleus (VLp). The subthalamic area is composed of the zona incerta, the STN, and white matter containing the fields of Forel (Fig. 45.2). The STN is connected to the GPe and the GPi via pathways that traverse the internal capsule. The zona incerta is the ventral extension of the nucleus reticularis thalami. Its rostral part is situated just dorsal to the STN. The fasciculus lenticularis runs in Forel's field H2 between the STN and the zona incerta, and then curves upward in Forel's field H to form the fasciculus thalamicus in Forel's field H1 before it enters the VLa.

The choice of the target structure depends on the presentation of the patient with a specific movement disorder but also on the surgeon's preference. The range of targets used today is much more limited than before. In summary, contemporary targets for treatment of movement disorders include the V.im (or VLp, according to Jones) for tremor, the GPi and the STN for parkinsonian symptoms, and the GPi for dystonia and ballism.

Thalamic subnuclei show a clear somatotopic organization. The concept of Hassler's thalamic homunculi is still

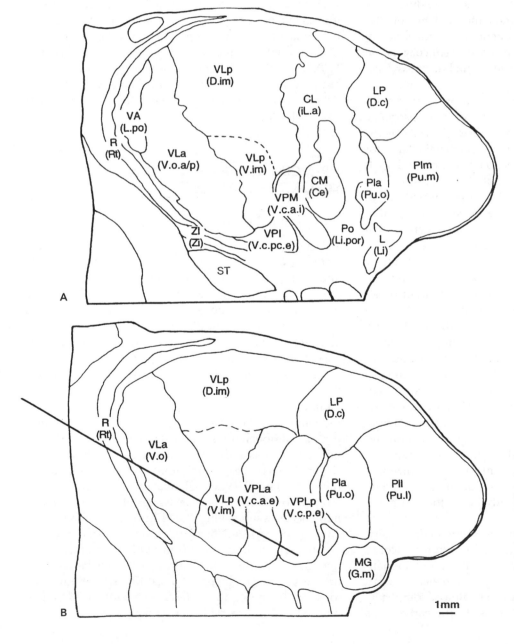

Figure 45.1 Camera lucida tracings of parasagittal sections of a human thalamus. Nomenclature of the thalamic nuclei according to Jones, with the original names of Hassler in parentheses (**A** is medial to **B**). (From Jones EG. Morphology, nomenclature, and connections of the thalamus and basal ganglia. In: Krauss JK, Jankovic J, Grossman, RG, eds. *Surgery for Parkinson's disease and movement disorders.* Philadelphia: Lippincott Williams & Wilkins, 2001:24–47, with permission.)

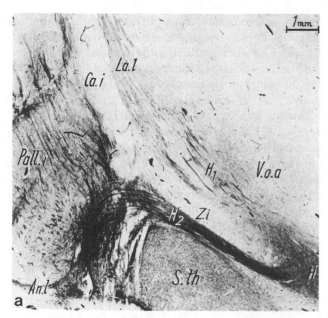

Figure 45.2 Morphology of the subthalamic area. Coronal section through the anterior thalamus of an 8-month-old fetus. An.l, ansa lenticularis; Ca.i, internal capsule; H, H1, and H2, Forel's fields; La.l, lamella lateralis thalami; Pall.i, globus pallidus pars interna; S.th, subthalamic nucleus; V.o.a, ventralis oralis anterior; Z.i, zona incerta. (From Hassler R, Mundinger F, Riechert T. *Stereotaxis in Parkinson syndrome.* Berlin, Heidelberg, New York: Springer, 1979, with permission.)

basically valid today. The leg is presented more lateral in the thalamic VLp than the arm. The x coordinate in a patient with tremor undergoing thalamic surgery, therefore, will differ depending on whether or not the patient also has prominent tremor of the leg. The somatotopy of the GPi is less clear than that of the thalamic VLp (19,20). With microelectrode techniques, investigators have shown that one cell often may respond to movement of multiple joints. Some investigators have found that most of the neurons in patients with PD responsive to passive manipulation or active movements of the limbs were in the lateral portion of the GPi with the upper limb and the axial body presented more frequently further lateral and in the ventral one-third, and the lower limb in the dorsal one-third. There is no clear somatotopy in the vertical axis for the distribution of tremor-related cells. Microelectrode recording studies in the STN have shown that all neurons with sensorimotor responses were in the dorsolateral region of the STN with arm-related neurons lateral to leg-related neurons, and presentation of the oromandibular musculature in the middle of the sensorimotor region, ventral to the arm and leg (21).

Techniques in Functional Stereotactic Neurosurgery

The principles of stereotactic surgery include the acquisition of data from various imaging modalities and their transfer to a Cartesian coordinate system (22). In functional stereotactic surgery, these coordinates are generally referenced to the stereotactic frame that is rigidly fixed to the patient's head. *Stereotaxis* has been derived from the Greek, meaning *three-dimensional arrangement*. The Cartesian coordinate system implies that any point in space can be determined by 3 coordinates (x, y, and z), which are defined with regard to 3 intersecting orthogonal planes. These 3 planes—the abscissa, ordina, and applicata—intersect at 1 point that is commonly defined as 0 (zero). By convention, the x coordinate defines the distance to the midsagittal plane (right to left), the y coordinate defines the distance to a reference point along the rostrocaudal axis (anterior to posterior), and the z coordinate defines the distance to a reference point in the coronal plain (superior to inferior). Because stereotactic positive-contrast ventriculography was the method of choice in functional stereotactic neurosurgery long before the advent of contemporary imaging methods, it generally has been accepted that it refers the coordinates of a target in the basal ganglia or in the thalamus to anatomic landmarks in the third ventricle. Commonly, the interconnecting line between the anterior commissure (AP) and the posterior commissure (PC), the intercommisural line, is used for this purpose. The general acceptance of the AC and PC as landmarks has resulted in the generation of stereotactic atlases, such as the Schaltenbrand-Bailey atlas and its newer edition, the Schaltenbrand-Wahren atlas (23,24). These atlases contain series of myelin-stained brain sections 1–4 mm thick in each of the 3 orthogonal planes. The atlas coordinates should be corrected in patients with shorter or longer intercommissural lines or widening of the third ventricle. Because these coordinates do not account for individual spatial variability, intraoperative physiologic confirmation and refinement of the target are necessary (25).

Functional stereotactic neurosurgery for treatment of movement disorders is performed using local anesthesia with few exceptions. Communication with the patient and neurologic assessment are essential during neurophysiologic confirmation of the target. Usually, any drugs for treatment of the movement disorders are withheld preoperatively. In almost all centers, PD patients are operated in the off state. This allows the surgeon to more easily monitor the efficacy of stimulation on such parkinsonian target symptoms as rigidity, tremor, and bradykinesia, which may guide the decision about whether an electrode should be repositioned or a lesion should be enlarged or additional lesions should be made. Furthermore, dyskinesias that can be provoked during target definition are considered useful hints at good surgical outcome both in the GPi and the STN. Careful intraoperative and perioperative monitoring of the patient's blood pressure is helpful for immediately recognizing and counteracting hypertension and hypotension. Monitored care by an anesthesiologist experienced in functional stereotactic surgery has proved to be valuable in our practice.

It is important when attaching the frame to the patient's head to avoid any rotation or tilt of the head relative to the frame axes. Several methods are available for stereotactic imaging. For decades, stereotactic ventriculography was used to identify the AC and the PC. To avoid parallax effects, ventriculography was ideally performed with fixed X-ray tubes with long projection lines (teleradiology). Today, ventriculography has been replaced by stereotactic computed tomography (CT) or magnetic resonance imaging (MRI). It has been demonstrated that CT- and MRI-guided localization of the commissures is accurate and even superior to ventriculography (26–28). CT is considered the most geometrically accurate imaging modality for stereotactic localization. CT imaging, compared to MRI, has the relative disadvantage of being inferior in the display of anatomic details. The geometric accuracy of magnetic resonance scanning can be comparable to that of CT scanning when gradient and magnetic field inhomogeneities are corrected. Under optimal conditions, the average difference in size between CT and MRI stereotactic coordinates of external fiducials, intracerebral target points, and anatomic landmarks is in the order of 1 pixel. Both with CT and MRI stereotactic imaging, it is important to obtain 1 mm or at least 2 mm axial scans through the third ventricle and the basal ganglia region. The imaging data can be transferred to a workstation where the axial scans are displayed simultaneously with coordinated reformatted sagittal and coronal images. The simultaneous and multiplanar display allows visualization and accurate confirmation of the localization of the commissures in

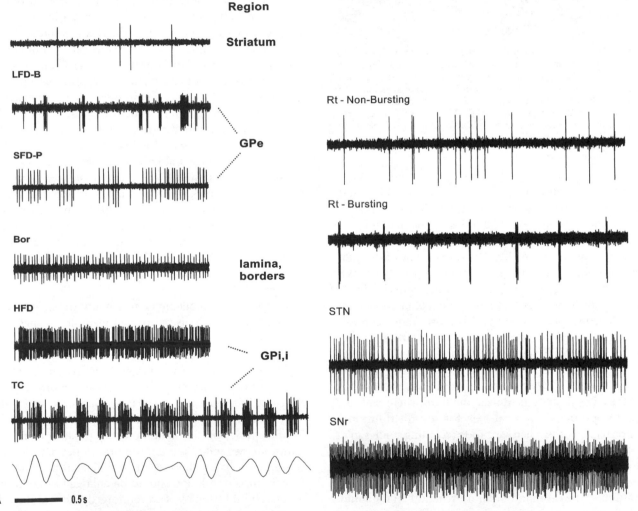

Figure 45.3 Microelectrode recording in Parkinson's disease surgery. **A:** Typical recordings of "signature" cell types in segments of globus pallidus. The trace below TC is the accelerometer attached to the dorsum of the contralateral hand. Bor, border cell; HFD, high-frequency discharge; LFD-B, low-frequency discharge with bursts; SFD-B, slow-frequency discharge with pauses; TC, tremor cell. **B:** Typical recordings of cell types encountered in trajectories targeting the subthalamic nucleus. The traces are 2 seconds in duration. Rt, thalamic reticular nucleus; STN, subthalamic nucleus; SNr, substantia nigra pars reticulata. (From Hutchison WD. Techniques of microelectrode recording in movement disorders surgery. In: Krauss JK, Jankovic J, Grossman, RG, eds. *Surgery for Parkinson's disease and movement disorders.* Philadelphia: Lippincott Williams & Wilkins, 2001:24–47, with permission.)

3 planes. Misalignment of the intercommissural line with regard to the 3 orthogonal axes of the stereotactic frame must be considered and corrected appropriately (29).

The basal ganglia and thalamic targets usually are reached through a frontal approach. The trajectory can be determined on the stereotactic imaging data to avoid the ventricles or cortical vessels. The cranial opening may be made with a twist drill or a burr hole. The dura is coagulated and incised in a cruciate fashion. A guiding cannula that allows passing of microelectrodes, macroelectrodes, and DBS electrodes is inserted into the brain at the crown of a gyrus. Microelectrode recording is an efficient and elegant technique, and it offers a unique opportunity for the electrophysiologic study of the basal ganglia. Microelectrode recording being necessary to enhance the precision and safety of targeting thalamic and basal ganglia nuclei in movement disorders surgery is a matter of debate. In our experience, microelectrode recording is useful in clinical routine, and it adds little operative time. Most microelectrodes have an impedance from 0.3 to 1.5 Mohm. Microelectrode recording allows detailed mapping of the target region and the trajectory to the target region (19–21,30). Furthermore, by active and passive movements of the patient's extremities, the sensorimotor regions of the target can be refined. We think that microelectrode recording is particularly helpful in GPi and STN surgery (Fig. 45.3). It allows precise definition of the nuclear borders. The number of pathways with a microelectrode depends on the preference of the surgeon and the quality of the signals. A technical variant is to obtain 5 parallel trajectories with electrode tips spaced by 1.5 to 2 mm. Microelectrode recording may be supplemented by microstimulation via the electrodes in situ. This technique may be used to determine thresholds for motor responses or stimulation of structures in the immediate vicinity of the electrode tip.

The target also can be confirmed and further refined with macrostimulation via the lesion-making electrode or via the DBS electrode. Upon insertion of the macroelectrode, a so-called *setzeffekt* consisting of temporary improvement of the movement disorder of the contralateral extremity may occur. This effect is most pronounced in thalamic surgery for tremor and may result in complete and prolonged disappearance of contralateral tremor. Macrostimulation is used to assess thresholds both for intrinsic responses (effects within the target) and extrinsic responses (effects on neighboring structures). Macrostimulation is typically performed at frequencies of 5 Hz and then 100 or 130 Hz. The voltage is increased incrementally from 0 V until a response is elicited. The occurrence of intrinsic and extrinsic responses is monitored and a protocol is established. According to the responses obtained, the electrode may be relocated and the stimulation may be repeated at the new choosen target.

Today, the technique of thermocontrolled radiofrequency lesioning is used almost exclusively. Lesioning electrodes are available in many different sizes and configurations. Radiofrequency electrodes used in movement disorders surgery most commonly have a diameter of 1–2 mm and a 1–4 mm uninsulated tip. Numerous variations among different surgeons are applied to how the lesions in thalamotomy or pallidotomy are created. We prefer to space lesions 1.5–2 mm apart along the same trajectory by subsequently withdrawing the electrode in pallidotomy. The lesions are created with the temperature controlled at 75°C for 60 seconds. However, other temperatures and times also are used. It is pivotal during lesioning to monitor the strength and mobility of the patient's extremities, speech, and visual fields. For the STN, smaller lesioning electrodes are useful. The predictability of radiofrequency lesions has been shown in experimental lesioning studies in egg white. However, although the lesion may be predicted accurately by such models, there is some variation in the size of the final lesion in clinical functional stereotactic surgery. The technical aspects of chronic DBS are discussed elsewhere in this volume.

PARKINSON'S DISEASE

Thalamotomy for Parkinson's Disease

Thalamotomy has been the mainstay in movement disorders surgery for PD for decades (31–33). It is performed today only rarely. Significant improvement or abolition of contralateral tremor is usually achieved in 80% to 90% of patients with VLp thalamotomy (Fig. 45.4). In general, if there is no relapse of tremor in the first few months, the effect of thalamotomy is long lasting and it may persist even with progression of the disease. Lesions that extend into the V.o.a (or the VLa according to Jones) also have an effect against rigidity. There is no effect on bradykinesia,

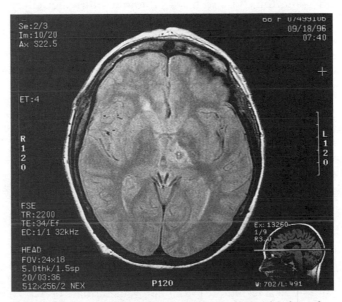

Figure 45.4 Axial FSE 2200/34 MR scans obtained 2 days after a left-sided VLp thalamotomy. Right-sided tremor at rest and intention tremor were completely abolished in this 68-year-old woman with Parkinson's disease and essential tremor.

however, and axial symptoms are also not improved. Contralateral dyskinesias often are eliminated by thalamotomy (34). Other studies have demonstrated that PD patients develop fewer or no dyskinesias contralateral to previous thalamotomy (31). When the results of unilateral thalamotomy were evaluated in a blinded fashion at a mean follow-up of 10.9 years, significant reduction of upper extremity tremor was observed contralateral to the stereotactic lesion when compared to the ipsilateral extremity (35). Usually there is no significant reduction of levodopa medication or total equivalent dose. Side effects of unilateral thalamotomy from 0.4% to 23% have been reported in a wide range of patients (36). Complications generally resolve rapidly during the postoperative period. Persistent side effects may include hemiparesis, facial weakness, paresthesias, numbness, and delayed onset of dystonia. The rate of complications may vary enormously from team to team.

In the past, bilateral thalamotomies were done either in the same operative session or were staged. Bilateral abolition or improvement of tremor and rigidity was achieved in about 70% of patients, but considerable variations were reported. The major problem with bilateral thalamotomy is the high occurrence of side effects. In particular, dysarthria has been described to be worsening in 18% to 60% of patients even when done within an interval of several months (36). Chronic DBS has been shown to be considerably safer in bilateral surgery.

With the typical rest tremor of PD, there often is only little postoperative improvement in functional disability. Nevertheless, patients may benefit remarkably in social performance. Nowadays, thalamic surgery is considered to be indicated only in a minority of PD patients. One of the major reasons is that it has been found that surgery in the STN and the GPi also has a profound antitremor effect. Thalamic DBS and thalamotomy were shown to be equally effective for the suppression of tremor, but thalamic stimulation had fewer adverse effects (37,38). The ideal candidate for thalamotomy would be an elderly PD patient with a long history of markedly asymmetric tremor with little or no effect of medication who does not display other parkinsonian features such as bradykinesia and gait disturbance.

Pallidotomy for Parkinson's Disease

Since its reintroduction in 1992, unilateral pallidotomy probably has been the most frequently performed procedure in movement disorders surgery around the world (15,39). Pallidotomy improves all cardinal PD symptoms, however, to a variable extent. Differences in outcome among different series are due to variations in patient selection, assessment of outcome criteria, medical therapy, and surgical technique (40). Improvements have been seen most consistently in the off state, whereas there were wide variations in the on state (41–46). In general, improvements on the Unified Parkinson's Disease Rating Scale

(UPDRS) have been described as ranging between 30% and 50%. The most immediate effect of pallidotomy is the abolition or marked improvement of contralateral and, to a certain extent, ipsilateral dyskinesias. Usually, there is no significant change of levodopa medication or total equivalent dose in the long-term period.

When the results of several larger studies on unilateral pallidotomy were summarized, bradykinesia was reported to be improved by 19% to 43% according to the UPDRS (40). There may be mild to moderate ipsilateral improvement that is, however, most often transient. In a study of 41 patients with advanced PD, objective improvement of off bradykinesia contralateral to pallidotomy at 3 months postoperatively was shown by significant improvement of both movement and reaction times (47). The improvement of rigidity on the side contralateral to pallidotomy ranged from 25% to 60% in most studies (40). The improvement of tremor at rest, in general, ranged between 30% and 70%, although the magnitude in reduction of tremor varied widely among different groups. Unilateral pallidotomy also improves axial symptoms of PD, such as gait disturbance and postural instability in the off state. Generally, the maximum improvement of postural control is seen at 3 months after pallidotomy with many variables remaining significantly improved at 12 months (48). Fluctuations are improved, and increased time spent by patients in the on state is reported by most groups. In particular, the relation of the percentage of on time without dyskinesias is altered, compared to the percentage of on time with dyskinesias. The improvement of dyskinesias is striking. Improvement of dyskinesia-related disability and pain accompanies the reduction of dyskinesia (49). Complications of unilateral pallidotomy include visual field defects, hemiparesis, and facial weakness. The frequency of persistent side effects may range between 4% and 14% among different groups. Most studies investigating neuropsychological outcome after unilateral pallidotomy have found minimal cognitive changes, compared to the robust improvements in motor function (50–52). There were generally mild to moderate declines in frontal lobe functioning and memory. In some studies, left-sided lesions were associated with impaired verbal learning and phonemic fluency, whereas right-sided lesions caused transient decreases in visuospatial abilities.

Bilateral pallidotomy has been performed much more infrequently (53). The additional benefit of a second, contralateral pallidotomy is usually less than that of the initial procedure if both procedures are staged. The occurrence of complications is clearly higher, compared to unilateral pallidotomy. Side effects of bilateral pallidotomy include changes in personality, behavior, executive functions and increased dysphagia, dysarthria, and falling. In a report on 12 unilateral and 8 bilateral (simultaneous) pallidotomies, significant declines in mean articulation rate and phonemic fluency were found only in the patients who underwent bilateral procedures (54).

A meta-analysis on pallidotomy for PD revealed that, at 1 year postoperatively, the mean improvement in the UPDRS motor score during off periods was 50.3% and the mean reported improvement in contralateral dyskinesias during on periods was 86.4% (39). Major adverse events, including intracerebral hemorrhages, contralateral weakness, and visual field defects, occurred in 5.3% of patients reported. The efficacy of unilateral pallidotomy has been confirmed in 2 randomized trials (41,55). In these studies, however, improvement by 31% and by 32% of the off motor UPDRS scores was more modest. Long-term studies have shown that reduction in limb dyskinesias and off-state tremor scores persisted on the side contralateral to pallidotomy at the end of 3 years, whereas other measures tended to deteriorate (56). In particular, there is a loss of the benefit on gait and on posture (57). Increasing symptoms on the nonoperated side may become an important source of disability.

The role of pallidotomy in the treatment of PD has changed tremendously. The option of performing DBS in simultaneous bilateral surgery has changed the concept regarding who should be considered an ideal candidate for unilateral pallidotomy. In most centers, bilateral pallidotomies are not performed. A randomized multicenter study showed that bilateral STN DBS is clearly more effective than unilateral pallidotomy in reducing parkinsonian symptoms in patients with advanced PD (58). Pallidal surgery for PD, in general, may be indicated in elderly patients with severe dyskinesias who tolerate poorly the reduction of levodopa medication because of depression and anhedonia.

Subthalamotomy for Parkinson's Disease

The STN was not considered a target for lesioning due to concerns regarding the occurrence of hemiballism/hemichorea for a long time. Now, it is the major target for DBS. The occurrence of hemiballism or hemichorea as a complication of functional stereotactic surgery has been known since the early prelevodopa era. Analysis of the literature of the classic period of functional neurosurgery, however, showed that only a small number of parkinsonian patients with hemiballism/hemichorea had a lesion involving the STN (59). Most patients with PD who developed hemiballism or hemichorea after STN lesioning showed only mild or transient hemiballism. It was hypothesized that the threshold for hemiballism/hemichorea might be higher in parkinsonian conditions than in the normal state (60). Thus, STN inactivation is thought to be less likely to induce hemiballism/hemichorea in PD patients.

There have been few studies on subthalamotomy for treatment of PD (60–65). As in STN DBS, it appears that the dorsolateral STN is the most appropriate target for radiofrequency lesioning. In a study of 11 patients with unilateral subthalamotomy, marked improvement in motor function was observed, and it was maintained during the follow-up period up to 1 year, and in some patients up to 24 months (60). Improvement was more striking contralateral to the lesion. Daily intake of levodopa equivalents were unchanged in most of the patients during the first 12 months. In general, dyskinesia scores did not change postoperatively. One patient developed a large infarction due to the operation and suffered from hemiballism/hemichorea, which was later alleviated by a pallidotomy. The occurrence of hemiballism after STN lesioning appears to be related to the size of the lesion (63). There are even fewer reports on bilateral lesioning of the STN (64,65). The risk profile of a bilateral STN lesioning is still unclear as of this writing, and it is difficult to predict whether it will be performed more widely. Functional imaging studies have shown that subthalamotomy reduces basal ganglia output through the GPi and the substantia nigra pars reticularis, and it also influences downstream neural activity in the pons and ventral thalamus (66).

TREMOR DISORDERS

In contrast to PD tremor, consideration must be given to different aspects in patients with other types of tremor. Tremor is frequently an isolated neurologic symptom in essential tremor (ET). In patients with tremor after severe craniocerebral trauma, multiple sclerosis, or stroke, however, tremor is usually only one of many symptoms, and the patient's functional abilities are further limited by other neurologic and psychologic disturbances. In ET, no morphologic cerebral lesions are present, whereas widespread damage may be found in the other tremor groups. Taking these considerations into account, it is obvious that the indications for surgery, the goals to be achieved, the nature and frequency of side effects, and the prospects of symptomatic and functional improvement differ considerably. Unfortunately, in the past many reports on stereotactic surgery have grouped all these heterogeneous entities in series under the general heading of *intention tremor*. This approach often precludes accurate assessment of the different types of tremor and does not allow comparison among different series and methods.

Essential Tremor

Although ET is a common tremor disorder, it is disabling only in a small percentage of patients. Patients with disabling tremor who do not experience adequate relief with medication or who do not tolerate medication are candidates for functional stereotactic surgery. Relief of ET after thalamic surgery has been thought to be related to disruption of abnormal thalamocortical synchronization.

The first thalamotomy for ET was reported in the early 1960s. Generally, the VLp has been used (32,67). Some surgeons have extended their lesions into the region of the zona incerta (68). Tremor control is achieved almost always in the short term. Studies on the long-term outcome are sparse. Mohadjer et al. reported good long-term improvement, defined as more than 50% benefit, in 69% of a larger population of patients at a mean follow-up of 8.6 years (68). Transient side effects were noted in 33% of patients. The cumulative frequency of persistent side effects was 9%. Persistent side effects, in general, were mild and included hypotonia, gait disturbance, and dysdiadochokinesis. In another report, ET was completely abolished in 4 of 6 patients at a mean follow-up of 5.9 years (32). Improvement of voice tremor was noted in 71% of patients in one series (67), and improvement of head tremor was found in 80% of patients in another series. In almost all studies, improvement of tremor was paralleled by improvement in functional disability. As in thalamotomy for PD tremor, bilateral thalamotomy in ET patients is burdened with a high risk of persistent dysarthria.

Unilateral VLp thalamotomy produces good long-term tremor control among patients with ET. It carries a slightly higher risk of permanent neurologic deficits than DBS, as has been shown in the study of Schuurman et al. (37). Chronic DBS is clearly the preferred procedure when bilateral procedures are required.

Posttraumatic Tremor

Severe, incapacitating, predominantly postural and kinetic tremors are commonly associated with posttraumatic midbrain syndromes (69,70). Tremor usually manifests with a delay of weeks or months after the accident. Occasionally, tremor also may be present at rest. The coarse, jerking 2.5–4 Hz tremor can be extremely violent and disabling with amplitudes of more than 12 cm. Tremors are bilateral in about one-third of patients. The mean age in this group of patients is much lower than that of patients with other types of tremor; the majority of patients are adolescents. The history of deceleration trauma and associated clinical findings indicate that most patients with posttraumatic tremor had suffered diffuse axonal injury. Therefore, usually a variety of other symptoms, such as psychological and cognitive deficits, oculomotor disturbances, and truncal and appendicular ataxia, are present. Medical treatment of posttraumatic tremor is notoriously difficult. Thalamotomies were first performed in the early 1960s for posttraumatic tremor. Larger series with longer follow-up periods were published mainly in the 1980s and 1990s (71–75). The data for more than 100 patients who were reported to have undergone ablative stereotactic surgery for posttraumatic tremor since 1960 are summarized in Table 45.1. Overall, immediate intraoperative or postoperative improvement of tremor was obtained in almost all instances. Amelioration of the tremor on follow-up examination was reported in 89% of patients. However, few studies have assessed true long-term follow-up, and in many cases the duration of follow-up was unclear or

was limited to 0.5–3 years postoperatively. Functional improvement, in general, paralleled the reduction of the kinetic tremors and was described in 87% of the patients in whom it was assessed. Both transient and persistent side effects were reported frequently. Transient side effects included worsening of preoperative dysarthria and dysphagia, gait disturbance, and contralateral motor deficits. In the multipatient studies on posttraumatic tremor, the frequency of transient side effects varied from 50% to 90%. Worsening of dysarthria was observed in 70% of patients in the early postoperative period in the series of Bullard and Nashold (73). Decreased velopharyngeal functioning, a decrease in the oronasal pressure differential, and decreased range of motion of the tongue were characteristic findings. Although many patients have a subsequent improvement of adverse effects in the first few weeks or months after the operation, postoperative morbidity tends to persist in a considerable proportion of patients. Overall, persistent side effects have been reported to occur in 37% of the patients with a range between 0% and 66% in different studies. In the series of 35 patients reported by Krauss et al., the primary target was the contralateral zona incerta alone in 12 patients and in combination with the basis of the VLp in 23 patients (71). In that study persistent improvement of tremor was found in 88% of the patients on long-term follow-up at a mean of 10.5 years. The tremor was absent or significantly reduced in 65% of the patients. Improvement of functional disability on long-term follow-up was seen in all except 4 patients. Persistent side effects were observed in 38% of patients. These side effects consisted mainly in the aggravation of preoperative symptoms with increased dysarthria in 11 patients (34%) and increased truncal ataxia in 3 patients (9%). Two patients developed postoperative hemiballism. Seven patients with preoperative dystonic postures had an increase in dystonia on long-term evaluation, and 7 other patients developed dystonic postures or hemidystonia during follow-up. It was unclear whether this effect was related to the surgical procedure or whether it presented a delayed aftermath of the trauma. Previous investigators observed that in cases with severe kinetic tremors, larger thalamic lesions were required to control the movement disorder than for other types of tremor (74). Stereotactic lesions in the zona incerta and in the basal VLp offer the advantage of keeping efficient lesions smaller in these patients (Fig. 45.5). Reduction of the lesion size may also minimize the risk of side effects.

VLp thalamotomy or lesioning of the subthalamic area is a highly effective treatment option for disabling persistent posttraumatic tremor. These patients, however, seem particularly prone to present with postoperative side effects. This predisposition is most probably related to the presence of widespread cerebral damage secondary to diffuse axonal injury. The experience with DBS is limited; nevertheless, DBS appears to be associated with fewer side effects than radiofrequency lesioning in posttraumatic tremor, and its effect can be titrated to balance between

TABLE 45.1

ABLATIVE FUNCTIONAL STEREOTACTIC SURGERY FOR POSTTRAUMATIC TREMOR: LITERATURE REVIEW

Author(s) and Year	Target	Cases	Immediate Improvement	Long-Term Follow-up	Last Follow-up, Mean Years (Range)	Symptomatic Improvement (%)	Functional Improvement (%)	Persistent Side Effects (%)
Cooper, 1960[a]	VL	2	2	1	1.3	1/1	1/1	NA
Spiegel et al., 1963	STR	1	1	1	NA	0/1	NA	NA
Fox and Kurtzke, 1966	VL	1	1	1	0.5	1/1	1/1	0/1
Samra et al., 1970	VL	5	5	NA	NA	5/5 (100)	NA	NA
Van Manen, 1974[b]	VL	2	2	2	7	1/2	NA	1/2
Eiras and García, 1980	GP, Vop	1	1	1	2.5	1/1	1/1	0/1
Andrew et al., 1982	VL	8	8	NA	NA	8/8 (100)	8/8 (100)	5/8 (63)
Kandel, 1982[b]	VL, STR, GP	10	NA	NA	NA	NA	NA	NA
Niizuma et al., 1982[b]	VL, Sub-Vim	3	3	NA	NA	NA	NA	1/8 (13)
Ohye et al., 1982	VL	8	8	NA	NA	NA	NA	0/5
Hirai et al., 1983	VL	5	4	NA	NA	NA	NA	NA
Bullard and Nashold, 1984	VL	7	7	7	1.5 (0.2 to 3)	7/7 (100)	6/7 (86)	3/7 (43)
Bullard and Nashold, 1988[c]	VL	10	10	8	1.3 (0.2 to 3)	8/8 (100)	7/8 (90)	4/8 (50)
Iwadate et al., 1989	VL	3	2	NA	NA	2/3 (66)	NA	NA
Richardson, 1989	VL	1	1	NA	NA	1/1	NA	NA
Goldman and Kelly, 1992	VL	4	4	4	3 (1.4 to 4.5)	3/4 (75)	3/4 (75)	0/4 (0)
Marks, 1993	VL	7	6	NA	NA	6/7 (86)	NA	1/7 (14)
Taira et al., 1993	VL	3	1	3	0.5	1/3 (33)	NA	2/3 (66)
Krauss et al., 1994	VL, Zi	35	35	32	10.5 (0.5 to 24)	28/32 (88)	26/29 (90)	12/32 (38)
Jankovic et al., 1995	VL	6	6	6	4	6/6 (100)	3/6 (50)	3/6 (50)
Shahzadi et al., 1995[b]	VL	11	11	NA	NA	NA	NA	6/11 (55)
Louis et al., 1996	VL	2	2	2	0.3 and 4	2/2	NA	NA
Sobstyl et al., 2004	VL	7	7	7	2	7/7	7/7	NA
Total		135	120/125 (98%)	65		88/99 (89%)	63/72 (87%)	38/103 (37%)

[a] The series of Cooper includes the cases of Gioino et al. [b] Information not available. [c] Only summarized/no detailed information available.
Stereotactic targets: AL, ansa lenticularis; CP, caudate and putamen; IC, internal capsule; pall (med, lat), pallidum (medial, lateral); SN, substantia nigra; SR, subthalamic region; VIM, ventralis intermedius thalami; VL, ventrolateral thalamus; ZI, zona incerta. Techniques: chem, injection of toxin; cryo, cooling via inserted probe; DBS, chronic deep-brain stimulation; EC, electrocoagulation; mech, mechanical lesion. (From Krauss JK, Jankovic J, Grossman, RG. Head injury and posttraumatic movement disorders: topic review. Neurosurgery 2002;50:927–939 [see for complete list of references], with permission.)

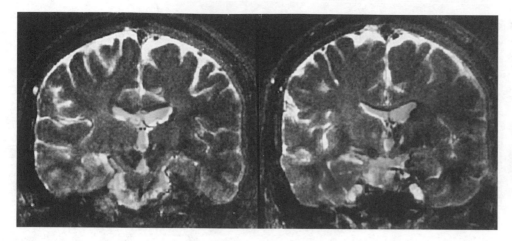

Figure 45.5 Coronal T2-weighted magnetic resonance images after functional stereotactic surgery for posttraumatic tremor. The images at 3 years postoperatively demonstrate the topographic localization of the small lesion at the base of the ventrolateral thalamus and the zona incerta, and its relationship to the adjacent nuclei. (From Krauss JK, Mundinger F. Functional stereotactic surgery for hemiballism. *J Neurosurg* 1996;85:278–286, with permission.)

improvement of tremor and induction of stimulation-induced increases in patients' neurologic deficits (70).

Tremor in Multiple Sclerosis

Functional stereotactic surgery for kinetic tremor in patients with multiple sclerosis presents several difficulties. These patients often are severely disabled, various neurologic symptoms are present, and the disease progresses insidiuously.

According to a review from 1992, on the effect of thalamotomy in a total of 131 patients pooled from different series, there was immediate postoperative improvement of tremor in 94% of cases (75). Good results were noted to persist on follow-up examinations in 65%; however, long-term follow-up was only exceptionally available. In 29% of patients, the tremor recurred. Persistent new postoperative deficits or worsening of preoperative symptoms were found in 22% of patients. Because of progression of the underlying disease, functional improvement was observed in only 44% of the patients. In a recent prospective case-controlled study, significant improvements in contralateral upper limb postural and kinetic tremors, spiral CT scores, and head tremor were detected at 3 months and at 12 months after unilateral thalamotomy (76). Tremor-related disability and finger-tapping speed were also significantly better 12 months after surgery, the latter having significantly worsened for the control group. A 3 Hz "filter" for postural upper limb tremor was detected by accelerometry and spectral analysis, above which tremor was always abolished but below which some residual tremor invariably remained. Both patients with and without surgery, however, showed significant deterioration in the expanded disability systems scores.

Patients with multiple sclerosis presenting with kinetic tremor should be carefully evaluated before they are considered candidates for thalamotomy. Notably, symptomatic improvement of tremor will not always translate in functional improvement. Chronic DBS has been used more and more frequently in this group of patients.

DYSTONIA

Surgical treatment of dystonia is experiencing a similar renaissance today, as did surgical treatment of PD some years ago (77). Considering surgical treatment of dystonia, various issues must be taken into account. The indications for different methods and the goals to be achieved depend on the distribution of dystonia, the severity, the etiology, the presence of other neurologic symptoms, and the patient's age. Particularly, the choice of the method depends also on whether a patient presents with hemidystonia, focal dystonia, or generalized dystonia. Hemidystonia, which is frequently secondary to contralateral caudatoputaminal lesions may be stable after delayed onset and progression over several years, whereas idiopathic dystonia may later spread progressively to other body parts and then limit the benefit of surgery. Current surgical options include lesioning and DBS of the GPi and the thalamus for hemidystonia and generalized dystonia, and intrathecal delivery of baclofen for severe truncal and generalized dystonia. These strategies will be discussed in the following sections. The outlines of surgical therapy for cervical dystonia (CD), the most common form of focal dystonia, are treated in separate sections later in this chapter. It also should be noted that a therapeutic option for severe blepharospasm that is refractory to botulinum toxin injection is surgical orbicularis oculi myectomy.

Functional Stereotactic Surgery for Dystonia

In the past, both thalamotomy and pallidotomy were used to treat dystonia (78–81). It had been the impression that pallidal targets are more suited for idiopathic dystonia, whereas thalamic targets are more suitable for secondary dystonia, which appears to be confirmed by more recent studies on radiofrequency lesioning and DBS (82,83). The focus on the treatment of dystonia has shifted more and more to DBS, again because of the lower risk of performing bilateral surgery in one session.

The target for thalamotomy for treatment of dystonia has been much more variable among different surgeons than have thalamic targets for tremor. Thalamotomy has involved the V.o.p, the V.o.a, the nucleus ventrooralis internus, the V.im, the subthalamic region, the centrum medianum/nucleus parafascicularis complex, and the pulvinar thalami. The comparison of the symptomatic and functional outcome of the reported series of thalamotomy is limited because of the heterogeneity of patients, variations of the target, differences in evaluation of outcome, and variable length of follow-up. Immediate postoperative improvement is less striking than in other movement disorders, such as PD or ET. Often, further amelioration can be observed within months after the operation. Postoperative improvement has been reported, in general, in 25% to 80% of patients with generalized dystonia, and in 33% to 100% of patients with hemidystonia (78,79,82). Andrew and colleagues found moderate or significant overall improvement in 25% of patients with generalized dystonia and in 100% of patients with hemidystonia; the benefit was more significant in secondary dystonia than in primary dystonia (78). Tasker et al. described that 68% of patients with secondary dystonia had more than 25% clinical improvement, whereas this was the case in only 50% of patients with primary dystonia (79). Patients with secondary dystonia also appeared to have more sustained improvement than patients with primary dystonia with thalamotomy. In the series of Tasker et al., 65% of patients with primary dystonia, but only 31% of patients with secondary dystonia, gradually lost the initial postoperative benefit. Immediate postoperative side effects were described in 7% to 47% of patients in different series. Transient side effects most commonly included confusion and contralateral weakness; as in PD, postoperative speech impairment has been observed more frequently after bilateral thalamotomies. Long-term follow-up rarely has been available. Cardoso et al. reported moderate or significant improvement in 50% of patients with secondary dystonia at a mean follow-up of 41 months, and in 43% of patients with primary dystonia at a mean of 33 months (81). Krauss et al. observed sustained moderate improvement in 3 of 6 patients with posttraumatic hemidystonia at a mean follow-up of 18 years (80). Recently, thalamotomy has been shown to be an effective treatment for writer's cramp (84).

Pallidotomy has been reintroduced for treatment of dystonia only within the past few years (82,83,85). In 16 patients with generalized dystonia or hemidystonia undergoing pallidotomy at Baylor College of Medicine, 14 patients demonstrated meaningful improvement. Eleven of these patients had bilateral procedures, staged in 3 and concurrent in 8 instances. Patients with genetic dystonias (both DYT1 positive and DYT1 negative) consistently demonstrated marked improvement, whereas improvement in secondary dystonias tended to be less dramatic and less consistent. It is difficult to compare the efficacy of unilateral versus concurrent bilateral procedures, as the decision was clinically based upon the anatomic distribution of the dystonia. Even more than after thalamotomy, improvement of dystonia is delayed. Whereas improvement of phasic dystonic movements may be seen early after surgery, tonic dystonic postures improve over a much longer time. At a mean of 1.5 years of follow-up, improvement was sustained (82). Persistent side effects were infrequent. Pallidotomy also has been shown to improve symptomatic dystonia resulting from other neurogenerative diseases such as Hallervorden-Spatz disease, Huntington's disease, and glutaric aciduria (86). The response of dystonia to pallidotomy may depend on etiology, according to the experience of different centers. It appears that patients with primary dystonia respond well to pallidotomy, whereas patients with secondary dystonia without structural lesions enjoy moderate improvement and patients with secondary dystonia and structural brain lesions often have only minimal benefit (87). Nevertheless, single patients with secondary dystonia may gain substantial benefit from pallidal surgery (88). In conclusion, the response of secondary hemidystonia to pallidal surgery (both lesioning and DBS) appears to be less predictable. Whereas a minority of patients may improve, most patients appear not to benefit.

Because of the relatively small number of patients with dystonia who are undergoing lesioning procedures, because of the variations in surgical methods, and because of the inconsistent outcome assessments, no definite recommendations about the best surgical options and ideal targets can be made at this time. DBS is being explored more extensively at many centers. The most problematic aspect is the high voltage that is needed in dystonia patients requiring early replacement of the pulse generators.

Intrathecal Baclofen Delivery

The mechanisms of actions by which intrathecal baclofen treatment alters dystonia may involve both spinal and cranial levels. Intrathecal baclofen has been used now for more than a decade in patients with generalized dystonia (89,90). Patients may be screened with bolus injections of baclofen via lumbar puncture or by continuous infusion via an external micropump and an intrathecal catheter. When the dystonia responds to the testing, a programmable subcutaneous pump is implanted and connected to an intrathecal catheter. This treatment modality results in reduction of dystonia and associated pain. Side effects may include infection and lethargy. In contrast to patients with spasticity, dystonia patients are more likely to respond to continuous infusion than to bolus injections. They require higher dosages than when treating spasticity, they are more likely to become resistent to the treatment, and they are less likely to experience substantial improvement in function.

CERVICAL DYSTONIA (SPASMODIC TORTICOLLIS)

The goals of treatment for CD are improving the abnormal neck posture and associated pain and preventing secondary complications such as development of contractures, cervical myelopathy, and radiculopathy (91). Medical treatment with anticholinergics and muscle relaxants often has limited benefit, and patients are frequently burdened by side effects. The treatment of choice for CD is undoubtedly the local injection of botulinum toxin type A into the dystonic muscles (92). The estimated frequency of primary nonresponders to botulinum toxin injections is 6% to 14% of patients with CD, and this approach loses its efficacy with continued use because of the development of immunoresistance in about another 3% to 10% of patients. Patients with secondary immunoresistance may benefit from newer types of botulinum toxin. Surgical treatment should be considered both in primary and in secondary nonresponders to botulinum toxin. It also may be considered an alternative in selected patients after years of successful trials with botulinum toxin because it can provide more permanent relief of the movement disorder.

Surgical Approaches and Strategies

Currently, surgery is performed mainly in patients who are primary or secondary nonresponders to botulinum toxin injections. Surgical treatment, in general, is indicated in those patients with functional disability caused by the dystonic movement disorder. Restriction of social activities because of embarassment related to CD is also a major driving force to seek more invasive therapies, particularly in younger patients. Surgical treatment of CD also can be used as an adjunct to conservative treatment to reduce drug dosages. Surgical options for patients with otherwise intractable CD are gaining increased attention

and acceptance. The operations most commonly used today aim at selectively weakening the dystonic muscles by nerve sectioning or myotomy. An alternative that has been reexplored is modification of basal ganglia activity. One of the crucial points of contemporary surgery for CD is tailoring the approach to the specific pattern of the individual patient, and this may involve several successive operative steps, and the use of different surgical techniques. In the past, operative procedures for treatment of CD were often performed as "standard" procedures, not taking into account the specific pattern of dystonic activity in the individual patient.

Today, extradural procedures are performed most frequently and, to a lesser extent, intradural nerve sectioning procedures. The primary goal of these techniques is to reduce the increased muscle tone. The denervation of muscles that are not involved in the production of dystonia should be avoided. The basic difference between intradural anterior cervical rhizotomy and extradural posterior ramisectomy is shown in Figure 45.6. Myotomies and myectomies are rarely used as a first step in patients with CD, but these techniques can be used as an adjunct to selective denervation or for treatment of dystonic activities in muscles that cannot be denervated completely with ease (91,93). Such muscles include the scalenes, the levator scapulae, and the omohyoid. In patients who present with painful dystonic activity of the trapezius, resulting in elevation and protraction of the shoulder or contributing to ipsilateral head tilt, partial myotomy and myectomy of the upper portion of the trapezius can be performed with an asleep–awake–asleep operative technique (93).

Microvascular decompression (MVD) of the spinal accessory nerve for treatment of CD has been used, as analogous with the therapeutic benefit of this procedure in other cranial neuropathies as hemifacial spasm (94). The existence of 2 pathogenetically different types of CD has been suggested by proponents of MVD. The first is

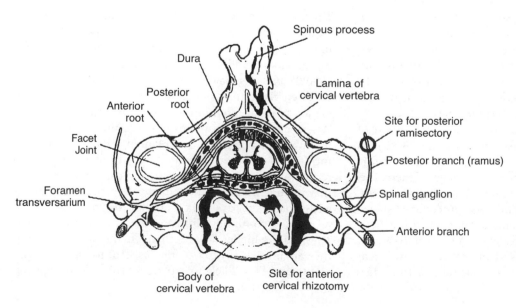

Figure 45.6 Schematic topographic anatomy of anterior cervical rhizotomy (intradural approach) and posterior ramisectomy (extradural approach). (From Krauss JK, Grossman RG. Principles and techniques of movement disorders surgery. In: Krauss JK, Jankovic J, Grossman, RG, eds. *Surgery for Parkinson's disease and movement disorders*. Philadelphia: Lippincott Williams & Wilkins, 2001:74–109, with permission.)

CD of "central" origin and the second is "spasmodic torticollis of 11th nerve origin." However, it is difficult to understand how MVD of the spinal accessory nerve should work, both regarding the pathophysiological concept of MVD and the fact that almost always muscles other than the sternocleidomastoid are involved in dystonic activity. Outcome data of MVD for treatment of CD are limited. Often, nerve sectionings were performed in addition to MVD (95). Jho and Jannetta claimed a cure of CD in 65% of their patients (13 of 20 patients), improvement considered as significant in 4 patients (20%), as moderate in 1 patient (5%), and as minimal in 2 patients on long-term follow-up between 5 and 10 years after MVD (94). In some series, high rates of surgical morbidity were described.

Intradural Section of Nerve Roots

In the past, intradural anterior cervical rhizotomy was the most common operation for CD (96,97). The "standard" procedure included bilateral intradural sectioning of the C1–3 anterior roots and of the caudal rootlets of the spinal accessory nerves. As mentioned, more restricted and selective sectioning is advisable to avoid postoperative side effects. For example, in a patient with rotational CD, unilateral anterior rhizotomy combined with contralateral spinal accessory nerve sectioning may be sufficient. Denervation with this approach, in general, is limited downward to the anterior root of C3 if it is performed bilaterally. The C4 root may be sectioned on one side, but that approach endangers functioning of the diaphragm.

Both the reported results and the complication rates in different series are highly variable. Most studies claimed useful postoperative improvement in 60% to 90% of their patients (96,97). Other series, however, have reported only modest results. Most often, it is unclear whether symptomatic amelioration of the abnormal postures or movements translated into improvement in functional disability with regard to the relatively high number of side effects. Bilateral rhizotomies are associated with a higher rate of postoperative neck weakness and dysphagia. Transient neck weakness has been estimated to occur in about 40% of patients and transient dysphagia in about 30% (98). A high variability of other complications has been described, including cerebrospinal fluid (CSF) fistulas, brainstem infarction, and infection.

Posterior Ramisectomy and Peripheral Denervation

Extradural sectioning of the posterior primary division of the cervical nerve roots is also known as *ramisectomy*. Bertrand coined the term *selective peripheral denervation* for the sectioning of the peripheral branch of the spinal accessory nerve to the sternocleidomastoid muscle combined with posterior ramisectomy from C1 to C6 (99). In contrast to anterior rhizotomy, there is no need for laminectomy

and opening of the dura in posterior ramisectomy, and denervation of laryngeal and pharyngeal muscles is largely avoided. The approach can be performed either unilaterally or bilaterally, depending on the pattern of dystonia. Beneficial results have been reported in the range of 70% to 90% of patients in most series, with only few persistent side effects (99–102). Side effects may include infection, paresthesias and hypesthesia in the territory of the major occipital nerve, pain, and transient dysphagia. In most studies, head tremor and phasic dystonic movements are improved to a lesser extent than are dystonic postures. It has been demonstrated that patients with no or minimal degenerative changes of the cervical spine had significant improvement in pain and severity of CD after selective denervation, whereas no difference was found in those with moderate or severe changes (103). Thus, it was concluded that effective early treatment of CD had a protective effect. A prospective study by Munchau et al. showed that reinervation is not infrequent after initially successful selective peripheral denervation (101). Occasionally, selective denervation can be useful in patients with fixed dystonic postures, with the goal being not to correct the head position but to alleviate accompanying pain (104).

Within the past few years, the concept of posterior ramisectomy and selective peripheral denervation has gained more widespread acceptance. In many institutions it has replaced intradural anterior rhizotomy. It appears that the efficacy of both procedures is comparable, however, that side effects are more rare and less severe with posterior ramisectomy.

Combination of Different Techniques

Surgical treatment combining several approaches and techniques can be successfully used in patients with CD (105–107). We have evaluated the symptomatic and functional outcome in a retrospective series of 46 consecutive patients with independent assessment using the Toronto Western Spasmodic Torticollis Rating Scale (TWSTRS). In this group, 76 surgical procedures were performed, including intradural denervation in 33 instances, extradural denervation in 21 instances, and muscle sections in 22 instances. Global improvement at long-term follow-up at a mean of 6.5 years postoperatively was rated as excellent in 21% of patients, as marked in 27%, as moderate in 21%, as mild in another 21%, and as nil in 11%. Almost all mean TWSTRS subscores for severity of CD, functional disability, and pain were significantly improved. Mild transient side effects were present in 10% of the patients and included swallowing difficulties, severe neck pain or headaches, psychotic decompensation, and cellulitis at the site of the skin incision. Persistent side effects, however, occurred only in 1 patient. In this series, there were no significant differences in the distribution of outcome scores between patients with idiopathic and secondary dystonia, nor were significant differences reported between patients who primarily did not respond to botulinum toxin injections and those who had developed secondary immunoresistance. There was a significant difference, however, with regard to the number of procedures performed. Patients with an excellent outcome had a higher number of surgical procedures on average than those patients who had achieved no benefit.

Functional Stereotactic Surgery for Cervical Dystonia

In the past, functional stereotactic surgery for treatment of CD was performed in several centers. With the refinement of peripheral techniques and the widespread use of botulinum toxin injections, however, this treatment modality was largely abandoned. The experience with pallidal surgery for dyskinesias and dystonia in patients with PD, the beneficial effect in dystonic movement disorders, and review of the history of functional stereotactic surgery of CD has prompted the reevaluation of the potential of basal ganglia surgery for treatment of CD. Between 1960 and the early 1980s, approximately 300 patients with CD were reported to have undergone functional stereotactic surgery (108). Overall, postoperative improvement was claimed in about 50% to 70% of patients in most studies. A delay in improvement varying between a few weeks and 2 years postoperatively often was described. Various thalamic nuclei were targeted according to different pathophysiologic concepts trying to account for the specific phenomenology of CD.

There is evidence that there is bilateral involvement in patients with CD regardless of the specific pattern of CD. PET investigations have shown higher glucose metabolism bilaterally in the lentiform nucleus in CD patients without significant differences concerning the laterality, specific pattern, or severity of CD in individual cases. Bilateral basal ganglia involvement also has been suggested by single-photon emission computed tomography (SPECT) studies. Also, bilateral rather than unilateral surgery is supported by accumulated knowledge on the innervation of neck muscles. Bilateral pallidal DBS has been shown to be promising in patients with severe complex CD and also in patients with cervical dyskinesias who undergo spinal surgery (109–111). Results have been stable more than 2 years postoperatively.

HEMIBALLISM AND HEMICHOREA

Hemiballism and hemichorea are relatively rare movement disorders. Hemiballism secondary to stroke most often has a favorable prognosis with spontaneous improvement over a few weeks. On the other hand, persistent hemiballism is well recognized. Surgical treatment is indicated in this subset of patients. In general, it should not be considered until 6 months after the onset of the movement disorder, except in patients with extremely violent hemiballism or in patients who do not tolerate medical therapy.

Early surgical treatment of hemiballism included several drastic measures, such as paralyzing limbs by alcohol injections, "stretching" of the brachial plexus, and even amputation of affected limbs. Over several decades, the mainstay of surgical treatment was manipulation of the motor cortex and the corticospinal tract. Such methods are only used exceptionally nowadays. Cervical cordotomy may be considered a last resort for patients who are not considered candidates for other treatment modalities.

Functional stereotactic surgery for treatment of hemiballism has been performed in a limited number of patients (60,81,112–115). We have identified a total of more than 60 patients published since 1950 in whom the diagnosis of hemiballism could be verified (115). Since the 1980s, only thalamic and pallidal targets have been used for treatment of hemiballism. Overall, immediate postoperative improvement was achieved in most patients, and for those patients in whom long-term follow-up was available, improvement has been sustained, in general (Table 45.2). Symptomatic and functional outcome was analyzed in a series of 14 patients with persistent hemiballism operated on over a period of 25 years (112). In 7 patients, concomitant hemichorea was present. Radiofrequency lesions were placed into the contralateral zona incerta and combined with lesions in the base of the VL thalamus in 13 patients. In 2 patients the GPi was targeted. Hemiballism was abolished or was considerably improved in the early postoperative period after 14 of 15 procedures. Lasting improvement at a mean of 11 years postoperatively was found in 12 of 13 patients (92%) available for long-term follow-up. Of these patients, 7 (54%) were free of any hyperkinesias, and 5 (39%) had minor residual predominantly hemichoreic hyperkinesias. In 6 patients who had presented preoperatively with hemichorea in addition to hemiballism, hemichorea was completely abolished in 3 in the long-term, whereas mild choreic movements persisted in the other 3 patients. Early postoperative side effects were present after 7 of the 15 procedures (47%). In general, these side effects were mild and included lateropulsion on walking, increase of preoperative hemiparesis, and confusion. Persistent morbidity was found in 3 patients. Mild dystonia in the extremities that had been affected by hemiballism previously was noted in 2 patients, and 1 patient had a mild hemiparesis. There was a highly significant reduction of functional disability on long-term follow-up. The Huntington's disease activities-of-daily-living scale was reduced from a preoperative mean of 83% of maximum disability to a mean of 30%. Residual disability was related most often to cardiovascular disease in older patients. Pallidotomy has been used more recently to effectively abate hemiballism (113,114). Bilateral ballism may be completely incapacitating and may require bilateral basal ganglia surgery. Under such circumstances, bilateral thalamotomy may be useful. Functional stereotactic surgery, in general, is not indicated for choreic dyskinesias in patients with Huntington's disease. Most patients tend to be more disabled by their behavioral and cognitive

TABLE 45.2

FUNCTIONAL STEREOTACTIC SURGERY FOR HEMIBALLISM: LITERATURE REVIEW

Author(s) and Year	No. of Cases	Stereotactic Targets	Technique	Improvement in Hemiballism (Early Postop)	Improvement in Hemiballism (Follow-up >1 yr)	Complications
Talairach et al., 1950	1	GP, IC, CP, AL	EC	1/1	1/1	1/1
Roeder and Orthner, 1956	1	GPi, AL	EC	1/1	b	0/1
Gurny, 1957	1	GP	Chem	1/1	b	b
Velasco-Suarez, 1957	1	GP, IC	Chem, mech	0/1	b	1/1
Martin and McCaul, 1959	1	VL	Chem	1/1	b	1/1
Andy, 1962	4	GPi, IC, SR	EC	4/4	1/1	2/4
Yasargil, 1962c	3	GPi, or VL, IC	EC	3/3	b	b
Spiegel et al., 1963	1	SN	EC	1/1	b	b
Gioino et al., 1966	5	GPi, or VL, SR	Chem	5/5	3/3	3/5
Cooper, 1969a,c	(4+5) 9	GPi, or VL, SR	Chem	c	c	b
Mundinger et al., 1970c	11	GPi, or VL, ZI	RF	b	7/11	b
Tsubokawa and Moriyasu, 1975	2	GPe	RF, chem	2/2	2/2	b
Kandel, 1982c	3	GPi, or VL, SR	Cryo	b	b	b
Levesque, 1992	1	VL	RF	1/1	b	1/1
Siegfried and Lippitz, 1994	1	VIM	DBS	1/1	1/1	b
Tsubokawa et al., 1995	2	VL, VIM	DBS	2/2	2/2	0/2
Cardoso et al., 1995	2	VL, VIM	RF	2/2	1/1	2/2
Krauss and Mundinger, 1996	14	VL, ZI, or GPi	RF	13/14	12/13	3/13
Suarez et al., 1997	1	GPi	RF	1/1	*	1/1
Vitek et al., 1999	1	GPi	RF	1/1	1/1	0/1
Alvarez et al., 2001	1	GPi	RF	1/1	1/1	0/1
Slavin et al., 2004	1	GPi	RF	1/1	*	1/1
Yamada et al., 2004	1	GPi	RF	1/1	*	0/1

[a] The series of Cooper includes the cases of Gioino et al. [b] Information not available. [c] Only summarized/no detailed information available. *Stereotactic targets:* AL, ansa lenticularis; CP, caudate and putamen; IC, internal capsule; pall (med, lat), pallidum (medial, lateral); SN, substantia nigra; SR, subthalamic region; VIM, ventralis intermedius thalami; VL, ventrolateral thalamus; ZI, zona incerta. *Techniques:* chem, injection of toxin; cryo, cooling via inserted probe; DBS, chronic deep-brain stimulation; EC, electrocoagulation; mech, mechanical lesion. (From Krauss JK, Mundinger F. Surgical treatment of hemiballism and hemichorea. In: Krauss JK, Jankovic J, Grossman RG, eds. *Surgery for Parkinson's disease and movement disorders.* Philadelphia: Lippincott Williams & Wilkins, 2001:397–403 [see for complete list of references], with permission.)

problems than by the choreic movement disorder. Several patients with Huntington's disease underwent pallidotomies in the 1950s and 1960s. Frequently, beneficial results with regard to the movement disorder were achieved. However, symptomatic improvement often was not paralleled by similar functional improvement.

Functional stereotactic surgery is a rewarding treatment modality in patients with persistent disabling hemiballism. Contemporary experiences with pallidal and thalamic ablative surgery have shown lasting symptomatic and functional improvement at a low frequency of mostly mild side effects. The question of which is the best target for hemiballism—the pallidum, the subthalamic region including the zona incerta, or the thalamus—cannot be settled with the available data.

TICS AND TOURETTE'S SYNDROME

In most patients with tics and Tourette's syndrome, the symptoms can be satisfactorily controlled, if necessary, with pharmacologic therapy and adjunct measures such as botulinum toxin injections. Few patients continue to be severely disabled by their motor and vocal tics or the concomitant behavioral disorder. Surgery might be considered primarily to alleviate severe tics or to improve obsessive–compulsive disorder (OCD) or self-injurious behavior (116). The evaluation of the effects of surgery, particularly over the long term, faces difficulties with regard to variability and to the waxing and waning of symptoms that occur spontaneously. The experience with functional stereotactic surgery for motor and vocal tics is limited. Encouraging results were reported in single case studies, whereas overall functional disabilities declined in other studies because of side effects. Hassler and Dieckmann reported their experiences with 15 patients on whom they had operated for Tourette's syndrome in the 1970s (117). Multiple lesions were made in the rostral interlaminar and medial thalamic nuclei, often bilaterally, in a staged fashion. Follow-up in 9 patients showed that tics in 4 were thought to be improved between 90% and 100%, whereas tics were improved in the other 5 patients by 50% to 80%. Some patients suffered severe adverse side effects, such as hemiparesis and personality changes. A review of the experiences with 17 consecutive patients treated between 1970 and 1998 in Freiburg, Germany, was published recently (118). Of 17 patients, 11 were available at a mean follow-up of 7 years. Lesions were placed in the zona incerta, the VL thalamus, and the thalamic lamella medialis. Patients underwent unilateral surgery based on asymmetry of tics, with later second-stage contralateral surgery in some instances. Alleviation of vocal tics was more significant than of motor tics. Both vocal and motor tics were relieved on long-term follow-up. Transient complications consisting of dysarthria, hemiparesis, hemiballism, and dystonia occurred in 68% of patients. One permanent complication was registered in the 6 patients followed up after unilateral surgery, whereas 2 of 5 patients had permanent disabling side effects after bilateral surgery.

For treatment of OCD in patients with Tourette's syndrome, several ablative surgical procedures have been used, including anterior cingulotomy, limbic leucotomy, and anterior capsulotomy (116). In general, such procedures have been described as effective in 33 to 61% of patients with OCD. Interestingly, although improvement of OCD in Tourette's syndrome was reported in several case reports after psychiatric surgery, the response of tics has been more variable (120,121).

Surgical treatment of Tourette's syndrome may be considered a treatment option in certain patients with severe disabling symptoms that are refractory to medical treatment. Surgery in such cases should be considered only as a part of an entire treatment plan and should be followed by appropriate neuropsychiatric programs. Experiences with DBS have shown promise (122).

SPASTICITY AND CHOREOATHETOSIS

Spasticity is a common sequelae of neurologic diseases. Although in some patients, spasticity is useful to some extent in compensating lost motor strength, in many other patients it may hinder useful function and can be associated with severe pain. When not controllable by physical therapy, medication, or botulinum toxin injections, spasticity can be improved by various surgical measures, such as neurostimulation, intrathecal pharmacotherapy, or selective ablative procedures. The choice of the procedure depends on the underlying pathology, associated symptoms, the distribution and pattern of spasticity, the degree of accompanying paresis, and the prospects of functional recovery.

Epidural spinal cord stimulation has been described to be useful for treatment of moderate degrees of spasticity. This method offers the possibility of a percutaneous trial of stimulation to assess whether or not there is a positive response. If relief occurs, the system can be internalized. The procedure involves chronic implantation of electrodes in the spinal epidural space via small partial laminectomies or percutaneous techniques and subcutaneous implantation of a programmable system for neurostimulation. The

electrodes may be placed at the level of the injury in patients with spinal cord trauma or over the upper spinal cord in children with spastic cerebral palsy. A meta-analysis of several published series including patients with different pathologies yielded good or very good results for reductions of spasticity in 40% of patients, fair results in 24%, no improvement in 36%; good or very good improvement of motor function was reported in 37% of patients, fair improvement in 14%, and no change in 49%; amelioration of bladder function was judged as good or very good in 48% of patients, fair in 17%, and was not seen in 35% (123). Although these data indicate efficacy of spinal cord stimulation in a certain proportion of patients with spasticity, a prospective double-blind study with a limited number of cases, consisting of 8 children with spastic cerebral palsy, failed to show significant improvement with this treatment modality (124). The most frequent complications consist of lead fracture and electrode displacement occurring in about 10% of patients and infections occurring in about 5% of patients (123). Several mechanisms have been proposed to explain the effect of spinal cord stimulation, including activation of inhibitory long-loop reflexes.

In patients with severe generalized spasticity, intrathecal application of baclofen via an implanted programmable pump may be considered (125). The efficacy of intrathecal baclofen infusion has been demonstrated in randomized, double-blind crossover studies (126). Before a pump is internalized, trials are performed with lumbar injections or infusion of baclofen. Large variations in efficacy thresholds have been observed among patients. Implantation of the pump is performed under general or local anesthesia. The pump is placed in a subcutaneous pocket in the abdomen and connected to an intrathecal silicon catheter inserted via lumbar puncture. The pump must be refilled every 2 to 3 months. In a study of 59 patients with severe spasticity of spinal origin, the mean Ashworth score, which measures the degree of hypertonicity, decreased significantly (127). Catheter-related problems occurred 19 times in 15 patients. The dose of baclofen had to be doubled in about 1 year. A recent study described that administration of intrathecal baclofen for more than 5 years in patients with severe spasticity of spinal origin resulted in improved clinical efficacy but not in disability or perceived health status (128). Pharmacologic tolerance can be managed with drug holidays. The most frequent adverse drug reactions include obstipation, dizziness, drowsiness, muscular hypotonia, and symptoms of drug withdrawal. Drug overdose can be treated with intravenous physostigmine.

Selective lesioning can be performed at the level of peripheral nerves, spinal roots, spinal cord, or dorsal root entry zone (DREZ) (129). Peripheral neurotomies are indicated when spasticity is localized to muscles or muscular groups supplied by a single or a few peripheral nerves that are easily accessible. Neurotomies of the tibial nerve at the popliteal region for so-called *spastic foot* and of the obturator nerve just below the subpubic canal for spastic flexion–adduction deformity of the hip are the most frequently performed peripheral procedures. Neurotomies also are performed for spasticity in the upper limb, including selective fascicular neurotomies in the musculocutaneous nerve and the median and ulnar nerves. Occasionally, neurotomies of brachial plexus branches have been performed for treating the spastic shoulder. Posterior rhizotomies are performed in children with cerebral palsy. There are several technical variants, such as selective posterior rhizotomy, sectorial posterior rhizotomy, partial posterior rhizotomy, and functional posterior rhizotomy. Overall, about 75% of patients have nearly normal muscle tone at 1 year postoperatively. Most children demonstrated improved stability in sitting or improvement of walking. In cases of fixed contractures, complementary orthopedic surgery was sometimes necessary. Lesioning of the DREZ is helpful both for severe spasticity and for associated pain (130). A refinement of this method, microDREZotomy, attempts to interrupt small nociceptive and large myotactic fibers, while sparing lemniscal fibers (129). DREZotomy can be performed for the lower limbs or for the upper limbs. Percutaneous techniques for rhizotomies have been described. Complementary orthopedic surgery may be necessary when deformities have become irreducible.

Functional ablative stereotactic surgery has been used in the past for choreoathetosis in children with cerebral palsy. The reported results have been highly variable, which may have been related partially to the methodologic assessment. Although some degree of improvement with targets in the VL thalamus and the subthalamic region was observed in the majority of patients, wide variations in outcome were reported. Significantly improved outcome has been described as ranging between 18% and 73% in different studies (131,132). In the past, the dentate nuclei were targeted for lesioning or chronic stimulation as treatment for spasticity and choreoathetosis. Cerebellar targets have been almost completely abandoned now. In a recent series of

33 pallidotomies in 24 patients with cerebral palsy, 67% had subjective improvement, and 42% had subjective and objective improvement (133). Many of those patients were described as enjoying functional gains, such as the ability to feed themselves or to maneuver their wheelchairs. The complication rate was 50% and included swallowing and speech difficulties. The permanent complication rate was 17.5%. Again, DBS is being explored as an alternative.

OTHER MOVEMENT DISORDERS

Hemifacial Spasm

Botulinum toxin injection is the therapeutic option that is most frequently employed for hemifacial spasm. The alternative, which renders permanent relief of hemifacial spasm, is MVD of the facial nerve via a lateral suboccipital approach. This technique was elaborated and refined by Jannetta for treatment of cranial nerve root compression. Exposure of the root exit zone is achieved with microneurosurgical techniques. After the offending vessel is identified, the vessel is mobilized and repositioned with small implants of Teflon or other nonresorbable materials placed between the facial nerve and the vessel. Both the integrity of the facial nerve and the vessel are preserved. In patients with typical or so-called *classic* hemifacial spasm, the causative vessel is usually found to be compressing the nerve from a caudal and anterior direction (Fig. 45.7). Usually, the causative vessel is identified as the posterior inferior cerebellar artery. In patients with so-called *atypical* hemifacial spasm, which is progression of the spasm from the lower face to the upper face, the side of compression appears to be rostral and posterior to the nerve and the root exit zone.

Complete or almost complete resolution of hemifacial spasm is reported in 80% to 90% of patients in more

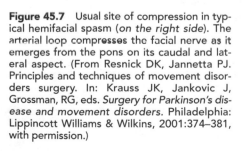

Figure 45.7 Usual site of compression in typical hemifacial spasm (*on the right side*). The arterial loop compresses the facial nerve as it emerges from the pons on its caudal and lateral aspect. (From Resnick DK, Jannetta PJ. Principles and techniques of movement disorders surgery. In: Krauss JK, Jankovic J, Grossman, RG, eds. *Surgery for Parkinson's disease and movement disorders*. Philadelphia: Lippincott Williams & Wilkins, 2001:374–381, with permission.)

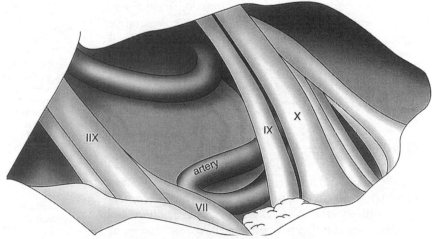

recent series (134,135). Recurrences were observed in 1% to 10% of patients over the long term. In the large series of 703 patients reported by Barker and Jannetta (134), excellent results, defined as *complete or nearly complete abolition of spasms,* were obtained in 86% of patients at 1 month postoperatively and in 79% at 10-year follow-up. Including patients who had reoperations for recurrence, the result for excellent improvement at 10-year follow-up increased to 84% of patients, whereas partial improvement was achieved in 7%, and failures occurred in 9%. Operative mortality was 0.1%, and operative complications included brainstem infarction in 0.3%, cerebellar hematoma in 0.5%, deafness in 2.7%, permanent facial weakness in 1.5%, and mild transient complications in 4.5%. The pattern of hemifacial spasm is an important predictor of operative success. Overall, only 70% of patients with atypical hemifacial spasm have an immediate relief of spasm. Also, long-term results of atypical hemifacial spasms are less gratifying. At 10 years postoperatively, only 59% of patients report excellent relief of symptoms. Sometimes, resolution of hemifacial spasm may be gradual (136).

Stiff-Man Syndrome

Stiff-man syndrome and progressive encephalomyelitis with rigidity and myoclonus (PERM) can be treated with intrathecal baclofen if there is no sufficient relief by oral medication (137,138). As for patients with spasticity or dystonia, intrathecal test boluses are given before pump implantation. Maintenance doses of baclofen vary greatly among patients. Particularly in patients with PERM, requirements may increase rapidly. In a series of 15 patients, 11 patients before intrathecal baclofen were either wheelchair bound or bedridden. Five patients achieved the ability to walk with crutches and 3 others walked freely. Symptoms of autonomic dysfunction also were alleviated after administration of intrathecal baclofen. Complications of intrathecal baclofen therapy for patients with stiff-man syndrome or PERM differ from those for patients with spasticity. Patients may experience severe sedation. Drug withdrawal may result in severe consequences. Only hours after drug administration is reduced or stopped, spasms may develop, occasionally associated with massive vegetative symptoms such as diaphoresis, tachycardia, tachypnea, and hyperthermia. Clinically, the picture may resemble that of myocardial infarction or gram-negative sepsis. In particular and because of these risks, intrathecal baclofen is the last-resort alternative to oral treatment in these patients.

CONCLUSIONS

Presently, there is an unprecedented choice among different surgical techniques and approaches in movement disorders surgery. Although the variables affecting outcome of different procedures and their risk profiles have been studied in more detail in the past few years, several questions remain unanswered and minimal data are available for comparing one procedure with the other. Neurosurgical trials are complicated by various confounding variables (139), and although the efficacy of various procedures has been clearly demonstrated, only a few studies fulfill the criteria of evidence-based medicine. Currently, the attention has shifted more and more to DBS as the treatment modality of choice for many movement disorders, especially against the background of the relatively disappointing clinical results seen with transplantation and other neurorestorative therapies.

Future achievements in neurobiology and further progress in technology will undoubtedly open new horizons for movement disorders surgery in the next few years. It is pivotal during this development not to ignore the achievements of established procedures. Recent studies have confirmed significant gain in quality of life after radiofrequency lesioning for advanced PD (140), and the efficacy of lesional surgery is associated with highly significant societal cost savings (141). Alternative techniques for creating lesions have evolved or they have been rediscovered but are being met with hesitancy. Thus far, gamma knife radiosurgery has been considered controversial as a tool for creating therapeutic lesions in movement disorders (142), but according to newer data this method might be useful in a subset of patients (143). Interesting new developments include staged lesioning through implanted DBS electrodes (144) and targeted distribution of substances to the basal ganglia via convection-enhanced delivery (145).

All contemporary surgical procedures for the treatment of movement disorders have their relative advantages and their specific limitations. While the combination of clinical symptoms may favor one approach in an individual patient, in other instances different alternatives are available.

REFERENCES

1. Alexander GE, Crutcher MD, Delong MR. Basal ganglia thalamocortical circuits: parallel substrates for motor, oculomotor, "prefrontal" and "limbic" functions. *Prog Brain Res* 1990; 85:119–146.
2. Marsden CD, Obeso JA. The functions of the basal ganglia and the paradox of stereotaxic surgery in Parkinson's disease. *Brain* 1994;117:877–897.
3. Mink JW. Basal ganglia motor control before and after surgery. In: Krauss JK, Jankovic J, Grossman RG, eds. *Surgery for Parkinson's disease and movement disorders.* Philadelphia: Lippincott Williams & Wilkins, 2001:56–73.
4. Guridi J, Luquin MR, Herrero MT, et al. The subthalamic nucleus: a possible target for stereotaxic surgery in Parkinson's disease. *Mov Disord* 1993;8:421–429.
5. Limousin P, Krack P, Pollak P, et al. Electrical stimulation of the subthalamic nucleus in advanced Parkinson's disease. *N Engl J Med* 1998;339:1105–1111.
6. Gildenberg PL. The history of stereotactic and functional neurosurgery. In: Gildenberg PL, Tasker RR, eds. *Textbook of stereotactic and functional neurosurgery.* New York: McGraw-Hill, 1998:5–19.
7. Krauss JK, Grossman RG. Historical review of pallidal surgery for treatment of parkinsonism and other movement disorders. In: Krauss JK, Grossman RG, Jankovic J, eds. *Pallidal surgery for the treatment of Parkinson's disease and movement disorders.* Philadelphia: Lippincott Raven, 1998:1–23.

8. Meyers R. The modification of alternating tremor, rigidity and festination by surgery of the basal ganglia. *Res Publ Assoc Res Nerv Ment Dis* 1942;21:602–665.

9. Meyers R. The surgery of the hyperkinetic disorders. In: Vinken PJ, Bruyn GW, eds. *Handbook of clinical neurology*, vol 6. Amsterdam: North Holland Publ, 1968:844–878.

10. Fenelon F. Essais de traitement neurochirurgical du syndrome parkisonien par intervention directe sur les voies extrapyramidales immediatement sousstriopallidales (ou lenticulaires). *Rev Neurol* 1950;83:437–440.

11. Spiegel EA, Wycis HT. Thalamotomy and pallidotomy for treatment of choreic movements. *Acta Neurochir* 1952;2:417–422.

12. Spiegel EA, Wycis HT, Marks M, et al. Stereotaxic apparatus for operations on the human brain. *Science* 1947;106:349–350.

13. Hassler R, Riechert T. Indikationen und Lokalisationsmethode der gezielten Hirnoperationen. *Nervenarzt* 1954;25:441–447.

14. Mundinger F, Riechert T. Die stereotaktischen Hirnoperationen zur Behandlung extrapyramidaler Bewegungsstörungen (Parkinsonismus und Hyperkinesen) und ihre Resultate. *Fortschr Neurol Psych* 1963;31:1–66, 69–120.

15. Laitinen LV, Bergenheim AT, Hariz MI. Leksell's posteroventral pallidotomy in the treatment of Parkinson's disease. *J Neurosurg* 1992;76:53–61.

16. Hassler R. Architectonic organization of the thalamic nuclei. In: Schaltenbrand G, Walker AE, eds. *Stereotaxy of the human brain*. Stuttgart, New York: Thieme, 1982:140–180.

17. Hassler R, Mundinger F, Riechert T. *Stereotaxis in Parkinson syndrome*. Berlin, Heidelberg, New York: Springer, 1979.

18. Jones EG. Morphology, nomenclature, and connections of the thalamus and basal ganglia. In: Krauss JK, Jankovic J, Grossman, RG, eds. *Surgery for Parkinson's disease and movement disorders*. Philadelphia: Lippincott Williams & Wilkins, 2001:24–47.

19. Taha JM, Favre J, Baumann TK, et al. Characteristics and somatotopic organization of kinesthetic cells in the globus pallidus of patients with Parkinson's disease. *J Neurosurg* 1996;85: 1005–1112.

20. Guridi J, Gorospe A, Ramos E, et al. Stereotactic targeting of the globus pallidus internus in Parkinson's disease: imaging versus electrophysiological mapping. *Neurosurgery* 1999;45:278–287.

21. Rodriguez-Oroz MC, Rodriguez M, Guridi J, et al. The subthalamic nucleus in Parkinson's disease: somatotopic organization and physiological characteristics. *Brain* 2001;124:1777–1790.

22. Krauss JK, Grossman RG. Principles and techniques of movement disorders surgery. In: Krauss JK, Jankovic J, Grossman, RG, eds. *Surgery for Parkinson's disease and movement disorders*. Philadelphia: Lippincott Williams & Wilkins, 2001:74–109.

23. Schaltenbrand G, Bailey P. *Introduction to stereotaxis with an atlas of the human brain*. Stuttgart, Germany: Thieme, 1959.

24. Schaltenbrand G, Wahren P. *Atlas for stereotaxy of the human brain*. Stuttgart, Germany: Thieme, 1977.

25. Kelly PJ, Derome P, Guiot G. Thalamic spatial variability and the surgical results of lesions placed with neurophysiologic control. *Surg Neurol* 1978;9:307–315.

26. Di Pierro CG, Francel PC, Jackson TR, et al. Optimizing accuracy in magnetic resonance image-guided stereotaxis: a technique with validation based on the anterior commissure-posterior commissure line. *J Neurosurg* 1999;90:94–100.

27. Holtzheimer PE 3rd, Roberts DW, Darcey TM. Magnetic resonance imaging versus computed tomography for target localization in functional stereotactic neurosurgery. *Neurosurgery* 1999;45:290–297.

28. Schuurman PR, de Bie RMA, Majoie CBL, et al. A prospective comparison between three-dimensional magnetic resonance imaging and ventriculography for target-coordinate determination in frame-based functional stereotactic neurosurgery. *J Neurosurg* 1999;91:911–914.

29. Krauss JK, King DE, Grossman RG. Alignment correction algorithm for transformation of stereotactic anterior commissure/posterior commissure-based coordinates into frame coordinates in image-guided functional neurosurgery. *Neurosurgery* 1998; 42:806–812.

30. Hutchison WD. Techniques of microelectrode recording in movement disorders surgery. In: Krauss JK, Jankovic J, Grossman, RG, eds. *Surgery for Parkinson's disease and movement*

disorders. Philadelphia: Lippincott Williams & Wilkins, 2001: 110–118.

31. Kelly PJ, Gillingham FJ. The long-term results of stereotaxic surgery and L-dopa therapy in patients with Parkinson's disease. *J Neurosurg* 1980;53:332–337.

32. Jankovic J, Cardoso F, Grossman RG, et al. Outcome after stereotactic thalamotomy for parkinsonian, essential, and other types of tremor. *Neurosurgery* 1995;37:680–687.

33. Linhares MN, Tasker RR. Microelectrode-guided thalamotomy for Parkinson's disease. *Neurosurgery* 2000;46:390–395.

34. Narabayashi H, Yokochi F, Nakajima Y. Levodopa-induced dyskinesias and thalamotomy. *J Neurol Neurosurg Psychiatry* 1984; 471:831–839.

35. Diederich N, Goetz CG, Stebbins GT, et al. Blinded evaluation confirms long-term asymmetric effect of unilateral thalamotomy or subthalamotomy on tremor in Parkinson's disease. *Neurology* 1992;42:1311–1314.

36. Tasker RR. Movement disorders. In: Apuzzo MLJ, ed. *Brain surgery: Complication avoidance and management*. New York: Churchill Livingstone, 1993:1509–1524.

37. Schuurman PR, Bosch DA, Bossuyt PM, et al. A comparison of continuous thalamic stimulation and thalamotomy for suppression of severe tremor. *N Engl J Med* 2000;342:461–468.

38. Tasker RR. Deep brain stimulation is preferable to thalamotomy for tremor suppression. *Surg Neurol* 1998;49:145–153.

39. Alkhani A, Lozano AM. Pallidotomy for Parkinson's disease: a review of contemporary literature. *J Neurosurg* 2001;94:43–49.

40. Payne BR, Bakay RAE, Vitek JL. Pallidotomy for treatment of Parkinson's disease. In: Krauss JK, Jankovic J, Grossman, RG, eds. *Surgery for Parkinson's disease and movement disorders*. Philadelphia: Lippincott Williams & Wilkins, 2001:161–169.

41. Vitek JL, Bakay RA, Freeman A, et al. Randomized trial of pallidotomy versus medical therapy for Parkinson's disease. *Ann Neurol* 2003;53:558–569.

42. Parkin SG, Gregory RP, Scott R, Bain P, et al. Unilateral and bilateral pallidotomy for idiopathic Parkinson's disease: a case series of 115 patients. *Mov Disord* 2002;17:682–692.

43. Lang AE, Lozano AM, Montgomery E, et al. Posteroventral medial pallidotomy in advanced Parkinson's disease. *N Engl J Med* 1997;337:1036–1042.

44. Kondziolka D, Bonaroti E, Baser S, et al. Outcomes after stereotactically guided pallidotomy for advanced Parkinson's disease. *J Neurosurg* 1999;90:197–202.

45. Krauss JK, Desaloms M, Lai EC, et al. Microelectrode-guided posteroventral pallidotomy for treatment of Parkinson's disease: postoperative magnetic resonance imaging findings. *J Neurosurg* 1997;87:358–367.

46. Lai EC, Jankovic J, Krauss JK, et al. Long-term efficacy of posteroventral pallidotomy in the treatment of Parkinson's disease. *Neurology* 2000;55:1218–1222.

47. Ondo WG, Jankovic J, Lai EC, et al. Assessment of motor function after stereotactic pallidotomy. *Neurology* 1998;50:266–270.

48. Roberts-Warrior D, Overby A, Jankovic J, et al. Postural control in Parkinson's disease after unilateral posteroventral pallidotomy. *Brain* 2000;123:2141–2149.

49. Jankovic J, Lai E, Ben-Arie L, et al. Levodopa-induced dyskinesias treated by pallidotomy. *J Neurol Sci* 1999;167:62–67.

50. Perrine K, Dogali M, Fazzini E, et al. Cognitive functioning after pallidotomy for refractory Parkinson's disease. *J Neurol Neurosurg Psychiatry* 1998;65:150–154.

51. Trépanier LL, Saint-Cyr JA, Lozano AM, et al. Neuropsychological consequences of posteroventral pallidotomy for the treatment of Parkinson's disease. *Neurology* 1998;51:207–215.

52. Rettig GM, York MK, Lai EC, et al. Neuropsychological outcome after unilateral pallidotomy for the treatment of Parkinson's disease. *J Neurol Neurosurg Psychiatry* 2000;69:326–336.

53. De Bie RM, Schuurman PR, Esselink RA, Bosch DA, Speelman JD. Bilateral pallidotomy in Parkinson's disease: a retrospective study. *Mov Disord* 2002;17:533–538.

54. Scott R, Gregory R, Hines N, et al. Neuropsychological, neurological and functional outcome following pallidotomy for Parkinson's disease: a consecutive series of eight simultaneous bilateral and twelve unilateral procedures. *Brain* 1998;121: 659–675.

55. De Bie RMA, Schuurman PR, Bosch DA, et al. Outcome of unilateral pallidotomy in advanced Parkinson's disease: cohort study of 32 patients. *J Neurol Neurosurg Psychiatry* 2001;71:375–382.

56. Pal PK, Samii A, Kishore A, et al. Long term outcome of unilateral pallidotomy: follow up of 15 patients for 3 years. *J Neurol Neurosurg Psychiatry* 2000;69:337–344.

57. Fine J, Duff J, Chen R, et al. Long-term follow-up of unilateral pallidotomy in advanced Parkinson's disease. *N Engl J Med* 2000;342:1708–1714.

58. Esselink RA, de Bie RM, de Haan RJ, et al. Unilateral pallidotomy versus bilateral subthalamic nucleus stimulation in PD: a randomized trial. *Neurology* 2004;62:201–207.

59. Guridi J, Obeso JA. The subthalamic nucleus, hemiballismus and Parkinson's disease: reappraisal of a neurosurgical dogma. *Brain* 2001;124:5–19.

60. Alvarez L, Macias R, Guridi J, et al. Dorsal subthalamotomy for Parkinson's disease. *Mov Disord* 2001;16:72–78.

61. Patel NK, Heywood P, O'Sullivan K, McCarter R, Love S, Gill SS. Unilateral subthalamotomy in the treatment of Parkinson's disease. *Brain* 2003;126:1136–1145.

62. Barlas O, Hanagasi HA, Imer M, et al. Do unilateral ablative lesions of the subthalamic nucleus in parkinsonian patients lead to hemiballism? *Mov Disord* 2001;16:306–310.

63. Tseng HM, Su PC, Liu HM. Persistent hemiballism after subthalamotomy: the size of the lesion matters more than the location. *Mov Disord* 2003;18:1209–1211.

64. Gill SS, Heywood P. Bilateral dorsolateral subthalamotomy for advanced Parkinson's disease. *Lancet* 1997;350:1224.

65. Alvarez L, Macias R, Lopez G, et al. Bilateral subthalamotomy in Parkinson's disease: initial and long-term response. *Brain* 2005;128:570–583.

66. Su PC, Ma Y, Fukuda M, et al. Metabolic changes following subthalamotomy for advanced Parkinson's disease. *Ann Neurol* 2001;50:514–520.

67. Goldman MS, Ahlskog JE, Kelly PJ. The symptomatic and functional outcome of stereotactic thalamotomy for medically intractable essential tremor. *J Neurosurg* 1992;76:924–928.

68. Mohadjer M, Goerke H, Milios E, et al. Long-term results of stereotaxy in the treatment of essential tremor. *Stereotact Funct Neurosurg* 1990;54:125–129.

69. Krauss JK, Wakhloo AK, Nobbe F, et al. MR pathological correlations of severe posttraumatic tremor. *Neurol Res* 1995;17:409–416.

70. Krauss JK, Jankovic. Head injury and posttraumatic movement disorders. *Neurosurgery* 2002;50:927–939.

71. Krauss JK, Mohadjer M, Nobbe F, et al. The treatment of posttraumatic tremor by stereotactic surgery. *J Neurosurg* 1994;80:810–819.

72. Sobstyl M, Zabek M, Koziara H, Kadziolka B. Stereotactic ventrolateral thalamotomy in the treatment of Holmes tremor. *Neurol Neurochir Pol* 2004;38:101–107.

73. Bullard DE, Nashold BS Jr. Stereotaxic thalamotomy for treatment of posttraumatic movement disorders. *J Neurosurg* 1984;61:316–321.

74. Hirai T, Miyazaki M, Nakajima H, et al. The correlation between tremor characteristics and the predicted volume of effective lesions in stereotaxic nucleus ventralis intermedius thalamotomy. *Brain* 1983;106:1001–1018.

75. Goldman MD, Kelly PJ. Symptomatic and functional outcome of stereotactic ventralis lateralis thalamotomy for intention tremor. *J Neurosurg* 1992;77:223–229.

76. Alusi SH, Aziz TZ, Glickman S, et al. Stereotactic lesional surgery for the treatment of tremor in multiple sclerosis: a prospective case-controlled study. *Brain* 2001;124:1576–1589.

77. Jankovic J. Re-emergence of surgery for dystonia. *J Neurol Neurosurg Psychiatry* 1998;65:434.

78. Andrew J, Fowler CJ, Harrison MJG. Stereotaxic thalamotomy in 55 cases of dystonia. *Brain* 1983;106:981–1000.

79. Tasker RR, Doorly T, Yamashiro K. Thalamotomy in generalized dystonia. *Adv Neurol* 1988;50:615–631.

80. Krauss JK, Mohadjer M, Braus DF, et al. Dystonia following head trauma: a report of nine patients and review of the literature. *Mov Disord* 1992;7:263–272.

81. Cardoso F, Jankovic J, Grossman RG, et al. Outcome after stereotactic thalamotomy for dystonia and hemiballismus. *Neurosurgery* 1995;36:501–508.

82. Ondo WG, Desaloms M, Krauss JK, et al. Pallidotomy and thalamotomy for dystonia. In: Krauss JK, Jankovic J, Grossman, RG, eds. *Surgery for Parkinson's disease and movement disorders.* Philadelphia: Lippincott Williams & Wilkins, 2001:299–306.

83. Yoshor D, Hamilton WJ, Ondo W, et al. Comparison of thalamotomy and pallidotomy for the treatment of dystonia. *Neurosurgery* 2001;48:818–826.

84. Taira T, Hori T. Stereotactic ventrooralis thalamotomy for task-specific focal hand dystonia (writer's cramp). *Stereotact Funct Neurosurg* 2003;80:88–91.

85. Ondo WG, Desaloms JM, Jankovic J, et al. Pallidotomy for generalized dystonia. *Mov Disord* 1998;13:693–698.

86. Rakocevic G, Lyons KE, Wilkinson SB, Overman JW, Pahwa R. Bilateral pallidotomy for severe dystonia in an 18-month-old child with glutaric aciduria. *Stereotact Funct Neurosurg* 2004;82:80–83.

87. Eltahawy HA, Saint-Cyr J, Giladi N, Lang AE, Lozano AM. Primary dystonia is more responsive than secondary dystonia to pallidal interventions: outcome after pallidotomy or pallidal deep brain stimulation. *Neurosurgery* 2004;54:613–619.

88. Loher TJ, Hasdemir MG, Burgunder JM, et al. Long-term follow-up study of chronic globus pallidus internus stimulation for posttraumatic hemidystonia. *J Neurosurg* 2000;92:457–460.

89. Albright AL. Intrathecal baclofen for treatment of dystonia. In: Krauss JK, Jankovic J, Grossman, RG, eds. *Surgery for Parkinson's disease and movement disorders.* Philadelphia: Lippincott Williams & Wilkins, 2001:316–322.

90. Albright AL, Barry MJ, Shafton DH, et al. Intrathecal baclofen for generalized dystonia. *Dev Med Child Neurol* 2001;43:652–657.

91. Krauss JK, Grossman RG, Jankovic J. Treatment options for surgery of cervical dystonia. In: Krauss JK, Jankovic J, Grossman, RG, eds. *Surgery for Parkinson's disease and movement disorders.* Philadelphia: Lippincott Williams & Wilkins, 2001:323–324.

92. Jankovic J, Hallett M. *Botulinum toxin treatment.* New York: Marcel Dekker, 1994.

93. Krauss JK, Koller R, Burgunder JM. Partial myotomy/myectomy of the trapezius muscle with an asleep-awake-asleep anesthetic technique for treatment of cervical dystonia. *J Neurosurg* 1999;91:889–891.

94. Jho HD, Jannetta PJ. Microvascular decompression for spasmodic torticollis. *Acta Neurochir* 1995;134:21–26.

95. Freckmann N, Hagenah R, Herrmann HD, et al. Bilateral microsurgical lysis of the spinal accessory nerve roots for treatment of spasmodic torticollis. *Acta Neurochir* 1986;83:47–53.

96. Hamby WB, Schiffer S. Spasmodic torticollis: results after cervical rhizotomy in 50 cases. *J Neurosurg* 1969;31:323–326.

97. Friedman AH, Nashold BS Jr, Sharp R, et al. Treatment of spasmodic torticollis with intradural selective rhizotomies. *J Neurosurg* 1993;78:46–53.

98. Colbassani HJ Jr, Wood JH. Management of spasmodic torticollis. *Surg Neurol* 1986;25:153–158.

99. Bertrand CM. Selective peripheral denervation for spasmodic torticollis: surgical technique, results, and observations in 260 cases. *Surg Neurol* 1993;40:96–103.

100. Braun V, Richter HP. Selective peripheral denervation for spasmodic torticollis: 13-year experience with 155 patients. *J Neurosurg* 2002;97(suppl 2):207–212.

101. Munchau A, Palmer JD, Dressler D, et al. Prospective study of selective peripheral denervation for botulinum-toxin resistant patients with cervical dystonia. *Brain* 2001;124:769–783.

102. Cohen-Gadol AA, Ahlskog JE, Matsumoto JY, Swenson MA, McClelland RL, Davis DH. Selective peripheral denervation for the treatment of intractable spasmodic torticollis: experience with 168 patients at the Mayo Clinic. *J Neurosurg* 2003;98:1247–1254.

103. Chawda SJ, Munchau A, Johnson D, et al. Pattern of premature degenerative changes of the cervical spine in patients with spasmodic torticollis and the impact on the outcome of selective peripheral denervation. *J Neurol Neurosurg Psychiatry* 2000;68:465–471.

104. Weigel R, Rittmann M, Krauss JK. Spontaneous craniocervical osseous fusion resulting from cervical dystonia. *J Neurosurg (Spine)* 2001;95:115–118.

105. Taira T, Hori T. A novel denervation procedure for idiopathic cervical dystonia. *Stereotact Funct Neurosurg* 2003;80:92–95.

106. Taira T, Kobayashi T, Hori T. Selective peripheral denervation of the levator scapulae muscle for laterocollic cervical dystonia. *J Clin Neurosci* 2003;10:449–452.

107. Krauss JK, Toups EG, Jankovic J, et al. Symptomatic and functional outcome of surgical treatment of cervical dystonia. *J Neurol Neurosurg Psychiatry* 1997;63:642–648.

108. Loher TJ, Pohle T, Krauss JK. Functional stereotactic surgery for treatment of cervical dystonia: review of the experience from the lesional era. *Stereotact Funct Neurosurg* 2004;82:1–13.

109. Krauss JK, Pohle T, Weber S, et al. Bilateral stimulation of globus pallidus internus for treatment of cervical dystonia. *Lancet* 1999;354:837–838.

110. Krauss JK, Loher TJ, Pohle T, et al. Pallidal deep brain stimulation in patients with cervical dystonia and severe cervical dyskinesias with cervical myelopathy. *J Neurol Neurosurg Psychiatry* 2002;72:249–256.

111. Eltahawy HA, Saint-Cyr J, Poon YY, Moro E, Lang AE, Lozano AM. Pallidal deep brain stimulation in cervical dystonia: clinical outcome in four cases. *Can J Neurol Sci* 2004;31:328–332.

112. Krauss JK, Mundinger F. Functional stereotactic surgery for hemiballism. *J Neurosurg* 1996;85:278–286.

113. Slavin KV, Baumann TK, Burchiel KJ. Treatment of hemiballismus with stereotactic pallidotomy. Case report and review of the literature. *Neurosurg Focus* 2004;17:E7.

114. Yamada K, Harada M, Goto S. Response of postapoplectic hemichorea/ballism to GPi pallidotomy: progressive improvement resulting in complete relief. *Mov Disord* 2004;19:1111–1114.

115. Krauss JK, Mundinger F. Surgical treatment of hemiballism and hemichorea. In: Krauss JK, Jankovic J, Grossman, RG, eds. *Surgery for Parkinson's disease and movement disorders.* Philadelphia: Lippincott Williams & Wilkins, 2001:397–403.

116. Rauch SL, Baer L, Cosgrove GR, et al. Neurosurgical treatment of Tourette's syndrome: a critical review. *Compr Psychiatry* 1995;36: 141–156.

117. Hassler R, Dieckmann G. Traitement stereotaxique des tics et cris inarticules ou coprolalique consideres comme phenomene d'obsession motrice au cours de maladies de Gilles de la Tourette. *Rev Neurol* 1970;123.89–106.

118. Babel TB, Warnke PC, Ostertag CB. Immediate and long term outcome after infrathalamic and thalamic lesioning for intractable Tourette's syndrome. *J Neurol Neurosurg Psychiatry* 2001;70:666–671.

119. Spangler WJ, Cosgrove GR, Ballantine HT, et al. Magnetic resonance image-guided stereotactic cingulotomy for intractable psychiatric disease. *Neurosurgery* 1996;38:1071–1078.

120. Kurlan R, Kersun J, Ballentine HT Jr, et al. Neurosurgical treatment of severe obsessive-compulsive disorder associated with Tourette's syndrome. *Mov Disord* 1990;5:152–155.

121. Baer L, Rauch SL, Jenike MA, et al. Cingulotomy in a case of concomitant obsessive-compulsive disorder and Tourette's syndrome. *Arch Gen Psychiatry* 1994;51:73–74.

122. Visser-Vandewalle V, Temel Y, Boon P, et al. Chronic bilateral thalamic stimulation: a new therapeutic approach in intractable Tourette syndrome. Report of three cases. *J Neurosurg* 2003; 99:1094–1100.

123. Gybels J, van Roost D. Spinal cord stimulation for spasticity. In: Sindou M, Abbott R, Keravel Y, eds. *Neurosurgery for spasticity.* Berlin, New York: Springer, 1991:73–81.

124. Hugenholtz H, Humphreys P, McIntyre WMJ, et al. Cervical spinal cord stimulation for spasticity in cerebral palsy. *Neurosurgery* 1988;22:707–714.

125. Ochs G, Struppler A, Meyerson BA, et al. Intrathecal baclofen for long-term treatment of spasticity: a multi-centre study. *J Neurol Neurosurg Psychiatry* 1989;52:933–939.

126. Penn RD, Savoy S, Corcos D, et al. Intrathecal baclofen for severe spinal spasticity. *N Engl J Med* 1989;320:1517–1521.

127. Ordia JI, Fischer E, Adamski E, et al. Chronic intrathecal delivery of baclofen by a programmable pump for the treatment of severe spasticity. *J Neurosurg* 1996;85:452–457.

128. Zahavi A, Geertzen JH, Middel B, Staal M, Rietman JS. Long term effect (more than five years) of intrathecal baclofen on impairment, disability, and quality of life in patients with severe spasticity of spinal origin. *J Neurol Neurosurg Psychiatry* 2004;75: 1553–1557.

129. Sindou MP, Mertens P. Ablative surgery for treatment of spasticity. In: Krauss JK, Jankovic J, Grossman, RG, eds. *Surgery for Parkinson's disease and movement disorders.* Philadelphia: Lippincott Williams & Wilkins, 2001:421–436.

130. Sindou M, Jeanmonod D. Microsurgical DREZ-otomy for the treatment of spasticity and pain in the lower limbs. *Neurosurgery* 1989;24:655–670.

131. Narabayashi H. Stereotaxic surgery for athetosis of the spastic state of cerebral palsy. *Confin Neurol* 1962;22:364–367.

132. Broggi G, Angelini L, Bono R, et al. Long term results of stereotactic thalamotomy for cerebral palsy. *Neurosurgery* 1983;12: 195–202.

133. Teo C. Functional stereotactic surgery of movement disorders in cerebral palsy. In: Krauss JK, Jankovic J, Grossman, RG, eds. *Surgery for Parkinson's disease and movement disorders.* Philadelphia: Lippincott Williams & Wilkins, 2001:410–420.

134. Barker FG, Jannetta PL, Bissonette DJ, et al. Microvascular decompression for hemifacial spasm. *J Neurosurg* 1995;82:201–210.

135. Payner TD, Tew JM. Recurrence of hemifacial spasm after microvascular decompression. *Neurosurgery* 1996;38:686–691.

136. Ishikawa M, Nakanishi T, Takamiya Y, et al. Delayed resolution of residual hemifacial spasm after microvascular decompression operations. *Neurosurgery* 2001;49:847–856.

137. Meinck HM, Tronnier V, Marquardt G. Surgical treatment of stiff man syndrome with intrathecal baclofen. In: Krauss JK, Jankovic J, Grossman RG, eds. *Surgery for Parkinson's disease and movement disorders.* Philadelphia: Lippincott Williams & Wilkins, 2001: 393–396.

138. Meinck HM, Tronnier V, Rieke K, et al. Intrathecal baclofen treatment for stiff-man syndrome: pump failure may be fatal. *Neurology* 1994;44:2209–2210.

139. Walter BL, Vitek JL. Surgical treatment for Parkinson's disease. *Lancet Neurol* 2004;3:719–728.

140. Gray A, McNamara I, Aziz T, et al. Quality of life outcomes following surgical treatment of Parkinson's disease. *Mov Disord* 2002;17:68–75.

141. Green AL, Joint C, Sethi H, Bain P, Aziz TZ. Cost analysis of unilateral and bilateral pallidotomy for Parkinson's disease. *J Clin Neurosci* 2004;11:829–834.

142. Okun MS, Stover NP, Subramanian T, et al. Complications of gamma knife surgery for Parkinson disease. *Arch Neurol* 2001;58:1995–2002.

143. Ohye C, Shibazaki T, Sato S. Gamma knife thalamotomy for movement disorders: evaluation of the thalamic lesion and clinical results. *J Neurosurg* 2005;102(suppl):234–240.

144. Raoul S, Faighel M, Rivier I, Verin M, Lajat Y, Damier P. Staged lesions through implanted deep brain stimulating electrodes: a new surgical procedure for treating tremor or dyskinesias. *Mov Disord* 2003;18:933–938.

145. Lonser RR, Corthesy ME, Morrison PF, Gogate N, Oldfield EH. Convection-enhanced selective excitotoxic ablation of the neurons of the globus pallidus internus for treatment of parkinsonism in nonhuman primates. *J Neurosurg* 1999;91: 294–302.

Being Realistic About Human Embryonic Stem Cell-Based Therapy for Parkinson's Disease

46

Sergey V. Anisimov   *Ana Sofia Correia*   *Jia-Yi Li*   *Patrik Brundin*

INTRODUCTION

Motor dysfunctions in Parkinson's disease (PD) are mainly caused by degeneration of dopaminergic (DAergic) neurons in the substantia nigra. Cell replacement therapy using the tissues of fetal ventral mesencephalon has proven to be beneficial for treating PD; however, numerous bioethical and logistical issues prevent wider application of the approach. Human embryonic stem cells (hESCs) are pluripotent and able to differentiate into various cell types, including DAergic neurons. These cells could, therefore, be used as an alternative source of DAergic neurons for cell replacement therapy in PD. Despite the existence of other optional sources of newly generated DAergic neurons (e.g., adult stem cells and neural progenitors), hESCs cells currently should be viewed as the most promising alternative. Though many problems and drawbacks are currently associated with the principal stages of this approach, further scientific research conducted in this direction should be encouraged. This review aims to provide a realistic and balanced view of the potential of hESCs in future cell-based treatment of PD.

Embryonic stem cells (ESCs) were first described in 1980 as cells derived from the inner cell mass of the late blastocyst stage of murine embryos (1,2). ESCs are truly pluripotent and able to differentiate into all cells present in adult organisms, such as the cells in the brain, blood, skin, skeleton, skeletal muscle, liver, and heart. Depending on the culture conditions, ESCs can propagate for an unlimited number of cell divisions as undifferentiated cells. The immortality of ESCs is thought to be caused by the high expression of telomerase that reconstructs each chromosome's telomeres after DNA replication during each cell division, and thus ESCs do not undergo senescence. Although ESCs can form cells constituting all adult tissues, they cannot form the "extraembryonic" tissues necessary for complete development, such as the placenta. For this reason, ESCs cannot become the origin of a new individual. Therefore, unlike a fertilized oocyte or the blastomere (cells derived from the first cleavage divisions), ESCs are not totipotent (3).

Thomson and colleagues (4) first isolated hESCs in 1998. Briefly, using immunosurgery they isolated the inner cell mass (ICM) from donated human blastocysts produced by *in vitro* fertilization (IVF) for clinical purposes. Isolated inner cell mass was plated on mitotically inactivated mouse embryonic fibroblasts with culture medium supplemented with vital growth factors and fetal bovine serum. These conditions allowed the ESCs to proliferate in an undifferentiated and pluripotent state. Two years later, Reubinoff, working in the group headed by Bongso, published the successful derivation of 2 more hESC lines from donated human blastocysts (5). The method described by Reubinoff et al. was similar to the one used by Thomson and his group. Since the publication of the first hESC lines by Thomson's and Bongso's groups, many other hESC lines have been derived.

Based on their capacity to grow indefinitely *in vitro* and to differentiate into every cell type of the human body, hESCs have been suggested as a source of specific cell types for transplantation therapies. Diseases involving the death or lost function of only one or a few cell types could be particularly suitable for hESC-based therapies. For example, PD primarily involves degeneration of nigrostriatal DAergic neurons. DAergic neurons already have been successfully derived from hESCs (6,7), but their ability to survive, integrate, and function when transplanted into an animal model of PD still has not been documented (8). Undoubtedly, this approach has great therapeutic potential. Nevertheless, many practical issues and potential biological hurdles should be addressed before it can become reality. This review discusses the current state of the hESC research field, the potential use of hESCs in PD, and the numerous problems associated with developing hESC grafting into a therapy for PD.

HUMAN EMBRYONIC STEM CELLS VERSUS EMBRYONIC/FETAL CELL MATERIAL: THE PATH AND THE PRINCIPLE

The possibility that PD could be treated with transplantation of DAergic neurons has captured the imagination of experimental and clinical scientists. Animal experiments with DAergic neurons derived from embryonic/fetal ventral mesencephalon, and the clinical trials performed so far, have been invaluable in furthering our understanding of the true potential of cell transplantation in PD patients. The studies have demonstrated that patients could clearly benefit from grafted DAergic neurons if certain criteria (related to the patient selection, cell handling, type of surgical technique, role of immunosuppression, and so on) are appropriately fulfilled. Thus, these studies serve as proof of the principle that DAergic neurons can be replaced in PD and under certain circumstances can exert antiparkinsonian effects (9–12), but they also show that the technique is difficult to reproduce consistently to obtain success in large series of patients (13,14).

For each potentially crucial parameter, several different approaches have been used in the different clinical trials that have been undertaken. There is significant variability in the clinical outcome, ranging from a considerable improvement in motor functions and quality of life for some patients, to no improvement for others (15–18). Unfortunately, the impact of most of the differences in technique among the various studies has not been monitored systematically. Therefore, it is difficult today to define an ideal transplantation protocol precisely. However, some parameters have clearly emerged as crucial. Some of the variability among patients is clearly dependent upon methodological factors, such as storage and handling of the cells before surgery, number and location of cells transplanted, techniques of immune suppression and implantation, and so on. Other aspects may be related to the type

and state of pathology in the patient, or even to stochastic events related to graft survival and integration. It appears that not every PD patient is suitable for cell transplantation. Factors contributing to the success of that could include genetic background, response to L-dopa, pathology and stage of the disease, age, general health, and so on. Therefore, the careful selection of patients susceptible for the transplantation is required (19,20). Taken together, minor differences in numerous factors actually contribute to large variations in cell transplantation clinical outcome (21). Despite the fact that no well-established ideal neural transplantation protocol exists for PD, some basic requirements for a successful graft can be suggested. Based on available data, it is clear that extensive DAergic reinnervation of the host striatum is necessary, and it has been proposed that a minimum of 100,000 grafted DAergic neurons need to survive in the putamen on each side of the brain (22). The number of embryos required to achieve this number of surviving cells depends on the age of the donor embryo, handling of the cells, and surgical technique. It is probably necessary with current technology to implant tissue from multiple donors, ranging from 2 to 4 on each side of the brain, into each patient (10,22,23).

Aside from problems with consistently obtaining symptomatic relief after transplantation in PD, an important side effect, *graft-induced dyskinesia*, appears in some graft recipients (13,14,18,24). Thus, about 15% to 50% of patients have exhibited involuntary movements after grafting, akin to those elicited by long-term levodopa treatment. Since it is not possible to predict with certainty which patients will develop graft-induced dyskinesias, and since pharmaceuticals cannot stop these dyskinesias, this side effect is a major drawback of the transplantation approach. It is unclear what mechanisms underlie graft-induced dyskinesias. A number of contributing factors have been suggested, including a presence of levodopa-induced dyskinesia prior to grafting (24), excessive level of dopamine (DA) release from the grafts (13), abnormal innervation of grafts, graft rejection, and presence of non-DAergic neurons in grafts (21,25,26).

Despite these important drawbacks, cell transplantation in PD still holds great promise. Several issues, such as patient selection and graft-induced dyskinesias, must be addressed in small systematic clinical trials before a wider clinical application can be considered. Even if all these issues are successfully resolved, the problems with unpredictable access to sufficient amounts of donor tissue for each patient and logistical problems associated with storage and handling must be successfully addressed. Furthermore, the ethical concerns regarding the use of cells obtained from aborted embryos restricts wider clinical application of this approach (27–29). Therefore, development of alternative sources of donor tissue is absolutely necessary. Such alternatives include adult stem cells derived from the patient's own body, either in a peripheral tissue or from a brain biopsy (30). It has been suggested that when treated with the appropriate factors while cultured *in vitro*, the adult neural stem cells can differentiate into *DAergic* neurons (31). However, despite the intensive research, there is currently no solid evidence that human adult stem cells are really able to give rise to DAergic neurons. Further studies are needed to prove the theoretical applicability of adult stem cells for derivation of DAergic neurons *in vitro*.

Another source of DAergic neurons could be hESCs purified from the inner cell mass of human blastocysts (5–6 days after fertilization). Such hESCs could be employed as an infinite source of self-renewing and pluripotent cells suitable for massive expansion and directed differentiation to DAergic neurons, followed by transplantation to the affected brain. The current status of research in the field of hESCs for the treatment of PD, the future potential of hESCs, and the principles of risk assessment associated with these applications are discussed in detail in this review.

IN VITRO NEURONAL DIFFERENTIATION OF EMBRYONIC STEM CELLS: PROGRESS, PERSPECTIVES, AND DRAWBACKS

To induce neuronal differentiation of hESCs, the systems developed so far rely on either of two major principles: the formation of embryoid bodies (EBs) (6,32–34) or the

coculturing of hESCs with a layer of feeder cells capable of inducing differentiation (7,35,36) (Fig. 46.1). In suspension cultures, ESCs aggregate and start differentiation that leads to the formation of the spherical EBs that contain precursor cells from all 3 germ layers (mesoderm, endoderm and ectoderm). The neuronal precursor cells within the EBs can then be isolated, forming aggregates termed *neurospheres*. Differentiation of the cells in the neurospheres into mature neurons can be induced by coculture systems and/or certain growth factors. Coculture of hESCs with mouse stromal cell lines (such as those called *PA6* and *MS5*) has demonstrated an ability to support neuronal differentiation of ESCs. The effects of the so-called *stromal cell–derived inducing activity* (SDIA) upon mouse ESCs was first described by Kawasaki et al. (37). It also has been applied to primate (38) and human (7) ESCs. In coculture with mouse stromal cells, hESC colonies tend to form neuronal rosettes, which are round structures within the colonies enriched in neuronal cells (7). The neuronal rosettes can then be isolated and differentiated in the presence of the specific differentiation-and survival-promoting factors in adhesion or suspension cultures (7). These growth-, differentiation-, and survival-promoting factors are normally known to be involved in *in vivo* development and maintenance of the nervous system. Transforming growth factor α (TGFα), for example, is expressed in the midbrain during early embryonic development of DAergic neurons and it has been suggested to direct the differentiation of hESCs into DAergic neurons (6). This factor is essential for

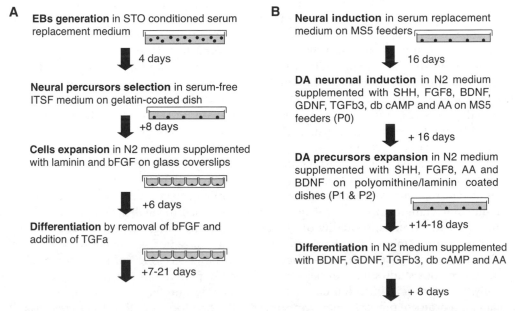

Figure 46.1 Schematic representation of the basic principles of the methods for the differentiation of hESCs into DAergic neurons. **A:** Method developed by Park et al., 2004. **B:** Method developed by Perrier et al. (Perrier AL, Tabar V, Barberi T, et al. Derivation of midbrain dopamine neurons from human embryonic stem cells. *Proc Natl Acad Sci USA* 2004;101:12,543–12,548). AA, ascorbic acid; BDNF, bone derived neurotrophic factor; bFGF, basic fibroblast growth factor; db cAMP, dibutyryl cAMP; FGF8, fibroblast growth factor 8; GDNF, glial derived neurotrophic factor; HH, sonic hedgehog; ITSF medium, insulin/transferrin/selenium/fibronectin medium; P 0, 1, 2, passages 0, 1 and 2; TGFα, transforming growth factor α.

both induction and survival of DAergic neurons *in vitro* and *in vivo* (39). After culturing in the presence of TGFα for 21 days, about 15% of the hESC-derived cells express tyrosine hydroxylase (TH; the key enzyme in the DA biosynthesis) and release DA. A more complex combination of factors was employed in the study by Perrier et al. (7). The differentiation of neuronal rosettes was induced by a sequential exposure to known patterning and differentiation factors of the midbrain DA system, including SHH, FGF8, BDNF, GDNF, TGFβ3, dibutyryl cAMP, and ascorbic acid. The sequential addition of combinations of these epigenetic factor aims to imitate the midbrain development *in vivo*, leading to the expression of midbrain transcription factors (such as Pax2, Aldh1, Lmx1b, En1, Nurr1, and Pitx3) in a sequence similar to that observed during development *in vivo*. After following the protocol for 50 days, more than 100 TH-positive neurons were generated from each undifferentiated hES cell initially plated (7). Numerous other studies aiming at further improvement and adaptation of the existing *in vitro* differentiation protocols have been performed (37,40–45).

The studies mentioned show that it is possible to derive DAergic neurons from hESCs *in vitro*. Many parameters, however, must be improved to make the protocols feasible for an actual therapy of PD. For example, it is generally accepted that to be suitable for a clinical therapy cells should be derived in a xeno-free system. Unfortunately, both Park's and Perrier's protocols (6,7) employ mouse stromal cell lines to initiate the neuronal differentiation (*see* Human Stem Cell-Related Ethical Considerations and Regulations). Moreover, so far there is no published study demonstrating that many hESC-derived DAergic neurons can survive grafting, integrate in the host brain, release DA, and decrease motor dysfunctions in animal models of PD. Besides the oxidative stress and the lack of trophic support responsible for low graft survival, the detachment of cells from the culture dishes followed by dissociation into single-cell suspension may considerably decrease the viability of cells before transplantation (46). Treatment with antioxidants and trophic factors as already applied to grafts of primary mesencephalic tissue (47,48; for review, see 49) could be tested to increase the survival of grafted hESC-derived DAergic neurons.

Besides the use of epigenetic factors, genetic modification of hESCs also may induce their differentiation into DAergic neurons. Nuclear receptor related-1 (Nurr1), a transcription factor known to be involved in differentiation of midbrain precursors into DAergic neurons, is a key candidate for application in differentiation of hESCs. Overexpression of Nurr1 in mouse ESCs results in a substantial increase in the proportion of TH⁺ neurons (43), especially after treatment with FGF8 and SHH. These neurons have electrophysiological properties typical for midbrain neurons and can reverse motor deficits after grafted to immunosuppressed rats (43). Another method for increasing the fraction of TH neurons would be to modify

the hESCs with a genetic construct containing an antibiotic resistance gene under the control of a lineage-restricted promoter (50). For example, a nearly homogeneous population of neurons was achieved by placing a neomyocin resistance gene in the Sox2 gene locus (Sox1 and Sox2 are expressed in the early neuroepithelium) in mouse ESCs. After inducing differentiation, the antibiotic was added, resulting in the selection of neuroepithelial progenitor cells expressing Sox2 (51).

The genetic manipulations are promising from the scientific point of view. However, they raise major safety issues from a clinical perspective. Because of the difficulty in controlling the incorporation of the transgene into the genome of a host cell, unexpected activation or inactivation of certain genes may occur. Unpredictable changes in the gene expression may lead, therefore, to the appearance of cells with high proliferative potential, capable of forming tumors following transplantation to the patient.

HUMAN STEM CELL-RELATED ETHICAL CONSIDERATIONS AND REGULATIONS

No matter how far from actual therapeutic application in humans, every hESC-related project rightfully raises a number of issues related to ethics and associated rules and regulations. Initially, relatively little effort was made to distinguish among studies aiming to develop treatments for humans (and thus directly falling under the rules and regulations of the corresponding supervising structures and offices) from those aimed at only studying stem cell biology *per se*. Coupled with the lack of immediate benefits in the clinical arena, the initial failure to carefully consider regulations coupled to clinical applications has caused delay in the actual progress in the field and a loss of momentum in the research. This has been particularly evident in the United States.

Although therapies based on adult stem cells also have raised widespread ethical concerns (52), controversies associated with studies employing embryonic cells are much greater. A strict governmental regulation is required to prevent the inappropriate use of human embryonic/fetal material. In most countries, specific status of personhood is not applied to the fetus, thus permitting the collections of embryonic cells. Moreover, ES cells used in the attempts to establish ES cell lines are derived from the human blastocysts seen as the side product of *in vitro* fertilization. Since the success rate of *in vitro* fertilization is far below 100%, a number of fertilized "reserve" eggs are obtained from the couple seeking treatment. It therefore could be seen as an ethical alternative for a couple to volunteer to dedicate their to-be-destroyed supernumerary blastocysts to scientific research or medical treatments.

One of the most important regulations restricting hESC applications is the decision (dated August 9, 2001) of the president of the United States to allow federal funds to be used for research only on existing hESC lines that satisfy certain criteria (see eligibility criteria at http://grants.nih .gov/grants/guide/notice-files/NOT-OD-02-006.html). Initially, some 60 hESC lines were considered to satisfy these criteria and thus were eligible for U.S. federal funding. An NIH Stem Cell Registry was created to provide up-to-date information on the subject, and it quickly has become an important resource for information related to hESC projects (http://stemcells.nih.gov/research/registry). Some hESC lines, however, were later withdrawn from the NIH Stem Cell Registry, whereas others were added. Even more importantly, some natural features in the biology of hESC lines prevent their indefinite application as an inexhaustible source of viable pluripotent cells for research and potential clinical applications. The karyotype of hESCs is not always stable (53), and each individual cell line can hardly be viewed as truly immortal and inalterable. Moreover, different hESC lines might vary regarding proliferation rate and their ability to maintain undifferentiated phenotype in preset conditions.

Major concerns associated with application of stem cells in clinical practice are the risks of having samples contaminated with microbial infections, nonhuman cell material or with genetic disorders from the donor. The U.S. Food and Drug Administration (FDA) Biological Response Modifiers Advisory Committee agreed in 2000 that the same standards used in blood banking and organ transplantation are appropriate for stem cell research. Most committee members also have supported screening the donor for certain genetic mutations that may predispose recipients to disease, but a consensus about which mutations were the most important could not be reached. This point raises additional bioethical issues related to the concept of eugenics. Laws and regulations are established in many countries to prevent inequality based on eugenics. The definition of a reasonable borderline between immoral practices of eugenics and protection of the recipient from developing a potentially severe disease is undoubtedly difficult.

The standard technique for maintaining established hESC lines in their undifferentiated state is to grow them on mouse embryonic fibroblasts (MEFs), known as *feeder cells*. In addition to vital cell–cell contacts, MEF cells excrete yet unidentified factors that support hESCs. The close contact entails risks of contaminating the human cells with immunogenic animal cells or potentially harmful murine viruses. The transmission of undetected animal infectious agents could cause diseases (xenozoonozes) that, in turn, theoretically could be transmitted from transplanted patients to the general public. This risk is of particular concern considering that patients might be immunosuppressed following hESC transplantation. Though there is no current evidence that viruses harmful to mice can cause diseases in humans, it is possible that they could change in a new host. Further elaborate studies of

potential animal viruses were required by the FDA, thus introducing more delay in moving the actual application of hESCs to the stage of clinical trials. The concerns were further justified by the recent study by Martin et al. (54), in which it was demonstrated that hESCs incorporate nonhuman Neu5Gc sialic acid isoform from nonhuman feeder cells and growth media components. Considering that most normal humans have circulating antibodies specific for Neu5Gc, contaminated hESCs could induce an immune response and compromise the transplant (54). Consequently, attempts to establish either feeder-free (55) or xeno-free protocols (56,57) have become important. In addition to being free of the risks of viral or cell contaminations, human feeder cells are more convenient in handling and can withstand higher numbers of passages. Among the last, mitotically inactivated adult human uterine endometrial cells, adult breast parenchymal cells, adult oviduct epithelial cells, and embryonic fibroblasts are employed. Though some hESC lines do not grow well after the switch from mouse to human feeder systems, others can be maintained on both (Fig. 46.2).

As an alternative to growing hESCs on feeders, it is also possible to use growth media enriched with factors secreted by MEFs (i.e., MEF-conditioned media). Although this approach eliminates the risk of contaminating hESCs with mouse cells, media enriched with mouse cell-derived secreted factors could still be viewed as contaminated by xenogeneic proteins, thus causing the risk of incorporating these to the human cells. For similar reasons, protocols that employ various serum replacements rather than fetal calf/bovine serum are considered more suitable for clinical applications (5,58,59).

So far, we have considered safety issues related only to propagating undifferentiated hESCs on cells derived from animals. In the next step (i.e., differentiation of the hESCs into DAergic neurons), some protocols also rely on mouse cells. As mentioned, using an intrinsic activity of murine stromal cells (such as PA6 cells), hESCs can be differentiated into DAergic neurons (36,37,60). In addition, several alternative protocols rely on promoting hESC differentiation by exposing them to media supplemented by growth factors/cytokines. Many of these, although used

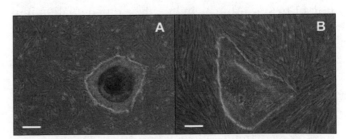

Figure 46.2 hESC line SA002 (present in the NIH Stem Cell Registry) growing over the layer of the feeder cells. **A:** Mouse embryonic fibroblasts (MEFs). **B:** Human foreskin fibroblasts. Scale bars: 100 μm.

extensively in research, are not FDA approved for human use. This effectively bans application of that growth factor for anything other than research associated with understanding the basic mechanisms of human stem cell biology. Using human recombinant growth factors to substitute nonhuman ones seems to be the direct solution to this problem.

IMMUNOSUPPRESSION: POTENTIAL CONSIDERATIONS AND DRAWBACKS

Grafts of hESC-derived DAergic neurons to patients with PD would in most cases be immunologically incompatible with the host. The only exception would be if the grafted cells were subjected to therapeutic nuclear transfer (61). In this case, the nucleus of the donor cells would be exchanged for a nucleus from one of the patient's cells. As a result, the hESCs used for grafting would be genetically identical to the patient. However, therapeutic nuclear transfer might not be a viable option for PD patients. First, some cases of PD are definitely genetically inherited (62,63) and transferring the mutant genes that caused neurodegeneration into the graft donor cells would be irrational. Second, therapeutic nuclear transfer is still technically difficult to perform, has a low success rate, and requires a large number of donor blastocysts (64). Therefore, it might not be a practical option. Consequently, most, if not all, grafts of hESCs in PD would by necessity be allogenic (i.e., within the same species but fully histoincompatible), possibly resulting in the necessity for continuous immunosuppression.

The brain is an immunologically privileged transplantation site (65,66). Previous studies demonstrated that this privilege may be attributed to one or more of the following: (a) presence of local immunosuppressive factors (67), (b) the existence of a blood–brain barrier (68), (c) the lack of a conventional lymphatic drainage (69), (d) the lack of classical antigen-presenting cells (70), and (e) the paucity of MHC antigen expression (71). Clearly, the immune-privileged state of intracerebral transplants depends at least in part on inadequate presentation of donor antigens to the host immune system. For example, after peripheral sensitization, well-established intracerebral grafts can undergo acute rejection (72–75), which suggests that they are not completely protected from the immune system. Thus, there is compelling evidence that the immune privilege in the brain is not absolute and that immune rejection has to be carefully considered when transplanting hESCs-derived DAergic neurons.

Animal studies demonstrate that neural allograft rejection may take a few weeks in rodents or could be delayed by weeks or even months, depending on the degree and type of histoincompatibility (72,74–78). In clinical trials employing allografted neural tissue in PD (9,13,14,17,22; for review, see 21) and Huntington's

disease (79), different immunosuppression protocols have been used. Early trials with grafts of embryonic DAergic neurons have relied on an extensive immunosuppression regimen with cyclosporine A, methylprednisolone, and azathioprine (24,80,81). The immunosuppression was maintained for several years in some patients. In those cases, positron emission tomography scans revealed [18]F L-dopa uptake, reflecting functionality of grafted cells, several years after surgery. However, in 2 more recent NIH-funded double-blind trials, patients were not given any immunosuppressive treatment (13) or were given only a low dose of cyclosporine A for 6 months (14). In the latter trials, there was some indication that the grafts were exerting functional effects in the short term. However, after cessation of the cyclosporine A treatment, these putative effects gradually disappeared, indicating a possible immune rejection of the grafts (for review, see 82). Undoubtedly, immune responses of the host may have an important effect upon long-term graft survival and function. Therefore, allografts of hESC-derived DAergic neurons are also likely to be at risk for immunorejection, and thus immunosuppression has to be carefully considered as part of any transplant protocol in the future.

TERATOMA FORMATION: RISKS AND PRECAUTIONS

To avoid teratoma formation, a complete elimination of any residual undifferentiated hESCs from donor cells is absolutely essential prior to grafting. Ideally, all the hESCs would be differentiated into specialized cell types. As mentioned, previous studies have shown that mouse, monkey, and human ESCs can differentiate into DAergic neurons under certain culture conditions (37,40–45). Dopaminergic neurons derived from mouse and monkey ESCs survive transplantation into brains with no teratoma formation (37,40,43,45,83,84). However, when nondifferentiated mouse ESCs were grafted into the striatum, 20% of grafted rats developed teratomas (85). Our studies on hESCs transplanted to the rat brain support the idea that the induction of the differentiation of these cells prior to implantation markedly reduces the likelihood of teratoma formation (Fig. 46.3). Therefore, the general consensus in the field of neural stem cell therapy is that some degree of differentiation *in vitro* is essential prior to grafting to avoid teratomas and to obtain functional neurons. On the other hand, if the stem cells are differentiated into neurons that have long and elaborate processes already *in vitro*, the survival rate after implantation into the brain is likely to be low. It is, therefore, essential to identify a window of opportunity within the differentiation protocol with (a) the highest possible content of DAergic neurons and DAergic neuron-fate committed cells that can support functional recovery, (b) an acceptable cell survival rate in the transplants, and (c) virtually no risk of teratoma formation (Fig. 46.4).

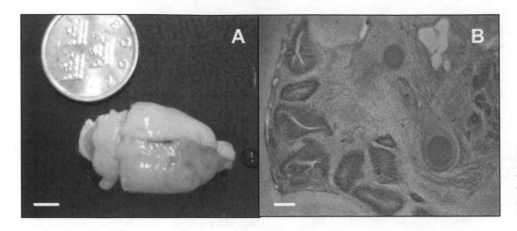

Figure 46.3 Macroscopic **(A)** and microscopic **(B)** evidence of teratoma formation in the brain of the rats transplanted with poorly differentiated hESCs. Scale bars: **(A)** 5 mm; **(B)** 100 μm.

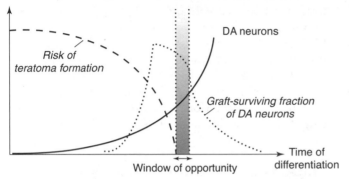

Figure 46.4 Balancing the parameters of hESCs grafting: a schematic representation. Solid line represents a fraction of the DAergic neurons in the mixed cell population; dotted line, ability of DAergic neurons to survive grafting procedure; dashed line, teratoma formation; shaded area, window of opportunity for performing a transplantation of hESC-derived DAergic neurons.

NEUROSURGICAL TECHNIQUE IMPACT ON THE OUTCOME OF HUMAN EMBRYONIC STEM CELL TRANSPLANTS

The optimal neurosurgical approach would be one that permits distribution of the hESC-derived DAergic neurons at multiple brain sites that require DAergic reinnervation. Extensive animal studies have shown that the functional recovery is much greater if DAergic neurons are implanted into the target regions of the nigrostriatal projections and not in the substantia nigra (i.e., the actual site of cell death in PD). Thus, the putamen and caudate nucleus, which normally are heavily innervated by DAergic neurons, and progressively lose these innervations during the course of PD, are primary targets for implantation. Most clinical trials with embryonic ventral mesencephalon have used stereotactic techniques to implant either cell suspensions or small tissue aggregates (13,80,86,87; also see 88). In a small number of cases, an open microsurgery technique has been used to access the head of the caudate nucleus via the lateral ventricle, thus allowing the placement of tissue chunks directly into the brain parenchyma (89,90). Because of higher morbidity, with side effects related to the surgical

trauma, this approach is not recommended. The advantage with the stereotactic approach is that multiple sites can be reached with relatively little trauma to the surrounding brain. If desired, the surgery can even be conducted under local instead of general anesthesia. When injecting cells stereotactically, the size of the implants is limited by the size of the injection cannula. Animal studies suggest that graft survival is compromised if the cannula is too large (e.g., 2.5 mm in outer diameter). To avoid excessive damage to the host brain, and thereby an inhospitable environment for the graft cells, the outer diameter of the cannula should not be larger than approximately 1 mm (91). Because the inner diameter is by necessity much smaller, in practice this means that it is difficult to inject cell aggregates that exceed approximately 500 μm in diameter. As mentioned, most hESC culture protocols involve growing the cells as monolayers or as small spheres. The disadvantage of growing hESC as monolayers is that the cells invariably suffer from severe damage when harvested from the culture dish and are transferred into the transplantation instrument. Early studies on cultured rat DAergic primary neurons demonstrated that the survival of the neurons was reduced when they had been grown *in vitro* for a prolonged period (7 days) compared to short periods (2 days) (92). However, as discussed, it appears essential that hESCs are relatively well differentiated before they are grafted as otherwise there is a high risk of teratoma formation and the chances of obtaining surviving DAergic neurons are reduced (Fig. 46.4). Thus, there is clearly a difficult paradox: hESC need prolonged culturing to be relatively well matured before grafting, but this may dramatically reduce survival upon transplantation. One solution to this problem could be to devise protocols in which the hESCs-derived DAergic neurons develop in small aggregates that can be grafted without any mechanical disruption. The validity of this approach was addressed in animal studies (93–95) in which reaggregates of cultured mesencephalic tissue–derived DAergic neurons or small pieces of mesencephalic tissue, rather than cell suspensions, were used for grafting. It would be important to ensure that the aggregates do not exceed a size that allows effective transfer of nutrients and metabolites.

This is particularly crucial following implantation into the brain, before the grafted hESC-derived aggregates have had an opportunity to establish a shared vascular network with the host brain. Previous studies suggest that a tissue aggregate diameter of approximately 600–1200 μm is feasible (96).

EMBRYONIC AND ADULT STEM CELLS: GRAFTING VERSUS DRAFTING

Both embryonic and adult human stem cells are currently considered a potential source of newly formed DAergic neurons. In discussions about the ethical issues of novel treatments, hESCs are clearly more controversial than are adult stem cells (97,98). Additionally, by virtue of being autologous, patient-derived adult stem cells do not cause problems of immune rejection. Furthermore, certain types of adult stem cells have been studied much longer than hESCs, resulting in a greater understanding of their basic biology. Differentiation of hematopoietic bone marrow stem cells, for example, is the best-known stem cell model to date, and those cells are used extensively in human subjects.

Regarding a potential cell therapy for PD, numerous pros and cons are associated with both hESCs and adult stem cells. First, although hESCs are pluripotent, adult stem cells appear already committed to a certain differentiation

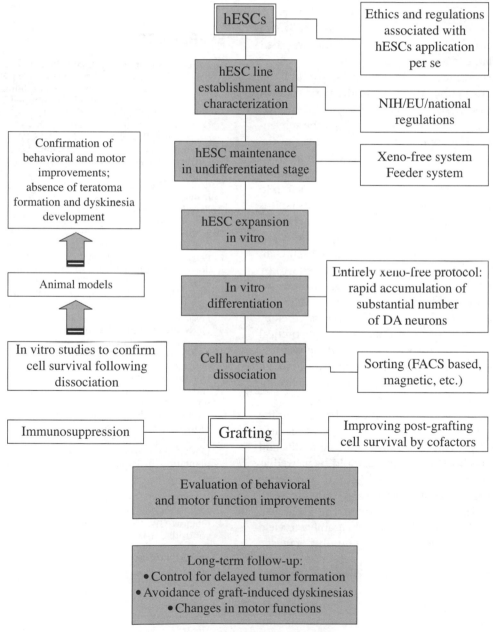

Figure 46.5 Application of hESC-derived DAergic neurons in cell transplantation therapy in PD: overview of research stages.

pathway. This latter view is controversial, and from 1999 to 2001 there were many studies claiming that adult stem cells also are pluripotent (99–102). This potential of adult stem cells to transdifferentiate to cells of another germ layer is currently being questioned (103–106). Second, there is a lack of cell culture protocols for most types of adult stem cells, which allows them to proliferate with relative efficiency.

Additionally, neural stem cells and progenitor cells are also considered a promising alternative source of DAergic neurons. The latter have demonstrated the ability to generate cells with several characteristics of DAergic neurons (96,107,108). With current protocols, however, the yield of DAergic neurons is low, and they survive poorly when grafted (107). Possibly, protocols designed to promote differentiation of hESCs into DAergic neurons also can be applied to these cells (109). Furthermore, targeted enhancement of the expression of certain genes, such as Bcl-X(L), in differentiating neural stem cells significantly improves their ability to yield viable DAergic neurons (110).

Another alternative for cell therapy in PD would be to recruit endogenous neural stem cells in the patient's own brain. Adult neurogenesis is a well-established phenomenon in certain mammalian brain regions (e.g., the subventricular zone of the forebrain and the dentate gyrus of the hippocampus). It is debatable whether newborn neurons occur in significant numbers in other brain regions and whether they have a significant impact on brain function in those cases in which they are present in low numbers. It is highly controversial whether neurogenesis occurs in the substantial nigra. Claims that newborn DAergic neurons can appear in the adult substantia nigra (111) have been challenged (112,113). The emerging consensus appears to be that under normal conditions no new DAergic neurons are generated in the adult substantia nigra, and it has to be concluded that the utilization of adult neurogenesis as a therapy for PD currently should be viewed as a purely theoretical possibility. Of course, this does not exclude the possibility that in the future it could be possible to develop a protocol promoting the formation of such cells following, for example, the infusion of a defined set of growth factors.

Taken together, it should be concluded that despite the existence of numerous optional sources of newly generated DAergic neurons (e.g., embryonic and adult stem cells and neural progenitors), hESCs currently should be viewed as the most promising. The ability of hESCs to proliferate and rapidly expand *in vitro* in relatively straightforward fashion is an indisputable advantage of the approach. Importantly, hESCs have already proven their ability to yield highly differentiated DAergic neurons in a number of *in vitro* protocols and to survive transplantation procedures. Though numerous problems and drawbacks are currently associated with many principal stages of the approach (bioethical, technological, and so on; Fig. 46.5), further scientific research conducted in this direction should be encouraged. With simplification and improvement of existing cell differentiation and cell transplantation protocols, and by addressing the

important safety issues mentioned, the joint efforts of the international scientific community would result in steady progress in this important field. It is hoped that this review has provided a realistic and balanced view of the potential of hESCs in future cell-based treatment of PD.

ACKNOWLEDGMENTS

This study was supported by a grant from the United States Army Medical Research Acquisition Activity (USAMRAA) Award No. W81XWH-04-1-0366, National Institute of Health Grant Number 1 R21 NS043717-01A1 and The Research Foundation of the Swedish Parkinson's Disease Association.

REFERENCES

1. Evans MJ, Kaufman MH. Establishment in culture of pluripotential cells from mouse embryos. *Nature* 1981;292:154–156.
2. Martin GR. Isolation of a pluripotent cell line from early mouse embryos cultured in medium conditioned by teratocarcinoma stem cells. *Proc Natl Acad Sci USA* 1981;78:7634–7638.
3. De Wert G, Mummery C. Human embryonic stem cells: research, ethics and policy. *Hum Reprod* 2003;18:672–682.
4. Thomson JA, Itskovitz-Eldor J, Shapiro SS, et al. Embryonic stem cell lines derived from human blastocysts. *Science* 1998;282:1145–1147.
5. Reubinoff BE, Pera MF, Fong CY, et al. Embryonic stem cell lines from human blastocysts: somatic differentiation in vitro. *Nat Biotechnol* 2000;18:399–404.
6. Park S, Lee KS, Lee YJ, et al. Generation of dopaminergic neurons in vitro from human embryonic stem cells treated with neurotrophic factors. *Neurosci Lett* 2004;359:99–103.
7. Perrier AL, Tabar V, Barberi T, et al. Derivation of midbrain dopamine neurons from human embryonic stem cells. *Proc Natl Acad Sci USA* 2004;101:12,543–12,548.
8. Park CH, Minn YK, Lee JY, et al. In vitro and in vivo analyses of human embryonic stem cell-derived dopamine neurons. *J Neurochem* 2005;92:1265–1276.
9. Lindvall O, Brundin P, Widner H, et al. Grafts of fetal dopamine neurons survive and improve motor function in Parkinson's disease. *Science* 1990;247:574–577.
10. Lindvall O, Widner H, Rehncrona S, et al. Transplantation of fetal dopamine neurons in Parkinson's disease: one-year clinical and neurophysiological observations in two patients with putaminal implants. *Ann Neurol* 1992;31:155–165.
11. Piccini P, Lindvall O, Bjorklund A, et al. Delayed recovery of movement-related cortical function in Parkinson's disease after striatal dopaminergic grafts. *Ann Neurol* 2000;48:689–695.
12. Lindvall O, Hagell P. Clinical observations after neural transplantation in Parkinson's disease. *Prog Brain Res* 2000;127:299–320.
13. Freed CR, Greene PE, Breeze RE, et al. Transplantation of embryonic dopamine neurons for severe Parkinson's disease. *N Engl J Med* 2001;344:710–719.
14. Olanow CW, Goetz CG, Kordower JH, et al. A double-blind controlled trial of bilateral fetal nigral transplantation in Parkinson's disease. *Ann Neurol* 2003;54:403–414.
15. Lindvall O, Sawle G, Widner H, et al. Evidence for long-term survival and function of dopaminergic grafts in progressive Parkinson's disease. *Ann Neurol* 1994;35:172–180.
16. Defer GL, Geny C, Ricolfi F, et al. Long-term outcome of unilaterally transplanted parkinsonian patients. I. Clinical approach. *Brain* 1996;119:41–50.
17. Hauser RA, Freeman TB, Snow BJ, et al. Long-term evaluation of bilateral fetal nigral transplantation in Parkinson disease. *Arch Neurol* 1999;56:179–187.

18. Freed CR, Leehey MA, Zawada M, et al. Do patients with Parkinson's disease benefit from embryonic dopamine cell transplantation? *J Neurol* 2003;250:III44–III46.

19. Lopez-Lozano JJ, Bravo G, Brera B, et al., and Clinica Puerta de Hierro Neural Transplantation Group. Long-term improvement in patients with severe Parkinson's disease after implantation of fetal ventral mesencephalic tissue in a cavity of the caudate nucleus: 5-year follow up in 10 patients. *J Neurosurg* 1997;86:931–942.

20. Rascol O, Goetz C, Koller W, et al. Treatment interventions for Parkinson's disease: an evidence based assessment. *Lancet* 2002;359:1589–1598.

21. Bjorklund A, Dunnett SB, Brundin P, et al. Neural transplantation for the treatment of Parkinson's disease. *Lancet Neurol* 2003;2:437–445.

22. Hagell P, Brundin P. Cell survival and clinical outcome following intrastriatal transplantation in Parkinson disease. *J Neuropathol Exp Neurol* 2001;60:741–752.

23. Cochen V, Ribeiro MJ, Nguyen JP, et al. Transplantation in Parkinson's disease: PET changes correlate with the amount of grafted tissue. *Mov Disord* 2003;18:928–932.

24. Hagell P, Piccini P, Bjorklund A, et al. Dyskinesias following neural transplantation in Parkinson's disease. *Nat Neurosci* 2002;5:627–628.

25. Isacson O, Bjorklund LM, Schumacher JM. Toward full restoration of synaptic and terminal function of the dopaminergic system in Parkinson's disease by stem cells. *Ann Neurol* 2003;53:S135–S146; discussion S146–S148.

26. Steece-Collier K, Collier TJ, Danielson PD, et al. Embryonic mesencephalic grafts increase levodopa-induced forelimb hyperkinesia in parkinsonian rats. *Mov Disord* 2003;18:1442–1454.

27. Boer GJ. Ethical issues in neurografting of human embryonic cells. *Theor Med Bioeth* 1999;20:461–475.

28. Hagell P. Restorative neurology in movement disorders. *J Neurosci Nurs* 2000;32:256–262.

29. Lindvall O. Stem cells for cell therapy in Parkinson's disease. *Pharmacol Res* 2003;47:279–287.

30. Galvin KA, Jones DG. Adult human neural stem cells for cell-replacement therapies in the central nervous system. *Med J Aust* 2002;177:316–318.

31. Daadi MM, Weiss S. Generation of tyrosine hydroxylase-producing neurons from precursors of the embryonic and adult forebrain. *J Neurosci* 1999;19:4484–4497.

32. Zhang SC, Wernig M, Duncan ID, et al. In vitro differentiation of transplantable neural precursors from human embryonic stem cells. *Nat Biotechnol* 2001;19:1129–1133.

33. Carpenter MK, Inokuma MS, Denham J, et al. Enrichment of neurons and neural precursors from human embryonic stem cells. *Exp Neurol* 2001;172:383–397.

34. Schulz TC, Palmarini GM, Noggle SA, et al. Directed neuronal differentiation of human embryonic stem cells. *BMC Neurosci* 2003;4:27.

35. Reubinoff BE, Itsykson P, Turetsky T, et al. Neural progenitors from human embryonic stem cells. *Nat Biotechnol* 2001;19:1134–1140.

36. Zeng X, Cai J, Chen J, et al. Dopaminergic differentiation of human embryonic stem cells. *Stem Cells* 2004;22:925–940.

37. Kawasaki H, Mizuseki K, Nishikawa S, et al. Induction of midbrain dopaminergic neurons from ES cells by stromal cell-derived inducing activity. *Neuron* 2000;28:31–40.

38. Mizuseki K, Sakamoto T, Watanabe K, et al. Generation of neural crest-derived peripheral neurons and floor plate cells from mouse and primate embryonic stem cells. *Proc Natl Acad Sci USA* 2003;100:5828–5833.

39. Farkas LM, Dunker N, Roussa E, et al. Transforming growth factor-beta(s) are essential for the development of midbrain dopaminergic neurons in vitro and in vivo. *J Neurosci* 2003;23:5178–5186.

40. Kawasaki H, Suemori H, Mizuseki K, et al. Generation of dopaminergic neurons and pigmented epithelia from primate ES cells by stromal cell-derived inducing activity. *Proc Natl Acad Sci USA* 2002;99:1580–1585.

41. Lee SH, Lumelsky N, Studer L, et al. Efficient generation of midbrain and hindbrain neurons from mouse embryonic stem cells. *Nat Biotechnol* 2000;18:675–679.

42. Wakayama T, Tabar V, Rodriguez I, et al. Differentiation of embryonic stem cell lines generated from adult somatic cells by nuclear transfer. *Science* 2001;292:740–743.

43. Kim JH, Auerbach JM, Rodriguez-Gomez JA, et al. Dopamine neurons derived from embryonic stem cells function in an animal model of Parkinson's disease. *Nature* 2002;418:50–56.

44. Barberi T, Klivenyi P, Calingasan NY, et al. Neural subtype specification of fertilization and nuclear transfer embryonic stem cells and application in parkinsonian mice. *Nat Biotechnol* 2003;21:1200–1207.

45. Takagi Y, Takahashi J, Saiki H, et al. Dopaminergic neurons generated from monkey embryonic stem cells function in a Parkinson primate model. *J Clin Invest* 2005;115:102–109.

46. Emgard M, Hallin U, Karlsson J, et al. Both apoptosis and necrosis occur early after intracerebral grafting of ventral mesencephalic tissue: a role for protease activation. *J Neurochem* 2003;86:1223–1232.

47. Mayer E, Fawcett JW, Dunnett SB. Basic fibroblast growth factor promotes the survival of embryonic ventral mesencephalic dopaminergic neurons. II. Effects on nigral transplants in vivo. *Neuroscience* 1993;56:389–398.

48. Sinclair SR, Svendsen CN, Torres EM, et al. GDNF enhances dopaminergic cell survival and fibre outgrowth in embryonic nigral grafts. *Neuroreport* 1996;7:2547–2552.

49. Brundin P, Karlsson J, Emgard M, et al. Improving the survival of grafted dopaminergic neurons: a review over current approaches. *Cell Transplant* 2000;9:179–195.

50. O'Shea KS. Directed differentiation of embryonic stem cells: genetic and epigenetic methods. *Wound Repair Regen* 2001;9:443–459.

51. Li M, Pevny L, Lovell-Badge R, et al. Generation of purified neural precursors from embryonic stem cells by lineage selection. *Curr Biol* 1998;8:9714.

52. Fruchtman S. Stem cell transplantation. *Mt Sinai J Med* 2003;70:166–170.

53. Draper JS, Moore HD, Ruban LN, et al. Culture and characterization of human embryonic stem cells. *Stem Cells Dev* 2004;13:325–336.

54. Martin MJ, Muotri A, Gage F, et al. Human embryonic stem cells express an immunogenic nonhuman sialic acid. *Nat Med* 2005;11:228–232.

55. Amit M, Shariki C, Margulets V, et al. Feeder layer- and serum-free culture of human embryonic stem cells. *Biol Reprod* 2004;70:837–845.

56. Amit M, Margulets V, Segev H, et al. Human feeder layers for human embryonic stem cells. *Biol Reprod* 2003;68:2150–2156.

57. Hovatta O, Mikkola M, Gertow K, et al. A culture system using human foreskin fibroblasts as feeder cells allows production of human embryonic stem cells. *Hum Reprod* 2003;18:1404–1409.

58. Xu C, Inokuma MS, Denham J, et al. Feeder-free growth of undifferentiated human embryonic stem cells. *Nat Biotechnol* 2001;19:971–974.

59. Passier R. Potential of human embryonic stem cells in regenerative medicine. *Horm Res* 2003;60:11–14.

60. Sasai Y. Generation of dopaminergic neurons from embryonic stem cells. *J Neurol* 2002;249:II41–II44.

61. Mayhall EA, Paffett-Lugassy N, Zon LI. The clinical potential of stem cells. *Curr Opin Cell Biol* 2004;16:713–720.

62. Mouradian MM. Recent advances in the genetics and pathogenesis of Parkinson disease. *Neurology* 2002;58:179–185.

63. Burke RE. Recent advances in research on Parkinson disease: synuclein and parkin. *Neurologist* 2004;10:75–81.

64. Gordon JW. Methods and strategies for gene transfer and engineering of the germ line. In: *The science and ethics of engineering the human germ line*. New York: John Wiley & Sons, Inc., 2003:121–152.

65. Barker CF, Billingham RE. Immunologically privileged sites. *Adv Immunol* 1977;25:1–54.

66. Widner H, Brundin P, Bjorklund A, et al. Immunological aspects of neural grafting in the mammalian central nervous system. *Prog Brain Res* 1988;78:303–307.

67. Massa PT. Specific suppression of major histocompatibility complex class I and class II genes in astrocytes by brain-enriched gangliosides. *J Exp Med* 1993;178:1357–1363.

68. Hart MN, Fabry Z. CNS antigen presentation. *Trends Neurosci* 1995;18:475–481.
69. Cserr HF, Knopf PM. Cervical lymphatics, the blood-brain barrier and the immunoreactivity of the brain: a new view. *Immunol Today* 1992;13:507–512.
70. Hart DN, Fabre JW. Demonstration and characterization of Ia-positive dendritic cells in the interstitial connective tissues of rat heart and other tissues, but not brain. *J Exp Med* 1981;154:347–361.
71. Bartlett PF, Kerr RS, Bailey KA. Expression of MHC antigens in the central nervous system. *Transplant Proc* 1989;21:3163–3165.
72. Mason DW, Charlton HM, Jones AJ, et al. The fate of allogeneic and xenogeneic neuronal tissue transplanted into the third ventricle of rodents. *Neuroscience* 1986;19:685–694.
73. Lund RD, Rao K, Kunz HW, et al. Instability of neural xenografts placed in neonatal rat brains. *Transplantation* 1988;46:216–223.
74. Duan WM, Widner H, Brundin P. Temporal pattern of host responses against intrastriatal grafts of syngeneic, allogeneic or xenogeneic embryonic neuronal tissue in rats. *Exp Brain Res* 1995;104:227–242.
75. Duan WM, Brundin P, Widner H. Addition of allogeneic spleen cells causes rejection of intrastriatal embryonic mesencephalic allografts in the rat. *Neuroscience* 1997;77:599–609.
76. Sloan DJ, Baker BJ, Puklavec M, Charlton HM. The effect of site of transplantation and histocompatibility differences on the survival of neural tissue transplanted to the CNS of defined inbred rat strains. *Prog Brain Res* 1990;82:141–152.
77. Lawrence JM, Morris RJ, Wilson DJ, et al. Mechanisms of allograft rejection in the rat brain. *Neuroscience* 1990;37:431–462.
78. Freed WJ, Dymecki J, Poltorak M, et al. Intraventricular brain allografts and xenografts: studies of survival and rejection with and without systemic sensitization. *Prog Brain Res* 1988;78:233–241.
79. Peschanski M, Bachoud-Levi AC, Hantraye P. Integrating fetal neural transplants into a therapeutic strategy: the example of Huntington's disease. *Brain* 2004;127:1219–1228.
80. Widner H, Tetrud J, Rehncrona S, et al. Bilateral fetal mesencephalic grafting in two patients with parkinsonism induced by 1-methyl-4-phenyl-1,2,3,6-tetrahydropyridine (MPTP). *N Engl J Med* 1992;327:1556–1563.
81. Brundin P, Pogarell O, Hagell P, et al. Bilateral caudate and putamen grafts of embryonic mesencephalic tissue treated with lazaroids in Parkinson's disease. *Brain* 2000;123:1380–1390.
82. Winkler C, Kirik D, Bjorklund A. Cell transplantation in Parkinson's disease: how can we make it work? *Trends Neurosci* 2005;28:86–92.
83. Morizane A, Takahashi J, Takagi Y, et al. Optimal conditions for in vivo induction of dopaminergic neurons from embryonic stem cells through stromal cell-derived inducing activity. *J Neurosci Res* 2002;69:934–939.
84. Nishimura F, Yoshikawa M, Kanda S, et al. Potential use of embryonic stem cells for the treatment of mouse parkinsonian models: improved behavior by transplantation of in vitro differentiated dopaminergic neurons from embryonic stem cells. *Stem Cells* 2003;21:171–180.
85. Bjorklund LM, Sanchez-Pernaute R, Chung S, et al. Embryonic stem cells develop into functional dopaminergic neurons after transplantation in a Parkinson rat model. *Proc Natl Acad Sci USA* 2002;99:2344–2349.
86. Molina H, Quinones-Molina R, Munoz J, et al. Neurotransplantation in Parkinson's disease: from open microsurgery to bilateral stereotactic approach: first clinical trial using microelectrode recording technique. *Stereotact Funct Neurosurg* 1994;62:204–208.
87. Kopyov OV, Jacques D, Lieberman A, et al. Clinical study of fetal mesencephalic intracerebral transplants for the treatment of Parkinson's disease. *Cell Transplant* 1996;5:327–337.
88. Olanow CW. Surgical therapy for Parkinson's disease. *Eur J Neurol* 2002;9:31–39.
89. Madrazo I, Leon V, Torres C, et al. Transplantation of fetal substantia nigra and adrenal medulla to the caudate nucleus in two patients with Parkinson's disease. *N Engl J Med* 1988;318:51.
90. Madrazo I, Franco-Bourland R, Ostrosky-Solis F, et al. Fetal homotransplants (ventral mesencephalon and adrenal tissue) to

the striatum of parkinsonian subjects. *Arch Neurol* 1990;47:1281–1285.
91. Brundin P. Dissection, preparation, and implantation of human embryonic brain tissue. In: Dunnett SB, Bjorklund A, ed. *Neural transplantation. A practical approach*. New York: Oxford University Press, 1992:139–160.
92. Brundin P, Barbin G, Strecker RE, et al. Survival and function of dissociated rat dopamine neurones grafted at different developmental stages or after being cultured in vitro. *Brain Res* 1988;467:233–243.
93. Strecker RE, Miao R, Loring JF. Survival and function of aggregate cultures of rat fetal dopamine neurons grafted in a rat model of Parkinson's disease. *Exp Brain Res* 1989;76:315–322.
94. Spector DH, Boss BD, Strecker RE. A model three-dimensional culture system for mammalian dopaminergic precursor cells: application for functional intracerebral transplantation. *Exp Neurol* 1993;124:253–264.
95. Freeman TB, Olanow CW, Hauser RA, et al. Bilateral fetal nigral transplantation into the postcommissural putamen in Parkinson's disease. *Ann Neurol* 1995;38:379–388.
96. Studer L, Tabar V, McKay RD. Transplantation of expanded mesencephalic precursors leads to recovery in parkinsonian rats. *Nat Neurosci* 1998;1:290–295.
97. Henon PR. Human embryonic or adult stem cells: an overview on ethics and perspectives for tissue engineering. *Adv Exp Med Biol* 2003;534:27–45.
98. Henningson CT, Stanislaus MA, Gewirtz AM. Embryonic and adult stem cell therapy. *J Allergy Clin Immunol* 2003;111:S745–S753.
99. Bjornson CR, Rietze RL, Reynolds BA, et al. Turning brain into blood: a hematopoietic fate adopted by adult neural stem cells in vivo. *Science* 1999;283:534–537.
100. Pittenger MF, Mackay AM, Beck SC, et al. Multilineage potential of adult human mesenchymal stem cells. *Science* 1999;284:385–389.
101. Alison MR, Poulsom R, Jeffery R, et al. Hepatocytes from non-hepatic adult stem cells. *Nature* 2000;406:257.
102. Clarke D, Frisen J. Differentiation potential of adult stem cells. *Curr Opin Genet Dev* 2001;11:575–580.
103. Wagers AJ, Sherwood RI, Christensen JL, et al. Little evidence for developmental plasticity of adult hematopoietic stem cells. *Science* 2002;297:2256–2259.
104. Eisenberg LM, Eisenberg CA. Stem cell plasticity, cell fusion, and transdifferentiation. *Birth Defects Res C Embryo Today* 2003;69:209–218.
105. Corti S, Locatelli F, Papadimitriou D, et al. Somatic stem cell research for neural repair: current evidence and emerging perspectives. *J Cell Mol Med* 2004;8:329–337.
106. Hoofnagle MH, Wamhoff BR, Owens GK. Lost in transdifferentiation. *J Clin Invest* 2004;113:1249–1251.
107. Storch A, Paul G, Csete M, et al. Long-term proliferation and dopaminergic differentiation of human mesencephalic neural precursor cells. *Exp Neurol* 2001;170:317–325.
108. Storch A, Lester HA, Boehm BO, et al. Functional characterization of dopaminergic neurons derived from rodent mesencephalic progenitor cells. *J Chem Neuroanat* 2003;26:133–142.
109. Kishi Y, Takahashi J, Koyanagi M, et al. Estrogen promotes differentiation and survival of dopaminergic neurons derived from human neural stem cells. *J Neurosci Res* 2005;79:279–286.
110. Liste I, Garcia-Garcia E, Martinez-Serrano A. The generation of dopaminergic neurons by human neural stem cells is enhanced by Bcl-XL, both in vitro and in vivo. *J Neurosci* 2004;24:10,786–10,795.
111. Zhao M, Momma S, Delfani K, et al. Evidence for neurogenesis in the adult mammalian substantia nigra. *Proc Natl Acad Sci USA* 2003;100:7925–7930.
112. Frielingsdorf H, Schwarz K, Brundin P, et al. No evidence for new dopaminergic neurons in the adult mammalian substantia nigra. *Proc Natl Acad Sci USA* 2004;101:10,177–10,182.
113. Cooper O, Isacson O. Intrastriatal transforming growth factor alpha delivery to a model of Parkinson's disease induces proliferation and migration of endogenous adult neural progenitor cells without differentiation into dopaminergic neurons. *J Neurosci* 2004;24:8924–8931.

Deep-Brain Stimulation for Movement Disorders

47

Pierre Pollak   *Paul Krack*

DEEP-BRAIN STIMULATION FOR MOVEMENT DISORDERS: HISTORICAL NOTES AND PERSONAL REMARKS

"Whatever happened to VIM thalamotomy for Parkinson's disease?" When Tasker asked this question in 1983 (1), functional stereotactic surgeons were a rare species. Psychosurgery had collapsed after the introduction of neuroleptics in the 1950s, and movement disorder surgery almost disappeared after the introduction of levodopa in the late 1960s. Later, when the revolution in imaging techniques completely transformed the field of surgery for brain tumors, all neurosurgeons began to perform stereotactic procedures, and many felt there was no more need for functional neurosurgery. Gildenberg despaired, "Whatever happened to stereotactic surgery?" (2). Since then, functional stereotactic surgery has made a remarkable comeback.

The revival of neurosurgery for movement disorders started in the mid-1980s when Laitinen et al. reintroduced Leksell's posteroventral pallidotomy and showed that this procedure almost eradicated levodopa-induced dyskinesias (3). This sparked a never-before-seen interest among neurosurgeons and movement disorder neurologists alike in surgical treatment (4), especially after interpretation of microrecording in normal monkeys and 1-methyl-4-phenyl-1,2,3,6-tetrahydropyridine (MPTP) monkeys provided a rational basis for pallidotomy (5). The introduction of ventralis intermedius nucleus (VIM) deep-brain stimulation (DBS) for tremor by the Grenoble Group went largely unnoticed at first, but with the expansion of applications and

targets, especially the subthalamic nucleus (STN), pallidotomy as a procedure became obsolete and DBS for movement disorders became the cornerstone of surgery for movement disorders.

Progress in understanding the pathophysiology of movement disorders, as well as technical progress in surgery and—especially—in imaging, often have been credited with the renaissance of functional stereotactic surgery for movement disorders. Other factors also were important but are not always considered.

> The importance in human stereotaxy of collaborative teamwork between clinicians of affiliated specialties, especially nonsurgical, for the analysis of clinical symptoms, decision-making, and evaluation of results cannot be overemphasized. (6)

Movement disorder surgery can only work in the long term if there is cooperation among movement disorder neurologists and functional stereotactic surgeons. Spiegel and Wycis, the pioneers of this field, illustrate this well, and the success of the Grenoble team also was based on this concept. The growing field of movement disorders was expanding in the 1980s, thanks to the impetus of two outstanding neurologists. Professor Stanley Fahn, alerted by reports of spectacular but nonreproducible results of movement disorder surgery has been and still is one of the most influential and critical voices promoting rigorous evaluation, rightly warning about placebo effects, and even advocating controlled studies using sham surgery (7–12). In the late 1980s, Professor David Marsden and Stan Fahn created the Movement Disorder Society, which promoted the use of videos, the use of standardized scales, and scientific interest in movement disorders, thereby creating a new neurological subspecialty. The impetus of this society cannot be underestimated. When the results of the Grenoble group on STN DBS in PD were presented for the first time in a 1994 international meeting in March 1994 at the 11th Parkinson's disease symposium in Roma, Prof Marsden publicly stated that this was the most important discovery since levodopa had been introduced. After having endured many aggressions by skeptical colleagues and severe drawbacks (among the first patients operated on in our center were 1 severe hematoma and 1 suicide), this encouragement from one of the most brilliant contemporary neurologists was a motivation for years to come.

There have been two milestones in the introduction of DBS for movement disorders. The first, the introduction of thalamic stimulation for tremor, was based on clinical research and empirical surgery, in the absence of animal models for tremor or basic research on the mechanisms of DBS (13). The second, the extension of this technique to the STN (14) and the globus pallidus pars interna (GPi) (15) for all parkinsonian motor symptoms, was driven mainly by progress in basal ganglia pathophysiology (16), but another important contribution was the empirical discovery of the dramatic effect of pallidotomy on levodopa-induced dyskinesia (3), not predicted by the new basal ganglia model but compatible with earlier findings of subthalamic dyskinesias in the animal model (17).

In 1987, Benabid et al. first proposed DBS of the VIM of the thalamus as an experimental treatment in a patient with severe PD tremor and a previous thalamotomy, based on the observation that intraoperative high-frequency electric stimulation used for electrophysiological definition of the target leads to tremor suppression (18). It was hoped that with a reversible technique the incidence of permanent side effects could be reduced, allowing for thalamic surgery with a low incidence of dysarthria, even when applied bilaterally. Indeed, the problem of thalamotomy is not a lack of efficacy, but it carries the risk of inducing pseudobulbar dysarthria, especially if surgery is performed bilaterally (19). The use of DBS for treatment of refractory pain was available (20,21) and already had been applied to various movement disorders in various targets and using different frequencies (22–31). Brice and McLellan stimulated the subthalamic area in 3 patients with multiple sclerosis (MS) tremor using 86–150 Hz (26). Andy used 50–125 Hz, 200 μs, 2–5 V stimulation in different thalamic targets, including VIM in PD tremor and a variety of other movement disorders, with a range of fair to excellent results (30). These case reports, however, did not gain much attention, were met with some skepticism (9,32), and could not always be reproduced (8). In this context, it was difficult to publish the reports of the effects of VIM stimulation on PD tremor as some editors judged that these effects were too spectacular not to represent placebo effects, especially as tremor is a variable sign. To

gain acceptance, it took not only some creativity and scientific observation but also rigorous evaluation and much perseverance. One of the premises was a systematic analysis of the frequency dependency of the antitremor effects of VIM stimulation. From the beginning of human stereotactic surgery, intraoperative stimulation has been a key technique for evaluating accurate electrode placement, mainly using the unwanted physiologic effects of stimulation as evidence of the electrode being out of target. It has been known from the beginning of human intraoperative electrophysiology in the sixties. That electrical stimulation could inhibit parkinsonian tremor in the same site where rhythmic activity synchronous to tremor was recorded and where thalamotomy would also suppress tremor, and this knowledge was used to define the target (33). Albe-Fessard, who had introduced microrecording and first described a tremorogenic rhythm in the thalamus (34), discussed the mechanisms of this tremor inhibition using stimulation (33):

> The fact that the stimulation of this rhythmogenic zone inhibits the tremor may seem a paradox. Whether we are dealing with a true inhibition or a desynchronization of the rhythmic centers by a stimulation at high frequency, we are today unable to decide. (33)

Several authors had stated that low-frequency stimulation can drive a tremor, whereas high-frequency stimulation can abolish tremor (33–36). In parkinsonism, 60 Hz of electrical stimulation of the VIM could either inhibit or facilitate the tremor (37–39). The most influential authors relied on microrecording rather than stimulation for targeting and, moreover, did not exceed 60 Hz for stimulation (37–40). This probably explains why surprisingly little detail about the stimulation parameters was included in the description of this surgery in the literature (41). Benabid et al. rediscovered and firmly established that tremor suppression with VIM stimulation is frequency dependent starting at around 50 Hz, but tremor suppression is reliably obtained only at frequencies above 100 Hz, with a peak effect around 200 Hz (13). This was done in the first patients with chronically implanted electrodes (i.e., outside the time constraints and risks of the operating room and thanks to the everlasting patience and cooperation of our patients). Indeed, without the help of the patients this technique could not have been developed. These first results also demonstrate that DBS is not only a therapeutic means but also a powerful tool for a better understanding of basal ganglia pathophysiology (42–44). The term *high-frequency stimulation* was coined to distinguish therapeutic stimulation frequencies of 100 Hz or higher from the lower frequencies generally used for intraoperative electrophysiological evaluation. The first open clinical trial of high-frequency VIM stimulation was promising and showed both long-term efficacy and safety, which allowed for bilateral procedures (13). Efficacy of high-frequency VIM stimulation was later confirmed in Parkinson's disease (PD) and essential tremor using blinded assessment and random assignment to on or off stimulation (45–46). A randomized trial comparing unilateral thalamotomy to unilateral thalamic stimulation showed a greater benefit in functional status and a lower incidence of permanent side effects in those patients who had been randomized for the stimulation technique (47). Long-term effects also have been confirmed (48,49).

In the 1990s, based on advancements in the understanding of the pathophysiology of basal ganglia (5,50), the surgical target of interest moved to the STN and GPi. Reports of improvement in the primate MPTP model of parkinsonism after lesions in the subthalamic nucleus (16) were published around the same time that Laitinen et al. published the results of a series of pallidotomies in patients with PD who showed improvement in akinesia, rigidity, and tremor (3). In fact, Laitinen had taken up as a target the posteroventrolateral part of the pallidum, which already had been successfully operated on in the sixties by Leksell before the advent of levodopa. These clinical data based on an empirical approach supported the new model of basal ganglia pathophysiology and the notion that excessive output from the sensorimotor pallidum contributed to parkinsonian motor signs. In addition, Laitinen was the first to report the dramatic effect of pallidotomy on levodopa-induced dyskinesia, and this was not predicted by the new model of basal ganglia pathophysiology. Now the stage was set for ongoing competition between two targets (the internal pallidum and the subthalamic nucleus GPi and STN) and two techniques (ablative surgery and DBS).

Over the next few years, multiple reports described the beneficial effects of pallidotomy on the clinical triad of parkinsonism and on levodopa-induced dyskinesia, which confirmed efficacy on contralateral symptoms (51–54). Because of common side effects associated with bilateral pallidotomies, however, physicians continued to search for alternative therapies. The subthalamic nucleus STN seemed to be a promising target, but as lesions of the STN were known for their potential to induce ballism, it seemed that the STN could not be explored with ablative surgery. DBS had been effective in improving different tremors when applied to the VIM, with DBS mimicking the effects of a lesion. It was, therefore, tempting also to apply this reversible technique to other targets, such as the STN or the GPi. The mechanism of action, however, remained unknown, and thus efficacy in one target could not simply be referred to another target. Benazzouz et al. finally found the missing link when they showed that DBS stimulation in the MPTP monkey could replicate the antiparkinsonian effects of an STN lesion (55). With awareness of these results, the Grenoble Group successfully applied STN DBS in PD patients. Based on the reports of efficacy in the MPTP model, which is a levodopa-sensitive model of PD, patients who were highly levodopa sensitive were selected. Because of the risk of inducing dyskinesia, these first patients were selected to have both relatively little dyskinesia and, as the surgery was experimental, an advanced stage of the disease.

In these patients, a first unilateral STN stimulation was administered, although improving contralateral symptoms did not improve any severe functional handicap related to axial symptoms, such as gait disturbance. However the anti-akinetic effect was spectacular after the first patient had been operated on bilaterally in this new target (14,56). As expected, STN stimulation-induced dyskinesias (57) ensued, and this side effect slowed the initial enthusiasm. However, it could be shown that reduction of levodopa was possible and that dyskinesia gradually improved with chronic STN stimulation (44,58). STN stimulation also was shown to have a marked effect on parkinsonian tremor (59). DBS also was applied to the internal pallidum, replicating the antiparkinsonian and antidyskinetic effects of a pallidal lesion, with the relative safety of the technique allowing for bilateral surgery (15). Based on its first experience with bilateral pallidal and subthalamic stimulation, the Grenoble Group started to prefer STN stimulation over GPi stimulation because its better antiakinetic effect allowed for marked reduction of levodopa (60). The antiparkinsonian effect of STN stimulation showed a good correlation with the antiparkinsonian effect of levodopa, and thus levodopa sensitivity has become a major selection criterion for STN surgery (60). The long-term effects of STN DBS in PD are well established now (61). Although today most centers performing DBS prefer the STN DBS to the GPi DBS in PD patients, this issue concerning the relative advantages and disadvantages of both targets is not settled yet (62). In the same way, although today DBS is generally preferred over ablative surgery because of its relative safety, with very few reports on bilateral lesions, the exact place of each technique in different clinical situations remains to be defined more precisely.

More recently, based on its major effects on levodopa-induced dyskinesia the pallidum also has been explored in dystonia. First, pallidotomy was shown to be effective in dystonia (63), and again the effects of a lesion could be replicated using DBS, which is relatively safe, thus allowing for bilateral procedures (64–66). Other, still more experimental indications also are being studied (67), and the application to DBS in movement disorders has opened the way for this technique to be used in other neurological or psychiatric diseases, such as epilepsy (68), Tourette's syndrome (69), cluster headache (70), obsessive–compulsive disorder (71), depression (72), and obesity (73).

PRINCIPLES OF STIMULATION

Mechanism of Deep-Brain Stimulation

There is still no consensus on the physiologic mechanism underlying the effects of DBS. The comparable effect of stimulation to ablation in the thalamus on tremor, and in the STN and internal segment of the globus pallidus (GPi) on the motor signs of PD have led many investigators to conclude that DBS acts to suppress neuronal activity, decreasing output from the stimulated site. Therefore, the starting hypothesis was that high-frequency electrical stimulation is neuroinhibitive (74). A more truthful mechanism should reconcile divergent data from in vivo and in vitro studies. It seems that DBS can activate fibers locally, which would deliver high-frequency synchronous bursts feeding the projection targets with either favorable gamma activity or a disrupted message.

In patients, frequency of stimulation is the crucial parameter, since no beneficial effect can be obtained below 50 Hz, and a plateau is reached with frequencies of 100–200 Hz (13,14). A depolarization block is possible, but the effective frequency of stimulation seems too low to induce such an effect, and the possibility for its maintenance in the long term is questionable, whereas the clinical effects of DBS seem permanent. The efficacy of a pulse width as narrow as 60 μs suggests that fibers are activated rather than cell bodies (75,76). By measuring the strength–duration time constant, Holsheimer et al. concluded that the primary targets of stimulation in VIM and GPi are probably large myelinated axons (77). A local stimulation of GABAergic fibers was intraoperatively shown in the Gpi (78). In the STN, stimulation at a frequency greater than 40 Hz significantly decreased the firing frequency and increased the burstlike activity in the firing pattern of STN neurons. An aftereffect was observed in cells that had been totally inhibited during high-frequency stimulation (79).

There are, however, various data that do not support an inhibitory action (80,81). Microdialysis studies in rat GPi showed increased levels of glutamate during STN stimulation, suggesting activation of glutamatergic output from the STN to the GPi (82). Studies in parkinsonian primates have demonstrated increased mean discharge rates of neurons in GPi during chronic stimulation in STN (83). Intraoperative stimulation in human GPe has been demonstrated to improve bradykinesia by activating GABAergic fibers projecting either to the GPi or the STN (84). Thus, projection axons from neurons in the stimulated structure would be tonically activated and would discharge independently of possibly inactivated somas, thereby increasing output from the structure during extracellular stimulation. However, long-term stimulation of a structure that would fire blanks may lead to an inactivated target.

In vitro studies on rat STN neurons using whole-cell, current-clamp techniques and online artifact suppression showed that stimulation at 10 Hz evoked 10-Hz single spikes but did not significantly modify ongoing STN activity. In contrast, at therapeutically relevant frequencies (80–185 Hz), stimulation had a dual effect: It fully suppressed STN spontaneous activity and generated a robust pattern of recurrent bursts of spikes, with each spike being time-locked to a stimulus pulse (85). The authors conclude that high-frequency stimulation drives the STN neuronal activity by directly activating the neuronal membrane.

In conclusion, the mechanisms underlying DBS therapy are unknown, and there are conflicting data suggesting inhibition or excitation of neurons. Even if local high-frequency stimulation inhibits neurons, it can also directly excite the cell and/or its axon. Therefore, the overall effects of DBS stimulation might be inhibition of intrinsic and synaptically mediated activity and its replacement by regular high-frequency firing (86). Stimulation drives neurons that behave as stable oscillators, yielding an average stable output that overrides spontaneous activity and introduces high-frequency regular spiking in the basal ganglia network. This pattern might remove the deleterious activity of the basal ganglia network, explaining the similarity between DBS and effects induced by lesioning. Also debated is the functional meaning of the target neurons driven to a high-frequency state of activity. The hypothesis of a high-frequency stimulation imposed on the projection structures of the stimulated area fits with models emphasizing the role of altered patterns of neuronal activity in the development of hypo- and hyperkinetic movement disorders. High-frequency stimulation would switch off a pathologically disrupted activity and impose a new type of discharge that would be endowed with beneficial effects, perhaps by feeding the system with a synchronous high-frequency nonsignificant message.

Does Chronic Stimulation Induce Tolerance or Lesion?

A main concern is the possible loss of effect of chronic stimulation owing to a progressive tolerance phenomenon. Using stimulation with charge-balanced biphasic pulses, as delivered by Medtronic implanted pulse generators (IPG), should minimize this issue. Usually, stimulation amplitude has to be increased in all patients during the first 1 to 3 months after electrode implantation (87). This could be related to the time of healing of the lesionlike effect induced by the implantation of the electrodes. In the long term, the voltage necessary to obtain a motor benefit remains relatively stable (13,61,88). The only exception concerns a few patients suffering from an intention component of severe action tremor and operated on in the VIM. It is wise in these patients who progressively lose the beneficial effects because of a true development of tolerance (89) not to continue increasing voltage over 3.6 V and to manage more or less prolonged periods of stimulation arrests. Tolerance could be due to a decreased biological response (habituation) of the neuronal network, which is responsible for the suppression of tremor, and/or to a new stimulation-induced behavior of this network, which could account for the rebound phenomenon, namely a temporary increased amplitude of tremor after turning off the stimulation (90,91). Concerning STN and GPi stimulation, such a tolerance with a rebound phenomenon has rarely occurred.

DBS does not work through a lesion since it is reversible when the stimulators are switched off, even years after surgery in most cases. Pathological studies show little tissue damage or very small gliosis at the tip of the electrode, which cannot explain the benefit (92–94). In some patients, the worsening of symptoms after hours of stimulation arrest is incomplete and would require perhaps days to reach the baseline preoperative level, which cannot be carried out for ethical reasons. In few patients, especially with tremor, stimulation can be stopped without recurrence of symptoms (95). This raises the possibility of changes of the tissue around the stimulating contact or long-term changes of functional or anatomical nature in the basal ganglia circuitry through neuronal plasticity. Using electron microscopy of explanted DBS electrodes, a foreign body multinucleate giant cell-type reaction was visualized (96).

Amount of Neuronal Tissue Involved by Stimulation

The amount of neuronal tissue involved by stimulation seems rather restricted and is estimated to spread at least to 2–3 mm from the electrode if intensities in the region of 2–3 mA are used with a chronic implanted macroelectrode (2–3 V with a mean impedance of 1000 Ω). Bipolar stimulation with 2 adjacent contacts spaced 1.5 mm apart, which would act more focally, induces about the same effect as monopolar stimulation with 1 contact but at a higher voltage. Further evidence that the effective current is localized arises from the observation of different effects obtained with 2 microelectrodes separated by 2 mm during surgery, as well as with 2 contacts of a chronic quadripolar electrode, with the middle one separated by 2–3 mm according to the electrode type (97). The intensity of the spreading current of monopolar stimulation decreases proportionally to the square of the distance (75,76). So, currents of very low intensities are recorded far from the emitting monopolar electrode but without relevant clinical effects.

Quality Control Issue

Since FDA approval was granted for deep-brain stimulation for advanced PD, dystonia, and tremor, DBS has been applied in many thousands of patients throughout the world. The FDA approval was based on published data that were gained in a few centers with dedicated teams. Doubts have been raised regarding whether the outcome of these few centers reflects what will be the reality after this technique is widely applied (10). A recent article has raised concerns about decline in the overall quality of DBS with the flood of new, inexperienced DBS centers. Patients were referred to two experienced teams because DBS performed in other centers had failed. Failures were related to misdiagnosis (some had never seen any movement-disorder neurologist), off-label indications in patients not fulfilling selection criteria (some were 80 or demented), mistargeting (1 electrode was found in the lateral ventricle), unrecognized

technical defects, or absence of access to follow-up (97a). We hope that this chapter will bring attention to the DBS quality-control issue; otherwise the baby may be thrown out with the bathwater and we will witness a new decline of functional stereotactic surgery.

Fair results from DBS require an adequate selection of surgical candidates, appropriate recognition of the target and placement of the electrodes in the intended positions, and expertise in the adjustment of stimulation and medication postoperatively. Failure to fulfill any of these crucial aspects will probably explain relatively poor results. It is mandatory to implement a multidisciplinary team, including neurologists involved in the field of movement disorders, neurosurgeons competent in functional stereotaxy, neuroradiologists, neurophysiologists, neuropsychologists, and psychiatrists. Complications and their avoidance are extremely dependent on the surgical team's experience (98,99). We recommend that the surgical procedures and follow-up be concentrated at relatively few centers, which will thereby acquire a high degree of experience.

SURGERY ISSUES

Imaging for Targeting

Each procedure is based on the stereotactic method for targeting the chosen neuronal structure. This varies according to each team. Most neurosurgeons use fiducials, which are attached, using various systems, to the skull of the patient. Numerous stereotactic head frames exist. The first step of targeting is imaging, which includes ventriculography, computed tomography (CT), and/or magnetic resonance imaging (MRI). Several groups continue to rely on ventriculography for direct visualization of the anterior commissure (AC) and posterior commmissure (PC) landmarks despite the inherent risks of ventriculostomy. The chief advantages of MRI include a noninvasive imaging modality, better resolution of the deep and superficial cerebral structures, and planning of the entry point (99a). Because of the problem of MRI distortion, many centers use MRI coregistered to CT (99b).

Following imaging, the coordinates of the target, either for an initial microelectrode recording (MER) track or for implantation of the DBS electrode, are determined. The coordinates are chosen either indirectly in relation to the intercommissural line (ICL) and the midcommissural point (MCP) or directly by targeting the structure of interest read from the MRI or CT, thanks to the progress in image resolution. Prospective comparison between 3D-MRI and ventriculography for determination of the AC, PC, and target showed shifts in the 1–3 mm range (100,101). Using direct targeting, T1-weighted images yield fair anatomical views that delineate the globus pallidus (102). However, nuclei inside the thalamus are not individualized. T2-weighted images with a long acquisition time are better for STN visualization (100,103–106). T2-weighted images show that the red nucleus (RN), the substantia nigra (SN) and the STN are relatively hypointense as compared to surrounding structures, although this signal does not perfectly fit with the anatomical structure (107). The use of the red nucleus as an internal fiducial marker for directly targeting the optimal region of STN stimulation was found reliable and approximates by more than 3 mm the position of the electrode contact that provides the optimal clinical results (108). The most important drawback to MRI is the potential for image distortion. Comparison of direct targeting and final MER-determined coordinates showed unacceptable distance errors of 2.6–3.9 mm (100,109,110). Thus, although direct targeting may be helpful, it can yield coordinates at some distance from the final MER target. What discrepancy between imaging-based targeting and MER can be considered acceptable? Since 2 MER tracks separated by 2 mm usually provide totally different results, in recordings as well as in clinical benefits or side effects induced by stimulation, precision within 1 mm is needed.

Most neurosurgeons assume that the electrode location, as noted on the coordinate system relative to the AC–PC line, is truly as intended, which ignores all possible deviation of the electrode from the intended track. The way to evaluate the quality of targeting would be to examine the distance from the initial to the final target. This can be done with an inframillimeter precision using ventriculography and teleradiography (with the X-ray tube far from the patient to decrease the magnification coefficient and distortion). Neurosurgeons do not exactly target where they intend to target with changes of about 1 to 3 mm. Teleradiography shows that even removing the stylet of the Medtronic electrode frequently induces a 1 mm displacement of the electrode, proving that the insertion of a stiff probe in a soft structure bathed in fluid, such as the brain, induces a slight shift despite the most accurate targeting. That is why functional electrophysiology is mandatory for achieving the precision necessary for optimal therapeutic benefit.

Electrode Recording

To identify the physiologically optimal target for DBS, MER (with impedances around 0.5 to 1.0 MΩ) or semi-microelectrodes (with impedances less than 0.1 MΩ) may be employed in a multitude of ways, according to the experience of each group. Without any doubt, in experienced hands, microrecording can precisely define the boundaries of the target. In the suitable implantation site, single-unit activities characteristic of the target (111–114) are recorded on several consecutive millimeters because the microelectrode goes through the main part of the neuronal structure. Individual strategies are reported from group to group. Since the anatomically precise determination of a target can be off by a few millimeters, some groups use a device allowing 5 simultaneous parallel trajectories in a concentric array, with 4 outer electrodes being separated by 2 mm

from a central electrode aimed at the theoretical target. Two to 5 microelectrodes are generally located in the target, but they were eventually replaced by the chronic Medtronic electrode, because it provides better results than the others. Using this device (the so-called *Ben's gun*) provides the advantage of comparing the effects of each electrode side by side and ensuring that the chronic electrode will be placed exactly at the same location as the microelectrode.

The effects of general anesthesia on MER are debatable, with some groups finding little changes, and others finding a decrease in frequency and patterns of discharges according to the drug used. More studies in animals and humans are needed to interpret data obtained from patients under general anesthesia. So far, the gold standard of MER should be considered to be MER performed under local anesthesia only.

Although MER being the cause of increased intracranial bleeding or contusion remains a controversial matter (115–124), it seems obvious that the risk of bleeding or contusion increases as the number of trajectories performed to delineate the target increases. A twice higher rate of hemorrhage in cases performed with MER as compared to macrostimulation alone has been reported (125). In the Palur et al. meta-analysis (125), it was noted that non-MER techniques were at least 5 times less likely to have hemorrhagic complications (126). In 2001, the DBS Study Group found that the number of microelectrode passes used to determine target location correlated with the risk of hemorrhage. However, the overall risk of bleeding in both MER and non-MER groups is relatively low, with an occurrence of 1% to 8% of cases (125–127). Without randomized comparative studies, it will not be possible to know if the additional information obtained with MER and multiple trajectories will lead to a better outcome and compensate for the likely increased risk. The number of patients required to allow a randomized study to have any significant statistical power, however, will probably prohibit this endeavor from taking place. The only correlation between MER strategy and outcome was with microstimulation-induced reduction in akinesia and emergence of microstimulation-induced dyskinesias in the STN of PD patients (128). Although the usefulness of MER may remain debatable, the use of stimulation in a nonanesthetized patient is necessary to localize the optimal target site.

Intraoperative Stimulation

Micro- and macrostimulation are both potentially useful intraoperative tools. Most groups find that their judicious use in the operating room may confirm optimal targeting and help avoid side effects due to chronic stimulation. In the suitable implantation site, high-frequency stimulation induces motor benefit at low intensities, as well as no side effects or side effects at far higher intensities in a patient under local anesthesia. The Paris group found suboptimal results in a group of PD patients operated on for STN stimulation under general anesthesia in comparison with the group under local anesthesia (129). General anesthesia allows assessment solely of motor contraction related to pyramidal tract stimulation. General anesthesia should only be used in patients with severe abnormal movement, such as some generalized or cervical dystonia or Tourette's syndrome. Generalized anesthesia may also be necessary for anxious or phobic patients.

To best approximate chronic stimulation effects, currents in the milliampere range should be used. Care must be taken to stimulate at high currents to avoid damaging the microelectrode tip or creating a brain lesion (caused by the higher current charge density of a microelectrode tip vs. a semimicroelectrode/DBS tip). Electrical variables used for stimulation during surgery are chosen according to those usually applied in chronic patients: monopolar stimulation with the cathode, a fixed rate of 130 Hz, a pulse width of 60 μs, and a variable intensity up to a few mA using a constant current stimulator. Despite the spreading inherent to stimulation, a relatively precise intraoperative mapping of the target area is possible since the clinical effects obtained with microelectrodes spaced only 2 mm apart are quite different.

The intraoperative effects of stimulation on tremor for the VIM target or on the parkinsonian triad for the STN target are usually dramatic and predictive of the final clinical benefit. In the GPi, the acute intraoperative effects induced by stimulation are less clear. GPe stimulation may acutely improve akinesia and induce dyskinesia, and GPi stimulation induces some parkinsonism relief but far less clearly than STN stimulation. Moreover, compared to STN stimulation, intraoperative GP stimulation is not predictive of outcome since long-term GPe stimulation does not improve parkinsonism and GPi-induced improvement progressively develops over weeks or months. Stimulation-induced side effects vary according to the target and should be interpreted with an anatomical and clinical reasoning in terms of anatomical-clinical correlation. They include motor contraction, eye deviation, abnormal movements, speech impairment, and the report by a cooperative patient of paresthesias, visual sensations, and vegetative or affective symptoms. Whereas the changes in tremor are easily quantifiable, at least if the examiner ensures that its amplitude remains constant, the assessment of akinesia in PD patients is difficult and greatly variable because of its dependence on the patient's motivation to perform repetitive movements and state of fatigue throughout the operation. That is why, in akinetic-rigid patients, we prefer to assess systematically rigidity by passive movements of the contralateral wrist (14), and then akinesia evaluation is carried out only to confirm stimulation-induced beneficial effects. Induction of dyskinesias contralaterally to the stimulated STN provides useful confirmation that an electrode has been placed in the correct location. Interestingly, it seems that patients with preoperative and severe levodopa-induced dyskinesias are more prone to exhibit stimulation-induced dyskinesias. Multiple track microrecordings previous to microstimulation with the same electrode help to map precisely the target borders and choose the sites of stimulation.

Intraoperative clinical testing should be done only by those who know both what to suspect and the details of a given patient's clinical profile. Ideally, that is someone with interest in the field and competency in the basic skills for systematic and careful assessments of benefits and side effects. Accurate interpretation of stimulation-induced effects requires substantial knowledge of and experience with parkinsonism, functional anatomy, and the evaluation of neurological symptoms and signs. The neurologist who evaluated the patient candidate preoperatively for surgery seems to be the person most prepared for intraoperative testing.

In summary, and concerning the most frequent type of DBS (i.e., STN stimulation for PD, at the sites where microelectrode recordings show neuronal discharges characteristic of the STN), electrical high-frequency stimulation induces a dramatic improvement in parkinsonian motor symptoms at low intensity and side effects at high intensity (wide therapeutic window). The amelioration of the symptoms can be accompanied by dyskinesias, which are a positive predictive factor for the outcome. The other unpleasant effects are induced by stimulating the surrounding areas of the STN.

Implanted Materials

Electrodes

Currently, there only one manufacturer of electrodes that is approved in the United States or elsewhere. Medtronic (Minneapolis, Minnesota, United States) offers 2 models of chronic electrodes, each with 4 cylindrical contacts (contact 0 distal to contact 3 proximal), 1.5 mm contact length, and 1.27 mm diameter. The contacts are separated by 1.5 mm for the model 3397 lead and by 0.5 mm for the model 3389. This reduces the overall span of the contacts from 10.5 mm to 7.5 mm, which seems reasonable given that in VIM, GPi, and STN the length of the efficient target region is less than 7.5 mm. Therefore, the model 3389 lead increases the spatial and stimulation resolution. The longer interval afforded by the model 3387 lead allows stimulation of a greater region outside the theoretical target and offers greater ability to compensate for a misplaced lead with regard to depth along the track. There are no data that directly compare the 3387 and 3389 models. The middle of the 4 contacts of the DBS electrode (between contacts 1 and 2) is positioned in the middle of the determined target for the VIM and STN and the tip of the electrode (contact 0) at the ventral border of the GPi.

Pulse Generator Implantation

According to each neurosurgical group, the attachment of the electrode to the extension lead and the connection of the latter to the IPG are made either immediately or in a staged fashion (typically over a 1- to 4-week period). Staged surgery has its advantages. In particular, it makes it possible to avoid a lengthy surgery for electrode implantation and to check electrode location with a postoperative MRI before IPG implantation. Currently, two models of IPG are available: the single-channel Soletra (almost identical to the Itrel II) and the dual-channel Kinetra. The latter is close to twice as large as the former but requires only one implantation site and one subcutaneous tunneling pass (130). In addition, there are other advantages, such as the absence of a current-multiplier circuit over 3.6 V, which lengthens battery life in high-voltage situations and makes the device more insensitive to magnets, which together prevent insensitivity to magnets, which prevents inadvertent arrests, the most frequent side effect of the Itrel. However, it seems that the increased size and weight of the Kinetra, compared to the Soletra, lead to a trend toward a higher rate of adverse surgery-related events. Different ways of securing the DBS electrode to the skull can be used: caps specific to the DBS electrode, titanium plates and screws, and methyl-metacrylate dental cement with a knot anchored in the bone. No electrode migration on large series of patients has been reported with the latter (89), in contract to the Medtronic cap (99). It is recommended that fluoroscopy be used to protect against lead migration during fixation, especially when using a cap.

Postoperative Imaging

Postoperative imaging is invaluable for documenting the absence of complications and the location of the electrode. The latter is useful for interpreting the clinical results of stimulation and for troubleshooting. Following insertion, the location of the lead should be confirmed by imaging (131). This may begin with intraoperative fluoroscopy or stereotactic X-rays. Most centers perform a postoperative imaging study consisting mainly of MRI (Figs. 47.1, 47.2, and 47.3). Yelnick et al. (132) have quantified the artifact created from a model 3389 lead. They show that the model 3389 electrode has an artifact on MRI of 3.5 mm in diameter instead of 1.27 mm and that the 4 contacts span 10.7 mm instead of 7.5 mm. The center of the artifact they reported concurred with the center of the electrode. A number of centers fuse the postoperative imaging study to the preoperative stereo MRI or CT to assess the final DBS electrode positioning (133). Postoperative T2-weighted MR images to localize STN also have been used.

Postoperative MRI before IPG implantation is safe. After implantation of the complete DBS system, potential MR-related complications include electrode or pulse generator movement or heating (134), the latter of which may result in an intraparenchymal lesion. No device failures were found as a result of postoperative MRI (130). However, heating at the lead tip may result in serious injury to the patient and it is therefore necessary to follow safety recommendations strictly (135,136) (see the following).

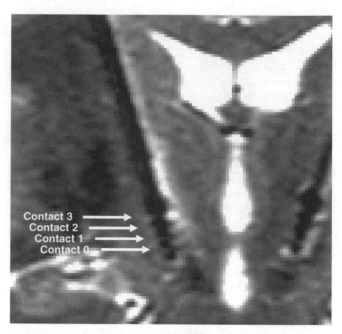

Figure 47.1   Postoperative T2-weighted MRI in the same coronal plane as electrodes. Model 3389 Medtronic electrodes are bilaterally implanted in the subthalamic nucleus. Although the electrodes appear larger than they actually are, the 4 contacts can be individualized.

Role of the Neurologist Before Surgery

The neurologist should play a major role in the management of patient candidates for DBS therapy. He or she should tell the patient objectively what to expect from DBS, what the risks are, and how to decide if and when to

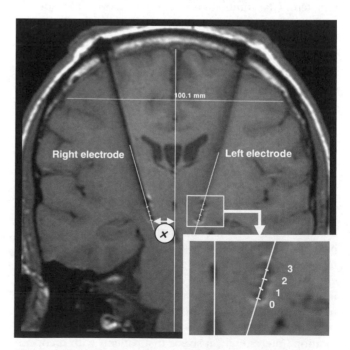

Figure 47.2   Postoperative coronal T1-weighted MRI. Model 3389 Medtronic electrodes are bilaterally implanted in the subthalamic nucleus. The artifact is less than in T2-weighted sequence. The laterality from midline can be measured (x) for each of the 4 contacts.

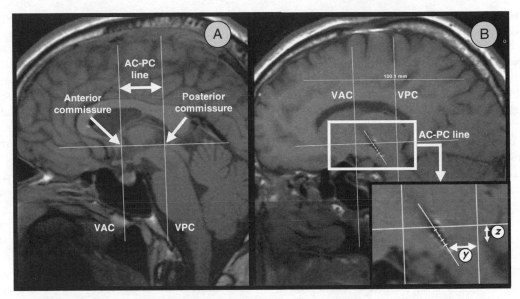

Figure 47.3 Postoperative sagittal T1-weighted MRI. Model 3389 Medtronic electrodes are bilaterally implanted in the subthalamic nucleus. The anterior commissure (AC)/posterior commissure (PC) lines and verticals are drawn on the midline slice **(A)**. On a lateral slice where the electrode tip is visualized **(B)**, the anteroposterior (*y*) and dorsoventral locations of the centers of each of the 4 contacts can be measured.

undergo an operation. As any probe implantation in the brain bears the risk of severe permanent morbidity in about 2% to 3% of patients, DBS should be proposed for patients with at least some difficulties in activities of daily living or socioprofessional activities. In comparison, operating on very disabled patients who have been dependent on caregivers for many years raises enormous psychological problems in relation to creating a renewed and independent life. Moreover, severely akinetic parkinsonian patients are more at risk for general health complications in the perioperative period. In generalized dystonia, adult patients with fixed postures and body deformation will not improve to the same extent as will children who have not finished their growth. Therefore, patients should not be operated on too late or too early. Personal, social, and professional considerations, as well as how the patient copes with the activities of daily living, are all taken into account by patients and their families when deciding on a suitable time for surgery.

In the weeks before surgery, the neurologist checks for the absence of a scalp infection and for use of any drugs that favor bleeding, such as aspirin, anti-inflammatory non-steroidal (AINS) drugs, anticoagulants, and lisuride. The patient should be made aware of what will happen during each step in the surgery. If operated on under local anesthesia, the patient should be prepared to participate when the site of implantation is determined during neurophysiological testing. Participation would include passive movement for evoked movement-related potentials, stimulation-induced effects on parkinsonian symptoms, and possible side effects such as motor contraction, paresthesias, eye deviation, and vegetative or emotional symptoms. An accurate

report of subjective side effects by a cooperative patient helps to achieve precise targeting (137). Because of the risk of intraoperative psychosis and confusion, especially in parkinsonian patients, it seems wise to simplify the antiparkinsonian drug therapy. Levodopa is favored, minor drugs generally are arrested, and the dosages of dopamine agonist drugs are decreased a few days or weeks before the date of electrode implantation, based on the drug pharmacokinetics.

Role of the Neurologist After Surgery

The setting of electrical variables after surgery requires that the neurologist develop and maintain the competence to manage this new therapy in combination with drugs. To avoid dyskinesias in parkinsonian patients stimulated in the STN, a slow and progressive increase in voltage is recommended while the levodopa dose is concurrently decreased, which is possible if taking into account the obtained antiparkinsonian effect (138). Whatever the targets, electrical parameters are adjusted based on clinical improvement and side effects. One can use a monopolar configuration with the active contact serving as the cathode, and the reference as the case of the stimulator, or a bipolar configuration with the reference as another contact. The latter focuses the effect of stimulation, which can be advantageous in the case of adverse effects or a narrow therapeutic window caused by a misplaced electrode. We tend to favor monopolar stimulation that is usually effective with a lower voltage than bipolar stimulation. Frequencies above 100 Hz, typically 130–185 Hz, are mainly effective. Pulse widths of 60–90 μs, rarely higher, are the most commonly used. Setting the narrowest pulse width minimizes consumption in comparison with a wider pulse width and a lower voltage for similar effects (139). Increasing the voltage higher than approximately 4.0 V generally means that the suitable target has not been attained. Such voltages usually induce adverse effects, whereas the beneficial effect has already reached a ceiling.

Electrical settings must be determined far from a drug-induced effect (i.e., in the worst off-motor period for PD patients) and checked afterward in the levodopa-induced dyskinesia period. It seems that patients with severe presurgical levodopa-induced dyskinesias are prone to developing STN stimulation-induced dyskinesias in the postsurgical period. Voltage must be increased slowly in such patients, and the progressive increase in the voltage threshold capable of inducing dyskinesias may take months and is facilitated by levodopa arrest (140). Postoperative GPi and thalamus stimulation is easier, both in PD and other movement disorders, and does not induce dyskinesias, thus allowing a rapid setting of chronic voltages. A complete stimulation setting includes individually testing each of the four contacts of the quadripolar electrode to determine the threshold voltages for both the beneficial and adverse effects on the disabling symptoms. Similar to what is observed during surgery, the best contact is the one with the lowest threshold for motor benefit and the highest for adverse effects. Refining this electrical setting fully is time-consuming, but it is done only once after surgery, once after the healing process, and generally once at a 3-month follow-up. Over the long term, the same results are usually obtained, and thus a new setting typically focuses only on the smallest possible variations for all types of parameters. Transient improvements often have been observed in the immediate postoperative period by simply implanting the DBS electrode at a given target site—the so-called *microlesion* effect. This makes setting stimulation parameters more difficult.

Clinical Issues Related to Implanted Materials

Before discharge from the hospital after a DBS procedure, the patient should know how to face certain circumstances related to the implanted system. Magnets close to the site of IPG implantation, and electromagnetic fields such as those of airport metal detectors, are to be avoided. In the case of body imaging for the purpose of diagnosis, scanner X imaging is preferred to MRI, which is theoretically contraindicated in patients with implanted pulse generators. However, Tronnier et al. (141) showed that MRI can be performed safely in patients with implanted neurostimulation systems with the tested deep-brain leads connected to an IPG. A conscientious explanation of the risks and benefits of MRI for patients with implanted devices is still recommended. Functional MRI (fMRI) during stimulation was reported with implanted thalamic electrodes (142,143). This findings demonstrate that fMRI can safely detect the activation of cortical and subcortical neuronal pathways

during stimulation and that stimulation does not interfere with imaging. Specific recommendations exist regarding MRI of implanted DBS systems (136,144–146). Patients should not be subjected to coils that extend down over the IPGs in the chest wall or abdomen; only a send/receive head coil should be used. MRIs should not be performed if there is a break in the system. The IPG should be set at 0 V and switched off.

Prevention of infection includes active treatment with antiseptic or antibiotic of any skin sore in the region of the implanted material. Patients must be referred immediately to the neurosurgeon. Antibiotics are given before any infected tooth extraction.

The problem of device–device interaction is common because of the frequency of heart pacemaker implantation. Case reports indicate that cardiac devices and IPGs may be implanted safely in the same patient. One patient suffered no neurological sequels following 10 cardioversions from an implantable cardioverter–defibrillator (147). Surgeons should try to maximize the distance between the implanted pulse generators to minimize potential for cross-talk (e.g., cardiac device in abdomen, bipolar sensing for cardiac pacemaker, bipolar neurostimulation) (148). No interaction occurred in 1 patient with thalamic stimulation and an implantable cardioverter–defibrillator (149). Diathermy along the lead track of DBS can lead to thermolesions at the electrode tip and is strictly forbidden (150).

The patient is taught how to switch the stimulator on and off with a magnet (all IPGs) or a therapy controller (for the Kinetra IPG) in case of thalamic stimulation for tremor with stimulation arrest at night. Since DBS can cause electrocardiogram (ECG) artefacts when monopolar settings are used, the IPG can be turned off transiently during ECG recording (151). If voltage cannot be increased rapidly after surgery and if the patient lives far from the neurology team, the Kinetra can be programmed by patients via a therapy self-controller, named *Therapy Access*, within limits set by the neurologist. The electrical parameters for STN stimulation frequently must be adjusted within the first 6 postoperative months, then once a year or occasionally in between, depending on the patient's state. However, few parkinsonian patients can understand perfectly the clinical circumstances in which to change voltage. Therapy Access also allows the patient to switch the Kinetra on and off and to get information when less than 15% of energy remains (IPG end of life). This permits the patient to anticipate the replacement of the Kinetra, and thus to prevent a recurrence of severe, even life-threatening, parkinsonism caused by sudden bilateral stimulation arrest in patients with advanced PD, from whom antiparkinsonian drugs have been withdrawn. Stimulators have to be changed every 3 to 8 years, with a range between 1 to 10 years, depending on the electrical energy used. GPi stimulation generally requires more energy for a shorter life expectancy than does thalamic or STN stimulation. The Itrel II or Soletra IPGs may switch off unexpectedly (for example, if a magnet is inadvertently placed close to the area of implantation), so patients must be taught how to check that the stimulation is working. This is done by listening for the stimulation frequency through a small radio set on the AM band. If the IPG is switched off, the patient should know how to switch it on with a magnet. The double-channel Kinetra IPG has the great advantage of being almost insensitive to magnets.

Surgical Complications

The real therapeutic value of DBS in advanced PD must take into account the risk of severe adverse effects leading to permanent neurological aftereffects. Intracranial hemorrhage associated with surgery occurred in 2% to 3% of cases (127,152). Risk factors might be age, number of electrode passes (127), and history of arterial hypertension (167). Perioperative mortality is less than 1% of cases.

Also noteworthy in this regard are complications related to the implant, such as infections, skin erosions, and lead breakage. This led to discontinuation of treatment in 6.1% of patients in a multicenter study with 4 years of follow-up (88). These side effects generally can be managed without permanent morbidity.

The Toronto group systematically reviewed the published literature describing patients with PD treated with bilateral STN stimulation from 38 studies and 34 neurosurgical centers in 13 countries. The outcomes for 471 patients showed a 1% to 2% incidence of severe adverse effects (death or permanent neurological deficits related to intracerebral hemorrhages). Of the patients, 19% had adverse effects related to stimulation that could be reversed by changing stimulation parameters. There was a 9% incidence of adverse effects related to the hardware (infections, lead and pulse generator problems) (153).

Globally, infection rates range from less than 1% to as high as 14% (154). Infections of the IPG site tend to present soon after surgery. Infections at the connector may be related to skin erosion and may present at variable times after implantation. Skin reactions and erosions above the device components are easily diagnosed by inspection of the area, which has to be done routinely by the neurologist at every follow-up. Any patients with suspected abnormalities must be sent to the neurosurgeon. Therapeutic strategies in cases of active infection involve mainly the removal of hardware, or antibiotics alone if there is no erosion, but with a high risk of failure (155). Reimplantation can be performed safely after resolution of infection and a sufficiently long period of antibiotics.

DBS electrode fracture, extension wire failure, consumption, and/or malfunction of the IPG (156) cause loss of efficacy for the patient. If the battery has run out, replacement of the IPG will solve the problem. If this is not the case, the impedances through the electrodes must be measured using the nominal setting with a higher tolerable voltage for greater accuracy. Impedances greater than 4000 Ω (Kinetra) or 2000 Ω (Soletra) suggest an open circuit with loss of connectivity. Impedances less than 100 Ω suggest a short circuit or migration of the DBS electrode into a CSF containing space. X-rays of the system may show a fracture in the DBS electrode or extension lead, or a disconnection (157). Replacement of the damaged DBS material is the only treatment for this type of malfunctioning. For a given center, most hardware-related problems frequently occurred in the first patients of a series and were less frequent afterward. This sheds light on the sophisticated nature of the procedure, which requires a lot of expertise for the neurosurgeon to acquire before getting into a routine with DBS surgery.

Other complications were frequent (Table 47.1) but transient or benign, without aftereffects. The transient confusion observed in some patients may be related to intracranial contusion or minimal bleeding, but such nonspecific factors as the long duration of brain surgery and the withdrawal of dopaminergic drugs can be implicated. Those patients became easily confused sometimes after changing the regularity of the levodopa intake due to the formal assessment protocol or to the transient levodopa arrest for MRI or surgery. Most patients with STN or GPi stimulation gained weight (158). Discomfort may appear about the extension lead, which can pull in the lateral region of the neck or about the stimulator in the subclavicular area. Scars may be unsightly, as can the bump made by the thickness of the cable connector in the parietal region of bald patients with thin scalps. New flat connectors minimize this side effect.

Optimal surgical positioning of the stimulating electrode helps to reduce the risk of stimulation-induced side effects that result mostly from unintended costimulation of adjacent fiber tracts or nuclei. Stimulation-induced side effects are fully reversible when stimulation is stopped and can be improved in most cases by changing stimulation parameters or electrode configuration. In some patients in whom the suppression of motor symptoms is not achieved without side effects, patient and physician may deliberately accept a mild degree of stimulation-induced adverse effects, which vary according to the anatomic location of the stimulated fibers or neuronal structure and should be interpreted in anatomoclinical terms. They include paresthesias, dysarthria, motor contraction, eye deviation, gaze deviation, nausea, dizziness, flushing, discontinuation of the effect of levodopa with worsening of akinesia, and—rarely—mood or behavior alterations.

Although adverse effects occur frequently, those inducing permanent neurological impairment are relatively rare, in the region of 3%. Therefore, in the face of clinically valuable improvement in motor function, the benefit-to-risk ratio of the DBS procedure seems favorable, at least in severely disabled patients. A careful selection of patient candidates for surgery should help maintain a relatively

TABLE 47.1		
ADVERSE EFFECTS RELATED TO DEEP-BRAIN SURGERY IN MOVEMENT DISORDERS		
Relation with the Surgical Stage	**Adverse Effects**	**Mean Rate**
Stereotactic frame and ventriculography	Seizure Mental confusion Extracerebral hematoma	About 1% when ventriculography is performed
Electrode implantation	Transient confusion or bradyphrenia	Up to 10% in PD
	Focal cerebral contusion or stroke; may be asymptomatic and only visualized on postoperative MRI	About 5%, half asymptomatic
	Intracerebral bleeding; may be asymptomatic if small	1 to 5% for all bleedings; 2%–3% with severe permanent aftereffects
	Intracranial extracerebral bleeding	
	Intracerebral abscess	Very rare
	Electrode fracture or failure (one or more of the 4 contacts) or migration	Unknown
	Misplaced lead	Frequently suboptimal; reimplantation to be considered after MRI checking
Connection lead and IPG	Superficial infection: aggressive antibiotherapy	1% to 15% for all types of infections
	Deep infection with cutaneous erosion: material removal and further replacement	
	Breaking or failure of extension lead	More frequent in patients with cervical dystonia
	Skin erosion, foreign body reaction, granuloma, seroma, and pain over the pulse generator	More frequent with Kinetra IPG
	IPG repositioning, pain over the extension lead or IPG region	All hardware problems in about 10% of cases
	IPG malfunction	Rare, rate unknown
Others	Transient general state complications, including aspiration pneumonia, pulmonary or urinary infection, thrombophlebitis, pulmonary embolism, etc.	5% of cases, mainly in PD patients; age and severity of akinesia are risk factors
Stimulation-induced	Eyelid-opening apraxia	15% in Parkinson's disease patients with STN stimulation
	Dysarthria, dysphagia Motor contraction, paresthesias Sweating, flushes Imbalance, dyskinesias Psychiatric symptoms	20% on the whole, mostly reversible

IPG, implanted pulse generator; PD, Parkinson's disease; MRI, magnetic resonance imaging; STN, subthalamic nucleus.

low level of morbidity. A skilled multidisciplinary team is needed to ensure the quality of patient selection, operative technique, intraoperative monitoring, and postoperative management.

PARKINSON'S DISEASE

There is widespread interest in the use of DBS for motor signs of PD, and large numbers of patients are regularly referred to surgical centers for consideration of DBS. Proper selection of patients who will reliably benefit is critical to the successful application of this procedure (159,160). Selecting patients for surgery requires careful evaluation of the motor signs of the disease and the effects and side effects of medical treatment, as well as the nonmotor cognitive, psychiatric, and behavioral aspects of this neuropsychiatric disease. In addition to disease-specific evaluation, a careful analysis of comorbidities, expectations of the patient, and individual socioeconomic status is necessary to explain the individual risk–benefit ratio to the patient. Patients will have to make decisions with their families, based on detailed information of the surgical procedure, knowing what potential benefits can be expected, and being aware of the risks and limitations that apply to individual situations. This time-consuming process of patient selection can be done only in the setting of a movement disorder center with specific neurological, neuropsychological, neuropsychiatric, neuroimaging, and—last but not least—neurosurgical expertise. Now that DBS has become an available treatment, general neurologists should be familiar with the main selection criteria.

CANDIDATES FOR DEEP-BRAIN STIMULATION

Whereas VIM stimulation has an impact on tremor only, stimulation of the STN or GPi improves akinesia, rigidity, tremor, and dyskinesias with a slightly different spectrum of effects. The target that will be best suited for an individual patient will be discussed in this section. Most basic considerations considered in this chapter will apply to all targets.

Age

The risks of surgery increase with age. It is common sense that elderly patients will have more surgical complications (e.g., brain surgery in old age is more likely to be complicated by brain hemorrhage), although this is difficult to prove for DBS based on published data, which tends to focus on highly levodopa-responsive young patients with a mean age that is generally below 60 years (although an age limit is not always clearly defined). Akinesia is a risk factor for deep vein thrombosis or pulmonary infection, and elderly patients are particularly fragile. The cognitive reserve also changes with old age. Although younger patients do tolerate DBS, even when performed bilaterally with minimal cognitive side effects (161), elderly patients are more likely to have postoperative cognitive or behavioral decompensation (162). The likelihood of comorbidities (whether recognized or not) will increase with age, thus increasing the risk of surgery. In the elderly patient, the nondopaminergic motor signs, such as dysarthria, dysphagia, postural instability, and gait disorders, are also more prominent, thus decreasing the potential benefit as nondopaminergic signs do not respond to surgery. Several studies found a less favorable outcome of bilateral STN stimulation in older (though not very old) compared to younger patients (163–165). The results of this comparison is probably explained by the coexistence of age-related reduced mobility on top of parkinsonian bradykinesia and comorbidities, such as cerebral small vessel disease or a decrease in cognitive reserve. Such comorbidities, even if largely asymptomatic, can lead to a higher prevalence of gait disorders, falls, and speech disorders that are resistant to levodopa. Expectancy of life is shorter in elderly patients, thereby also influencing the risk–benefit ratio. Although no specific age cutoff has been defined in many clinical DBS studies, most have excluded patients above age 75 years, and thus efficacy and safety of DBS in elderly patients over age 75 years has not been studied. We tend to consider age under 70 years as a relative contraindication and age above 75 years as an absolute contraindication, but some rare exceptions to this rule may be discussed in those patients with a biological age that seems younger than a chronological age, and in whom the risk–benefit ratio is otherwise favorable.

Comorbidities

When assessing comorbidities, one should bear in mind that PD is not restricted to the dopaminergic system but rather to a diffuse neurodegenerative disease (166). Thus comorbidities that may be well compensated in the absence of such neurodegeneration are more likely to become symptomatic or to decompensate. Based on common sense, all DBS centers do exclude patients with serious medical comorbidities as for any elective brain surgery, and it is therefore not surprising that almost no systematic studies are available that specifically correlate complication rates or outcome with presurgical comorbidity. One study showed a more than tenfold increase in cerebral hemorrhage in patients with preoperative vascular hypertension (167), emphasizing the importance of taking into account general health problems when estimating the risk–benefit ratio in surgical candidates. Preoperative MRI screening allows for identification of structural lesions that may increase the risk of surgery or decrease its benefit (such as relevant white matter lesions) and features of atypical parkinsonism that also will likely affect the outcome. One study retrospectively evaluated exclusion criteria in 98 patients hospitalized for surgical screening. This report did not account for patients who had been excluded from presurgical screening on the basis of more overt medical and neurological comorbidities. The authors considered that 30% ($n = 29$) of the subjects were not suitable for surgery. The most frequent exclusion was neuropsychological and psychiatric dysfunction ($n = 14$), followed by abnormalities in MRI scans ($n = 9$) or nonneurological conditions ($n = 2$) (168). Although formal studies are lacking, serious systemic comorbidities or evolving malignancies with markedly reduced life expectancy, such as unstable heart disease, active infection, marked subcortical arteriosclerotic encephalopathy, or other disabling cerebrovascular disease, should be regarded as contraindications to DBS (160).

Neuropsychological and Neuropsychiatric Evaluation

Although transient postoperative cognitive side effects are relatively common (61), surgery for DBS has relatively few permanent cognitive side effects in well-selected young and nondemented patients, even when performed bilaterally (161,169–171). However, elderly patients or those with preoperative cognitive deterioration are at risk for permanent postoperative cognitive deterioration (61,162,172–174). A thorough screening for cognitive deficits is mandatory. Neuropsychological evaluation with a special emphasis on memory and executive function is highly recommended (175,176). For evaluation of overall cognitive function, the Mattis Dementia Rating Scale (MDRS) (range 0–144) is an appropriate tool in degenerative diseases involving subcortical structures, given the inclusion of tests evaluating attention and executive functions. A cutoff score of 130 usually distinguishes demented from nondemented patients (175). To investigate verbal memory, the Grober Buschke Verbal Learning Test is an appropriate procedure because it distinguishes the executive component of memory (free recall) from the hippocampal consolidation component (cued recall and recognition). The executive component is usually impaired in nondemented PD patients, but the hippocampal component is preserved. Total recall (sum of free and cued recall) lower than 40/48 indicates a memory disorder that is abnormally severe for a nondemented PD patient (175). In case of borderline scores or complaints of relevant cognitive deterioration, it is useful to repeat the evaluation after 1 year to ascertain that cognitive function is stable. It also must be ascertained that cognitive dysfunction is not related to antiparkinsonian medication, especially anticholinergics or depression.

Mood changes and behavioral side effects are common after DBS surgery for STN or GPi (176–183) and occur especially in the first postoperative weeks or months (61,184). As for cognitive side effects, most available data concern the STN rather than the GPi, which is at least partly explained by the fact that most published series deal with this target. In addition, contrary to GPi stimulation, STN stimulation allows for and requires major manipulations in dopaminergic medication that also can be responsible for changes in mood or behavioral side effects (138,176,185). VIM stimulation seems to be much safer as far as behavioral side effects are concerned.

PD is a neuropsychiatric disorder (186). Psychiatric symptoms that are disease related must be distinguished from the psychiatric side effects of medication (187). It has been shown clearly that those patients with preoperative psychiatric disorders are most prone to develop postoperative psychiatric complications (188). Although psychiatric symptoms that are disease related, such as apathy, are prone to be exacerbated after surgery in the context of a dopaminergic withdrawal syndrome (61,138), the symptoms outside the spectrum of the dopamine dysregulation syndrome (187) may possibly be improved if dopaminergic treatment can be reduced after surgery (189). Ongoing severe depression with suicidal ideation should be considered as an absolute contraindication to surgery because of the risk of suicide (184,190).

Motor Evaluation

The signs that can be improved with STN or GPi stimulation are the off-period related motor parkinsonian signs (akinesia, rigidity, tremor) and painful off-period dystonia as well as on-period dyskinesia (14,44,59,60,61,127,181,191). VIM stimulation improves off-period parkinsonian tremor (13,45,47). DBS of any target does no better than levodopa at its peak effect. (Provided adequate doses are being used for chronic treatment and the levodopa test, the preceding statement does not apply to a first-ever levodopa test in a de novo patient.) In other words, DBS at best can improve those signs that can be improved by levodopa as well as the motor side effects of levodopa. DBS is therefore considered only if (a) it has been ascertained that medical treatment is adequate in an individual patient and (b) that despite optimal treatment there is a relevant disability directly related to motor complications of dopaminergic treatment. Several reports have shown a good correlation of improvement of parkinsonism with levodopa or STN stimulation (60,163,164,192). It is thus mandatory to evaluate carefully the effects and side effects of levodopa in each surgical candidate to explain to the patient what the signs and symptoms are that can potentially be improved with DBS.

Off-period motor signs are generally evaluated in defined off (i.e., the off period in the morning after 12 hours without dopaminergic treatment). It must be acknowledged, however, that in this condition the off-period motor signs may not be at their worst for several reasons. For example, some patients have a major sleep benefit. In addition, long-acting agonists taken even 12 hours earlier are still active, and the long-term effects of levodopa, during the day, after taking suprathreshold doses of levodopa, can cause patients to experience a rebound off that can be much more disabling than an early-morning off period. Evaluation of defined off may, therefore, not reflect the full disability. In some patients it may be useful to evaluate a worst-off condition either during a hospitalization or an outpatient visit, by asking the patient to prepare by not taking his or her regular medication.

One of the best predictors of outcome, other than the magnitude of the motor response to levodopa, is the quality of the on period (193). Patients having no complaints related to parkinsonism at the peak effect of levodopa who are simultaneously disabled by dyskinesias and/or off periods can, therefore, be considered as the best candidates for surgery. Thus, in our opinion it is important to use a suprathreshold dose of levodopa (e.g., 1.5 times the equivalent dose of morning medication) to ascertain the "best on" motor condition. The patient and examiner should agree that the "best on" is obtained at the moment of evaluation. Dyskinesias can be quantified using the United Parkinson's Disease Rating Scale (UPDRS) Part IV anamnestic item, but an objective evaluation during the levodopa test seems preferable. Objective assessment is preferable (44,194,195), but unfortunately the present version of the UPDRS lacks objective evaluation of dyskinesias, so presently no widely used scale for assessment of dyskinesias is available. When assessing dyskinesia severity, one has to be aware that off-period dystonia is not necessarily present during each off period and that diphasic dyskinesia tends to worsen in duration and severity in the course of a day, thus emphasizing the utility of a combined subjective and objective evaluation.

The selection of patients can be based either on the UPDRS motor score (Part III) or on individual items of the UPDRS, taking into account the duration and severity of a sign or symptom in the off period, the related disability, the response to levodopa, and the severity and duration of on-period dyskinesias (UPDRS Part IV, plus plus objective dyskinesia assessment). As recommended by the Core Assessment Program for Surgical Interventional Therapies in Parkinson's Disease (CAPSIT-PD) protocol (194), a patient should have a disease duration of at least 5 years before being considered for surgery so that atypical forms of parkinsonism become evident. In everyday practice, patients often ask for surgery from the day of diagnosis. Some are ready to accept the risks of surgery while not accepting even minor side effects of levodopa. Generally, these patients are not ready (yet) to accept their disease, and practitioners must emphasize that DBS is as much a symptomatic treatment as levodopa, and DBS has no impact on the neurodegenerative process. Poor acceptance of the disease can contribute to failure of treatment with medication or with DBS.

Another potential indication for STN stimulation could be disabling psychiatric symptoms induced by (adequate) dopaminergic treatment. Indeed there are first reports of single cases with improvement of dopaminergic dysregulation syndrome after subthalamic stimulation allowing for substantial reduction of dopaminergic treatment (189), but this requires further evaluation.

Socioeconomic Status, Expectancy, and Cooperation

Disability depends to some extent on individual social and personal status, and patient selection must be individualized according to each patient's professional activities, interpersonal relationships, and expectations of functionality. For example, a patient who is married and has a dedicated husband or wife constantly present may more easily accept an occasional off period with loss of autonomy than will a patient with the same motor features living on his or her own. Patients who are working may have to take increasingly high doses of medication to be able to pursue their physical activities at the same pace as a nondisabled person, thereby exacerbating a vicious circle with increasingly severe dyskinesias, rebound off periods, dopamine dependency, and psychiatric side effects. On the other hand, surgery may allow some patients to resume or pursue their professional activities (196). Patients' expectations are not always realistic, and each evaluator is responsible, after careful assessment of the individual risk–benefit ratio, for providing a realistic explanation of the potentially functional benefits of surgery. Surgery and postoperative adaptation to drugs and stimulation parameters require a great deal of patient cooperation. Any severe personality disorder that prevents a minimum of cooperation is likely to be an absolute contraindication to this type of elective surgery.

TARGETS FOR DEEP-BRAIN STIMULATION

DBS can be applied to three different targets (thalamus, GPi, STN) to improve parkinsonian signs. Results of surgery differ, depending on the target. Although presently the STN is the preferred target for most patients in most centers, all three targets may be relevant, depending on patient profiles. The three targets are discussed separately in the following subsections.

Thalamic Deep-Brain Stimulation

Most neurosurgeons are still using the Hasslerian nomenclature for the thalamic nuclei (197,198), although that does not agree with the nomenclature based on experimental animal studies (199). The ventral intermedius nucleus (VIM) is situated posteriorly to the V.o. complex (comprising the ventralis oralis anterior [V.o.a] and the ventralis oralis posterior [V.o.p] nucleus) and anteriorly to the sensory nucleus (ventralis posterior nucleus [VP]). The electrophysiologically defined VIM (200,201) is the target for thalamic lesions (202) or thalamic DBS for PD tremor (13). Intraoperative recording in VIM shows the presence of tremor-synchronous bursts and kinesthetic cells, anterior to cutaneous receptive cells. Intraoperative high-frequency stimulation (>100 Hz) within VIM induces tremor arrest with low threshold. Increasing the current using a well-localized electrode can lead to sensory side effects (posterior spread to sensory nucleus) and/or dysarthria with lateral current spread to the internal capsule. As the electrode generally is located at the anterior border of the lower part of the VIM, it cannot be excluded that anterior current spread to V.o.p or ventral spread to fibers may also contribute to the antitremoric effect (203). Presently, resolution of MRI does not allow direct visualization of the VIM and indirect landmarks (therefore, anterior commissure, posterior commissure, height of the thalamus, and width of the third ventricle are used) (204). MRI visualization of the medial dorsal nucleus and the internal capsule also can guide the targeting (201). Cytoarchitectonic definition of nuclei is difficult to determine in the motor thalamus, which explains the presence of different nomenclatures, and thus it is best to define the nuclei based on their subcortical afferents. However, knowledge obtained in studies of monkeys and applied to human brains has led to different conclusions (203). It is thought that VIM receives receive cerebellar afferents (205,206) and that the more anterior V.o.p receives either cerebellar (206) or pallidal (205) afferents. VIM DBS has an effect almost exclusively on tremor. Akinesia is not improved with either thalamic DBS or thalamic lesioning (199). VIM DBS has little impact on rigidity and dyskinesias, except if the electrodes are implanted more anteriorly and/or more medially (207). This is akin to thalamotomies that have an antidyskinetic effect only if the lesion extends more anteriorly than VIM, including V.o.p and V.o.a (ventrooralis anterior nucleus, according to Hassler's nomenclature) (208,209). These antidyskinetic and antirigidity effects of anterior thalamotomies are likely explained by inclusion of the thalamic territory that receives its subcortical afferents from the basal ganglia.

Globus Pallidus Pars Interna Deep-Brain Stimulation

Targeting of GPi is based primarily on MRI and may be refined using intraoperative electrophysiology. Using adequate technique, MRI allows visualization of the boundaries of the globus pallidus internus, globus pallidus externus, and lamina medullaris interna. The pallidocapsular border, the medial putaminal border, and the optical tract can be used as additional landmarks. Given the significant variability of the position of the pallidal structures, especially for laterality, relying on an atlas or on the commissures is inadequate for targeting. The anatomic target is the middle of the visualized posteroventral pallidum, which corresponds to the sensorimotor part of this nucleus (102). Intraoperative macrostimulation allows for estimation of the location of the medial internal capsule (induction of motor contraction and/or dysarthria) and the ventral optic tract (induction of a subjective visual flash). Testing of antiparkinsonian effects of intraoperative macrostimulation is also useful (191). In the awake patient, a reliable localization of the electrode is possible using these means. Even if a patient requires general anesthesia capsular effects can be seen, and visual-evoked potentials allow location of the optic tract. After the target is chosen, mapping through microelectrodes can be used to identify the somatosensory region of the target and to confirm the boundaries of the target and its distance to the internal capsule and optic tract. A map is then generated to determine the final placement of the stimulating electrode. However, the usefulness of microelectrode mapping, although it has its advocates (210,211) is heavily criticized by others, based mainly on the increased risk of intraoperative hemorrhage related to multiple passes with microelectrodes (98,122,212).

Subthalamic Nucleus Deep-Brain Stimulation

The STN can be visualized easily and directly on MRI on T2-weighted coronal slices (97), allowing for direct targeting based on MRI (131). Compared to the GPi, there is relatively little variability in the localization of this more medial structure in relation to the anterior and posterior commissures that can be used for indirect targeting (204). The anterior border of the red nucleus, lying very close to the STN, is another useful internal landmark (103,108,213). The STN is a small target with a volume of about 160 mm^3, compared to 480 mm^3 for the GPi (214). This small target is surrounded by many eloquent structures, and precise targeting is required for optimal benefit. Intraoperative stimulation of the STN area in the parkinsonian patient under local anesthesia allows a precise definition of the target (137). Stimulation-related side effects help to identify neighboring fibers that must be avoided (corticobulbar and corticospinal fibers anterolaterally, third nerve fibers medioventrally, medial lemniscus posteroventrally). Intraoperative stimulation-induced antiparkinsonian effects and dyskinesias

define the sensorimotor part of the STN (128,137). Although improvement of segmental akinesia and observation of dyskinesias induced by stimulation during the operation are the best predictors of good outcome (128), evaluation of akinesia can be difficult, and for this reason we also rely on assessment in rigidity (137).We consider intraoperative stimulation to be a mandatory step in determining the precise location of the final electrode. Whenever possible, STN surgery should be performed under local anesthesia with the aim of optimal targeting based on the prodyskinetic and antiparkinsonian effects of intraoperative stimulation. If a patient cannot tolerate local anesthesia, the threshold for such stimulation-induced side effects as ocular deviation or motor contraction can be evaluated in the absence of muscle relaxation. Some centers have reported good outcomes using general anesthesia, but accepting general anesthesia nevertheless means accepting the risk of suboptimal outcome (129). Therefore, we use a physiotherapist to help decrease discomfort related to immobility and off-period dystonia (215).

Continual contact during surgery is also gratefully acknowledged by patients (215). In patients with severe parkinsonism, off-period panic attacks, or off-period painful dystonia, the use of an apomorphine pump during surgery greatly improves the patient's comfort. Many centers also use microrecording to define this small target. As the STN is surrounded by fibers, it is relatively easy to define its boundaries. The most useful criteria for selecting a trajectory are (a) the length of an individual trajectory displaying typical STN activity, (b) the bursting pattern of activity, and (c) motor responses typical of the sensorimotor part of the nucleus (216). The sensorimotor part of the nucleus is localized dorsolaterally (217) and, accordingly, the most effective electrodes are localized near the dorsolateral border zone of the STN (218).

RESULTS OF VENTRALIS INTERMEDIUS NUCLEUS DEEP-BRAIN STIMULATION

In 1987 Benabid et al. first proposed VIM stimulation contralateral to thalamotomy, with the aim of reducing the morbidity of bilateral thalamic surgery (18). The preliminary results were encouraging, and this group started to perform VIM stimulation as a first surgical option, abandoning thalamotomy. PD tremor was controlled in 85% of the patients, a figure similar to that of thalamotomy, but the morbidity was lower, especially the incidence of dysarthria, allowing for bilateral thalamic surgery (13,89). An effect on levodopa-induced dsykinesia was reported in some patients (219), but this effect was not found to be significant in other studies. Efficacy of VIM stimulation was confirmed in PD, and essential tremor, using blinded assessment and random assignment to on or off stimulation (45,46). A randomized trial comparing unilateral thalamotomy to unilateral thalamic DBS showed a greater benefit in functional status and a lower incidence of permanent side effects in those patients who had been randomized for the stimulation technique (47). Long-term effects also have been confirmed (48,49). There is substantial agreement that, similar to thalamotomy, thalamic stimulation is highly effective in the relief of PD tremor (220). However, VIM stimulation does not significantly influence bradykinesia, rigidity, on-period dyskinesia, or off-period painful dystonia. Even if patients are selected initially for having tremor-predominant PD, motor fluctuations and dyskinesias eventually may become major problems after several years of evolution, despite ongoing successful tremor control (58). In a series of 15 patients operated on in the VIM for PD tremor 8 years (±5 years) after onset of the disease, STN implantation was carried out 10 years (±4 years) later. Duration of follow-up after beginning STN stimulation was 24 months (±20 months). The UPDRS motor score, tremor score, difficulties in performance of activities of daily living, and levodopa equivalent daily dose decreased significantly after STN stimulation (221). STN stimulation seems a better option for PD patients with tremor, even for PD patients with tremor as the most disabling symptom. Compared to STN DBS, however, there are also some advantages. VIM DBS does not induce dyskinesias, and it does not require postoperative adaptation of medication. It can be performed unilaterally, whereas STN DBS is generally performed bilaterally. A unilateral VIM stimulation is considered relatively safe. Patients suffering mainly from tremor often have a more benign disease course. Tremor suppression often requires high doses of levodopa with higher risk of psychosis in the elderly. For these reasons, some experts consider that age may be less critical when considering VIM DBS in elderly patients suffering mainly from disabling tremor (160). In our experience, indications for VIM DBS in PD have become exceedingly rare for several reasons: (a) disabling tremor as the only sign of PD is rare; (b) we rarely see PD tremor that does not respond to the combination of high doses of levodopa in association with clozapine (clozapine is an excellent antipsychotic, and thus allows introduction of high doses of levodopa while having a major antitremor effect of its own); and (c) elderly patients who have a pure tremor resistant to levodopa in association with clozapine often have comorbidity that increases the risk of surgery.

The different side effects of VIM stimulation are specific to this thalamic target and surrounding structures. Increasing voltage too much can induce paresthesias, and a further increase will induce pain. Motor side effects are dysarthria and contralateral tetanic muscle contraction of the face and limbs. More rarely, a contralateral cerebellar syndrome or ataxic gait can be induced. Stimulation arrest can result in rebound tremor (91).

Although VIM DBS is highly effective on PD tremor, activities of daily living and diability are improved to a lesser extent as tremor is not the only symptom of the disease (48,222). According to evidence-based criteria, VIM DBS as an adjunct to levodopa is presently considered to be investigational (223).

RESULTS OF PALLIDAL DEEP-BRAIN STIMULATION

Pallidal DBS improves levodopa-induced dyskinesias and the cardinal motor symptoms of PD, including akinesia, rigidity, tremor, and gait (15,43,60,127,181,191,224–238). Painful off-period dystonia is also improved (43,238). The antidyskinetic effects of GPi stimulation are immediate, dramatic, and long lasting, whereas the effects on off-period motor symptoms are more moderate (generally about 40% improvement in UPDRS motor score at 12 months) and tend to decline progressively after surgery (230,234,236,239) to the extent that some patients have had to be reoperated in the STN (236,239). This is all the more intriguing as the group that has obtained the best antiparkinsonian effects ever reported after surgery (56% improvement in UPDRS at 3 months) has more recently reported decline in antiparkinsonian effects in the long term (236). Does this reflect tolerance to DBS or suboptimal electrode placement in a complex structure? A recent multicenter study was reassuring as the outcome at 3 to 4 years was stable. Of 26 patients, 2 had been reimplanted in the STN in the hope of a better outcome, but the 20 patients who reached 3- to 4-year follow-up were improved by 44% at 1 year and still by 39% at 3 to 4 years (88). This argues for a suboptimal placement in those patients in whom results are not stable over time. The GPi is indeed a complex structure with effects that are highly variable and partly opposite depending on the exact location of the electrode (43,240,241). Stimulation of the dorsal GPi/GPe induces good acute antiparkinsonian effects (43,242), but these are not long lasting (243). Stimulation of the ventral GPi or below the GPi induce excellent antirigidity and antidyskinetic effects, but stimulation of this area also leads to inhibition of levodopa effects (244), or even worsening of akinesia in the off-drug condition (242,245). Intraoperative target definition is more difficult for the GPi than for the STN, which is a smaller target surrounded by eloquent structures. The optimal target is the same as for pallidotomy, and well-located electrodes can have stable effects lasting for at least 3 years (246). Although many series of unilateral pallidotomies have been published, there are relatively few articles reporting the long-term outcome of pallidotomy. The available data show that the antidyskinetic effects are long lasting but that the antiparkinsonian effects are less stable (53,247,248). In contrast to DBS, pallidotomy is not reversible, and it is therefore more difficult to know whether this represents progression of the disease or partial loss of benefit. The fact that the antidyskinetic effects are long lasting, however, argues rather for a decrease in antiparkinsonian effects over time.

Side effects related to surgery or hardware problems are discussed in a previous section of this chapter. In selected young and nondemented patients, GPi DBS has few overall cognitive side effects (161,171,249). However, cognitive decline may occur in elderly patients after surgery (172) Mania (180) and a dysexecutive syndrome (179) have been reported in direct relation to GPi stimulation. Manic psychosis and pathological gambling could occur, due to necessary increase in dopaminergic therapy 3 years after GPi DBS. On the other hand, these adverse effects were reversible after STN DBS allowing for decrease in dopaminergic drugs (236). Other side effects include dysarthria, freezing of gait, gait ignition failure (43,226,230), worsening of on-period parkinsonism related to inhibition of levodopa effects (245), and loss of efficacy in the long term (236,239).

Several reports comparing STN and GPi stimulation find a better antiakinetic effect of STN compared to GPi stimulation (60,88,127,181,232). In these studies, levodopa is reduced in STN DBS only. The only prospective study planned for comparing these two targets in a randomized way (10 patients in an STN group, 10 patients in a GPi group, evaluation at 12 months) also found a trend for better improvement of akinesia with STN compared to GPi ($p = 0.06$) (237). On the other hand, side effects have been more frequent in STN DBS (88,181,237). There are several unanswered questions, and the question remains open to debate (62,250,251). Fewer data are available for pallidal stimulation compared to subthalamic stimulation. According to evidence-based criteria, pallidal stimulation is considered to be efficacious and possibly useful, whereas subthalamic nucleus stimulation is considered to be efficacious and clinically useful as an adjunct to levodopa (223). In the United States, there are several ongoing large, prospective, double-blinded, randomized studies comparing both targets. It is hoped that the potential confounding problems related to initial lack of experience in targeting and postoperative management, as well as publication bias, will be resolved with the help of these studies. Some authors believe that based on the risk–benefit ratio of GPi DBS versus STN DBS, with a slightly better antiakinetic effect of STN DBS but a better antidyskinetic effect and lower side effects of pallidal DBS, pallidal deep-brain stimulation may make a triumphant return (62). The comparison between targets will have to take into account not only the short-term motor benefit and side effects but also the long-term overall outcome. In the meantime, while awaiting the results of future studies and taking into account the published data on long-term outcome of DBS in both targets (61,88,236, 252–255), we continue to prefer the STN.

RESULTS OF SUBTHALAMIC NUCLEUS DEEP-BRAIN STIMULATION

The effects of STN stimulation are mainly contralateral (14,256), and unilateral STN stimulation does not provide maximal improvement in walking (14,257). Although PD can manifest clinically as a unilateral disease in early stages, there is always bilateral neurodegeneration of the presynaptic dopaminergic system. By the time patients develop motor complications, the disease is usually bilateral, but marked asymmetry may persist. Subthalamic stimulation can induce dyskinesias and therefore requires a postoperative decrease in dopaminergic treatment (57). Levodopa is effective bilaterally but cannot be administered asymmetrically in asymmetric disease. Decreasing the medication can reveal symptoms that had been masked by the long-term effects of levodopa (258). Therefore, unilateral subthalamic stimulation would be difficult to manage because medication would have to be adapted differently for both sides. For these reasons, subthalamic nucleus stimulation is generally performed bilaterally, and there are virtually no published reports on unilateral subthalamic stimulation. After unilateral STN lesioning, dopaminergic treatment is not reduced and dyskinesias do not improve. Surprisingly, lesion-induced dyskinesias were not considered to be problematic after unilateral subthalamic lesions (259).

Bilateral subthalamic nucleus stimulation has been studied in idiopathic, levodopa-sensitive young (mostly <70 years) PD patients suffering from motor complications of levodopa therapy. In such patients, almost all studies report postoperative improvement in off-period motor scores between 40% and 70% (60,127,163, 164, 181,229,252,253,260–276). One study has separately analyzed outcome depending on age. In 52 consecutive patients, improvement in UPDRS motor scores was 62% in those who were younger than 60 years ($n = 15$), 37% in the group of patients ($n = 24$) ages 60 to 70 years, and only 22% in those more than 70 years (mean 74 ± 3; $n = 13$) (165). In a recent review, the average improvement 12 months after surgery was found to be 56% (153). After 12 months of subthalamic nucleus stimulation, when compared with preoperative off-medication subscores, the mean improvement was 81% in tremor, 63% in rigidity, 52% in bradykinesia, 64% in gait, and 69% in postural instability (153). Contrary to other parkinsonian signs, speech is generally not improved with STN stimulation (62,88,260). Although in individual patients dysarthria (which only rarely shows an excellent levodopa response) can improve, dysarthria related to electrical current diffusion to corticobulbar fibers also can worsen speech, which explains the mitigated overall effects of subthalamic stimulation on speech (277). Some groups have reported a smaller improvement in UPDRS motor scores (10,278). Whereas the results of Pahwa et al. (277a) were largely explained by patient selection (lower response to levodopa) and a surgical learning curve (278), Ford et al. (10) believe that their more modest results represent a more realistic estimate of the effect of DBS on PD based on the fact that they used a double-blinded evaluation of the motor UPDRS as their main outcome criterion. However, their data differ greatly from the vast majority of published outcomes (including double-blind, crossover evaluations

(127,279), not only in the double-blind evaluation but also in nonblinded assessment of several secondary outcome measures, including activities of daily living (no benefit) and postoperative decrease in dopaminergic treatment (30%). This chapter, however, raises the issue of publication bias. Published data do not necessarily reflect the outcome of those centers that do not publish and that may be less experienced in diagnosing and treating PD, performing stereotactic surgery, or managing patients with DBS after surgery. Ford et al. are from a center that is well-known for treating movement disorders. If in the hands of Ford et al. subthalamic DBS does not improve activities of daily living, this should discourage widespread propagation of this difficult technique. In the United States, the Food and Drug Administration has approved DBS for PD, essential tremor, and dystonia based on published results. As revealed by a recent study (280,97a), not all centers performing DBS rely on movement disorder neurologists for diagnosis, on neuropsychologists for cognitive evaluation, or on skilled surgeons or neurologists trained in DBS. The history of medicine has shown more than once that uncritical application of new developments can discredit techniques that are useful, even when the latter are applied according to the state of the art.

In our experience, on-period motor signs are not improved with subthalamic stimulation, provided care is taken to use an individually adapted suprathreshold dose of levodopa to carry out the levodopa test (61,260). Many authors, however, report a 30% to 40% improvement in on-period motor scores (88,261) related to improvement in tremor and rigidity (88). This difference in outcome measurements reflects differences in evaluation techniques that are likely to be explained by the fact that not all authors use suprathreshold doses of levodopa as a levodopa challenge, but rather they evaluate while the patient is receiving optimal medication therapy, including levodopa, dopamine agonists, and other antiparkinsonian medication (261). Using a suprathreshold dose of levodopa to obtain a "best on" is useful when trying to predict the maximal potential benefit of surgery in an individual patient. Using the usual early-morning dose more closely reflects the everyday situation of the patient; thus, a patient who often has a tremor while in an on period may have a benefit from surgery that is not restricted to an off period.

Effects of STN stimulation on levodopa-induced dyskinesias have been assessed using different methods. The most frequent assessment tool is anamnestic data using UPDRS items for duration and disability of dyskinesia (items 32 and 33) (60,61). Another measure of the duration of dyskinesia is the assessment, based on patient diaries, of time spent in the on state without dyskinesias (88,127). Dyskinesia scales evaluating the severity of dyskinesias in different body parts also have been used (44,88,260). Using a dyskinesia scale is more objective, but giving a suprathreshold levodopa dose to induce dyskinesia can be an artificial situation in some patients in whom levodopa has been markedly reduced or even completely stopped. Therefore, the anamnestic data from patient diaries on duration and severity better reflect everyday life. Dyskinesias are improved on all assessments in all published reports whatever the evaluation tool, and duration and severity of UPDRS items are improved by about 75% on average (153). One study separately assessing off-period dystonia, diphasic dyskinesia, and peak-dose dyskinesia found the highest improvement in off-period dystonia and the least improvement in peak-dose dyskinesias. STN stimulation has a direct effect on off-period dystonia, whereas the reversal of peak-dose dyskinesia mainly reflects desensitization (280,281) after levodopa withdrawal. As for off-period dystonia, there may also be some direct effects on dyskinesia, especially diphasic dyskinesia (44).

Off-period dystonia and pain related to off-period dystonia are improved with subthalamic stimulation (44,61,88). Improvement in off-period dystonia is a direct effect of subthalamic stimulation in the same way as are improvement in akinesia, rigidity, and tremor (44), whereas improvement of on-period dyskinesias is mainly an indirect effect, related to a decrease in dopaminergic medication (44,58,281).

Activities of daily living in off-drug conditions, as measured by UPDRS Part II, improve to the same extent as improvement in motor symptoms (61). Although on-period dyskinesias improve, activities of daily living in on-drug conditions remain unchanged (61), indicating that dyskinesias on average do not have a major impact on activities of daily living, in contrast to parkinsonism. Activities of daily living, as measured by the Schwab and England scale, also improve only in the off-drug condition (61). Patients in preoperative off-drug condition who depend on a caregiver can become independent in their activities of daily living after surgery with chronic subthalamic stimulation, with the off-drug scores being close to the on-drug scores (61). Improvement of sleep architecture (282) and quality (283) have been reported with an increase in total sleep time (by as much as 47%) resulting indirectly from nighttime akinesia and early-morning dystonia (282). Subthalamic stimulation can be effective for decreasing detrusor hyperreflexia (284,285).

Data concerning cognitive or behavioral deterioration must be viewed with caution as most studies suffer from small sample sizes and generally do not include PD control groups (176,286). In this context, an article analyzing postoperative behavioral side effects and preoperative history of behavioral side effects found that those patients displaying behavioral abnormalities after surgery generally had a history of exactly the same behavioral abnormalities before surgery, thus illustrating that not every reported abnormal behavior should be seen as directly related to stimulation and even less as a specific side effect of a specific target (188). Analysis of long-term follow-up after STN surgery shows that immediately after surgery there is a high prevalence of confusion and behavioral side effects, but in the long term, cognitive and psychiatric side effects are relatively rare (61). The side effects in the first weeks or months are multifactorial. They can be related to surgery or to changes in medication and stimulation, and sometimes they are reactions to a life event. A side effect occurring several months or years after surgery can be related either to treatment or to progression of the disease, and sometimes it may be completely independent of PD and its treatment. Apathy is a frequent finding in PD patients on chronic subthalamic stimulation (61,184). Although apathy is part of PD (287), in our experience severe apathy or abulia can occur related to postoperative withdrawal of dopaminergic medication, especially in patients with an addiction to levodopa (60). In these patients, apathy responds to an increase in dopaminergic medication (184,188). In the long term, follow-up apathy can increase and progressive worsening of frontal executive function with progression of the disease may be a contributing factor (61).

Switching on stimulation, acutely, using high stimulation parameters, can lead to such acute changes in behavior as acute sadness (288), hypomania (61), impulsive aggressive behavior (61,289,290), or hilarity (291), all of which are rapidly reversible upon stimulation arrest. Most authors have related these side effects to surrounding structures, assuming a different and specific topography for the different behaviors (288–290), but it could be that these changes in mood are related to a release of behavioral patterns related to an abrupt change in subthalamic limbic activity (291,292) in the same way as ballism is explained by acute disinhibition of the sensorimotor area of the subthalamic nucleus. Pathologic behaviors that are induced by acute changes in stimulation parameters are rapidly reversible upon stimulation arrest. Postoperative transient hypomania is a frequent finding (61,184), and some cases of full-blown mania also have been reported (183,293). We consider hypomania to be a specific effect of stimulation of the limbic STN. In the postoperative period, the interaction among the short-term psychotropic effects of dopaminergic treatment (185); the ongoing long-term effects of dopaminergic treatment in the first weeks after reduction of treatment (258); and the transient lesionlike effects of surgery related to an edema surrounding the electrode contribute to the psychotropic effects of subthalamic stimulation (185).

The publication of acute stimulation-induced depression (294) using an electrode close to the STN, as well as reports on suicides after STN surgery (188,190,260), have raised much concern. In our first series of 20 patients treated with subthalamic stimulation, 1 patient committed suicide (260). Meanwhile, we have operated on more than 250 patients, and the suicide rate decreased from 5% to less than 0.5% with approximately 1000 patient years of follow-up and 1 suicide also on the wait list with approximately 500 patient years (unpublished data). This raises the issue of extrapolating data from uncontrolled studies. Selection bias is another issue. The patient who had committed suicide in our series had been suicidal and severely depressed 3 months before surgery. During the preoperative evaluation, his depression had improved and he was not suicidal then, which was probably related to the expectations he had concerning outcome. Indeed, he had hoped not only to have substantial improvement of his very severe PD but also to reestablish relations with his wife. Although after surgery with improvement in parkinsonism his depression further improved, he committed suicide 6 months after surgery. Although the mean scores of the Beck Depression Inventory improve for most patients after surgery (184), this improvement is only minor and likely reflects improvement in somatic items. Globally, depression does not seem to change with subthalamic stimulation. Indeed, those patients who were found to be depressed after surgery were the same ones who were already depressed before surgery (184). Preoperative depression and a history of repeat surgery were found to be risk factors for postoperative suicide, also pointing to selection bias (190). Depression is a frequent finding in the patient population requesting surgery (188), and patients with suicidal ideation are at risk, require optimal antidepressant treatment, and need a close psychiatric follow-up. L-dopa withdrawal and reactive depression also may play a role in patients at risk. The majority of the observed neuropsychiatric symptoms are considered to be transient, treatable, and potentially preventable (176).

Data concerning neuropsychological consequences of STN stimulation usually show no global cognitive deterioration in the short term in selected young and nondemented patients (161,176,249,295). Isolated studies note minor improvements or deteriorations in a few neuropsychological tests (176), but the impact of these findings on overall cognitive function is only minor. However, elderly patients with reduced cognitive reserve or patients with preoperative cognitive decline (162,173) can show global cognitive deterioration. Postoperative dementia also can occur as a consequence of surgical complications (61). In the long term, there is a progression of the dysexecutive syndrome, which can lead to dementia. This is not related to subthalamic stimulation but to progression of the disease (61). The most common side effect of subthalamic stimulation is weight gain, occurring in the vast majority of patients (61,158), whereas patients on medication tend to lose weight. On average, weight gain is about 4 kg, and this weight gain often corresponds to a return to previous weight. In individual patients, however, weight gain can be a major problem.

Side effects of stimulation that can be related either to the target or to current diffusion surrounding fibers are dysarthria, apraxia of eyelid opening, titanic motor contraction leading to fixed dystonic postures, disabling dyskinesia, freezing of gait, imbalance, gaze deviation or ipsilateral eye deviation, dysesthesia, vegetative side effects such as ipsilateral mydriasis, or ipsilateral sweating. These side effects are reversible on stimulation arrest, but sometimes tolerable side effects are accepted as a compromise to gain maximal benefit.

Quality of life is an interesting outcome measure as it takes into account not only the motor benefits but also changes in pain, sleep, mood, autonomy, and social adaptation, as well as the impact of side effects, whether cognitive, motor, or behavioral. One study has used a generic measure of health-related quality of life showing improvements in physical and psychosocial dimensions. The most improved aspects included body care, movement, sleep and rest, ambulation, social interactions, and recreation and pastimes (296). Several studies focused on disease-specific aspects of health-related quality of life (297–303) and consistently showed greater improvements in subscores of mobility, activities of daily living, stigma, emotional well-being, and bodily discomfort, whereas social support, cognition, and communication were less improved (304). The quality of life of caregivers also was improved (303).

Improvement of motor symptoms and dyskinesias, and a decrease in dopaminergic medication, are largely sustained in the long term (61,88,253,254,275,279). Mild worsening of akinesia, mainly of such axial features as speech, postural reflexes, and freezing, occurred over time (61). There also was progressive worsening of apathy and frontal dysexecutive syndrome, and some patients developed dementia. There is no indication of tolerance as effects are stable over 5 years with no increase in stimulation parameters after the first year (61). Progression of symptoms over time closely resembles the natural history of PD on medical treatment but without the motor complications (305,306), and these changes are therefore believed to represent progression of the disease rather than side effects of stimulation. This is compatible with a longitudinal positron emission tomography (PET) study showing continuous decline of dopaminergic function in patients with advanced PD under clinically effective bilateral STN stimulation, with rates of progression that are within the range of previous studies in nonstimulated patients (307). According to evidence-based criteria, subthalamic nucleus stimulation is considered as efficacious and clinically useful as an adjunct to levodopa (223).

POSTOPERATIVE MANAGEMENT: DEEP-BRAIN STIMULATION

Setting stimulation parameters has become a subspecialty of its own among movement disorder neurologists and functional stereotactic surgeons. Follow-up for patients with DBS requires specialized and detailed knowledge of movement disorders, including psychiatric aspects, psychological reactions to surgical intervention, medical treatments, medication–stimulation interactions, side effects

and limitations, technical aspects of stimulators, effects and limitations of stimulation of different targets, potential placebo effects of stimulation, evolution of neurodegenerative diseases, variability of signs and symptoms over time, and so on. Patients with DBS need lifelong follow-up, and this must be done by neurologists and surgeons with the appropriate knowledge and skills (99,138, 308–312). With the number of DBS procedures increasing throughout the world, there is presently a need for training in this new subspecialty.

Postoperative antiparkinsonian treatment should be restarted as soon as possible after electrode implantation to relieve discomfort related to off periods and to limit the risks of acute dopaminergic withdrawal. The postoperative dopaminergic medication must be adapted to the clinical state. Prolonged levodopa withdrawal can induce an akinetic state in some patients, which requires rapid uptake of the preoperative levodopa dose, whereas other patients may have a lesionlike effect with improvement in parkinsonism that allows for a decrease in medication. Rapid titration of dopaminergic treatment in the first days following surgery is facilitated with primary use of levodopa instead of long-acting agonist drugs. Close follow-up is necessary for avoiding such general health complications as postoperative aspiration pneumonia or deep vein thrombosis or local infection from the implanted material. As in the immediate postoperative phase, heparin is contraindicated and compression stockings and physiotherapy are important for every akinetic patient. In case of postoperative psychosis, introduction of clozapine on a transient basis may be useful. Postoperative management of antiparkinsonian treatment asks for close cooperation among neurologists and neurosurgeons.

The neurologist is responsible for adaptation of stimulation parameters as there can be interactions between stimulation and medication. For optimal management of stimulation parameters, information on the exact electrode position is required. Postoperative MRI immediately following surgery (and, ideally, before implantation of the neurostimulator, otherwise strict MRI safety procedures must be respected) is highly recommended to confirm electrode location and to rule out adverse intracranial events. To rule out technical problems of the implanted material, measurements of the impedance of all electrode contacts must be documented before beginning to program stimulation parameters.

Whatever the target, and whatever the disease, in the postoperative period an evaluation of the effects and side effects of each of the 4 contacts of each implanted quadripolar electrode must be documented. This evaluation will serve as a reference for all future adaptations of DBS parameters. The determination of which contact to use for chronic stimulation requires a careful evaluation of beneficial effects and side effects, while taking into account the therapeutic window. The target symptoms may differ, depending on the target nucleus selected for stimulation and on the disease. In PD, the target symptoms are off-period tremor for VIM, off-period dystonia, rigidity, tremor and bradykinesia for both STN and GPi, on-period dyskinesia for GPi, and induction of dyskinesia for STN. In essential tremor the only target symptom is tremor, and in dystonia the focus is on mobile dystonia and dystonic tremor more than on fixed dystonic postures. Each contact of the quadripolar electrode can be programmed as anode or cathode in bipolar settings or as cathode for monopolar stimulation against the neurostimulator case as an anode. Monopolar stimulation is generally selected for current delivery. The most effective contact is used, but if monopolar stimulation using a single contact is not sufficiently effective, the 2 adjacent contacts with the best therapeutic window can be combined as anodes in a monopolar setting. Bipolar stimulation between 2 adjacent contacts allows for a more focused stimulation, which may be useful if current diffusion to a neighboring structure leads to side effects, generally indicating suboptimal placement. During the initial assessment, it is suggested that the pulse and frequency be held constant while incrementing the amplitude in steps of 0.5 V up to side effects that would prevent chronic stimulation. The threshold for such side effects can be slightly lower in the immediate postoperative period related to local edema facilitating current spread. Parkinsonian signs also may be improved in the immediate postoperative period, and thus evaluation of antiparkinsonian effects may be more difficult. Therefore, it may be useful to assess antiparkinsonian effects and threshold of side effects again several weeks after surgery and some groups delay the initial programming session to save time of programming. Some groups begin programming weeks after surgery, which avoids the initial postoperative programming and saves time. To start programming, monopolar stimulations using a single contact with a pulse width of 60 μs and a frequency of 130 Hz are generally used in all 3 targets. The voltage is then increased, depending on the effects and side effects of stimulation.

Postoperative Management: Ventralis Intermedius Nucleus Deep-Brain Stimulation

PD tremor is a rest tremor that at least transiently diminishes in amplitude or completely disappears at movement onset. If severe, it also may be present during posture or even during movement. Rest tremor can be intermittent and is facilitated by activation, such as speaking or mental activity. A typical facilitating maneuver is to ask the patient to count aloud backward. It is important to know the variability and maximal amplitude of tremor before setting electrical parameters. Immediately after surgery, there may be an important thalamotomy-like effect and, in this case, low voltage can control the tremor that may reoccur after a variable delay with disappearance of postoperative edema surrounding the electrode. In individual patients, an electrode that is perfectly located or a small contusion may have a permanent antitremor effect, and rare individuals in whom tremor disappears during surgery will never require a neurostimulator. VIM stimulation—in contrast to STN stimulation—does not induce delayed side effects such as dyskinesia or behavioral changes and, therefore, current can be increased rapidly until complete tremor suppression or occurrence of unacceptable side effects. The most frequent side effect of thalamic stimulation is paresthesias, by diffusion of the current to the ventral posterolateral nucleus of the thalamus (VPL). Electrodes located in the most ventral part of the VIM usually have the lowest threshold for inducing paresthesias. This should not lead to exclusion of these contacts as they are usually the most effective ones on tremor. As paresthesias are usually transient, disappearing within seconds, they are not a problem if they are not too unpleasant. If paresthesias persist for more than a minute or are unpleasant, stimulation should be increased only after a delay. Indeed, the threshold for paresthesias varies over time. Painful dysesthesia without tremor suppression indicates that the electrode has been located too posteriorly. Dysarthria is a problem if electrodes are localized too laterally. Corticobulbar fibers in the posterior limb of the internal capsule are close to the target. If dysarthria is a problem, bipolar stimulation may be useful to avoid diffusion to the internal capsule. Cerebellar signs, such as contralateral limb ataxia, ataxic gait, or cerebellar dysarthria, also can be induced if current intensity is increased too much, and speech worsening can be seen in the context of a cerebellar syndrome. It is therefore important to evaluate gait and speech and to perform the finger–nose test. Importantly, patients can be aware of a worsening of speech before the evaluator, as they better realize an increased effort to articulate. The current also can diffuse to the pyramidal tract, inducing contraction of the contralateral face or hand, and more rarely the lower limb. The threshold for small twitches of the face or hand has to be carefully ascertained as, contrary to sensory side effects, contractions do not disappear with time but can sometimes worsen, inducing progressive speech disorder or hand deformities. The voltage for chronic stimulation should be chosen 10% to 15% below the threshold to induce dysarthria or any visible contraction. During follow-up, some tolerance (requires more and more voltage to control tremor) and rebound effect (tremor much worse than before when stimulation was switched off) can occur (91,313). To avoid tolerance or rebound tremor, those patients who can tolerate their rest tremor at night should be asked to stop VIM stimulation overnight. This can be facilitated by using an extra dose of levodopa at bedtime or some sedative drugs (311). Some patients will develop symptoms other than tremor, such as bradykinesia, gait problems, and dyskinesias, that will not respond to VIM stimulation but will require adaptation of antiparkinsonian drugs. In the event of severe motor complications, those patients can be reimplanted in another target, such as the subthalamic nucleus (221).

Postoperative Management: Pallidal Deep-Brain Stimulation

Dyskinesia

GPi DBS has a direct antidyskinetic effect when posteroventral electrodes are used in on-drug condition. Induction of dyskinesias in off-drug condition using high-frequency stimulation suggests electrode positioning in dorsal GPi or in the Gpe (43,84,242). Although induction of dyskinesias can be accompanied with a marked antiakinetic effect, in our experience this antiakinetic effect does not last and, to the contrary, using such electrodes will progressively worsen akinesia (243). To assess the antidyskinetic effect of GPi stimulation, patients must be assessed in on-drug condition. If GPi stimulation completely stops levodopa-induced dyskinesias, a worsening of akinesia may be seen. Such worsening of akinesia must be assessed through careful screening. It would be preferable to accept minor residual dyskinesias rather than a worsening of akinesia or so-called inhibition of levodopa effect (244,245). Assessment of the antiparkinsonian effects must be done off medication. GPi stimulation improves akinesia, rigidity, tremor, and off dystonia. These antiparkinsonian effects must be looked for on the ventral contacts located in the GPi, those contacts that also reduce dyskinesias in the on-drug condition. Induction of dyskinesias indicates dorsal location of the electrodes at the border zone of GPi and GPe or in the Gpe, and stimulation of these contacts is not effective on parkinsonian signs in the long term.

Dysarthria can be a side effect of pallidal stimulation related to diffusion to the medially located posterior arm of the internal capsule containing corticobulbar fibers. If dysarthria is a problem in bilateral stimulation, the threshold to induce dysarthria must be detected separately for both sides. A decrease in stimulation parameters may then be necessary. The patient often notices difficulty of speech before the examiner actually can hear obvious dysarthria. Stimulation parameters should be set 10% below the threshold for inducing dysarthria, whether subjective or objective. Tetanic contraction imitating dystonic postures of the contralateral part of the body—generally located in the middle or lower part of the face, or in the hand, more rarely in the arm or lower limb—is related to diffusion to the first motoneuron descending in the internal capsule to the cranial nerves and spinal cord. Such tetanic contraction can be accompanied by an increase in reflexes, clonus, or even a Babinski's sign mimicking a pyramidal syndrome. Whereas high-frequency stimulation (>50 Hz) induces tetanic contraction, low-frequency stimulation (2–5 Hz) will induce muscle twitches synchronous to the low-frequency stimulation. If there is any doubt whether a dystonic posture is a pyramidal side effect or a true dystonia (either off dystonia or diphasic dystonia), it may be useful to stimulate with 2–3 Hz. Rhythmic 2–3 Hz muscle twitches will then indicate diffusion to the first motoneuron. To induce low-frequency muscle twitches, much higher stimulation parameters are needed compared to those that induce tetanic contraction.

Weight gain is a common side effect of pallidal surgery. Patients should be informed about potential weight gain before surgery and encouraged to lose weight if they are obese before surgery. Nutritional counseling can be useful, especially for those patients who gain more than 3 kg within the first 3 months after surgery and those who tend to be overweight. Phosphenes in the contralateral visual field are related to current diffusion to the optic tract that passes just below the GPi. Unless the threshold to induce phosphenes is very low, this side effect tends to adapt rapidly. Changes in mood and executive function, although exceedingly rare, have been reported, probably indicating a mispositioning of electrodes too anteriorly in the associative and limbic parts of the GPi (179,180,182). If behavioral symptoms can be related to stimulation, a decrease in stimulation parameters is recommended. Ocular deviation (314) and dysesthesias are exceedingly rare with GPi stimulation and also show some tendency to develop tolerance. Thus, these side effects are generally not a problem with chronic stimulation. Reemerging motor symptoms should prompt an adjustment of stimulation parameters, including a change in electrode configuration, amplitude, frequency, and pulse width. Medication adjustment may be necessary. In a few patients, loss of effect from GPi stimulation has led to successful reoperation in the STN (236,239).

Postoperative Management: Subthalamic Nucleus Deep-Brain Stimulation

The subthalamic nucleus is a very small target. With correct electrode localization, all parkinsonian signs are improved using relatively small current amplitudes. On the other hand, this small target is surrounded by corticobulbar, corticospinal, oculomotor, sensory, and autonomic fibers. Whereas these eloquent structures are helpful during intraoperative targeting, misplaced electrodes can lead to side effects related to these bypassing fibers. Moreover, due to their small size, the motor, associative, and limbic territories of this target are close, explaining some of the potential effects and side effects on mood and behavior specific to the target. Stimulation of electrodes that are perfectly located within the sensorimotor part of the STN will lead to stimulation-induced dyskinesias, especially if levodopa-induced dyskinesias are severe before surgery (138). Although dyskinesias induced by STN stimulation predict a good long-term outcome (164), in the short term such dyskinesias can be difficult to handle and require major changes in dopaminergic medication. The subthalamic nucleus is currently the most frequently used target in PD, but the management of patients with subthalamic stimulation is more complicated and more time-consuming in the postoperative period compared to other targets (138). This is mainly because of the drug-stimulation interactions that require progressive adaptation of both medication and stimulation parameters. However in the long term, the effects seem more stable (61,236), and this justifies the choice of this complex target, in addition to prompting a better antiakinetic effect, lower energy consumption, and the possibility of sparing medication (60). A further advantage may be the possibility of improving levodopa-induced behavioral side effects in the long term, an indirect benefit that is related to the possibility of reducing dopaminergic medication (189).

The antiparkinsonian effects must be assessed in the off-drug condition. Whereas the effects on tremor and rigidity are almost time-locked to the onset of stimulation, the effects on akinesia and also the induction of dyskinesia may appear after some delay, generally minutes to hours. To avoid disabling stimulation-induced dyskinesia, the amplitude is therefore only gradually increased. The strategy is to increase the amplitudes until parkinsonian signs improve to the same level as with levodopa or up to the threshold for adverse effects. Side effects related to diffusion will limit a further increase, whereas occurrence of dyskinesias will ask for a more gradual increase and a further decrease in dopaminergic medication. The rapidity and degree of drug reduction depend on the degree of the antiparkinsonian effects of stimulation and the presence of disabling dyskinesias. In the immediate postoperative period, we prefer stopping agonist drugs as levodopa is easier to titrate due to its shorter half-life. In addition to the short-term effects, the long-term effects of dopaminergic medication also must be taken into account. After a marked decrease in dopaminergic medication, the loss of long-term effects will lead to a resurgence of motor and nonmotor signs of parkinsonism over the following weeks, requiring either a further increase in stimulation parameters or dopaminergic medication. At this stage, dopamine agonists are useful again to obtain a nonpulsatile treatment. The choice of L-dopa versus a dopamine agonist also will depend on the prevalence of disabling dyskinesias (agonists preferred), apathy (agonists preferred), or a dopamine dysregulation syndrome (L-dopa preferred). These strategies are discussed in more detail in the text that follows.

So-called *apraxia of eyelid opening*, a bilateral involuntary closure of the eyelids without the lowering of the eyebrows, is typical for blepharospasm, mainly characterized by prolonged effort to reopen the eyelids with visible contraction of the frontalis muscle, and one of the most frequent side effects of subthalamic stimulation (61). This side effect is related to lateral current diffusion to the corticonuclear fibers to the facial nerve to the upper part of the face (315). About half of the fibers to the upper part of the face descend to the ipsilateral facial nerve, the other half cross contralaterally. For this reason, side effects related to current diffusion are bilateral in the upper part of the face, whereas they are almost exclusively found contralaterally in the lower part of the face, manifesting mainly as perioral contractions. This apraxia of eyelid opening shows a good response to pretarsal injections of

botulinum toxin (138). Dysarthria can be a side effect of subthalamic stimulation related to lower facial contraction but also to diffusion to the laterally located corticobulbar fibers, the latter inducing dysarthria without clinically detectable muscle contractions. The thresholds for dysarthria and visible facial contraction are generally close, and even minor muscle contractions in the lower part of the face must be looked for carefully. Stimulation parameters should be set 10% below the threshold to induce dysarthria, whether subjective or objective. High-frequency stimulation can also induce tetanic muscle contraction imitating dystonic postures of the contralateral limbs related to current diffusion to the laterally located corticospinal tract. Tetanic muscle contraction induces abnormal postures, typically a flexion of the fingers leading to a hand posture (main creuse) that can be confused easily with the typical hand posture related to off dystonia in PD. The contraction in the upper limbs always predominates in the flexors of the fingers, hands, and elbows. Lower limb contractions are less frequent. Such tetanic contraction can be accompanied with an increase in reflexes, clonus, or even a Babinski's sign mimicking a pyramidal syndrome. Motor contractions can appear after several months of stimulation, and we also have observed intermittent contractions that can mimic dyskinesia or even focal seizures. Whereas high-frequency stimulation (>50 Hz) induces tetanic contraction, low-frequency stimulation (2–5 Hz) will induce muscle twitches synchronous to the low-frequency stimulation. If there is any doubt as to whether a dystonic posture is a pyramidal side effect or a true dystonia, it may be useful to stimulate at low frequency. Rhythmic 2–3 Hz muscle twitches will then indicate diffusion to the first motoneuron. To induce low-frequency muscle twitches, much higher stimulation parameters are needed compared to those that induce tetanic contraction. Inhibition of levodopa effects, a decrease in dyskinesia, and a worsening of gait, especially of freezing of gait, and a worsening of balance have been observed using electrodes located above the STN, despite improvement in rigidity. These side effects are identical to those observed when stimulating an electrode located below the GPi in the ansa lenticularis (43,244) and are likely related to stimulation of pallidothalamic fibers in the zona incerta (316). Diplopia related to adduction of the ipsilateral eye that can be accompanied with downward or more rarely upward deviation, sometimes also with a widening of the ipsilateral palpebral fissure, is a sign of current diffusion to the third cranial nerve from electrodes that are located too medially and too caudally (317). Using bipolar stimulation of electrode contacts that are located more dorsally may help to avoid this side effect. Conjugate contralateral eye deviation is a common side effect and does not indicate misplacement of the electrode. There is rapid tolerance, especially in bilateral stimulation. Horizontal gaze palsy is a rare phenomenon related to electrodes that are misplaced too medially. Ipsilateral mydriasis and homolateral sudation of the head are vegetative side effects related to anteromedial placement, and these side effects show rapid tolerance. Contralateral paresthesias is a common side effect related to posterior diffusion to the medial lemniscus. This side effect tends to disappear rapidly with chronic stimulation. Subthalamic stimulation tends to improve off-period related sensory phenomena and pain. However, related to a decrease in dopaminergic medication, a restless legs syndrome may be unmasked requiring a further increase in dopaminergic medication (318).

Weight gain is the most common side effect of subthalamic stimulation. Patients gain on average 5 kg. They should be informed about potential weight gain before surgery and encouraged to lose weight if they are obese before surgery. Nutritional counseling can be useful, especially for those patients who gain more than 3 kg within the first 3 months after surgery and who tend to be overweight.

Many behavioral problems have been reported in PD patients after surgery. However, PD is a neuropsychiatric disorder (186) and most of the postsurgical behavioral disorders can be explained by preexisting personality disorders and decompensation of previous psychiatric disorders (188). The most common problem encountered is postoperative transient confusion (61) with or without psychosis, which may require transient treatment with clozapine in case of relevant hallucinations, delusions, or agitation. Both levodopa and subthalamic stimulation do have psychotropic effects in addition to the motor effects (185). In the postoperative period, both treatments must be adapted not only to the motor state but also to the behavioral and affective states. An excess of treatment (levodopa and stimulation) will lead not only to dyskinesias but frequently induces hypomania or even rarely can lead to full-blown manic states (183,293,319). To the contrary, if the dopaminergic treatment is reduced too much, dyskinesias disappear and an apathy inherent to PD is frequently unmasked (60,162,188), requiring another increase in dopaminergic treatment (184). Apathy frequently appears as an isolated problem without depression (320) and generally responds to dopaminergic treatment. In the long term, however, apathy is the most frequent behavioral abnormality (61). Apathy is inherent to PD (287), and in the long term the natural history with cognitive decline may contribute to this problem. Depression also has been described after surgery (188,270,321,322). Depression can be reactive in a population at risk, whereas depression can also appear in the context of dopaminergic withdrawal, and this depression can also respond to an increase in dopaminergic medication (184).

Suicide has been reported after surgery (61,190). Risk factors for suicide are preoperative depression and repeat surgery, indicating a selection bias (190). The prevalence of depression in typical surgical candidate was found to be 60% (323). In our series of more than 250 patients with bilateral subthalamic stimulation, there was 1 suicide 6 months after surgery and 1 suicide on the waiting list.

The patient who committed suicide after surgery had been severely depressed and suicidal before surgery. Globally, in the long term, depression scores do not change (184). In the long term, it is generally possible to balance both treatments and behavioral disorders, which are relatively rare (184).

Before surgery on high doses of dopaminergic treatment, the typical surgical candidate is often hypomanic, and some patients do have a dopamine dysregulation syndrome. Since after surgery dopaminergic treatment can be reduced, and since apathy scores systematically increase (320), one would expect an improvement of levodopa-induced behavioral abnormalities. Indeed, such improvement has been reported (189). In conclusion, it seems obvious that PD patients do require a modulation of their dopaminergic treatment not only in response to their motor state, but medication also must be adapted to mood and behavior (176). Furthermore, factors related to psychosocial adjustment must be taken into account, including psychological "reactive" changes in response to motor and functional changes, unrealistic expectations, limited social support, changes in identity or interpersonal relationships, or the loss of the "sick role" of the patient within the family (324).

Apart from behavioral disorders that are related to psychosocial adjustment or to changes in dopaminergic treatment, some rare cases with acute behavioral disorders directly linked to stimulation have been reported, such as impulsive aggressive behavior (184,289,290), hilarity (291), or acute depression (288). These abnormal behaviors always appear to occur from minutes to a few hours after an increase in stimulation parameters, and they reverse rapidly with a decrease in voltage. Interpretation is challenging, but these rare events have been explained in part by current diffusion outside the subthalamic nucleus. Even though these behaviors differ among patients, we believe they are specific side effects related to stimulation of the limbic part of the subthalamic nucleus, just as hemiballism is a side effect related to stimulation of the sensorimotor part of the subthalamic nucleus. What they do have in common is an acute disinhibition or release of a behavioral program that is pathologically exacerbated. Indeed, a transient mild disinhibited behavior in a hypomanic context is frequently observed in the first days or weeks after surgery. Those who are in charge of programming the neurostimulator must be aware of the potential for such acute changes in mood or behavior, which may signal the delayed appearance of disabling dyskinesias and the concomitant need for a progressive increase in stimulation intensity, and these changes also may indicate the need for an observation period of several hours after each important increase (more than 0.3 V) in voltage. This causes no problem in management if stimulation parameters are adapted after surgery in an inpatient setting in the morning with the possibility of seeing the patient again in the afternoon. In an outpatient setting, a patient should remain near the hospital for a few hours after surgery, especially if he or she lives far from the care center.

TREMOR

Patient Selection

Almost all types of tremors are reported to have improved by thalamotomy. Since thalamic stimulation, which allows a bilateral procedure if necessary, has been shown to be safer than thalamotomy in a randomized study (47), it is also suitable for different forms of tremor that often cannot be treated with medication. Therefore, it can be applied for essential tremor (ET), cerebellar or multiple sclerosis (MS) tremor, Holmes' tremor, primary writing tremor, or tremor in neuropathies (325). Monosymptomatic tremor at rest is usually related to tremor-dominant PD and thus is likely to be associated with the development of akinetic-rigid symptoms and levodopa-induced dyskinesias throughout the development of the disease. Therefore, STN or GPi surgery seems to be a better indication for rest tremor (59,121,221,326). As for other movement disorders, the appropriate selection of patients is critical for the outcome of surgical relief of tremors. Considering the risks of any stereotactic intervention, the following must apply: (a) motor symptoms lead to a relevant disability in activities of daily living, despite optimal medical treatment; (b) biological age of the patient must present no contraindications for neurosurgery; and (c) the patient is neither demented nor severely depressed.

The outcome of surgery for tremor depends on the clinical type and distribution. Distal limb tremors are easier to treat than proximal limb tremors. Intention tremor is more difficult to treat than rest or postural tremor.

Targets for Tremors

In the treatment of tremors, the area stimulated or lesioned within the thalamus is assumed to be the ventral intermediate nucleus (VIM), as defined by Hassler (1,327,328) and considered to receive mainly cerebellar outputs. The VIM corresponds to the posterior part of the ventrolateral nucleus lying just anterior to the sensory nucleus (38,200,329). Most neurosurgeons agree that the optimal electrode location for thalamic DBS in ET corresponds to the anterior margin of the VIM (330,331). This site of effective stimulation has been histologically confirmed (332). Can this thalamic VIM target be advocated for the treatment of all tremors, whatever the origin? Problems of insufficient efficacy or secondary tolerance may arise in severe kinetic tremors (89,333) related to lesions of the cerebellar outflow pathway, mainly located in the midbrain and usually due to MS (334) or vascular or traumatic lesions. However, VIM stimulation can be greatly effective when the rhythmic component of tremor prevails over cerebellar ataxia (335). Therefore, other targets have been proposed. In the absence of randomized series of patients with the same type of tremor operated in two different targets, any definitive recommendation is impossible. The posterior subthalamic white matter region, including the zona incerta (ZI) and the prelemniscal radiation (PRL), has been advocated for parkinsonian tremor (336) and for severe ET involving the proximal arm (337). This tentative target was situated in the area lateral to the red nucleus and posteromedial to the subthalamic nucleus. The same target was effectively stimulated for tremor related to MS (338). This subthalamic region was bilaterally stimulated to arrest tremor and head titubation, without dysarthria, disequilibrium, or tolerance at 1 year (339). Holmes' tremor and tremors due to posttraumatic lesions in the region of the midbrain have been improved by implanting 2 electrodes separated by 2 mm to stimulate the nucleus ventralis anterior (V.o.a) and the nucleus ventralis posterior (V.o.p), as well as the VIM, thus affecting both the cerebellar receiving area (VIM) and the pallidal receiving area (V.o.a/V.o.p) (340). Poststroke tremor also was better improved by V.o.a than by VIM stimulation (341). This stimulates enlarged lesions to control dystonic or intention tremors, whereas stimulating the sole VIM lesion was sufficient to control distal hand ET. Stimulation of the STN itself could improve a patient with medically refractory cervical dystonia and ET resulting in dystonic head tremor and action tremor of the hands (342). Combined VIM and STN stimulation improved 1 patient with Holmes' tremor (343).

As discussed, albeit highly effective on parkinsonian rest tremor, there is no future for VIM surgery in PD. Moreover, STN stimulation can improve both postural and rest tremors, as seen in patients with a combination of PD and ET (344). Because of the simplicity of managing PD patients with VIM stimulation, compared to managing them with STN stimulation, the only exception could concern elderly fragile patients with pure unilateral rest hand tremor.

The target of stimulation in patients with dystonic tremor is debated. Although VIM stimulation is effective on the rhythmic component of the movement disorder, the dystonic component can worsen after surgery. This is why the posterolateral GPi could be the target of choice, although months are often required to achieve the antitremoric effect.

Clinical Results

We will not cover the exhaustive results of VIM stimulation in tremors of various origins, since they have already been discussed in the previous edition of this book. DBS for rest parkinsonian tremor has been discussed in the PD section. Multiple studies of VIM stimulation have shown that it is efficacious in the treatment of ET hand tremor, often with secondary improvement in voice and head tremor (345). VIM stimulation greatly decreases or suppresses ET in almost all patients (13,45,48,89). Bilateral VIM simulation is also effective for isolated head tremor in patients with ET (346). Bilateral thalamic DBS is more effective than unilateral DBS at controlling bilateral appendicular and head or voice tremors of ET (345,347).

If stimulation is ineffective, one should suspect a misplaced electrode. Secondary recurrence of tremor is observed in some patients, especially those with severe intentional proximal tremor. This is why most patients are asked to arrest stimulation at night (90) to avoid a tolerance phenomenon that can mitigate long-term benefit (95,348). However, long-term studies have indicated that a majority of patients continue to experience improvement in tremor and activities of daily living (349,350). Improvement in quality of life also has been reported (351). VIM stimulation can be done contralaterally to a previous thalamotomy or bilaterally at the same session.

Benefit from VIM stimulation in severe kinetic tremors caused by lesions is less than for typical ET. Tremor is frequently not the sole manifestation of the lesion, which explains the lesser degree of improvement in activities of daily living and handicap (352). Moreover, proximal and intention tremors, typical of these postlesion tremors, especially in MS, may not be completely suppressed by VIM stimulation or subjected to secondary tolerance (353). That is why other targets of stimulation have been proposed, as well as thalamotomy, which seem to be a more efficacious surgical treatment for intractable MS tremor at the price of a higher incidence of persistent neurological adverse effects than DBS (354).

VIM stimulation induces some side effects that are mild and accepted by patients. Dysarthria is the most common side effect, occurring in 20% of patients, almost all of whom are bilaterally stimulated (13,355). A feeling of unsteadiness occurred in 10% of patients, and limb numbness occurred in 6%. Balance was improved in a few patients, as reported elsewhere (356,357). Neither the patients nor their families reported neuropsychological disturbances. No changes in formal neuropsychological tests were noted except for lexical verbal fluency (350,358). However, subtle cognitive morbidity may exist (359), with age and a large pulse width as risk factors (360). Suddenly switching on the stimulator frequently induced transient and mild contralateral cheiro-oral paresthesias lasting a few seconds (361). All these side effects disappeared instantaneously when stimulation was stopped or decreased. Long-term hardware complications are the same as for other targets or other indications of DBS.

Patient Management

Setting electrical parameters is relatively easy to do in patients operated on for tremor. As the decrease in tremor amplitude is almost synchronous with stimulation, the contact allowing the best tremor control with the lowest voltage is chosen. Increasing frequency from 130 Hz up to 185 Hz may lead to better tremor control. In the VIM, adverse effects limiting increase in voltage are motor contraction (lateral spreading of current), dysarthria, and especially paresthesias (posterior spreading). Moreover, some tolerance develops for paresthesias, allowing a progressive increase in voltage with time, contrary to motor contraction. Chronic electrical parameters are set within a period of a few postoperative weeks, due to the healing process and the parallel disappearance of the lesionlike effect. In the long term, either no change or a mild increase in voltage is necessary. One should avoid progressively increasing voltage in relation to the development of tolerance with a rebound phenomenon (high-amplitude severe tremor at stimulation arrest). In our experience, this can occur with voltages higher than 4.0 volts. Period of stimulation arrest may limit this phenomenon. If tremor is well controlled, the antitremoric drug dose can be progressively decreased or arrested.

DYSTONIA

Pharmacological treatments of dystonia have limited efficacy, and botulinum toxin injections are useful only in restricted (e.g., face, neck) topographies. Stereotactic brain surgery has been applied for decades. Thalamotomy and pallidotomy may induce variable and unstable responses and unacceptable adverse effects, including speech difficulties and cognitive disturbances. Bilateral procedures are generally required for generalized dystonia or dystonia with a wide distribution of muscle contractions. This is why DBS, which has a better index of safety than lesioning, especially when applied bilaterally, is becoming a recognized treatment option. Coubes et al. pioneered bilateral GPi stimulation in generalized dystonia. A strong improvement of dystonia and functional disability was initially reported in 7 patients with DYT1-positive generalized dystonia (65). Within the past few years, DBS has been used more and more to treat various forms of dystonia (362,363).

Patient Selection

Despite the scarcity of good-quality controlled studies, it seems that all types of dystonias can respond to DBS, the preferred target being the GPi. On the whole, primary dystonias and tardive dystonic syndromes (364) respond most dramatically to treatment with DBS, whereas secondary dystonia tends to be less responsive (365,366). This is why the presence of basal ganglia abnormalities on the preoperative MRI is an indicator of a lesser response to surgery. In patients with primary dystonia, the most improved were those with DYT1, those who were non-DYT1 mutation carriers with generalized dystonia, and those with cervical dystonia. Small studies showed variable benefit in secondary dystonia, such as posttraumatic hemidystonia, panthotenate kinase-associated neurodegeneration (PKAN), or kinesigenic paroxysmal choreoathetosis. Mobile forms of the disorder or myoclonic dystonia are better improved than fixed postures. This explains why early surgery in childhood before the end of growth may benefit more from DBS than from late surgery with definitive deformities. Appendicular and axial dystonia respond better to surgery than oromandibular or speech dystonia. Benefit is generally maintained at long-term, but the progression of the disease process may mitigate this benefit according to the etiology of dystonia.

Targets for Dystonia

Reports over three decades of improvement in dystonia by thalamotomy or pallidotomy combined with the striking improvement of levodopa-induced dyskinesias in PD by deep-brain stimulation of the GPi has encouraged the use of this therapy for generalized and severe segmental dystonia in children and adults. In movement disorders related to basal ganglia dysfunction, there is a disrupted activity in the main outflow nucleus, the GPi, relayed to the motor areas of the thalamus whose outflow is consequently also disrupted. It is interesting and paradoxical that elimination of this abnormal activity with destruction of the motor GPi or superimposition of high-frequency stimulation is usually well tolerated and can improve almost all types of movement disorders. Indeed, having no motor pallidum appears to be preferable to having a pallidum generating and transmitting pathologic inputs to downstream targets.

There are no comparative studies to precisely know the most suitable target for dystonia (367). From small, usually uncontrolled studies, it seems that stimulation of the posterolateral ventral GPi, corresponding to the sensorimotor part of the structure leads to the best results. The most adequate location within the globus pallidus remains unknown. Stimulation of the GPe/GPi junction has induced excellent results (Jérôme Yelnik, personal communication, 2004), and a somatotopic organization in the GPi was found with a location more anterior for the inferior limb and more posterior for the superior limb (368). However, this was noticed only on the right side, which casts doubt on the relevance of this finding. Before DBS was fashionable, lesions of the thalamus, especially large lesions encompassing the whole ventral lateral nucleus, could greatly improve dystonia. Thalamic stimulation seems to improve dystonic patients to a lesser degree than does GPi stimulation, perhaps because the volume of stimulation around the active contact is not large enough or does not include the anterior part of the ventral lateral nucleus, which receives the basal ganglia loop from the GPi. Some authors reason that the optimal target for secondary dystonias is still unclear, but some patients appear to benefit more from thalamic stimulation (363,369,370). Nevertheless, analysis of the literature favors the GPi target (371,372), and GPi stimulation could produce a marked effect even in patients who had previously undergone thalamotomy or pallidotomy (373,374). Subthalamic nucleus stimulation was ineffective in patients with heredodegenerative forms of advanced stage dystonia (375), but Chou et al. (342) reported improvement in a patient with cervical dystonia and ET. A favorable outcome was reported orally in primary generalized dystonia.

Clinical Results

In 1999, Coubes et al. reported that bilateral GPi stimulation induced dramatic improvement in an 8-year-old girl who had suffered since the age of 3 from severe non-DYT1 generalized dystonia, and who progressively became totally dependent and bedridden (64). In 2000, impressive improvement of dystonia and functional disability was reported in 7 children with DYT1-generalized dystonia by the same group (65). Afterward, in an uncontrolled study, Coubes et al. showed that the long-term efficacy and safety of bilateral GPi stimulation were maintained in 31 children and adults with primary generalized dystonia with and without the DYT1 mutation (376). The efficacy of stimulation improved with time. After 2 years, compared with preoperative values, the mean clinical and functional Burke-Fahn-Marsden Dystonia Rating Scale (BFMDRS) scores had improved by 79% and 65%, respectively. Children displayed greater improvements in the clinical scores than did adult patients. This great benefit was shown by other groups in small studies with heterogeneous patient groups (377–379). Dystonic movements of the axis and limbs responded to DBS to a greater extent than did oromandibular dystonia and fixed dystonic postures. In a prospective controlled study of bilateral GPi stimulation in primary generalized dystonia, Vidailhet et al. reported significant improvement in the dystonia movement score by 54% and in the disability score by 50% at month 12, but with a great variability among patients. General health and physical functioning subscores of health-related quality of life (SF-36 scale) were significantly improved at month 12. All adverse effects resolved without permanent sequelae (66).

Pallidal DBS has been shown also to be effective in primary nongeneralized dystonia, especially complex cervical dystonia (378,380–382). Using a blinded assessment, Kiss et al. found an improvement of 79% in the total Toronto Western Spasmodic Torticollis Rating Scale (TWSTRS) scores with major benefit of pain and disability subscores (383). Others also reported fair reduction in the TWSTRS total scores, with improvement in pain occurring soon after DBS surgery. Motor improvement was delayed and prolonged over several months (384). The Short-Form Health Survey (SF-36) showed an improvement in health status by an average of 36% in 8 different health categories (385). However, the improvement in cervical dystonic tremor could be disappointing (377). Isolated patients with Meige syndrome were successfully treated with bilateral GPi stimulation (386,387), as was a patient with Meige syndrome associated with spasmodic dysphonia and cervical dystonia

(374). Myoclonus-dystonia syndrome also can be greatly improved by GPi stimulation (388,389). GPi stimulation failed to improve a patient with severe sporadic rapid onset dystonia-parkinsonism syndrome (390). Stimulation of the VIM was found effective and maintained over 4 years in a patient with dystonic paroxysmal nonkinesigenic dyskinesias (391).

There have been recent reports of positive effects of pallidal stimulation in secondary dystonia, although efficacy is generally more limited. One year after surgery, the Montpellier group found an improvement in the clinical score of 31% in the group with secondary dystonia of various causes, whereas patients with primary dystonia improved by more than 70% (392). In patients with dystonia secondary to birth injury, the mean improvement in BFMDRS score was 23% at 2 years postoperatively, which was not significant (393). GPi DBS was also found to be beneficial in delayed onset posttraumatic cervical dystonia and posttraumatic hemidystonia with 4 years of follow-up (394,394a). A disappearance of self-mutilating behavior was noted after pallidal stimulation for the control of dystonic movements in patients with Lesch-Nyhan syndrome (394b). A sustained beneficial effect of bilateral GPi stimulation was reported in 6 patients with PKAN, exhibiting early onset, progressive, severe generalized dystonia. The 74% mean global motor improvement and the 53% disability improvement on the BFMDRS were similar to those observed in primary dystonia (395,396). However, the benefit on speech intelligibility was more critical, and some PKAN patients with more extended lesions may be only moderately improved. Moreover, secondary worsening of the disease may limit this therapy (377).

In patients with medically refractory tardive dystonia, bilateral GPi stimulation was associated with a rapid (within hours to days) and substantial improvement of dystonia and functional disability (397,398). However, failure of GPi stimulation has been reported in 1 patient with tardive dystonia (377).

One characteristic of GPi stimulation-induced effects is the progressive and delayed nature of improvement (399,400). Involuntary movements (mobile dystonia, myoclonus) improve first. Fixed dystonic postures progressively improve over a period of up to a year or more after surgery (363). The beginning of improvement is generally rapid, within hours or a few days (365,383,385). Within about 6 months, 95% percent of the final improvement is attained, with no significant improvement after 1 year postoperatively (354).

In conclusion, despite a favorable and sometimes impressive benefit from surgery in dystonic syndromes, the variable results among patients make the continuation of research mandatory. Controlled studies, in homogeneous groups of either primary or secondary dystonia are essential for determining the optimal selection criteria for surgical procedures in dystonia and for evaluating their long-term results.

Patient Management

The main difficulty of setting electrical parameters for the treatment of dystonia is the lack of acute beneficial effect contrary to VIM stimulation for tremor or STN stimulation for parkinsonism. The most ventral contact of quadripolar electrodes are generally chosen since dorsal contacts may be located in the GPe and may be ineffective and even deleterious (401,402). The most common adverse effects are caused by current spreading ventrally to the optic tracts, leading to visual flashes, and spreading medially to the corticobulbar and corticospinal tracts, leading to dysarthria or motor contraction. Use of a maximal voltage at least 15% below the threshold of these adverse effects is recommended. A frequency of 130 Hz is generally applied. Rarely, 50 Hz was reported to be effective (402,403), and lower frequencies are ineffective. Frequencies above 130 Hz can lead to more favorable effects (404). The range of voltage is wide, from 1 V to 5 V, and most authors agree that energy consumption is higher than in PD (405). The pulse width setting is debated. Whereas the Montpellier group advocates using 450 μs, other authors have shown fair results with 60 μs pulse width (66). However, because of the need for high currents, pulse widths of 90 μs or 120 μs are frequently used. To date, the optimal parameters are still to be determined. As for all DBS procedures, frequent adjustment in the stimulation parameters is necessary in the first 3 months, although a high voltage close to the chronic one can be set a few days after surgery. All stimulation-induced side effects are reversible on adjustment of the DBS settings. Because more energy is needed for stimulation than in other movement disorders, such as PD, more frequent battery replacements are necessary, which results in relatively higher costs for chronic DBS (363).

An increased risk of lead fracture and migration in dystonia compared with other movement disorders following DBS has been reported, perhaps related to the postoperative persistence of cervical abnormal movements (406).

OTHER MOVEMENT DISORDERS

Gilles de la Tourette's Syndrome

Temel et al. reviewed the literature from 1960 until 2003 on lesioning procedures of diverse target sites carried out in 65 patients with Gilles de la Tourette syndrome (GTS) (407). Based on the results of thalamotomies described by Hassler in 1970, bilateral thalamic stimulation was performed in 3 patients with intractable Gilles de la Tourette's syndrome (GTS). The target for stimulation was chosen at the level of the centromedian nucleus, substantia periventricularis, and nucleus ventrooralis internus. After a follow-up period from 8 months to 5 years, all major motor and vocal tics had disappeared, and no serious complications had occurred. When stimulation was applied at the voltage necessary to achieve an optimal result on the tics, a slight sedative effect was noted in all 3 patients. Stimulation-induced changes in sexual behavior were noted in 2 patients (408). A study on stimulation of the posterolateral GPi by the same group is ongoing. Stimulation of the latter target could also greatly improve tics (409) or the self-mutilating behavior in a patient with Lesch-Nyhan syndrome (394a). Considering the role of the dysfunction of limbic striato-pallido-thalamo-cortical systems in GTS, Houeto et al. reported the results of stimulating the output basal ganglia subnuclei belonging to this loop, namely, the centromedian-parafascicular complex of the thalamus, the anteromedial part of the globus pallidus (GPi), or both (67). A patient with a severe form of GTS was studied using a double-blind protocol including 2 phases without stimulation; the therapeutic benefit had persisted for 24 months after the operation. Stimulation improved the severity and frequency of tics by about 70%, markedly ameliorated coprolalia, and eliminated self-injurious behavior when either the thalamus, the GPi, or both were stimulated, indicating that there was no potentiation between the targets. Improvement of tics was delayed. The limbic parts of the GPi or thalamus seem to be candidate targets for treatment of severe forms of GTS by DBS.

Treatment of GTS is still investigational, and controlled studies with stimulation of a well-defined target are needed.

Choreas and Other Dyskinesias

There are few case reports of effective DBS treatment of choreic movements. One patient with hemichorea-hemiballism due to a striatal lesion was successfully treated by thalamic stimulation contralateral to the abnormal movements (410). Bilateral GPi stimulation was performed in a patient with Huntington's disease (HD) with severe chorea (411). Stimulation at 40 Hz and 130 Hz improved chorea, but stimulation at 130 Hz worsened bradykinesia slightly overall, whereas 40 Hz had little effect. A patient with senile chorea was treated successfully with stimulation of the left GPi and, subsequently, the left ventralis oralis posterior nucleus of the thalamus (412). GPi stimulation at 60 Hz improved a patient with tardive dyskinesia of the choreiform oro-facial-laryngeal type (413). Bilateral stimulation of the motor thalamus (V.o.p nucleus) improved the trunk spasms of a patient with a severe form of chorea-acanthocytosis, but no clear effect was observed on dysarthria nor on hypotonia (414). Three patients suffering from chronic neuropathic pain and movement disorders were stimulated in the center of the median-parafascicular complex of the thalamus, which improved foot choreoathetotic movements in 1 patient, rest tremor in another, and stump dyskinesias in another (415). Finally, bilateral GPi stimulation arrested restless legs syndrome associated with generalized dystonia in 1 patient (416). Thus, it seems that disrupting the output of the basal ganglia by stimulation either in the GPi or the thalamus can improve many types of movement disorders.

It is a pity that most studies were not controlled, all the more so since DBS allows the blinded evaluation of periods of sham or true stimulation.

CONCLUSION

DBS had an outstanding impact on the renewal of the surgical treatment of movement disorders. Although only a minority of patients can benefit from DBS, it generally induces a major improvement in quality of life in severely disabled patients, provided DBS is carried out by a multidisciplinary team with considerable expertise (280). It turns out that DBS is more than a new surgical treatment for movement disorders. It is a new therapeutic concept that acts as a focal neuromodulator capable of altering the activity of a restricted brain area. DBS might improve any signs or symptoms associated with a dysfunction of a brain network provided that a major part of this network is included in the target hit by the neurosurgeon. For example, DBS in psychosurgery may have the same success as in movement disorders, along with advancement in neurosciences and brain imaging of psychiatric disorders.

REFERENCES

1. Tasker RR, Siqueira J, P, Organ LW. What happened to VIM thalamotomy for Parkinson's disease? *Appl Neurophysiol* 1983;46:68–83.
2. Gildenberg PL. Whatever happened to stereotactic surgery? *Neurosurgery* 1987;20:983–987.
3. Laitinen LV, Bergenheim AT, Hariz MI. Leksell's posteroventral pallidotomy in the treatment of Parkinson's disease. *J Neurosurg* 1992;76:53–61.
4. Hariz MI. From functional neurosurgery to "interventional" neurology: survey of publications on thalamotomy, pallidotomy, and deep brain stimulation for Parkinson's disease from 1966 to 2001. *Mov Disord* 2003;18:845–852.
5. Alexander GE, Crutcher MD, DeLong MR. Basal ganglia-thalamocortical circuits: parallel substrates for motor, oculomotor, "prefrontal" and "limbic" functions. [Review]. *Prog Brain Res* 1990;85:119–146.
6. Narabayashi H. The future of stereotaxy. In: Schaltenbrand G, Walker AE, eds. Stereotaxy of the human brain: anatomical, physiological and clinical applications. Stuttgart, Germany: Georg Thieme, 1982:686–689.
7. Madrazo I, Drucker-Colin R, Diaz V, Martinez-Mata J, Torres C, Becerril JJ. Open microsurgical autograft of adrenal medulla to the right caudate nucleus in two patients with intractable Parkinson's disease. *N Engl J Med* 1987;316:831–834.
8. Goetz CG, Penn RD, Tanner CM. Efficacy of cervical cord stimulation in dystonia. *Adv Neurol* 1988;50:645–649.
9. Marsden CD, Fahn S. Surgical approaches to the dyskinesias: afterword. In: Marsden CD, Fahn S, eds. *Movement disorders*. London: Butterworths, 1982:345–347.
10. Ford B, Winfield L, Pullman SL, et al. Subthalamic nucleus stimulation in advanced Parkinson's disease: blinded assessments at one year follow up. *J Neurol Neurosurg Psychiatry* 2004;75:1255–1259.
11. Fahn S, Elton RL. Unified Parkinson's disease rating scale. In: Fahn S, Marsden CD, Calne D, Goldstein M, eds. *Recent developments in Parkinson's disease*. Florham Park, NJ: Macmillan Health Care Information, 1987:153–163.
12. Freed CR, Greene PE, Breeze RE, et al. Transplantation of embryonic neurons for severe Parkinson's disease. *N Engl J Med* 2001;344:710–719.

13. Benabid AL, Pollak P, Gervason C, et al. Long-term suppression of tremor by chronic stimulation of the ventral intermediate thalamic nucleus. *Lancet* 1991;337:403–406.
14. Limousin P, Pollak P, Benazzouz A, et al. Effect on parkinsonian signs and symptoms of bilateral subthalamic nucleus stimulation. *Lancet* 1995;345:91–95.
15. Siegfried J, Lippitz B. Bilateral chronic electrostimulation of ventroposterolateral pallidum: a new therapeutic approach for alleviating all parkinsonian symptoms. *Neurosurgery* 1994;35:1126–1130.
16. Bergman H, Wichmann T, DeLong MR. Reversal of experimental parkinsonism by lesions of the subthalamic nucleus. *Science* 1990;249:1436–1438.
17. Mettler FA, Carpenter MB. The modification of subthalamic hyperkinesia in primates. *Trans Amer Neur Assoc* 1949;74:81.
18. Benabid AL, Pollak P, Louveau A, Henry S, de Rougemont J. Combined (thalamotomy and stimulation) stereotactic surgery of the VIM thalamic nucleus for bilateral Parkinson's disease. *Appl Neurophysiol* 1987;30:344–346.
19. Gillingham FJ, Kalyanaraman S, Donaldson AA. Bilateral stereotactic lesions in the management of parkinsonism. *J Neurosurg* 1966;24:449–453.
20. Hosobuchi Y, Adams JE, Rutkin B. Chronic thalamic stimulation for the control of facial anesthesia dolorosa. *Arch Neurol* 1973;29:158–161.
21. Hosobuchi Y. Subcortical electrical stimulation for control of intractable pain in humans. *J Neurosurg* 1986;64:543–553.
22. Bechtereva NP, Bondartchuk AN, Smirnov VM, Meliutcheva LA, Shandurina AN. Method of electrostimulation of the deep brain structures in treatment of some chronic diseases. *Confin Neurol* 1975;37:136–140.
23. Cooper IS, Riklan M, Amin I, Waltz JM, Cullinan T. Chronic cerebellum stimulation in cerebral palsy. *Neurology* 1976;26:744–753.
24. Mundinger F. Neue stereotaktisch-funktionelle Behandlungsmethode des Torticollis spasmodicus mit Hirnstimulatoren. *Med Klinik* 1977;72:1982–1986.
25. Gildenberg PL. Treatment of spasmodic torticollis with dorsal column stimulation. *Acta Neurochir* 1977;24(suppl):65–66.
26. Brice J, McLellan L. Suppression of intention tremor by contingent deep-brain stimulation. *Lancet* 1980;ii:1221–1222.
27. Mazars G, Merienne L, Cioloca G. Control of dyskinesia due to sensory deafferentation by means of thalamic stimulation. *Acta Neurochir Suppl* 1980;30:239–243.
28. Mundinger F, Neumuller H. Programmed stimulation for control of chronic pain and motor diseases. *Appl Neurophysiol* 1982;45:102–111.
29. Waltz JM. *Surgical approach to dystonia.* In: Marsden CD, Fahns, S, eds. *Movement disorders. Vol. Neurology 2.* London: Butterworth, 1982:300–307.
30. Andy OJ. Thalamic stimulation for control of movement disorders. *Appl Neurophysiol* 1983;46:107–111.
31. Siegfried J. Effets de la stimulation du noyau sensitif du thalamus sur les dyskinésies et la spasticité. *Rev Neurol* 1986;142:380–383.
32. McLellan DL. Cerebellar and deep brain stimulation in movement disorders. In: Marsden CD, Fahn S, eds. *Movement Disorders.* London: Butterworths, 1982:334–344.
33. Albe-Fessard D. Electrophysiological methods for the identification of thalamic nuclei. *Z Neurol* 1973;205:15–28.
34. Albe-Fessard D, Arfel G, Guiot G, et al. Dérivations d'activités spontanées et évoquées dans les structures cérébrales profondes de l'homme. *Rev Neurol* 1962;106:89–105.
35. French LA, Story J, Galicich JH, Schultz EA. Some aspects of stimulation and recording from the basal ganglia in patients with abnormal movements. *Confin Neurol* 1962;22:265–273.
36. Nashold BS, Slaughter DG. Some observations on tremors. In: Gillingham FJ, ed. *Third symposium on Parkinson's disease.* Edinburgh, Scotland: Livingstone Ltd., 1969:241–246.
37. Narabayashi H. Tremor: its generating mechanism and treatment. In: Vinken PJ, Bruyn GW, Klawans HL, eds. *Handbook of clinical neurology, vol. 5 (49): Extrapyramidal disorders.* Amsterdam, The Netherlands: Elsevier Science Publishers, 1986:597–607.
38. Ohye C, Maeda T, Narabayashi H. Physiologically defined VIM nucleus: its special reference to control of tremor. *Appl Neurophysiol* 1976;39:285–295.
39. Tasker RR, Organ LW, Hawrylyshyn PA. *The thalamus and midbrain of man: a physiological atlas using electrical stimulation.* Springfield,IL: Charles C Thomas, 1982.
40. Taren J, Guiot G, Derome P, Trigo JC. Hazards of stereotaxic thalamectomy: added safety factor in corroborating X-ray target localization with neurophysiological methods. *J Neurosurg* 1968;29:173–182.
41. Gildenberg PL. History repeats itself. *Stereotact Funct Neurosurg* 2003;80:61–75.
42. Limousin P, Greene J, Pollak P, Rothwell J, Benabid AL, Frackowiak R. Changes in cerebral activity pattern due to subthalamic nucleus or internal pallidum stimulation in Parkinson's disease. *Ann Neurol* 1997;42:283–291.
43. Krack P, Pollak P, Limousin P, et al. Opposite motor effects of pallidal stimulation in Parkinson's disease. *Ann Neurol* 1998;43:180–192.
44. Krack P, Pollak P, Limousin P, Benazzouz A, Deuschl G, Benabid AL. From off-period dystonia to peak-dose chorea: the clinical spectrum of varying subthalamic nucleus activity. *Brain* 1999;122:1133–1146.
45. Koller W, Pahwa R, Busenbark K, et al. High-frequency unilateral thalamic stimulation in the treatment of essential and parkinsonian tremor. *Ann Neurol* 1997;42:292–299.
46. Ondo W, Jankovic J, Schwartz K, Almaguer M, Simpson RK. Unilateral thalamic deep brain stimulation for refractory essential tremor and Parkinson's disease tremor. *Neurology* 1998;51:1063–1069.
47. Schuurman PR, Bosch DA, Bossuyt PMM, et al. A comparison of continuous thalamic stimulation and thalamotomy for suppression of severe tremor. *N Engl J Med* 2000;342:461–468.
48. Limousin P, Speelman JD, Gielen F, Janssens M, and the study collaborators. Multicenter European study of thalamic stimulation in parkinsonian and essential tremor. *J Neurol Neurosurg Psychiatry* 1999;66:289–296.
49. Rehncrona S, Johnels B, Widner H, Törnqvist AL, Hariz M, Sydow O. Long-term efficacy of thalamic deep brain stimulation for tremor: double-blind assessments. *Mov Disord* 2003;18:163–170.
50. Albin RL, Young AB, Penney JB. The functional anatomy of basal ganglia disorders. *TINS* 1989;12:366–375.
51. Baron MS, Vitek JL, Bakay RAE, et al. Treatment of advanced Parkinson's disease by posterior GPi pallidotomy: 1-year results of a pilot study. *Ann Neurol* 1996;40:355–366.
52. De Bie RMA, de Haan RJ, Nijssen PCG, et al. Unilateral pallidotomy in Parkinson's disease: a randomised, single-blind, multicentre trial. *Lancet* 1999;354:1665–1669.
53. Fine J, Duff J, Chen R, et al. Long-term follow-up of unilateral pallidotomy in advanced Parkinson's disease. *N Engl J Med* 2000;342:1708–1714.
54. Vitek JL, Bakay RAE, Freeman A, et al. Randomized trial of pallidotomy versus medical therapy for Parkinson's disease. *Ann Neurol* 2003;53:558–569.
55. Benazzouz A, Gross C, Féger J, Boraud T, Bioulac B. Reversal of rigidity and improvement in motor performance by subthalamic high-frequency stimulation in MPTP-treated monkeys. *Eur J Neurosci* 1993;5:382–389.
56. Pollak P, Benabid AL, Gross C, et al. Effets de la stimulation du noyau sousthalamique dans la maladie de Parkinson. *Rev Neurol* 1993;149:175–176.
57. Limousin P, Pollak P, Hoffmann D, Benazzouz A, Benabid AL. Abnormal involuntary movements induced by subthalamic nucleus stimulation in parkinsonian patients. *Mov Disord* 1996;11:231–235.
58. Krack P, Limousin P, Benabid AL, Pollak P. Chronic stimulation of subthalamic nucleus improves levodopa-induced dyskinesias in Parkinson's disease. *Lancet* 1997;350:1676.
59. Krack P, Pollak P, Limousin P, Benazzouz A, Benabid AL. Stimulation of subthalamic nucleus alleviates tremor in Parkinson's disease. *Lancet* 1997;350:1675.
60. Krack P, Pollak P, Limousin P, et al. Subthalamic nucleus or internal pallidal stimulation in young onset Parkinson's disease. *Brain* 1998;121:451–457.
61. Krack P, Batir A, Van Blercom N, et al. Five-year follow-up of bilateral stimulation of the subthalamic nucleus in advanced Parkinson's disease. *N Engl J Med* 2003;349:1925–1934.

62. Okun MS, Foote KD. Subthalamic nucleus vs globus pallidus interna deep brain stimulation, the rematch: will pallidal deep brain stimulation make a triumphant return? *Arch Neurol* 2005;62:533–536.

63. Lozano AM, Kumar R, Gross RE, et al. Globus pallidus internus pallidotomy for generalized dystonia. *Mov Disord* 1997;12:865–870.

64. Coubes P, Echenne B, Roubertie A, et al. Traitement de la dystonie généralisée à début précoce par stimulation chronique bilatérale des globus pallidus internes: a propos d'un cas. *Neurochirurgie* 1999;45:139–144.

65. Coubes P, Roubertie A, Vayssiere N, Hemm S, Echenne B. Treatment of DYT1-generalised dystonia by stimulation of the internal globus pallidus. *Lancet* 2000;355:2220–2221.

66. Vidailhet M, Vercueil L, Houeto JL, et al., for the French Stimulation du Pallidum Interne dans la Dystonie (SPIDY) Study Group. Bilateral deep-brain stimulation of the globus pallidus in primary generalized dystonia. *N Engl J Med* 2005;352:459–467.

67. Houeto JL, Karachi C, Mallet L, et al. Tourette's syndrome and deep brain stimulation. *J Neurol Neurosurg Psychiatry* 2005;76:992–995.

68. Benabid AL, Minotti L, Koudsié A, De Saint Martin A, Hirsch E. Antiepileptic effect of high-frequency stimulation of the subthalamic nucleus (corpus luysi) in a case of medically intractable epilepsy caused by focal dysplasia: a 30-month follow-up: technical case report. *Neurosurgery* 2002;50:1385–1392.

69. Vandewalle V, van der Linden C, Groenewegen HJ, Caemaert J. Stereotactic treatment of Gilles de la Tourette syndrome by high frequency stimulation of thalamus. *Lancet* 1999;353:724.

70. Leone M, Franzini A, Bussone G. Stereotactic stimulation of posterior hypothalamic gray matter in a patient with intractable cluster headache. *N Engl J Med* 2001;345:1428–1429.

71. Nuttin B, Cosyns P, Demeulemeester H, Gybels J, Meyerson B. Electrical stimulation in anterior limbs of internal capsules in patients with obsessive-compulsive disorder. *Lancet* 1999;354:1526.

72. Mayberg HS, Lozano AM, Voon V, et al. Deep brain stimulation for treatment-resistant depression. *Neuron* 2005;45:651–660.

73. Benabid AL, Koudsie A, Pollak P, et al. Future prospects of brain stimulation. *Neurol Res* 2000;22:237–246.

74. Benazzouz A, Hallett M. Mechanism of action of deep brain stimulation. *Neurology* 2000;55(suppl 6):S13–S16.

75. Tehovnik EJ. Electrical stimulation of neural tissue to evoke behavioral responses. *J Neurosci Methods* 1996;65:1–17.

76. Ranck JB. Which elements are excited in electrical stimulation of mammalian central nervous system: a review. *Brain Res* 1975;98:417–440.

77. Holsheimer J, Demeulemeester H, Nuttin B, de Sutter P. Identification of the target neuronal elements in electrical deep brain stimulation. *Eur J Neurosci* 2000;12:4573–4577.

78. Dostrovsky JO, Levy R, Wu JP, Hutchison WD, Tasker RR, Lozano AM. Microstimulation-induced inhibition of neuronal firing in human globus pallidus. *J Neurophysiol* 2000;84:570–574.

79. Welter ML, Houeto JL, Bonnet AM, et al. Effects of high-frequency stimulation on subthalamic neuronal activity in parkinsonian patients. *Arch Neurol* 2004;61:89–96.

80. Vitek JL. Mechanisms of deep brain stimulation: excitation or inhibition. *Mov Disord* 2002;17(suppl 3):69–72.

81. McIntyre CC, Savasta M, Kerkerian-Le Goff L, Vitek JL. Uncovering the mechanism(s) of action of deep brain stimulation: activation, inhibition, or both. *Clin Neurophysiol* 2004;115:1239–1248.

82. Windels F, Bruet N, Poupard A, Feuerstein C, Bertrand A, Savasta M. Influence of the frequency parameter on extracellular glutamate and gamma-aminobutyric acid in substantia nigra and globus pallidus during electrical stimulation of subthalamic nucleus in rats. *J Neurosci Res* 2003;72:259–267.

83. Hashimoto T, Elder CM, Okun MS, Patrick SK, Vitek JL. Stimulation of the subthalamic nucleus changes the firing pattern of pallidal neurons. *J Neurosci* 2003;23:1916–1923.

84. Vitek JL, Hashimoto T, Peoples J, DeLong MR, Bakay RA. Acute stimulation in the external segment of the globus pallidus improves parkinsonian motor signs. *Mov Disord* 2004;19:907–915.

85. Garcia L, D'Alessandro G, Bioulac B, et al. High-frequency stimulation in Parkinson's disease: more or less? *Trends Neurosci* 2005;28:209–216.

86. Filali M, Hutchinson WD, Palter VN, Lozano AM, Dostrovsky JO. Stimulation-induced inhibition of neuronal firing in human subthalamic nucleus. *Exp Brain Res* 2004;156:274–281.

87. Benabid AL, Pollak P, Hoffmann D, LeBas JF, Dong Ming G. Chronic high-frequency thalamic stimulation in Parkinson's disease. In: Koller WC, Paulson G, eds. *Therapy of Parkinsons disease.* New York: Marcel Dekker, 1995:381–401.

88. Rodriguez-Oroz MC, Obeso JA, Lang AE, et al. Bilateral deep brain stimulation in Parkinson's disease: a multicentre study with 4 years follow-up. *Brain* 2005;128:2240–2249.

89. Benabid AL, Pollak P, Gao D, et al. Chronic electrical stimulation of the ventralis intermedius nucleus of the thalamus as a treatment of movement disorders. *J Neurosurg* 1996;84:203–214.

90. Pollak P, Benabid AL, Gervason CL, Hoffmann D, Seigneuret E, Perret J. Long-term effects of chronic stimulation of the ventral intermediate thalamic nucleus in different types of tremor. In: Narabayashi H, Nagatsu T, Yanagisawa N, Mizuno Y, eds. *Parkinson's disease: From basic research to treatment.* New York: Raven Press, 1993:408–413.

91. Hariz MI, Shamsgovara P, Johansson F, Hariz GM, Fodstad H. Tolerance and tremor rebound following long-term chronic thalamic stimulation for parkinsonian and essential tremor. *Stereotact Funct Neurosurg* 1999;72:208–218.

92. Caparros Lefebvre D, Ruchoux MM, Blond S, Petit H, Percheron G. Long-term thalamic stimulation in Parkinson's disease: post-mortem anatomoclinical study. *Neurology* 1994;44:1856–1860.

93. Haberler C, Alesch F, Mazal PR, et al. No tissue damage by chronic deep brain stimulation in Parkinson's disease. *Ann Neurol* 2000;48:372–376.

94. Henderson JM, O'Sullivan DJ, Pell M, et al. Lesion of thalamic centromedian-parafascicular complex after chronic deep brain stimulation. *Neurology* 2001;56:1576–1579.

95. Kumar R, Lozano A, Sime E, Lang A. Long-term follow-up of thalamic deep brain stimulation for essential and parkinsonian tremor. *Neurology* 2003;61:1601–1604.

96. Moss J, Ryder T, Aziz TZ, Graeber MB, Bain PG. Electron microscopy of tissue adherent to explanted electrodes in dystonia and Parkinson's disease. *Brain* 2004;127:2755–2763.

97. Pollak P, Benabid AL, Limousin P, et al. Subthalamic nucleus stimulation alleviates akinesia and rigidity in Parkinsonian patients. In: Battistin L, Scarlato G, Caraceni T, Ruggieri S, eds. *Advances in neurology, vol. 69: Parkinson's disease.* Philadelphia: Lippincott-Raven, 1996:591–594.

97a. Okun MS, Tagliati M, Pourar M. et al. Management of referred deep brain stimulation failures. *Arch Neurol* 2005;62:1250–1255.

98. Hariz MI. Complications of deep brain stimulation surgery. *Mov Disord* 2002;17(suppl 3):162–166.

99. Blomstedt P, Hariz MI. Hardware-related complications of deep brain stimulation: a ten year experience. *Acta Neurochir (Wien)* 2005;147:1061–1064.

99a. Dormont D, Cornu P, Pidoux B, et al. Chronic thalamic stimulation with three-dimensional MR stereotactic guidance. *AM J Neuroradiol* 1997;18:1093–1107.

99b. Gillar CA, Dewey RB, Ginsburg MI, et al. Stereotactic pallidotomy and thalamotomy using individual variations of anatomic landmarks for localization. *Neurosurgery* 1998;42:56–62.

100. Cuny E, Guehl D, Burbaud P, Gross C, Dousset V, Rougier A. Lack of agreement between direct magnetic resonance imaging and statistical determination of a subthalamic target: the role of electrophysiological guidance. *J Neurosurg* 2002;97:591–597.

101. Schuurman PR, De Bie RMA, Majoie CBL, Speelman JD, Bosch DA. A prospective comparison between three-dimensional magnetic resonance imaging and ventriculography for target-coordinate determination in frame-based functional stereotactic neurosurgery. *J Neurosurg* 1999;91:911–914.

102. Hirabayashi H, Tengvar M, Hariz MI. Stereotactic imaging of the pallidal target. *Mov Disord* 2002;17(suppl 3):130–134.

103. Bejjani BP, Dormont D, Pidoux B, et al. Bilateral subthalamic stimulation for Parkinson's disease by using three-dimensional stereotactic magnetic resonance imaging and electrophysiological guidance. *J Neurosurg* 2000;92:615–625.

104. Aziz T, Nandi D, Parkin S, et al. Targeting the subthalamic nucleus. *Stereotact and Funct Neurosurg* 2001;77:87–90.

105. Benabid AL, Koudsie A, Benazzouz A, et al. Subthalamic stimulation for Parkinson's disease. *Arch Med Res* 2000;31:282–289.
106. Lemaire JJ, Durif F, Boire JY, Debilly B, Irthum B, Chazal J. Direct stereotactic MRI location in the globus pallidus for chronic stimulation in Parkinson's disease. *Acta Neurochir (Wien)* 1999; 141:759–765; discussion, 766.
107. Dormont D, Ricciardi KG, Tande D, et al. Is the subthalamic nucleus hypointense on T2-weighted images? A correlation study using MR imaging and stereotactic atlas data. *AJNR* 2004;25:1516–1523.
108. Andrade-Souza YM, Schwalb JM, Hamani C, et al. Comparison of three methods of targeting the subthalamic nucleus for chronic stimulation in Parkinson's disease. *Neurosurgery* 2005;56(suppl 2):360–368.
109. Zonenshayn M, Rezai AR, Mogilner AY, Beric A, Sterio D, Kelly PJ. Comparison of anatomic and neurophysiological methods for subthalamic nucleus targeting. *Neurosurgery* 2000;47:282–294.
110. Guridi J, Rodriguez-Oroz MC, Ramos E, Linazasoro G, Obeso JA. Discrepancy between imaging and neurophysiology in deep brain stimulation of medial pallidum and subthalamic nucleus in Parkinson's disease. *Neurologia* 2002;17:183–192.
111. Hutchison WD, Lozano AM, Tasker RR, Lang AE, Dostrovsky JO. Identification and characterization of neurons with tremor-frequency activity in human globus pallidus. *Exp Brain Res* 1997;113:557–563.
112. Hutchison WD, Allan RJ, Opitz H, et al. Neurophysiological identification of the subthalamic nucleus in surgery for Parkinson's disease. *Ann Neurol* 1998;44:622–628.
113. Lozano A, Hutchison W, Kiss Z, Tasker R, Davis K, Dostrovsky J. Methods for microelectrode-guided posteroventral pallidotomy. *J Neurosurg* 1996;84:194–202.
114. Ohye C, Shibazaki T, Hirato M, Kawashima Y, Matsumura M. Strategy of selective VIM thalamotomy guided by microrecording. *Stereotact Funct Neurosurg* 54,55 1990;54:186–191.
115. Hariz M, Fodstad H. Do microelectrode techniques increase accuracy or decrease risks in pallidotomy and deep brain stimulation? A critical review of the literature. *Stereotact and Funct Neurosurg* 1999;72:157–169.
116. Starr PA, Vitek J, Bakay AE. Ablative surgery and deep brain stimulation for Parkinson's disease. *Neurosurgery* 1999;43:989–1015.
117. Gross RE, Lombardi WJ, Hutchison WD, et al. Variability in lesion location after microelectrode-guided pallidotomy for Parkinson's disease: anatomical, physiological, and technical factors that determine lesion distribution. *J Neurosurg* 1999;90:468–477.
118. Giller CA, Dewey RB, Ginsburg MI, Mendelsohn DB, Berk AM. Stereotactic pallidotomy and thalamotomy using individual variations of anatomic landmarks for localization. *Neurosurgery* 1998;42:56–62.
119. Tsao K, Wilkinson S, Overman J, Koller WC, Batnitzky S, Gordon MA. Pallidotomy lesion locations: significance of microelectrode refinement. *Neurosurgery* 1998;43:506–512; discussion, 512–513.
120. Alterman RL, Sterio D, Beric A, Kelly PJ. Microelectrode recording during posteroventral pallidotomy: impact on target selection and complications. *Neurosurgery* 1999;44:315–321; discussion, 321–323.
121. Lozano AM, Lang AE, Hutchison WD. Pallidotomy for tremor. *Mov Disord* 1998;13(suppl 3):107–110.
122. Hariz MI, Bergenheim AT, Fodstad H. Crusade for microelectrode guidance in pallidotomy. [Comment on Vitek JL, Bakay RA, Hashimoto T, et al. Microelectrode-guided pallidotomy: technical approach and its application in medically intractable Parkinson's disease. *J Neurosurg* 1998;88:1027–1043.] *J Neurosurg* 1999;90:175–179.
123. Carlson JD, Pearlstein RD, Buchholz J, Iacono RP, Maeda G. Regional metabolic changes in the pedunculopontine nucleus of unilateral 6-hydoxydopamine Parkinson's model rats. *Brain Res* 1999;828:12–19.
124. Guridi J, Gorospe A, Ramos E, Linazasoro G, Rodriguez MC, Obeso JA. Stereotactic targeting of the globus pallidus internus in Parkinson's disease. imaging versus electrophysiological mapping. *Neurosurgery* 1999;45:278–287; discussion, 287–289.
125. Palur RS, Berk C, Schulzer M, Honey CR. A metaanalysis comparing the results of pallidotomy performed using microelectrode recording or macroelectrode stimulation. *J Neurosurg* 2002;96:1058–1062.
126. Hariz MI. Safety and risk of microelectrode recording in surgery for movement disorders. *Stereotact Funct Neurosurg* 2002;78:146–157.
127. Deep-Brain Stimulation for Parkinson's Disease Study Group. Deep-brain stimulation of the subthalamic nucleus or the pars interna of the globus pallidus in Parkinson's disease. *N Engl J Med* 2001;345:956–963.
128. Houeto JL, Welter ML, Bejjani PB, et al. Subthalamic stimulation in Parkinson's disease: intraoperative predictive factors. *Arch Neurol* 2003;60:690–694.
129. Maltete D, Navarro S, Welter ML, et al. Subthalamic stimulation in Parkinson disease: with or without anesthesia? *Arch Neurol* 2004;61:390–392.
130. Vesper J, Chabardes S, Fraix V, Sunde N, Ostergaard K, for the Kinetra Study Group. Dual channel deep brain stimulation system (Kinetra) for Parkinson's disease and essential tremor: a prospective multicenter open label clinical study. *J Neurol Neurosurg Psychiatry* 2002;73:275–280.
131. Hariz MI, Krack P, Melvill R, et al. A quick and universal method for stereotactic visualization of the subthalamic nucleus before and after implantation of deep brain stimulation electrodes. *Stereotact Funct Neurosurg* 2003;80:96–101.
132. Yelnik J, Damier P, Demeret S, et al. Localization of stimulating electrodes in patients with Parkinson disease by using a three-dimensional atlas-magnetic resonance imaging coregistration method. *J Neurosurg* 2003;99:89–99.
133. Ferroli P, Franzini A, Marras C, Maccagnano E, D'Incerti L, Broggi G. A simple method to assess accuracy of deep brain stimulation electrode placement: pre-operative stereotactic CT + postoperative MR image fusion. *Stereotact Funct Neurosurg* 2004;82:14–19.
134. Kainz W, Neubauer G, Uberbacher R, Alesch F, Chan DD. Temperature measurement on neurological pulse generators during MR scans. *Biomed Eng Online* 2002;1:2.
135. Spiegel J, Fuss G, Backens M, et al. Transient dystonia following magnetic resonance imaging in a patient with deep brain stimulation electrodes for the treatment of Parkinson disease: case report. *J Neurosurg* 2003;99:772–774.
136. Rezai AR, Phillips M, Baker KB, et al. Neurostimulation system used for deep brain stimulation (DBS): MR safety issues and implications of failing to follow safety recommendations. *Invest Radiol* 2004;39:300–303.
137. Pollak P, Krack P, Fraix V, et al. Intraoperative micro- and macrostimulation of the subthalamic nucleus in Parkinson's disease. *Mov Disord* 2002;17(suppl 3):S155–S161.
138. Krack P, Fraix V, Mendes A, Benabid AL, Pollak P. Postoperative management of subthalamic nucleus stimulation for Parkinson's disease. *Mov Disord* 2002;17(suppl 3):188–197.
139. Moro E, Esselink RJA, Xie J, Hommel M, Benabid AL, Pollak P. The impact on Parkinson's disease of electical parameter settings in STN stimulation. *Neurology* 2002;59:706–713.
140. Moro E, Esselink RJ, Benabid AL, Pollak P. Response to levodopa in parkinsonian patients with bilateral subthalamic nucleus stimulation. *Brain* 2002;125:2408–2417.
141. Tronnier VM, Staubert A, Hahnel S, Sarem-Aslani A. Magnetic resonance imaging with implanted neurostimulators: an in vitro and in vivo study. *Neurosurgery* 1999;44:118–126; discussion, 125–126.
142. Rezai AR, Lozano AM, Crawley AP, et al. Thalamic stimulation and functional magnetic resonance imaging: localization of cortical and subcortical activation with implanted electrodes: technical note. *J Neurosurg* 1999;90:583–590.
143. Jech R, Urgosik D, Tintera J, et al. Functional magnetic resonance imaging during deep brain stimulation: a pilot study in four patients with Parkinson's disease. *Mov Disord* 2001;16:1126–1132.
144. Rezai AR, Finelli D, Nyenhuis JA, et al. Neurostimulation systems for deep brain stimulation: in vitro evaluation of magnetic resonance imaging-related heating at 1.5 tesla. *J Magn Reson Imaging* 2002;15:241–250.

145. Sharan A, Rezai AR, Nyenhuis JA, et al. MR safety in patients with implanted deep brain stimulation systems (DBS). *Acta Neurochir* 2005;87(suppl):141–145.

146. Uitti RJ, Tsuboi Y, Pooley RA, et al. Magnetic resonance imaging and deep brain stimulation. *Neurosurgery* 2002;51:1423–1428.

147. Rosenow JM, Tarkin H, Zias E, Sorbera C, Mogilner A. Simultaneous use of bilateral subthalamic nucleus stimulators and an implantable cardiac defibrillator: case report. *J Neurosurg* 2003;99:167–169.

148. Capelle HH, Simpson RK, Kronenbuerger M, Michaelsen J, Tronnier V, Krauss JK. Long-term deep brain stimulation in elderly patients with cardiac pacemakers. *J Neurosurg* 2005;102:53–59.

149. Obwegeser AA, Uitti RJ, Turk MF, et al. Simultaneous thalamic deep brain stimulation and implantable cardioverter-defibrillator. *Mayo Clin Proc* 2001;76:87–89.

150. Nutt JG, Anderson VC, Peacock JH, Hammerstad JP, Burchiel KJ. DBS and diathermy interaction induces severe CNS damage. *Neurology* 2001;56:1384–1386.

151. Constantoyannis C, Heilbron B, Honey CR. Electrocardiogram artifacts caused by deep brain stimulation. *Can J Neurol Sci* 2004;31:343–346.

152. Umemura A, Jaggi JL, Hurtig HI, et al. deep brain stimulation for movement disorders: morbidity and mortality in 109 patients. *J Neurosurg* 2003;98:779–784.

153. Hamani C, Richter E, Schwalb JM, Lozano AM. Bilateral subthalamic nucleus stimulation for Parkinson's disease: a systematic review of the clinical literature. *Neurosurgery* 2005;56:1313–1324.

154. Oh MY, Abosch A, Kim SH, Lang AE, Lozano AM. Long-term hardware-related complications of deep brain stimulation. *Neurosurgery* 2002;50:1268–1276.

155. Beric A, Kelly PJ, Rezai A, et al. Complications of deep brain stimulation surgery. *Stereotact Funct Neurosurg* 2001;77:73–78.

156. Alesch F. Sudden failure of dual channel pulse generators. *Mov Disord* 2005;20:64–66.

157. Schwalb JM, Riina HA, Skolnick B, Jaggi JL, Simuni T, Baltuch GH. Revision of deep brain stimulator for tremor: technical note. *J Neurosurg* 2001;94:1010–1012.

158. Macia F, Perlemoine C, Coman I, et al. Parkinson's disease patients with bilateral subthalamic deep brain stimulation gain weight. *Mov Disord* 2004;19:206–212.

159. Lang AE, Widner H. deep brain stimulation for Parkinson's disease: patient selection and evaluation. *Mov Disord* 2002;17(suppl 3):S94–S101.

160. Lang AE, Houeto JL, Krack P, et al. Deep brain stimulation: pre-operative issues. *Mov Disord* 2006;(suppl 14):S171–S196.

161. Ardouin C, Pillon B, Peiffer E, et al. Bilateral subthalamic or pallidal stimulation for Parkinson's disease affects neither memory nor executive functions: a consecutive series of 62 patients. *Ann Neurol* 1999;46:217–223.

162. Saint-Cyr JA, Trépanier LL, Kumar R, Lozano AM, Lang AE. Neuropsychological consequences of chronic bilateral stimulation of the subthalamic nucleus in Parkinson's disease. *Brain* 2000;123:2091–2108.

163. Charles PD, Van Blercom N, Krack P, et al. Predictors of effective bilateral subthalamic nucleus stimulation for Parkinson's disease. *Neurology* 2002;59:932–934.

164. Welter ML, Houeto JL, Tezenas du Montcel S, et al. Clinical predictive factors of subthalamic stimulation in Parkinson's disease. *Brain* 2002;125:575–583.

165. Russmann H, Ghika J, Villemure JG, et al. Subthalamic nucleus deep brain stimulation in Parkinson's disease patients over age 70 years. *Neurology* 2004;63:1952–1954.

166. Braak H, Del Tredici K, Rub U, de Vos RA, Jansen Steur EN, Braak E. Staging of brain pathology related to sporadic Parkinson's disease. *Neurobiol Aging* 2003;24:197–211.

167. Gorgulho A, De Salles AA, Frighetto L, Behnke E. Incidence of hemorrhage associated with electrophysiological studies performed using macroelectrodes and microelectrodes in functional neurosurgery. *J Neurosurg* 2005;102:888–896.

168. Lopiano L, Rizzone M, Bergamasco B, et al. Deep brain stimulation of the subthalamic nucleus in PD: an analysis of the exclusion causes. *J Neurol Sci* 2002;195:167–170.

169. Alegret M, Junqué C, Valldeoriola F, et al. Effects of bilateral subthalamic nucleus stimulation on cognitive function in Parkinson's disease. *Arch Neurol* 2001;58:1223–1227.

170. Troster AI, Fields JA, Wiklinson SB, et al. Unilateral pallidal stimulation for Parkinson's disease: neurobehavioral functioning before and 3 months after electrode implantation. *Neurology* 1997;49:1078–1083.

171. Fields JA, Troster AI, Wilkinson SB, Pahwa R, Koller WC. Cognitive outcome following staged bilateral pallidal stimulation for the treatment of Parkinson's disease. *Clin Neurol Neurosurg* 1999;101:182–188.

172. Vingerhoets G, van der Linden C, Lannoo E, et al. Cognitive outcome after unilateral pallidal stimulation in Parkinson's disease. *J Neurol Neurosurg Psychiatry* 1999;66:297–304.

173. Hariz M, Johansson F, Shamsgovara P, Johansson E, Hariz GM, Fagerlund M. Bilateral subthalamic nucleus stimulation in a parkinsonian patient with preoperative deficits in speech and cognition: persistent improvement in mobility but increased dependency: a case study. *Mov Disord* 2000;15:136–139.

174. Jarraya B, Bonnet AM, Duyckaerts C, et al. Parkinson's disease, subthalamic stimulation, and selection of candidates: a pathological study. *Mov Disord* 2003;18:1517–1520.

175. Pillon B. Neuropsychological assessment for management of patients with deep brain stimulation. *Mov Disord* 2002;17(suppl 3):S116–S122.

176. Voon V, Kubu CS, Krack P, Houeto JL, Troster AI. Deep-brain stimulation: neuropsychological and neuropsychiatric issues. *Mov Disord* 2006;21(suppl 14):S305–S327.

177. Trépanier LL, Kumar R, Lozano A, Lang AE, Saint-Cyr JA. Neuropsychological outcome of neurosurgical therapies in Parkinson's disease: a comparison of GPi pallidotomy and deep brain stimulation of GPi or STN. *Brain Cogn* 2000;42:324–347.

178. Miyawaki E, Troster AI. Introduction to neurobehavioral issues in pallidotomy and pallidal stimulation. *Brain Cogn* 2000;42:309–312.

179. Dujardin K, Krystkowiak P, Defebvre L, Blond S, Destee A. A case of severe dysexecutive syndrome consecutive to chronic bilateral pallidal stimulation. *Neuropsychologia* 2000;38:1305–1315.

180. Miyawaki E, Perlmutter JS, Troster AI, Videen TO, Koller WC. The behavioral complications of pallidal stimulation: a case report. *Brain Cogn* 2000;42:417–434.

181. Volkmann J, Allert N, Voges J, Weiss PH, Freund HJ, Sturm V. Safety and efficacy of pallidal or subthalamic nucleus stimulation in advanced PD. *Neurology* 2001;56:548–551.

182. Roane DM, Yu M, Feinberg TE, Rogers JD. Hypersexuality after pallidal surgery in Parkinson's disease. *Neuropsychiatry Neuropsychol Behav Neurol* 2002;15:247–251.

183. Herzog J, Reiff J, Krack P, et al. Manic episode with psychotic symptoms induced by subthalamic nucleus stimulation in a patient with Parkinson's disease. *Mov Disord* 2003;18:1382–1384.

184. Funkiewiez A, Ardouin C, Caputo E, et al. Long-term effects of bilateral subthalamic nucleus stimulation on cognitive function, mood and behaviour in Parkinson's disease. *J Neurol Neurosurg Psychiatry* 2004;75:834–839.

185. Funkiewiez A, Ardouin C, Krack P, et al. Acute psychotropic effects of bilateral subthalamic nucleus stimulation and levodopa in Parkinson's disease. *Mov Disord* 2003;18:524–530.

186. Agid Y, Arnulf I, Bejjani P, et al. Parkinson's disease is a neuropsychiatric disorder. *Adv Neurol* 2003;91:365–370.

187. Lawrence AD, Evans AH, Lees AJ. Compulsive use of dopamine replacement therapy in Parkinson's disease: reward systems gone awry? *Lancet Neurol* 2003;2:595–604.

188. Houeto JL, Mesnage V, Mallet L, et al. Behavioural disorders, Parkinson's disease and subthalamic stimulation. *J Neurol Neurosurg Psychiatry* 2002;72:701–707.

189. Witjas T, Baunez C, Henry JM, et al. Addiction in Parkinson's disease: impact of subthalamic nucleus deep brain stimulation. *Mov Disord* 2005;20:1052–1055.

190. Burkhard PR, Vingerhoets FJ, Berney A, Bogousslavsky J, Villemure JG, Ghika J. Suicide after successful deep brain stimulation for movement disorders. *Neurology* 2004;14:2170–2172.

191. Volkmann J, Sturm V, Weiss P, et al. Bilateral high-frequency stimulation of the internal globus pallidus in advanced Parkinson's disease. *Ann Neurol* 1998;44:953–961.

192. Pinter MM, Alesch F, Murg M, Helscher RJ, Binder H. Apomorphine test: a predictor for motor responsiveness to deep brain stimulation of the subthalamic nucleus. *J Neurol* 1999;246:907–913.

193. Fraix V, Hoveto JL, Lagrange C, et al. Clinical and economic results of bilateral subthalamic nucleus stimulation in Parkinson's disease. *J Neurol Neurosurg Psychiatry* 2006;77:443–449.

194. Defer GL, Widner H, Marié RM, Rémy P, Levivier M, and the Conference Participants. Core assessment program for surgical interventional theapies in Parkinson's disease (CAPSIT-PD). *Mov Disord* 1999;14:572–584.

195. Metman LV, Myre B, Verwey N, et al. Test-retest reliability of UPDRS-III, dyskinesia scales, and timed motor tests in patients with advanced Parkinson's disease: an argument against multiple baseline assessments *Mov Disord* 2004;19:1079–1084.

196. Mesnage V, Houeto JL, Welter ML, et al. Parkinson's disease: neurosurgery at an earlier stage? *J Neurol Neurosurg Psychiatry* 2002;73:778–779.

197. Hassler R. Anatomy of the thalamus. In: Schaltenbrand G, Baily P, eds. *Introduction to stereotaxis with an atlas of the human brain.* Stuttgart, Germany: Thieme, 1959:230–290.

198. Schaltenbrand G, Wahren W. *Atlas for stereotaxy of the human brain: with an accompanying guide.* 2nd ed. Stuttgart, Germany: Thieme, 1977.

199. Speelman JD, Schuurman R, DeBie RMA, Esselink RAJ, Bosch DA. Stereotactic neurosurgery for tremor. *Mov Disord* 2002;17 (suppl 3):84–88.

200. Ohye C, Shibazaki T, Hirai T, Wada H, Hirato M, Kawashima Y. Further physiological observations on the ventralis intermedius neurons in the human thalamus. *J Neurophysiol* 1989;61:488–500.

201. Garonzik IM, Hua SE, Ohara S, Lenz FA. Intraoperative micro-electrode and semi-microelectrode recording during the physiological localization of the thalamic nucleus ventral intermediate. *Mov Disord* 2002;17(suppl 3):S135–S144.

202. Speelman JD, Schuurman PR, De Bie RMA, Bosch DA. Thalamic surgery and tremor. *Mov Disord* 1998;13(suppl 3):103–106.

203. Krack P, Dostrovsky J, Ilinsky I, et al. Surgery of the motor thalamus: problems with the present nomenclatures. *Mov Disord* 2002;17(suppl 3):2–8.

204. Benabid AL, Koudsie A, Benazzouz A, Le Bas JF, Pollak P. Imaging of subthalamic nucleus and ventralis intermedius of the thalamus. *Mov Disord* 2002;17(suppl 3).S123–S129.

205. Macchi G, Jones EG. Toward an agreement on terminology of nuclear and subnuclear divisions of the motor thalamus. *J Neurosurg* 1997;86:670–685.

206. Ilinsky IA, Kultas-Ilinsky K. Motor thalamic circuits in primates with emphasis on the area targeted in treatment of movement disorders. *Mov Disord* 2002;17(suppl 3):9–14.

207. Caparros-Lefebvre D, Blond S, Feltin M-P, Pollak P, Benabid AL. Improvement of levodopa induced dyskinesias by thalamic deep brain stimulation is related to slight variation in electrode placement: possible involvement of the centre median and parafascicularis complex. *J Neurol Neurosurg Psychiatry* 1999;67:308–314.

208. Narabayashi H, Yokochi F, Nakajima Y. Levodopa-induced dyskinesia and thalamotomy. *J Neurol Neurosurg Psychiatry* 1984;47:831–839.

209. Goto S, Kunitoku N, Hamasaki T, Nishikawa S, Ushio Y. Abolition of postapoplectic hemichorea by Vo-complex thalamotomy: long-term follow-up study. *Mov Disord* 2001;16:771–774.

210. Vitek JL, Bakay RA, Hashimoto T, et al. Microelectrode-guided pallidotomy: technical approach and its application in medically intractable Parkinson's disease. *J Neurosurg* 1998;88:1027–1043.

211. Lozano AM, Hutchison WD. Microelectrode recordings in the pallidum. *Mov Disord* 2002;17(suppl 3):150–154.

212. Carroll CB, Scott R, Davies LE, Aziz T. The pallidotomy debate. *Br J Neurosurg* 1998;12:146–150.

213. Zhu XL, Hamel W, Schrader B, et al. Magnetic resonance imaging-based morphometry and landmark correlation of basal ganglia nuclei. *Acta Neurochir* 2002;144:959–969.

214. Yelnik J. Functional anatomy of the basal ganglia. *Mov Disord* 2002;17(suppl 3):15–21.

215. Chevrier E, Fraix V, Krack P, Chabardes S, Benabid AL, Pollak P. Is there a role for physiotherapy during deep brain stimulation surgery in patients with Parkinson's disease? *Eur J Neurol* 2006;13:496–498.

216. Benazzouz A, Breit S, Koudsie A, Pollak P, Krack P, Benabid AL. Intraoperative microrecordings of the subthalamic nucleus in Parkinson's disease. *Mov Disord* 2002;17(suppl 3):S145–S149.

217. Rodriguez-Oroz MC, Rodriguez M, Guridi J, et al. The subthalamic nucleus in Parkinson's disease: somatotopic organization and physiological characteristics. *Brain* 2001;124:1777–1790.

218. Herzog J, Fietzek U, Hamel W, et al. Most effective stimulation site in subthalamic deep brain stimulation for Parkinson's disease. *Mov Disord* 2004;19:1050–1054.

219. Caparros Lefebvre D, Blond S, Vermersch P, Pecheux N, Guieu JD. Chronic thalamic stimulation improves tremor and levodopa induced dyskinesias in Parkinson's disease. *J Neurol Neurosurg Psychiatry* 1993;56:268–273.

220. Walter BL, Vitek JL. Surgical treatment for Parkinson's disease (review). *Lancet Neurol* 2004;3:719–728.

221. Fraix V, Pollak P, Moro E, et al. Subthalamic nucleus stimulation in tremor dominant parkinsonian patients with previous thalamic surgery. *J Neurol Neurosurg Psychiatry* 2005;76:246–248.

222. Hariz GM, Lindberg M, Hariz MI, Bergenheim T. Does the ADL part of the unified Parkinson's disease rating scale measure ADL? An evaluation in patients after pallidotomy and thalamic deep brain stimulation. *Mov Disord* 2003;18:373–381.

223. Goetz CG, Poewe W, Rascol O, Sampaio C. Evidence-based medical review update: pharmacological and surgical treatments of Parkinson's disease: 2001 to 2004. *Mov Disord* 2005;20:523–539.

224. Pahwa R, Wilkinson S, Smith D, Lyons K, Miyawaki E, Koller WC. High-frequency stimulation of the globus pallidus for the treatment of Parkinson's disease. *Neurology* 1997;49:249–253.

225. Gross C, Rougier A, Guehl D, Boraud T, Julien J, Bioulac B. High-frequency stimulation of the globus pallidus internalis in Parkinson's disease: a study of seven cases. *J Neurosurg* 1997;87:491–498.

226. Tronnier VM, Fogel W, Kronenbuerger M, Steinvorth S. Pallidal stimulation: an alternative to pallidotomy? *Neurosurgery* 1997;87:700–705.

227. Siegfried J, Wellis G. Chronic electrostimulation of ventroposterolateral pallidum: follow-up. *Acta Neurochir (Wien)* 1997;68(suppl):11–13.

228. Durif F, Lemaire JJ, Debilly B, Dordain G. Acute and chronic effects of anteromedial globus pallidus stimulation in Parkinson's disease. *J Neurol Neurosurg Psychiatry* 1999;67:315–321.

229. Burchiel KJ, Andersen VC, Favre J, Hammerstad JP. Comparison of pallidal versus subthalamic nucleus deep brain stimulation: results of a randomized, blinded pilot study. *Neurosurgery* 1999;45:1375–1382; discussion, 1382–1384.

230. Ghika J, Villemure JG, Fankhauser H, Favre J, Assal G, Ghika-Scmid F. Efficiency and safety of bilateral contemporaneous pallidal stimulation (deep brain stimulation) in levodopa-responsive patients with Parkinson's disease with severe motor fluctuations: a 2-year follow-up review. *J Neurosurg* 1998;89:713–718.

231. Kumar R, Lang AE, Rodriguez-Oroz MC, et al. Deep brain stimulation of the globus pallidus pars interna in advanced Parkinson's disease. *Neurology* 2000;55(suppl 6):S34–S39.

232. Scotto di Luzio AE, Ammannati F, Marini P, Sorbi S, Mennonna P. Which target for DBS in Parkinson's disease? Subthalamic nucleus versus globus pallidus internus. *Neurol Sci* 2001;22:87–88.

233. Defebvre LJP, Krystkowiak P, Blatt JL, et al. Influence of pallidal stimulation and levodopa on gait and preparatory postural adjustments in Parkinson's disease. *Mov Disord* 2002;17:76–83.

234. Durif F, Lemaire JJ, Debilly B, Dordain G. Long-term follow-up of globus pallidus chronic stimulation in advanced Parkinson's disease. *Mov Disord* 2002;17:803–807.

235. Loher TJ, Burgunder JM, Pohle T, Weber S, Sommerhalder R, Krause JK. Long-term pallidal deep brain stimulation in patients with advanced Parkinson disease: 1-year follow-up study. *J Neurosurg* 2002;96:844–853.

236. Volkmann J, Allert N, Voges J, Sturm V, Schnitzler A, Freund HJ. Long-term results of bilateral pallidal stimulation in Parkinson's disease. *Ann Neurol* 2004;55:871–875.

237. Anderson VC, Burchiel K, Hogarth P, Favre J, Hammerstad JP. Pallidal vs subthalamic nucleus deep brain stimulation in Parkinson's disease. *Arch Neurol* 2005;62:554–560.

238. Loher TJ, Burgunder JM, Weber S, Sommerhalder R, Krauss JK. Effect of chronic pallidal deep brain stimulation on off period dystonia and sensory symptoms in advanced Parkinson's disease. *J Neurol Neurosurg Psychiatry* 2002;73:395–399.

239. Houeto JL, Bejjani PB, Damier P, et al. Failure of long-term pallidal stimulation corrected by subthalamic stimulation in PD. *Neurology* 2000;55:728–730.

240. Yelnik J, Damier P, Bejjani BPFC, et al. Functional mapping of the human globus pallidus: contrasting effect of stimulation in the internal and external pallidum in Parkinson's disease. *Neuroscience* 2000;101:77–87.

241. Peppe A, Pierantozzi M, Altibrandi MG, et al. Bilateral GPi DBS is useful to reduce abnormal involuntary movements in advanced Parkinson's disease patients, but its action is related to modality and site of stimulation. *Eur J Neurol* 2001;8:579–586.

242. Bejjani B, Damier P, Arnulf I, et al. Pallidal stimulation for Parkinson's disease: two targets? *Neurology* 1997;49:1564–1569.

243. Krack P, Pollak P, Limousin P, Hoffman D, Benazzouz A, Benabid AL. Decrease in akinesia seems to result from chronic electrical stimulation in the external (GPe) rather than internal (GPi) pallidum: reply. *Mov Disord* 1999;14:537–539.

244. Krack P, Pollak P, Limousin P, Benabid AL. Levodopa-inhibiting effect of pallidal surgery. *Ann Neurol* 1997;42:129.

245. Krack P, Pollak P, Limousin P, Hoffmann D, Benazzouz A, Benabid AL. Inhibition of levodopa-effects by internal pallidal stimulation. *Mov Disord* 1998;13:648–652.

246. Wallace BA, Foote KD, Krack P, Koudsie A, Benabid AL, Pollak P. Pallidal deep brain stimulation for PD: correlation of long-term clinical outcome and active lead location [abstract]. *Mov Disord* 2002;17(suppl 5):S206.

247. Hariz MI, Bergenheim AT. A 10-year follow-up review of patients who underwent Leksell's posteroventral pallidotomy for Parkinson's disease. *J Neurosurg* 2001;94:552–558.

248. Baron MS, Vitek JL, Bakay RAE, et al. Treatment of advanced Parkinson's disease by unilateral posterior GPi pallidotomy: 4-year results of a pilot study. *Mov Disord* 2000;15:230–237.

249. Pillon B, Ardouin C, Damier P, et al. Neuropsychological changes between "off" and "on" STN or GPi stimulation in Parkinson's disease. *Neurology* 2000;55:411–418.

250. Vitek JL. Deep brain stimulation for Parkinson's disease: a critical re-evaluation of STN versus GPi DBS. *Stereotact Funct Neurosurg* 2002;78:119–131.

251. Minguez-Castellanos A, Escamilla-Sevilla F, Katati MJ, et al. Different patterns of medication change after subthalamic or pallidal stimulation for Parkinson's disease: target related effect or selection bias? *J Neurol Neurosurg Psychiatry* 2005;76:34–39.

252. Vingerhoets FJ, Villemure JG, Temperli P, Pollo C, Pralong E, Ghika J. Subthalamic DBS replaces levodopa in Parkinson's disease: two-year follow-up. *Neurology* 2002;58:396–401.

253. Herzog J, Volkmann J, Krack P, et al. Two-year follow-up of subthalamic deep brain stimulation in Parkinson's disease. *Mov Disord* 2003;18:1332–1337.

254. Kleiner-Fisman G, Fisman DN, Sime E, Saint-Cyr JA, Lozano A, Lang AE. Long-term follow up of bilateral deep brain stimulation of the subthalamic nucleus in patients with advanced Parkinson disease. *J Neurosurg* 2004;99:489–495.

255. Visser-Vandewalle V, van der Linden C, Temel Y, et al. Long-term effects of bilateral subthalamic nucleus stimulation in advanced Parkinson disease: a four year follow-up study. *Parkinsonism Relat Disord* 2005;11:157–165.

256. Kumar RLA, Sime E, Halket E, Lang AE. Comparative effects of unilateral and bilateral subthalamic nucleus deep brain stimulation. *Neurology* 1999;53:561–566.

257. Bastian AJ, Kelly VE, Revilla FJ, Perlmutter JS, Mink JW. Different effects of unilateral versus bilateral subthalamic nucleus stimulation on walking and reaching in Parkinson's disease. *Mov Disord* 2003;18:1000–1007.

258. Fahn S, Oakes D, Shoulson I, et al., for the Parkinson Study Group. Levodopa and the progression of Parkinson's disease. *N Engl J Med* 2004;351:2547–2549.

259. Alvarez L, Macias R, Guridi J, et al. Dorsal subthalamotomy for Parkinson's disease. *Mov Disord* 2001;16:72–78.

260. Limousin P, Krack P, Pollak P, et al. Electrical stimulation of the subthalamic nucleus in advanced Parkinson's disease. *N Engl J Med* 1998;339:1105–1111.

261. Kumar R, Lozano AM, Kim YJ, et al. Double-blind evaluation of subthalamic nucleus deep brain stimulation in advanced Parkinson's disease. *Neurology* 1998;51:850–855.

262. Moro E, Scerrati M, Romito LMA, Roselli R, Tonali P, Albanese A. Chronic subthalamic nucleus stimulation reduces medication requirements in Parkinson's disease. *Neurology* 1999;53:85–90.

263. Pinter MM, Alesch F, Murg M, Seiwald M, Helscher RJ, Binder H. Deep brain stimulation of the subthalamic nucleus for control of extrapyramidal features in advanced idiopathic Parkinson's disease: one year follow-up. *J Neural Transm* 1999;106:693–709.

264. Rodriguez-Oroz MC, Gorospe LM, Guridi J, et al. Bilateral deep brain stimulation of the subthalamic nucleus in Parkinson's disease. *Neurology* 2000;55(suppl 6):S45–S51.

265. Houeto JL, Damier P, Bejjani PB, et al. Subthalamic stimulation in Parkinson disease: a multidisciplinary approach. *Arch Neurol* 2000;57:461–465.

266. Molinuevo JL, Valldeoriola F, Tolosa E, Rumià J. Levodopa withdrawal after bilateral subthalamic nucleus stimulation in advanced Parkinson's disease. *Arch Neurol* 2000;57:983–988.

267. Valldeoriola F, Pilleri M, Tolosa E, Molinuevo JL, Rumia J, Ferrer E. Bilateral subthalamic stimulation monotherapy in advanced Parkinson's disease: long-term follow-up of patients. *Mov Disord* 2002;17:125–132.

268. Lopiano L, Rizzone M, Bergamasco B, et al. Deep brain stimulation of the subthalamic nucleus: clinical effectiveness and safety. *Neurology* 2001;56:552–554.

269. Ostergaard K, Sunde N, Dupont E. Effects of bilateral stimulation of the subthalamic nucleus in patients with severe Parkinson's disease and motor fluctuations. *Mov Disord* 2002;17:693–700.

270. Thobois S, Mertens P, Guenot M, et al. Subthalamic nucleus stimulation in Parkinson's disease. *J Neurol* 2002;249:529–534.

271. Simuni T, Jaggi JL, Mulholland H, et al. Bilateral stimulation of the subthalamic nucleus in patients with Parkinson disease: a study of efficacy and safety. *J Neurosurg* 2002;96:666–672.

272. Voges J, Volkmann J, Allert N, et al. Bilateral high-frequency stimulation in the subthalamic nucleus for the treatment of Parkinson's disease: correlation of therapeutic effect with anatomical electrode position. *J Neurosurg* 2002;96:269–279.

273. Romito LM, Scerrati M, Contarino MF, Bentivoglio AR, Tonali P, Albanese A. Long-term follow up of subthalamic nucleus stimulation in Parkinson's disease. *Neurology* 2002;58:1546–1550.

274. Figueiras-Mendez R, Regidor I, Riva-Meana C, Magarinos-Ascone CM. Further supporting evidence of beneficial subthalamic stimulation in Parkinson's patients. *Neurology* 2002;58:469–470.

275. Schobach WM, Chastan N, Welter ML, et al. Stimulation of the subthalamic nucleus in Parkinson's disease: a 5 year follow up. *J Neurol Neurosurg Psychiatry* 2005;76:1640–1644.

276. Peppe A, Pierantozzi M, Bassi A, et al. Stimulation of the subthalamic nucleus compared with the globus pallidus internus in patients with Parkinson disease. *J Neurosurg* 2004;101:195–200.

277. Pinto S, Gentil M, Krack P, et al. Changes induced by levodopa and subthalamic nucleus stimulation on parkinsonian speech. *Mov Disord* 2005. Epub. 2005;20:1507–1515.

277a. Pahwa R, Wilkinson SB, Overman J, et al. Bilateral subthalamic stimulation in patients with Parkinson disease: long-term follow up. *J Neurosurg* 2003;99:71–77.

278. Rodriquez-Oroz MC, Gorospe A, Guridi J, et al. Bilateral deep brain stimulation of the subthalamic nucleus in Parkinson's disease. *Neurology* 2000;55(suppl 6):S45–S51.

279. Rodriguez-Oroz MC, Zamarbide I, Guridi J, Palmero MR, Obeso JA. Efficacy of deep brain stimulation of the subthalamic nucleus in Parkinson's disease 4 years after surgery: double blind and open label evaluation. *J Neurol Neurosurg Psychiatry* 2004; 75:1382–1385.

280. Russman H, Ghika J, Combrement P, et al. L-dopa-induced dyskinesia improvement after STN-DBS depends upon medication reduction. *Neurology* 2004;63:153–155.

281. Bejjani BP, Arnulf I, Demeret S, et al. Levodopa-induced dyskinesias in Parkinson's disease: is sensitization reversible? *Ann Neurol* 2000;47:655–658.

282. Arnulf I, Bejjani B, Garma L, et al. Improvement of sleep architecture in PD with subthalamic nucleus stimulation. *Neurology* 2000;55:1732–1734.

283. Hjort N, Ostergaard K, Dupont E. Improvement of sleep quality in patients with advanced Parkinson's disease treated with deep brain stimulation of the subthalamic nucleus. *Mov Disord* 2004;19:196–199.

284. Finazzi-Agro E, Peppe A, D'Amico A, et al. Effects of subthalamic nucleus stimulation on urodynamic findings in patients with Parkinson's disease. *J Urol* 2003;169:1388–1391.

285. Seif C, Herzog J, van der Horst C, et al. Effect of subthalamic deep brain stimulation on the function of the urinary bladder. *Ann Neurol* 2004;55:118–120.

286. Burn DJ, Tröster AI. Neuropsychiatric complications of medical and surgical therapies for Parkinson's disease. *J Geriatr Psychiatry Neurol* 2004;17:172–180.

287. Czernecki V, Pillon B, Houeto JL, et al. Does bilateral stimulation of the subthalamic nucleus aggravate apathy in Parkinson's disease? *J Neurol Neurosurg Psychiatry* 2005;76:775–779.

288. Bejjani BP, Damier P, Arnulf I, et al. Transient acute depression induced by high-frequency deep-brain stimulation. *N Engl J Med* 1999;340:1476–1480.

289. Bejjani BP, Houeto JL, Hariz M, et al. Aggressive behavior induced by intraoperative stimulation in the triangle of Sano. *Neurology* 2002;59:1425–1427.

290. Sensi M, Eleopra R, Cavallo MA, et al. Explosive-aggressive behavior related to bilateral subthalamic stimulation. *Parkinsonism Relat Disord* 2004;10:247–251.

291. Krack P, Kumar R, Ardouin C, et al. Mirthful laughter induced by subthalamic nucleus stimulation. *Mov Disord* 2001;16:867–875.

292. Krack P, Ardouin C, Funkiewiez A, et al. What is the influence of STN stimulation on the limbic loop? In: Kultas-Ilinsky K, Ilinsky IA, eds. *Basal ganglia and thalamus in health and movement disorders.* New York: Kluwer Academic/Plenum Publishers, 2001:333–340.

293. Romito LM, Raja M, Daniele A, Contarino MF, et al. Transient mania with hypersexuality after surgery for high frequency stimulation of the subthalamic nucleus in Parkinson's disease. *Mov Disord* 2002;17:1371–1374.

294. Bejjani BP, Damier P, Arnulf I, Bonnet AM, Agid Y, and the DBS group. Acute major depression induced by subthalamic deep brain stimulation. *Mov Disord* 1998;13(suppl 2):123.

295. Dujardin K, Defebvre L, Krystkowiak P, Blond S, Destée A. Influence of chronic bilateral stimulation of the subthalamic nucleus on cognitive function in Parkinson's disease. *J Neurol* 2001;248:603–611.

296. Spottke EA, Volkmann J, Lorenz D, et al. Evaluation of health-care utilization and health status of patients with Parkinson's disease treated with deep brain stimulation of the subthalamic nucleus. *J Neurol* 2002;249:759–766.

297. Lagrange E, Krack P, Moro E, et al. Bilateral subthalamic nucleus stimulation improves health-related quality of life in PD. *Neurology* 2002;59:1976–1978.

298. Esselink RAJ, De Bie RMA, de Haan RJ, et al. Unilateral pallidotomy versus bilateral subthalamic nucleus stimulation in PD: a randomized trial. *Neurology* 2004;62:201–207.

299. Martinez-Martin P, Valldeoriola F, Tolosa E, et al. Bilateral subthalamic nucleus stimulation and quality of life in advanced Parkinson's disease. *Mov Disord* 2002;17:372–377.

300. Patel NK, Plaha P, O'Sullivan K, McCarter R, Heywood P, Gill SS. MRI directed bilateral stimulation of the subthalamic nucleus in patients with Parkinson's disease. *J Neurol Neurosurg Psychiatry* 2003;74:1631–1637.

301. Just H, Ostergaard K. Health-related quality of life in patients with advanced Parkinson's disease treated with deep brain stimulation of the subthalamic nuclei. *Mov Disord* 2002;17:539–545.

302. Tröster AI, Fields JA, Wilkinson S, Pahwa R, Koller WC, Lyons KE. Effect of motor improvement on quality of life following subthalamic stimulation is mediated by changes in depressive symptomatology. *Stereotact Funct Neurosurg* 2003;80:43–47.

303. Lezcano E, Gomez-Esteban JC, Zarranz JJ, et al. Improvement in quality of life in patients with advanced Parkinson's disease following bilateral deep-brain stimulation in subthalamic nucleus. *Eur J Neurol* 2004;11:451–454.

304. Diamond A, Jankovic J. The effect of deep brain stimulation on quality of life in movement disorders. *J Neurol Neurosurg Psychiatry* 2005;76:1188–1193.

305. Klawans HL. Individual manifestations of Parkinson's disease after ten or more years of levodopa. *Mov Disord* 1986;3:187–192.

306. Hely MA, Morris JGL, Reid WGJ, Trafficante R. Sydney multicenter study of Parkinson's disease: non-L-dopa-responsive problems dominate at 15 years. *Mov Disord* 2005;20:190–199.

307. Hilker R, Portman AT, Voges J, et al. Disease progression continues in patients with advanced Parkinson's disease and effective

308. Volkmann J, Herzog J, Kopper F, Deuschl G. Introduction to the programming of deep brain stimulators. *Mov Disord* 2002;17(suppl 3):S181–S187.

309. Joint C, Nandi D, Parkin S, Gregory R, Aziz T. Hardware-related problems of deep brain stimulation. *Mov Disord* 2002;17 (suppl 3):175–180.

310. Kumar R. Methods for programming and patients management with deep brain stimulation of the globus pallidus for the treatment of advanced Parkinson's disease and dystonia. *Mov Disord* 2002;17(suppl 3):198–207.

311. Dowsey Limousin P. Postoperative management of Vim DBS for tremor. *Mov Disord* 2002;17(suppl 3):208–211.

312. Deuschl G, Herzog J, Kleiner-Fisman G, et al. Deep brain stimulation: Postoperative issues. *Mov Disord* 2006;21(suppl 14): S219–S237.

313. Pollak P, Benabid AL, Limousin P, Benazzouz A, Hoffmann D, Perret J. Chronic intracerebral stimulation in Parkinson's disease. *Adv Neurol* 1997;74:213–220.

314. Anagnostu E, Sporer B, Steude U, Kempermann U, Büttner U, Bötzel K. Contraversive eye deviation during deep brain stimulation of the globus pallidus internus. *Neurology* 2001;56: 1396–1399.

315. Tommasi G, Krack P, Fraix V, Batir A, Benabid AL, Pollak P. Subthalamic nucleus stimulation and apraxia of eyelid opening in patients with Parkinson's disease [asbtract]. *Mov Disord* 2005;20(suppl 10):154.

316. Gere J, Krack P, Fraix V, Lebas JF, Benabid AL, Pollak P. Worsening of parkinsonism outside the subthalamic nucleus [asbtract]. *Mov Disord* 2005;20(suppl 10):151.

317. Bejjani BP, Arnulf I, Houeto JL, et al. Concurrent excitatory and inhibitory effects of high frequency stimulation: an oculomotor study. *J Neurol Neurosurg Psychiatry* 2002;72:517–522.

318. Kedia S, Moro E, Tagliati M, Lang AE, Kumar R. Emergence of restless legs syndrome during subthalamic stimulation for Parkinson disease: emergence of restless legs syndrome during subthalamic stimulation for Parkinson disease. *Neurology* 2004;63:2410–2412.

319. Kulisevsky J, Berthier ML, Gironell A, Pascual-Sedano B, Molet J, Parés P. Mania following deep brain stimulation for Parkinson's disease. *Neurology* 2002;59:1421–1424.

320. Ardouin C, Batir A, Krack P, Funkiewiez A, Benabid AL, Pollak P. Effect of STN stimulation on mood, motivation and personality in PD patients [abstract]. *Mov Disord* 2004;19(suppl 9): S176–S177.

321. Berney A, Vingerhoets F, Perrin A, et al. Effect on mood of subthalamic DBS for Parkinson's disease: a consecutive series of 24 patients. *Neurology* 2002;59:1427–1429.

322. Doshi PK, Chhaya N, Bhatt MH. Depression leading to attempted suicide after bilateral subthalamic nucleus stimulation for Parkinson's disease. *Mov Disord* 2002;17:1084–1085.

323. Voon V, Saint-Cyr J, Lozano AM, Moro E, Poon YY, Lang AE. Psychiatric symptoms in patients with Parkinson disease presenting for deep brain stimulation surgery. *J Neurosurg* 2005;103: 246–251.

324. Voon V, Moro E, Saint-Cyr JA, Lozano AM, Lang AE. Psychiatric symptoms following surgery for Parkinson's disease with an emphasis on subthalamic stimulation. *Adv Neurol* 2005;96: 130–147.

325. Deuschl G, Bain P. Deep brain stimulation for tremor: patient selection and evaluation. *Mov Disord* 2002;17(suppl 3):102–111.

326. Krack P, Benazzouz A, Pollak P, et al. Treatment of tremor in Parkinson's disease by subthalamic nucleus stimulation. *Mov Disord* 1998;13:907–914.

327. Nagaseki Y, Shibazaki T, Hirai T, et al. Long-term follow-up results of selective VIM-thalamotomy. *J Neurosurg* 1986;65:296–302.

328. Blond S, Caparros-Lefebvre D, Parker F, et al. Control of tremor and involuntary movement disorders by chronic stereotactic stimulation of the ventral intermediate thalamic nucleus. *J Neurosurg* 1992;77:62–68.

329. Lenz FA, Normand SL, Kwan HC, et al. Statistical prediction of the optimal site for thalamotomy in parkinsonian tremor. *Mov Disord* 1995;10:318–328.

subthalamic nucleus stimulation. *J Neurol Neurosurg Psychiatry* 2005;76:1217–1221.

330. Papavassiliou E, Rau G, Heath S, et al. Thalamic deep brain stimulation for essential tremor: relation of lead location to outcome. *Neurosurgery* 2004;54:1120–1129.

331. Benabid AL, Lebas JF, Grand S, et al. Deep brain stimulation for Parkinson's disease. In: Schapira AHV, Olanow CW, eds. *Principles of treatment in Parkinson's disease*. Philadelphia: Butterworth Heinemann Elsevier, 2005:169–191.

332. Gross RE, Jones EG, Dostrovsky JO, Bergeron C, Lang AE, Lozano AM. Histological analysis of the location of effective thalamic stimulation for tremor: case report. *J Neurosurg* 2004;100:547–552.

333. Geny C, Nguyen JP, Cesaro P, Goujon C, Brugieres P, Degos JD. Thalamic stimulation for severe action tremor after lesion of the superior cerebellar peduncle. *J Neurol Neurosurg Psychiatry* 1995;59:641–642.

334. Montgomery EB, Baker KB, Kinkel RP, Barnett G. Chronic thalamic stimulation for the teratment of multiple sclerosis. *Neurology* 1999;53:625–628.

335. Berk C, Carr J, Sinden M, Martzke J, Honey CR. Thalamic deep brain stimulation for the treatment of tremor due to multiple sclerosis: a prospective study of tremor and quality of life. *J Neurosurg* 2002;97:815–820.

336. Kitagawa M, Murata J, Uesugi H, et al. Two-year follow-up of chronic stimulation of the posterior subthalamic white matter for tremor-dominant Parkinson's disease. *Neurosurgery* 2005;56:281–289.

337. Murata J, Kitagawa M, Uesugi H, et al. Electrical stimulation of the posterior subthalamic area for the treatment of intractable proximal tremor. *J Neurosurg* 2003;99:708–715.

338. Nandi D, Chir M, Liu X, et al. Electrophysiological confirmation of the zona incerta as a target for surgical treatment of disabling involuntary arm movements in multiple sclerosis: use of local field potentials. *J Clin Neurosci* 2002;9:64–68.

339. Plaha P, Patel NK, Gill SS. Stimulation of the subthalamic region for essential tremor. *J Neurosurg* 2004;101:48–54.

340. Foote KD, Okun MS. Ventralis intermedius plus ventralis oralis anterior and posterior deep brain stimulation for posttraumatic Holmes tremor: two leads may be better than one: technical note. *Neurosurgery* 2005;56(suppl 2):445.

341. Yamamoto T, Katayama Y, Kano T, Kobayashi K, Oshima H, Fukaya C. Deep brain stimulation for the treatment of parkinsonian, essential, and poststroke tremor: a suitable stimulation method and changes in effective stimulation intensity. *J Neurosurg* 2004;101:201–209.

342. Chou KL, Hurtig HI, Jaggi JL, Baltuch GH. Bilateral subthalamic nucleus deep brain stimulation in a patient with cervical dystonia and essential tremor. *Mov Disord* 2005;20:377–380.

343. Romanelli P, Bronte-Stewart H, Courtney T, Heit G. Possible necessity for deep brain stimulation of both the ventralis intermedius and subthalamic nuclei to resolve Holmes tremor: case report. *J Neurosurg* 2003;99:566–571.

344. Stover NP, Okun MS, Evatt ML, Raju DV, Bakay RA, Vitek JL. Stimulation of the subthalamic nucleus in a patient with Parkinson disease and essential tremor. *Arch Neurol* 2005;62:141–143.

345. Lyons KE, Pahwa R. Deep brain stimulation and essential tremor. *J Clin Neurophysiol* 2004;21:2–5.

346. Berk C, Honey CR. Bilateral thalamic deep brain stimulation for the treatment of head tremor: report of two cases. *J Neurosurg* 2002;96:615–618.

347. Ondo W, Almaguer M, Jankovic J, Simpson RK. Thalamic deep brain stimulation: comparison between unilateral and bilateral placement. *Arch Neurol* 2001;58:218–222.

348. Koller WC, Lyons KE, Wilkinson SB, Troster AI, Pahwa R. Long-term safety and efficacy of unilateral deep brain stimulation of the thalamus in essential tremor. *Mov Disord* 2001;16:464–468.

349. Sydow O, Thobois S, Alesch F, Speelman JD, and study collaborators. Multicentre European study of thalamic stimulation in essential tremor: a six year follow up. *J Neurol Neurosurg Psychiatry* 2003;74:1387–1391.

350. Pahwa R, Lyons KE, Wilkinson SB, et al. Long-term evaluation of deep brain stimulation of the thalamus. *J Neurosurg* 2006;104:506–512.

351. Hariz GM, Lindberg M, Bergenheim AT. Impact of thalamic deep brain stimulation on disability and health-related quality of life in patients with essential tremor. *J Neurol Neurosurg Psychiatry* 2002;72:47–52.

352. Hooper J, Taylor R, Pentland B, Whittle IR. A prospective study of thalamic deep brain stimulation for the treatment of movement disorders in multiple sclerosis. *Br J Neurosurg* 2002;16:102–109.

353. Wishart HA, Roberts DW, Roth RM, et al. Chronic deep brain stimulation for the treatment of tremor in multiple sclerosis: review and case reports. *J Neurol Neurosurg Psychiatry* 2003;74:1392–1397.

354. Bittar RG, Hyam J, Nandi D, et al. Thalamotomy versus thalamic stimulation for multiple sclerosis tremor. *J Clin Neurosci* 2005;12:638–642.

355. Obwegeser AA, Uitti RJ, Witte RJ, Lucas JA, Turk MF, Wharen RE. Quantitative and qualtitative outcome measures after thalamic deep brain stimulation to treat disabling tremors. *Neurosurgery* 2001;48:274–281; discussion, 281–284.

356. Burleigh AL, Horak FB, Burchiel KJ, Nutt JG. Effects of thalamic stimulation on tremor, balance, and step initiation: a single subject study. *Mov Disord* 1993;8:519–524.

357. Pinter MM, Murg M, Alesch F, Freundl B, Helscher RJ, Binder H. Does deep brain stimulation of the nucleus ventralis intermedius affect postural control and locomotion in Parkinson's disease? *Mov Disord* 1999;14:958–963.

358. Troster AI, Fields JA, Pahwa R, et al. Neuropsychological and quality of life outcome after thalamic stimulation for essential tremor. *Neurology* 1999;53:1774–1780.

359. Schuurman PR, Bruins J, Merkus MP, Bosch DA, Speelman JD. A comparison of neuropsychological effects of thalamotomy and thalamic stimulation. *Neurology* 2002;59:1232–1239.

360. Woods SP, Fields JA, Lyons KE, Pahwa R, Troster AI. Pulse width is associated with cognitive decline after thalamic stimulation for essential tremor. *Parkinsonism Relat Disord* 2003;9:295–300.

361. Hubble JP, Busenbark KL, Wilkinson S, Penn RD, Lyons K, Koller WC. Deep brain stimulation for essential tremor. *Neurology* 1996;46:1150–1153.

362. Lozano AM, Abosch A. Pallidal stimulation for dystonia. *Adv Neurol* 2004;94:301–308.

363. Krauss JK, Yianni J, Loher TJ, Aziz TZ. Deep brain stimulation for dystonia. *J Clin Neurophysiol* 2004;21:18–30.

364. Eltahawy HA, Feinstein A, Khan F, Saint-Cyr J, Lang AE, Lozano AM. Bilateral globus pallidus internus deep brain stimulation in tardive dyskinesia: a case report. *Mov Disord* 2004;19:969–972.

365. Vercueil L, Krack P, Pollak P. Results of deep brain stimulation for dystonia: a critical reappraisal. *Mov Disord* 2002;17(suppl 3):89–93.

366. Eltahawy HA, Saint-Cyr J, Giladi N, Lang AE, Lozano AM. Primary dystonia is more responsive than secondary dystonia in pallidal interventions: outcome after pallidotomy or pallidal stimulation. *Neurosurgery* 2004;54:613–619.

367. Volkmann J, Benecke R. Deep brain stimulation for dystonia: patient selection and evaluation. *Mov Disord* 2002;17(suppl 3):112–115.

368. Vayssiere N, van der Gaag N, Cif L, et al. Deep brain stimulation for dystonia confirming a somatotopic organization in the globus pallidus internus. *J Neurosurg* 2004;101:181–188.

369. Trottenberg T, Meissner W, Kabus C, et al. Neurostimulation of the ventral intermediate thalamic nucleus in inherited myoclonus-dystonia syndrome. *Mov Disord* 2001;16:769–771.

370. Ghika J, Villemure JG, Miklossy J, et al. Postanoxic generalized dystonia improved by bilateral Voa thalamic deep brain stimulation. *Neurology* 2002;58:311–313.

371. Vercueil L, Pollak P, Fraix V, et al. Deep brain stimulation in the treatment of severe dystonia. *J Neurol* 2001;248:695–700.

372. Trottenberg T, Paul G, Meissner W, Maier-Hauff K, Taschner C, Kupsch A. Pallidal and thalamic neurostimulation in severe tardive dystonia. *J Neurol Neurosurg Psychiatry* 2001;70:557–559.

373. Katayama Y, Fukaya C, Kobayashi K, Oshima H, Yamamoto T. Chronic stimulation of the globus pallidus internus for control of primary generalized dystonia. *Acta Neurochir Suppl* 2003;87:125–128.

374. Muta D, Goto S, Nishikawa S, et al. Bilateral pallidal stimulation for idiopathic segmental axial dystonia advanced from Meige

syndrome refractory to bilateral thalamotomy. *Mov Disord* 2001;16:774–777.

375. Detante O, Vercueil L, Krack P, Chabardes S, Benabid AL, Pollak P. Off-period dystonia in Parkinson's disease but not generalized dystonia is improved by high-frequency stimulation of the subthalamic nucleus. *Adv Neurol* 2004;94:309–314.

376. Coubes P, Cif L, El Fertit H, et al. Electrical stimulation of the globus pallidus internus in patients with primary generalized dystonia: long-term results. *J Neurosurg* 2004;101:189–194.

377. Krause M, Fogel W, Kloss M, Rasche D, Volkmann J, Tronnier V. Pallidal stimulation for dystonia. *Neurosurgery* 2004;55:1361–1368.

378. Yianni J, Bain P, Giladi N, et al. Globus pallidus internus deep brain stimulation for dystonic conditions: a prospective audit. *Mov Disord* 2003;18:436–442.

379. Zorzi G, Marras C, Nardocci N, et al. Stimulation of the globus pallidus internus for childhood-onset dystonia. *Mov Disord* 2005;20:1194–1200.

380. Krauss JK, Pohle T, Weber S, Ozdoba C, Burgunder JM. Bilateral stimulation of globus pallidus internus for treatment of cervical dystonia. *Lancet* 1999;354:837–838.

381. Krauss JK, Loher TJ, Pohle T, et al. Pallidal deep brain stimulation in patients with cervical dystonia and severe cervical dyskinesias with cervical myelopathy. *J Neurol Neurosurg Psychiatry* 2002;72:249–256.

382. Parkin S, Aziz T, Gregory R, Bain P. Bilateral internal globus pallidus stimulation for the treatment of spasmodic torticollis. *Mov Disord* 2001;16:489–493.

383. Kiss ZH, Doig K, Eliasziw M, Ranawaya R, Suchowersky O. The Canadian multicenter trial of pallidal deep brain stimulation for cervical dystonia: preliminary results in three patients. *Neurosurg Focus* 2004;17:E5.

384. Eltahawy HA, Saint-Cyr J, Poon YY, Lang AE, Lozano AM. Pallidal deep brain stimulation in cervical dystonia: clinical outcome in four cases. *Can J Neurol Sci* 2004;31:328–332.

385. Bereznai B, Steude U, Seelos K, Bötzel K. Chronic high-frequency globus pallidus internus stimulation in different types of dystonia: a clinical, video, and MRI report of six patients presenting with segmental, cervical, and generalized dystonia. *Mov Disord* 2002;17:138–144.

386. Houser M, Waltz T. Meige syndrome and pallidal deep brain stimulation. *Mov Disord* 2005;20:1203–1205.

387. Foote KD, Sanchez JC, Okun MS. Staged deep brain stimulation for refractory craniofacial dystonia with blepharospasm: case report and physiology. *Neurosurgery* 2005;56:E415.

388. Cif L, Valente EM, Hemm S, et al. Deep brain stimulation in myoclonus-dystonia syndrome. *Mov Disord* 2004;19:724–727.

389. Magarinos-Ascone CM, Regidor I, Martinez-Castrillo JC, Gomez-Galan M, Figueras-Mendez R. Pallidal stimulation relieves myoclonus-dystonia syndrome. *J Neurol Neurosurg Psychiatry* 2005;76:989–991.

390. Deutschlander A, Asmus F, Gasser T, Steude U, Botzel K. Sporadic rapid-onset dystonia-parkinsonism syndrome: failure of bilateral pallidal stimulation. *Mov Disord* 2005;20:254–257.

391. Loher TJ, Krauss JK, Burgunder JM, Taub E, Siegfried J. Chronic thalamic stimulation for treatment of dystonic paroxysmal nonkinesigenic dyskinesia. *Neurology* 2001;56:268–270.

392. Cif L, El Fertit H, Vayssiere N, et al. Treatment of dystonic syndromes by chronic electrical stimulation of the internal globus pallidus. *J Neurosurg Sci* 2003;47:52–55.

393. Krauss JK, Loher TJ, Weigel R, Capelle HH, Weber S, Burgunder JM. Chronic stimulation of the globus pallidus internus for the treatment of non-DYT1 generalized dystonia and choreoathetosis. *J Neurosurg* 2003;98:785–792.

394. Chang JW, Choi JY, Lee BW, Kang UJ, Chung SS. Unilateral globus pallidus internus stimulation improves delayed onset post-traumatic cervical dystonia with an ipsilateral focal basal ganglia lesion. *J Neurol Neurosurg Psychiatry* 2002;73:588–590.

394a. Loher TJ, Hasdemir MG, Bergunder JM, Krauss JK. Long-term follow-up study of chronic globus pallidus internus stimulation for posttraumatic hemidystonia. *J Neurosurg* 2000;92:457–460.

394b. Taira T, Kobayashi T, Hori T. Disappearance of self-mutilating behavior in a patient with Lesch-Nyhan Syndrome after bilateral

chronic stimulation of the globus pallidus internus: case report. *J Neurosurg* 2003;98:414–416.

395. Castelnau P, Cif L, Valente EM, et al. Pallidal stimulation improves pantothenate kinase-associated neurodegeneration. *Ann Neurol* 2005;57:738–741.

396. Umemura A, Jaggi JL, Dolinskas CA, Stern MB, Baltuch GH. Pallidal deep brain stimulation for longstanding severe generalized dystonia in Hallervorden-Spatz syndrome: case report. *J Neurosurg* 2004;100:706–709.

397. Trottenberg T, Volkmann J, Deuschl G, et al. Treatment of severe tardive dystonia with pallidal deep brain stimulation. *Neurology* 2005;64:344–346.

398. Franzini A, Marras C, Ferroli P, et al. Long-term high-frequency bilateral pallidal stimulation for neuroleptic-induced tardive dystonia: report of two cases. *J Neurosurg* 2005;102:721–725.

399. Krauss JK, Yianni J, Loher TJ, Aziz TZ. Deep brain stimulation for dystonia. *J Clin Neurophysiol* 2004;21:18–30.

400. Yianni J, Bain PG, Gregory RP, et al. Post-operative progress of dystonia patients following globus pallidus internus deep brain stimulation. *Eur J Neurol* 2003;10:239–247.

401. Kumar R. Methods for programming and patient management with deep brain stimulation of the globus pallidus for the treatment of advanced Parkinson's disease and dystonia. *Mov Disord* 2005;17(suppl 3):198–207.

402. Goto S, Mita S, Ushio Y. Bilateral pallidal stimulation for cervical dystonia: an optimal paradigm from our experiences. *Stereotact Funct Neurosurg* 2002;79:221–227.

403. Kumar R, Dagher A, Hutchison WD, Lang AE, Lozano AM. Globus pallidus deep brain stimulation for generalized dystonia: clinical and PET investigation. *Neurology* 1999;53:871–874.

404. Kupsch A, Kuehn A, Klaffke S, et al. Deep brain stimulation in dystonia. *J Neurol* 2003;250(suppl 1):47–52.

405. Vesper J, Klostermann F, Funk T, Stockhammer F, Brock M. Deep brain stimulation of the globus pallidus internus (GPI) for torsion dystonia: a report of two cases. *Acta Neurochir* 2002;79(suppl 2):83–88.

406. Yianni J, Nandi D, Shad A, Bain P, Gregory R, Aziz T. Increased risk of lead fracture and migration in dystonia compared with other movement disorders following deep brain stimulation. *J Clin Neurosci* 2004;11:243–245.

407. Temel Y, Visser-Vandewalle V. Surgery in Tourette syndrome. *Mov Disord* 2004;19:3–14.

408. Visser-Vandewalle V, Temel Y, Boon P, et al. Chronic bilateral thalamic stimulation: a new therapeutic approach in intractable Tourette syndrome: report of three cases. *J Neurosurg* 2003;99:1094–1100.

409. Diederich NJ, Kalteis K, Stamenkovic M, Pieri V, Alesch F. Efficient internal pallidal stimulation in Gilles de la Tourette syndrome: a case report. *Mov Disord* 2005;20:1496–1499.

410. Nakano N, Uchiyama T, Okuda T, et al. Successful long-term deep brain stimulation for hemichorea-hemiballism in a patient with diabetes. Case report. *J Neurosurg* 2005;102:1137–1141.

411. Moro E, Lang AE, Strafella AP, et al. Bilateral globus pallidus stimulation for Huntington's disease. *Ann Neurol* 2004;56:290–294.

412. Yianni J, Nandi D, Bradley K, et al. Senile chorea treated by deep brain stimulation: a clinical, neurophysiological and functional imaging study. *Mov Disord* 2004;19:597–602.

413. Schrader C, Peschel T, Petermeyer M, Dengler R, Hellwig D. Unilateral deep brain stimulation of the internal globus pallidus alleviates tardive dyskinesia. *Mov Disord* 2004;19:583–585.

414. Burbaud P, Rougier A, Ferrer X, et al. Improvement of severe trunk spasms by bilateral high-frequency stimulation of the motor thalamus in a patient with chorea-acanthocytosis. *Mov Disord* 2002;17:204–207.

415. Krauss JK, Pohle T, Weigel R, Burgunder JM. Deep brain stimulation of the centre median-parafascicular complex in patients with movement disorders. *J Neurol Neurosurg Psychiatry* 2002;72:546–548.

416. Okun MS, Fernandez HH, Foote KD. Deep brain stimulation of the GPi treats restless legs syndrome associated with dystonia. *Mov Disord* 2005;20:500–501.

Clinical Rating Scales in Movement Disorders

Katie Kompoliti   *Cynthia L. Comella*   *Christopher G. Goetz*

PRINCIPLES OF SCALE DEVELOPMENT AND USAGE

Over the past two decades, extensive research has focused on the natural history, genetics, and treatment of movement disorders, including Parkinson's disease (PD), Huntington's disease, dystonia, and Gilles de la Tourette's syndrome. Both the care of patients and research associated with movement disorders demand the availability of reliable and valid clinical rating instruments. The ability to measure movement disorder characteristics over time allows for comparison of outcomes, helps the interpretation of results, and minimizes errors of measurement. Clearly, a study with a reliable and valid outcome measure is more powerful in detecting meaningful differences among groups than the same study without such measures.

Measurement is the assignment of numerals to symptoms, behaviors, or clinical signs according to agreed-upon rules. Scales are the means used in clinical medicine for assigning numbers to observable qualities (1). The scales used in clinical medicine can be classified as nominal, ordinal, interval, or ratio scales. In *nominal* or categorical scales, the basic relationships described are equality or difference and, therefore, signs are present or absent. In an *ordinal* scale, an attribute is classified according to its rank order. However, the steps in the scale are not necessarily presumed to be equal. The basic relationship described in an ordinal scale is greater or less. *Interval* scales, like ordinal scales, order behaviors, but all steps in the scale are presumed to be equal, so the difference between 30 and 35 is the same as the difference between 60 and 65. The basic relationship described in an interval scale is equality or difference of intervals. True interval scales are rare in neurology. *Ratio* scales have equal intervals, but in addition they have a true (nonarbitrary) zero—for example, the Kelvin temperature scale is a ratio scale since it is based on absolute zero.

The ability of scales to produce consistent results and, thereby, to be useful instruments in monitoring patients and conducting research, depends upon their *psychometric* properties. Reliability is the extent to which a measure yields the same results on repeated trials. This is the proportion of variation in any given measurement that is due to true variation and not error. Reliability can be classified as *intrarater* and *interrater* reliability. The former refers to the reproducibility of a single examiner's rating on separate occasions (test–retest), the latter to the reproducibility of ratings when multiple examiners independently examine the same patient. *Dimensionality* refers to the ability of a rating instrument to measure several subdomains of a particular construct. Dimensionality and internal consistency of a scale are important in forming composite measures of tic severity or of subscale scores. *Internal consistency* is the extent to which the items making up a composite score measure the same latent factor. *Validity* is the extent to which an instrument measures what it is designed to measure (1).

Rating scales in movement disorders focus on two primary concepts of dysfunction: impairment and disability.

Whereas *impairment* relates to objective deficits, *disability* refers to the impact of disease on patient function. As such, items usually rated by the investigator and based on the neurological examination assess impairment, whereas interviews that involve the patient's, caregiver's, and investigator's assessments of activities of daily living or quality of life rate disability. Some scales are uniquely impairment ratings, others are uniquely disability assessments, and many combine the two in separate sections, allowing a total score to estimate a global level of disease severity. Global scales that combine the two concepts also exist.

For all scales, movement disorders pose a number of implicit challenges. First, even within a single diagnosis, there are a variety of movements, and multiple variables, such as frequency of movements, number of different types of movements, intensity, complexity, body distribution, suppressibility and interference, can be elements that affect severity ratings. Second, symptoms vary spontaneously and under certain environmental conditions, such as stress or excitement. Third, patients with some movement disorders are able to suppress voluntarily some of their symptoms for minutes to hours. These factors complicate the evaluation of movement disorders, and rating scales that are accurate measures of movement disorders must accommodate these factors to the maximum. In some instances, strategies such as videotaping or controlling the time of day or the environment of evaluation have helped to control these confounding influences. Finally, rater and subject bias are important limiting issues in rating scales. In scales that rely on the subject's impression of the movement disorder, personal expectations, affective illness, and educational level can strongly impact the ratings, and even in objective evaluations the raters may be influenced by their own expectations of change or stability. Efforts to remove investigator bias from ratings through computer-generated testing or examinations by raters who otherwise have no contact with the patient are useful in research paradigms but have little application to clinical practice. In this chapter, rating scales for PD, other parkinsonian syndromes, tremor, dystonia, Huntington's disease, Gilles de la Tourette's syndrome, and functional movement disorders are discussed.

PARKINSON'S DISEASE

Unified Parkinson's Disease Rating Scale

The *Unified Parkinson's Disease Rating Scale* (*UPDRS*) is the international gold standard of clinical rating scales for PD. It combines assessments of impairment and disability derived from several earlier scales and is currently the most widely applied scale in clinical trials (2). The UPDRS is a 4-part scale, but the predominant areas of clinical focus are Part II (activities of daily living) and Part III (objective motor ratings). These sections can be assessed for both the on and the off periods. Each item is rated using a 5-point system, in which 0 is normal and 4 represents severe abnormality. In Part II, 13 activities are assessed, ranging from speech, salivation, and swallowing to handwriting, eating, dressing, turning in bed, and walking. Part III has 14 components, but several are rated separately for more than one body area (tremor, rigidity, finger taps, and hand movements). As such, the range for Part II is 0–52, whereas the range for Part III is 0–96.

In addition to its wide usage, the scale has passed a number of psychometric tests. Martínez-Martín and colleagues (5) showed its high internal consistency (Cronbach = s alpha = 0.96), and interrater reliability was satisfactory for all items (*kappa* values always at least 0.40). There was a statistically significant correlation between UPDRS score and Hoehn and Yahr stage ($rs = 0.71$, $p < 0.001$) and UPDRS and timed finger tapping (3). Richards et al. (4) also examined interrater reliability among 3 neurologists experienced with the scale and found that interclass correlation coefficients for the total motor section of the UPDRS, as well as for several of the individual items, was high (0.40–0.92). Only speech and facial expression items had poor agreements.

In spite of these excellent psychometric dimensions, the length of the UPDRS has disturbed several investigators and prompted attempts to eliminate duplicative items. To this end, factor analyses have examined the actual domains assessed by the items of the motor section of the UPDRS. Among 294 patients assessed in the on state, Stebbins et al. (5) found that the scale had 6 clinically distinct factors: 3 bradykinesia factors (axial/gait, right and left); 1 rigidity measure; and 2 tremor measures (rest and postural). These same 6 factors retain their independence in both the on and off states.

Van Hilten et al. (6) examined Parts II and III (total of 27 items) and suggested that the UPDRS could be reduced to 16 items (8 items in each part) without loss of reliability or validity. The authors suggested dropping salivation, falling, freezing, tremor, and sensory symptoms from Part II and dropping hand movements, pronation/supination, leg agility, facial expression, posture, and action tremor from Part III. Their factor analysis of the motor section suggested only 3 factors, the first dealing predominantly with extremity bradykinesia, the second with midline functions, and the third with tremor. However, because they did not apply their ratings using the prescribed UPDRS directions and did not assess left and right sides independently, these results are difficult to apply to the actual UPDRS. Other attempts to reduce items have been suggested (see the following).

An important element of any scale's success is its uniformity of usage and communication. To enhance the standardized application of the scale, a teaching tape of the motor subsection of the UPDRS is available (7). This tape provides examples of PD patients fitting each rating possibility as reviewed by a panel of 3 movement disorder specialists with extensive experience in the use of the scale.

Furthermore, the tape includes a series of complete UPDRS motor examinations for investigators and trainees to self-administer and report their internal concordance and agreement with the rating panel when they use the UPDRS for publishable studies. The rate of agreement among the 3 experts was always statistically significant for the selected samples with Kendell's coefficient of concordance ranging between 0.97 and 0.62. This tape is available through the Movement Disorder Society.

Based on a 2002 critique of the UPDRS (2), the Movement Disorder Society is sponsoring a rewriting effort to revise the UPDRS and to provide a new version that addresses several issues: greater emphasis on mild impairments and disabilities, greater cultural sensitivity, clearer wording and resolution of ambiguities, and added emphasis on nonmotor components of PD. This new version is undergoing clinimetric testing (8).

Hoehn and Yahr Stage Scale

The *Hoehn and Yahr* (*HY*) *scale* is a widely used clinical rating measure that combines impairment and disability assessment to divide patients into 5 broad stages, based on 2 primary issues: (a) unilateral versus bilateral signs and (b) the absence, presence, and severity of balance/gait difficulties (9). Among the scale's advantages are the fact that it is simple and quick to complete, involving a single 1–5 integer designation. It has been successfully applied by raters without movement disorder expertise, as well as by specialists (10). Further, HY captures typical patterns of PD progression with and without dopaminergic therapy (11). Progression in HY stage correlates with motor decline on the UPDRS and deterioration in quality of life, as measured by several different instruments (12). HY stage also correlates with neuroimaging measures of PD-related pathology, such as beta-CIT SPECT scanning and 18F-fluorodopa positron emission tomography (PET) scanning (13,14). The limited clinimetric analyses conducted to date support its scientific and clinical credibility (11,15).

On the other hand, because of its simplicity, the scale is not comprehensive, and by focusing on the issues of unilateral versus bilateral disease and the presence or absence of postural reflex impairment, it leaves other aspects of PD unassessed. By combining disability and impairment, ambiguities exist, and all clinical presentations of PD are not covered. Because the scale has only 5 scores, effective pharmacological or surgical interventions, even when they induce significant changes in UPDRS, often fail to show HY changes (see reference 13). Attempts to rectify weaknesses have included the introduction of widely used 1.5 and 2.5 increments to the scale, but this adaptation has not been clinimetrically tested and introduces unresolved analytic problems (16). Though still frequently used as an outcome measure in clinical trials, the HY scale has been largely replaced by the UDPRS as a primary outcome measure of treatment efficacy. Instead, it is currently utilized to generally describe populations of patients and as an inclusion/exclusion criterion in baseline assessments during clinical trials. Because it is a categorical scale, populational descriptions must be reported as medians and ranges, not as means with standard deviations, and comparisons must utilize nonparametric statistical tools. The time to development of a given HY stage has been used successfully to distinguish patients with PD from other parkinsonism-plus syndromes, and this measure potentially could be incorporated into interventional studies designed to test delay in clinical progression (17).

Other Scales

Parkinsonism

The *Short Parkinson's Rating Scale* (*SPES*) is based on the the UPDRS but has fewer items and uses a 0–3 rating (18). Similar to the UPDRS, it assesses mental function, activities of daily living, motor findings, and complications of therapy. It involves approximately 7–10 minutes and was developed to be efficiently applied, particularly to a practice situation. Excellent correlation was established between SPES scores and UPDRS scores, and a factor analysis identified 4 primary factors: rigidity, tremor, activities of daily living, and bradykinesia/postural stability. This scale has been incorporated in a larger-scale development program: Scales for Outcome in Parkinson's Disease (SCOPA) (19).

The *Core Assessment Program for Intracerebral Transplanation* (*CAPIT*) and its modifications are conglomerations of different scales, including the UPDRS and HY, developed by international investigators to capture the essential elements to test efficacy of neurotransplantation surgery in PD (20). The CAPIT introduced the widely adopted operational examination of patients in "practically defined off," meaning early morning function after no medications for 12 hours and at least 1 hour after initial rising from bed. Clearly, this off is not the absolute nadir of function for most patients, but these restrictions allow a standard protocol for off assessment that is clear and easy to standardize across multiple centers. To contrast with "practically defined off," the CAPIT calls for a second UPDRS to be performed during the "best on" state. This level of function refers to the point at which clinician and patient agree that function is optimized. In most instances, patients are very clear of the time when they arrive at this state. A few other tasks are attached to the CAPIT evaluation: timed motor tasks and a dyskinesia assessment developed by Obeso (see the following). Finally, a levodopa challenge test is administered in the "practically defined off" state, with regularly repeated timed motor tasks and dyskinesia assessments every 20 minutes throughout the time of levodopa activity. This provides an "area under the curve" assessment of function that demonstrates both duration and intensity of improvements in motor disability.

The *Core Assessment Program for Surgical Interventional Therapies in Parkinson's Disease* (*CAPSIT*) is a more recent modification that added additional cognitive and behavioral assessments along with some modifications in the CAPIT protocol aimed at simplifying elements of the motor examination (21).

Global Disability and Quality of Life

The *Schwab and England Activities of Daily Living Scale* is a questionnaire that measures the patient's perception of functional independence (22). It is not specific to PD but has been widely applied to this condition. The scale includes general statements intended as anchors and ranging from normal (100%) to completely independent, able to do all chores but with some degree of slowness (90%), and so forth until 0% (completely bedridden and vegetative functions are not functioning). The scale is easy to apply, and all numeric values are possible so that parametric analyses can be applied to differences among groups. Its scores also correlate well with UPDRS ratings.

The *Parkinson's Disease Questionnaire-39 (PDQ-39)* is a 39-item questionnaire aimed at assessing numerous areas of health-related quality of life (23). It is self-completed by patients and is designed as a series of statements that patients endorse with 1 of 5 options (0 = never, 1 = occasional . . . 4 = always). Its scores correlate with other measures of parkinsonian impairments, and the scale has been incorporated into several pharmaceutical trials. The *Parkinson's Disease Quality of Life Questionnaire* has 37 questions aggregated into 4 divisions: parkinsonism, systemic symptoms, emotional functioning, and social functioning (24). Constructed in a fashion similar to the PDQ-39, patients respond to a series of statements with endorsements that range from never to always. This scale has been less widely used internationally than the PDQ-39.

Dyskinesias and Motor Fluctuations

Patients with moderate and advanced PD often develop involuntary movements, termed dyskinesias, and an erratic or uneven response to medication, termed *motor fluctuations*. Because the problems are intermittent and may not be witnessed by the investigator, many scales rely on patient-derived data.

For dyskinesias, the *UPDRS Part IV (Motor Complications)* section has a series of questions on duration of dyskinesia, patient perception of disability, and the presence of pain and dystonia (2). Though widely used, the clinimetric dimensions of this part of the UPDRS have not been established. The information is rather general and does not provide definitions for dyskinesia, so the risk that tremor will be misconstrued for dyskinesias lurks within this scale. The new version of the UPDRS has clear definitions of dyskinesia for patients and incorporates information from patient, caregiver, and rater, with all questions on dyskinesia rated with the standard 0–4 options that characterize the rest of the scale (8).

In contrast, the modified version of the *Abnormal Involuntary Movement Scale* is a purely objective scale that rates dyskinesia across body parts by severity. It was

originally developed for the evaluation of tardive dyskinesia but has been widely used in PD research efforts (25). This scale rates 7 body areas at rest with 0–4 severity rating, and it also has 3 global assessments: overall severity, incapacitation for the patient, and patient awareness of dyskinesias. It is a simple and quick scale to complete but does not distinguish between choreic and dystonic dyskinesias and does not involve activation maneuvers that often increase dyskinesia and provide information on severity that is likely more relevant to activities of daily living.

To deal with functional disability, the modified *Rush Dyskinesia Rating Scale (RDRS)* rates patients during activities of daily living, such as drinking, dressing, and walking (26). This scale has a teaching tape that accompanies the scale with several patient examples of the ratings. It is an adaptation of the *Obeso Dyskinesia Scale* (27), which combines examiner-based ratings with patient-based historical ratings on function. The RDRS is based on objective observation only and rates the interference by dyskinesia with the patient's ability to carry out activities. The scale's clinimetric properties have been examined, and both physicians and nurse coordinators use the scale with high inter- and intrarater reliability.

For evaluating motor fluctuations, the *UPDRS Part IV* has questions that estimate the amount of time spent with poor medication response off and the types of off function, whether predictable, unpredictable, gradual in onset or sudden. *Home-based diaries* that patients utilize to document their motor states have been developed and utilized in both research and practice settings. In most instances, patients choose among 4 categories: sleep, off, on without troublesome dyskinesia, and on with troublesome dyskinesias, although a 3-part breakdown into leep, Good Time (on without troublesome dyskinesia) and Bad Time (combined off and on with troublesome dyskinesia) has been utilized effectively (28). Training tapes for on and off definitions are available, but clinical situations and definitions vary widely among patients (29).

Other Domains of Interest

The increasing appreciation of nonmotor elements of PD has prompted the need for ratings of several elements that are not assessed in detail within any of the preceding scales. As part of the new version of the UPDRS10, an appendix has been developed to guide investigators and clinicians on scales that can assess various nonmotor aspects of PD in greater detail than do screening questions. In this appendix, recommended scales are designated if they have been studied clinimetrically and have been considered valid, reliable, and sensitive, as well as having been used specifically in the study of PD by more than the group that published the original description. With these criteria, the *Pittsburgh Sleep Quality Index (PSQI)* is recommended to assess insomnia and quality of nighttime sleep; the *Epworth Sleepiness Scale*

(*ESS*) is recommended to assess daytime sleepiness; and the *Hamilton Depression Scale* and the *Hospital Anxiety and Depression Scale* are recommended for the assessment of depression.

DYSTONIA

Dystonia is categorized by body distribution into focal (involving a single body area), segmental (involvement of 2 or more contiguous body areas), and generalized (involving at least 1 leg, the trunk, and some other body area). Dystonia rating scales, likewise, have been developed specifically to assess these categories of dystonia, with separate scales for generalized dystonia and for each body region affected.

The changeable quality of dystonia has made the development of reliable rating scales problematic and has necessitated the development of standardized examination protocols that include dystonia-activating maneuvers, such as writing, chewing, and speaking. The state-dependent character of dystonia has resulted in the addition of items that are intended to capture the effects of sensory inputs or to measure the duration of time that dystonia is present during the examination. Most rating scales additionally provide a uniform examination protocol to ensure consistent and complete assessments of patients.

Fahn-Marsden Dystonia Rating Scale

The *Fahn-Marsden Dystonia Rating Scale* (*F-M*) has been a standard instrument used to assess the severity of generalized dystonia (30). The F-M has two parts: (a) a movement scale based on the motor features of dystonia and (b) a disability scale based on a patient's subjective impairment in activities of daily living. The movement scale has two separate factors and assesses nine body regions: eyes, mouth, speech/swallowing, neck, bilateral arms-2, bilateral legs-2, and trunk). The factors include a severity factor that measures the intensity of movement and is tailored to each body area and a provocative factor that assesses the circumstances of rest or activity that elicit the dystonia in each area. The final score for each body area is the product of the two factors, with the exception of eyes, mouth, and neck, which are further multiplied by 0.5. The maximal score of the F-M movement scale is 120. The disability scale assesses a variety of functions (speech, handwriting, feeding, eating/swallowing, hygiene, dressing, and walking) rated from 0 (normal) to 4 (severe), with a maximal score of 30. The psychometric properties of the F-M have been assessed in one study using 10 patients and 4 raters. This study demonstrated good to excellent interrater agreement and validity as assessed by a good correlation of the movement scale with the global dystonia severity scale and the dystonia disability scale. A subsequent study assessing the F-M in 100 patients using 25 dystonia experts showed good to

excellent agreement for the total score but only fair agreement (weighted *kappa* of 0.37 to 0.62) for dystonia in the eyes, jaw, and face (31).

Unified Dystonia Rating Scale

The Unified Dystonia Rating Scale was developed in 1997 at a consensus conference of dystonia experts and was intended to address the potential limitations of the F-M scale by subdividing body regions and separately assessing a duration factor measuring the time dystonia was present during the examination (31). This scale rates 14 body regions for dystonia severity and duration, with each scored from 0 to 4. The total score for the UDRS is 112. Similar to the F-M, testing in a large number of dystonia patients showed good to excellent interrater agreement, with the lowest agreement for face, eyes, jaws, and speech.

Neither the F-M nor the UDRS have been tested for clinical responsiveness to therapeutic interventions or reproducibility. The F-M has been used regularly as an outcome for pharmacological and surgical studies of generalized dystonia. The UDRS has been used as a measure of efficacy following surgical interventions. Although applicable to generalized dystonia, neither scale is considered useful for focal dystonia.

Toronto Western Spasmodic Torticollis scale

The instruments used to assess the severity of cervical dystonia, a common focal dystonia involving the neck, are numerous and include objective and subjective rating scales and quantitative measures (32). Several clinical rating scales have been developed, including the Columbia torticollis scale, the Tsui scale, and the *Toronto Western Spasmodic Torticollis Scale* (*TWSTRS*) (33–36). The TWSTRS (36) is currently the most widely used. The TWSTRS consists of 3 subscales: motor severity, activities of daily living, and pain. The motor severity scale is a 10 item rater assessment that evaluates the severity of head posture in several axes of movement (turning, tilting, anterocollis, retrocollis, shoulder elevation), the effect of sensory tricks, range of motion, and the duration of dystonia during the examination. The TWSTRS subsection for motor severity has been evaluated for interrater reliability and validity (36), and a teaching tape has been developed to ensure consistency across raters for multicenter trials (37). The TWSTRS has been used extensively in clinical trials of pharmacological and surgical interventions.

Rating scales for blepharospasm have not been extensively evaluated. Most currently useded scales are modifications of a blepharospasm rating scale developed by Fahn (38). Rating scales to assess the severity of limb dystonias and occupational dystonias (writer's cramp, musician's dystonia) have been particularly problematic. Most studies use patient-derived assessments or electrophysiological tests. The *writer's cramp rating scale* (*WCRS*) and *arm dystonia disability scale*

(*ADDS*) (38–40) but never tested for clinometric properties. For many limb and occupational dystonias, customized rating scales are developed that are specifically tailored to evaluate the particular tasks affected by the dystonia. (41).

CHOREA

Unified Huntington's Disease Rating Scale

The *Unified Hungtington's Disease Rating Scale* (*UHDRS*) was developed by the Huntington Study Group to describe clinical performance and functional capacity in patients with Huntington's disease. It assesses 4 main domains of impairment in Huntington's disease in a semiquantitative way: motor performance, cognitive performance, behavioral abnormalities, and functional capacity (42). The scale assesses relevant clinical features of Huntington's disease to allow comparisons of inter- and intraindividual clinical signs, disease progression, and effects of therapy.

The motor section of the UHDRS assesses motor features of Huntington's disease with standardized ratings of oculomotor function, dysarthria, chorea, dystonia, gait, and postural stability. Each item is rated using a 4-point system, in which 0 is normal and 4 represents severe abnormality. The total motor impairment score is the sum of all the individual motor ratings, with higher scores indicating more severe motor impairment than lower scores.

Cognition is assessed by the verbal-fluency Symbol Digit Modalities Test and the Stroop Interference Test (42,43), with results reported as the raw number of correct answers. The Stroop Interference Test is recorded as the number of correct answers given in color naming, word reading, and interference in a 45-second period.

The behavioral assessment measures the frequency and severity of symptoms related to affect, thought content, and copying styles. The total behavioral score is the sum of all responses. The total score, however, may not be as useful as the individual subscale scores for mood, behavior, psychosis, and obsessiveness, which are created by summing the responses to the corresponding questions (42,43). The examiner is asked to provide a clinical impression as to whether the patient, at the time of the evaluation, is confused, demented, depressed, or requires treatment for depression. Higher scores on the behavior subscale indicate more severe disturbance.

Functional assessments include the Huntington Disease Functional Capacity Scale, the Independence Scale, and a checklist of common daily tasks. The Huntington Disease Functional Capacity Scale is reported as the total functional capacity score, and its items include ability to maintain occupation, ability to manage one's finances, ability to perform domestic chores, degree of independence with activities of daily living, and level of care required. Each item is rated on a 0- to 2- or 3-point system. Higher scores indicate better functioning than lower scores (42,43). The Independence

Scale assesses the level of the subject's independence on a 10- to 100-point system, with 10 being a patient who is tube fed and in total bed care and 100 a patient who needs no special care. The functional assessment checklist includes 25 yes or no questions concerning common daily tasks. A score of 1 is given for each yes reply, and 0 is given for each no reply. Higher scores indicate better functioning (42,43).

The UHDRS has been found to have a high degree of internal consistency in each of its 4 components. Cronbach's *alpha* values were 0.95 for the motor scale, 0.90 for the cognitive tests, 0.83 for the behavioral scale, and 0.95 for the functional checklist (42). There were significant intercorrelations between the domains of the UHDRS, with the exception of the total behavioral score. The poor correlation of the behavioral score with the other sections of the UHDRS may reflect the heterogeneous, episodic character of the behavioral abnormalities and their responsiveness to treatment (42,43). However, the mood subscale correlates with better motor performance, reflecting the predominance of mood disorders in early Huntington's disease. Additionally, the psychotic and obsessive subscales correlate with functional impairment, reflecting the predominance of these symptoms in advanced disease (42). The intraclass correlation coefficient was 0.94 for the total motor score, 0.82 for the chorea score, and 0.62 for the dystonia score (42).

A factor analysis of the UHDRS has yielded 15 factors accounting for 77% of the variance. The Total Functional Capacity score declined at a rate of 0.72 units per year, and the Independent Scale score declined at a rate of 4.52 units per year. In multivariate analysis, longer disease duration and better cognitive status at baseline were associated with a less rapid rate of decline in the Total Functional Capacity score, and depression at baseline was associated with a more rapid decline in the Independence Scale (44). In summary, UHDRS is a useful clinical tool to follow disease progression and may be useful in assessing clinical changes in the setting of experimental interventions.

GILLES DE LA TOURETTE'S SYNDROME

Although many clinical manifestations of Gilles de la Tourette's syndrome (GTS) are visible or audible, there is considerable difficulty in objectively quantifying them. One factor contributing to this difficulty is the significant variety of tics that can affect an individual at any given time. To assess severity, one must consider multiple variables, such as frequency, number of tic types, intensity, complexity, body distribution, suppressibility, and interference. Second, symptoms vary spontaneously. Third, patients are able to suppress voluntarily their symptoms for minutes to hours. Situational stimuli also can change tic expression. Even in the physician's office, they increase when the examiner leaves the room. Hence an assessment measure can focus on objective observation or subjective report, each having strengths and weaknesses. As suggested from the preceding data, information from multiple informants may be required to assess the multitude of clinical manifestations of tic disorders. As a result of the multidimensionality of GTS, it has been difficult to develop a single scale that can give a quantification of the disease in a simple, accurate, and comprehensive way. The approaches to creating a GTS scale include use of historical information, direct observation, or both.

Combined Historical and Objective Rating Scales

Shapiro Tourette Syndrome Severity Scale

The *Shapiro Tourette Syndrome Severity Scale* (*STSSS*) was developed by Shapiro and Shapiro for use in a clinical trial of Pimozide (45). STSSS is a composite clinician rating of severity comprising 5 factors: the degree to which tics are noticeable to others, whether they elicit comments of curiosity, whether other individuals consider the patient odd or bizarre, whether tics interfere with functioning, and whether the patient is incapacitated, homebound, or hospitalized. The scores for the 5 items are summed and converted into a global severity rating. STSSS is simple to use, valid, and highly reliable when used by physicians and provides an overall index of severity (46). Limitations include failure to assess the wide range of tic characteristics; weighting and focus primarily on the social disabilities associated with GTS; and lack of anchor points for determining the degree of severity for each of the 5 factors.

Tourette Syndrome Global Scale

The *Tourette Syndrome Global Scale* (*TSGS*) is a multidimensional scale of GTS symptoms and social functioning comprising 8 individually rated dimensions. The tic domain consists of 4 dimensions: simple motor tics, complex motor tics, simple phonic tics, and complex phonic tics. Each dimension is rated for frequency (on a scale of 0 to 5) and degree of disruption (on a scale of 1 to 5). For each tic category, frequency and disruption scores are multiplied and summed to yield a total severity score. The social function domain contains 3 dimensions: behavioral problems, motor restlessness, and level of school and occupational functioning. The social dimensions are rated on a continuous scale of 0 (no impairment) to 25 (severe impairment). The tic and social functioning scores are then inserted into a mathematical formula that yields a global score. These 2 scores contribute equally to the global score and can be used separately (47). The TSGS has a high interrater agreement for both scores as assessed on 23 patients seen in an outpatient setting (47). One of the problems with this scale is that by multiplying frequency by disruption scores it may exaggerate small differences in tic severity and may cause the social functioning domain to be underweighted (48). Furthermore, by combining information from completely different dimensions in a manner without any empirical justification, the scale fails to assess several important tic

characteristics, such as number of tic types and complexity. Finally, its reliability and validity properties have been documented with only a small number of patients (49).

Yale Global Tic Severity Scale

The *Yale Global Tic Severity Scale* (YGTSS) was developed in response to the criticism of TSGS and is designed for use by an experienced clinician following a semistructured interview with multiple informants. YGTSS includes separate rating of severity for motor and phonic tics along 5 dimensions: number, frequency, intensity, complexity, and interference. It also includes a checklist for specific types of motor and vocal tics. An independent rating of impairment, which focuses on the impact of the tic disorder over the previous week, is added to the total tic score to obtain a final score (50). Data from 105 GTS patients revealed high internal consistency of the items, convergent validity with other scales, including the Shapiro Tourette Severity Scale (STSS), Tourette Syndrome Global Scale (TSGS), and Tourette Syndrome-Global Clinical Impression (TS-GCI), and evidence of discriminant validity (50). Other favorable features of YGTSS are ease of administration; measurement of tic behaviors only and their impact, rather than attempting to assess a broader range of maladaptive behaviors; separate ratings for the severity of motor and phonic tic behaviors; and slightly better psychometric properties than the other scales. Disadvantages include lack of differentiation of historical information from observations made by the examiner and lack of inclusion of specific tic characteristics such as tic distribution, type, and suppression. The amount of time required to collect the necessary information is 15 to 20 minutes, as opposed to 5 to 10 minutes for the Shapiro Tourette Severity Scale (STSS).

Hopkins Motor and Vocal Tic Scale

The *Hopkins Motor and Vocal Tic Scale* (HMVTS) consists of a series of visual analogue scales (10 cm) on which both parent and physician separately rank each tic (motor and vocal), taking into consideration the frequency, intensity, interference, and impairment. The range of the scale is 0 (no tics) to 10 (most severe), and it can be roughly subdivided into 4 ranges: mild, moderate, moderately severe, and severe. Based on ratings for all individual tics present over the preceding week, the rater derives 3 final scores for both motor and vocal symptoms: 1 based on parent information, 1 based on rater observation, and 1 for overall assessment. Final scores use a 5-point scale: 1 for no tics; 2 for mild tics; 3 for moderate tics; 4 for moderately severe tics; 5 for severe tics. The Hopkins Motor and Vocal Tic Scale was created in response to the need for a simple, accurate, comprehensive rating scale. It focuses both on the tics themselves and on impairment from them. It is quick and simple to administer, was found to be effective in evaluating overall severity, and showed good interrater reliability. The Yale Global Tic Severity Scale (YGTSS), Shapiro Tourette's Syndrome Severity Scale (STSSS), Clinical Global Impression Scale (CGI-S), and Hopkins

Motor and Vocal Tic Severity Scale were found to be equally effective in determining overall severity and have shown good interrater reliability (51).

Videotape-Based Rating Scales

Goetz et al. (52) developed a filming protocol for a double-blind crossover study of the efficacy of clonidine in GTS, which was later revised in a study of talipexole in GTS (53). During this protocol, an 8-minute audio and video recording was taken during each visit with far (full frontal body views) and near (head and shoulders only) views for 2 minutes each, during quiet conversation with the examiner in the room and during relaxation with the patient alone in the room. At the completion of the study, segments of the videotapes for each patient were randomized and rated by 3 blinded observers. For each rated tape, a 1-minute segment from the middle of the near taping with the examiner out of the room was reviewed 3 times to count normal eye blinks per minute, a total number of eye, face, head, neck, and shoulder tics, as well as vocalizations per minute. A 1-minute segment from the middle of the full body video was used to determine the total number of body areas showing tics and the number of body tics. The intensity was determined by rating the worst tic viewed during the videotape according to a 100-point scale with 5 anchor points at 25-point intervals.

Other videotape-based rating scales have videotaped patients under different stimulus conditions (45,46,54) or with the patient unaware of being videotaped through a one-way mirror (55).

Symptom Checklists and Global Scales

Symptom checklists were developed to help obtain detailed information about a patient's condition for research purposes and to assist parents in making daily or weekly ratings of tic behaviors. They incorporate assessment of tic severity and fluctuation, impact on the family, and the extent of the patient's and family's coping with the disease. They include the Tourette Syndrome Symptom List (TSSL), the Tourette Syndrome Questionnaire (TSQ), the Motor tic, Obsessions and compulsions, Vocal tic Evaluation Survey (MOVES), and the 1987 Ohio Tourette Survey (56).

Global scales were introduced to assess the impact of GTS symptoms on daily functioning. They include the Global Clinical Impression Scales (GCI-S), the Global Assessment Scale (GAS), and the Children's Global Assessment Scale (CGAS) (56).

TREMOR

Measuring tremor clinically is difficult because tremors behave in different and often complex ways. Tremor is influenced by a variety of factors, including natural fluctuations;

the patient's physical, emotional, and mental state; and various environmental triggers. Therefore, it is difficult to develop a tool that would allow measurements of a movement disorder that is rarely stable.

The clinical rating scale for tremor developed by Sweet et al. (57) was designed specifically for essential tremor. This scale assigned different point values to different body parts. The number of points for the presence of tremor in each region was then multiplied by a factor (1 to 3) reflecting severity. A score for functional impairment was added to the sum of these products. For this functional score and in a fashion similar to what was done for severity of tremor, a weighted number was assigned to various activities, namely handling a cup, handling food, using the hands, swallowing, talking, and walking. This scale did not include ratings for rest tremor; lacked specific definitions for mild, moderate, and marked severity; did not account for specific activities; and did not assess the functional impact of tremor on a patient's daily activities.

Fahn et al. developed a new clinical rating scale assessing rest, postural, and action tremor. This scale also evaluated voice tremor, as well as handwriting and other tasks, such as hygiene and dressing. Functional disability and tremor impact also were scored. A uniform rather than a weighted score was used, and the severity was based on 5 points rather than 4. Interrater reliability of this scale has been assessed in 10 tremor patients with variable severity and was found to be good (58).

Bain et al. devised a scale that assesses the severity (0–10) of tremor in different body parts for different tremor components. For each body part, tremor is assessed (a) during rest, action, and movement and (b) during writing and spiral drawing (59–61). This scale was assessed at specific anatomical sites for both inter- and intrarater reliability, and the scores obtained with the scale were compared with the results of upper limb accelerometry, an activities-of-daily-living questionnaire, and estimates of the tremor-induced impairment in writing and drawing specimens (62). The same authors have proposed objective functional performance tests: (a) pouring water from one cup into another (a bimanual kinetic tremor test); (b) holding a full cup of water for 1 minute (test for unilateral postural tremor); (c) the 9-hole pegboard test (test for upper limb function); and (d) the Gibson Spiral Maze test (measuring the number of times a patient's drawn line crosses the boundaries of a printed spiral) (63). All of these tests are unvalidated, insensitive to extreme (very fine or very severe) tremors, and influenced by factors other than tremor.

Louis et al. developed a detailed tremor examination that incorporated multiple test items, in addition to writing and a clinical rating scale. The Washington Heights-Inwood Genetic Study of Essential Tremor (WHIGET) Rating Scale consists of a 26-item, 10-minute tremor examination designed to elicit tremor during 2 different postures, 5 different tasks, and 2 different positions at rest (64). Tasks included pouring water between 2 cups, drinking water from a cup, using a spoon to drink water, finger-to-nose movement, and drawing spirals. Each task is first performed with the dominant arm and then with the nondominant arm. Each item is rated on a 0- to 4-point scale, with 0 being no tremor and 4 being extremely large-amplitude jerky tremor. A teaching videotape has been developed to assess the interrater reliability of the WHIGET tremor scale among different raters (65). WHIGET has been found to have a substantial interrater reliability (weighted *kappa* = 0.62–0.78) and a high degree of test–retest stability ($r = 0.98$, $p < 0.00001$) (66), as well as high validity (67). WHIGET also has been validated against a quantitative computerized tremor analysis (67).

MYOCLONUS

The Unified Myoclonus Rating Scale (UMRS) (68) is a quantitative 73-item scale developed by the Myoclonus Study Group and is a revised version of the scale introduced initially by Truong and Fahn (69). UMRS contains a patient questionnaire, a handwriting and spiral drawing sample, rating instructions, a score sheet, and a videotape protocol (approximately 8 minutes). The scale consists of 8 sections: (a) patient questionnaire (11 items); (b) myoclonus at rest (frequency and amplitude, 16 items); (c) stimulus sensitivity of myoclonus (17 items); (d) severity of myoclonus with action (frequency and amplitude, 20 items); (e) performance on functional tests (5 items); (f) physician rating of patient's global disability (1 item); (g) presence of negative myoclonus (1 item); (h) severity of negative myoclonus (1 item). Each item is rated on a scale of 0 to 4, with the exception of sections 3 and 7 (in which stimulus sensitivity and negative myoclonus, respectively, are either present, rated 1, or absent, rated 0), and section 8, which is rated 0 to 3 (68).

UMRS has been found to have excellent interrater reliability. Cronbach's α values for sections 1–5 of the UMRS were section 1: 0.92; section 2: frequency 0.80, amplitude 0.74; section 3: 0.90; section 4: frequency 0.85, amplitude 0.86; and section 5 0.89 (68). UMRS appears to be sensitive to changes in myoclonus of all severities. For the purpose of clinical trials, the most useful primary endpoints are the change in scores of action myoclonus (section 4) and functional performance (section 5). Although some treatments also may improve myoclonus at rest (section 2) and stimulus sensitivity (section 3), these parameters may be less important contributors to global disability.

REFERENCES

1. Rocca NG. Statistical and methodologic considerations in scale construction. In: Munsat TL, ed. *Quantification of neurologic deficit*. Boston, MA: Butterworth, 1989:49–67.
2. The Unified Parkinson's Disease Rating Scale (UPDRS): status and recommendations. *Mov Disord* 2003;18:738–750.
3. Martinez-Martin P, Gil-Nagel A, Gracia LM, et al., and the Cooperative Multicentric Group. Unified Parkinson's Disease Rating Scale characteristics and structure. *Mov Disord* 1994;9:76–83.
4. Richards M, Marder K, Cote L, et al. Interrater reliability of the Unified Parkinson's Disease Rating Scale motor examination. *Mov Disord* 1994;9:89–91.
5. Stebbins GT, Goetz CG. Factor structure of the Unified Parkinson's Disease Rating Scale: motor examination section. *Mov Disord* 1998;13:633–636.
6. Van Hilten JJ, van der Zwan AD, Zwinderman AH, et al. Rating impairment and disability in Parkinson's disease: evaluation of the Unified Parkinson's Disease Rating Scale. *Mov Disord* 1994;9:84–88.
7. Goetz CG, Stebbins GT, Chmura TA, et al. Teaching tape for the motor section of the unified Parkinson's disease rating scale (see comments). *Mov Disord* 1995;10:263–266.
8. Goetz CG, Fahn S, Martinez-Martin P, et al. The Movement Disorders Society-sponsored new version of UPDRS: description and early clinimetric data. *Mov Disord* 2006. In press.
9. Hoehn NM, Yahr MD. Parkinsonism: onset, progression and mortality. *Neurology* 1967;17:427–442.
10. Geminiani G, Cesana BM, Tamma F, et al. Interobserver reliability between neurologists in training of Parkinson's disease rating scales: a multicenter study. *Mov Disord* 1991;6:330–335.
11. Goetz CG, Poewe W, Rascol O, et al. Movement Disorder Society Task Force report on the Hoehn and Yahr staging scale: status and recommendations. *Mov Disord* 2004;19:1020–1028.
12. Welsh M, McDermott MP, Holloway RG, et al. Development and testing of the Parkinson's disease quality of life scale. *Mov Disord* 2003;18:637–645.
13. Eidelberg D, Moeller JR, Ishikawa T, et al. Assessment of disease severity in parkinsonism with fluorine-18-fluorodeoxyglucose and PET. *J Nucl Med* 1995;36:378–383.
14. Staffen W, Mair A, Unterrainer J, et al. Measuring the progression of idiopathic Parkinson's disease with [123I] beta-CIT SPECT. *J Neural Transm* 2000;107:543–552.
15. Ginanneschi A, Degl'Innocenti F, Maurello MT, et al. Evaluation of Parkinson's disease: a new approach to disability. *Neuroepidemiology* 1991;10:282–287.
16. Jankovic J, McDermott M, Carter J, et al., and the Parkinson Study Group. Variable expression of Parkinson's disease: a base-line analysis of the DATATOP cohort. *Neurology* 1990;40:1529–1534.
17. Muller J, Wenning GK, Jellinger K, et al. Progression of Hoehn and Yahr stages in parkinsonian disorders: a clinicopathologic study. *Neurology* 2000;55:888–891.
18. Rabey JM, Bass H, Bonuccelli U, et al. Evaluation of the Short Parkinson's Evaluation Scale: a new friendly scale for the evaluation of Parkinson's disease in clinical drug trials. *Clin Neuropharmacol* 1997;20:322–337.
19. Marinus J, Visser M, Stiggelbout AM, et al. A short scale for the assessment of motor impairments and disabilities in Parkinson's disease: the SPES/SCOPA. *J Neurol Neurosurg Psychiatry* 2004;75: 388–395.
20. Langston JW, Widner H, Goetz CG, et al. Core assessment program for intracerebral transplantations (CAPIT). *Mov Disord* 1992;7:2–13.
21. Defer GL, Widner H, Marie RM, et al. Core assessment program for surgical interventional therapies in Parkinson's disease (CAPSIT-PD). *Mov Disord* 1999;14:572–584.
22. Schwab JF, England AC. Projection technique for evaluating surgery in Parkinson's disease. In: Billingham FH, Donaldson MC, eds. *Third symposium on Parkinson's disease*. Edinburgh, Scotland: Livingstone, 1969:152–157.
23. Peto V, Jenkinson C, Fitzpatrick R, et al. The development and validation of a short measure of functioning and well being for individuals with Parkinson's disease. *Qual Life Res* 1995;4: 241–248.
24. De Boer AG, Wijker W, Speelman JD, et al. Quality of life in patients with Parkinson's disease: development of a questionnaire. *J Neurol Neurosurg Psychiatry* 1996;61:70–74.
25. Guy W. *ECDEU assessment manual for psychopharmacology*. Washington, DC: Government Printing Office, 1976.
26. Goetz CG, Stebbins GT, Shale HM, et al. Utility of an objective dyskinesia rating scale for Parkinson's disease: inter- and intrarater reliability assessment (see comments). *Mov Disord* 1994;9:390–394.

27. Obeso JA, Grandas F, Vaamonde J, et al. Motor complications associated with chronic levodopa therapy in Parkinson's disease. *Neurology* 1989;39(suppl 2):11–19.

28. Hauser RA, Deckers F, Lehert P. Parkinson's disease home diary: further validation and implications for clinical trials. *Mov Disord* 2004;19:1409–1413.

29. Goetz CG, Stebbins GT, Blasucci LM, et al. Efficacy of a patient-training videotape on motor fluctuations for on-off diaries in Parkinson's disease. *Mov Disord* 1997;12:1039–1041.

30. Burke RE, Fahn S, Marsden CD, et al. Validity and reliability of a rating scale for the primary torsion dystonias. *Neurology* 1985;35:73–77.

31. Comella CL, Leurgans S, Wuu J, et al. Rating scales for dystonia: a multicenter assessment. *Mov Disord* 2003;18:303–312.

32. Lindeboom R, de Haan RJ, Aramideh M, et al. Treatment outcomes in cervical dystonia: a clinimetric study. *Mov Disord* 1996;11:371–376.

33. Tsui JK, Eisen A, Caine CB. Botulinum toxin in spasmodic torticollis. *Adv Neurol* 1988;50:593-597.

34. Tarsy D. Comparison of clinical rating scales in treatment of cervical dystonia with botulinum toxin. *Mov Disord* 1997;12:100–102.

35. Greene P, Kang U, Fahn S, et al. Double-blind, placebo-controlled trial of botulinum toxin injections for the treatment of spasmodic torticollis. *Neurology* 1990;40:1213–1218.

36. Consky ES, Lang AE. Clinical assessments of patients with cervical dystonia. In: Jankovic J, Hallett M, eds. *Therapy with botulinum toxin.* New York: Marcel Dekker, 1994:211–237.

37. Comella CL, Stebbins GT, Goetz CG, et al. Teaching tape for the motor section of the Toronto Western Spasmodic Torticollis Scale. *Mov Disord* 1997;12:570–575.

38. Fahn S. Assessment of the primary dystonias. In: Munsat TL, ed. *Quantification of neurologic deficit.* London, England: Butterworths, 1989:241–270.

39. Priori A, Pesenti A, Cappellari A, et al. Limb immobilization for the treatment of focal occupational dystonia. *Neurology* 2001;57:405–409.

40. Wissel J, Kabus C, Wenzel R, et al. Botulinum toxin in writer's cramp: objective response evaluation in 31 patients. *J Neurol Neurosurg Psychiatry* 1996;61:172–175.

41. Jabusch HC, Vauth H, Altenmuller E. Quantification of focal dystonia in pianists using scale analysis. *Mov Disord* 2004;19: 171–180.

42. Huntington Study Group. Unified Huntington's Disease Rating Scale: reliability and consistency. *Mov Disord* 1996;11:136–142.

43. Siesling S, van Vugt JP, Zwinderman KA, et al. Unified Huntington's disease rating scale: a follow up. *Mov Disord* 1998;13:915–919.

44. Marder K, Zhao H, Myers RH, et al., and the Huntington Study Group. Rate of functional decline in Huntington's disease. *Neurology* 2000;54:452–458.

45. Shapiro AK, Shapiro E. Controlled study of pimozide vs. placebo in Tourette's syndrome. *J Am Acad Child Psychiatry* 1984;23:161–173.

46. Shapiro AK, Shapiro ES, Young JG, et al. Measurement in tic disorders. In: Shapiro AK, Shapiro ES, Young JG, Feinberg TE, eds. *Gilles de la Tourette syndrome.* New York: Raven Press, 1988:451–480.

47. Harcherik DF, Leckman JF, Detlor J, et al. A new instrument for clinical studies of Tourette's syndrome. *J Am Acad Child Psychiatry* 1984;23:153–160.

48. Kurlan R, McDermott MP. Rating tic severity. In: Kurlan R, ed. *Handbook of Tourette's syndrome and related tic and behavioral disorders.* New York: Dekker, 1993:199–220.

49. Leckman JF, Towbin KE, Ort SI, et al. Clinical assessment of tic disorder severity. In: Cohen DJ, Bruun R, Leckman JF, eds. *Tourette's syndrome and tic disorders.* New York: Wiley & Sons, 1988.

50. Leckman JF, Riddle MA, Hardin MT, et al. The Yale Global Tic Severity Scale: initial testing of a clinician-rated scale of tic severity. *J Am Acad Child Adolesc Psychiatry* 1989;28:566–573.

51. Walkup JT, Rosenberg LA, Brown J, et al. The validity of instruments measuring tic severity in Tourette's syndrome. *J Am Acad Child Adolesc Psychiatry* 1992;31:472–477.

52. Goetz CG, Tanner CM, Wilson RS, et al. Clonidine and Gilles de la Tourette's syndrome: double-blind study using objective rating methods. *Ann Neurol* 1987;21:307–310.

53. Goetz CG, Stebbins GT, Thelen JA. Talipexole and adult Gilles de la Tourette's syndrome: double-blind, placebo-controlled clinical trial. *Mov Disord* 1994;9:315–317.

54. Leckman JF, Hardin MT, Riddle MA, et al. Clonidine treatment of Gilles de la Tourette's syndrome. *Arch Gen Psychiatry* 1991;48: 324–328.

55. Peterson AL, Azrin NH. An evaluation of behavioral treatments for Tourette syndrome. *Behav Res Ther* 1992;30:167–174.

56. Kompoliti K, Goetz CG. Tourette syndrome: clinical rating and quantitative assessment of tics. *Neurol Clin* 1997;15:239–254.

57. Sweet RD, Blumberg J, Lee JE, et al. Propranolol treatment of essential tremor. *Neurology* 1974;24:64–67.

58. Fahn S, Tolosa E, Marin C. Clinical rating scale for tremor. In: Jankovic J, Tolosa E, eds. *Parkinson's disease and movement disorders,* 2nd ed. Baltimore, MD: Williams and Wilkins, 1993: 271–280.

59. Bain PG. Clinical measurement of tremor. *Mov Disord* 1998; 13(suppl 3):77–80.

60. Bain P. A combined clinical and neurophysiological approach to the study of patients with tremor. *J Neurol Neurosurg Psychiatry* 1993;56:839–844.

61. Bain PG, Mally J, Gresty M, et al. Assessing the impact of essential tremor on upper limb function. *J Neurol* 1993;241:54–61.

62. Bain PG, Findley LJ, Atchison P, et al. Assessing tremor severity. *J Neurol Neurosurg Psychiatry* 1993;56:868–873.

63. Bain PG. Tremor assessment and quality of life measurements. *Neurology* 2000;54(suppl 4):S26–29.

64. Louis ED, Wendt KJ, Albert SM, et al. Validity of a performance-based test of function in essential tremor. *Arch Neurol* 1999;56: 841–846.

65. Louis ED, Barnes L, Wendt KJ, et al. A teaching videotape for the assessment of essential tremor. *Mov Disord* 2001;16:89–93.

66. Louis ED, Ford B, Bismuth B. Reliability between two observers using a protocol for diagnosing essential tremor. *Mov Disord* 1998;13:287–293.

67. Louis ED, Barnes LF, Wendt KJ, et al. Validity and test-retest reliability of a disability questionnaire for essential tremor. *Mov Disord* 2000;15:516–523.

68. Frucht SJ, Leurgans SE, Hallett M, et al. The Unified Myoclonus Rating Scale. *Adv Neurol* 2002;89:361–376.

69. Truong DD, Fahn S. Therapeutic trial with glycine in myoclonus. *Mov Disord* 1988;3:222–232.

Subject Index

Figures are indicated by page numbers followed by *f*. Tables are indicated by page numbers followed by *t*.